D0773225

DISCARDED.

NOTE: MAY CONTAIN OUTDATED INFORMATION.

To borrow: send email to library@sharp.com with your *name, phone, email barcode of the book or CD*. Item will be due back in 4 weeks.

Principles of Diabetes Mellitus

Second Edition

Leonid Poretsky

Editor

WR
810
P957
2010

Principles of Diabetes Mellitus

Second Edition

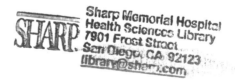
Sharp Memorial Hospital
Health Sciences Library
7901 Frost Street
San Diego, CA 92123
library@sharp.com

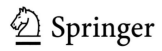 Springer

Editor
Leonid Poretsky
Division of Endocrinology and Metabolism
Beth Israel Medical Center
317 East 17th Street
New York, NY 10003
USA
lporetsk@chpnet.org

8 239 38/

4/3/12

ISBN 978-0-387-09840-1   e-ISBN 978-0-387-09841-8
DOI 10.1007/978-0-387-09841-8
Springer New York Dordrecht Heidelberg London

Library of Congress Control Number: 2009939995

© Springer Science+Business Media, LLC 2010
All rights reserved. This work may not be translated or copied in whole or in part without the written permission of the publisher (Springer Science+Business Media, LLC, 233 Spring Street, New York, NY 10013, USA), except for brief excerpts in connection with reviews or scholarly analysis. Use in connection with any form of information storage and retrieval, electronic adaptation, computer software, or by similar or dissimilar methodology now known or hereafter developed is forbidden.
The use in this publication of trade names, trademarks, service marks, and similar terms, even if they are not identified as such, is not to be taken as an expression of opinion as to whether or not they are subject to proprietary rights.
While the advice and information in this book are believed to be true and accurate at the date of going to press, neither the authors nor the editors nor the publisher can accept any legal responsibility for any errors or omissions that may be made. The publisher makes no warranty, express or implied, with respect to the material contained herein.

Printed on acid-free paper

Springer is part of Springer Science+Business Media (www.springer.com)

Preface to the Second Edition

Seven years have elapsed since the first edition of the *Principles of Diabetes Mellitus* appeared. It is sobering to realize how much new important information on the subject of this textbook has been developed during this relatively short period of time. Hence, the second edition.

Every chapter has been updated in terms of both material it covers as well as the references and the websites where additional useful information can be found. Several new chapters have been added. These chapters cover such topics as the role of brain in glucose metabolism, the role of incretins in the pathogenesis and therapy of diabetes, the relationship between diabetes and cancer and between diabetes and human immunodeficiency virus infection, diabetes among minorities, and hospital management of diabetes. Many authors who contributed to the first edition worked on the second edition as well, but many new writers joined the "crew." We thank *all* of the authors of the first edition for their role in preparing this textbook.

The goals of this text are outlined in the preface to the first edition, which follows. We hope that our readers will continue to find *Principles of Diabetes Mellitus* both useful and enjoyable.

New York
2009

Leonid Poretsky

Preface to the First Edition

Diabetes mellitus is a very common disease. Described initially in the Egyptian papyrus *Ebers* in 1500 BC and now affecting approximately 150,000,000 people worldwide, with its prevalence rising rapidly, diabetes continues to mystify and fascinate both practitioners and investigators by its elusive causes and multitude of manifestations.

A neurosurgeon operating on a patient with a life-threatening brain tumor, an obstetrician delivering a baby, a psychiatrist trying to penetrate deep into a patient's emotional life – all will encounter diabetes from their very early days of medical practice. This disease will significantly affect the choice of therapeutic approaches throughout their careers, regardless of their specialty. Hence, there is need for every student of medicine, whatever his or her ultimate career goals, to understand and learn to manage diabetes.

Many excellent diabetes textbooks exist. Most of them, however, are written for endocrinologists. This textbook is written not only for endocrinologists, but also for other specialists, primary care physicians, housestaff, and particularly for medical students.

The needs of the latter group are well understood by the authors of this text, most of whom have been medical students and all of whom continue to teach medical students on a regular basis. The main challenge for a medical student is to "digest" a large amount of complicated, rapidly changing information under heavy time pressure. Therefore, a book written for medical students must be up-to-date and cover all aspects of the disease, from its pathogenesis on the molecular and cellular levels to its most modern therapy. Such textbook must also be concise, clear, and easy to use. To achieve these goals, we have made liberal use of illustrations and tables, provided a summary after each chapter, and added website addresses where additional information can be found to the lists of references. Each chapter is written to stand on its own, and readers who wish to explore a particular subject should not have to search through many chapters. This may have resulted in redundancies noticeable to readers of the entire text, but the pages where the most detailed discussion of a given topic can be found are highlighted in the index in bold print.

We hope that these features will make *Principles of Diabetes Mellitus* user-friendly. We also hope that readers will find this volume useful for studies of diabetes throughout their professional lives: first in medical school, then during the years of residency, and, finally, as they enter their chosen specialty.

The authors would like to dedicate this book to those from whom we learned and continue to learn about diabetes: our teachers, who inspired us to undertake studies of the challenging diabetes problems and then supported us throughout these studies; our students, who lead us to ponder new questions; and finally, our patients, who live with the disease every moment of every day and in some ways know more about it than we do.

We thank Jill Gregory for her expert help with illustrations and Anthony J. DiCarlo for help with computer programming. We also gratefully acknowledge the efforts of Marilyn Small Jefferson, who helped coordinate the work of 61 writers, and without whose patience, diligence, and dedication this book would not have been possible.

New York, 2002   Leonid Poretsky

Contents

Contributors

Zinoviy Abelev, M.D. Division of Endocrinology and Metabolism, Beth Israel Medical Center, New York, NY 10003, USA

Martin J. Abrahamson, M.D. FACP Joslin Diabetes Center, Harvard Medical School, Boston, MA, USA

Bianca Alfonso, M.D. Division of Endocrinology and Metabolism, Beth Israel Medical Center, New York, NY, USA

Omar Ali, M.D. Medical College of Wisconsin, Milwaukee, WI, USA

Mazen Alsahli, M.D. Division of Endocrinology, Department of Medicine, University of Rochester School of Medicine, Rochester, NY, USA

Kalliopi M. Arampatzi, M.D. Division of Endocrinology, Diabetes, and Metabolism, Beth Israel Deaconess Medical Center, Boston, MA, USA

Bradley W. Bakotic, DPM, DO Podiatric Pathology, DermPath Diagnostics, Pompano Beach, FL, USA; Barry University School of Podiatric Medicine, Miami Shores, FL, USA; New York College of Podiatric Medicine, New York, NY, USA

Mary Ann Banerji, M.D. Downstate Medical Center, State University of New York, Brooklyn, NY, USA

Rajiv Bhambri, M.D. Division of Endocrinology, Metabolism and Nutrition, UMDNJ-Robert Wood Johnson Medical School, New Brunswick, NJ, USA

Henry C. Bodenheimer Jr., M.D. Department of Medicine, Beth Israel Medical Center and Albert Einstein College of Medicine, New York, NY, USA

Barry J. Brass, M.D., Ph.D.* Division of Endocrinology and Metabolism, Albert Einstein College of Medicine, Beth Israel Medical Center, New York, NY 10003, USA

David J. Brillon, M.D. Division of Endocrinology, Diabetes and Metabolism, Weill Cornell Medical College, New York, NY, USA

Kevin Brown, M.D. Division of Endocrinology, Diabetes and Nutrition, University of Maryland School of Medicine, Baltimore, MD, USA

Agustin Busta, M.D. Division of Endocrinology and Metabolism, Beth Israel Medical Center and Albert Einstein College of Medicine, New York, NY, USA

Enrique Caballero, M.D. Joslin Diabetes Center, Harvard Medical School, Boston, MA 02215, USA

Rochelle L. Chaiken, M.D. VP Medical Affairs, Pfizer Inc., SUNY Downstate Medical Center, New York, State University of New York, Brooklyn, NY, USA

Shadi Chamany, M.D., M.P.H. New York City Department of Health and Mental Hygiene, New York, NY, USA

Russell L. Chin, M.D.   Peripheral Neuropathy Center, Weill Cornell Medical College, New York, NY, USA

Sara Choudhry, M.D.   Division of Endocrinology, Diabetes and Hypertension, Department of Medicine, State University of New York, Downstate Medical Center, Brooklyn, NY, USA

Ronald J. Christopher, Ph.D.   Takeda San Diego, Inc., San Diego, CA, USA

Theodore P. Ciaraldi, Ph.D.   Department of Medicine, VA San Diego Healthcare System, University of California, San Diego, CA, USA

Pejman Cohan, M.D.   University of California at Los Angeles School of Medicine, Los Angeles, CA, USA

Samantha DeMauro-Jablonski, M.D.   Division of Endocrinology and Metabolism, University of Pittsburgh Physicians, Pittsburgh, PA, USA

Richard B. Devereux, M.D.   Laboratory of Echocardiography, New York Presbyterian Hospital, Weill Medical College of Cornell University, New York, NY, USA

Michael E. DiSanto, Ph.D.   Department of Urology, Montefiore Medical Center/Albert Einstein College of Medicine, Bronx, NY, USA

Rosalia Doyle, RD, MS, CDE   Division of Endocrinology, Department of Medicine, Friedman Diabetes Institute, Beth Israel Medical Center, New York, NY, USA

Alan Dubrow, M.D.   Division of Nephrology, Beth Israel Medical Center, Albert Einstein College of Medicine, New York, NY, USA

Faith Ebel, MPH, RD, MS   Laparoscopic and Bariatric Surgery, Weill Medical College of Cornell University, New York, NY, USA

Donald A. Feinfeld, M.D.*   Department of Surgery, Division of Nephrology, Beth Israel Medical Center, Albert Einstein College of Medicine, New York, NY, USA

Yun Feng, M.D.   Department of Medicine, Beth Israel Medical Center, New York, NY, USA

Stephen J. Ferrando, M.D.   Division of Psychosomatic Medicine, Department of Psychiatry, Payne Whitney Clinic, New York-Presbyterian Hospital, Weill Cornell Medical College, New York, NY, USA

Adrienne M. Fleckman, M.D.   Department of Medicine, Albert Einstein College of Medicine, Beth Israel Medical Center, New York, NY, USA

Vivian Fonseca, M.D.   Section of Endocrinology, Tullis Tulane Alumni Chair in Diabetes and Tulane University Health Sciences Center, New Orleans, LA, USA

Emily Jane Gallagher, M.D.   Division of Endocrinology, Diabetes & Bone Disease, Department of Medicine, Mount Sinai School of Medicine, New York, NY, USA

Om P. Ganda, M.D.   Joslin Diabetes Center, Beth-Israel Deaconess Medical Center, Harvard Medical School, Boston, MA, USA

Yana B. Garger, M.D.   Department of Medicine, Beth Israel Medical Center, New York, NY, USA

John E. Gerich, M.D.   Department of Medicine, University of Rochester School of Medicine, Rochester, NY 14642, USA

George Grunberger, M.D., FACP, FACE   Grunberger Diabetes Institute, Wayne State University School of Medicine, Detroit, MI, USA

Chiara Guglielmi, M.D.   Department of Endocrinology and Diabetes, University Campus Bio-Medico, Rome, Italy

Yuriy Gurevich, D.O. Division of Endocrinology and Metabolism, Beth Israel Medical Center, New York, NY, USA

Nancy Habib, B.S. Department of Surgery, Beth Israel Medical Center, Albert Einstein College of Medicine, New York, NY, USA

Nikolas B. Harbord, M.D. Beth Israel Medical Center, Albert Einstein College of Medicine, New York, NY, USA

Abhijith Hegde, M.D. Attending, Pulmonary, Critical Care and Sleep Medicine, Danbury Office of Physician Services, Danbury Hospital, Danbury, CT, USA

Susan Herzlinger, M.D. Joslin Diabetes Center, Harvard Medical School, Boston, MA, USA

Edward S. Horton, M.D. Joslin Diabetes Center, Harvard Medical School, Boston, MA, USA

Stanley Hsu, M.D. Division of Gastroenterology and Liver Disease, Saint Luke's Roosevelt Hospital, Columbia University College of Physician and Surgeons, New York, NY, USA

William C. Hsu, M.D. Joslin Diabetes Center, Harvard Medical School, Boston, MA, USA, cmantzor@bidmc.harvard.edu

Silvio E. Inzucchi, M.D. Section of Endocrinology, Yale University School of Medicine, Yale Diabetes Center, Yale-New Haven Hospital, New Haven, CT, USA

Jennifer John-Kalarickal, M.D. Tulane University Health Science Center, New Orleans, LA, USA

Prajesh M. Joshi Department of Medicine, Beth Israel Medical Center, New York, NY, USA

Jeffrey S. Kirk, M.D. Department of Surgery, Beth Israel Medical Center, New York, NY, USA

Orville Kolterman, M.D. Amylin Pharmaceuticals, Inc., San Diego, CA, USA

Donald P. Kotler, M.D. Division of Gastroenterology and Liver Disease, Saint Luke's Roosevelt Hospital, Columbia University College of Physician and Surgeons, New York, NY, USA

Jennifer L. Kraker, M.D., M.S. Division of Psychosomatic Medicine, Department of Psychiatry, Payne Whitney Clinic, New York-Presbyterian Hospital, Weill Cornell Medical College, New York, NY, USA

Marina Krymskaya, N.P. Division of Endocrinology, Department of Medicine, Gerald J. Friedman Diabetes Institute, Beth Israel Medical Center, New York, NY, USA

Ketan Laud, M.D. Vitreoretinal Fellow, Vitreous Retina Macula Consultants of New York/Columbia University, New York, NY, USA

Ho Won Lee, D.V.M., Ph.D. Division of Endocrinology, Diabetes and Hypertension, Department of Medicine, State University of New York, Downstate Medical Center, Brooklyn, NY, USA

Bumsup Lee, D.V.M., Ph.D. Takeda San Diego, Inc., San Diego, CA, USA

Derek LeRoith, M.D., Ph.D. Division of Endocrinology, Diabetes & Bone Disease, Department of Medicine, Mount Sinai School of Medicine, New York, NY, USA

James P. Leu, M.D. Division of Endocrinology and Metabolism, Department of Medicine, Montefiore Medical Center and Albert Einstein College of Medicine, Bronx, NY, USA

Albert C. Leung, M.D. Department of Urology, Montefiore Medical Center/Albert Einstein College of Medicine, Bronx, NY, USA

Emilia Pauline Liao, M.D. Division of Endocrinology and Metabolism, Albert Einstein College of Medicine, Beth Israel Medical Center, New York, NY, USA

Omar H. Llaguna, M.D., M.P.T.   Department of Surgery, Beth Israel Medical Center, New York, NY, USA

Christos S. Mantzoros, M.D., D.Sc.   Division of Endocrinology, Diabetes, and Metabolism, Beth Israel Deaconess Medical Center, Harvard Medical School, Boston, MA, USA

Ellen S. Marmur, M.D.   Department of Dermatology, The Mount Sinai Medical Center, New York, NY, USA

Paulo José Forcina Martins, Ph.D.   Department of Psychiatry, Obesity Research Center, University of Cincinnati, Cincinnati, OH 45237, USA

Barry M. Mason, M.D.   Department of Urology, Montefiore Medical Center/Albert Einstein College of Medicine, Bronx, NY, USA

Samy I. McFarlane, M.D., M.P.H., M.B.A.   Division of Endocrinology, Diabetes and Hypertension, State University of New York, Downstate Medical Center and Kings County Hospital Center, Brooklyn, NY, USA

Graham T. McMahon, M.D., M.M.Sc.   Division of Endocrinology, Diabetes and Hypertension, Brigham and Women's Hospital, Boston, MA 02115, USA

Arnold Melman, M.D.   Department of Urology, Montefiore Medical Center/Albert Einstein College of Medicine, Bronx, NY, USA

Maria A. Mendoza, R.N.   Jacobi Medical Center, City University of New York, New York, NY, USA

Douglas Meyer, M.D.*   Division of Digestive Diseases, Beth Israel Medical Center, Albert Einstein College of Medicine, New York, NY, USA

Kathleen Mulligan, Ph.D.   Division of Endocrinology and Metabolism, University of California, San Francisco, CA, USA

Ruslan Novosyadlyy, M.D., Ph.D.   Division of Endocrinology, Diabetes & Bone Disease, Department of Medicine, Mount Sinai School of Medicine, New York, NY, USA

Silvana Obici, M.D.   Department of Psychiatry, Obesity Research Center, University of Cincinnati, Cincinnati, OH 45237, USA

Ashutosh S. Pareek, D.O.   Department of Medicine, Beth Israel Medical Center, New York, NY, USA

Grishma Parikh, M.D.   Division of Endocrinology and Metabolism, Beth Israel Medical Center, New York, NY, USA

Parini Patel, M.D.   Division of Endocrinology and Metabolism, Beth Israel Medical Center, New York, NY, USA

Anne L. Peters, M.D., CDE   University of Southern California Keck School of Medicine, Los Angeles, CA, USA

Leonid Poretsky, M.D.   Division of Endocrinology and Metabolism, Albert Einstein College of Medicine, Beth Israel Medical Center, New York, NY, USA

Paolo Pozzilli, M.B.B.S., M.D.   Department of Endocrinology and Diabetes, University Campus Bio-Medico, Rome, Italy; Centre for Diabetes and Metabolic Medicine, Barts and The London School of Medicine and Dentistry, London, UK

Madhu N. Rao, M.D.   Division of Endocrinology and Metabolism, University of California, San Francisco, CA, USA

Elliot J. Rayfield, M.D.   Mount Sinai School of Medicine, New York, NY, USA

Carla M. Romero, M.D.   Department of Medicine, Beth Israel Medical Center, New York, NY, USA

Michael Rubin, M.D. Electromyography Laboratory, Department of Neurology, Weill Cornell Medical College, New York Presbyterian Hospital, New York, NY, USA

Steve H. Salzman, M.D. Division of Pulmonary and Critical Care Medicine, Winthrop-University Hospital, Mineola, NY, USA

Morris Schambelan, M.D. Division of Endocrinology and Metabolism, University of California, San Francisco, CA, USA

Adina E. Schneider, M.D. Division of Endocrinology and Metabolism, Mount Sinai School of Medicine, New York, NY, USA

Stephen H. Schneider, M.D. Division of Endocrinology, Metabolism and Nutrition, UMDNJ-Robert Wood Johnson Medical School, New Brunswick, NJ, USA

Brock E. Schroeder, Ph.D. Amylin Pharmaceuticals, Inc., San Diego, CA, USA

Amit K. Seth, M.D. Beth Israel Medical Center, New York, NY, USA

Uri Shabto, M.D. Department of Ophthalmology, The New York Eye and Ear Infirmary, New York, NY, USA

Dennis Shavelson, D.P.M. Beth Israel Medical Center and Weill Medical College of Cornell University, New York, NY, USA

Muhammad Z. Shrayyef, M.D. Dalhousie University, Moncton Hospital, Moncton, NB, Canada

Anil Shrestha, M.D. Division of Endocrinology and Metabolism, Beth Israel Medical Center, New York, NY, USA

Alan R. Shuldiner, M.D. Division of Endocrinology, Diabetes and Nutrition, University of Maryland School of Medicine, Baltimore, MD, USA; Geriatric Research and Education Clinical Center, Veterans Administration Medical Center, Baltimore, MD, USA

John S. Steinberg, DPM Department of Plastic Surgery, Georgetown University School of Medicine, Washington, DC, USA

Markus Stoffel, M.D. Institute of Molecular Systems Biology, Swiss Federal Institute of Technology, Zurich 8093, Switzerland

Gladys Witt Strain, Ph.D., RD Laparoscopic and Bariatric Surgery, Weill Medical College of Cornell University, New York, NY, USA

Gary E. Striker, M.D. Division of Nephrology, Departments of Medicine and Geriatrics, Mount Sinai School of Medicine, New York, NY, USA

Marina Strizhevsky, M.D. Division of Endocrinology and Metabolism, Beth Israel Medical Center, New York, NY, USA

Jennifer K. Svahn, M.D. Department of Surgery, Division of Vascular Surgery, Beth Israel Medical Center, New York, NY, USA

Bahman P. Tabaei, M.P.H. New York City Department of Health and Mental Hygiene, New York, NY, USA

Koji Takeuchi, Ph.D. Pharmacology Research Laboratories, Takeda Pharmaceutical Company Limited, Osaka, Japan

Marsha C. Tolentino, M.D. Division of Endocrinology and Metabolism, Beth Israel Medical Center, New York, NY, USA

Mathew C. Varghese, M.D., M.P.H. Department of Dermatology, New York Presbyterian Hospital, Weill Medical College of Cornell University, New York, NY, USA

George I. Varghese, M.D. School of Medicine, State University of New York at Stony Brook, Stony Brook, NY, USA

Sefton Vergano, M.D. Division of Endocrinology, Metabolism and Nutrition, UMDNJ-Robert Wood Johnson Medical School, New Brunswick, NJ, USA

Helen Vlassara, M.D. Division of Experimental Diabetes and Aging, Division of Geriatrics, Mount Sinai School of Medicine, New York, NY, USA

Monique Welbeck, N.P. Division of Endocrinology and Metabolism, Friedman Diabetes Institute, Beth Israel Medical Center, New York, NY, USA

James F. Winchester, M.D., FRCP (Glas), FACP Division of Nephrology and Hypertension, Department of Medicine, Beth Israel Medical Center, Albert Einstein College of Medicine, New York, NY, USA

Nathaniel Winer, M.D. Division of Endocrinology, Diabetes and Hypertension, Department of Medicine, State University of New York, Downstate Medical Center, Brooklyn, NY, USA

Shoshana Yakar, M.D. Division of Endocrinology, Diabetes & Bone Disease, Department of Medicine, Mount Sinai School of Medicine, New York, NY, USA

Vincent Yen, M.D. Saint Vincent's Medical Center, New York Medical College, New York, NY, USA

Jacek Zajac, M.D. Division of Endocrinology and Metabolism, Beth Israel Medical Center, New York, NY, USA

Joel Zonszein, M.D. Division of Endocrinology and Metabolism, Department of Medicine, Montefiore Medical Center and Albert Einstein College of Medicine, Bronx, NY, USA

Susan B. Zweig, M.D. Division of Endocrinology and Metabolism, Beth Israel Medical Center, New York, NY, USA

Part I

Chapter 1
The Main Events in the History of Diabetes Mellitus

Jacek Zajac, Anil Shrestha, Parini Patel, and Leonid Poretsky

In Antiquity

A medical condition producing excessive thirst, continuous urination, and severe weight loss has interested medical authors for over three millennia. Unfortunately, until the early part of twentieth century the prognosis for a patient with this condition was no better than it was over 3000 years ago. Since the ancient physicians described almost exclusively cases of what is today known as type 1 diabetes mellitus, the outcome was invariably fatal.

Ebers Papyrus, which was written around 1500 BC, excavated in 1862 AD from an ancient grave in Thebes, Egypt, and published by Egyptologist Georg Ebers in 1874, describes, among various other ailments and their remedies, a condition of "too great emptying of the urine" – perhaps, the reference to diabetes mellitus. For the treatment of this condition, ancient Egyptian physicians were advocating the use of wheat grains, fruit, and sweet beer.[1,2]

Physicians in India at around the same time developed what can be described as the first clinical test for diabetes. They observed that the urine from people with diabetes attracted ants and flies. They named the condition "madhumeha" or "honey urine." Indian physicians also noted that patients with "madhumeha" suffered from extreme thirst and foul breath (probably, because of ketosis). Although the polyuria associated with diabetes was well recognized, ancient clinicians could not distinguish between the polyuria due to what we now call diabetes mellitus from the polyuria due to other conditions.[3]

Around 230 BC, Apollonius of Memphis for the first time used the term "diabetes," which in Greek means "to pass through" (dia – through, betes – to go). He and his contemporaries considered diabetes a disease of the kidneys and recommended, among other ineffective treatments, such measures as bloodletting and dehydration.[3]

The first complete clinical description of diabetes appears to have been made by Aulus Cornelius Celsus (30 BC–50 AD). Often called "Cicero medicorum" for his elegant Latin, Celsus included the description of diabetes in his monumental eight-volume work entitled *De medicina*.[4,5]

Aretaeus of Cappadocia, a Greek physician who practiced in Rome and Alexandria in the second century AD, was the first to distinguish between what we now call diabetes mellitus and diabetes insipidus. In his work *On the Causes and Indications of Acute and Chronic Diseases*, he gave detailed account of diabetes mellitus and made several astute observations, noting, for example, that the onset of diabetes commonly follows acute illness, injury, or emotional stress. Aretaeus wrote:

> Diabetes is a dreadful affliction, not very frequent among men, being a melting down of the flesh and limbs into urine. The patients never stop making water and the flow is incessant, like the opening of the aqueducts. Life is short, unpleasant and painful, thirst unquenchable, drinking excessive and disproportionate to the large quantity of urine, for yet more urine is passed. . . . If for a while they abstain from drinking, their mouths become parched and their bodies dry; the viscera seem scorched up, the patients are affected by nausea, restlessness and a burning thirst, and within a short time they expire.[4,6]

Although the term "diabetes mellitus" was not firmly established until the nineteenth century, we will refer to this disease using its modern name throughout this chapter, even for the earlier periods.

L. Poretsky (✉)
Division of Endocrinology and Metabolism, Albert Einstein College of Medicine, Beth Israel Medical Center, New York, NY, USA
e-mail: lporetsk@chpnet.org

L. Poretsky (ed.), *Principles of Diabetes Mellitus*, DOI 10.1007/978-0-387-09841-8_1,
© Springer Science+Business Media, LLC 2010

Both Aretaeus and the renowned Roman physician Galen observed that diabetes was a rare disease. In fact, Galen mentioned that he encountered only two such cases in his entire career.[6] Galen attributed the development of diabetes to weakness of the kidney and gave it a name "diarrhea of the urine" ("diarrhea urinosa").[4]

In the fifth century AD, Sushruta and Charaka, two Indian physicians, were the first to differentiate between the two types of diabetes mellitus, observing that thin individuals with diabetes developed diabetes at a younger age in contrast to heavier individuals with diabetes, who had a later onset and lived longer period of time after the diagnosis. In seventh century AD in China, Li Hsuan noted that the patients with diabetes were prone to boils and lung infections. He prescribed avoidance of sex and wine as treatment for diabetes. Avicenna, or Ibn-Sina (980–1037 AD), a court physician to Caliphs of Baghdad, compiled an exhaustive medical text ("Canon Avicennae"), which included a detailed description of diabetes. Its clinical features, such as sweet urine and increased appetite, and complications, such as diabetic gangrene and sexual dysfunction, were described by Avicenna in detail.[7]

Renaissance and After

The origin of current understanding of some aspects of diabetes can be traced to discoveries made in Europe between sixteenth and eighteenth centuries. Aureolus Theophrastus Bombastus von Hohenheim, a Swiss physician better known as Paracelsus (1494–1541), allowed the urine of patients with diabetes to evaporate and observed a white residue. He incorrectly thought that this residue consisted of salt and proceeded to attribute excessive thirst and urination in these patients to salt deposition in the kidneys.[8] In 1670, Thomas Willis in Oxford noticed the sweet taste of urine of patients with diabetes. Thomas Cawley, in 1788, was the first to suggest the link between the pancreas and diabetes after he observed that people with pancreatic injury developed diabetes.[8]

In 1776, British physiologist Matthew Dobson (1713–1784) in his *Experiments and Observations on the Urine in Diabetics* was the first to show that the sweet-tasting substance in the urine of patients with diabetes was sugar. He also noted the sweet taste of serum in these individuals and thus discovered hyperglycemia. Dobson put forward the theory that the diabetes was a systemic disease, rather than one of the kidneys.[9]

The Nineteenth and the Early Twentieth Century: Discovery of Insulin

The important elements of current understanding of diabetes mellitus can be traced to nineteenth century when modern scientific disciplines, including biochemistry and experimental physiology, acquired prominence in biological studies.

In 1815, Eugene Chevreul in Paris proved that the sugar in urine of individuals with diabetes was glucose. Von Fehling developed quantitative test for glucose in urine in 1848.[9] Thus, in the nineteenth century, glucosuria became an accepted diagnostic criterion for diabetes.

Claude Bernard (1813–1878), professor of physiology at Sorbonne University, was one of the most prominent and prolific experimental physiologists in nineteenth-century Europe. Because of the scope of Bernard's interests, Louis Pasteur referred to him as "Physiology itself."[10] In the course of his work on the physiology of gastrointestinal tract, Bernard developed an experimental operation during which the pancreatic ducts were ligated. Degeneration of the pancreas followed. This technique proved invaluable for later experiments searching for pancreatic substance which controlled glucose level. In addition to developing the technique for pancreatic duct ligation, Bernard also discovered that the liver stored glycogen and secreted sugary substance into the blood. He assumed that it was an excess of this secretion that caused diabetes. Bernard's theory of sugar over-secretion leading to diabetes received wide acceptance.[11]

At the same time as researchers were looking for the cause of diabetes, clinicians were further advancing the understanding of diabetes mellitus as a systemic disease with various manifestations and complications. William Prout (1785–1850) was the first to describe diabetic coma and Wilhelm Petters in 1857 demonstrated the presence of acetone in the urine of patients with diabetes. Adolf Kussmaul (1822–1902) proposed that acetonemia was the cause of diabetic coma. Henry Noyes in 1869 described retinopathy in a person with advanced diabetes. M. Troiser in 1871 observed diabetes in patients with hemochromatosis, naming it "bronze diabetes."[12]

John Rollo (1749–1809), surgeon general to the British Army, added the term "mellitus" (derived from the Greek word for honey) to "diabetes" in order to distinguish it from diabetes insipidus. In 1797, Rollo developed a high-protein, low-carbohydrate diet consisting of rancid meats, blood pudding, and mixture of milk and lime water for patients with diabetes.[13] It has been suggested that he prescribed anorexic agents, such as antimony, digitalis, and opium to suppress appetite in patients with diabetes.

During the years prior to insulin discovery, diabetes treatment mostly consisted of starvation diets. Frederick Allen (1879–1964), a leading American diabetologist of the time, believed that, since diabetes patients could not utilize the food efficiently, limiting the amount of food would improve the disease. The dietary restriction treatment was harsh and death from starvation was not uncommon in patients with type 1 diabetes on this therapy. On the other hand, it is easy to understand why outcomes of low-calorie diets were often quite good in patients with type 2 diabetes.[12,14]

Discovery of insulin by Frederick Banting and Charles Best was the final step in identifying the substance whose deficiency had been postulated to be responsible for development of diabetes. This milestone, however, was preceded by a number of earlier significant advances.

Oscar Minkowski (1858–1931) and Joseph von Mering (1849–1908), working in Strasbourg in 1889, observed that the dogs whose pancreas was removed developed severe thirst, excessive urination, and weight loss with increased appetite. Minkowski, suspecting that such symptoms were caused by diabetes, tested the urine of these dogs and found glucose. Since Minkowski was working in the laboratory of Bernard Naunyn (1839–1925), who was interested in carbohydrate metabolism and was a leading authority on diabetes at the time, Minkowski's research received enthusiastic endorsement by Naunyn. Work on pancreatic extraction ensued, but the investigators were not able to obtain presumed antidiabetic substance. They suspected that digestive juices produced by pancreas might have interfered with their ability to purify this substance. To prove that the absence of exocrine pancreatic secretion was not related to the development of diabetes, they ligated dog's pancreatic duct. This procedure led to the development of digestive problems but not the diabetes.[12,15]

In 1893 a very important contribution was made by French investigator Edouard Hedon (1863–1933) in Montpellier, who showed that the total pancreatectomy was necessary for the development of diabetes. After removing the pancreas, he grafted a small piece of it under the skin. No evidence of diabetes in experimental animals was present at this stage. However, removal of the graft caused the symptoms of diabetes to develop immediately. Similar results were independently obtained by Minkowski. It was becoming clear that the internal secretion of the pancreas was pivotal to the pathogenesis of diabetes mellitus.[15]

In 1893, French scientist Gustave–Edouard Laguesse (1861–1927) suggested that tiny islands of pancreatic tissue described in 1869 by Paul Langerhans might be the source of the substance involved in blood glucose control. Paul Langerhans (1847–1888), distinguished German pathologist, was a student of Rudolf Virchow. In his doctoral thesis, at the age of 22, he described small groupings of pancreatic cells that were not drained by pancreatic ducts. In 1909, the Belgian physician Jean de Mayer named the presumed substance produced by the islets of Langerhans "insulin."[16]

A number of researchers worked on isolating the active component of internal pancreatic secretion. In 1902, John Rennie and Thomas Fraser in Aberdeen, Scotland, extracted a substance from the endocrine pancreas of codfish (*Gadus callurious*) whose endocrine and exocrine pancreata are anatomically separate. They injected the extract into the dog that soon died, presumably from severe hypoglycemia. In 1907, Georg Ludwig Zuelzer (1870–1949), a German physician, removed pancreas from the dog and then injected the dog with pancreatic extract. His experiments resulted in lowered amount of glucosuria and raised blood pH. Zuelzer patented the extract in the United States under the name "acomatol." In 1908, he used it successfully to rescue a comatose diabetic patient, but, owing to likely contamination of the extract by other substances, the treatment produced severe complications and led to withdrawal of further funding of Zuelzer's work by Schering. Zuelzer continued his investigations, however, and developed a new extract for Hoffman–La Roche. The new extract produced convulsive reaction, most likely caused by hypoglycemia.[12,15] Nicolas Constantin Paulesco (1869–1931), professor of Physiology at Bucharest University in Romania, was also involved in research on pancreatic extracts. In 1916 in the course of his first experiment, he injected the diabetic dog with the pancreatic extract. The injection resulted in the death of the animal with symptoms of hypoglycemia. During the experiment, dog's blood glucose fell from 140 to 26 mg%. Because of World War I, Paulesco did not publish the report of his experiments until 1921.[12]

Frederick Grant Banting (1891–1941) was a young (and not very successful) orthopedic surgeon when he developed interest in diabetes. A war veteran, wounded in France in 1918, he was decorated with Military Cross for heroism. After returning from Europe, he briefly practiced orthopedic surgery and then took the position as a demonstrator in Physiology at the University of Western Ontario, Canada.[17] On October 31, 1920, Banting wrote in his notebook:

> Diabetus (sic!). Ligate pancreatic ducts of the dog. Keep dog alive till acini degenerate leaving Islets. Try to isolate the internal secretion of these to relieve glycosurea[17]

The technique of pancreatic duct ligation, leading to pancreatic degeneration, was developed and used for pancreatic function studies by Claude Bernard, as discussed earlier. Banting approached John J.R. MacLeod, professor of Physiology at the University of Toronto, who agreed to provide Banting with limited space in his laboratory for the eight-week summer period in 1921. McLeod assigned a physiology student Charles Best (1899–1978) to assist Banting with the experiments (Best apparently won the opportunity to work alongside Banting on the toss of coin with another student).[17]

In July 1921, after initial delays caused by insufficient ligature of the pancreatic ducts, Banting and Best were able to harvest atrophied pancreatic glands from the dogs, chop them up, grind the tissue in the mortar, strain the solution, and inject the extract into the vein of pancreatectomized (diabetic) dog. When it was clear that the dog's condition improved, they proceeded to repeat the experiments with other diabetic dogs, with similar dramatic results. They also experimented with fresh pancreata, fetal calf pancreata, and different routes of administration (rectal, subcutaneous, and intravenous).

At the end of 1921, biochemist James Collip joined the team of Banting and Best and was instrumental in developing better extraction and purification techniques.[12] First report of successful animal experiments with Banting's pancreatic extracts was presented at Physiological Journal Club of Toronto on November 14, 1921 and American Physiological Society later that year.[18]

On January 11, 1922, Banting and Best injected Leonard Thompson, a 14-year old boy being treated for diabetes at Toronto General Hospital, with their extract. At the time Thompson's weight was only 64 lb. After having 15 cm^3 of "thick brown" substance injected into the buttocks, Thompson became acutely ill upon developing abscesses at the injection sites. Second injection, using a much improved preparation made with Collip's method, followed on January 23. This time the patient's blood glucose fell from 520 to 120 mg/dl within about 24 h and urinary ketones disappeared. Thompson received ongoing therapy and lived for another 13 years but died of pneumonia at the age of 27.[19]

On May 3, 1922, McLeod presented results of Toronto group's research to the Association of American Physicians and received standing ovation.[19] Banting and Best were not present at the meeting. In 1923, the Nobel Prize was awarded for discovery of insulin, but only to Banting and MacLeod, who shared their portions of the prize with Best and Collip, respectively.[12] The new proposed antidiabetic substance was named by Banting "isletin." The name was later changed by MacLeod to "insulin." MacLeod apparently did not know that this name had already been coined by de Mayer in 1909. Later, Banting and Best fully acknowledged this fact.[19]

In April 1922, Banting and Best accepted the offer by Eli Lilly Company to work on purification and large-scale commercial production of insulin. The Board of Governors of the University of Toronto and Eli Lilly signed the agreement, providing that Lilly would pay royalties to the University of Toronto to support research in exchange for manufacturing rights for North and South America.[20]

The announcement of insulin discovery was greeted with tremendous enthusiasm around the world. Press was bringing numerous reports of miraculous cures. Previously doomed patients were getting the new lease on life. Indeed, Ted Ryder, one of the first four children to receive insulin in 1922 in Toronto, died at the age of 76 in 1993.

Over the years, insulin purification methods improved and new insulin formulations were developed. Protamine–zinc insulin, a long-acting insulin, was introduced in the 1930s; Neutral Protamine Hagedorn (NPH) was introduced in the 1940s; and Lente series of insulin in the 1950s.[20]

Among the people who first witnessed the introduction of insulin into clinical use was a Portuguese physician Ernesto Roma, who was visiting Boston shortly after insulin became available. Upon returning to Portugal he founded the world's first organization for people with diabetes – the *Portuguese Association for Protection of Poor Diabetics*. The association provided insulin free of charge to the poor. Subsequently, the *British Diabetic Association* was founded in 1934 by Robin Lawrence, a physician with diabetes whose life was saved by insulin, and the writer H.G. Wells, who had diabetes.[21] A few years later, at a meeting of the American College of Physicians in 1937, a small group of physicians with interest in diabetes met for lunch. They felt that diabetes management was inadequately covered at regular meetings. They realized a need of a platform to share their experiences. After two years of deliberations, in April 2, 1940, delegates from local societies in the United States met and founded the *National Diabetes Association*. Both the first president of the association Dr. Cecil Striker and the vice-president Dr. Herman O. Mosenthal were very instrumental in the founding of the association. Subsequently, as per Dr. Mosenthal's suggestion, the association was renamed *American Diabetes Association* to include the Canadian physicians, there being no such association in Canada at the time as well as to pay homage to the country where insulin was discovered.[22]

In 1922, August Krogh of Denmark, winner of the Nobel Prize for his studies of capillaries, was lecturing in the United States, accompanied by his wife Marie, who had recently been diagnosed with diabetes. Krogh and his wife were informed by famous diabetologist of the time Eliot P. Joslin about new diabetes treatment developed in Toronto by Banting's group. Marie and August Krogh decided to visit Toronto and stayed as John McLeod's guests. After return to Denmark, Krogh, with H.C. Hagedorn, founded Nordisk Insulin Company, a not-for-profit concern that, together with Novo Company, was responsible for making Denmark the main insulin-producing country outside of the United States.[23]

Oral Agents in Diabetes

Oral hypoglycemic agents were discovered following the fortuitous observations of hypoglycemia as a side effect of various investigative substances. In 1918, while investigating biological effects of guanidine, C.K. Watanabe noted that guanidine, under certain condition, can cause hypoglycemia. Watanabe injected guanidine subcutaneously into rabbits, initially causing hyperglycemia followed by hypoglycemia within several hours. Inspired by these findings, E. Frank, M. Nothmann, and A. Wagner tried to modify the guanidine molecule. Several guanidine derivatives were studied, including monoguanidines and biguanidines. The biguanidines were found to have greatest hypoglycemic effect. The first commercially available guanidine derivative decamethyl–diguanidine was introduced in 1928 and marketed in Europe under the name Synthalin. In the United States, phenylethyl–biguanidine was introduced for treatment of diabetes in 1957 and was available for clinical use in 1959 under the name Phenformin. Synthalin was discontinued from the use because of liver and kidney toxicity.[24]

Celestino Ruiz and L.L. Silva of Argentina noted the hypoglycemic properties of certain sulfonamide derivatives in 1939. In 1942, in occupied France, Professor of Pharmacology at Montpellier University M.J. Janbon discovered that the sulfonylurea agent tested for the treatment of typhoid fever produced bizarre toxic side effects. Janbon correctly attributed these effects, which included confusion, cramps, and coma, to hypoglycemia.[6,24] This compound was then administered to diabetic patients, lowering their blood glucose. The researchers explored the potential mechanism of action of the substance and found that it became ineffective if experimental animal had been pancreatectomized. After well-publicized research by German investigators Hans Franke and Joachim Fuchs, sulfonylureas were studied extensively. Franke and Fuchs discovered hypoglycemic actions of sulfonylureas during testing of the new long-acting sulfonamide antibiotic. Chemists at Hoechst manufactured a compound D 860, which was marketed in the United States as tolbutamide in 1956. This compound became the first commercially available sulfonylurea agent.[24]

Many chemical substances have been studied for their hypoglycemic effect but extremely few have made it to the market. As an example, from 1962 to 1977, Boehringer–Mannheim and Hoechst studied 8000 different chemicals for hypoglycemic properties, of which 6000 produced hypoglycemia in laboratory animals. Out of these, only five made it as far as clinical tests and ultimately only one, HB 419 (glibenclamide/glyburide), was marketed.[24]

In addition to biguanides and sulfonylureas, a number of other classes of oral hypoglycemic agents were ultimately discovered and are currently in clinical use. These are discussed in detail in Chapter 44.

Use of Radioimmunoassay for Measurement of Circulating Insulin Level

One of the most important milestones in the understanding of pathophysiology of diabetes was the development of radioimmunoassay (RIA) by Rosalyn Sussman Yalow (b. 1921) and Salomon A. Berson (1919–1972).

During her graduate studies at the University of Chicago, Yalow, a nuclear physicist, worked on the development of the device to measure radioactive substances. In 1947, she became a consultant in Nuclear Physics at Veteran Administration Hospital in the Bronx, New York. She became a full-time faculty member at the Bronx VA Hospital in 1950. Here Yalow worked with Salomon A. Berson investigating the use of radioactive isotopes in physiologic systems. Yalow and Berson developed the technique called radioimmunoassay (RIA), which allowed quantification of very small amounts of biological substances. The first report of the new technique in 1959 was largely ignored.[25]

The RIA is based on a principle of competition between the radiolabeled compound of interest and unlabeled compound in the patient's serum for limited number of binding sites on the antibody against this compound. After the incubation period, which allows for equilibrium to develop, the antibody–antigen complexes are precipitated and the amount of radioactive label attached to the antibody is measured. Because of the competition for binding sites on the antibody, the higher the concentration of unlabeled compound in the patient's serum, the smaller the amount of labeled compound that bind to the precipitated antibody.[26]

In 1959, using their method, Yalow and Berson demonstrated that patients with diabetes did not always suffer from deficiency of insulin in their blood. Thus, insulin was the first hormone measured with the new technique.[25]

For this groundbreaking work, Rosalyn Yalow was awarded many honors, including Nobel Prize in 1977, which she accepted on behalf of herself and Berson, who had died 5 years earlier. The Nobel Prize Committee called the RIA the most valuable advance in basic clinical research in the previous two decades.[25]

Yalow and Berson never patented the RIA technique, instead sparing no effort to make it more popular and accessible for use by both the clinicians and the investigators.

Recombinant DNA Technology and the Synthesis of Human Insulin

The groundwork for the production of large quantities of human insulin was laid by Frederick Sanger (b. 1918), who published the structural formula of bovine insulin in 1955 while working at Cambridge University. He received Nobel Prize for this work in 1958.[24] Dorothy Hodgkin (1910–1994) described the three-dimensional structure of porcine insulin in 1969 at Oxford using X-ray crystallography.[27]

Prior to the development of recombinant DNA technology, patients with diabetes mostly received bovine or porcine insulin. Although bovine insulin differs from human insulin only by three amino acids and porcine only by one amino acid, these differences are sufficient for human immune system to produce antibodies against insulin, neutralizing its action and causing local inflammatory reactions. The pharmacokinetics of insulin is altered by its binding to antibodies, resulting in increased half-life of the circulating insulin and prolongation of its action. These considerations and growing demand for insulin, coupled with the difficulties in animal insulin production (it is estimated that 8000 lb of animal pancreatic tissue is needed to produce 1 lb of insulin), prompted work on developing alternative sources of insulin.[28]

The gene coding for human insulin was cloned in 1978 by Genentech. It is located on the short arm of chromosome 11. Once incorporated in the bacterial plasmid of *E. coli*, the human insulin gene became active, resulting in the production of alpha and beta chains of insulin, which were then combined to construct complete insulin molecule.[29]

In 1978, Genentech, Inc. and City of Hope National Medical Center, a private research institution in Duarte, California, announced the successful laboratory production of human insulin using recombinant DNA technology. This was achieved by a team of scientists led by Robert Crea, Keichi Itakura, David Goeddel, Dennis Kleid, and Arthur Riggs. Insulin thus became the first genetically manufactured drug to be approved by the FDA.[28]

In July 1996, the FDA approved the first recombinant DNA human insulin analog, the insulin lispro. At present more than 300 human insulin molecule analogs have been identified, including about 70 animal insulins, 80 chemically modified insulins, and 150 biosynthetic insulins.

In January 2006, FDA approved inhaled form of insulin marketed under the name of Exubera. This was the first noninjectable form of insulin available to patients with diabetes. The device did not become popular for a variety of reasons and was withdrawn from the market by the company in 2007.

Glucose Monitoring by Physicians and Patients

Although, the chemical tests to detect sugar in blood and urine were discovered in the early nineteenth century, the concept of self-monitoring was not conceived until the 1960s. In 1965, Ames introduced a product called dextrostix created by Ernest C. Adams, at Ames Co. This was a paper strip that developed a blue color after a drop of blood was placed on it for 1 min. This blue strip was then washed with water and its color was compared with the color chart to estimate the blood glucose levels. This technique did not allow estimation of fingerstick glucose accurately. Hence, a meter that would measure the light reflected back from a test strip and would give a numerical value to it was designed. Tom Clemens, the inventor of the first blood glucose meter, started working on it in 1966 and built several prototypes for field trials in 1968. The meter became available on the market in 1970. Initially used in doctors' offices, meters and strips gradually gained popularity for patient use. Over the years, glucometer models have become smaller in size, require less blood, and have acquired a variety of user-friendly options such as memory and computer download features.[30]

An important laboratory test that has changed our approach to management of diabetes is hemoglobin A1c (HbA1c) measurement. Hemoglobin A1c was identified as one of the larger fraction of the minor components of normal adult hemoglobin in the 1950s. In 1966, Holmquist and Shroeder showed that the β-globin chain contained an unidentified compound attached to it.[31] About 2 years later, Bookchin and Gallop reported that a hexose moiety was linked to the N-terminal of β-globin chain of the hemoglobin A1c.[32] At the same time, Samuel Rahbar independently reported an abnormally fast-moving hemoglobin fraction that was present in hemoglobin of patients with diabetes in Iran.[33] Subsequently, while working as an international post-doctoral fellow at Albert Einstein College of Medicine in New York in 1969, he and his colleagues reported that this fast-moving hemoglobin in patients with diabetes was identical to the HbA1c.[34] In 1975, Tattersall et al. studied twins concordant and discordant for diabetes and suggested that hemoglobin A1c was an acquired manifestation of the metabolic abnormality in diabetes.[35] In 1976, Koenig and colleagues demonstrated that HbA1c concentration was an indicator of fasting blood glucose concentrations. HbA1c concentrations decreased as diabetes control improved with treatment.[36] Today, HbA1c measurements and use of glucometers have revolutionized management of diabetes and enhanced our understanding of effects of glycemic control on diabetes-related outcomes.

Landmark Clinical Trials in Diabetes

One of the major questions in diabetes therapy, which had remained unresolved until recently, was that of the relationship between glycemic control and development of the complications of diabetes. The evidence supporting the role of metabolic abnormalities in the development of diabetic complications had long been known. It was not clear, however, if meticulous glycemic control could prevent the development of these complications.

Two very important studies were conducted to answer this question.

Diabetes Control and Complications Trial (DCCT) was a large multicenter diabetes study conducted by NIH from 1983 to 1993. The study was designed to evaluate whether tight glucose control can prevent or reduce the rate of progression of long-term complications of diabetes. DCCT involved 1441 volunteers 13–39 years of age in 29 centers in the United States. They all had type 1 diabetes for at least 1 year but no longer than 15 years. The subjects were divided into two groups. The Primary Prevention group consisted of patients with type 1 diabetes of 1–5 years duration and no complications of diabetes. The subjects in the Secondary Intervention group had type 1 diabetes for 1–15 years. They also had mild diabetic nephropathy and retinopathy. Patients in both groups were randomized to receive either intensive or conventional therapy. The goal of intensive therapy was to keep pre-meal blood glucose between 70 and 120 mg/dl and post-meal glucose less than 180 mg/dl. In the conventional treatment group, the aim was to keep the patients free of diabetic symptoms.[37] At the conclusion, the study showed that the hemoglobin A1c (a measure of glycemic control within previous 3 months) in the intensively treated patients was almost 2% lower than in those treated conventionally. The average blood glucose level in the intensive treatment group was 155 mg/dl, as compared to average blood glucose of 231 mg/dl in the conventional treatment group. Intensive therapy resulted in 76% reduction in retinopathy, 34% reduction in the development of early nephropathy, and 69% reduction in the development of neuropathy. In the Secondary Intervention group, intensive therapy resulted in 54% reduction in progression of established eye disease. The risk of hypoglycemia, however, was increased three times in those receiving intensive therapy; this group also experienced weight gain 1.6 times more frequently.[37]

After completion of the DCCT, researchers continued to follow DCCT subjects to assess long-term implications of intensive glycemic control during the observational Epidemiology of Diabetes Interventions and Complications (EDIC) study. After the DCCT study, the conventional treatment group was offered intensive management of diabetes and then asked to follow up with their health-care providers. During the fourth year after the DCCT, the gap in glycosylated hemoglobin values between the conventional therapy and the intensive therapy group narrowed from average 9.1 and 7.2% to 8.2 and 7.9%, respectively ($p < 0.001$). However, the proportion of patients who had progression of retinopathy was significantly lower in the intensive treatment group (odds reduction 75%). The proportion of patients with an increase in urinary albumin was significantly lower in the intensive treatment group.[38] Furthermore, during the 11-year post-DCCT follow-up, the intensive treatment group continued to exhibit a 57% reduction in risk of nonfatal myocardial infarction, stroke, or death from cardiovascular disease compared to the conventional treatment group. This occurred in spite of very minor differences in glycosylated hemoglobin values ($8.0 \pm 1.2\%$ vs. $8.2 \pm 1.2\%$, respectively; $p = 0.03$). The pathophysiological mechanism responsible for this sustained beneficial effect of tight glycemic control remains unclear and is now referred to as "metabolic memory."[39]

The United Kingdom Prospective Diabetes Study (UKPDS), completed in 1998, was the largest study of patients with type 2 diabetes mellitus. The study was designed to observe the effects of glycemic control on long-term complications of diabetes. Researchers enrolled 5102 patients with newly diagnosed type 2 diabetes and followed them for a median of 11 years. Intensive treatment (insulin or oral agents or both) was compared to conventional therapy (diet and, if necessary, pharmacological therapy). Median level of HbA1c in intensively treated group was 7.0%; it was 7.9% in conventionally treated group. Intensive treatment significantly decreased risk (by 12%) of aggregated diabetes-related endpoints (sudden death, death from hyperglycemia or hypoglycemia, fatal or nonfatal myocardial infarction, angina, heart failure, stroke, renal failure, amputation, vitreous hemorrhage, retinal photocoagulation, blindness, or cataract extraction). Risk reduction for progression of retinopathy was 21% and for appearance of microalbuminuria was 30%. However, individual cardiovascular events did not decrease significantly.[40] Tight blood pressure control (mean blood pressure 144/82 mmHg) compared to less tight control (mean blood pressure 154/87 mmHg) significantly reduced the risk of microvascular and macrovascular complications by 37 and 34%, respectively.[41] Adding metformin to the diet in overweight patients lowered the risk of any diabetes-related endpoints, diabetes-related death, and all-cause mortality and did not induce weight gain.[42]

Collectively, DCCT and UKPDS, along with other studies (discussed in detail in Chapters 39 and 45), established that improvement in the control of metabolic abnormalities decreases the risk of the development of dreaded complications responsible for severe and chronic disabilities associated with the disease, such as blindness and renal failure. However, the effects of tight glycemic control on cardiovascular outcomes remain unclear.

ACCORD (Action to Control Cardiovascular Risk in Diabetes) trial sponsored by the National Heart, Lung and Kidney Institute is being conducted to study effects of tight glycemic control, blood pressure treatment, and lipid control on cardiovascular outcomes in individuals with type 2 diabetes. In February 2008, the ACCORD investigators halted the intensive glycemic control arm (hemoglobin A1c goal less than 6%) because of increased risk of death in this arm. Although details of this study are not published, at the time of this writing it appears that this group consisted of individuals who had type 2 diabetes for an average of 10 years with at least two risk factors for heart disease other than diabetes or a previous history of heart disease. Among 10,251 participants, the rates of death in intensive and conventional group were 257 and 203, respectively, over 4 years of treatment. The incidence of deaths in this study (11 deaths/1000 patients per year in conventional treatment group versus 14 deaths/1000 patients per year in intensive treatment group over 4 years) is lower than death rates found in similar population in other studies. At this point, the cause for increased death is not clear and is under investigation. The other treatment arms are being continued and the study is scheduled to conclude in June 2009.[43]

Patients with diabetes are typically counseled to lose weight and exercise. However, long-term consequences of intentional weight loss are unknown. Look AHEAD is the first randomized controlled trial to assess whether weight reduction, combined with increased physical activity in overweight individuals with type 2 diabetes, reduces cardiovascular morbidity and mortality. The study began in 2001 and is scheduled to conclude in 2012.[44]

Attempts to Cure Diabetes: Whole Pancreas and Pancreatic Islet Cell Transplantation

Majority of the treatment methods available for the management of diabetes offer means of controlling the disease. The ultimate goal of the physicians treating patients with diabetes is to achieve cure. There have been many attempts to develop the safe and effective methods of curing diabetes. Although very intensive research is being conducted in this field, current protocols still have only limited applications.

In 1966, University of Minnesota surgeons performed the first cadaver pancreas transplant. The first living donor transplant was performed in 1978. With improved surgical techniques, newer immunosuppressive agents, and healthier recipients, the graft survival rate has remarkably improved. In experienced centers, the 1- and 5-year pancreas graft survival rates have increased significantly from 29 and 11% (1976–1985) to 73 and 46% (1996–2006), respectively.[45] Although the risk of the procedure and the rates of the graft failure have declined, the complications associated with prolonged immunosuppression limit the use of this procedure to a small number of patients with type 1 diabetes.

In 1972, Paul Lacy and coworkers published the paper on methods of isolation of intact pancreatic islet cells.[46] First attempts at islet cell transplants were performed in animals with experimental diabetes and resulted in the reversal of hyperglycemia.

First autologous islet cell transplant was performed by surgeons at the University of Minnesota in 1977.[47] Autologous islet cell transplants are reported to have 75% long-term success rate. Autologous transplants are usually used in the setting of chronic pancreatitis requiring removal of pancreas.

Success with autologous cell transplants has foreshadowed the recent very promising developments in the field of allogeneic islet cell transplants. Early experience with human allogeneic transplants was not promising. It is thought that the poor success rate with the early allogeneic transplants was related to the use of immuno-suppressants like prednisone, which is diabetogenic. That may have been compounded by insufficient number of islets used for transplantation.

In 1999, a group of researchers from Edmonton in Alberta, Canada, reported successful experience (defined by insulin independence up to a median time of 11 months) in seven patients with type 1 diabetes mellitus that had a history of severe recurrent hypoglycemia and poor metabolic control. These patients received islet cell transplants from non-HLA (human leukocyte antigen)-matched cadaveric pancreata, with the use of glucocorticoid-free immunosuppressive regimen.[48] A 5-year follow-up from the same center reported data on 65 patients who received islet cell transplant as of November 2004. Majority (80%) had c-peptide present, but only a minority (10%) maintained insulin independence. The median duration of insulin independence was 15 months.

The HbA1c was lower in patients who were off insulin or on insulin but c-peptide positive and higher in those who lost all graft function. Furthermore, the hypoglycemic episodes and the amplitude of glycemic excursions improved post-transplant.[49]

The most serious limitation to the use of donor islet cells is the shortage of available donors. This limitation has led to a search for alternative islet cell sources. Porcine cells have been suggested as a potential source of islet cells for the transplant. The development of transgenic pigs (expressing human genes to diminish immunological reaction) might decrease the need for immunosuppression after the transplant procedure. The disadvantage of using cells from transgenic pigs involves the risk of cross-species infection with porcine retroviruses, which can adapt to human hosts. These concerns have led the FDA to halt trials of porcine xenografts until those patients who have already received grafts are assessed for possible infections.[50]

Other possible sources of islet cells under investigation are human pancreatic duct cells, fetal pancreatic stem cells, and embryonic stem cells.[50]

Diabetes Prevention

In 1921 Eliot P. Joslin wrote:

> It is proper at the present time to devote not alone to treatment but still more to prevention of diabetes. The results may not be as striking or immediate, but they are sure to come and to be important.

Studies have clearly demonstrated that diet and exercise improve glycemic control and some patients with diabetes treated with diet and exercise alone enter a sustained remission state lasting up to 5 years. Data from two NHANES (National Health and Nutrition Examination Survey) surveys show that among adults aged 20–74 years, the prevalence of obesity increased from 15.0% (in the 1976–1980 survey) to 32.9% (in the 2003–2004 survey). Thirty-four percent of adults aged 20–70 are overweight.[51] This can be partly attributed to a significant increase in total calories and carbohydrate consumption in the past 30 years.[52]

The Physician Health Study has demonstrated inverse relationship between physical activity and rate of development of diabetes.[53] Similar results were reported from Nurses' Health Study.[54] National Health Interview Survey completed in 1990 has shown that diabetic individuals were less likely to participate in regular physical exercise than were people without diabetes.[55]

Several clinical studies present the evidence suggesting that diet and exercise can reduce the incidence of type 2 diabetes. Tuomilehto and coworkers demonstrated that the individuals on a consistent diet and exercise program had 10% incidence of diabetes during 4 years of follow-up compared to 22% for patients in the control group who met only once a year with the dietician and the physician.[56] A 6-year randomized trial conducted by Pan and colleagues demonstrated that exercise resulted in 46% reduction in the incidence of diabetes in patients with impaired glucose tolerance.[57] Helmrich and coworkers administered questionnaires evaluating the pattern of physical activity to 5990 male alumni of University of Pennsylvania. The researchers found that the leisure time activity (like walking, stair climbing, and participation in sports) during 14-year follow-up was inversely related to the risk of development of type 2 diabetes. The protective effect was strongest among the people at the highest risk for diabetes.[58] Study by Manson and coworkers followed 87,253 women (aged 34–59) free of diabetes, cardiovascular disease, or cancer for 8 years. Women who engaged in vigorous exercise at least once per week, after adjusting for age, family history, body mass index, and other factors, had 46% relative risk reduction for development of diabetes.[54]

In 1993, National Institute of Diabetes and Digestive and Kidney Diseases initiated a multicenter study with the objective of developing methods to prevent new cases of type 2 diabetes in adults. The study was named Diabetes Prevention Program (DPP). DPP was a 27-center randomized clinical trial designed to evaluate the safety and efficacy of interventions that may delay or prevent development of diabetes in people with increased risk. Three thousand two hundred and thirty-four obese patients with impaired glucose tolerance and fasting plasma glucose of 5.3–6.9 mmol/l were randomized into three groups: intensive lifestyle modification, standard care plus metformin, and standard care plus placebo. Trial was terminated 1 year prematurely because the data had clearly addressed main research objectives. Results of DPP were reported in 2001. About 29% of DPP control subjects developed diabetes during the average follow-up period of 3 years. In contrast, 14% of the diet and exercise subgroup and 22% in metformin arm developed diabetes. Volunteers in the diet and exercise arm achieved average weight loss of about 5% during the duration of the study.[59]

A Diabetes Prevention Trial (DPT-1) was conducted to determine if subcutaneous or oral insulin administration can delay or prevent diabetes in nondiabetic relatives of patients with diabetes. This was a large multicenter study sponsored by the National Institute of Diabetes and Digestive and Kidney Diseases in cooperation with the National Center for Research Resources, the Juvenile Diabetes Foundation International, and the American Diabetes Association. There was no decrease in incidence of development of type 1 diabetes with parenteral or oral insulin administration.[60,61]

Genome-Wide Association Studies

The susceptibility to develop diabetes is determined by a combination of genetic and environmental factors. Given the polygenic etiology of type 2 diabetes, the genes responsible for the disease are not yet identified. However, with the completion of the Human Genome Project in 2003 and the International HapMap Project in 2005, researchers are now able to quickly analyze the whole genome for single-nucleotide polymorphisms (SNPs) in large populations. Genomic areas with variations in SNPs between populations with and without diabetes are then studied in greater details. The most comprehensive genome-wide association study for type 2 diabetes was reported in April 2007 by three groups working in close collaboration – US–Finnish team, US–Swiss team, and a British group. These studies identified four new genetic variants and confirmed existence of another six.[62–64] The significance of these variants is currently under investigation. Once new genetic associations are recognized, the information can be utilized to better understand pathophysiology of diabetes and develop better strategies to detect, treat, and prevent the disease.

Summary

Diabetes mellitus has been observed and reported throughout written history since at least 1500 BC. It is only relatively recently that the perception of this disease has changed. Type 1 diabetes no longer carries the stigma of inevitably fast progressing and deadly disease. Intensive scientific research worldwide has brought new insight into this disease with modern management methods. Yet, much remains to be done and the cure has remained elusive. With improving standard of living and increasing affluence, the western world is now witnessing the rising epidemic of obesity predisposing to type 2 diabetes. As the disease itself and its complications impose great social and economical burdens, attention of medical professionals should increasingly be directed toward raising awareness of diabetes and promoting healthy lifestyle to prevent the development of this disease. Ultimately, with effective strategies for prevention and cure of diabetes, this disease will be eliminated.

Diabetes Timeline

Circa 1500 BC, Ebers Papyrus	First written reference to diabetes by ancient Egyptian physicians
230 BC, Apollonius of Memphis	The name diabetes (from Greek "to pass through") given to the disease
First century AD, Aulus Cornelius Celsus	First clinical description of diabetes
Fifth century AD, Susruta and Charaka, India	First distinction between type 1 and type 2 diabetes mellitus
1776, Mathew Dobson, England	Determined that the sweet-tasting substance in the urine of diabetic individuals is sugar

Diabetes Timeline (continued)

1788, Thomas Cowley, England	First link between diabetes and pancreas
1869, Paul Langerhans, Germany	Discovery of small cell clusters in the pancreas, not drained by the pancreatic ducts. These cell clusters later named "islets of Langerhans"
1889, Oscar Minkowski, Joseph von Mehring, Germany	Removal of the pancreas in the dogs causing immediate development of diabetes
1893, Edouard Laguesse, France	Islets of Langerhans might be the source of anti-diabetic substance
1907, Georg Zuelzer, Germany	Pancreatic extract "acomatol," produced by Zuelzer, decreased glucosuria and raised blood pH in diabetic dogs
1921–1922, Frederick Banting, Charles Best, James Collip, and John J.R. Macleod, Canada	Dog's pancreatic extracts shown to decrease glucosuria. First successful clinical use of refined pancreatic extract for diabetic patient. Eli Lilly Company begins the work on the commercial development of insulin
1928, Germany	Synthalin–a guanidine derivative administered orally for treatment of diabetes
1939, C. Ruiz, L.L. Silva, Argentina	Hypoglycemic properties of sulfonamide antibiotics observed for the first time
1958, Frederic Sanger, Great Britain	Nobel prize for the structural formula of bovine insulin
1959, Rosalyn Yalow and Salomon Berson, USA	Development of radioimmunoassay. Rosalyn Yalow received Nobel Prize for RIA in 1977
1966, University of Minnesota, USA	First transplant of the pancreas performed
1969, Dorothy Hodgkin, Great Britain	Description of the three-dimensional structure of porcine insulin using X-ray crystallography
1978, Robert Crea, David Goeddel, USA	Human insulin production using recombinant DNA technology
1993, Diabetes Control and Complications Trial, USA	Relation of the metabolic control of type 1 diabetes to the development of diabetic complications
1998, United Kingdom Prospective Diabetes Study, Great Britain	Relation of the metabolic control of type 2 diabetes to the development of diabetic complications
2001, Diabetes Prevention Program, USA	Relation of diet and exercise to the rate of development of type 2 diabetes in high-risk population
2003, Human Genome Project	Sequencing of human genome
2007, First Genome-Wide Association Studies for Diabetes	Novel loci identified in association with type 2 diabetes

Internet Resources

1. http://nobelprize.org
2. http://www.genome.gov/
3. http://utdol.com
4. www.crystalinks.com/egyptmedicine.html – ancient Egyptian medicine, Ebers papyrus
5. www.uic.edu – Claude Bernard
6. www.britannica.com – Claude Bernard
7. www.nobel.se – August Krogh
8. http://web.mit.edu/invent/iow/yalow.html
9. www.gene.com – press release September 6, 1978
10. http://www.mendosa.com/history.htm
11. Prevalence of Overweight and Obesity Among Adults: United States, 2003–2004. National Center for Health Statistics www.cdc.gov
12. www.niddk.nih.gov – results of Diabetes Prevention Program, Diabetes Prevention Trial.

References

1. Papaspyros NS. The history of diabetes. In: Verlag GT, ed. *The History of Diabetes Mellitus*. Stuttgart: Thieme; 1964:4.
2. http://www.crystalinks.com/egyptmedicine.html – ancient Egyptian medicine, Ebers papyrus.
3. Papaspyros NS. The history of diabetes. In: Verlag GT, ed. *The History of Diabetes Mellitus*. Stuttgart: Thieme; 1964:4–5.
4. Medvei VC. The Greco – Roman period. In: Medvei VC, ed. *The History of Clinical Endocrinology: A Comprehensive Account of Endocrinology from Earliest Times to the Present Day*. New York: Parthenon Publishing; 1993:34, 37.
5. Southgate TM. De medicina. *JAMA*. 1999;10:921.
6. Sanders LJ. From Thebes to Toronto and the 21st century: an incredible journey. *Diabetes Spect*. 2002;15:56–60.
7. Medvei VC. Mediaeval scene. In: Medvei VC, ed. *The History of Clinical Endocrinology: A Comprehensive Account of Endocrinology from Earliest Times to the Present Day*. New York: Parthenon Publishing; 1993:46, 49.
8. Medvei VC. The 16th century and the Renaissance. In: Medvei VC, ed. *The History of Clinical Endocrinology: A Comprehensive Account of Endocrinology from Earliest Times to the Present Day*. New York: Parthenon Publishing; 1993:55–56.
9. Medvei VC. The 18th century and the beginning of the 19th century. In: Medvei VC, ed. *The History of Clinical Endocrinology: A Comprehensive Account of Endocrinology from Earliest Times to the Present Day*. New York: Parthenon Publishing; 1993:97.
10. www.uic.edu – Claude Bernard.
11. www.britannica.com – Claude Bernard.
12. Medvei VC. Story of insulin. In: Medvei VC, ed. *The History of Clinical Endocrinology: A Comprehensive Account of Endocrinology from Earliest Times to the Present Day*. New York: Parthenon Publishing; 1993:249–251.
13. Schullian DM. John Rollo's patient. *J Hist Med*. 1965;2:163–164.
14. Bliss M. A long prelude. In: Bliss M, ed. *The Discovery of Insulin*. Chicago: The University of Chicago Press; 1982:33–39.
15. Minkowski O. Introduction and translation by R. Levine. Historical development of the theory of pancreatic diabetes. *Diabetes*. 1989;38:1–6.
16. Medvei VC. The birth of endocrinology. In: Medvei VC, ed. *The History of Clinical Endocrinology: A Comprehensive Account of Endocrinology from Earliest Times to the Present Day*. New York: Parthenon Publishing; 1993:151.
17. Bliss M. Banting's idea. In: Bliss M, ed. *The Discovery of Insulin*. Chicago: University of Chicago Press; 2007:45–58.
18. Bliss M. A mysterious something. In: Bliss M, ed. *The Discovery of Insulin*. Chicago: University of Chicago Press; 2007: 84–103.
19. Bliss M. Triumph. In: Bliss M, ed. *The Discovery of Insulin*. Chicago: University of Chicago Press; 1982:104–128.
20. MacCracken J. From ants to analogues. Puzzles and promises in diabetes management. *Postgrad Med*. 1997;4:138–150.
21. Pratt P. *History of Insulin. Hutchinson Family Encyclopedia*. online edition. Oxford: Helicon Publishing Ltd.; 2000.
22. Born DM. *The Journey and the Dream: A History of the American Diabetes Association*. Alexandria, VA: American Diabetes Association; 1990:1–14.
23. www.nobel.se – August Krogh.
24. Medvei VC. Present trends and outlook for the future – Part III. In: Medvei VC, ed. *The History of Clinical Endocrinology: A Comprehensive Account of Endocrinology from Earliest Times to the Present Day*. New York: Parthenon Publishing; 1993: 380–383.
25. http://web.mit.edu/invent/iow/yalow.html.
26. Segre GV, Brown EN. Measurement of hormones. In: Wilson JD, Foster DW, Kronenberg HM, Larsen PR, eds. *Williams Textbook of Endocrinology*. 9th ed. Philadelphia, PA: WB Saunders; 1998:44–45.
27. Medvei VC. Chronological tables. In: Medvei VC, ed. *The History of Clinical Endocrinology: A Comprehensive Account of Endocrinology from Earliest Times to the Present Day*. New York: Parthenon Publishing; 1993:495.
28. www.gene.com – press release September 6, 1978.
29. Galloway J, deShazo R. Insulin chemistry and pharmacology: insulin allergy, resistance, and lipodystrophy. In: Rifkin H, Porte D Jr, eds. *Diabetes Mellitus. Theory and Practice*. 4th ed. New York: Elsevier; 1990:498.
30. http://www.mendosa.com/history.htm.
31. Holmquist WR, Schroeder WA. A new N-terminal blocking group involving a Schiff base in hemoglobin A1c. *Biochemistry*. 1966;5:2489–2503.
32. Bookchin RM, Gallop PM. Structure of hemoglobin A1c: nature of the N-terminal β chain blocking Group. *Biochem Biophys Res Commun*. 1968;32:86–93.
33. Samuel R. An abnormal hemoglobin in red cells of diabetics. *Clin Chim Acta*. 1968;22:296–298.
34. Rahbar S, Blumenfeld O, Ranney HM. Studies of an unusual hemoglobin in patients with diabetes mellitus. *Biochem Biophys Res Commun*. 1969;36:838–843.
35. Tattersall RB, Pyke DA, Ranney HM, Bruckheimer SM. Hemoglobin components in diabetes mellitus: studies in identical twins. *N Engl J Med*. 1975;293:1171–1173.
36. Koenig RJ, Peterson CM, Jones RL, Saudek C, Lehrman M, Cermani A. Correlation of glucose regulation and hemoglobin A1c in diabetes mellitus. *N Engl J Med*. 1976;295:417–420.
37. The Diabetes Control and Complications Trial Research Group. The effect of intensive treatment of diabetes on the development and progression of long-term complications in insulin-dependent diabetes mellitus. *N Engl J Med*. 1993;329: 997–986.

38. The Diabetes Control and Complications Trial/Epidemiology of Diabetes Interventions and Complications Research Group. Retinopathy and nephropathy in patients with type 1 diabetes four years after a trial of intensive therapy. *N Engl J Med.* 2000;342:381–389.

39. The Diabetes Control and Complications Trial/Epidemiology of Diabetes Interventions and Complications Research Group. Intensive diabetes treatment and cardiovascular disease in patients with type 1 diabetes. *N Engl J Med.* 2005;353:2643–2653.

40. UK Prospective Diabetes Study Group. Intensive blood-glucose control with sulphonylurea or insulin compared with conventional treatment and risk of complications in patients with type 2 diabetes (UKPDS 33). *Lancet.* 1998;352:837–853.

41. UK Prospective Diabetes Study Group. Association of systolic blood pressure with macrovascular and microvascular complications of type 2 diabetes (UKPDS 36): prospective observational study. *BMJ.* 2000;321:412–419.

42. UK Prospective Diabetes Study Group. Effects of intensive blood-glucose control with metformin on complications in overweight patients with type 2 Diabetes (UKPDS 34). *Lancet.* 1998;325:854–865.

43. ACCORD trial, press release, February 6, 2008 http://public.nhlbi.nih.gov/Newsroom/Home/NewsRoom.aspx.

44. The Look AHEAD Research Group. The Look AHEAD study: a description of the lifestyle intervention and the evidence supporting it. *Obesity.* 2006;14:737–752.

45. Gruessner RWG, Sutherland D, Kandaswamy R, et al. Lessons learned from > 500 pancreas transplants alone at a single institution. *Am J Transplant.* 2007;7:249.

46. Lacy PE, Kostianovsky M. Methods for the isolation of intact islets of Langerhans from rat pancreas. *Diabetes.* 1967;16:35–39.

47. Wahoff DC, Papalois BE, Najarian JS, et al. Autologous islet cell transplant to prevent diabetes after pancreatic resection. *Ann Surg.* 1995;222:562–579.

48. Shapiro JAM, Lakey JRT, Ryan EA, et al. Islet transplantation in seven patients with type 1 diabetes mellitus using a glucocorticoid-free immunosuppressive regimen. *N Engl J Med.* 2000;343:230–23.

49. Ryan EA, Paty BW, Senior PA, et al. Five-year follow-up after clinical islet transplantation. *Diabetes.* 2005;54:2060–2068.

50. Serup P, Madsen DO, Mandrup–Poulsen T. Islet and stem cell transplantation for treating diabetes. *Brit Med J.* 2001;322:29–32.

51. Prevalence of overweight and obesity among adults: United States, 2003–2004. National Center for Health Statistics www.cdc.gov.

52. Morbidity and Mortality Weekly Report. Center of diabetes control and prevention. *MMWR.* 2004;53:80–82.

53. Manson JE, Nathan DM, Krolewski AS, Stampfer MJ, Willett WC, Hennekens CH. A prospective study of exercise and incidence of diabetes among U.S. male physicians. *JAMA.* 1992;268:63–67.

54. Manson JE, Rimm EB, Stampfer MJ, et al. A prospective study of physical activity and incidence of non insulin-dependent diabetes mellitus in women. *Lancet.* 1991;338:774–777.

55. U.S. Department of Health and Human Services: Healthy People 2000: Summary Report. Washington, DC: U.S. Department of Health and Human Services (DHHS Publ. PHSSs 91-50213); 1992:6–8, 55, 91–92.

56. Tuomilehto J, Lindstrom J, Eriksson JG, et al. Finnish Diabetes Prevention Study Group. Prevention of type 2 diabetes mellitus by changes in lifestyle among subjects with impaired glucose tolerance. *N Engl J Med.* 2001;344:1343–1350.

57. Pan XR, Li GW, Wang JX, et al. Effects of diet and exercise in preventing NIDDM in people with impaired glucose tolerance: the Da Qing IGT and Diabetes Study. *Diabetes Care.* 1997;20:537–544.

58. Helmrich SP, Ragland DR, Leung RW, Paffenbarger RS. Physical activity and reduced occurrence of non-insulin-dependent diabetes mellitus. *N Engl J Med.* 1991;325:147–152.

59. www.niddk.nih.gov – results of Diabetes Prevention Program, Diabetes Prevention Trial.

60. Diabetes Prevention Trial – Type 1 Diabetes Group. Effects of insulin in relatives of patients with type 1 diabetes mellitus. *N Engl J Med.* 2002;346:1685–1691.

61. Diabetes Prevention Trial – Type 1 Diabetes Group. Effects of oral insulin in relatives of patients with type 1 diabetes. *Diabetes Care.* 2005;28:1068–1076.

62. Scott LJ, Mohlke KL, Bonnycastle LL, et al. A genome-wide association study of type 2 diabetes in Finns detects multiple susceptibility variants. *Science.* 2007;316:1341–1345.

63. Saxena R, Voight BF, Lyssenko V, et al. Genome-wide association analysis identifies loci for type 2 diabetes and triglyceride levels. *Science.* 2007;316:1331–1336.

64. Zeggini E, Weedon MN, Lindgren CM, et al. The welcome trust case control consortium (WTCCC), McCarthy MI, Hattersley AT. *Science.* 2007;316:1336–1341.

Part II
Physiology of Glucose Metabolism

Chapter 2
Normal Glucose Homeostasis

Muhammad Z. Shrayyef and John E. Gerich

Glucose: From Origins to Fates

Arterial plasma glucose values throughout a 24-h period average approximately 90 mg/dl, with a maximal concentration usually not exceeding 165 mg/dl such as after meal ingestion[1] and remaining above 55 mg/dl such as after exercise[2] or a moderate fast (60 h).[3] This relative stability contrasts with the situation for other substrates such as glycerol, lactate, free fatty acids, and ketone bodies whose fluctuations are much wider (Table 2.1).[4]

This narrow range defining normoglycemia is maintained through an intricate regulatory and counterregulatory neuro-hormonal system: A decrement in plasma glucose as little as 20 mg/dl (from 90 to 70 mg/dl) will suppress the release of insulin and will decrease glucose uptake in certain areas in the brain (e.g., hypothalamus where glucose sensors are located); this will activate the sympathetic nervous system and trigger the release of counterregulatory hormones (glucagon, catecholamines, cortisol, and growth hormone).[5] All these changes will increase glucose release into plasma and decrease its removal so as to restore normoglycemia. On the other hand, a 10 mg/dl increment in plasma glucose will stimulate insulin release and suppress glucagon secretion to prevent further increments and restore normoglycemia.

Glucose in plasma either comes from dietary sources or is either the result of the breakdown of glycogen in liver (glycogenolysis) or the formation of glucose in liver and kidney from other carbons compounds (precursors) such as lactate, pyruvate, amino acids, and glycerol (gluconeogenesis).

In humans, glucose removed from plasma may have different fates in different tissues and under different conditions (e.g., postabsorptive vs. postprandial), but the pathways for its disposal are relatively limited. It (1) may be immediately stored as glycogen or (2) may undergo glycolysis, which can be *non-oxidative* producing pyruvate (which can be reduced to lactate or transaminated to form alanine) or *oxidative* through conversion to acetyl CoA which is further oxidized through the tricarboxylic acid cycle to form carbon dioxide and water. Non-oxidative glycolysis carbons undergo gluconeogenesis and the newly formed glucose is either stored as glycogen or released back into plasma (Fig. 2.1).

Importance of Glucose Homeostasis

Although free fatty acids are the main fuel for most organs, glucose is the obligate metabolic fuel for the brain under physiologic conditions. This occurs because of low circulating concentrations of other possible alternative substrates (e.g., ketone bodies) or because of limitations of transport across the blood-brain barriers (e.g., free fatty acids).[6] After prolonged fasting, because of an increase in their circulating concentration, ketone bodies may be used by the brain to a significant extent.[7]

J.E. Gerich (✉)
Department of Medicine, University of Rochester School of Medicine, Rochester, NY 14642, USA
e-mail: johngerich@compuserve.com

L. Poretsky (ed.), *Principles of Diabetes Mellitus*, DOI 10.1007/978-0-387-09841-8_2,
© Springer Science+Business Media, LLC 2010

Table 2.1 Circulating substrates and regulatory hormones after overnight, moderate, and prolonged fasting

	Overnight fast (12–16 h)	Moderate fast (30–60 h)	Prolonged fast (>1 week)
Substrates (mmol/l)			
Glucose	5.0	4.0	3.0
Free fatty acids	0.5	1.0	1.5
Glycerol	0.05	0.1	0.2
3-Hydroxybutyrate	0.02	0.5	1.0
Lactate	0.8	0.8	0.7
Glutamine	0.6	0.5	0.4
Alanine	0.3	0.2	0.2
Hormones			
Insulin (pmol/l)	60	40	20
Glucagon (ng/l)	100	150	150
Cortisol (mmol/l)	0.3	0.5	0.9
Growth hormone (ng/l)	<2	4	8
Triiodothyronine (nmol/l)	1.8	1.6	0.9
Epinephrine (nmol/l)	0.2	0.4	0.6

This table was published in Gerich[4]. Copyright © Elsevier. Used with permission.

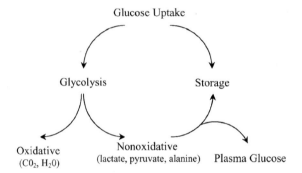

Fig. 2.1 Routes of postprandial glucose disposal. From Woerle et al.[18]. Copyright © 2003. The American Physiological Society. Used with permission

Brain cannot synthesize glucose or store as glycogen more than a few minutes supply. Thus brain is dependent on a continuous supply of glucose from plasma.

At plasma glucose concentrations 20 mg/dl below normal levels, glucose transport becomes rate-limiting for brain glucose utilization.[6] Glucose plasma concentrations below 55 mg/dl impair cerebral function,[8] whereas more severe and prolonged hypoglycemia causes convulsions, permanent brain damage, and even death. On the other hand, even mildly elevated plasma glucose concentrations which occur in patients with impaired glucose tolerance increase risk for cardiovascular morbidity.[9–11]

General Considerations

Relative Changes in Glucose Fluxes

Plasma glucose concentrations are determined by the relative rates at which glucose enters and leaves the circulation. Thus, the plasma glucose will increase only if the rate of entry exceeds its rate of exit and, conversely, plasma glucose level will decrease only if rates of exit exceed the rates of entry. To maintain relatively stable plasma glucose concentrations, increases in rates of glucose delivery into the systemic circulation (e.g., when meal is ingested) require a comparable increase in rates of glucose removal from the circulation.[12] For example, during vigorous exercise, fever, or trauma when the body's utilization of glucose increases, there is normally a compensatory increase in glucose delivery.[2]

Changes in glucose clearance, an index of efficiency of glucose removal from the circulation, by itself do not affect plasma glucose concentrations independent of changes in rates of glucose entry and exit.

Factors Influencing Glucose Fluxes

The most important factors on a moment to moment basis are the hormones (insulin, glucagon, and cate-cholamines), the sympathetic nervous system activity as well as the concentration of other substrates (FFA). On a more prolonged time basis (hours–days), other hormones (cortisol and growth hormone), nutritional factors (e.g., diet composition), exercise and physical fitness, along with concomitant changes in the sensitivity to hormones become important.[4] Cortisol, growth hormone, and catecholamines affect glucose homeostasis by altering insulin sensitivity and also by changes in the availability of alternative substrates.

Fasting vs. Postprandial States

The mechanisms delivering glucose into the circulation (i.e., glycogenolysis vs. gluconeogenesis) and the sites for glucose disposal will vary depending on duration of fasting. For example, as fasting is prolonged, the proportion of gluconeogenesis increases and the contribution of hepatic glycogen stores decreases. Moreover, the relative contribution of the kidney increases. In regard to utilization, after an overnight fast, there is no net storage of glucose and all glucose taken up by tissues is either completely oxidized or converted to lactate.

Actions of Key Regulatory Factors

Insulin

Insulin regulates glucose metabolism by direct and indirect actions. Through binding to its receptors in the liver, kidney, muscle, and adipose tissue, insulin activates its signaling pathway which involves a complex cascade of protein kinases and regulatory proteins of which IRS-1 and IRS-2 are the most important (Table 2.2). This causes (1) suppression of glucose release from liver and kidney,[13] (2) translocation of glucose transporters in muscle and adipose tissue to increase their glucose uptake,[14] and (3) inhibition of release of FFA into the circulation due to suppression of the activity of *hormone-sensitive lipase* and a simultaneous increase in their clearance from the circulation.[15] Although insulin does not increase glucose transport into liver, it promotes glycogen accumulation by inhibiting *glucose-6-phosphatase* ② and *phosphorylase* ① (glycogenolysis enzymes) while stimulating *glycogen synthase* ③.[16]

The effect of insulin on circulating FFA levels indirectly reduces glucose release into circulation and promotes glucose removal since FFA stimulate gluconeogenesis and reduce glucose transport into cells.[15]

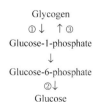

Table 2.2 Mechanism of action of key metabolic regulators

	Glucose production	Glucose utilization	Lipolysis
Insulin	↓	↑	↓
Glucagon	↑	–	–
Epinephrine	↑	↓	↑
Cortisol	↑	↓	↑
Growth hormone	↑	↓	↑
FFA	↑	↓	–

The main regulator of insulin secretion is the plasma glucose concentration: Increased plasma glucose after meal ingestion results in three-to fourfold increase in plasma insulin within 30–60 min whereas a decrease plasma glucose below 50 mg/dl will result in 80–90% reduction in plasma insulin levels. Acute increases in amino acids, and to a lesser extent, FFA also increase insulin secretion.[4,16–18]

After meal ingestion, intestinal factors called incretins (e.g., gastrointestinal-inhibitory peptide [GIP] and glucagon-like peptide [GLP-1]) augment insulin secretion. This is why plasma insulin concentrations increase to a greater extent after oral glucose load than after intravenous glucose despite identical plasma glucose concentrations.[18,19]

Metabolic processes vary in their sensitivity to insulin and their dose-response characteristics. At basal levels observed in the postabsorptive state (∼5–10 μU/ml), insulin is already inhibiting glucose and FFA release 30–50% (counteracting the effect of glucagon and the sympathetic nervous system) while having a trivial effect on tissue glucose uptake. Maximal suppression of glucose and FFA release normally is observed with plasma insulin concentrations seen postprandially (∼40–50 μU/ml), whereas maximal stimulation of tissue glucose uptake requires plasma insulin concentrations greater than 300 μU/ml levels not seen under normal physiological conditions except in extremely insulin resistant individuals in whom, of course, such level would not produce maximal effect.[4,17,18,20]

Glucagon

Glucagon, a hormone secreted from the α cells of the endocrine pancreas, is the major counterpart to insulin in the moment to moment regulation of plasma glucose. The control of its secretion is multifactorial.[21] The main factors are direct effects of glucose and insulin. In humans, neural signals and substrates other than glucose, e.g., FFA and amino acids, play a minor role. Glucagon secretion is inhibited by hyperglycemia and stimulated by hypoglycemia.

Glucagon acts exclusively on the liver where it binds to its receptors and activates *adenylate cyclase*. As a result, intracellular cAMP level increases, enhancing glycogenolysis as a result of *phosphorylase* stimulation.[22,23] This response wanes after several hours and is followed by an increase in gluconeogenesis due to a complex process involving both increased substrate uptake and enzyme activation.[4,19–21,24] Thus, the main immediate action of glucagon to increase plasma glucose level is through stimulation of hepatic glycogenolysis.[24]

Catecholamines

Catecholamine release is mediated through changes in sympathetic nervous system, being increased during stress and hypoglycemia. Catecholamines inhibit insulin secretion while decreasing insulin action. Acting as both hormones (epinephrine) and neurotransmitters (norepinephrine), they are potent hyperglycemic factors whose actions, unlike those of glucagon, are sustained and affect both glucose release and glucose removal.[20,25,26]

For the most part, metabolic actions of catecholamines are mediated through beta 2 adrenergic receptors: At the liver, they directly increase glycogenolysis via cAMP activation of *phosphorylase* and, to a lesser extent, augment gluconeogenesis indirectly through increasing gluconeogenic substrate availability and plasma FFA.[24,26]

At the kidney level, they are potent stimulators of gluconeogenesis both directly and indirectly as in the liver and are actually more potent stimulators of renal glucose release than hepatic glucose release.[27] In skeletal muscles, they reduce glucose uptake and stimulate glycogenolysis which results in an increase in release of lactate – the major gluconeogenic precursor. In adipose tissue, catecholamines stimulate lypolysis via activation of *hormone-sensitive lipase* which results in an increase in the release of FFA and glycerol, another key gluconeogenic precursor.[24–26,28]

Growth Hormone and Cortisol

In contrast to glucagon and catecholamines which act almost immediately, the metabolic actions of growth hormone and cortisol generally take several hours to become evident. These can be summarized as being antagonistic to the action of insulin (i.e., they reduce the ability of insulin to suppress glucose release, stimulate glucose uptake, and inhibit lipolysis).[25,29] Both hormones increase the synthesis of gluconeogenic enzymes and reduce glucose transport.[29–31] In addition, cortisol can impair insulin secretion.[31] Accordingly, the mechanisms for deterioration in glucose tolerance during immunosuppressive glucocorticoid treatment involve induction of insulin resistance and prevention of an appropriate compensatory increase in insulin secretion.[31]

It is important to note that counterregulatory hormones work via different intracellular mechanisms which reinforce/synergize with one another. Simultaneously small increases in their plasma levels will have greater effect than large increases in plasma levels of only one hormone.[8]

FFA

FFA are the predominant fuel used by most tissues of the body, the major exceptions being the brain, renal medulla, and blood cells.[32–34] Increases in plasma FFA have many potentially important metabolic consequences[35,36]: stimulation of hepatic and renal gluconeogenesis; inhibition of muscle glucose transport; and competition with glucose as an oxidative fuel. The major regulators of circulating FFA levels are the sympathetic nervous system and growth hormone[32] (which increase plasma FFA levels), insulin (which reduces plasma FFA levels by suppressing lipolysis and increasing FFA clearance), and hyperglycemia. There is evidence for heterogeneity of adipose depots with visceral fat being more metabolically active than subcutaneous fat.[32,36]

Incretins: The Entero-insular Axis

The concept that certain factors secreted from the intestinal mucosa in response to nutrients can stimulate the pancreas to release insulin was first introduced to explain the phenomenon of greater increase in plasma insulin levels in response to oral glucose load compared with the same load of glucose given intravenously (Table 2.3). The term *incretin* was used to denote these factors.[37] The first incretin hormone identified, was called *gastric inhibitory polypeptide* (GIP) based on its ability to inhibit gastric acid secretion in dogs.[37] Another peptide was discovered later and named *glucagon-like peptide-1* based on its homology to glucagon.[38] Both peptides are

Table 2.3 Effects of GLP1 and GIP on different tissues

Effects on	GLP1	GIP
Pancreas	↑Insulin secretion	↑Insulin secretion
	↓Glucagon secretion	–
Peripheral	↓Hepatic glucose release	–
	↑Muscle glucose uptake	–
Gastric	Delay gastric emptying	Inhibit secretions only at suraphysiologic levels
CNS	↑ Satiety, ↓ appetite, ↓ weight	–

secreted from intestinal endocrine mucosa (L and K cells) within minutes of nutrient ingestion and have short half-life (minutes) due to the rapid inactivation by a proteolytic enzyme called dipeptidyl peptidase-4 (DPP-4).

GLP-1 and GIP inhibit glucagon secretion;[39] only GLP-1 delays gastric emptying and only GLP-1, possibly through a neural mechanism, promotes satiety, decreasing food intake and leading to weight loss.[37]

Upper Gastrointestinal Function and Glycemic Homeostasis

Recent studies indicate that gastric emptying is a major physiologic determinant of postprandial glycemia by controlling the nutrient delivery into the small intestine: It accounts for ∼35% of the variance in peak blood glucose concentrations after ingestion of oral glucose in healthy volunteers[40,41] or patients with type 2 diabetes.[40,42] It is delayed in acute hyperglycemia[14,43] and accelerated during hypoglycemia.[44]

Effect of Meal Composition on Glucose Metabolism

In healthy humans, adding protein or fat to oral glucose was found to lower postprandial glucose concentrations by slowing the gastric emptying and stimulating incretins. Protein also enhances non-glucose-dependent insulin release.[45,46]

Glucose Transport Pathways

Due to its hydrophilic nature, glucose diffuses slowly across the lipid bilayer of the cell membrane and needs specific transporter proteins to facilitate its entry into cells. Glucose flux varies among tissues depending to a large extent on the characteristics of the transporters in that specific tissue and whether the process is sensitive to insulin or not.[47,48] Insulin regulates the steady-state concentration of glucose transporters by promoting their synthesis and also acutely accelerates the uptake of glucose, promoting mobilization of the transporters to the cell membrane.[48]

There are two distinct families of transport proteins.[49] (1) *Facilitative GLUT family:* These transporters promote facilitated diffusion of glucose, a process that is not energy dependent and that follows Michaelis–Menton kinetics.[50] The high-affinity transporters (GLUT 1, 3, 4) have a Michaelis–Menton constant (K_m) below the normal range of blood glucose concentrations and are capable of providing glucose transport under basal conditions for many cells.[49] GLUT3 is the major neuronal transporter (lowest K_m) whereas GLUT4 mediates insulin-stimulated glucose uptake by skeletal muscle, heart, and adipose tissues. Insulin and exercise promote GLUT3 expression on cell surface.[49,51] The low-affinity transporters (GLUT2) are present on ß-cells and in tissues exposed to large glucose fluxes, such as intestine, liver, and kidney.[49] (2) *SGLT family:* These transporters utilize the electrochemical sodium gradient to transport glucose against concentration gradients[49,52] and are prominent in intestine and kidney. SGLT1 is responsible for the dietary uptake of glucose from the small intestine lumen whereas SGLT2 plays a major role in glucose reabsorption from proximal renal tubule.[49,52]

Glucose Production and Hepatorenal Glucose Reciprocity

A considerable body of evidence indicates that somehow release of glucose by the liver and kidney are interrelated so that a reduction in release by one organ is associated by an increase by the other to further maintain optimal glucose homeostasis. This relationship is referred to as hepatorenal glucose reciprocity.[53]

Until recently, it was widely thought that the liver was the sole source of glucose except during acidosis and after prolonged fasting. During the past few years, numerous reports[54–62] indicated that the kidney is responsible on an average for about 20% of glucose released into the circulation in overnight fasted normal human volunteers. Moreover, a number of studies have shown that kidney increased its glucose release (gluconeogenesis) to compensate for restricted (physiologic) or impaired (pathologic) hepatic glucose release.[53]

Physiologic examples of the phenomena occur postprandially and after prolonged fasting. After meal ingestion, the hepatic glucose release is suppressed ~80%, while renal glucose release increases and actually exceeds hepatic glucose release (HGR) for several hours[63] to allow for hepatic glycogen repletion.[53] Also after prolonged fasting (60 h), renal glucose release increases fourfold while hepatic glucose release decreases by ~45%.[59] Examples of renal compensation with pathologic process are the following: (1) *Hepatic Diseases:* Hypoglycemia is extremely uncommon in patients with severe liver disease in the absence of other factors (infection, heart failure). Studies using an animal model for liver failure have demonstrated that there is a compensatory increase in renal glucose release to compensate for the reduced hepatic glucose release.[53,64–66] In humans, during the period of hepatic transplantation when patients have no functioning liver, hypoglycemia does not occur; overall glucose release into the circulation either decreases minimally or not at all, and there is an increase in renal glucose release.[67,68] (2) *Acidosis:* Acidosis stimulates renal glucose release[69] while inhibiting hepatic glucose release.[70] In patients with respiratory acidosis, an increase in net renal glucose release has been demonstrated inversely proportional to blood pH.[71] (3) *Glucose Counterregulation in Diabetes:* Patients with type 1[5] and prolonged type 2[72] diabetes lose their glucagon response and become dependent on catecholamine responses. Catecholamines are the major hormonal factor responsible for the increase in renal glucose release during hypoglycemia.[73] Consequently, type 1 diabetic patients with both reduced glucagon and epinephrine responses have decreases in both hepatic and renal glucose release during hypoglycemia.[74] In patients with type 2 diabetes, who have reduced plasma glucagon responses, compensatory increases in hepatic glucose release during recovery from hypoglycemia are reduced, whereas renal glucose release is increased.[75]

The Postabsorptive State

The period after 14–16 h overnight fast is commonly referred to as the postabsorptive state. During this time plasma glucose concentrations average about 85 mg/dl (70–100 mg/dl) and are relatively stable since rates of glucose release into the circulation approximate the rates of glucose exit from the circulation (~10 μg/kg/min).[4]

Glucose Production

The liver is responsible for approximately 80% of glucose release into the circulation in the postabsorptive state.[76] Under these conditions, ~50% of the glucose entering the circulation is due to glycogenolysis and the reminder (~5.0 μmol/kg/min) to gluconeogenesis[77] (Table 2.4). The proportion owing to gluconeogenesis rapidly increases with the duration of fasting, as glycogen stores become depleted; by 24 h from the last meal, gluconeogenesis accounts for about 70% of all glucose released into the circulation, and by 48 h, it accounts for over 90% of all glucose released into the circulation.[3,77]

The kidney normally contains little glycogen and renal cells that could make glycogen lack glucose-6-phosphatase. Consequently, virtually all the glucose released by the kidney is the result of gluconeogenesis.[76] Although the liver releases about four times as much as the kidney under postabsorptive conditions, both organs release about the same amount (2.5–3.0 μmol/kg/min) from gluconeogenesis and the proportion of overall glucose release owing to renal gluconeogenesis increases even further with prolonged fasting.[60]

The liver releases glucose both by glycogenolysis and gluconeogenesis and can be considered to be the sole source of glucose due to glycogenolysis. In overnight fasted people, the liver contains about 75 g of glycogen.[78] Thus, if it releases glycogen at a rate of 63 mg/min (5 μmol/kg/min), glycogen stores would be totally depleted in about 20 h and the sole source of glucose released into the circulation at this point would be gluconeogenesis.[4]

Table 2.4 Summary of postabsorptive glucose release

	Rate (μmol/kg/min)	% of total
I. Glucose release	10.0	100
A. Hepatic	8.0	80
1. Glycogenolysis	5.0	50
2. Gluconeogenesis	3.0	30
Lactate	1.3	13
Alanine	0.8	8
Other amino acids	0.2	2
Glycerol	0.4	4
Glutamine	0.3	3
B. Renal	2.0	20
1. Glycogenolysis	0	0
2. Gluconeogenesis	2.0	20
Lactate	1.2	12
Glutamine	0.4	4
Glycerol	0.2	2
Other amino acids	0.1	1
Alanine	0.1	1

Regulation of Glucose Production: Hepatic vs. Renal

Glucose release by the liver and kidney are regulated differently. Insulin suppresses glucose release by both organs (1) directly by affecting enzyme activation/deactivation and (2) indirectly through gluconeogenic substrate availability and gluconeogenic activators (e.g., suppression of FFA and glucagon).[13]

Glucagon, which increases both glycogenolysis and gluconeogenesis in the liver, however, has no effect on the kidney.[55] Epinephrine, which can directly activate hepatic glycogenolysis, appears to increase glucose release, predominantly by directly stimulating renal gluconeogenesis and, to a lesser extent, by increasing availability of gluconeogenic precursors/activators (e.g., glycerol and FFA).[27,56]

The major precursors for gluconeogenesis are lactate, glycerol, glutamine, and alanine.[4] Most amino acids released from skeletal muscle protein are converted to alanine and glutamine for transport through plasma to liver and kidney: alanine being selectively used by liver, glutamine being preferentially used in the kidney, while lactate and glycerol used to roughly comparable extent by both organs. In the resting postabsorptive state, lactate is the major gluconeogenic precursor, accounting for about half of all gluconeogenesis.[4]

Glucose Utilization

Although the postabsorptive state is often considered to represent a steady state, it is actually a pseudo-steady state, since rates of glucose removal slightly, and undetectably, exceed rates of glucose release so that if fasting is prolonged, plasma glucose levels gradually decrease; by 20–24 h of fasting they may be 15–20% lower (Fig. 2.2). However, even after 72 h of fasting, they are usually maintained above 50 mg/dl.[3]

In the postabsorptive state, there is no net storage of glucose; consequently, glucose taken up by tissues is either completely oxidized to CO_2 or released back into the circulation as lactate, alanine, and glutamine[79] for reincorporation into glucose via gluconeogenesis (Table 2.5).

Most glucose used by the body can be accounted for by six tissues: the brain (45–60%), skeletal muscle (15–20%), kidney (10–15%), blood cells (5–10%), splanchnic organs (3–6%), and adipose tissue (2–4%).[4]

Glucose taken up by the brain is completely oxidized whereas that taken up by the kidney, blood cells, splanchnic tissues, and muscle mainly undergoes glycolysis. Recall that most of the body energy requirements are met by oxidation of FFA which compete with glucose as the fuel of choice in certain organs (e.g., skeletal muscles, heart, and possibly kidney).[35]

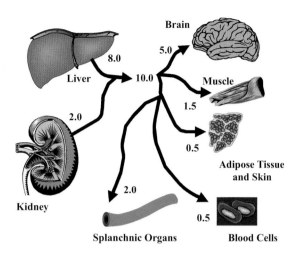

Fig. 2.2 Glucose utilization and production in the postabsorptive state. The liver and kidney contribute approximately 8.0 and 2.0 μmol/kg/min, respectively; top, the total release of glucose into the circulation (10 μmol/kg/min); the brain, splanchnic tissue, muscle, adipose tissue, and blood cells account for approximately 5.0, 2.0, 1.5, 0.5, and 0.5 μmol/kg/min, respectively. This figure was published in *Endocrinology* Volume 1 edited by LJ DeGroot and JL Jameson, chapter entitled "Hypoglycemia" authored by John Gerich, p. 923. Copyright © Elsevier 2001. Used with permission

Table 2.5   Glucose disposal in the postabsorptive state

	Rate (μmol/kg/min)	% of total
Overall	10	100
Oxidation	~7	~70
Glycolysis	~3	~30
Tissues		
Brain	5	~50
Skeletal muscle	2	~20
Splanchnic organs	1	~10
Kidney	1	~10
Adipose tissue	0.5	~5
Blood cells	0.5	~5

Glucose uptake by brain, blood cells, renal medulla, and splanchnic tissue occurs largely independent of insulin, and plasma insulin concentrations are low in the postabsorptive state (<10 μU/ml). Under these conditions, amount of glucose removed from the circulation is determined almost exclusively by tissue demands, the mass action effect of the plasma glucose concentration per se, and the number and characteristics of the glucose transporters in specific tissue rather than by insulin. Insulin may be viewed as playing a permissive role, while counterregulatory hormones that antagonize the action of insulin (e.g., cortisol, growth hormone, epinephrine, and thyroid hormones) can be viewed as modulating the sensitivity of tissue to the effect of insulin on tissue glucose uptake and utilization.[4,8]

Prolonged Fasting

With prolongation of fasting, plasma insulin levels decrease while those of glucagon, catecholamines, growth hormone, and cortisol increase (Table 2.6). Consequently, plasma FFA, glycerol, and the ketone bodies – products of FFA oxidation (beta hydroxybutyrate) – increase. Since hepatic glycogen stores become depleted by 60 h, virtually all of the glucose release at this time is due to gluconeogenesis. Initially, hepatic gluconeogenesis decreases while renal gluconeogenesis increases, with an overall result of a decrease in overall glucose release

Table 2.6 Glucose release and disposal after prolonged fasting (~60 h)

	Glucose disposal[a]		Glucose release[a]
Overall	6.0	Overall	6.0
Oxidation	4.8	Gluconeogenesis	5.5
Glycolysis	1.2	Glycogenolysis	0.5
Tissues		Tissues	
Brain	3.5	Liver	2.7
Skeletal muscle	1.0	Kidney	2.8
Splanchnic organs	0.5		
Kidney	0.4		
Adipose tissue	0.2		
Blood cells	0.4		

[a] μmol/kg/min.

and a slight increase in gluconeogenesis. With more prolonged fasting, there is a further decrease in glucose release as gluconeogenesis decreases.[59]

Although more glycerol is available for gluconeogenesis, less lactate is available due to decreased production by glycolysis, and less amino acids are available because muscle proteolysis decreases. These changes limit gluconeogenesis despite increase in plasma FFA and counterregulatory hormones which promote gluconeogenesis.

Initially during the course of the fast, decreases in glucose release are slightly greater than decreases in glucose uptake so that plasma glucose levels decrease slowly. However, eventually, the rates of uptake and release approximate one another so that a new pseudo-steady state is established after 60–70 h with plasma glucose levels usually averaging 55–65 mg/dl.[59]

These changes during prolonged fasting are relevant to changes seen in chronically ill patients who often are anorexic, malnourished, and miss meals in hospital because of diagnostic or therapeutic procedures. Because of the limitations on gluconeogenesis, such patients, i.e., those with chronic renal failure, severe liver disease, or heart failure, are prone to develop hypoglycemia during infections or other situations which increase the body's glucose utilization.[4,59]

Suppression of insulin secretion with prolonged fasting forms the basis for the 72 h fast for the diagnosis of insulinoma. In such patients, insulin secretion is not appropriately reduced and this leads to the development of hypoglycemia (i.e., plasma glucose levels <45 mg/dl).[4]

The Postprandial State

Complete assimilation of the constituents of a mixed meal containing fat, protein, and carbohydrate and restoration of the postabsorptive state takes at least 6 h,[80] whereas assimilation of a pure carbohydrate load is generally complete within 4–5 h. Despite these time differences, there is little evidence that the fate of ingested carbohydrate differs markedly under the two conditions.[80] Because people usually eat at least three times a day, the majority of the day is spent in the postprandial state.

Various factors can affect the extent of circulating glucose excursions after meal ingestion. These include the time and the degree of physical activity since the last meal; the composition and form (liquid vs. solid); rate of gastric emptying; digestion within the lumen of the small intestine; absorption into the portal vein; extraction by the liver; suppression of endogenous glucose release; and finally the uptake, storage, oxidation, and glycolysis of glucose in posthepatic tissues.[81]

From a practical point of view, however, the major factors influencing postprandial glucose homeostasis are those that affect suppression of endogenous glucose release and those that affect hepatic and posthepatic tissue glucose uptake.

Glucose taken up by tissues postprandially can be either immediately stored or undergoes glycolysis. Therefore, initial direct storage of glucose (glucose to glucose-6-phosphate to glycogen) can be calculated as the difference between whole body glucose uptake and whole body glycolysis. Since postprandial de novo lipogenesis and adipose tissue glucose storage are negligible in humans, virtually all of this storage should represent glycogen formation.[80,82]

Of the glucose undergoing glycolysis, some will be oxidized; the remainder will undergo non-oxidative glycolysis leading to the formation of pyruvate, lactate, and alanine. These 3-carbon compounds will then be available to undergo gluconeogenesis and either be stored in glycogen via the indirect pathway or be released into plasma as glucose.[18]

Figure 2.3 depicts the pathways for disposal of a mixed meal containing 78 g of glucose.[18] During the 6-h postprandial period, a total of ~98 g of glucose were disposed of. This was more than the glucose contained in the meal due to persistent endogenous glucose release (~21 g): Splanchnic tissues initially took up ~23 g, and an additional ~75 g were removed from the systemic circulation. Direct glucose storage accounted for ~32 g and glycolysis ~66 g (oxidative ~43 g and non-oxidative ~23 g). About 11 g of glucose appeared in plasma as a result of gluconeogenesis. This indicates that glycolysis is the main initial postprandial fate of glucose, accounting for ~66% of overall disposal. Oxidation and storage each account for about 45%. The majority of glycogen is formed via the direct pathway (~73%).

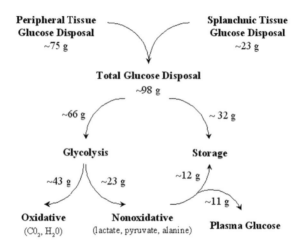

Fig. 2.3 Summary of sites and routes of postprandial glucose disposal. From Woerle et al.[18]. Copyright © 2003. The American Physiological Society. Used with permission

Changes in Plasma Hormone and Substrate Concentration

After ingestion of 75 g glucose, plasma glucose levels increase to a peak in 30–60 min, usually not exceeding 160 mg/dl and gradually return to or slightly below postabsorptive values by 3–4 h (Fig. 2.4). Although plasma glucose levels have returned to postabsorptive levels, glucose fluxes and organ glucose exchange have not. Plasma insulin concentrations follow a similar profile to those of plasma glucose and average only about three- to fourfold basal values during this period.

Plasma glucagon concentrations change reciprocally to those of insulin and are generally suppressed by about 50%. Early insulin release (i.e., that accruing within 30–60 min) plays a critical role in maintaining normal postprandial glucose homeostasis.[81]

Plasma FFA and glycerol levels decrease due to inhibition of lipolysis while plasma lactate concentrations increase as a result of increased glycolysis in liver, muscle, adipose tissue, and kidney. After ingestion of a mixed meal containing protein, the circulating concentrations of several amino acids increase.[18]

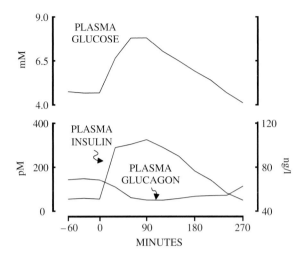

Fig. 2.4 Changes in plasma glucose, insulin, and glucagon after ingestion of a 75 g oral glucose load in normal volunteers

Changes in Rates of Glucose Entry into and Exit from Plasma

Rates of glucose appearance in plasma represent the sum of orally ingested glucose escaping first pass splanchnic (hepatic) extraction and the residual release of endogenous glucose by liver and kidney (Figs. 2.5 and 2.6). Appearance of ingested glucose in the systemic circulation is detected as early as 15 min. Glucose concentration reaches a peak at 60–80 min and gradually decreases thereafter.[18]

On average during a 4–5 h postprandial period about 75% of the glucose molecules in plasma represent those from the meal. Endogenous glucose release by the liver decreases rapidly and is suppressed nearly 80% during the 5 h postprandial period. As a result, nearly 25 g less glucose due to endogenous production reaches the systemic circulation during this interval. In contrast to the liver, recent studies indicate that endogenous renal glucose release is not suppressed and actually increases during this period so that it exceeds hepatic glucose release.[83] This increase in renal glucose release would permit more complete suppression of hepatic glucose release and facilitate more efficient hepatic glycogen replenishment.[83]

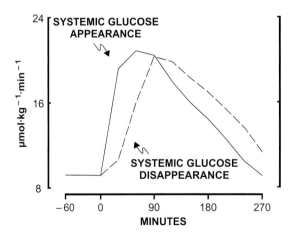

Fig. 2.5 Changes in rates of glucose entry into and removal from plasma after ingestion of a 75 g oral glucose load in normal volunteers

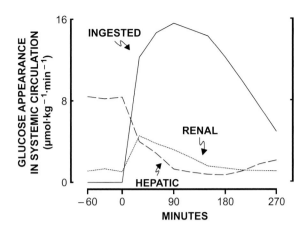

Fig. 2.6 Changes in rates of entry of glucose into the circulation from ingested glucose, liver, and kidney

Tissues Responsible for Disposal of Ingested Glucose

Based on a survey of published studies, a consensus view of the disposal of a hypothetical meal containing 100 g carbohydrate is depicted in Fig. 2.7. About 30% of the ingested glucose (~33 g) is initially extracted by splanchnic tissues.[12,80,84–89] Most is taken up by the liver and immediately incorporated into glycogen via "direct pathway" to hepatic glycogen.[90,91] A significant portion of glucose taken up by the liver probably undergoes glycolysis and is released as lactate which is eventually taken up by the liver where it undergoes gluconeogenesis and is subsequently incorporated into glycogen via "indirect pathway."[12,91–93] Inhibition of glucose-6-phosphatase causes the glucose-6-phosphate made from this lactate to enter glycogen rather than being released into the circulation as free glucose.

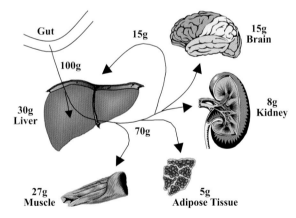

Fig. 2.7 Postprandial glucose disposal. Of 100 g glucose ingested 30% is taken up by the liver and 70% is released into the systemic circulation. Of this 70 g, 15 g (~20%) is extracted by the liver, 15 g (~20%) is taken up by the brain, 27 g (~40%) is taken up by skeletal muscle, and the remaining 20% is taken up by kidney, adipose tissue, skin, and blood cells

Of the remaining 70 g glucose, which enters the systemic circulation, 25–30 g is taken up by skeletal muscle,[12,80,84,85,87,89,94] initially to be oxidized in place of FFA and later (after 2–3 h) to be stored as glycogen.[82,95] Relatively little of the glucose taken up by muscle is released into the circulation as lactate and alanine.[12,96]

About 15 g (~20% of the ingested glucose entering the circulation) is taken up by brain as a substitute for the endogenously produced glucose that normally would have been taken up during this period. Recall that endogenous release of glucose from the liver is markedly reduced postprandially.

Another 15 g is extracted from the systemic circulation by the liver either as intact glucose (direct pathway) or as lactate, alanine, and glutamine, whose carbon backbone originated from ingested glucose, for further glycogen formation (indirect pathway).[92] Thus, ultimately splanchnic tissues dispose of nearly half of the ingested glucose.[97]

The kidney may take up as much as 8 g (~10% of the ingested glucose entering the circulation).[83] This would leave 5–10 g (7–15%) of the ingested glucose reaching the systemic circulation) to be taken up by adipose and other tissues.[82]

Summary

For both the fasting and postprandial states, factors which affect the rate of entry of glucose into the circulation are more important for maintaining normal glucose homeostasis than those which affect the rate of removal of glucose from the circulation. In the postabsorptive state gluconeogenesis and glycogenolysis contribute equally to glucose release. The liver is responsible for all of glycogenolysis and half of gluconeogenesis. In the postprandial state almost all endogenous glucose release is via gluconeogenesis.

The regulation of glucose entry into the circulation is complex, being influenced by hormones, the sympathetic nervous system, and substrates (i.e., free fatty acid concentrations and availability of gluconeogenic precursors). Of these, insulin and glucagon are most important both in the fasting and in the postprandial state. In the latter, incretins which form the entero-insular axis contribute by altering gastric emptying and insulin and glucagon secretion. Finally, recent studies have provided evidence for hepatorenal reciprocity, meaning that, under a variety of conditions, reciprocal changes occur in hepatic and renal glucose release so as to maintain overall glucose release relatively constant.

References

1. Rizza R, Gerich J, Haymond M, et al. Control of blood sugar in insulin-dependent diabetes: comparison of an artificial endocrine pancreas, subcutaneous insulin infusion and intensified conventional insulin therapy. *N Engl J Med*. 1980;303:1313–1318.
2. Wahren J, Felig P, Hagenfeldt L. Physical exercise and fuel homeostasis in diabetes mellitus. *Diabetologia*. 1978;14:213–222.
3. Consoli A, Kennedy F, Miles J, Gerich J. Determination of Krebs cycle metabolic carbon exchange in vivo and its use to estimate the individual contributions of gluconeogenesis and glycogenolysis to overall glucose output in man. *J Clin Invest*. 1987;80:1303–1310.
4. Gerich J. Control of glycaemia. *Baillieres Clin Endocrinol Metab*. 1993;7:551–586.
5. Gerich J. Glucose counterregulation and its impact on diabetes mellitus. *Diabetes*. 1988;37:1608–1617.
6. Siesjo BK. Hypoglycemia, brain metabolism, and brain damage. *Diabetes Metab Rev*. 1988;4:113–144.
7. Owen O, Morgan A, Kemp H, Sullivan J, Herrera M, Cahill G. Brain metabolism during fasting. *J Clin Invest*. 1967;46: 1589–1595.
8. Mitrakou A, Ryan C, Veneman T, et al. Hierarchy of glycemic thresholds for counterregulatory hormone secretion, symptoms, and cerebral dysfunction. *Am J Physiol*. 1991;260:E67–E74.
9. Jarrett RJ, Keen H. Hyperglycaemia and diabetes mellitus. *Lancet*. 1976;2:1009–1012.
10. Tominaga M, Eguchi H, Manaka H, Igarashi K, Kato T, Sekikawa A. Impaired glucose tolerance is a risk factor for cardiovascular disease, but not impaired fasting glucose. The Funagata Diabetes Study. *Diabetes Care*. 1999;22:920–924.
11. Tchobroutsky G. Relation of diabetic control to development of microvascular complications. *Diabetologia*. 1978;15:143–152.
12. Kelley D, Mitrakou A, Marsh H, et al. Skeletal muscle glycolysis, oxidation, and storage of an oral glucose load. *J Clin Invest*. 1988;81:1563–1571.
13. Meyer C, Dostou J, Nadkarni V, Gerich J. Effects of physiological hyperinsulinemia on systemic, renal and hepatic substrate metabolism. *Am J Physiol*. 1998;275:F915–F921.
14. Oster-Jorgensen E, Pedersen SA, Larsen ML. The influence of induced hyperglycaemia on gastric emptying rate in healthy humans. *Scand J Clin Lab Invest*. 1990;50:831–836.
15. Meyer C, Nadkarni V, Stumvoll M, Gerich J. Human kidney free fatty acid and glucose uptake: evidence for a renal glucose-fatty acid cycle. *Am J Physiol*. 1997;273:E650–E654.
16. Gerich JE. Physiology of glucose homeostasis. *Diabetes Obes Metab*. 2000;2:345–350.
17. Stumvoll M, Mitrakou A, Pimenta W, et al. Assessment of insulin secretion from the oral glucose tolerance test in white patients with type 2 diabetes. *Diabetes Care*. 2000;23:1440–1441.

18. Woerle HJ, Meyer C, Dostou JM, et al. Pathways for glucose disposal after meal ingestion in humans. *Am J Physiol Endocrinol Metab*. 2003;284:E716–E725.

19. Gosmanov NR, Szoke E, Israelian Z, et al. Role of the decrement in intraislet insulin for the glucagon response to hypoglycemia in humans. *Diabetes Care*. 2005;28:1124–1131.

20. Bolli G, Gottesman I, Cryer P, Gerich J. Glucose counterregulation during prolonged hypoglycemia in normal humans. *Am J Physiol*. 1984;247:E206–E214.

21. Gromada J, Franklin I, Wollheim CB. Alpha-cells of the endocrine pancreas: 35 years of research but the enigma remains. *Endocr Rev*. 2007;28:84–116.

22. Magnusson I, Rothman D, Gerard D, Katz L, Shulman G. Contribution of hepatic glycogenolysis to glucose production in humans in response to a physiological increase in plasma glucagon concentration. *Diabetes*. 1995;44:185–189.

23. Gerich J. Physiology of glucagon. *Int Rev Physiol*. 1981;24:244–275.

24. Lecavalier L, Bolli G, Cryer P, Gerich J. Contributions of gluconeogenesis and glycogenolysis during glucose counterregulation in normal humans. *Am J Physiol*. 1989;256:E844–E851.

25. Gerich J, Cryer P, Rizza R. Hormonal mechanisms in acute glucose counterregulation: the relative roles of glucagon, epinephrine, norepinephrine, growth hormone and cortisol. *Metabolism*. 1980;29(Suppl 1):1164–1175.

26. Rizza R, Cryer P, Haymond M, Gerich J. Adrenergic mechanisms of catecholamine action on glucose homeostasis in man. *Metabolism*. 1980;29(Suppl):1155–1163.

27. Stumvoll M, Chintalapudi U, Perriello G, Welle S, Gutierrez O, Gerich J. Uptake and release of glucose by the human kidney: postabsorptive rates and responses to epinephrine. *J Clin Invest*. 1995;96:2528–2533.

28. DeFeo P, Perriello G, Torlone E, et al. Contribution of adrenergic mechanisms to glucose counterregulation in humans. *Am J Physiol*. 1991;261:E725–E736.

29. Rizza R, Mandarino L, Gerich J. Effects of growth hormone on insulin action in man: mechanisms of insulin resistance, impaired suppression of glucose production and impaired stimulation of glucose utilization. *Diabetes*. 1982;31:663–669.

30. DeFeo P, Perriello G, Torlone E, et al. Demonstration of a role of growth hormone in glucose counterregulation. *Am J Physiol*. 1989;256:E835–E843.

31. DeFeo P, Perriello G, Torlone E, et al. Contribution of cortisol to glucose counterregulation in humans. *Am J Physiol*. 1989;257:E35–E42.

32. Fanelli C, Calderone S, Epifano L, et al. Demonstration of a critical role for free fatty acids in mediating counterregulatory stimulation of gluconeogenesis and suppression of glucose utilization in humans. *J Clin Invest*. 1993;92:1617–1622.

33. Cahill G. Starvation in man. *N Engl J Med*. 1970;282:668–675.

34. Havel R. Caloric homeostasis and disorders of fuel transport. *N Engl J Med*. 1972;287:1186–1192.

35. Boden G. Role of fatty acids in the pathogenesis of insulin resistance and NIDDM. *Diabetes*. 1997;46:3–10.

36. McGarry J. Glucose-fatty acid interactions in health and disease. *Am J Clin Nutr*. 1998;67(3 Suppl):500S–504S.

37. Baggio LL, Drucker DJ. Biology of incretins: GLP-1 and GIP. *Gastroenterology*. 2007;132:2131–2157.

38. Brown JC, Dryburgh JR, Ross SA, Dupre J. Identification and actions of gastric inhibitory polypeptide. *Recent Prog Horm Res*. 1975;31:487–532.

39. Nauck MA, Heimesaat MM, Behle K, et al. Effects of glucagon-like peptide 1 on counterregulatory hormone responses, cognitive functions, and insulin secretion during hyperinsulinemic, stepped hypoglycemic clamp experiments in healthy volunteers. *J Clin Endocrinol Metab*. 2002;87:1239–1246.

40. Rayner CK, Samsom M, Jones KL, Horowitz M. Relationships of upper gastrointestinal motor and sensory function with glycemic control. *Diabetes Care*. 2001;24:371–381.

41. Horowitz M, Edelbroek MA, Wishart JM, Straathof JW. Relationship between oral glucose tolerance and gastric emptying in normal healthy subjects. *Diabetologia*. 1993;36:857–862.

42. Jones KL, Horowitz M, Carney BI, Wishart JM, Guha S, Green L. Gastric emptying in early noninsulin-dependent diabetes mellitus. *J Nucl Med*. 1996;37:1643–1648.

43. MacGregor IL, Gueller R, Watts HD, Meyer JH. The effect of acute hyperglycemia on gastric emptying in man. *Gastroenterology*. 1976;70:190–196.

44. Bjornsson ES, Urbanavicius V, Eliasson B, Attvall S, Smith U, Abrahamsson H. Effects of hyperglycemia on interdigestive gastrointestinal motility in humans. *Scand J Gastroenterol*. 1994;29:1096–1104.

45. Karamanlis A, Chaikomin R, Doran S, et al. Effects of protein on glycemic and incretin responses and gastric emptying after oral glucose in healthy subjects. *Am J Clin Nutr*. 2007;86:1364–1368.

46. Gentilcore D, Chaikomin R, Jones KL, et al. Effects of fat on gastric emptying of and the glycemic, insulin, and incretin responses to a carbohydrate meal in type 2 diabetes. *J Clin Endocrinol Metab*. 2006;91:2062–2067.

47. Mueckler M. Family of glucose-transporter genes implications for glucose homeostasis and diabetes. *Diabetes*. 1990;39:6–11.

48. Cushman S, Wardzala L. Potential mechanism of insulin action on glucose transport in the isolated rat adipose cell. Apparent translocation of intracellular transport systems to the plasma membrane. *J Biochem*. 1980;255:4728–4762.

49. Bouche C, Serdy S, Kahn CR, Goldfine AB. The cellular fate of glucose and its relevance in type 2 diabetes. *Endocr Rev*. 2004;25:807–830.

50. Gottesman I, Mandarino L, Gerich J. Use of glucose uptake and glucose clearance for the evaluation of insulin action in vivo. *Diabetes*. 1984;33:184–191.

51. Rodnick KJ, Piper RC, Slot JW, James DE. Interaction of insulin and exercise on glucose transport in muscle. *Diabetes Care*. 1992;15:1679–1689.
52. Wright EM. Renal Na(+)-glucose cotransporters. *Am J Physiol Renal Physiol*. 2001;280:F10–F18.
53. Gerich J. Hepatorenal glucose reciprocity in physiologic and pathologic conditions. *Diab Nutr Metab*. 2002;15:298–302.
54. Meyer C, Stumvoll M, Nadkarni V, Dostou J, Mitrakou A, Gerich J. Abnormal renal and hepatic glucose metabolism in type 2 diabetes mellitus. *J Clin Invest*. 1998;102:619–624.
55. Stumvoll M, Meyer C, Kreider M, Perriello G, Gerich J. Effects of glucagon on renal and hepatic glutamine gluconeogenesis in normal postabsorptive humans. *Metabolism*. 1998;47:1227–1232.
56. Stumvoll M, Meyer C, Perriello G, Kreider M, Welle S, Gerich J. Human kidney and liver gluconeogenesis: evidence for organ substrate selectivity. *Am J Physiol*. 1998;274:E817–E826.
57. Cersosimo E, Garlick P, Ferretti J. Renal glucose production during insulin-induced hypoglycemia in humans. *Diabetes*. 1999;48:261–266.
58. Cersosimo E, Garlick P, Ferretti J. Insulin regulation of renal glucose metabolism in humans. *Am J Physiol*. 1999;276:E78–E84.
59. Ekberg K, Landau B, Wajngot A, et al. Contributions by kidney and liver to glucose production in the postabsorptive state and after 60 h of fasting. *Diabetes*. 1999;48:292–298.
60. Cersosimo E, Garlick P, Ferretti J. Regulation of splanchnic and renal substrate supply by insulin in humans. *Metabolism*. 2000;49:676–683.
61. Cersosimo E, Garlick P, Ferretti J. Renal substrate metabolism and gluconeogenesis during hypoglycemia in humans. *Diabetes*. 2000;49:1186–1193.
62. Moller N, Rizza R, Ford G, Nair K. Assessment of postabsorptive renal glucose metabolism in humans with multiple glucose tracers. *Diabetes*. 2001;50:747–751.
63. Meyer C, Dostou J, Welle S, Gerich J. Role of human liver, kidney and skeletal muscle in postprandial glucose homeostasis. *Am J Physiol Endocrinol Metab*. 2002;282:E419–E427.
64. Garcia-Ruiz J, Moreno F, Sanchez-Medina F, Mayor F. Stimulation of rat kidney phosphoenolpyruvate carboxykinase activity in experimental liver disease induced by galactosamine. *FEBS Lett*. 1973;34:13–16.
65. Bergman H, Drury DR. The relationship of kidney function to the glucose utilization of the extra abdominal tissues. *Am J Physiol*. 1938;124:279–284.
66. Drury D, Wick A, MacKay E. Formation of glucose by the kidney. *Am J Physiol*. 1950;165:655–661.
67. Joseph S, Heaton N, Potter D, Pernet A, Umpleby M, Amiel S. Renal glucose production compensates for the liver during the anhepatic phase of liver transplantation. *Diabetes*. 2000;49:450–456.
68. Battezzati A, Fattorini A, Caumo A, et al. Non-hepatic glucose production in humans. *Diabetes*. 1999;48(Suppl 1):A49 (Abstract).
69. Schoolwerth A, Smith B, Culpepper R. Renal gluconeogenesis. *Min Electr Metab*. 1988;14:347–361.
70. Iles R, Cohen R, Rist A, Baron P. The mechanism of inhibition by acidosis of gluconeogenesis from lactate in rat liver. *Biochem J*. 1977;164:185–191.
71. Aber G, Morris L, Housley E. Gluconeogenesis by the human kidney. *Nature*. 1966;212:1589–1590.
72. Gerich J. Hypoglycaemia and counterregulation in type 2 diabetes. *Lancet*. 2000;356:1946–1947.
73. Meyer C, Dostou J, Gerich J. Role of the human kidney in glucose counterregulation. *Diabetes*. 1999;48:943–948.
74. Cersosimo E, Garlick P, Ferretti J. Abnormal glucose handling by the kidney in response to hypoglycemia in type 1 diabetes. *Diabetes*. 2001;50:2087–2093.
75. Woerle HJ, Meyer C, Popa E, Cryer P, Gerich J. Renal compensation for impaired hepatic glucose release during hypoglycemia in type 2 diabetes. *Diabetologia*. 2001;44(Suppl 1):A67 (Abstract).
76. Stumvoll M, Meyer C, Mitrakou A, Nadkarni V, Gerich J. Renal glucose production and utilization: new aspects in humans. *Diabetologia*. 1997;40:749–757.
77. Landau B, Wahren J, Chandramouli V, Schuman W, Ekberg K, Kalhan S. Contributions of gluconeogenesis to glucose production in the fasted state. *J Clin Invest*. 1996;98:378–385.
78. Nilsson L, Hultman E. Liver glycogen in man – the effect of total starvation or a carbohydrate-poor diet followed by refeeding. *Scand J Clin Lab Invest*. 1973;32:325–330.
79. Perriello G, Jorde R, Nurjhan N, et al. Estimation of the glucose-alanine-lactate-glutamine cycles in postabsorptive man: role of the skeletal muscle. *Am J Physiol*. 1995;269:E443–E450.
80. McMahon M, Marsh H, Rizza R. Comparison of the pattern of postprandial carbohydrate metabolism after ingestion of a glucose drink or a mixed meal. *J Clin Endocrinol Metab*. 1989;68:647–653.
81. Dinneen S, Gerich J, Rizza R. Carbohydrate metabolism in noninsulin-dependent diabetes mellitus. *N Engl J Med*. 1992;327:707–713.
82. Marin P, Hogh-Kristiansen I, Jansson S, Krotkiewski M, Holm G, Bjorntorp P. Uptake of glucose carbon in muscle glycogen and adipose tissue triglycerides in vivo in humans. *Am J Physiol*. 1992;263:E473–E480.
83. Meyer C, Dostou J, Welle S, Gerich J. Role of liver, kidney and skeletal muscle in the disposition of an oral glucose load. *Diabetes*. 1999;48(Suppl 1):A289 (Abstract).
84. Kelley D, Mokan M, Veneman T. Impaired postprandial glucose utilization in non-insulin-dependent diabetes mellitus. *Metabolism*. 1994;43:1549–1557.

85. Butler P, Kryshak E, Rizza R. Mechanism of growth hormone-induced postprandial carbohydrate intolerance in humans. *Am J Physiol*. 1991;260:E513–E520.
86. Ferrannini E, Bjorkman O, Reichard G, et al. The disposal of an oral glucose load in healthy subjects: a quantitative study. *Diabetes*. 1985;34:580–588.
87. Jackson R, Roshania R, Hawa M, Sim B, DiSilvio L. Impact of glucose ingestion on hepatic and peripheral glucose metabolism in man: an analysis based on simultaneous use of the forearm and double isotope techniques. *J Clin Endocrinol Metab*. 1986;63:541–549.
88. McMahon M, Marsh H, Rizza R. Effects of basal insulin supplementation on disposition of a mixed meal in obese patients with NIDDM. *Diabetes*. 1989;38:291–303.
89. Mitrakou A, Kelley D, Mokan M, et al. Role of reduced suppression of glucose production and diminished early insulin release in impaired glucose tolerance. *N Engl J Med*. 1992;326:22–29.
90. Beckmann N, Fried R, Turkalj I, Seelig J, Keller U, Stalder G. Noninvasive observation of hepatic glycogen formation in man by 13C MRS after oral and intravenous glucose administration. *Magn Reson Med*. 1993;29:583–590.
91. Petersen K, Cline G, Gerard D, Magnusson I, Rothman D, Shulman G. Contribution of net hepatic glycogen synthesis to disposal of an oral glucose load in humans. *Metabolism*. 2001;50:598–601.
92. Taylor R, Magnusson I, Rothman D. Direct assessment of liver glycogen storage by 13C nuclear magnetic resonance spectroscopy and regulation of glucose homeostasis after a mixed meal in normal subjects. *J Clin Invest*. 1996;97:126–132.
93. Mitrakou A, Jones R, Okuda Y, et al. Pathway and carbon sources for hepatic glycogen repletion in the dog. *Am J Physiol*. 1991;260:E194–E202.
94. Firth R, Bell P, Marsh H, Hansen I, Rizza R. Postprandial hyperglycemia in patients with noninsulin-dependent diabetes mellitus. Role of hepatic and extrahepatic tissues. *J Clin Invest*. 1986;77:1525–1532.
95. Taylor R, Price T, Katz L, Shulman R, Shulman G. Direct measurement of change in muscle glycogen concentration after a mixed meal in normal subjects. *Am J Physiol*. 1993;265:E224–E229.
96. Radziuk J, Inculet R. The effects of ingested and intravenous glucose on forearm uptake of glucose and glucogenic substrate in normal man. *Diabetes*. 1983;32:977–981.
97. Ferrannini E, Wahren J, Felig P, DeFronzo R. The role of fractional glucose extraction in the regulation of splanchnic glucose metabolism in normal and diabetic man. *Metabolism*. 1980;29:28–35.

Chapter 3
Endocrine Pancreas

Barry J. Brass, Zinoviy Abelev, Emilia Pauline Liao, and Leonid Poretsky

Introduction

The endocrine pancreas is composed of the islets of Langerhans, which comprise approximately two million clusters of cells dispersed within the acinar tissue of the exocrine pancreas. Whereas the exocrine pancreas is responsible for secreting digestive enzymes for nutrient absorption, the endocrine pancreas regulates nutrient homeostasis and metabolism, including uptake, storage, and release of metabolic fuels. In adults, the islets constitute between 1 and 2% of pancreatic mass. At least four cell types have been identified in the islets: α-cells, β-cells, δ-cells, and pancreatic polypeptide (PP) cells. β-Cells constitute the majority of islet cells and are concentrated in the anterior head, body, and tail of the pancreas. In contrast, the posterior portion of the head, which is derived from the primordial ventral bud (versus the dorsal bud for the remainder of the pancreas), consists of mostly PP cells (Table 3.1). Recently, another subgroup of endocrine cells (epsilon cells) producing hormone ghrelin was discovered in pancreas of mice.[1,2]

Insulin and glucagon play opposing roles in glucose and nutrient homeostasis. While insulin promotes energy storage, glucagon promotes catabolism, making energy available to tissues when food is not available. In the liver, high insulin:glucagon ratio (such that occurs following a meal) stimulates glycogen synthesis and inhibits glycogenolysis, gluconeogenesis, fatty acid oxidation, and ketone production. In adipose tissue, high insulin:glucagon ratio favors fatty acid and glucose uptake and triglyceride formation. Conversely, low insulin:glucagon ratio signals energy utilization, resulting in glycogenolysis, gluconeogenesis, and fatty acid oxidation. Amylin is cosecreted with insulin and appears to play a role in the regulation of gut physiology. Glucagon-like peptides (GLP) 1 and 2 also play roles in nutrient metabolism. GLP-1 stimulates production and release of insulin and somatostatin, and inhibits glucagon. GLP-1 also has effects on the stomach, brain, and heart. GLP-2 stimulates mucosal growth and nutrient absorption, and inhibits motility in the intestine. Pancreatic polypeptide (PP) levels rise after a mixed meal, and PP is often elevated in patients with pancreatic neuroendocrine tumors, but its physiologic action is not known.

The islets receive a disproportionately large (5–10 times more) amount of blood supply, compared to a similar volume of exocrine tissue. The posterior head is supplied by the superior mesenteric artery, and the remainder of the pancreas is supplied by the celiac artery. Insulin-secreting cells are centrally located within the islets and the direction of blood flow from center to periphery allows insulin-secreting cells to exert a tonic inhibitory effect on glucagon secretion. The islets have a complex innervation and capillary network to receive signals from other hormones, allowing the islet to integrate the hormonal response and function as a coordinated secretory unit. This chapter will discuss the interactions of various factors involved in the regulation of nutrient metabolism by the endocrine pancreas.

L. Poretsky (✉)

Division of Endocrinology and Metabolism, Albert Einstein College of Medicine, Beth Israel Medical Center, New York, NY 10003, USA

e-mail: lporetsk@chpnet.org

L. Poretsky (ed.), *Principles of Diabetes Mellitus*, DOI 10.1007/978-0-387-09841-8_3,
© Springer Science+Business Media, LLC 2010

Table 3.1 Islet cell types

Cell type	Percentage of total	Hormone
Alpha (α)	15–20	Glucagon, ghrelin
Beta (β)	65–80	Insulin, amylin
Delta (δ)	3–10	Somatostatin
PP	1	Pancreatic polypeptide
Epsilon (ε)	1	Ghrelin

Insulin Synthesis

Insulin is synthesized in the pancreas within the beta cells (β-cells) of the islets of Langerhans. Insulin, one of the smallest proteins in the human body, is built from 51 amino acids. It consists of two polypeptide chains (A and B) linked by disulfide bonds. Another disulfide bond exists within the A chain. Insulin mRNA is translated as a single sequence precursor called preproinsulin in the rough endoplasmic reticulum of β-cells. It is composed of 110 amino acids and is relatively inactive. Almost immediately, preproinsulin is being converted to proinsulin by the removal of its signal peptide (Fig. 3.1).

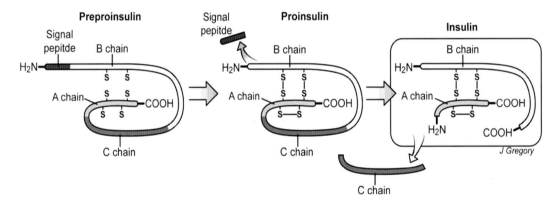

Fig. 3.1 Conversion of preproinsulin to insulin

Theoretically, there are several ways in which proinsulin may be secreted from the β-cell, but none of them involves the regulated secretory pathway. The clathrin-coated microvesicles that bud from the maturing secretory vesicle contain a small fraction of the synthesized proinsulin. Some of these vesicles fuse with endosomes, and their contents are cycled to the cell membrane and released. This is referred to as the constitutive-like (CL) pathway. Other vesicles fuse directly with the cell membrane prior to vesicle maturation and release their contents. This is referred to as the constitutive pathway (Fig. 3.2). The process of secretory vesicle maturation is highly efficient and less than 15% of the total insulin is secreted as proinsulin. This figure is much higher under conditions in which insulin secretion is less well regulated as in patients with type 2 diabetes mellitus or with insulinomas.

Proinsulin is converted to insulin by the action of two prohormone-converting enzymes (PC1/3 and PC2), which become activated in the *trans* Golgi network. These enzymes excise pairs of basic amino acids that are subsequently removed by exoprotease carboxypeptidase E. This results in the formation of an insulin molecule and the C-peptide, a 31-amino acid residue. Partially processed proinsulin, called des-31,32 proinsulin, is secreted to some extent in the process of exocytosis and makes up a large proportion of the circulating proinsulin. As proinsulin processing proceeds, the interior of the granules becomes acidic by the action of vesicular proton pumps, creating conditions for the optimum crystallization of insulin within the granules.

C-peptide is secreted with insulin in equimolar amounts and serves as a useful marker of insulin secretion. It had been presumed that C-peptide had no biological activity; however, reports have appeared describing biologic

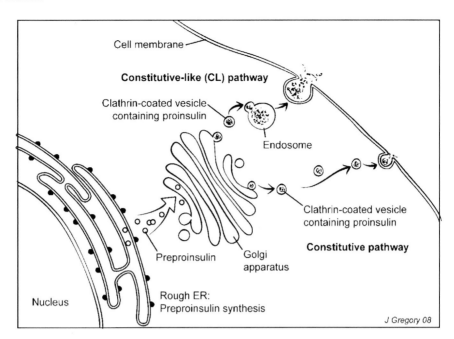

Fig. 3.2 Insulin biosynthesis and secretion

effects of C-peptide. Those include enhancement of glucose transport and utilization, improvements in micro-circulation in muscle, skin, retina, and nerve, stimulation of renal tubular Na[+], K[+] ATPase, and stimulation of islet cell proliferation. As a result, C-peptide has been demonstrated to increase renal and nerve blood flow,[3,4] as well as blood flow in both resting and exercising muscles.[5,6] It also affects relocation of skin blood flow from shunt channels to nutritive blood flow.[7] Some clinical trials showed that short-term C-peptide infusion in type 1 diabetic patients exerts beneficial effects on microvascular function by improving both myocardial blood flow and blood volume.[8]

The proposed actions of C-peptide raise the possibility that combined insulin and C-peptide therapy in patients with type 1 diabetes may more effectively alleviate the progression of diabetes-related complications, including the stabilization (or even reversal) of diabetic neuropathy, nephropathy, and retinopathy.[9–11] However, C-peptide receptors have not been demonstrated, and physiologic actions of C-peptide would require novel interactions with membrane bilayers or other cellular constituents. Recently completed clinical trial of C-peptide among patients with type 1 diabetes and diabetic neuropathy showed some improvement in nerve functions, including nerve conduction velocity and vibration perception.[12,13]

The Insulin Gene and Insulinopathies

The human insulin gene is a single-copy gene located on the short arm of chromosome 11 in band 15. Unlike other members of the insulin gene family which include IGF-I and IGF-II and which are synthesized by most tissues, insulin is produced only by islet β-cells. The selective expression of the insulin gene is brought about by the actions of transactivating factors that bind to specific DNA recognition sequences.

Several families in whom structurally abnormal insulin is produced have been identified. The disorder is inherited in an autosomal fashion and presents with mild hyperinsulinemia and glucose intolerance. The hyper-insulinemia is likely due to impaired receptor binding, leading to reduced insulin clearance. In all cases, a single nucleotide substitution leads to a single amino acid replacement. In another type of variant, an amino acid sub-stitution at the proconvertase cleavage site leads to increased proinsulin secretion via the constitutive secretory pathway.[14]

It is unlikely that variations in either coding or noncoding sequences of the insulin gene are associated with a significant number of cases of diabetes. However, it is possible that variants in promoter regions or defects in regulatory proteins will lead to decreased insulin gene expression and to diabetes of the MODY type (see Chapter 14).

Insulin Release and Second Messenger Signal Transduction

Neurotransmitters and hormones bind to specific cell surface receptors activating second messenger systems that regulate insulin secretion (Fig. 3.3). Cyclic AMP generated by binding of glucagon-like peptide-1 (GLP-1), vasoactive intestinal peptide (VIP), pituitary adenylate cyclase-activating peptide (PACAP), and gastric inhibitory peptide (GIP) to their respective stimulatory G protein-coupled receptors magnifies glucose-stimulated insulin secretion. Conversely, norepinephrine binding to its inhibitory G protein-coupled receptor inhibits cyclic AMP formation and consequently inhibits insulin secretion.

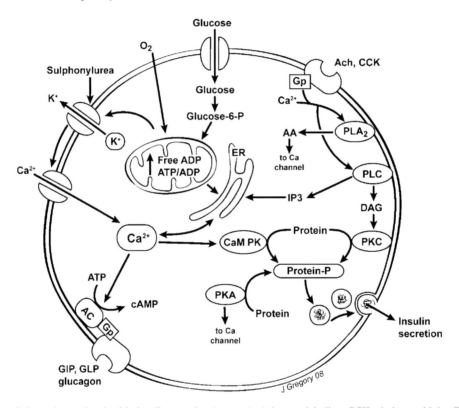

Fig. 3.3 Intracellular pathways involved in insulin secretion (see text). Ach, acetylcholine; CCK, cholecystokinin; Gp, G protein; GK, glucokinase; PLA$_2$, phospholipase A$_2$; AA, arachidonic acid; PLC, phospholipase C; CaM PK, calcium calmodulin-dependent protein kinase; ER, endoplasmic reticulum; P, phosphate; GIP, gastric inhibitory peptide; GLP, glucagon-like peptide. Adapted with permission from Liang et al.[44]

Cyclic AMP increases [Ca^{++}]$_c$ both directly, by activating L-type calcium channels, and indirectly, by activating protein kinase A which phosphorylates and closes potassium channels depolarizing the plasma membrane potential. In addition, cyclic AMP sensitizes the insulin secretory machinery by shifting the dose–response curve of calcium-induced insulin secretion to lower calcium concentrations. Protein kinase A also rapidly phosphorylates a set of proteins that potentiate insulin secretion. Finally, cyclic AMP stimulates insulin gene transcription both directly, by binding to a cyclic AMP response element of the insulin promoter, and indirectly, by phosphorylating (via protein kinase A) a cyclic AMP response element-binding protein.

Three phospholipases in β-cells (phospholipase A_2, C, and D) play a role in regulating insulin secretion. Binding of acetylcholine to its G protein-coupled receptor activates phospholipase C that hydrolyzes membrane-bound phospholipids to inositol triphosphate (IP_3) and diacylglycerol (DAG). IP_3 binds to specific receptors on intracellular membrane-bound structures releasing calcium from intracellular stores and increasing the $[Ca^{++}]_c$. DAG-activated protein kinase C phosphorylates proteins that elicit a variety of cellular responses amplifying glucose-stimulated insulin secretion. In addition, DAG stimulates insulin secretion by increasing the fusogenic potential of cell membranes and by activating DAG lipase, which liberates arachidonic acid from phospholipids.

Arachidonic acid is a 20-carbon unsaturated fatty acid containing four double bonds that exists for the most part esterified in membrane phospholipids. It is released from the plasma membrane by the action of phospholipase A2 upon binding of acetylcholine to its G protein-coupled receptor. This is independent of its release by the action of DAG lipase. Arachidonic acid interacts with the voltage-dependent calcium channels and amplifies insulin secretion by shifting the activation curve of the channels to potentials that are more negative. Arachidonic acid also activates protein kinase C and mobilizes calcium from intracellular stores.

Phosphatidic acid is released from membrane phospholipids upon binding of acetylcholine to its receptor with subsequent activation of phospholipase D. Increased phosphatidic acid levels stimulate insulin secretion by a yet to be determined mechanism.

The resting membrane potential of β-cells is determined primarily by potassium conductance through ATP-dependent K^+ channels. When the cells are exposed to 3 mM glucose (below the threshold for stimulated insulin secretion), the membrane potential is between –60 and –70 mV. As the glucose concentration is increased, the K^+ channels begin to close. This elicits an oscillatory pattern in which periods of more negative potentials are interspersed with plateaus of membrane depolarization upon which spikes of calcium-dependent action potentials are superimposed. As the glucose concentration increases, the duration of the depolarized plateaus increases as well, and the interplateau durations decrease until, at a concentration of 20 mM, the depolarization is continuous. Membrane depolarization opens voltage-gated calcium channels increasing $[Ca^{++}]_c$ and leading to insulin secretion. Two other potassium channels, the delayed rectifier K^+ channel and the Ca^{++}-dependent K^+ channel, function to repolarize the membrane potential. As mentioned above, sulfonylureas bind to and close the ATP-dependent K^+ channels providing the mechanism by which these agents stimulate insulin secretion.

A second source of increased $[Ca^{++}]_c$ is release of calcium from intracellular stores. The endoplasmic reticulum contains a large number of low-affinity calcium-binding sites. Two specific receptors, the IP_3 receptor and the ryanodine receptor, serve as intracellular channels for mobilizing stored calcium. The IP_3 receptor can be phosphorylated by cyclic AMP-dependent protein kinase, protein kinase C, and calcium calmodulin-dependent protein kinase II, providing mechanisms by which several second messenger systems affect insulin secretion. Calcium itself activates the ryanodine receptor, and it has been proposed that this calcium-induced calcium release may be important in the calcium oscillations observed in β-cells.

Insulin Secretion

The total amount of insulin secreted at any given time reflects the sum of the insulin secreted by individual islets. The human pancreas secretes about 30 units of insulin per day in normal adults. The average fasting insulin concentration is 10 μU/ml and rarely rises above 100 μU/ml in normal subjects following a meal. The concept of insulin resistance is demonstrated by Fig. 3.4. Insulin resistance[15] is defined as impaired insulin-stimulated glucose disposal. Obese subjects who are insulin resistant require a higher concentration of insulin to maintain normoglycemia. Insulin-resistant subjects who have beta cell dysfunction and are unable to make this compensatory insulin response will develop hyperglycemia and type 2 diabetes.

Stimulated insulin secretion, either by an ingested meal or by an intravenously administered glucose, results in a biphasic insulin response (Fig. 3.5). The first phase is rapid in onset, has a sharp peak, and lasts for about 10 min. The second phase is a prolonged plateau that lasts for as long as the blood glucose remains elevated. As the figure shows, the first phase of secretion is lost in patients with type 2 diabetes. However, in the same diabetic subjects, the first phase response to intravenously administered arginine is intact, demonstrating that

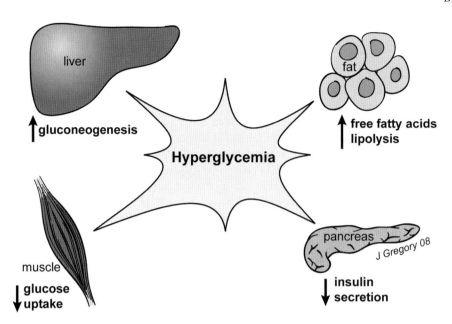

Fig. 3.4 Mechanism of hyperglycemia

the loss of the glucose-stimulated first phase secretion is due to failure to transduce a glucose-associated signal. Sustained levels of high glucose stimulation result in a reversible desensitization of the beta cell response to glucose ("glucose toxicity") but not to other stimuli.

A plausible explanation for biphasic insulin secretion is that the first phase represents release of insulin from a population of secretory vesicles that are "docked" and "primed" at the β-cell membrane and awaiting a glucose-dependent calcium signal for immediate release. The second phase represents replenishment of exocytosis-competent secretory vesicles.

While glucose concentration is the most potent stimulus for insulin secretion, it is not the only determinant. Just as insulin affects the uptake and storage of fatty acids and amino acids (as well as glucose), fatty acids and amino acids also exert an influence on insulin secretion. Extrapancreatic hormones and neural activity also coordinate and magnify the effects of nutrients on pancreatic hormone secretion. Thus, there are four main factors that are responsible for regulating insulin secretion: (1) concentrations of nutrients (including glucose, free fatty acids, amino acids) bathing the islets; (2) activity of autonomic nerves innervating the islets; (3) endocrine hormonal inputs (glucagon, etc); and (4) interactions between the islet cells.

Nutrients and Insulin Secretion

The principal role of the pancreatic hormones is to regulate the uptake and release of metabolic fuels from the hormone-sensitive tissues, liver, muscle, and fat. After meals, when nutrient levels in the blood are high, insulin secretion is stimulated, glucagon secretion is inhibited, and the high insulin to glucagon ratio promotes nutrient storage. At times of fasting, when stored fuel energy is needed, insulin secretion is inhibited, glucagon secretion is stimulated, and the low insulin to glucagon ratio promotes nutrient release from storage.

Glucose and the Fuel Hypothesis of Insulin Secretion

Insulin is secreted at a rate that depends in part on the concentration of glucose in the blood. It was originally theorized that increased blood concentrations of glucose led to greater receptor occupancy on islet cells, which

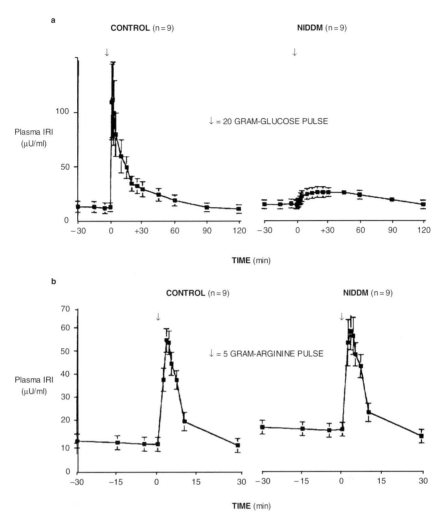

Fig. 3.5 The *top panel* shows the first phase of insulin secretion in response to intravenous insulin in normal subjects (*left plot*) and the loss of the first phase in diabetic subjects (*right plot*). The *bottom panel* shows the intact insulin secretory response to intravenous arginine in normal subjects and individuals with diabetes. From Poitout and Robertson[45] with permission

subsequently resulted in greater insulin secretion. This view was abandoned in light of a large body of evidence, demonstrating that insulin secretion is proportional to the rate at which glucose is metabolized within the islet β-cells.[16] This forms the basis of the well-accepted "fuel hypothesis" (Fig. 3.6), which states that the intracellular glucose concentration determines the rate of glucose metabolism, and the rate of glucose metabolism determines the rate of insulin secretion.

Details of this mechanism have been well worked out. Metabolism of glucose increases the ratio of the concentrations of ATP to ADP. ATP interacts with ATP-dependent potassium channels closing the channels. Potassium channel closure depolarizes the plasma membrane potential, which in turn opens L-type voltage-gated calcium channels. The cytoplasmic calcium concentration, $[Ca^{++}]_c$, rises and calcium activates protein kinases and interacts with the cell's secretory machinery leading to exocytosis of insulin-laden secretory vesicles, i.e., insulin secretion.

This cellular pathway explains the mechanism of action of sulfonylureas, the first class of drugs used to enhance insulin secretion in patients with type 2 diabetes mellitus. Sulfonylureas bind to the ATP-dependent potassium channel complex, closing the channels. Subsequent membrane depolarization and calcium channel opening raises intracellular calcium concentrations and increases insulin secretion.

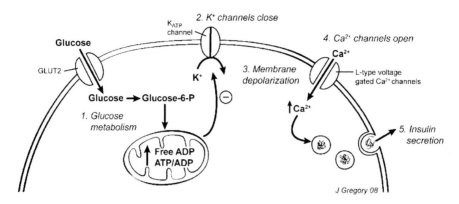

Fig. 3.6 Schematic view of the fuel hypothesis (see text above)

Glucose enters the β-cell through facilitated glucose transporters, GLUT-2, which are constitutively expressed in the plasma membrane of islet cells. As a result, changes in plasma glucose are reflected by changes in the free glucose concentration within islet cells. Glucose is trapped within the β-cell by the first step in glycolysis, the phosphorylation of glucose to glucose-6-P. This reaction, catalyzed by glucokinase, is the rate-limiting step in glycolysis, and since insulin secretion is proportional to the rate of glucose metabolism, it can be said that the combined actions of GLUT-2 and glucokinase form a physiologic "glucose sensor."

The mechanism outlined above does not account for all of the insulin secretion stimulated by glucose. It has been shown that the mitochondrial metabolism of glycolytically derived pyruvate causes insulin secretion independently of increased $[Ca^{++}]_c$.[17] The exact nature of the mitochondrial signals is unknown and is the subject of intensive investigation and debate. There is strong evidence that mitochondrially derived glutamate provides the signal for insulin secretion in insulinoma cell lines. However, several labs have shown that this does not appear to be the case in native islets. It is anticipated that further elucidation of the mechanism of insulin secretion will lead to new therapies.

The total amount of insulin secreted at any given time reflects the sum of the insulin secreted by individual islets. In type 2 diabetes, an inadequate insulin secretory response reflects inadequate insulin secretion from the individual β-cells of the individual islets. This is referred to as beta cell dysfunction. Figure 3.7 shows the concentrations of insulin, C-peptide, and glucose in the blood of normal and diabetic subjects over a 24-h period.[18] The subjects were fed three standard meals a day composed of 50% carbohydrate, 15% protein, and 35% fat. In the normal subjects, insulin and C-peptide concentrations rose to a sharp peak after meals and then

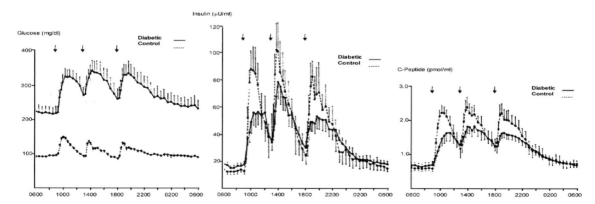

Fig. 3.7 Blood glucose, insulin, and C-peptide levels over a 24-h period in normal subjects and in subjects with type 2 diabetes. Postprandial insulin and C-peptide levels are higher in normal subjects. Glucose levels are lower. From Polansky et al.[46] with permission

rapidly declined. Glucose rose to approximately 50% above basal levels and then returned to baseline within 1–2 h. In subjects with type 2 diabetes, insulin and C-peptide peaked less sharply and rose to lower levels. Glucose levels were higher and their peaks were more prolonged.

Lipids and Insulin Secretion

Nonesterified fatty acids (NEFA), also known as free fatty acids (FFAs), are an important energy source for many tissues of the body. In addition, they are metabolized in β-cells where they also serve as important signaling molecules regulating β-cell function. Acute exposure to free fatty acids increases both basal insulin secretion and glucose-stimulated insulin secretion. Chronically elevated levels of free fatty acids, such as those seen in patients with type 2 diabetes mellitus, may have deleterious effects on β-cell function and may have an etiologic role in both the β-cell dysfunction and the insulin resistance of type 2 diabetes mellitus.[19]

The cellular events leading to the fatty acid-induced enhancement of glucose-stimulated insulin secretion are illustrated in Fig. 3.8. High glucose and insulin lead to Krebs cycle activation, resulting in increased citrate and acetyl-CoA, which are converted to malonyl-CoA via acetyl-CoA carboxylase. Malonyl-CoA is a potent inhibitor of carnitine palmitoyltransferase I (CPT-I), the outer mitochondrial membrane enzyme that transports fatty acyl-CoA into the mitochondria, thereby playing a central role in the balance between mitochondrial glucose and fatty acid metabolism. Inhibition of CPT-I results in an increase in cytoplasmic fatty acyl-CoA, which acts as a signaling molecule having several actions that ultimately increase insulin secretion. Fatty acyl-CoA also increases insulin vesicle trafficking, alters ion channel activity, and promotes vesicle docking and fusion with the cell membrane.

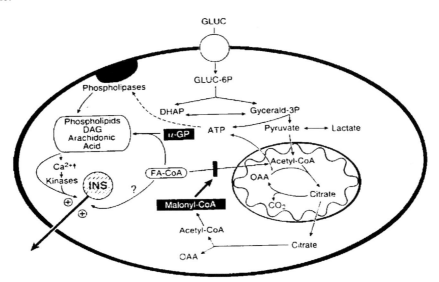

Fig. 3.8 Glucose inhibits the oxidation of fatty acyl-CoA by increasing the production of malonyl-CoA which blocks transport of fatty acyl-CoA into the mitochondria. This ensures that cytoplasmic fatty acyl-CoA is available to enhance insulin secretion. From Newgard and McGarry[16] with permission

The accumulation of lipids in muscle leads to insulin resistance.[20] Since fatty acids enhance insulin secretion, it may be that this enhancement arose as an adaptation to protect against the hyperglycemia that would otherwise have resulted from fatty acid-mediated insulin resistance. The breakdown of this balance may occur in type 2 diabetes mellitus. In early type 2 diabetes, the disease is characterized by prolonged elevation of FFA along with insulin resistance, basal hyperinsulinemia, and exaggerated postprandial insulin secretion. It may be speculated that prolonged exposure to elevated fatty acids causes a decompensation in which β-cell dysfunction cannot overcome the effects of insulin resistance.

Forty years ago, Randle hypothesized that free fatty acids compete with glucose as substrate oxidation and that increased FFA oxidation may cause insulin resistance via elevation of intramitochondrial acetyl-CoA/CoA and NADH/NAD ratios, with subsequent inactivation of pyruvate dehydrogenase.[21] This would lead to increased citrate, inhibition of phosphofructokinase, and increased glucose-6-phosphate (G6P). Increased G6P inhibits hexokinase II, which ultimately decreases glucose uptake. More recent studies have challenged this view. Shulman et al. showed that increased plasma FFA led to 50% reduction in insulin-stimulated rates of muscle glycogen synthesis, which was preceded by a fall (not increase) in G6P. Inhibition of glucose transport and phosphorylation led to reduction in rates of glucose oxidation and muscle glycogen synthesis.[22]

Higher circulating FFA (NA/IL/Hep) produces higher levels of insulin and C-peptide. Experiments using animal models of diabetes support this view. In the male Zucker diabetic fatty rat, there is a pronounced increase in plasma fatty acids, triglycerides, and islet triglycerides that occurs before hyperglycemia appears. Diet restriction as sole therapy reduces hyperlipidemia, islet hypertriglyceridemia and improves β-cell function while preventing hyperglycemia. In another experiment using rats, circulating FFA was rapidly increased by infusing intralipid. It was found that elevated fatty acids enhanced glucose-stimulated insulin secretion at 3 and 6 hours of exposure but suppressed it at 48 h. Carpentier et al.[23] showed essentially the same results in healthy young men. Observations such as these raise the possibility that in diabetes-prone individuals, chronically elevated fatty acids play a role in the β-cell dysfunction of clinical diabetes. However, data are not definitely conclusive that FFAs are the link between insulin resistance and beta cell dysfunction.

Neural Regulation of Insulin Secretion

The pancreatic islets are richly innervated by autonomic and sensory nerves.[24] Insulin secretion is enhanced by stimulation of parasympathetic nerves and inhibited by stimulation of sympathetic nerves. Sensory pathways are for the most part inhibitory. Additional neural pathways mediate direct entero-pancreatic interactions.

The cephalic phase of insulin secretion refers to the first 3–4 min of insulin secretion triggered not by blood-borne nutrients but by the sight, smell, and anticipation of food. The cephalic phase has been demonstrated in a number of ways: by imaginary feeding under hypnosis, by the ingestion of nonnutrient sweeteners, and by the rise in blood insulin levels prior to the rise in blood glucose after ingestion of a glucose load.

The neural effector pathways begin in the ventro-medial hypothalamus and dorsal motor nucleus of the vagus. The cephalic phase is abolished by vagotomy or by ganglionic blockade with muscarinic antagonists, demonstrating that it is mediated by cholinergic neurons of the parasympathetic nervous system (Fig. 3.9).[25]

The question of the physiologic importance of the cephalic phase has been raised since it accounts for only 1–3% of the total insulin response to a meal (or about 25% above baseline). Pancreatic polypeptide, on contrary, is almost entirely under vagal control and increases 100% above baseline during tasting or chewing food. Therefore, the pancreatic polypeptide response during cephalic phase is a sensitive marker of vagal activation by food stimuli.[26] The significance of the cephalic phase of insulin release was demonstrated with the use of trimethaphan, a nondepolarizing antagonist at the nicotinic acetylcholine receptor, that was accompanied by impaired reduction of glucose levels at half an hour to an hour, typical sign of glucose intolerance.[27] On the other hand, replacement of insulin in subjects with type 2 diabetes in the first 15 min after food ingestion improves glucose tolerance. These data imply that cephalic phase plays a role in glucoregulation, causing insulin to lower blood glucose in response to an ingested glucose load. Increase in insulin during the first 10–15 min after meal intake, inversely correlating to the change in glycemia between 25 and 60 min, suggests a relationship between postprandial blood glucose and neurally mediated preabsorptive insulin secretion.

The insulin output of an individual islet derives from the coordinated function of many β-cells. Within islet cells, oscillatory patterns can be seen in oxygen consumption, production of ATP, and concentrations of cytosolic calcium. Electrical coupling by gap junctions serves to help coordinate activity. In addition, insulin secretion from the pancreas as a whole is pulsatile, suggesting synchronization between the islets as well. Blockade of

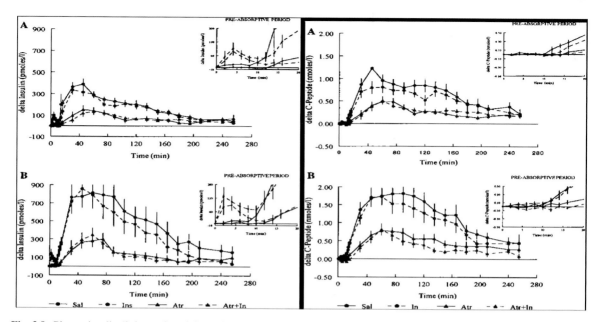

Fig. 3.9 Plasma insulin (*left panel*) and C-peptide (*right panel*) levels expressed as difference from baseline in normal-weight (**a**) and obese (**b**) subjects after ingestion of mixed-nutrient meal during saline (Sal), insulin (Ins), atropine (Atr), and atropine and insulin infusions (Atr + Ins). Adapted with permission from Teff and Townsend[25]

pancreatic ganglia abolishes this synchronization. The clinical importance of oscillatory insulin secretion is suggested by its loss in patients with impaired glucose tolerance and type 2 diabetes.

Parasympathetic Nerves

The parasympathetic nerves innervating the islets originate in the dorsal motor nuclei of the vagus. Preganglionic fibers traverse the vagus in the bulbar outflow tract and the hepatic and gastric branches of the vagus. They enter the pancreas and terminate in intrapancreatic ganglia from which postganglionic fibers emerge to innervate the islets. The postganglionic nerve terminals contain the classical neurotransmitter acetylcholine and the neuropeptides gastrin-releasing peptide (GRP), vasoactive intestinal polypeptide (VIP), and pituitary adenylate cyclase-activating polypeptide (PACAP).[28]

Vagal activation stimulates insulin secretion. Stimulation of the postganglionic fibers releases acetylcholine, which binds to M3 muscarinic receptors on islet cells. The hormones secreted by the other three islet cell types, glucagon, somatostatin, and pancreatic polypeptide, are also stimulated by acetylcholine via M3 receptors. In β-cells, binding of acetylcholine to its receptor stimulates phospholipase C (PLC) activation via a G protein-coupled mechanism. This stimulates phosphoinositide hydrolysis to IP$_3$ and diacylglycerol (DAG). Phospholipase A$_2$ (PLA$_2$) is also activated producing arachidonic acid. Insulin secretion is stimulated by subsequent increase in [Ca^{++}]$_c$ and protein phosphorylation. The mechanisms by which PLC and PLA$_2$ stimulate insulin secretion are discussed in section "Insulin Release and Second Messenger Signal Transduction". The intracellular pathways by which acetylcholine stimulates secretion of the other islet hormones have not been elucidated.

VIP, PACAP, and GRP stimulate insulin secretion upon binding to their respective G protein-coupled receptors. VIP and PACAP exert their effects by stimulating adenylate cyclase and increasing levels of cAMP. GRP binding to its receptor activates PLC and phospholipase D (PLD). The mechanisms by which cAMP and PLD stimulate insulin secretion are discussed in section "Insulin Release and Second Messenger Signal Transduction."

Sympathetic Nerves

At times of physiologic stress (such as prolonged fasting, exercise, hypoglycemia, or hypovolemia), maintaining blood glucose levels becomes vitally important. Glucose output by the liver plays the main role in this process stimulated in part by the counter-regulatory hormones cortisol, epinephrine, and growth hormone. In addition, activation of local sympathetic nerves stimulates glucagon secretion, while insulin secretion is concurrently inhibited. The decreased insulin to glucagon ratio provides the signal for hepatic glucose production and output.

The adrenergic nerves innervating the islets are postganglionic fibers whose cell bodies are located in the celiac ganglion and paravertebral sympathetic ganglia. The preganglionic nerves originate in the hypothalamus, leave the spinal cord at the level of C8 to L3, and traverse the lesser and greater splanchnic nerves to reach the postganglionic cell bodies. The postganglionic nerve terminals contain the classical sympathetic neurotransmitter, norepinephrine, along with the neuropeptides galanin and neuropeptide Y (NPY).

Norepinephrine inhibition of glucose-stimulated insulin secretion is mediated by $\alpha2$-adrenoreceptors. It is not known whether the inhibition of basal insulin secretion is also mediated by norepinephrine. Sympathetic activation also stimulates glucagon and pancreatic polypeptide secretion, while somatostatin secretion is inhibited.

The norepinephrine-induced inhibition of insulin secretion is mediated by several signaling pathways: First, $\alpha2$-adrenoreceptor activation leads to hyperpolarization of the β-cell through opening of the ATP-dependent potassium channels. This prevents opening of the voltage-gated calcium channels, thereby preventing increased $[Ca^{++}]_c$ and subsequent exocytosis of secretory granules. Second, the formation of cyclic AMP is inhibited, and third, there is an inhibitory action on the distal exocytotic machinery.[29]

The concept that sympathetic neuropeptides inhibit glucose-stimulated insulin secretion derives from animal experiments in which sympathetic stimulation leads to inhibition of secretion under conditions in which $\alpha2$-adrenoreceptors are blocked. The mediators of this inhibition are the neuropeptides galanin and NPY. Binding of these neuropeptides to their respective receptors activates pathways similar to those activated by norepinephrine.

Sensory and Other Nerves

The islets are extensively innervated with sensory afferents containing the neuropeptides calcitonin gene-related peptide (CGRP) and substance P (SP). The afferent fibers leave the pancreas along with the sympathetic fibers of the splanchnic nerve and participate in reflexes whose effectors are the autonomic nerves. CGRP has an inhibitory effect on insulin secretion mediated by a decrease in islet cyclic AMP probably reflecting $\alpha2$-adrenoreceptor activation. The CGRP neurons also stimulate glucagon secretion and thus likely participate in the islet's reflex response to hypoglycemia. The actions of SP neurons are less well characterized and both stimulatory and inhibitory effects have been demonstrated.

Other nerves that innervate the islets and affect insulin secretion include neurons that contain nitric oxide synthase (NOS) and cholecystokinin (CCK). The NOS neurons stimulate insulin secretion. The CCK neurons stimulate insulin secretion via mechanisms that involve PLC and PL2 pathways. In addition, nerves originating in the duodenal ganglia directly innervate islets, suggesting the existence of direct entero-pancreatic neural mechanisms.

Glucagon and Glucagon-Like Peptides

Glucagon and the glucagon-like peptides, GLP-1 and GLP-2, are the products of a single gene and are derived from differential posttranslational processing of a single proglucagon protein. Glucagon is produced by the alpha cells of the pancreatic islets, and the GLPs are produced by entero-endocrine cells of the small and large intestine. Glucagon and GLP-1 have important roles in maintaining glucose homeostasis.

Glucagon

Glucagon is synthesized in alpha cells of pancreatic islets as a 160-amino acid prohormone (proglucagon), which is encoded by the preproglucagon gene on chromosome 2. The proglucagon is then split into four peptides, of which glucagon, the 29-amino acid polypeptide with the molecular weight of 3485 Da, is biologically active[30] (Fig. 3.10). The whole process takes about 60–90 min.

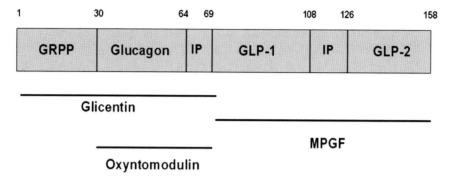

Fig. 3.10 Structure of the mammalian preproglucagon product. GRPP, glicentin-related pancreatic peptide; IP, intervening peptide; GLP-2, glucagon-related peptide-2; MPGF, major proglucagon fragment. Reprinted with permission of Dr. Michael W. King at http://themedicalbiochemistrypage.org/insulin.html

Additional peptides are derived from the preproproteins including glicentin, oxyntomodulin, and the major proglucagon fragment (MPGF) that comprises amino acids 72–158.

Glucagon plays a central role in the maintenance of basal blood glucose levels. Hypoglycemia stimulates and hyperglycemia suppresses glucagon secretion. Glucagon levels rise with fasting and exercise. During times of nutrient need, blood glucose levels are maintained by hepatic glucose production stimulated by low insulin–glucagon ratios. The binding of glucagon to its G protein-coupled receptor on hepatocytes increases intracellular levels of cAMP, leading to activation of protein kinase A, phosphorylase kinase, and phosphorylase. Glycogen synthase is inactivated. The result is stimulation of gluconeogenesis and glycogenolysis and inhibition of glycolysis. Increased hepatic fatty acid oxidation and ketone body formation provide additional energy substrate (Fig. 3.11). In adipocytes, glucagon acts via increased cAMP to stimulate lipolysis, liberating fatty acids into the circulation. In addition, glucose uptake into adipocytes is inhibited, thereby decreasing triglyceride synthesis.

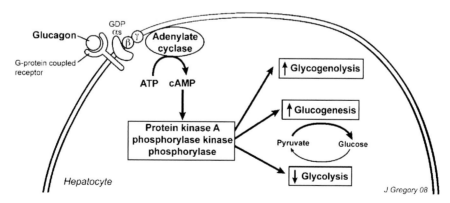

Fig. 3.11 Mechanism of glucagon action

Positive regulators of glucagon secretion include sympathetic nerve stimulation, epinephrine, CCK, PACAP, and GIP. Insulin released by β-cells tonically suppresses glucagon secretion. Conversely, during hypoglycemia, insulin levels are low, releasing glucagon from tonic suppression. Glucagon is one of the first hormones secreted in response to falling glucose concentrations and is crucial for normal glucose counter-regulation.[31] Additionally, glucose suppresses glucagon secretion by inducing β-cell release of the inhibitory neurotransmitter γ-aminobutyric acid (GABA).

Table 3.2 below provides a summary of both stimulating and inhibiting regulators of glucagon secretion.

Table 3.2 Major regulators of glucagon secretion

Stimulators	Inhibitors
Decreased plasma glucose levels	Elevated plasma glucose levels
Catecholamines	Insulin[a]
Gastrin	Somatostatin[a]
Cholecystokinin	Increased levels of circulating
Gastric inhibitory polypeptide	fatty acids
Amino acids (such as arginine,[b] alanine,[c] cysteine,[c] serine,[c] glycine[c])	γ-Aminobutyric acid (GABA)
Glucocorticoids	
Pituitary adenylate cyclase-activating peptide (PACAP)[47]	
Sympathetic and parasympathetic stimulation	

[a] Direct inhibition of α-cells.
[b] Stimulates both glucagon and insulin release.
[c] Stimulates mainly glucagon release.

Glucagon-Like Peptides

L cells of the small intestine synthesize an identical proglucagon molecule whose alternate processing results in the formation of several polypeptides, of which glucagon-like peptides 1 and 2 are probably of most physiologic importance.

GLP-1

The majority of GLP-1-producing cells are in the terminal ileum and proximal colon. Proglucagon synthesis in the gut is stimulated by nutrient intake, and GLP-1 levels in the blood increase rapidly after a meal. The activity of GLP-1 is largely regulated by its rate of degradation, with its half-life being very short, approximately 1 min. GLP-1 binding to its G protein-coupled receptor on β-cells increases glucose-stimulated insulin secretion via both increased cyclic AMP and increased intracellular calcium.

GLP-1 infused into healthy subjects decreases gastric emptying, causes a sensation of satiety, and decreases appetite. Thus, in addition to enhancing insulin secretion, GLP-1 has effects outside of the pancreas that serve to limit postprandial hyperglycemia. In rodents, intracerebroventricularly administered GLP-1 inhibits food intake demonstrating CNS actions. Infusion of the GLP-1 antagonist exendin into healthy subjects increases blood glucose and reduces glucose-stimulated insulin secretion.[32] The multiple actions of GLP-1 in lowering blood glucose make the development of a GLP-1-like agent modified for a longer half-life, an interesting approach to be used in the treatment of diabetes mellitus. For additional information on GLP-1, please see Chapter 4.

Somatostatin

Somatostatin was originally identified in 1973 in hypothalamic extracts as a 14-amino acid peptide that inhibits the release of growth hormone from dispersed rat pituitary cells. Since then, somatostatin and its receptors have been found in all neuroendocrine tissues, as well as in the central and peripheral nervous systems. A single somatostatin gene codes for two biologically active peptides of 14 and 28 amino acids, named somatostatin-14 and somatostatin-28, respectively. In addition to acting as hormones, the peptides act as neurotransmitters, neuromodulators, and local paracrine regulators. Their diverse physiologic actions include modulation of secretion, neurotransmission, smooth muscle contractility, and cell proliferation.

There are five different somatostatin receptors designated sst1, sst2A, sst3, sst4, and sst5. All subtypes have been found in the brain.[33] In contrast, peripheral tissues vary in the subtype expressed (Table 3.3).

Table 3.3 Subtypes of somatostatin receptors

Subtype	Chromosomal location	Distribution in tissues
sst1	14	Brain, lungs, stomach, Jejunum, kidneys, liver, pancreas
sst2	17	Brain, kidneys
sst3	22	Brain, pancreas
sst4	20	Brain, lungs
sst5	16	Brain, heart, adrenal glands, placenta, pituitary, skeletal muscles, small intestine

Adapted with permission from Lamberts et al.[48].

All types of somatostatin receptors are members of the G protein-coupled receptor family, and all inhibit adenylate cyclase activity. Other effectors linked to the ssts via G proteins include voltage-sensitive calcium channels, potassium channels, ser/thr phosphatases, and tyrosine phosphatases.

Somatostatin is produced in neurons of the hypothalamic periventricular area that terminate near the pituitary portal capillaries. Release of somatostatin by these neurons inhibits growth hormone secretion by cells of the anterior pituitary. Elsewhere in the brain, somatostatin acts as a neurotransmitter or a neuromodulator. It is stored in synaptic vesicles, released by a calcium-dependent mechanism upon depolarization, and produces postsynaptic hyperpolarization upon its release.

In the gastrointestinal tract, somatostatin is found in the stomach, the duodenum, submucosal neurons, and the mesenteric plexus of the intestinal tract. It is produced both by gastrointestinal endocrine D cells and by visceral autonomic neurons. Thus it has paracrine and hormonal functions as well as act as a neurotransmitter. It inhibits the secretion of a variety of hormones including insulin, VIP, GIP, gastrin, cholecystokinin, secretin, motilin, and GLP-1 and reduces gastrointestinal motility, gallbladder contraction, and blood flow. Its concentration in the blood increases after meals as a consequence of both gastrointestinal and pancreatic secretion.

Intravenous administration of somatostatin inhibits insulin secretion as well as exocrine pancreatic secretion. However, the precise role of somatostatin in islet function has not been determined. Sst2A receptors are present on islet β-cells and α-cells, suggesting that somatostatin may have a direct role in regulating insulin and glucagon secretion.

Islet Amyloid Polypeptide (IAPP)

IAPP is a 37-amino acid protein that is the principal component of islet amyloid deposits. These deposits are formed in normal islets during aging but are more abundant in the islets of individuals with type 2 diabetes. The amino acid sequences of IAPP from normal and diabetic subjects are identical, and consequently the increased deposition of amyloid deposits in diabetes is not due to structural abnormalities in the amyloid protein.

IAPP is localized in the secretory vesicles of β-cells and is cosecreted with insulin. Levels of IAPP are in the range of 0.2–3.0% of that of insulin in islets, and the amount cosecreted with insulin is about 5.0%. Several hormonal effects of IAPP have been proposed, but the data in support of a precise physiologic role for IAPP are far from compelling. Studies showing that amidated IAPP inhibits insulin-stimulated glucose disposal used non-physiologically high concentrations of IAPP. Other studies showed IAPP having complementary action to insulin. Still other studies showed that extremely high concentrations of IAPP inhibit insulin secretion.

Ghrelin

Recently, a new peptide hormone ghrelin was discovered in alpha cells of the Langerhans' islets as well as in epsilon cells. The latter constitute a newly detected endocrine cell type and originate from neurogenin 3-expressing precursor cells.[34] Ghrelin (meaning "to grow" in reference to the Proto-Indo-European word "ghre") was originally found in a rat stomach as an endogenous ligand for growth hormone secretagogue receptor. It is mainly produced in the stomach with fundus being the predominant harbor of the ghrelin-containing cells. Lower levels of ghrelin were also found in other compartments of the gastrointestinal tract, including the duodenum, the jejunum, the ileum, and the colon. Ghrelin receptors are mainly expressed in the hypothalamus and pituitary, first-trimester human placenta, and germ cells. The ghrelin mRNA expression in the glomeruli of the kidneys, and direct correlation of ghrelin plasma concentration in patients with advanced renal disease, suggests that kidneys are the main organ participating in ghrelin clearance.[35]

Ghrelin and other growth hormone secretagogues (GHSs) kindle the release of growth hormone from the pituitary gland.[36] Additionally, ghrelin stimulates appetite and increases fat mass by activating cells on the hypothalamic arcuate nucleus,[37] a region known to control food intake, and promoting the mesolimbic cholinergic–dopaminergic reward link.[38,39] Plasma ghrelin concentration is increased during fasting and diminished with regular feeding,[40] implicating that either ghrelin may serve as one of the first signals for food intake or its secretion is controlled by some nutritional factors in blood (Fig. 3.12). Plasma ghrelin levels are lower

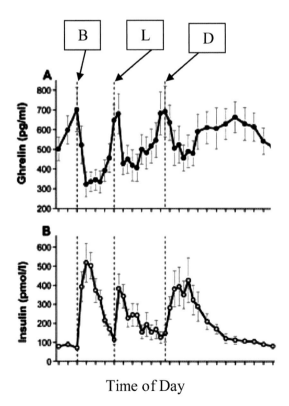

Fig. 3.12 Average plasma ghrelin (**a**) and insulin (**b**) concentrations during a 24-h period in 10 human subjects consuming breakfast (B), lunch (L), and dinner (D) at the times indicated. Blood concentrations of ghrelin are lowest shortly after meal and rise during fast, just prior to the next meal. Adapted with permission from Cummings et al.[40]

in obese patients compared to lean controls.[41] Bariatric surgical procedures, including laparoscopic Roux-en-Y gastric bypass and gastric banding, are associated with significantly suppressed ghrelin levels, possibly contributing to the weight-reducing effect of the procedure.[42] However, patients who underwent gastric bypass, were found to have lower levels of ghrelin and more profound suppression of its fluctuations in relation to meals in comparison to the patients who underwent laparoscopic gastric banding. These findings can explain more sustained long term weight loss in a former group.[43]

Summary

The endocrine pancreas has a central role in maintaining energy homeostasis by regulating nutrient uptake and release by the hormone-sensitive storage tissues, liver, fat, and muscle. When the circulating levels of nutrient fuels, such as glucose and FFA, are high, energy metabolism within islet β-cells is increased, and intracellular signals that increase insulin secretion are generated. At the same time, glucagon secretion from islet α-cells is inhibited. Thus, high insulin to glucagon ratio signals nutrient storage, and a low ratio signals nutrient release. The islet response is further regulated by autonomic and sensory nerves and by blood-borne hormones produced at distant sites of the gastrointestinal tract.

Type 2 diabetes mellitus is a condition marked by both insulin resistance and β-cell dysfunction in which insulin secretion is inadequate to fully signal storage of circulating nutrient fuels. β-cell dysfunction is the descriptive term for the condition in which there is a breakdown in the intracellular chain of events that leads to insulin secretion. This is manifested by blunted peaks of insulin secretion in response to meals and by an inappropriately high concentration of circulating proinsulin. In addition, there is dysregulation involving the autonomic nervous system so that both inter-islet communication and intra-islet stimulation of secretion are lost.

Both obesity and type 2 diabetes are characterized by insulin resistance. However, in non-diabetic individuals, insulin resistance is compensated for by increased insulin secretion. Only when β-cell dysfunction is also present does type 2 diabetes mellitus result.

References

1. Wierup N, Svensson H, Mulder H, Sundler F. The ghrelin cell: a novel developmentally regulated islet cell in the human pancreas. *Regul Pept*. 2002;107:63–69.
2. Wierup N, Yang S, McEvilly RJ, Mulder H, Sundler F. Ghrelin is expressed in a novel endocrine cell type in developing rat islets and inhibits insulin secretion from INS-1 (832/13) cells. *J Histochem Cytochem*. 2004;52:301–310.
3. Johansson B-L, Sjöberg S, Wahren J. The influence of human C-peptide on renal function and glucose utilization in type 1 (insulin-dependent) diabetic patients. *Diabetologia*. 1992;35:121–128.
4. Cotter M, Cameron N. The effects of insulin C-peptide on nerve function in diabetic rats are blocked by nitric oxide synthase inhibition (Abstract). *Diabetologia*. 2001;44(1):A46.
5. Ekberg K, Johansson B-L, Wahren J. Stimulation of blood flow by C-peptide in patients with type 1 diabetes. *Diabetologia*. 2001;44(1):A323.
6. Fernqvist-Forbes E, Johansson B-L, Eriksson M. Effects of C-peptide on forearm blood flow and brachial artery dilatation in patients with type 1 diabetes. *Acta Physiol Scand*. 2001;172:159–165.
7. Forst T, Kunt T, Pohlmann T, Goitom K, Engelbach M, Beyer J, Pfützner A. Biological activity of C-peptide on the skin microcirculation in patients with insulin dependent diabetes mellitus. *J Clin Invest*. 1998;101:2036–2041.
8. Hansen A, Johansson B, Wahren J, von Bibra H. C-peptide exerts beneficial effects on myocardial blood flow and function in patients with type 1 diabetes. *Diabetes*. 2002;51:3077–3082.
9. Marques R, Fontaine M, Rogers J. C-peptide: much more than a byproduct of insulin biosynthesis. *Pancreas*. 2004;29(3):231–238.
10. Kamiya H, Zhang W, Ekberg K, Wahren J, Sima A. C-peptide reverses nociceptive neuropathy in type 1 diabetes. *Diabetes*. 2006;55:3581–3587.
11. Samnegård B, Jacobson S, Jaremko G, et al. C-peptide prevents glomerular hypertrophy and mesangial matrix expansion in diabetic rats. *Nephrol Dial Transplant*. 2005;20(3):532–538.
12. Ekberg K, Brismar T, Johansson B-L, Jonsson B, Lindström P, Wahren J. Amelioration of sensory nerve dysfunction by C-peptide in patients with type 1 diabetes. *Diabetes*. 2003;52(2):536–541.

13. Ekberg K, Brismar T, Johansson B-L, et al. C-peptide replacement therapy and sensory nerve function in type 1 diabetic neuropathy. *Diabetes Care*. 2007;30(1):71–76.
14. Carroll R, Hammer R, Chan S, et al. A mutant human proinsulin is secreted from islets of Langerhans in increased amounts via an unregulated pathway. *Proc Natl Acad Sci USA*. 1988;85:8943–8947.
15. Reaven G. Role of insulin resistance in human disease. Banting lecture 1988. *Diabetes*. 1988;37:1595–1607.
16. Newgard C, McGary J. Metabolic coupling factors in pancreatic ß-cell signal transduction. *Annu Rev Biochem*. 1995;64:689–719.
17. Heart E, Corkey R, Wikstrom J, Shirihai O, Corkey B. Glucose-dependent increase in mitochondrial membrane potential, but not cytoplasmic calcium, correlates with insulin secretion in single islet cells. *Am J Physiol Endocrinol Metab*. 2006;290:E143–E148.
18. Polonsky K, Given B, Hirsch L, et al. Abnormal patterns of insulin secretion in non-insulin-dependent diabetes mellitus. *N Engl J Med*. 1988;318:1231–1239.
19. Bergman R, Ader M. Free fatty acids and pathogenesis of type 2 diabetes mellitus. *Trends Endocrinol Metab*. 2000;11:351–356.
20. Schmitz-Peiffer C. Signaling aspects of insulin resistance in skeletal muscle: mechanisms induced by lipid oversupply. *Cell Signal*. 2000;12:583–594.
21. Randle P, Garland P, Hales C, Newsholme E. The glucose fatty-acid cycle: its role in insulin sensitivity and the metabolic disturbances of diabetes mellitus. *Lancet*. 1963;1:785–789.
22. Fisher J, Nolte L, Kawanaka K, Han Dong-Ho, Jones T, Holloszy J. Glucose transport rate and glycogen synthase activity both limit skeletal muscle glycogen accumulation. *Am J Physiol Endocrinol Metab*. 2002;282:E1214–E1221.
23. Carpentier A, Mittelman SD, Lamarche B, et al. Acute enhancement of insulin secretion by FFA in humans is lost with prolonged FFA elevation. *Am J Physiol*. 1999;276:E1055–E1066.
24. Ahren B. Autonomic regulation of islet hormone secretion – implications for health and disease. *Diabetologia*. 2000;43:393–410.
25. Teff K, Townsend R. Early phase insulin infusion and muscarinic blockade in obese and lean subjects. *Am J Physiol Regul Integr Comp Physiol*. 1999;277:R198–R208.
26. Teff K. Nutritional implications of the cephalic-phase reflexes: endocrine responses. *Appetite*. 2000;34(2):206–213.
27. Ahrén B, Holst J. The cephalic insulin response to meal ingestion in humans is dependent on both cholinergic and noncholinergic mechanisms and is important for postprandial glycemia. *Diabetes*. 2001;50(5):1030–1038.
28. Ahrén B, Wierup N, Sundler F. Neuropeptides and the regulation of islet function. *Diabetes*. 2006;55:S98–S107.
29. Cheng H, Straub S, Sharp G. Protein acylation in the inhibition of insulin secretion by norepinephrine, somatostatin, galanin, and PGE$_2$. *Am J Physiol Endocrinol Metab*. 2003;285:E287–E294.
30. Patzelt C, Schiltz E. Conversion of proglucagon in pancreatic alpha cells: the major endproducts are glucagon and a single peptide, the major proglucagon fragment, that contains two glucagon-like sequences. *Proc Natl Acad Sci USA*. 1984;81(16):5007–5011.
31. Heptulla R, Tamborlane W, Ma TY, et al. Oral glucose augments the counterregulatory hormone response during insulin-induced hypoglycemia in humans. *J Clin Endocrinol Metab*. 2001;86:645–648.
32. Edwards C, Todd J, Mahmoudi M. Glucagon-like peptide 1 has a physiological role in the control of postprandial glucose in humans: studies with the antagonist exendin 9–39. *Diabetes*. 1999;48:86–93.
33. Raulf F, Perez J, Hoyer D, Bruns C. Differential expression of five somatostatin receptor subtypes, SSTR1-5, in the CNS and peripheral tissue. *Digestion*. 1994;55(3):46–53.
34. Heller RS, Jenny M, Collombat P, et al. Genetic determinants of pancreatic epsilon-cell development. *Dev Biol*. 2005;286(1):217–224.
35. Yoshimoto A, Mori K, Sugawara A, et al. Plasma ghrelin and desacyl ghrelin concentrations in renal failure. *J Am Soc Nephrol*. 2002;13:2748–2752.
36. Kojima M, Kangawa K. Ghrelin: structure and function. *Physiol Rev*. 2005;85:495–522 doi:10.1152/physrev.00012.2004.
37. Hewson A, Dickson S. Systemic administration of ghrelin induces Fos and Egr-1 proteins in the hypothalamic arcuate nucleus of fasted and fed rats. *J Neuroendocrinol*. 2000;12(11):1047–1049.
38. Jerlhag E, Egecioglu E, Dickson S, Andersson M, Svensson L, Engel JA. Ghrelin stimulates locomotor activity and accumbal dopamine-overflow via central cholinergic systems in mice: implications for its involvement in brain reward. *Addict Biol*. 2004;111:45–54.
39. Jerlhag E, Egecioglu E, Dickson S, Douhan A, Svensson L, Engel J. Ghrelin administration into tegmental areas stimulates locomotor activity and increases extracellular concentration of dopamine in the nucleus accumbens. *Addict Biol*. 2007;12:6–16.
40. Cummings D, Purnell J, Scott Frayo R, Schmidova K, Wisse B, Weigle D. A preprandial rise in plasma ghrelin levels suggests a role in meal initiation in humans. *Diabetes*. 2001;50:1714–1719.
41. Shiiya T, Nakazato M, Mizuta M, et al. Plasma ghrelin levels in lean and obese humans and the effect of glucose on ghrelin secretion. *J Clin Endocrinol Metab*. 2002;87:240–244.
42. Cummings D, Weigle D, Scott Frayo R, et al. Plasma ghrelin levels after diet-induced weight loss or gastric bypass surgery. *N Engl J Med*. 2002;346:1623–1630.
43. Leonetti F, Silecchia G, Iacobellis G, et al. Different plasma ghrelin levels after laparoscopic gastric bypass and adjustable gastric banding in morbid obese subjects. *J Clin Endocrinol Metab*. 2003;88(9):4227–4231.
44. Liang Y, et al. Mechanisms of action of nonglucose insulin secretagogues. *Ann Rev Nutr*. 1994;14:59–81.

45. Poitout V, Robertson RP. An integrated view of ß-cell dysfunction in type-II diabetes. *Ann Rev Med*. 1996;47:69–83.
46. Polansky KS, Given BD, Hirsch I, et al. Abnormal patterns of insulin secretion in non-insulin-dependent diabetes mellitus. *N Engl J Med*. 1988;318:1231–1239.
47. Filipsson K, Tornøe K, Holst J, Ahré NB. Pituitary adenylate cyclase-activating polypeptide stimulates insulin and glucagon secretion in humans. *J Clin Endocrinol Metab*. 1997;82:3093–3098.
48. Lamberts SW, van der Lely AJ, de Herder WW, Hofland LJ. Octreotide. *N Engl J Med*. 1996;334:246.

Chapter 4
The Role of Incretins in Insulin Secretion

Brock E. Schroeder and Orville Kolterman

Overview of Glucose Regulation and Insulin Secretion

The maintenance of the plasma glucose concentration is a critical bodily function. Hyperglycemia is associated with long-term micro- and macrovascular complications, while hypoglycemia can lead to serious injury to the brain, which is dependent on plasma glucose as a fuel source. At any given time the body's plasma glucose concentration is a balance between the relative rates of glucose appearance and disappearance. These rates are regulated by several key organs through the actions of multiple hormonal signals. A brief introduction follows; however, for more detailed information, see Chapter 2.

During fasting and before meals, glucose appearance is regulated largely by glucagon-induced hepatic glucose output. Binding of glucagon to receptors in the liver leads to both glycogenolysis and gluconeogenesis. Glucose disappearance is regulated by peripheral glucose uptake – primarily by the brain, muscle, and splanchnic organs. Together, these processes normally keep plasma glucose regulated between approximately 70 and 100 mg/dl during the fasting state.

During a meal and in the postprandial period, meal-derived glucose is the major determinant of glucose appearance. Glucose absorption in the gut leads to a rise in plasma glucose. This increase in plasma glucose stimulates insulin secretion from β-cells in the pancreas. Meal-induced increases in plasma insulin – 3 to 4-fold within 30–60 min of a meal – stimulate glucose uptake by peripheral tissues, keeping 2-h postprandial plasma glucose concentrations below approximately 140 mg/dl in healthy individuals.

The mechanisms underlying glucose-stimulated insulin secretion from β-cells are complex and involve the integration of signals from multiple internal and external stimuli. Under normal circumstances, glucose elevation induces a biphasic pattern of insulin release.[1,2] Within a few minutes of plasma glucose increases, first-phase insulin release occurs. This phase, which lasts for approximately 10 min, is thought to reflect a "readily releasable" pool of insulin stored within β-cell secretory vesicles. A longer-lasting second-phase of insulin release follows – reflecting release of both stored insulin as well as newly produced insulin – and lasts as long as plasma glucose remains elevated.

These processes describe a general framework of glucose-induced insulin secretion; however, our current understanding of the mechanisms underlying insulin secretion, as mentioned above, involves an integrated and complex regulatory system. A key to this understanding has been the identification of the "incretin" hormones and elucidation of the role they play in the regulation of glucose-dependent insulin release.

O. Kolterman (✉)
Amylin Pharmaceuticals, Inc., San Diego, CA 92121, USA
e-mail: laura.featherstone@amylin.com

L. Poretsky (ed.), *Principles of Diabetes Mellitus*, DOI 10.1007/978-0-387-09841-8_4,
© Springer Science+Business Media, LLC 2010

Incretin Hormones: Introduction and History

In the 1960s, several groups first described what has become known as the "incretin effect," based upon observations that glucose administered orally elicits an augmented insulin secretory response compared to an equivalent glucose load administered intravenously (IV).[3,4] Elrick and colleagues[4] first described an experiment in subjects without diabetes in which the mean increase in plasma insulin during the first hour after glucose administration was 37% greater following oral glucose than following IV glucose. This increase occurred despite higher mean blood glucose concentrations in the IV administration group. During the second hour following glucose administration, the elevated plasma insulin concentrations were maintained in the oral glucose group (in fact, plasma insulin increased ~55% compared to the first hour), while plasma insulin returned toward fasting concentrations in the IV administration group.

Perley and Kipnis[3] confirmed these findings, demonstrating that oral glucose administration elicited an approximately 60–70% greater insulin secretory response than an equivalent IV glucose load (see Fig. 4.1a, b).

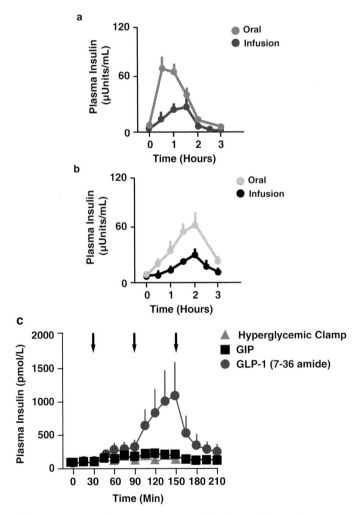

Fig. 4.1 (**a**, **b**) Plasma insulin responses to oral or infused glucose in healthy individuals (**a**) and patients with type 2 diabetes (**b**). Data from Perley and Kipnis[3]. (**c**) Insulinotropic effects of GLP-1, but not GIP, infusion in patients with type 2 diabetes under hyperglycemic clamp conditions. *Arrows* indicate start of low, then high-dose administrations of GLP-1 or GIP, followed by end of administration. Data from Nauck et al.[41]. All data points, Mean ± SE

In addition, they noted that the timing of insulin secretion was also different between the two groups: maximal plasma insulin concentrations were reached earlier (~30–60 min) following oral glucose administration than following IV administration (~90–120 min). Perley and Kipnis also demonstrated for the first time that patients with type 2 diabetes (T2DM) exhibit the incretin effect; however, they noted that patients with diabetes exhibited a decreased insulin response to oral glucose, a concept which will be explored in much greater detail below.

The findings described above indicate that insulin secretion following meals is not accounted for solely by changes in blood glucose concentration. In fact, it has been estimated that approximately 60% of insulin secreted in response to a meal is due to the incretin effect.[5] The discovery of the incretin effect led to a search for mechanisms triggered by oral glucose administration which might play a role in mediating insulin secretion. While a number of factors were initially proposed,[3] currently the incretin effect is attributed largely to two hormones secreted by specialized endocrine cells in the gut: glucose-dependent insulinotropic peptide (GIP, also termed gastric inhibitory polypeptide) and glucagon-like peptide-1 (GLP-1).

Glucose-Dependent Insulinotropic Peptide (GIP)

GIP is a peptide hormone, 42-amino acids in length, processed from a 153-amino acid precursor. It is secreted by the endocrine K-cells of the gut,[6] which are located in highest density in the duodenum and upper intestinal tract. Secretion of GIP increases by approximately 10-fold in response to meal ingestion.[7,8] The insulinotropic effects of GIP are stimulated via activation of specific G protein-coupled receptors on pancreatic β-cells.[9] Following secretion, GIP is rapidly metabolized by the ubiquitous enzyme dipeptidyl peptidase-4 (DPP-4),[10,11] and has a half-life of approximately 7 min.[11]

GIP Function Overview

The insulinotropic properties of GIP were identified first in 1973,[12] and since have been characterized in islet cells, isolated pancreas, and in vivo in healthy humans.[13–17] The insulinotropic effect of GIP is glucose-dependent, and is absent at glucose concentrations under 140 mg/dl.[18] Physiologically, it has been estimated that GIP-dependent insulin secretion accounts for approximately 20–50% of the incretin effect.[19,20] Multiple groups have shown that inhibiting GIP function causes reduced insulin secretion and impaired glucose regulation in animals models.[20,21] Furthermore, mice with genetic deletions of the GIP receptor develop glucose intolerance.[22]

In addition to its incretin effects, a number of other effects of GIP have been identified. These include the following:

(1) GIP has both proliferative and anti-apoptotic effects on β-cells.[23–26] The physiological importance of these findings and potential effects in humans are not known at present.
(2) Evidence for a role of GIP signaling in obesity has come from a variety of studies. GIP receptors are expressed on adipocytes[27] and GIP has been implicated in lipid metabolism in a variety of studies.[28–30] Mice with genetic disruption of the GIP receptor are resistant to diet-induced obesity and have reduced adiposity following high-fat feeding.[22,31] Furthermore, when GIP receptors were disrupted in ob/ob mice (a mouse model of obesity), these mice experienced less weight gain, decreased fat, and increased energy expenditure.[31] While in theory antagonism of GIP signaling may have beneficial effects on obesity, the benefits are likely outweighed by the negative effects on glucose tolerance.
(3) GIP receptors are also expressed on bone and stimulation of this pathway elicits new bone formation.[32] Conversely, young mice lacking GIP receptors have reduced bone size and mass.[33] The potential for clinical application of GIP effects on bone is unknown at present.

Glucagon-Like Peptide-1 (GLP-1)

While early studies conclusively demonstrated that GIP elicited insulin secretion, Ebert and colleagues[34] showed that removal of GIP from the gut did not eliminate the incretin effect. This finding provided strong evidence for the existence of additional gut-derived factors with insulinotropic properties. The second incretin hormone identified is GLP-1, a product of the proglucagon gene (the same precursor gene which codes for glucagon when expressed in the pancreas). GLP-1 is rapidly secreted from the L-cells of the lower gut following meal ingestion.[35] A truncated version of GLP-1 (amino acids 7–36; GLP-1$_{7-36}$) has been shown to be the predominant form of bioactive GLP-1 in circulation following meals.[36–38] Like GIP, GLP-1 is rapidly metabolized by the enzyme DPP-4 following release (resulting in the inactive fragment GLP-1$_{9-36}$),[10,11,39,40] and has a half-life of only 2 min in circulation.[11]

Following a meal, the concentration of GLP-1 rises by about 3-fold.[38] This increase is notably less than that of GIP following a meal; however, GLP-1 has been shown to be the more potent insulinotropic compound.[41] In fact, GLP-1 is one of the most potent insulin-releasing substances known.[42] GLP-1 exerts its activity via interaction with specific GLP-1 receptors on β-cells (despite its name, GLP-1 does not bind to the glucagon receptor). GLP-1 receptors are G protein-coupled receptors which belong to the same family as the GIP receptor[9,43] and, as described below, the intracellular signaling cascade, which follows incretin binding, elicits insulin release.

GLP-1 Function Overview

The insulinotropic effects of GLP-1 have been identified by several groups in both humans[16,44–46] and animal models.[37,47,48] Similar to GIP, GLP-1-induced insulin release is glucose-dependent,[46,49] such that increased insulin secretion only occurs in the presence of elevated glucose concentrations. This characteristic has been important in the development of incretin-based therapeutics, as the glucose dependence greatly reduces the risk of treatment-induced hypoglycemia. In animal experiments, treatment with a GLP-1 receptor-specific antagonist (exendin 9–39) increased both fasting and postprandial glucose concentrations and lowered insulin concentrations following an oral glucose load.[50–52] These studies also showed that GLP-1 signaling is responsible for a considerable proportion (as much as 60%) of the insulin response to an oral glucose load. Lending further support to the physiological role of GLP-1, mice with a genetic deletion of the GLP-1 receptor have diminished circulating insulin and increased plasma glucose following an oral glucose challenge.[53] In humans, administration of the GLP-1-receptor antagonist exendin 9–39 caused an approximately 35% increase in postprandial glucose,[54] suggesting that GLP-1 is essential for normal glucose tolerance. Lastly, GLP-1 has been shown to contribute to first-phase insulin secretion[55] – the robust insulin secretion that occurs during the first 10 min following glucose administration. Because first-phase insulin secretion is characteristically absent in patients with T2DM, the ability of GLP-1 to affect first-phase insulin release is an important therapeutic consideration.

In addition to glucose-dependent insulinotropic effects, GLP-1 is known to have several other important functions which affect glucoregulation. These include the following:

(1) GLP-1 suppresses the secretion of glucagon by pancreatic α-cells in a glucose-dependent manner,[41,56,57] which leads to a reduction in hepatic glucose production. This effect reinforces the insulin-induced suppression of glucagon release that occurs during the fed state, helping to regulate postprandial glucose control.

(2) GLP-1 delays gastric emptying.[58–60] Slowing nutrient entry into the gut moderates plasma glucose increases in the post-meal period. The delay in gastric emptying is thought to be mediated via GLP-1 receptors in the brain, which lead to stimulation of the parasympathetic vagus nerve.[61] In addition, GLP-1 reduces the production of gastric acid, helping to regulate digestion of stomach contents.[59,62]

(3) A number of lines of evidence suggest that GLP-1 plays a role in the central nervous system control of food intake. First, GLP-1 receptors are present in a number of brain regions implicated in the control of food intake including the hypothalamus and area postrema.[63,64] These regions lack a blood–brain barrier, permitting

GLP-1 to access the brain directly from the circulation. In rodents, direct intracerebroventricular injection of GLP-1 produced a dose-dependent reduction in food intake,[53,63–66] while repeated intracerebroventricular administration resulted in long-term reductions in food intake and body weight.[67] Conversely, administration of a GLP-1 antagonist increased food intake and resulted in weight gain.[68] GLP-1 has also been shown to reduce appetite and caloric intake in studies of healthy humans[69] and in patients with T2DM.[70] Moreover, chronic GLP-1 administration is associated with weight loss,[71] an effect which was attributed to reduced appetite in this study.

(4) Lastly, GLP-1 has been shown to have trophic effects on β-cells.[72] In animal studies, GLP-1 administration resulted in islet neogenesis, β-cell proliferation, and an increase in β-cell mass.[73–77] GLP-1 has also been shown to enhance the proliferation of new β-cells from pancreatic progenitor cells.[78–80] Finally, GLP-1 has been reported to inhibit apoptosis of β-cells.[81,82] These results suggest that GLP-1 may be beneficial in patients with T2DM by protecting existing β-cells and/or influencing proliferation of new β-cells; however, effects in humans have not been established.

Incretin-Induced Insulin Secretion: Mechanism of Action

Before considering the mechanisms of action underlying incretin-induced insulin secretion, it is important to understand the basic cellular physiology underlying glucose-induced insulin secretion in β-cells. The details of the regulation of insulin secretion by glucose are reviewed in Chapters 2 and 3 as well by other authors (for example, see review by Henquin[83]). Briefly, glucose enters β-cells via facilitated transport (Glut2 transporters[84]), where it is metabolized, and adenosine triphosphate (ATP) is generated. The ensuing increase in the intracellular ATP/adenosine diphosphate (ADP) ratio causes inhibition of ATP-sensitive potassium channels (K_{ATP}). Potassium efflux through K_{ATP} channels normally keeps the β-cell membrane polarized (negative resting voltage); thus, when K_{ATP} channels are inhibited, the cell membrane is depolarized (moves toward a neutral or positive resting voltage) in the immediate vicinity of the K_{ATP} channels. This depolarization activates voltage-dependent calcium channels (VDCCs), allowing calcium to enter the cell. Calcium entry leads to insulin secretory vesicle exocytosis and insulin release.[85] Under normal circumstances, delayed rectifier voltage-dependent potassium channels (K_V) then open, allowing potassium to leave the cell. This efflux repolarizes the cell membrane and halts the insulin release.

The cellular and molecular mechanisms by which GLP-1 and GIP elicit insulin secretion overlap considerably and include (see Fig. 4.2) the following:

(1) K_{ATP} Channel Modulation. Both GLP-1 and GIP bind to G protein-coupled receptors and activate adenylate cyclase, which catalyzes the conversion of ATP to the cellular second messenger $3'$–$5'$-cyclic adenosine monophosphate (cAMP). These initial steps begin a series of cellular actions by which GLP-1 and GIP are thought to exert insulinotropic effects. The first downstream mechanism involves modulation of K_{ATP} channels. A number of groups have shown that both GLP-1 and GIP cause closure of K_{ATP} channels.[86–90] As described above, inhibition of K_{ATP} channels facilitates membrane depolarization which induces downstream insulin release. The mechanism underlying the effect on K_{ATP} channels is thought to involve cAMP-dependent protein kinase (PKA); inhibition of PKA reverses the effects of both incretin hormones on K_{ATP} channels[86,91] (but see also Suga and colleagues[88]). Furthermore, in mouse models with a genetic mutation causing an absence of K_{ATP} channels, GLP-1- and GIP-induced insulin secretion is diminished.[92,93] These results provide further evidence that K_{ATP} channel modulation represents an important component of incretin-induced insulin secretion.

Interestingly, GLP-1 action at the K_{ATP} channel may play an important role in the glucose-dependence of GLP-1-dependent insulin secretion. In the absence of elevated glucose concentrations, GLP-1 cannot inhibit K_{ATP} channels enough to affect exocytosis. However, when GLP-1 is administered with a sulfonylurea, which directly inhibits K_{ATP} channels in a glucose-independent manner, GLP-1 dependent insulin secretion is augmented.[94,95] This effect – uncoupling the glucose dependence of GLP-1 – has consequences in GLP-1-based therapy which are detailed later in this chapter.

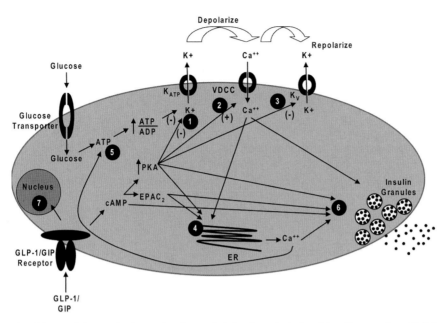

Fig. 4.2 Schematic of intracellular mechanisms of action underlying incretin-induced insulin secretion. GLP-1 receptor activation leads cAMP generation and PKA activation, leading to (1) inhibition of K_{ATP} channels, which depolarizes β-cells leading to increased excitability and downstream insulin release; (2) increased VDCC activity, leading to an increase in intracellular calcium; (3) inhibition of K_v channels, delaying repolarization and extending β-cell excitability. (4) Additional calcium is released from intracellular stores via PKA, $EPAC_2$, and calcium entry through VDCCs. (5) Intracellular calcium increases stimulate mitochondrial ATP production, increasing the ATP/ADP ratio, and leading to additional effects on K_{ATP} channels. (6) Multiple intracellular steps involving PKA, $EPAC_2$, calcium, and cAMP lead to the priming and mobilization of insulin granules for release. (7) Receptor activation leads to new insulin synthesis as well as increases in the transcription of genes involved in insulin synthesis

(2) Calcium Efflux Through VDCCs. Gromada and colleagues[89,90] have demonstrated that GLP-1 and GIP administration also increase VDCC activity, leading to increased calcium entry into β-cells and insulin exocytosis. As with K_{ATP} channel effects, PKA activation appears to underlie the effects on VDCC current changes.[89,90,96]

(3) K_v Channel Modulation. As described above, K_v channels are integral in restoring cell membrane potential following depolarization and thereby limiting calcium entry and further exocytosis of insulin-containing granules. GLP-1 receptor activation has been shown to inhibit K_v channel currents by approximately 40% in rat pancreatic β-cells.[97] GIP has been reported to have similar effects on K_v channel currents.[7] Thus, inhibiting K_v channel currents may lead to prolonged exocytosis. The effects on K_v channels appear to be dependent on PKA signaling as well as the phosphatidylinositol-3 kinase pathway.[98] In addition to effects on K_v channel currents, GIP has also been reported to affect cell surface expression and modulation of K_v channels.[99]

(4) Intracellular Calcium Stores. In addition to the direct and indirect effects that GLP-1 and GIP have on calcium entry into the cell through VDCCs, additional calcium is released from intracellular stores such as the endoplasmic reticulum (ER). This process is thought to be dependent on converging intracellular signals. For example, GLP-1-stimulated PKA[100] and cAMP-regulated guanine nucleotide exchange factor-II (Epac2, also termed cAMP-GEFII)[101] sensitize calcium channels in the ER. Intracellular calcium release is then initiated by the transient increase in calcium entering the cell through VDCCs,[101–105] the net result being a further increase in intracellular calcium as well as a wider spatial distribution of intracellular calcium. GIP has been reported to have similar effects.[7] The entire process, termed "calcium-induced calcium release," is thought to contribute to exocytosis of insulin granules located in subcellular regions not located in the immediate vicinity of the VDCCs.[7,106,107] Thus, calcium-induced calcium release may play a prominent role in the postprandial state, allowing for an even greater incretin-induced insulin secretory response.

(5) Mitochondrial ATP synthesis. In addition to stimulating exocytosis, the increase in calcium-induced intracellular calcium release described above has also been shown to affect mitochondrial ATP production.[108] Amplified ATP production may lead to further effects on K_{ATP} channels in a feed-forward manner.[107]

(6) cAMP-associated Insulin Granule Mobilization. The insulinotropic activity of GLP-1 results in part from calcium influx through VDCCs (described above). However, only a small fraction of insulin-containing granules (less than 1%[109]) belong to what is termed the "readily releasable pool,"[90,110] meaning that they are located close enough to VDCCs that they undergo exocytosis soon after VDCC opening. The remaining insulin-containing granules must be "primed" by series of cellular steps involving cAMP, calcium, and both PKA and Epac2.[90,111,112] These steps involve granule mobilization (via PKA) and increases in the size of granules (via Epac2), both processes which are influenced by GLP-1 and GIP signaling. The increased availability of insulin-containing granules for exocytosis has been estimated to account for as much as 70% of the insulinotropic activity of GLP-1 and GIP.[89,113]

(7) Insulin Biosynthesis. In addition to effecting acute changes in insulin release, both GLP-1 and GIP simulate insulin synthesis and gene transcription in β-cells.[114–116] This process ensures that adequate insulin remains available for secretion. Moreover, GLP-1 has been shown to upregulate the transcription of genes involved in insulin secretion.[117]

Incretins and Type 2 Diabetes Mellitus

It is generally accepted that two key pathophysiological defects contribute to the metabolic irregularities observed in T2DM: first, progressive β-cell dysfunction with associated insulin secretory deficits; and second, peripheral insulin resistance. Both defects play a fundamental role in the chronic progression of hyperglycemia and both are targets of therapeutic intervention. While β-cell loss – in excess of 50% on average at the time of T2DM diagnosis[118] – certainly influences insulin secretion deficits, the discovery and continued research into incretin hormones and the incretin effect has shed light on new pathways that may play a role in the progression of T2DM as well as new therapeutic options. Patients with T2DM have been shown to have a significantly reduced incretin effect.[119] Theoretically, this deficit could be caused by impaired secretion of GIP or GLP-1, accelerated metabolism of the hormones, or defective responsiveness to either.

GIP in Type 2 Diabetes

In contrast to its effects in healthy humans, the role of GIP in patients with T2DM is unclear. Decreased GIP secretion in T2DM has been reported by one group;[120] however, the majority of published studies have reported normal or even increased GIP secretion in T2DM.[121,122] Importantly, a number of groups have reported that the insulinotropic effects of GIP are lost or nearly lost in T2DM[41,123–126] (see Fig. 4.1c), even when GIP is administered at supraphysiological concentrations.[41] These results indicate that patients with T2DM have a defective responsiveness to GIP. Genetic factors may underlie this effect, as first-degree relatives of patients with T2DM have diminished GIP-induced insulin secretion compared to normal patients.[127] While a conclusive explanation regarding the loss of the insulinotropic activity of GIP in T2DM has not been determined, some evidence indicates that GIP receptor downregulation and desensitization may be responsible.[128,129]

GLP-1 in Type 2 Diabetes

Unlike GIP, GLP-1 secretion has been demonstrated to be deficient in patients with T2DM.[121,130] Whether this defect is a primary causative factor in the pathogenesis of diabetes or a secondary effect has not been conclusively determined; however, studies of identical twins in which only one twin has T2DM have demonstrated that GLP-1 secretion is impaired only in the sibling with diabetes.[131] This result suggests that GLP-1 secretion deficits are secondary to the development of T2DM.

While GLP-1 secretion is abnormal in patients with T2DM, cellular responsiveness to GLP-1 is not diminished[41] (see Fig. 4.1c). Thus, unlike with GIP, therapeutic replacement of GLP-1 holds promise for pharmacologic development. A number of proof-of-concept studies demonstrated the therapeutic potential of GLP-1 in patients with T2DM. First, GLP-1 infusion consistently has been shown to induce insulin release.[41,46] Second, GLP-1 maintained its effects on gastric emptying and glucagon release in patients with T2DM.[41,59,132] The glucoregulatory outcomes of GLP-1 infusion have also been investigated. Acute infusion studies (leading to pharmacological plasma concentrations of GLP-1) have demonstrated beneficial effects on both fasting and postprandial blood glucose concentrations.[45,46,132] Longer-term experiments have shown normalized blood glucose, improved hemoglobin A1C (A1C), and body weight loss.[71,133–136]

While early GLP-1 infusion studies conclusively demonstrated the potential for GLP-1-based therapy for T2DM, the pharmacotherapeutic value of GLP-1 is significantly limited by its rapid degradation by the enzyme DPP-4. As described earlier, the half-life of GLP-1 in circulation is approximately 2 min. As a result, the benefits of GLP-1 therapy would only be possible with continuous infusion.

Leveraging the Glucoregulatory Effects of GLP-1

In response to this important clinical challenge, the GLP-1 signaling pathway has been leveraged by two distinct pharmacologic approaches. The first approach involves utilizing peptides that have glucoregulatory effects similar to GLP-1 itself, but are resistant to degradation by DPP-4. These peptides have been termed "incretin mimetics." The second approach involves utilizing a variety of small molecules to inhibit the enzymatic activity of DPP-4, thereby increasing endogenous concentrations of GLP-1. These small molecules have been termed "DPP-4 inhibitors."

Incretin Mimetics

Exenatide

At present, exenatide is the only incretin mimetic which has been approved by the US Food and Drug Administration [FDA] and European Medicines Agency [EMEA]. Liraglutide has been approved by the EMEA, but was under review by the FDA at the time of publication of this book. The vast majority of published clinical data on incretin mimetics have focused on exenatide; consequently, the bulk of the description of incretin mimetics presented here will focus on exenatide.

Exenatide is a synthetic version of exendin-4 (not to be confused with exendin 9-39, a GLP-1 antagonist), a peptide first identified and isolated from the salivary secretions of the Gila Monster (*Heloderma suspectum*).[137] Exenatide shares approximately 50% sequence identity with human GLP-1 and binds to the mammalian GLP-1 receptor;[137–139] however, the unique amino acid sequence renders exenatide resistant to degradation from DPP-4, resulting in detectable concentrations persisting for more than 10 h in the circulation after a single subcutaneous dose.[140]

Exenatide shares many of the same glucoregulatory actions as GLP-1. In both human and animal studies, exenatide enhanced glucose-dependent insulin secretion, suppressed the inappropriate glucagon secretion seen in T2DM in a glucose-dependent manner, and slowed gastric emptying.[141–145] These effects contribute to a lowering of both fasting and postprandial glucose.[140,143] Importantly, though inappropriate glucagon secretion during hyperglycemia is suppressed by exenatide, hypoglycemia-induced glucagon secretion is unimpaired.[146] Like GLP-1, intravenous infusion of exenatide also has been shown to acutely improve β-cell function, as measured by the restoration of first- and second-phase insulin secretion in patients with T2DM following intravenous glucose administration.[147] In this study, exenatide rapidly restored normal glucose-stimulated insulin secretion in patients with T2DM. Both in vivo animal models and human clinical trials have demonstrated that exenatide reduces food intake and body weight, reproducing the effects of GLP-1 infusion in clinical studies.[145,148–150] Lastly, exenatide has been shown to promote β-cell proliferation and neogenesis in animal models.[75,80,151,152]

The safety and efficacy of exenatide have been investigated in long-term pivotal clinical trials. Patients with T2DM who were inadequately controlled with metformin and/or a sulfonylurea were treated with placebo, 5 or 10 μg exenatide twice daily (BID).[153–156] After 30 weeks of exposure to exenatide, significant changes from baseline in mean A1C and body weight were reported. Exenatide 10 μg was associated with A1C changes from baseline of approximately –1%, with average body weight changes from baseline of –2 to –3 kg.[153–156] In open-label extensions of these placebo-controlled trials, patients received 10 μg exenatide BID for up to 3 years. In the 3-year completer population, mean A1C change from baseline of –1.0% was reported,[157] demonstrating sustained glycemic control. Body weight loss was progressive, with an average change of –5.3 kg in the completer population after 3 years (see Fig. 4.3). In these open-label extension studies, improvements in several cardiovascular (CV) risk factors also were reported after 82 weeks of exenatide treatment. Plasma triglycerides (–39 mg/dl), diastolic blood pressure (–2.7 mmHg), and C-reactive protein (–44%) were all decreased, while plasma HDL cholesterol (+4.6 mg/dl) was increased.[158]

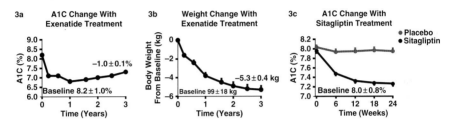

Fig. 4.3 Independent clinical trials of incretin-based therapies. (**a, b**) In a 3-year open-label extension of placebo-controlled clinical trials, exenatide treatment led to sustained improvements in A1C (**a**) and progressive weight loss (**b**). Data from Klonoff et al.[157]. (**c**) In an independent trial with a distinct study design, sitagliptin therapy led to improvements in A1C over 24 weeks. Data from Charbonnel et al.[178]. All data points, Mean ± SE, Baselines, Mean ± SD

Exenatide therapy is associated with gastrointestinal side effects. In the three large placebo-controlled trials, nausea, mostly transient, was reported by 41–45% of patients treated with exenatide, compared to approximately 18% in patients receiving placebo.[154–156,159] Most nausea were mild to moderate and declined over the duration of the trial, while severe nausea was uncommon (occurring in less than 5% of subjects).[154–156,159] Importantly, exenatide-associated reductions in body weight have been shown to be independent of nausea.[158]

Because the insulinotropic effects of the GLP-1 pathway are glucose-dependent, exenatide should not have an intrinsic risk for hypoglycemia. Indeed, the risk of hypoglycemia was not increased when exenatide was administered on a background of metformin in patients with T2DM.[155] Moreover, compared to insulin glargine and metformin, the risks of both overall and nocturnal hypoglycemia in patients with T2DM treated with exenatide and metformin were reduced despite similar improvements in A1C.[160] When exenatide was administered to patients also taking a sulfonylurea, however, the risk of mild-to-moderate hypoglycemia was increased.[154,156] This effect is not unexpected, given the aforementioned ability of sulfonylureas to uncouple the glucose-dependence of GLP-1 agonism. Hypoglycemia risk can be mitigated by decreasing the dose of sulfonylurea at the time of exenatide treatment initiation.[156]

A once weekly formulation of exenatide is currently in late-phase development. In a 15-week placebo-controlled study in patients with T2DM, a 2.0 mg/week dose ($n = 15$) exerted a potent effect on hemoglobin A1C (–1.7%) and a robust effect on weight (–3.8 kg).[161] This study suggests that once weekly exenatide may provide 24-h glycemic control with reduction in body weight. Larger long-term Phase 3 clinical trials are currently underway.

Liraglutide

Liraglutide is an acylated analog of GLP-1 currently in Phase 3 of clinical development. By binding to serum albumin, the half-life of liraglutide is increased to approximately 13 h in circulation, allowing for once-daily injections in patients with T2DM.[162] In trials published to date, liraglutide has been shown to induce glucose-dependent insulin secretion, reduce glucagon secretion, improve fasting and postprandial plasma glucose, and slow gastric emptying in patients with T2DM.[163-168] In multi-dose studies lasting 12–14 weeks, liraglutide has been reported to reduce A1C (–1.5% at highest dose) and lower body weight (–3 kg at highest dose) in patients with T2DM.[169] Adverse events have been reported to be primarily gastrointestinal in nature.[165,167,168,170]

DPP-4 Inhibitors

As described above, GLP-1 undergoes rapid degradation in the circulation by DPP-4, limiting the therapeutic potential of exogenously administered GLP-1. However, the half-life of endogenous GLP-1 ($\sim$2 min) can be increased by pharmacologically inhibiting the DPP-4 enzyme.[171] Several DPP-4 inhibitors have been developed for the treatment of patients with T2DM.[172,173] These small molecule agents inhibit the proteolytic cleavage of GLP-1 as well as a number of other peptides that are natural substrates for DPP-4 cleavage. These include GIP as well as a wide range of other peptides including chemokines, glucagon secretin family hormones, pancreatic polypeptide proteins, and neuropeptides. A membrane-bound form of DPP-4, also known as CD26, plays a role in cell signaling and is involved in immune function, ion transport, the regulation of extracellular matrix binding, and cell–cell signaling.[174] The functional effect of inhibiting cleavage of these other peptides in unclear at this time. Two DPP-4 inhibitors, sitagliptin and vildagliptin, have a substantial amount of published clinical data available, and are discussed here.

Sitagliptin

Sitagliptin is the first DPP-4 inhibitor to be approved by regulatory authorities for the treatment of T2DM. Sitagliptin treatment results in an approximately 80% inhibition of DPP-4 activity in the circulation, leading to a 2-fold increase in the plasma concentration of postprandial GLP-1 in healthy human subjects.[175] Following an oral glucose tolerance test in patients with T2DM, sitagliptin increased the active form of GLP-1, as well as insulin and C-peptide, while reducing plasma glucose and glucagon concentrations.[176] Sitagliptin has not been shown to affect gastric emptying or food intake. To date, there are no published data assessing phasic insulin secretion during treatment with DPP-4 inhibitors.

In 24-week clinical trials, patients with T2DM who were unable to achieve adequate glycemic control with metformin, glimepiride, pioglitazone, or diet and exercise experienced significant improvements in A1C (–0.7 to –0.8%, placebo corrected) and fasting plasma glucose with sitagliptin treatment[177-181] (see Fig. 4.3). Body weight was unchanged in these trials. Unlike therapy with incretin mimetics, such as exenatide, which leads to weight loss, administration of DPP-4 inhibitors are not associated with weight reductions. This difference may be explained by the relatively modest increases in postprandial GLP-1 concentrations induced by DPP-4 inhibitors compared with larger pharmacological increases in GLP-1-receptor agonism induced by incretin mimetics. Thus, the relative effect at the GLP-1 receptor may be higher following treatment with incretin mimetics. In a long-term comparator trial, sitagliptin demonstrated non-inferiority versus the sulfonylurea glipizide over 52 weeks in patients with T2DM unable to achieve adequate glycemic control with metformin alone. Sitagliptin treatment was associated with neutral effects on body weight and a lower incidence of hypoglycemia compared to glipizide treatment.[182] In the clinical development of sitagliptin, the most commonly reported adverse events were nasopharyngitis, upper respiratory tract infection, and headache.[178-180] As expected, when sitagliptin is coadministered with a sulfonylurea, the incidence of hypoglycemia is increased.[181]

Vildagliptin

Vildagliptin is a DPP-4 inhibitor in Phase 3 of clinical development. In a 12-week clinical trial in patients with T2DM who were not undergoing treatment with oral antidiabetic agents, patients treated with vildagliptin experienced improvements in hemoglobin A1C, fasting plasma glucose, 4-h postprandial plasma glucose, and insulin concentrations.[173] No significant changes in patient body weight were reported. In a 52-week clinical trial, patients with T2DM who were not achieving glycemic control with metformin alone reported improvements in glycemic control with vildagliptin treatment.[183] In a similar 24-week clinical study, vildagliptin improved hemoglobin A1C and fasting plasma glucose, in association with neutral effects on body weight.[184] When examined in a monotherapy setting, 24 weeks of vildagliptin treatment was reported to improve A1C and fasting plasma glucose, with neutral effects on body weight;[185] however, vildagliptin failed to demonstrate non-inferiority compared to metformin in this study. The most frequently reported adverse events in vildagliptin clinical studies were headache, upper respiratory tract infection, nasopharyngitis, and symptomatic mild hypoglycemia.[173,185]

Conclusion

The discovery of the incretin effect in the 1960s has led to an enhanced understanding of the importance of gut hormones in normal glucose homeostasis. Notably, the finding that the incretin effect is diminished or absent in T2DM has led to the development of several novel therapeutic options for patients with T2DM. Two distinct classes of medications – incretin mimetics and DPP-4 inhibitors – leverage the incretin pathway to improve blood glucose control. Both classes of compounds have been shown to increase insulin secretion and reduce the paradoxically elevated glucagon concentrations in patients with diabetes. Additional effects demonstrated with incretin mimetics such as exenatide include restoration of first-phase insulin response to IV glucose, slowing of gastric emptying, and reduction of food intake, often resulting in weight loss (Table 4.1). Diabetes treatments based on the multiple pharmacologic effects of incretin hormones can address the multihormonal and multifaceted nature of T2DM and help overcome the clinical barriers present with many traditional therapies.

Table 4.1   Mechanisms of action and clinical results of incretin mimetics and DPP-4 inhibitors

	Incretin mimetics	DPP-4 inhibitors
Mechanism of action		
Increase meal-stimulated insulin secretion	√	√
Restore first-phase insulin response	√	–
Suppression of inappropriate postprandial glucagon secretion	√	√
Slow gastric emptying	√	–
Reduce food intake	√	–
Clinical results		
Improved glycemic control (A1C)	√	√
Improved postprandial glucose control	√	√
Body weight reduction	√	–

References

1. Rorsman P, Renstrom E. Insulin granule dynamics in pancreatic beta cells. *Diabetologia.* 2003;46:1029–1045.
2. Rorsman P, Eliasson L, Renstrom E, Gromada J, Barg S, Gopel S. The cell physiology of biphasic insulin secretion. *News Physiol Sci.* 2000;15:72–77.
3. Perley MJ, Kipnis DM. Plasma insulin responses to oral and intravenous glucose: studies in normal and diabetic subjects. *J Clin Invest.* 1967;46:1954–1962.
4. Elrick H, Stimmler L, Hlad CJ, Arai Y. Plasma insulin responses to oral and intravenous glucose administration. *J Clin Endocrinol Metab.* 1964;24:1076–1082.
5. Nauck MA, Homberger E, Siegel EG, Allen RC, Eaton RP, Ebert R, et al. Incretin effects of increasing glucose loads in man calculated from venous insulin and C-peptide responses. *J Clin Endocrinol Metab.* 1986;63:492–498.
6. Buchan AM, Polak JM, Capella C, Solcia E, Pearse AG. Electroimmunocytochemical evidence for the K cell localization of gastric inhibitory polypeptide (GIP) in man. *Histochemistry.* 1978;56:37–44.

7. Holst JJ, Gromada J. Role of incretin hormones in the regulation of insulin secretion in diabetic and nondiabetic humans. *Am J Physiol Endocrinol Metab*. 2004;287:E199–E206.

8. Orskov C, Wettergren A, Holst JJ. Secretion of the incretin hormones glucagon-like peptide-1 and gastric inhibitory polypeptide correlates with insulin secretion in normal man throughout the day. *Scand J Gastroenterol*. 1996;31:665–670.

9. Mayo KE, Miller LJ, Bataille D, Dalle S, Goke B, Thorens B, et al. International union of pharmacology. XXXV. The glucagon receptor family. *Pharmacol Rev*. 2003;55:167–194.

10. Kieffer TJ, McIntosh CH, Pederson RA. Degradation of glucose-dependent insulinotropic polypeptide and truncated glucagon-like peptide 1 in vitro and in vivo by dipeptidyl peptidase IV. *Endocrinology*. 1995;136:3585–3596.

11. Deacon CF, Nauck MA, Meier J, Hucking K, Holst JJ. Degradation of endogenous and exogenous gastric inhibitory polypeptide in healthy and in type 2 diabetic subjects as revealed using a new assay for the intact peptide. *J Clin Endocrinol Metab*. 2000;85:3575–3581.

12. Dupre J, Ross SA, Watson D, Brown JC. Stimulation of insulin secretion by gastric inhibitory polypeptide in man. *J Clin Endocrinol Metab*. 1973;37:826–828.

13. Siegel EG, Creutzfeldt W. Stimulation of insulin release in isolated rat islets by GIP in physiological concentrations and its relation to islet cyclic AMP content. *Diabetologia*. 1985;28:857–861.

14. Pederson RA, Brown JC. Interaction of gastric inhibitory polypeptide, glucose, and arginine on insulin and glucagon secretion from the perfused rat pancreas. *Endocrinology*. 1978;103:610–615.

15. Andersen DK, Elahi D, Brown JC, Tobin JD, Andres R. Oral glucose augmentation of insulin secretion. Interactions of gastric inhibitory polypeptide with ambient glucose and insulin levels. *J Clin Invest*. 1978;62:152–161.

16. Nauck MA, Bartels E, Orskov C, Ebert R, Creutzfeldt W. Additive insulinotropic effects of exogenous synthetic human gastric inhibitory polypeptide and glucagon-like peptide-1-(7-36) amide infused at near-physiological insulinotropic hormone and glucose concentrations. *J Clin Endocrinol Metab*. 1993;76:912–917.

17. Nauck M, Schmidt WE, Ebert R, Strietzel J, Cantor P, Hoffmann G, et al. Insulinotropic properties of synthetic human gastric inhibitory polypeptide in man: interactions with glucose, phenylalanine, and cholecystokinin-8. *J Clin Endocrinol Metab*. 1989;69:654–662.

18. Vilsboll T, Krarup T, Madsbad S, Holst JJ. Both GLP-1 and GIP are insulinotropic at basal and postprandial glucose levels and contribute nearly equally to the incretin effect of a meal in healthy subjects. *Regul Pept*. 2003;114:115–121.

19. Ebert R, Creutzfeldt W. Influence of gastric inhibitory polypeptide antiserum on glucose-induced insulin secretion in rats. *Endocrinology*. 1982;111:1601–1606.

20. Lewis JT, Dayanandan B, Habener JF, Kieffer TJ. Glucose-dependent insulinotropic polypeptide confers early phase insulin release to oral glucose in rats: demonstration by a receptor antagonist. *Endocrinology*. 2000;141:3710–3716.

21. Tseng CC, Kieffer TJ, Jarboe LA, Usdin TB, Wolfe MM. Postprandial stimulation of insulin release by glucose-dependent insulinotropic polypeptide (GIP) – effect of a specific glucose-dependent insulinotropic polypeptide receptor antagonist in the rat. *J Clin Invest*. 1996;98:2440–2445.

22. Miyawaki K, Yamada Y, Yano H, Niwa H, Ban N, Ihara Y, et al. Glucose intolerance caused by a defect in the entero-insular axis: a study in gastric inhibitory polypeptide receptor knockout mice. *Proc Natl Acad Sci USA*. 1999;96:14843–14847.

23. Winter KD, Ehses JA, Eeson G, Kim S-J, Nian C, Warnock G, et al. Effects of glucose-dependent insulinotropic polypeptide on the phosphorylation of protein kinase B (PKB/AKT) and its contribution to pancreatic beta-cell survival. *J Invest Med*. 2007;55:S124.

24. Trumper A, Trumper K, Trusheim H, Arnold R, Goke B, Horsch D. Glucose-dependent insulinotropic polypeptide is a growth factor for beta (INS-1) cells by pleiotropic signaling. *Mol Endocrinol*. 2001;15:1559–1570.

25. Trumper A, Trumper K, Horsch D. Mechanisms of mitogenic and anti-apoptotic signaling by glucose-dependent insulinotropic polypeptide in beta(INS-1)-cells. *J Endocrinol*. 2002;174:233–246.

26. Ehses JA, Casilla VR, Doty T, Pospisilik JA, Winter KD, Demuth HU, et al. Glucose-dependent insulinotropic polypeptide promotes beta-(INS-1) cell survival via cyclic adenosine monophosphate-mediated caspase-3 inhibition and regulation of p38 mitogen-activated protein kinase. *Endocrinology*. 2003;144:4433–4445.

27. Usdin TB, Mezey E, Button DC, Brownstein MJ, Bonner TI. Gastric inhibitory polypeptide receptor, a member of the secretin-vasoactive intestinal peptide receptor family, is widely distributed in peripheral organs and the brain. *Endocrinology*. 1993;133:2861–2870.

28. Eckel RH, Fujimoto WY, Brunzell JD. Gastric inhibitory polypeptide enhanced lipoprotein lipase activity in cultured preadipocytes. *Diabetes*. 1979;28:1141–1142.

29. Oben J, Morgan L, Fletcher J, Marks V. Effect of the entero-pancreatic hormones, gastric inhibitory polypeptide and glucagon-like polypeptide-1(7-36) amide, on fatty acid synthesis in explants of rat adipose tissue. *J Endocrinol*. 1991;130:267–272.

30. Beck B, Max JP. Gastric inhibitory polypeptide enhancement of the insulin effect on fatty acid incorporation into adipose tissue in the rat. *Regul Pept*. 1983;7:3–8.

31. Miyawaki K, Yamada Y, Ban N, Ihara Y, Tsukiyama K, Zhou H, et al. Inhibition of gastric inhibitory polypeptide signaling prevents obesity. *Nat Med*. 2002;8:738–742.

32. Bollag RJ, Zhong Q, Phillips P, Min L, Zhong L, Cameron R, et al. Osteoblast-derived cells express functional glucose-dependent insulinotropic peptide receptors. *Endocrinology*. 2000;141:1228–1235.

33. Xie D, Cheng H, Hamrick M, Zhong Q, Ding KH, Correa D, et al. Glucose-dependent insulinotropic polypeptide receptor knockout mice have altered bone turnover. *Bone*. 2005;37:759–769.

34. Ebert R, Unger H, Creutzfeldt W. Preservation of incretin activity after removal of gastric inhibitory polypeptide (GIP) from rat gut extracts by immunoadsorption. *Diabetologia*. 1983;24:449–454.

35. Holst JJ. Enteroglucagon. *Annu Rev Physiol*. 1997;59:257–271.

36. Orskov C, Holst JJ, Poulsen SS, Kirkegaard P. Pancreatic and intestinal processing of proglucagon in man. *Diabetologia*. 1987;30:874–881.

37. Holst JJ, Orskov C, Nielsen OV, Schwartz TW. Truncated glucagon-like peptide I, an insulin-releasing hormone from the distal gut. *FEBS Lett*. 1987;211:169–174.

38. Kreymann B, Yiangou Y, Kanse S, Williams G, Ghatei MA, Bloom SR. Isolation and characterisation of GLP-1 7-36 amide from rat intestine. Elevated levels in diabetic rats. *FEBS Lett*. 1988;242:167–170.

39. Mentlein R, Gallwitz B, Schmidt WE. Dipeptidyl-peptidase IV hydrolyses gastric inhibitory polypeptide, glucagon-like peptide-1(7-36)amide, peptide histidine methionine and is responsible for their degradation in human serum. *Eur J Biochem*. 1993;214:829–835.

40. Deacon CF, Nauck MA, Toft-Nielsen M, Pridal L, Willms B, Holst JJ. Both subcutaneously and intravenously administered glucagon-like peptide I are rapidly degraded from the NH2-terminus in type II diabetic patients and in healthy subjects. *Diabetes*. 1995;44:1126–1131.

41. Nauck MA, Heimesaat MM, Orskov C, Holst JJ, Ebert R, Creutzfeldt W. Preserved incretin activity of glucagon-like peptide 1 [7-36 amide] but not of synthetic human gastric inhibitory polypeptide in patients with type-2 diabetes mellitus. *J Clin Invest*. 1993;91:301–307.

42. Fehmann HC, Göke R, Göke B. Cell and molecular biology of the incretin hormones glucagon-like peptide-I and glucose-dependent insulin releasing polypeptide. *Endocrine Rev*. 1995;16:390–410.

43. Thorens B. Expression cloning of the pancreatic cell receptor for the gluco-incretin hormone glucagon-like peptide 1. *Proc Natl Acad Sci USA*. 1992;89:8641–8645.

44. Kreymann B, Williams G, Ghatei MA, Bloom SR. Glucagon-like peptide-1 7-36: a physiological incretin in man. *Lancet*. 1987;2:1300–1304.

45. Gutniak M, Orskow C, Holst JJ, Ahrén B, Efendic S. Antidiabetogenic effect of glucagon-like peptide-1 (7-36)amide in normal subjects and patients with diabetes mellitus. *N Engl J Med*. 1992;326:1316–1322.

46. Nathan DM, Schreiber E, Fogel H, Mojsov S, Habener JF. Insulinotropic action of glucagonlike peptide-I-(7-37) in diabetic and nondiabetic subjects. *Diabetes Care*. 1992;15:270–276.

47. Mojsov S, Weir GC, Habener JF. Insulinotropin: glucagon-like peptide I (7-37) co-encoded in the glucagon gene is a potent stimulator of insulin release in the perfused rat pancreas. *J Clin Invest*. 1987;79:616–619.

48. Goke R, Wagner B, Fehmann HC, Göke B. Glucose-dependency of the insulin stimulatory effect of glucagon-like peptide-1 (7-36) amide on the rat pancreas. *Res Exp Med (Berl)*. 1993;193:97–103.

49. Qualmann C, Nauck MA, Holst JJ, Orskov C, Creutzfeldt W. Insulinotropic actions of intravenous glucagon-like peptide-1 (GLP-1) [7-36 amide] in the fasting state in healthy subjects. *Acta Diabetol*. 1995;32:13–16.

50. Kolligs F, Fehmann HC, Göke R, Göke B. Reduction of the incretin effect in rats by the glucagon-like peptide 1 receptor antagonist exendin (9-39) amide. *Diabetes*. 1995;44:16–19.

51. D'Alessio DA, Vogel R, Prigeon R, Laschansky E, Koerker D, Eng J, et al. Elimination of the action of glucagon-like peptide 1 causes an impairment of glucose tolerance after nutrient ingestion by healthy baboons. *J Clin Invest*. 1996;97:133–138.

52. Baggio L, Kieffer TJ, Drucker DJ. Glucagon-like peptide-1, but not glucose-dependent insulinotropic peptide, regulates fasting glycemia and nonenteral glucose clearance in mice. *Endocrinology*. 2000;141:3703–3709.

53. Scrocchi LA, Brown TJ, MaClusky N, Brubaker PL, Auerbach AB, Joyner AL, et al. Glucose intolerance but normal satiety in mice with a null mutation in the glucagon-like peptide 1 receptor gene. *Nat Med*. 1996;2:1254–1258.

54. Edwards CMB, Todd JF, Mahmoudi M, Wang ZL, Wang RM, Ghatei MA, et al. Glucagon-like peptide 1 has a physiological role in the control of postprandial glucose in humans – studies with the antagonist exendin 9-39. *Diabetes*. 1999;48:86–93.

55. Otonkoski T, Hayek A. Constitution of a biphasic insulin response to glucose in human fetal pancreatic beta-cells with glucagon-like peptide 1. *J Clin Endocrinol Metab*. 1995;80:3779–3783.

56. Orskov C, Holst JJ, Nielsen OV. Effect of truncated glucagon-like peptide-1 [proglucagon-(78-107) amide] on endocrine secretion from pig pancreas, antrum, and nonantral stomach. *Endocrinology*. 1988;123:2009–2013.

57. Kawai K, Suzuki S, Ohashi S, Mukai H, Ohmori H, Murayama Y, et al. Comparison of the effects of glucagon-like peptide-1-(1-37) and -(7-37) and glucagon on islet hormone release from isolated perfused canine and rat pancreases. *Endocrinology*. 1989;124:1768–1773.

58. Wettergren A, Schjoldager B, Mortensen PE, Myhre J, Christiansen J, Holst JJ. Truncated GLP-1 (proglucagon 78-107-amide) inhibits gastric and pancreatic functions in man. *Dig Dis Sci*. 1993;38:665–673.

59. Willms B, Werner J, Holst JJ, Orskov C, Creutzfeldt W, Nauck MA. Gastric emptying glucose responses, and insulin secretion after a liquid test meal: effects of exogenous glucagon-like peptide-1 (GLP-1)-(7-36) amide in type 2 (noninsulin-dependent) diabetic patients. *J Clin Endocrinol Metab*. 1996;81:327–332.

60. Young AA, Gedulin BR, Rink TJ. Dose-responses for the slowing of gastric emptying in a rodent model by glucagon-like peptide (7-36)NH2, amylin, cholecystokinin, and other possible regulators of nutrient uptake. *Metabolism*. 1996;45:1–3.

61. Imeryuz N, Yegen BC, Bozkurt A, Coskun T, Villanueva-Penacarrillo ML, Ulusoy NB. Glucagon-like peptide-1 inhibits gastric emptying via vagal afferent-mediated central mechanisms. *Am J Physiol*. 1997;273:G920–G927.

62. Schjoldager BT, Mortensen PE, Christiansen J, Orskov C, Holst JJ. GLP-1 (glucagon-like peptide 1) and truncated GLP-1, fragments of human proglucagon, inhibit gastric acid secretion in humans. *Dig Dis Sci*. 1989;34:703–708.

63. Turton MD, O'Shea D, Gunn I, Beak SA, Edwards CM, Meeran K, et al. A role for glucagon-like peptide-1 in the central regulation of feeding. *Nature*. 1996;379:69–72.

64. Shughrue PJ, Lane MV, Merchenthaler I. Glucagon-like peptide-1 receptor (GLP1-R) mRNA in the rat hypothalamus. *Endocrinology*. 1996;137:5159–5162.

65. Donahey JCK, van Dijk G, Woods SC, Seeley RJ. Intraventricular GLP-1 reduces short- but not long-term food intake or body weight in lean and obese rats. *Brain Res*. 1998;779:75–83.

66. Conlon JM, Samson WK, Dobbs RE, Orci L, Unger RH. Glucagon-like polypeptides in canine brain. *Diabetes*. 1979;28:700–702.

67. Davis HR, Mullins DE, Pines JM, Hoos LM, France CF, Compton DS, et al. Effect of chronic central administration of glucagon-like peptide-1 (7-36) amide on food consumption and body weight in normal and obese rats. *Obes Res*. 1998;6:147–156.

68. Meeran K, O'shea D, Edwards CMB, Turton MD, Heath MM, Gunn I, et al. Repeated intracerebroventricular administration of glucagon-like peptide-1-(7-36) amide or exendin-(9-39) alters body weight in the rat. *Endocrinology*. 1999;140:244–250.

69. Flint A, Raben A, Astrup A, Holst JJ. Glucagon-like peptide 1 promotes satiety and suppresses energy intake in humans. *J Clin Invest*. 1998;101:515–520.

70. Gutzwiller JP, Drewe J, Göke B, Schmidt H, Rohrer B, Lareida J, et al. Glucagon-like peptide-1 promotes satiety and reduces food intake in patients with diabetes mellitus type 2. *Am J Physiol*. 1999;45:R1541–R1544.

71. Zander M, Madsbad S, Madsen JL, Holst JJ. Effect of 6-week course of glucagon-like peptide 1 on glycaemic control, insulin sensitivity, and beta-cell function in type 2 diabetes: a parallel-group study. *Lancet*. 2002;359:824–830.

72. Egan JM, Bulotta A, Hui H, Perfetti R. GLP-1 receptor agonists are growth and differentiation factors for pancreatic islet beta cells. *Diabetes Metab Res Rev*. 2003;19:115–123.

73. Edvell A, Lindstrom P. Initiation of increased pancreatic islet growth in young normoglycemic mice (Umea +/?). *Endocrinology*. 1999;140:778–783.

74. Perfetti R, Zhou J, Doyle ME, Egan JM. Glucagon-like peptide-1 induces cell proliferation and pancreatic-duodenum homeobox-1 expression and increases endocrine cell mass in the pancreas of old, glucose-intolerant rats. *Endocrinology*. 2000;141:4600–4605.

75. Xu G, Stoffers DA, Habener JF, Bonner-Weir S. Exendin-4 stimulates both beta-cell replication and neogenesis, resulting in increased beta-cell mass and improved glucose tolerance in diabetic rats. *Diabetes*. 1999;48:2270–2276.

76. Stoffers DA, Kieffer TJ, Hussain MA, Drucker DJ, Bonner-Weir S, Habener JF, et al. Insulinotropic glucagon-like peptide 1 agonists stimulate expression of homeodomain protein IDX-1 and increase islet size in mouse pancreas. *Diabetes*. 2000;49:741–748.

77. Farilla L, Hui H, Bertolotto C, Kang E, Bulotta A, Di Mario U, et al. Glucagon-like peptide-1 promotes islet cell growth and inhibits apoptosis in zucker diabetic rats. *Endocrinology*. 2002;143:4397–4408.

78. Abraham EJ, Leech CA, Lin JC, Zulewski H, Habener JF. Insulinotropic hormone glucagon-like peptide-1 differentiation of human pancreatic islet-derived progenitor cells into insulin-producing cells. *Endocrinology*. 2002;143:3152–3161.

79. Hardikar AA, Wang XY, Williams LJ, Kwok J, Wong R, Yao M, et al. Functional maturation of fetal porcine beta-cells by glucagon-like peptide 1 and cholecystokinin. *Endocrinology*. 2002;143:3505–3514.

80. Zhou J, Wang X, Pineyro MA, Egan JM. Glucagon-like peptide 1 and exendin-4 convert pancreatic AR42J cells into glucagon- and insulin-producing cells. *Diabetes*. 1999;48:2358–2366.

81. Farilla L, Bulotta A, Hirshberg B, Li Calzi S, Khoury N, Noushmehr H, et al. GLP-1 inhibits cell apoptosis and improves glucose responsiveness of freshly isolated human islets. *Endocrinology*. 2003;144:5149–5158.

82. Li Y, Hansotia T, Yusta B, Ris F, Halban PA, Drucker DJ. Glucagon-like peptide-1 receptor signaling modulates beta cell apoptosis. *J Biol Chem*. 2003;278:471–478.

83. Henquin JC. Triggering and amplifying pathways of regulation of insulin secretion by glucose. *Diabetes*. 2000;49:1751–1760.

84. Steiner DF, James DE. Cellular and molecular biology of the beta-cell. *Diabetologia*. 1992;35:S41–S48.

85. Ashcroft FM, Proks P, Smith PA, Ammala C, Bokvist K, Rorsman P. Stimulus-secretion coupling in pancreatic beta cells. *J Cell Biochem*. 1994;55:54–65.

86. Holz GG, Kuhtreiber WM, Habener JF. Pancreatic beta-cells are rendered glucose-competent by the insulinotropic hormone glucagon-like peptide-1(7-37). *Nature*. 1993;361:362–365.

87. Light PE, Manning Fox JE, Riedel MJ, Wheeler MB. Glucagon-like peptide-1 inhibits pancreatic ATP-sensitive potassium channels via a protein kinase A- and ADP-dependent mechanism. *Mol Endocrinol*. 2002;16:2135–2144.

88. Suga S, Kanno T, Ogawa Y, Takeo T, Kamimura N, Wakui M. cAMP-independent decrease of ATP-sensitive K+ channel activity by GLP-1 in rat pancreatic beta-cells. *Pflugers Arch*. 2000;440:566–572.

89. Gromada J, Ding WG, Barg S, Renstrom E, Rorsman P. Multisite regulation of insulin secretion by cAMP-increasing agonists: evidence that glucagon-like peptide 1 and glucagon act via distinct receptors. *Pflugers Arch*. 1997;434:515–524.

90. Gromada J, Bokvist K, Ding WG, Holst JJ, Nielsen JH, Rorsman P. Glucagon-like peptide 1(7-36) amide stimulates exocytosis in human pancreatic beta-cells by both proximal and distal regulatory steps in stimulus-secretion coupling. *Diabetes*. 1998;47:57–65.

91. Ding WG, Gromada J. Protein kinase A-dependent stimulation of exocytosis in mouse pancreatic beta-cells by glucose-dependent insulinotropic polypeptide. *Diabetes*. 1997;46:615–621.

92. Nakazaki M, Crane A, Hu M, Seghers V, Ullrich S, Aguilar-Bryan L, et al. cAMP-activated protein kinase-independent potentiation of insulin secretion by cAMP is impaired in SUR1 null islets. *Diabetes*. 2002;51:3440–3449.

93. Shiota C, Larsson O, Shelton KD, Shiota M, Efanov AM, Hoy M, et al. Sulfonylurea receptor type 1 knock-out mice have intact feeding-stimulated insulin secretion despite marked impairment in their response to glucose. *J Biol Chem*. 2002;277:37176–37182.

94. de Heer J, Holst JJ. Sulfonylurea compounds uncouple the glucose dependence of the insulinotropic effect of glucagon-like peptide 1. *Diabetes*. 2007;56:438–443.

95. Gutniak MK, Juntti-Berggren L, Hellstrom PM, Guenifi A, Holst JJ, Efendic S. Glucagon-like peptide I enhances the insulinotropic effect of glibenclamide in NIDDM patients and in the perfused rat pancreas. *Diabetes Care*. 1996;19: 857–863.

96. Ammala C, Ashcroft FM, Rorsman P. Calcium-independent potentiation of insulin release by cyclic AMP in single beta-cells. *Nature*. 1993;363:356–358.

97. MacDonald PE, Salapatek AM, Wheeler MB. Glucagon-like peptide-1 receptor activation antagonizes voltage-dependent repolarizing K(+) currents in beta-cells: a possible glucose-dependent insulinotropic mechanism. *Diabetes*. 2002;51(Suppl 3):S443–S447.

98. MacDonald PE, Wang X, Xia F, El-Kholy W, Targonsky E, Tsushima RG, et al. Antagonism of rat beta-cell voltage-dependent K+ currents by exendin-4 requires dual activation of the cAMP/PKA and PI3 kinase signalling pathways. *J Biol Chem*. 2003;278:52446–52453.

99. Kim SJ, Choi WS, Han JS, Warnock G, Fedida D, McIntosh CH. A novel mechanism for the suppression of a voltage-gated potassium channel by glucose-dependent insulinotropic polypeptide: protein kinase A-dependent endocytosis. *J Biol Chem*. 2005;280:28692–28700.

100. Yada T, Itoh K, Kakei M, Tanaka H. Glucose metabolism by rat pancreatic beta-cells produces dual change in cytosolic Ca2+. *Jpn J Physiol*. 1993;43:S115–S118.

101. Kang G, Chepurny OG, Holz GG. cAMP-regulated guanine nucleotide exchange factor II (Epac2) mediates Ca2+-induced Ca2+ release in INS-1 pancreatic beta-cells. *J Physiol*. 2001;536:375–385.

102. Gromada J, Dissing S, Bokvist K, Renstrom E, Frokjaer-Jensen J, Wulff BS, et al. Glucagon-like peptide I increases cytoplasmic calcium in insulin-secreting beta TC3-cells by enhancement of intracellular calcium mobilization. *Diabetes*. 1995;44:767–774.

103. Kang G, Joseph JW, Chepurny OG, Monaco M, Wheeler MB, Bos JL, et al. Epac-selective cAMP analog 8-pCPT-2′-O-Me-cAMP as a stimulus for Ca2+-induced Ca2+ release and exocytosis in pancreatic beta-cells. *J Biol Chem*. 2003;278:8279–8285.

104. Islam MS, Leibiger I, Leibiger B, Rossi D, Sorrentino V, Ekstrom TJ, et al. In situ activation of the type 2 ryanodine receptor in pancreatic beta cells requires cAMP-dependent phosphorylation. *Proc Natl Acad Sci USA*. 1998;95: 6145–6150.

105. Liu YJ, Grapengiesser E, Gylfe E, Hellman B. Crosstalk between the cAMP and inositol trisphosphate-signalling pathways in pancreatic beta-cells. *Arch Biochem Biophys*. 1996;334:295–302.

106. Kang G, Holz GG. Amplification of exocytosis by Ca(2+)-induced Ca(2+) release in INS-1 pancreatic beta cells. *J Physiol*. 2003;546:175–189.

107. Holz G. New insights concerning the glucose-dependent insulin secretagogue action of glucagon-like peptide-1 in pancreatic beta-cells. *Horm Metab Res*. 2004;36:787–794.

108. Tsuboi T, da Silva Xavier G, Holz GG, Jouaville LS, Thomas AP, Rutter GA. Glucagon-like peptide-1 mobilizes intracellular Ca2+ and stimulates mitochondrial ATP synthesis in pancreatic MIN6 beta-cells. *Biochem J*. 2003;369:287–299.

109. Eliasson L, Renstrom E, Ding WG, Proks P, Rorsman P. Rapid ATP-dependent priming of secretory granules precedes Ca(2+)-induced exocytosis in mouse pancreatic B-cells. *J Physiol*. 1997;503(Pt 2):399–412.

110. Eliasson L, Ma X, Renstrom E, Barg S, Berggren PO, Galvanovskis J, et al. SUR1 regulates PKA-independent cAMP-induced granule priming in mouse pancreatic B-cells. *J Gen Physiol*. 2003;121:181–197.

111. Renstrom E, Eliasson L, Rorsman P. Protein kinase A-dependent and -independent stimulation of exocytosis by cAMP in mouse pancreatic B-cells. *J Physiol*. 1997;502(Pt 1):105–118.

112. Hisatomi M, Hidaka H, Niki I. Ca2+/calmodulin and cyclic 3,5′ adenosine monophosphate control movement of secretory granules through protein phosphorylation/dephosphorylation in the pancreatic beta-cell. *Endocrinology*. 1996;137: 4644–4649.

113. Gromada J, Holst JJ, Rorsman P. Cellular regulation of islet hormone secretion by the incretin hormone glucagon-like peptide 1. *Pflugers Arch Eur J Physiol*. 1998;435:583–594.

114. Fehmann HC, Habener JF. Insulinotropic hormone glucagon-like peptide-I(7-37) stimulation of proinsulin gene expression and proinsulin biosynthesis in insulinoma beta TC-1 cells. *Endocrinology*. 1992;130:159–166.

115. Drucker DJ, Philippe J, Mojsov S, Chick WL, Habener JF. Glucagon-like peptide I stimulates insulin gene expression and increases cyclic AMP levels in a rat islet cell line. *Proc Natl Acad Sci USA*. 1987;84:3434–3438.

116. Wang Y, Montrose-Rafizadeh C, Adams L, Raygada M, Nadiv O, Egan JM. GIP regulates glucose transporters, hexokinases, and glucose-induced insulin secretion in RIN 1046-38 cells. *Mol Cell Endocrinol*. 1996;116:81–87.

117. Buteau J, Roduit R, Susini S, Prentki M. Glucagon-like peptide-1 promotes DNA synthesis, activates phosphatidylinositol 3-kinase and increases transcription factor pancreatic and duodenal homeobox gene 1 (PDX-1) DNA binding activity in beta (INS-1)-cells. *Diabetologia*. 1999;42:856–864.

118. U.K. Prospective Diabetes Study Group. U.K. Prospective Diabetes Study 16. Overview of 6 years' therapy of type II diabetes: a progressive disease. U.K. Prospective Diabetes Study Group. *Diabetes*. 1995;44:1249–1258.

119. Nauck M, Stockmann F, Ebert R, Creutzfeldt W. Reduced incretin effect in type 2 (non-insulin-dependent) diabetes. *Diabetologia*. 1986;29:46–52.

120. Creutzfeldt W, Ebert R, Nauck M, Stockmann F. Disturbances of the entero-insular axis. *Scand J Gastroenterol Suppl*. 1983;82:111–119.

121. Toft-Nielsen MB, Damholt MB, Madsbad S, Hilsted LM, Hughes TE, Michelsen BK, et al. Determinants of the impaired secretion of glucagon-like peptide-1 in type 2 diabetic patients. *J Clin Endocrinol Metab*. 2001;86:3717–3723.

122. Vilsboll T, Krarup T, Deacon CF, Madsbad S, Holst JJ. Reduced postprandial concentrations of intact biologically active glucagon-like peptide 1 in type 2 diabetic patients. *Diabetes*. 2001;50:609–613.

123. Amland PF, Jorde R, Aanderud S, Burhol PG, Giercksky KE. Effects of intravenously infused porcine GIP on serum insulin, plasma C-peptide, and pancreatic polypeptide in non-insulin-dependent diabetes in the fasting state. *Scand J Gastroenterol*. 1985;20:315–320.

124. Elahi D, McAloon-Dyke M, Fukagawa NK, Meneilly GS, Sclater AL, Minaker KL, et al. The insulinotropic actions of glucose-dependent insulinotropic polypeptide (GIP) and glucagon-like peptide-1 (7-37) in normal and diabetic subjects. *Regul Pept*. 1994;51:63–74.

125. Krarup T, Saurbrey N, Moody AJ, Kuhl C, Madsbad S. Effect of porcine gastric inhibitory polypeptide on beta-cell function in type I and type II diabetes mellitus. *Metabolism*. 1987;36:677–682.

126. Jones IR, Owens DR, Moody AJ, Luzio SD, Morris T, Hayes TM. The effects of glucose-dependent insulinotropic polypeptide infused at physiological concentrations in normal subjects and type 2 (non-insulin-dependent) diabetic patients on glucose tolerance and B-cell secretion. *Diabetologia*. 1987;30:707–712.

127. Meier JJ, Hucking K, Holst JJ, Deacon CF, Schmiegel WH, Nauck MA. Reduced insulinotropic effect of gastric inhibitory polypeptide in first-degree relatives of patients with type 2 diabetes. *Diabetes*. 2001;50:2497–2504.

128. Lynn FC, Pamir N, Ng EH, McIntosh CH, Kieffer TJ, Pederson RA. Defective glucose-dependent insulinotropic polypeptide receptor expression in diabetic fatty Zucker rats. *Diabetes*. 2001;50:1004–1011.

129. Lynn FC, Thompson SA, Pospisilik JA, Ehses JA, Hinke SA, Pamir N, et al. A novel pathway for regulation of glucose-dependent insulinotropic polypeptide (GIP) receptor expression in beta cells. *FASEB J*. 2003;17:91–93.

130. Toft-Nielsen M-B, Damholt MB, Hilsted L, Hughes TE, Krarup T, Madsbad S, et al. GLP-1 secretion is decreased in NIDDM patients compared to matched control subjects with normal glucose tolerance. *Diabetologia*. 1999;42:A40.

131. Vaag AA, Holst JJ, Volund A, BeckNielsen H. Gut incretin hormones in identical twins discordant for non-insulin-dependent diabetes mellitus (NIDDM) – evidence for decreased glucagon-like peptide 1 secretion during oral glucose ingestion in NIDDM twins. *Eur J Endocrinol*. 1996;135:425–432.

132. Nauck MA, Kleine N, Orskov C, Holst JJ, Willms B, Creutzfeldt W. Normalization of fasting hyperglycaemia by exogenous glucagon-like peptide 1 (7-36 amide) in type 2 (non-insulin-dependent) diabetic patients. *Diabetologia*. 1993;36:741–744.

133. Nauck MA, Holst JJ, Willms B. Glucagon-like peptide 1 and its potential in the treatment of non-insulin-dependent diabetes mellitus. *Horm Metab Res*. 1997;29:411–416.

134. Larsen J, Hylleberg B, Ng K, Damsbo P. Glucagon-like peptide-1 infusion must be maintained for 24 h/day to obtain acceptable glycemia in type 2 diabetic patients who are poorly controlled on sulphonylurea treatment. *Diabetes Care*. 2001;24:1416–1421.

135. Todd JF, Edwards CM, Ghatei MA, Mather HM, Bloom SR. Subcutaneous glucagon-like peptide-1 improves postprandial glycaemic control over a 3-week period in patients with early type 2 diabetes. *Clin Sci (Colch)*. 1998;95:325–329.

136. Nauck MA, Wollschlager D, Werner J, Holst JJ, Orskov C, Creutzfeldt W, et al. Effects of subcutaneous glucagon-like peptide 1 (GLP-1 [7-36 amide]) in patients with NIDDM. *Diabetologia*. 1996;39:1546–1553.

137. Eng J, Kleinman WA, Singh L, Singh G, Raufman JP. Isolation and characterization of exendin-4, an exendin-3 analogue, from Heloderma suspectum venom. Further evidence for an exendin receptor on dispersed acini from guinea pig pancreas. *J Biol Chem*. 1992;267:7402–7405.

138. Goke R, Fehmann HC, Linn T, Schmidt H, Krause M, Eng J, et al. Exendin-4 is a high potency agonist and truncated exendin-(9-39)-amide an antagonist at the glucagon-like peptide 1-(7-36)-amide receptor of insulin-secreting beta-cells. *J Biol Chem*. 1993;268:19650–19655.

139. Thorens B, Porret A, Buhler L, Deng SP, Morel P, Widmann C. Cloning and functional expression of the human islet GLP-1 receptor. Demonstration that exendin-4 is an agonist and exendin-(9-39) an antagonist of the receptor. *Diabetes*. 1993;42:1678–1682.

140. Kolterman OG, Kim DD, Shen L, Ruggles JA, Nielsen LL, Fineman MS, et al. Pharmacokinetics, pharmacodynamics, and safety of exenatide in patients with type 2 diabetes mellitus. *Am J Health Syst Pharm*. 2005;62:173–181.

141. Parkes DG, Pittner R, Jodka C, Smith P, Young A. Insulinotropic actions of exendin-4 and glucagon-like peptide-1 in vivo and in vitro. *Metabolism*. 2001;50:583–589.

142. Egan JM, Clocquet AR, Elahi D. The insulinotropic effect of acute exendin-4 administered to humans: comparison of nondiabetic state to type 2 diabetes. *J Clin Endocrinol Metab*. 2002;87:1282–1290.

143. Kolterman OG, Buse JB, Fineman MS, Gaines E, Heintz S, Bicsak TA, et al. Synthetic exendin-4 (exenatide) significantly reduces postprandial and fasting plasma glucose in subjects with type 2 diabetes. *J Clin Endocrinol Metab*. 2003;88:3082–3089.

144. Gedulin B, Jodka C, Hoyt J. Exendin-4 (AC2993) decreases glucagon secretion during hyperglycemic clamps in diabetic fatty Zucker rats. *Diabetes*. 1999;48(Suppl 1):A199 (Abstract 0864).

145. Nielsen LL, Young AA, Parkes DG. Pharmacology of exenatide (synthetic exendin-4): a potential therapeutic for improved glycemic control of type 2 diabetes. *Regul Pept*. 2004;117:77–88.

146. Degn KB, Brock B, Juhl CB, Djurhuus CB, Grubert J, Kim D, et al. Effect of intravenous infusion of exenatide (synthetic exendin-4) on glucose-dependent insulin secretion and counterregulation during hypoglycemia. *Diabetes*. 2004;53:2397–2403.

147. Fehse F, Trautmann M, Holst JJ, Halseth AE, Nanayakkara N, Nielsen LL, et al. Exenatide augments first and second phase insulin secretion in response to intravenous glucose in subjects with type 2 diabetes. *J Clin Endocrinol Metab*. 2005;90:5991–5997.

148. Szayna M, Doyle ME, Betkey JA, Holloway HW, Spencer RG, Greig NH, et al. Exendin-4 decelerates food intake, weight gain, and fat deposition in Zucker rats. *Endocrinology*. 2000;141:1936–1941.

149. Young AA, Gedulin BR, Bhavsar S, Bodkin N, Jodka C, Hansen B, et al. Glucose-lowering and insulin-sensitizing actions of exendin-4: studies in obese diabetic (*ob/ob, db/db*) mice, diabetic fatty Zucker rats and diabetic rhesus monkeys (*Macaca mulatta*). *Diabetes*. 1999;48:1026–1034.

150. Bhavsar S, Watkins J, Young A. Comparison of central and peripheral effects of exendin-4 and GLP-1 on food intake in rats. Program and Abstracts: 80th Annual Meeting of the Endocrine Society; 1998:433 (Abstract P3–223).

151. Tourrel C, Bailbe D, Meile MJ, Kergoat M, Portha B. Glucagon-like peptide-1 and exendin-4 stimulate beta-cell neogenesis in streptozotocin-treated newborn rats resulting in persistently improved glucose homeostasis at adult age. *Diabetes*. 2001;50:1562–1570.

152. Tourrel C, Bailbe D, Lacorne M, Meile MJ, Kergoat M, Portha B. Persistent improvement of type 2 diabetes in the Goto-Kakizaki rat model by expansion of the beta-cell mass during the prediabetic period with glucagon-like peptide-1 or exendin-4. *Diabetes*. 2002;51:1443–1452.

153. Keating GM. Exenatide. *Drugs*. 2005;65:1681–1692.

154. Buse JB, Henry RR, Han J, Kim DD, Fineman MS, Baron AD. Effects of exenatide (exendin-4) on glycemic control over 30 weeks in sulfonylurea-treated patients with type 2 diabetes. *Diabetes Care*. 2004;27:2628–2635.

155. DeFronzo RA, Ratner RE, Han J, Kim DD, Fineman MS, Baron AD. Effects of exenatide (exendin-4) on glycemic control and weight over 30 weeks in metformin-treated patients with type 2 diabetes. *Diabetes Care*. 2005;28:1092–1100.

156. Kendall DM, Riddle MC, Rosenstock J, Zhuang D, Kim DD, Fineman MS, et al. Effects of exenatide (exendin-4) on glycemic control over 30 weeks in patients with type 2 diabetes treated with metformin and a sulfonylurea. *Diabetes Care*. 2005;28:1083–1091.

157. Klonoff DC, Buse JB, Nielsen LL, Guan X, Bowlus CL, Holcombe JH, et al. Exenatide effects on diabetes, obesity, cardiovascular risk factors and hepatic biomarkers in patients with type 2 diabetes treated for at least 3 years. *Curr Med Res Opin*. 2007;24:275–286.

158. Blonde L, Klein EJ, Han J, Zhang B, Mac SM, Poon TH, et al. Interim analysis of the effects of exenatide treatment on A1C, weight and cardiovascular risk factors over 82 weeks in 314 overweight patients with type 2 diabetes. *Diabetes Obes Metab*. 2006;8:436–447.

159. Amylin Pharmaceuticals Inc. *Byetta ® Exenatide Injection [Prescribing Information]*. San Diego, CA: Amylin Pharmaceuticals, Inc.; 2007.

160. Trautmann ME, Burger J, Johns D, Brodows R, Okerson T, Roberts A, et al. Less hypoglycemia with exenatide versus insulin glargine, despite similar HbA1C improvement, in patients with T2DM adjunctively treated with metformin. *Diabetes*. 2007;56(Suppl 1):A45 (Abstract 172-OR).

161. Kim D, MacConell L, Zhuang D, Kothare PA, Trautmann M, Fineman M, et al. Effects of once-weekly dosing of a long-acting release formulation of exenatide on glucose control and body weight in subjects with type 2 diabetes. *Diabetes Care*. 2007;30:1487–1493.

162. Agerso H, Jensen LB, Elbrond B, Rolan P, Zdravkovic M. The pharmacokinetics, pharmacodynamics, safety and tolerability of NN2211, a new long-acting GLP-1 derivative, in healthy men. *Diabetologia*. 2002;45:195–202.

163. Degn KB, Juhl CB, Sturis J, Jakobsen G, Brock B, Chandramouli V, et al. One week's treatment with the long-acting glucagon-like peptide 1 derivative liraglutide (NN2211) Markedly improves 24-h glycemia and alpha- and beta-cell function and reduces endogenous glucose release in patients with type 2 diabetes. *Diabetes*. 2004;53:1187–1194.

164. Chang AM, Jakobsen G, Sturis J, Smith MJ, Bloem CJ, An B, et al. The GLP-1 derivative NN2211 restores beta-cell sensitivity to glucose in type 2 diabetic patients after a single dose. *Diabetes*. 2003;52:1786–1791.

165. Harder H, Nielsen L, Thi TD, Astrup A. The effect of liraglutide, a long-acting glucagon-like peptide 1 derivative, on glycemic control, body composition, and 24-h energy expenditure in patients with type 2 diabetes. *Diabetes Care*. 2004;27:1915–1921.

166. Juhl CB, Hollingdal M, Sturis J, Jakobsen G, Agerso H, Veldhuis J, et al. Bedtime administration of NN2211, a long-acting GLP-1 derivative, substantially reduces fasting and postprandial glycemia in type 2 diabetes. *Diabetes*. 2002;51:424–429.

167. Madsbad S, Schmitz O, Ranstam J, Jakobsen G, Matthews DR. Improved glycemic control with no weight increase in patients with type 2 diabetes after once-daily treatment with the long-acting glucagon-like peptide 1 analog liraglutide (NN2211): a 12-week, double-blind, randomized, controlled trial. *Diabetes Care*. 2004;27:1335–1342.

168. Nauck MA, Hompesch M, Filipczak R, Le TD, Zdravkovic M, Gumprecht J. Five weeks of treatment with the GLP-1 analogue liraglutide improves glycaemic control and lowers body weight in subjects with type 2 diabetes. *Exp Clin Endocrinol Diabetes*. 2006;114:417–423.

169. Vilsboll T, Zdravkovic M, Le-Thi T, Krarup T, Schmitz O, Courreges JP, et al. Liraglutide, a long-acting human GLP-1 analog, given as monotherapy significantly improves glycemic control and lowers body weight without risk of hypoglycemia in patients with type 2 diabetes mellitus. *Diabetes Care*. 2007;30:1608–1610.

170. Feinglos MN, Saad MF, Pi-Sunyer FX, An B, Santiago O. Effects of liraglutide (NN2211), a long-acting GLP-1 analogue, on glycaemic control and bodyweight in subjects with Type 2 diabetes. *Diabetes Med*. 2005;22:1016–1023.

171. Holst JJ. Therapy of type 2 diabetes mellitus based on the actions of glucagon-like peptide-1. *Diabetes Metab Res Rev*. 2002;18:430–441.

172. Ahren B, Landin-Olsson M, Jansson PA, Svensson M, Holmes D, Schweizer A. Inhibition of dipeptidyl peptidase-4 reduces glycemia, sustains insulin levels, and reduces glucagon levels in type 2 diabetes. *J Clin Endocrinol Metab*. 2004;89:2078–2084.

173. Ristic S, Byiers S, Foley J, Holmes D. Improved glycaemic control with dipeptidyl peptidase-4 inhibition in patients with type 2 diabetes: vildagliptin (LAF237) dose response. *Diabetes Obes Metab*. 2005;7:692–698.

174. McIntosh CH, Demuth HU, Kim SJ, Pospisilik JA, Pederson RA. Applications of dipeptidyl peptidase IV inhibitors in diabetes mellitus. *Int J Biochem Cell Biol*. 2006;38:860–872.

175. Herman GA, Stevens C, Van Dyck K, Bergman A, Yi B, De Smet M, et al. Pharmacokinetics and pharmacodynamics of sitagliptin, an inhibitor of dipeptidyl peptidase IV, in healthy subjects: results from two randomized, double-blind, placebo-controlled studies with single oral doses. *Clin Pharmacol Ther*. 2005;78:675–688.

176. Herman GA, Zhao P-L, Dietrich G, Color G, Schrodter A, Keymeulen B, et al. The DPP-IV inhibitor MK-0341 enhances active GLP-1 and reduces glucose following an OGTT in type 2 diabetics. *Diabetes*. 2004;53(Suppl 2):A82 (Abstract 353-OR).

177. Aschner P, Kipnes MS, Lunceford JK, Sancez M, Mickel C, Williams-Herman D, et al. Effect of the dipeptidyl peptidase-4 inhibitor sitagliptin as monotherapy on glycemic control in patients with type 2 diabetes. *Diabetes Care*. 2006;29:2632–2637.

178. Charbonnel B, Karasik A, Liu J, Wu M, Meininger G. Sitagliptin Study 020 Group. Efficacy and safety of the dipeptidyl peptidase-4 inhibitor sitagliptin added to ongoing metformin therapy in patients with type 2 diabetes inadequately controlled with metformin alone. *Diabetes Care*. 2006;29:2638–2643.

179. Rosenstock J, Brazg R, Andryuk PJ, Lu K, Stein P. Efficacy and safety of the dipeptidyl peptidase-4 inhibitor sitagliptin added to ongoing pioglitazone therapy in patients with type 2 diabetes: a 24-week, multicenter, randomized, double-blind, placebo-controlled, parallel-group study. *Clin Ther*. 2006;28:1556–1568.

180. Goldstein B, Feinglos M, Lunceford J, Johnson J, Williams-Herman DE, for the Sitagliptin 036 Study Group*. Effect of initial combination therapy with sitagliptin, a dipeptidyl peptidase-4 inhibitor, and metformin on glycemic control in patients with type 2 diabetes. *Diabetes Care*. 2007;30:1979–1987.

181. Hermansen K, Kipnes M, Luo E, Fanurik D, Khatami H, Stein P. Efficacy and safety of the dipeptidyl peptidase-4 inhibitor, sitagliptin, in patients with type 2 diabetes mellitus inadequately controlled on glimepiride alone or on glimepiride and metformin. *Diabetes Obes Metab*. 2007;9:733–745.

182. Nauck MA, Meininger G, Sheng D, Terranella L, Stein PP, Sitagliptin Study 024 Group. Efficacy and safety of the dipeptidyl peptidase-4 inhibitor, sitagliptin, compared with the sulfonylurea, glipizide, in patients with type 2 diabetes inadequately controlled on metformin alone: a randomized, double-blind, non-inferiority trial. *Diabetes Obes Metab*. 2007;9:194–205.

183. Ahren B, Pacini G, Foley JE, Schweizer A. Improved meal-related beta-cell function and insulin sensitivity by the dipeptidyl peptidase-IV inhibitor vildagliptin in metformin-treated patients with type 2 diabetes over 1 year. *Diabetes Care*. 2005;28:1936–1940.

184. Bosi E, Camisasca RP, Collober C, Rochotte E, Garber AJ. Effects of vildagliptin on glucose control over 24 weeks in patients with type 2 diabetes inadequately controlled with metformin. *Diabetes Care*. 2007;30:890–895.

185. Pi-Sunyer FX, Schweizer A, Mills D, Dejager S. Efficacy and tolerability of vildagliptin monotherapy in drug-naive patients with type 2 diabetes. *Diabetes Res Clin Pract*. 2007;76:132–138.

Chapter 5
Cellular Mechanisms of Insulin Action

Theodore P. Ciaraldi

Introduction

Insulin is a highly pleiotropic hormone, with predominantly anabolic actions in a variety of tissues. Selectivity of final responses to insulin arises both from cell-specific expression of final effector proteins and by activation of different signaling pathways. We will consider first an overview of mechanisms of insulin action in normal human physiology, introducing the pathways, players, and principles involved, before returning to consider how these elements are modulated in type 2 diabetes. While the critical initial studies in this area were performed in animal and cell systems and later confirmed in humans, for the consideration of pathophysiology we will concentrate on the literature concerning insulin action in humans. This is intended to be an overview of the field; readers will be directed to reviews on specific topics.

Figure 5.1 presents a simplified schematic representation of the major pathways of insulin signaling. The organizing principles to note are that insulin signaling is characterized by the following features: (1) presence of phosphorylation/dephosphorylation cascades, (2) phosphorylation of specific sites creates recognition domains that permit the formation of multimolecular complexes, (3) complex formation involves scaffolding or adaptor proteins, and (4) these multimolecular complexes often target enzymes to specific intracellular locales where critical substrates reside.

Normal Physiology

The Insulin Receptor

The insulin receptor is a heterotetrameric protein consisting of two identical α-subunits and two β-subunits, linked by sulfhydryl bonds.[1] The α-subunits are totally extracellular and contain the hormone recognition domain (Fig. 5.2). The β-subunits are primarily intracellular. Most importantly, the β-subunit contains an intrinsic tyrosine kinase activity, placing the insulin receptor in the large family of receptor tyrosine kinases. The vast majority of studies indicate that this tyrosine kinase activity is essential for the normal signaling function of the insulin receptor.[2] Binding of insulin to the receptor generates a conformational change in the α-subunit that is transmitted to the β-subunit, activating the intrinsic kinase activity. The next event is ordered *trans*-phosphorylation of three tyrosine residues in the kinase regulatory region on the adjacent β-subunit (Y1146/Y1150/Y1151), further activating the kinase activity. Other tyrosines on the receptor are then phosphorylated, including Y960 in the juxtamembrane domain and Y1316/Y1322 in the C-terminus, creating recognition sites. These recognition sites permit high-affinity association with other substrates, which are subsequently tyrosine phosphorylated, propagating the phosphorylation cascade.

T.P. Ciaraldi (✉)

Department of Medicine, VA San Diego Healthcare System, University of California, San Diego, CA, USA

e-mail: tciaraldi@ucsd.edu

L. Poretsky (ed.), *Principles of Diabetes Mellitus*, DOI 10.1007/978-0-387-09841-8_5,
© Springer Science+Business Media, LLC 2010

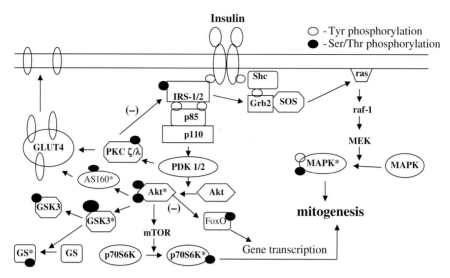

Fig. 5.1 Pathways of insulin signaling. All events initiate from the insulin receptor after hormone binding. Phosphorylation of IRS-1/2 leads to the control of both metabolism, represented by glucose uptake and glycogen synthase, and mitogenesis. The Shc/Grb2/ras/MAPK pathway regulates mitogenesis. Key: AS160, Akt substrate of 160 kDa; FoxO, Forkhead box "other"; GLUT4, glucose transporter 4; GS, glycogen synthase; GSK3, glycogen synthase kinase 3; Grb2–IRS, insulin receptor substrate; MAPK, mitogen-activated protein kinase; mTOR, mammalian target of rapamycin; PDK, phosphoinositide-dependent kinase; PKC, protein kinase C; Shc, Src homology 2/α-collagen related; SOS, son of sevenless
*Activated form of enzyme

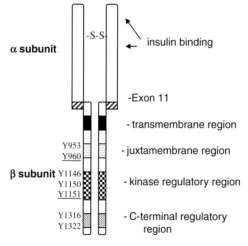

Fig. 5.2 Insulin receptor structure. Regions of differing function are indicated by *shading*. Critical potential tyrosine phosphorylation sites are identified

Insulin Receptor Substrates

Insulin receptor substrates are, by definition, molecules phosphorylated by the insulin receptor kinase. They are most often adaptor or scaffolding proteins which have no catalytic activity but, by means of multiple recognition domains, act to form multimolecular complexes, bringing enzymes and substrates into proximity or to the proper intracellular localization. Best characterized and most specific for insulin action are the insulin receptor substrates, IRSs. At least four different IRS molecules have been identified, of varying tissue distribution.[3] The common structural features of the IRS proteins are the presence of a pleckstrin homology (PH) domain, a phosphotyrosine-binding (PTB) domain, and multiple tyrosines available for phosphorylation (Fig. 5.3). IRS-1 and IRS-2 each contains 21 tyrosine residues in their COOH-terminus that are potential phosphorylation sites. Another insulin receptor substrate, Shc, lacks the PH domain and has a single tyrosine phosphorylation site.

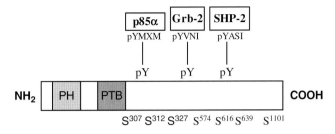

Fig. 5.3 Representative recognition domains and regulatory serine phosphorylation sites in IRS-1

These varying domains provide the means by which insulin signaling is organized and specificity is provided for substrate recognition and complex formation. The PH domain binds specific lipid products with high affinity (Table 5.1), which would target the molecule to the inner surface of the plasma membrane, bringing it into close proximity to the insulin receptor. The PTB domain recognizes the phosphotyrosine residue present in an NPXpY sequence motif, such as that formed in the juxtamembrane region of the receptor after phosphorylation of tyrosine 960 (Fig. 5.2). Association of the protein with the insulin receptor through these interactions is transitory. During this association the substrate is phosphorylated, then released to propagate the signaling cascade. The next level of specificity is provided by Src homology-2 (SH2) domains, which recognize specific amino acid motifs containing a phosphotyrosine. While there is some flexibility, the pY-SH2 association is of higher affinity than that involving the PTB domain. Beyond tyrosine phosphorylation, it is important to note that IRS-1 and IRS-2 have numerous (~70) potential serine/threonine phosphorylation sites.[4] Serine phosphorylation of IRS-1, as an example, is stimulated by a number of factors and mediated by a variety of kinases. Serine phosphorylation of IRS-1 can have a number of impacts, such as impairing the ability of IRS-1 to associate with and be tyrosine phosphorylated by the IR,[5] reducing association with phosphatidylinositol 3-kinase[6] and targeting to protoeasomal mediated degradation[7] (Table 5.2).

Table 5.1 Recognition domains important in insulin signaling

Domain	Recognition site	Present in
PH	Lipids: PIP3	IRS-1, Shc
PTB	Phosphotyrosine: NPXpY	IRS-1
SH2	Phosphotyrosine: ex, pYMXM	Grb-2, p85α
SH3	Proline-rich region: ex, PXXP	Grb-2, p85α

Phosphatidylinositol 3-Kinase

Key among the molecules that can associate with the IRS proteins is phosphatidylinositol 3'-kinase (PI 3-kinase). PI 3-kinase is a lipid kinase that phosphorylates the 3-position of the inositol ring in phosphatidylinositol. A major product is phosphatidylinositol-3',4',5'-trisphosphate ($PtIns^{3-5} P_3$), an important lipid second messenger. PI 3-kinase consists of a regulatory subunit and a catalytic subunit. As many as eight isoforms of the regulatory subunit, including alternative splicing forms, have been identified, which vary in their tissue distribution. The most ubiquitously expressed form is p85α. The regulatory subunit is not phosphorylated itself but associates with IRS proteins through its SH2 domains after IRS-1/2 phosphorylation. The SH2 domains of p85 recognize phosphotyrosines in YMXM and YXXM motifs.[17] The p110 catalytic subunit is then recruited to p85 and activated. Complex formation and kinase activation have been disturbed by a number of complementary approaches such as the use of chemical inhibitors of PI 3-kinase (e.g., wortmannin), expression of dominant-negative or interfering proteins, or reduction of the expression of endogenous proteins. The common result is that a number of insulin responses are reduced or eliminated; these include stimulation of glucose transport, antilipolysis,

Table 5.2 Regulatory serine phosphorylation of IRS-1

Site	Kinase	Impact on insulin signaling	References
Ser[307]	Akt/PKB, mTOR S6K1, JNK	↑ – initial ↓ – prolonged	Danielsson et al.[8]
Ser[312]	PKCθ	↓ – pY-IRS-1	Gao et al.[9,10] and Jiang et al.[11]
Ser[327]	GSK3	↓ – pY-IRS-1 ↓ – PI 3-K activity	Liberman and Eldar-Finkelman[12]
Ser[574]	PKCζ	↓ – PI 3-K activity	Gual et al.[4]
Ser[616]	MAPK, mTOR cPKC, PKCζ		Gao et al.[9], Gual et al.[13], and Mothe and Van Obberghen[14]
Ser[639]	MAPK, S6K1 mTOR	↓ – pY-IRS-1 ↓ – PI 3-K activity	Bouzarki et al.[6], Gual et al.[13], and Mothe and Van Obberghen[14]
Ser[1101]	PKCθ, S6K1	↓ – pY-IRS-1 ↓ – pSAkt	Li et al.[15] and Tremblay et al.[16]

Numbering for human sequence.
Key: JNK, c-jun NH_2-terminal kinase; GSK3, glycogen synthase kinase-3; MAPK, p42/44 mitogen-activated PK; S6K1, p70 ribosomal S6 kinase.

activation of glycogen synthase, and stimulation of protein and DNA synthesis, indicating that PI 3-kinase is essential for many of insulin's actions.[18]

A number of growth factors have been shown to stimulate PI 3-kinase activity yet do not generate the metabolic responses seen with insulin. For most growth factors, such as EGF, p85 can associate directly with the growth factor receptor, thus targeting PI 3-kinase to the proximity of the inner surface of the plasma membrane.[19] This association does not occur with the insulin receptor. Rather, IRS-1/2 is recruited from its primarily cytoplasmic distribution in resting cells to be phosphorylated by the insulin receptor. Binding to the receptor, mediated by the PTB domain, is weak and phosphorylated IRS-1/2 is released to intracellular membranous pools, where it complexes with the components of PI 3-kinase. In this manner insulin-stimulated PI 3-kinase is targeted to different sites than after stimulation by other growth factors, and $PtIns(3,4,5)P_3$ delivered to specific effectors.

Pathways Downstream of PI 3-Kinase

With regard to insulin action, the key effector or target of PIP3 generated by PI 3-kinase is $3'$-phosphoinositide-dependent kinase (PDK1), a serine kinase that is activated by binding of $PtIns(3,4,5)P_3$ to its C-terminal PTH domain.[20] Major substrates for PDK1 include the atypical forms of protein kinase C (aPKC), PKC ζ and λ.[21] PDK1-mediated phosphorylation of aPKCs activates these enzymes. This activation is associated with insulin stimulation of glucose transport and GLUT4 translocation[22] as well as stimulation of MAPK,[23] implicating aPKCs as important elements in insulin signaling. Besides this positive intermediary role, aPKCs can also phosphorylate IRS-1, impairing stimulation of PI 3-kinase activity[24] (Table 5.2). Thus PKC ζ/λ can participate in a negative feedback loop to limit insulin action. The classic, lipid-dependent PKC forms are also stimulated by insulin.[21] In this instance the result is negative, as classic PKCs also phosphorylate IRS-1, interfering with signaling.[25]

The other important substrate for PDK1 is yet another serine kinase, designated both Akt and protein kinase B (PKB), which exists in three isoforms. Akt contains an N-terminal PH domain (26). Activation of Akt requires both binding of $PtIns(3,4,5)P_3$ to the PH domain and phosphorylation by PDK1. Phosphorylation on two sites, Ser473 and Thr308, is required for full activation. A number of studies implicate Akt/PKB in stimulation of glucose transport,[26] while others cast doubt on the absolute requirement for Akt in that role.[21,27] It is clear that glycogen synthase kinase 3 is a direct substrate for Akt,[28] providing one pathway for insulin to stimulate glycogen synthesis.

Another direct substrate of Akt that is important in insulin signaling has been named AS160, Akt substrate of 160 kDa.[29] AS160 contains a Rab GTPase-activating protein (GAP) domain. Insulin stimulates the phosphorylation of AS160, deactivating the GAP and resulting in increased glucose transport activity (see below). Indeed,

AS160 phosphorylation appears to be required for insulin-responsive glucose transport.[29] AS160 is also phosphorylated by the AMP-activated protein kinase (AMPK), which is stimulated by muscle contractions.[30] Thus AS160 can serve to integrate the glucose transport responses to insulin and exercise.[31]

Also directly downstream of Akt is the p70 ribosomal S6 kinase (Fig. 5.1). Akt acts primarily on mammalian target of rapamycin (mTOR), which subsequently stimulates p70S6K to phosphorylate ribosomal protein S6 and accelerate translation of mRNA. p70S6K may also have some involvement in metabolic signaling, as blockade of p70S6K activation by rapamycin partially inhibits insulin action on glycogen synthesis.[32]

One means by which the PI 3-kinase/Akt pathway can regulate gene expression is through the Forkhead box "other" (FoxO) transcription factors. Akt can phosphorylate FoxO, resulting in nuclear exclusion of the protein and a reduction in transcription.[33] In the liver this results in suppression of PEPCK and other genes involved in gluconeogenesis.

Phosphatases and Insulin Signaling

Dephosphorylation events also play an important role in insulin action, either to propagate or terminate the signal. Protein tyrosine phosphatases (PTPases) of interest can be placed in two categories: membrane associated and cytoplasmic. The leukocyte antigen-related phosphatase (LAR) is an example of the membrane-associated PTPases.[34] LAR has been shown to associate with the phosphorylated insulin receptor and preferentially dephosphorylate a tyrosine in the kinase regulatory region (Y1150), reducing kinase activity.[35] Cytoplasmic phosphatases include PTP-1B and SH2-containing protein phosphatase-2 (designated as SH-PTP-2, SHP-2, or syp). PTP-1B has been shown to associate with the insulin receptor and dephosphorylate both the receptor and IRS-1, reducing association of the latter with p85 and stimulation of PI 3-kinase activity.[36] SH-PTP-2 has been shown to associate with the insulin receptor, via phosphotyrosines in the C-terminal region[37] and dephosphorylate the receptor, though IRS-1 is the preferential substrate.[38] SH-PTP-2 can also associate with Shc.

Insulin signaling through PI 3-kinase can be terminated or attenuated by lipid phosphatases.[39] The most common of these, PTEN (phosphatase and tensin homolog deleted on chromosome 10) and SHIP2 (SH2-containing inositol 5′-phosphatase), dephosphorylate the lipid mediators generated by PI 3-kinase. PTEN acts on both PtIns(3,4,5)P$_3$ and PtIns(3,4)P$_2$, removing the phosphate from the 3′-position, while SHIP2 has substrate specificity for only PtIns(3,4,5)P$_3$.

Akt itself is also subject to inactivating dephosphorylation. Two recently discovered phosphatases, PHLPP1 & PHLPP2 (PH domain leucine-rich repeat protein phosphatase), dephosphorylate Akt at Ser473.[40] Interestingly, though the two related proteins (50% amino acid identity) act on the same site in Akt, they display isoform specificity. PHLPP1 dephosphorylates Akt2 while PHLPP2 recognizes Akt1,[40] influencing different substrates downstream of Akt.

Non-PI 3-Kinase Pathways

While many of insulin's actions occur through activation of PI 3-kinase, other pathways are also employed. The best characterized is one shared with other growth factors leading to activation of members of the mitogen-activated protein kinase (MAPK) family of serine/threonine kinases. The prime mediator is Shc. Upon tyrosine phosphorylation by the insulin receptor, Shc is able to complex with another adaptor protein, Grb-2, through the SH2 domain on Grb-2. Grb-2 exists in a constitutive complex with the guanine nucleotide exchange factor son of sevenless (SOS). The Grb-2/SOS complex resides in the cytoplasm but upon binding to Shc associated with the insulin receptor is recruited to the inner surface of the plasma membrane. There SOS is brought into proximity with the membrane-localized small G protein *ras*,[41] activating *ras* and its associated phosphorylation cascade, leading to phosphorylation/activation of the p42/p44 forms of MAPK (Fig. 5.1). The MAPK pathway represents the major, though not only,[42] mechanism mediating nuclear effects of insulin on gene expression. The accumulation of evidence supports the conclusion that this pathway has no involvement in the acute metabolic responses to insulin.

Beyond these pathways, new work has revealed additional processes including: activation of heterotrimeric G proteins,[29] the cbl–CAP pathway,[43] and insulin activation of the stress-activated p38 MAP kinase.[44] As the physiologic significance of these pathways has not yet been verified in humans, they have been omitted from the current presentation.

Representative Final Responses

Glucose Transport

Glucose entry into the primary insulin target tissues (skeletal muscle, heart, adipose tissue, and liver) occurs by facilitated diffusion, mediated by a family of transport proteins. Up to 12 members of this family have been identified, designated GLUT1-12.[45] With regard to insulin action, the most important are GLUT1 and GLUT4. GLUT1 is near ubiquitous in expression and resides primarily on the cell surface. GLUT4 is present in adipose tissue and cardiac and skeletal muscles and distributed mainly in a specific population of intracellular vesicles.[46] There is a constitutive recycling of GLUT4 between the plasma membrane and intracellular vesicles. Insulin action on glucose uptake involves a multistep process: translocation of GLUT4-containing vesicles to the plasma membrane, fusion of the vesicles with the membrane, insertion of GLUT4 into the membrane, and activation of the transporters.[46] Insulin primarily accelerates the rate of GLUT4 exocytosis, though transporter endocytosis is slowed as well. The previously mentioned Akt substrate AS160 acts to constitutively retain GLUT4-containing vesicles in the cytoplasm; phosphorylation of AS160 releases this restraint, augmenting GLUT4 exocytosis. There appear to be multiple intracellular populations of GLUT4, subject to distinct control, as insulin stimulation and contraction of skeletal muscle cause loss of GLUT4 from distinct pools.[47] Considering the multiple steps involved in the glucose transport response, it is not surprising that multiple signaling pathways are also involved. That PI 3-kinase is necessary for the response is broadly accepted, but the relative importance of Akt/PKB and aPKC isoforms is still under debate. Recent evidence also suggests that PI 3-kinase is not sufficient for the full transport response and there are PI 3-kinase-independent signaling pathways involved as well.

Glycogen Synthesis

The ability of insulin to increase nonoxidative glucose utilization into muscle involves stimulation of glucose transport as well as activation of glycogen synthase (GS), the key enzyme catalyzing glycogen synthesis. Glycogen synthase activity is regulated by allosteric and covalent (phosphorylation/dephosphorylation) mechanisms.[48] While a number of kinases and phosphatases can act on GS, the most important enzymes with regard to insulin action are protein phosphatase-1 (PP1) and glycogen synthase kinase 3 (GSK3). PP1 activates GS while GSK3 deactivates the enzyme. Insulin stimulates PP1 through a PI 3-kinase-dependent mechanism.[49] The main target of insulin is the portion of PP1 activity that is localized with the glycogen particle. Insulin also removes a tonic inhibition of GS by suppressing GSK3 activity. Serine phosphorylation of GSK3 by Akt (Fig. 5.1) reduces GSK3 activity, resulting in an augmentation of the effect on PP1. The relative importance of PP1 and GSK3 in mediating insulin action on GS may vary in a tissue-specific manner.

Pathophysiology of Insulin Action in Diabetes

Each of the elements involved in the pathways leading to insulin regulation of metabolism could represent a site of possible defects in insulin-resistant states. Diabetes-related differences could arise at several levels: the presence of mutations, which influence protein turnover or activity, alterations in protein expression, or posttranslational modifications, which modify activity.

Insulin Receptor Regulation

Mutations of the insulin receptor that influence primarily intrinsic kinase activity are exceedingly rare and are usually associated with syndromes of extreme insulin resistance. In more typical cases of type 2 diabetes, a reduction in insulin receptor binding and receptor protein expression has been a common finding in skeletal muscle[50,51] and adipose tissue.[52] This downregulation of insulin receptors may be an acquired defect, resulting from hyperinsulinemia, as similar reductions were observed in obese, nondiabetic individuals.[52] More importantly, insulin receptor tyrosine kinase activity, especially toward the receptor itself, has been repeatedly shown to be impaired in tissues from diabetic subjects.[53,54] This defect in insulin-stimulated receptor autophosphorylation exists even when results are normalized to the amount of receptor protein. Thus the insulin-stimulated kinase activity of the receptor is impaired in diabetes. A possible cause for defects in receptor kinase activity could be augmented serine phosphorylation. However, in one report, phosphorylation of the serine and threonine residues most important for suppression of receptor kinase activity was normal in diabetic skeletal muscle.[55] Impaired receptor kinase activity may also be an acquired defect, as kinase activity in adipose tissue of obese diabetic subjects is improved by weight loss.[56] Under the usual conditions of hyperinsulinemia and hyperglycemia present in diabetes, it is clear that the initial events in insulin signaling, hormone recognition, and receptor kinase activation are impaired and can contribute to insulin resistance.

Insulin Receptor Substrates

A number of single nucleotide polymorphisms (SNPs) have been identified in the human IRS-1 gene.[57] One of these, G972R, displays reduced functionality when expressed in cells[58] and is associated with obesity.[59] However, the allele frequency of each of these polymorphisms is similar in nondiabetic and diabetic populations.[57,59] A polymorphism has also been identified in the human IRS-2 gene, the frequency of this polymorphism, however, is also not associated with diabetes.[60,61]

Protein expression of IRS-1 has been reported to be reduced in adipose tissue of diabetic subjects, while that of IRS-2 was normal.[62] As a result, the relative importance of IRS-2 as a docking protein for PI 3-kinase was increased. Others have found IRS-1 expression to be normal in adipose tissue.[63] Normal expression of IRS-1 in skeletal muscle of diabetic individuals has been reported by several laboratories.[64] A common observation is that insulin-stimulated tyrosine phosphorylation of IRS-1 is impaired in type 2 diabetes. This is true for both adipose tissue[65] and skeletal muscle[66,67] and the magnitude of the defect agrees with the extent of whole body insulin resistance. Thus, defects in IRS-1 phosphorylation and function appear to play an important role in insulin resistance.

Serine phosphorylation of the IRS proteins, with IRS-1 as the most studied example, is emerging as a key regulatory process.[4] Many of the kinases that phosphorylate IRS-1 (Table 5.2) are activated by pro-inflammatory cytokines such as TNF-α, IL-1, and IL-6. In one example of this process, insulin resistance resulting from the elevated circulating lipid levels characteristic of diabetes has been linked to the intracellular accumulation of lipid metabolites that can activate inhibitor kappaB kinase (IKK)[4] and PKCtheta,[68] which phosphorylate IRS-1 and reduce IRS-1 associated PI 3-kinase activity. Inhibiting IKKβ activity with high-dose aspirin therapy protects against fatty acid-induced insulin resistance in humans.[69]

Phosphatidylinositol 3-Kinase

A single polymorphism has been identified in the p110β catalytic subunit[70] that appears with the same frequency in nondiabetic and diabetic populations. A polymorphism resulting in a Met to Ile substitution at amino acid 326 in the p85α regulatory subunit has been reported by several groups.[71,72] In a population of Pima Indians the presence of this polymorphism is not associated with changes in insulin-stimulated glucose disposal, yet those expressing M326I have an impaired insulin response.[71] Individuals heterozygous for M326I appear with equal frequency in nondiabetic and diabetic populations, while those homozygous for the polymorphism do display glucose intolerance.[72]

While the importance of mutations in the components of PI 3-kinase to insulin resistance appears limited, posttranslational regulatory mechanisms are critical. Insulin-stimulated PI 3-kinase activity is reduced by ~50% in both skeletal muscle[64,66,67] and adipose tissue[65] from type 2 diabetic subjects. Impairments in PI 3-kinase activity are also seen in nondiabetic obese individuals,[73] suggesting that dis-regulation of PI 3-kinase activity may appear early in the development of insulin resistance.

Pathways Downstream of PI 3-Kinase

There is, to date, a limited literature about the influence of diabetes on signaling events downstream of PI 3-kinase. Insulin-stimulated phosphorylation and activation of Akt/PKB is reduced in adipose tissue from type 2 diabetic subjects.[65] In skeletal muscle the story is mixed; two groups report that, at physiologic insulin levels, total Akt/PKB activity is normal in diabetic subjects,[66,67] even as PI 3-kinase activity is impaired. One of these groups did find Akt/PKB activity to be reduced at supraphysiologic insulin levels.[66] Such a discrepancy, together with defects in final insulin action, highlights the importance of studying the localization and function of specific Akt isoforms. Activity of PKCθ was found to be elevated in skeletal muscle from diabetic patients.[74] Changes of this nature would be consistent with the postulate that classic PKC isoforms impede insulin action.

The only PI 3-kinase-independent pathway to be studied to date in diabetic individuals is activation of MAPK. Insulin-stimulated phosphorylation and activation of MAPK in skeletal muscle was found to be normal.[73] Retention of normal mitogenic responses in the face of hyperinsulinemia could contribute to proliferative effects involved in the development of diabetic complications.

Phosphatases

In adipose tissue PTP-1B protein expression is elevated, even as specific activity of the enzyme is reduced,[75] resulting in no net change in enzyme activity. Several groups have reported that basal PTPase activity in the particulate fraction, as well as protein expression, is reduced in diabetic muscle,[76–78] while others found activity to be elevated.[79] A common observation was that the insulin effect on PTPase activity was lost in diabetic muscle.[77,79] Further complicating understanding of the potential role of PTP1B in human diabetes is the fact that, while a number of SNPs in the PTP1B gene have been associated with type 2 diabetes[80] in some studies, other large-scale studies have failed to find such associations.[81,82] Evidence about PTEN and SHIP2 expression and activity in human tissues is lacking, but associations between certain SNPs in the genes for both proteins and type 2 diabetes have been reported in some populations[83] and not others.[84] Lastly, elevated expression of PHLPP1 has been found in cells cultured from the skeletal muscle of type 2 diabetic subjects, together with impaired insulin-stimulated phosphorylation of Akt2 on Ser473.[85]

Effectors

Glucose Transporters

A number of polymorphisms have been identified in the GLUT4 gene. None of them have been linked to or found to be associated with type 2 diabetes in a variety of populations.[86,87] Interestingly, an association found between a polymorphism in the human GLUT1 gene and that in type 2 diabetes[87] was significant for obese women. Regulation of GLUT4 protein expression in diabetes occurs in a strongly tissue-specific manner. The total cellular complement of GLUT4 is reduced by 40–50% in subcutaneous adipocytes from diabetic subjects.[88] The magnitude of this impairment is sufficient to account for the reduction in maximal insulin-stimulated adipocyte glucose transport in the same subjects. A different situation exists in skeletal muscle, where the total cellular complement of GLUT4 is the same in nondiabetic and diabetic muscle.[89] Thus, in muscle, GLUT4 content is not the determinant of muscle glucose uptake. These differences in GLUT4 expression suggest tissue-specific mechanisms for defective glucose uptake. In adipocytes it is the reduced intracellular GLUT4 pool that is responsible in large part for impaired transport, while in skeletal muscle the problem lies at the level of late steps in signal transduction or GLUT4 translocation to the cell surface. A number of laboratories, using different and complementary approaches, have verified that insulin-stimulated GLUT4 translocation is indeed impaired in diabetic muscle.[90,91] This resistance is specific to insulin signaling, for translocation in response to muscle contraction is intact in diabetes, as is the glucose transport response.[92] A candidate for the site of impaired signaling leading to GLUT4 translocation is AS160, as insulin stimulation of its phosphorylation has been reported to be impaired in skeletal muscle from type 2 diabetic subjects, even as AS160 protein expression was normal.[93]

Glycogen Synthesis

Skeletal muscle glycogen synthesis is impaired in type 2 diabetes, in both the fasting state and in response to insulin. These defects are reflected at the level of glycogen synthase activity, which is also reduced.[94] Impairments in GS activity are not due to mutations in the GS gene.[95] Expression of immunoreactive GS protein is also normal in diabetic muscle,[96] rather differences exist in the activation state of GS. While both the frequency of PPI polymorphisms and mRNA expression are normal in diabetes,[97] glycogen synthase phosphatase activity has been reported to be lower in insulin-resistant, though not necessarily diabetic, individuals.[98] On the other side of the equation, deactivation of GS, both the protein expression and total activity of GSK3 have been found to be elevated in diabetic skeletal muscle.[99] While GSK3 responds in a qualitatively normal manner to insulin with regard to both serine phosphorylation and a reduction in activity, there is still augmented activity compared to nondiabetic muscle. This diabetes-related qualitative overexpression of GSK3 could account for a large portion of the decrement in GS activity in diabetic muscle. Yet there is no apparent insulin resistance for regulation of GSK3 activity, which would be consistent with normal Ak/PKB activity in the same subjects.[67]

Summary

A highly complex system has developed to transmit insulin signals from the cell surface to metabolic and mitogenic responses. Such a multiplicity of signaling pathways provides flexibility, redundancy, and specificity. Tissue selectivity of insulin responsiveness is modulated, in large part, by the cell-specific expression of different elements of the signaling pathways or of final effectors. Despite this complexity, there are several principles in the organization of insulin signaling. These principles are (1) phosphorylation/dephosphorylation cascades initiated by the insulin receptor kinase, (2) formation of multimolecular complexes involving specific recognition domains on adapter proteins, and (3) targeting of signaling and effector molecules to appropriate intracellular locales. Impaired insulin action in type 2 diabetes most often involves defects in insulin receptor kinase and PI 3-kinase activation. It is unlikely that mutations in individual elements of insulin signaling are responsible for the majority of instances of insulin resistance. Such mutations, however, may represent susceptibility factors, reflecting the polygenic nature of diabetes.

References

1. Ottensmeyer FP, Beniac DR, Luo RZ, et al. Mechanism of transmembrane signaling: insulin binding and the insulin receptor. *Biochemistry*. 2000;39:12103–12112.
2. Ellis L, Tavare JM, Levine BA. Insulin receptor tyrosine kinase structure and function. *Biochem Soc Trans*. 1991;43:426–432.
3. Lee YH, White MF. Insulin receptor substrate proteins and diabetes. *Arch Pharm Res*. 2004;27:361–370.
4. Gual P, Le Marchand-Brustel Y, Tanti J-F. Positive and negative regulation of insulin signaling through IRS-1 phosphorylation. *Biochimie*. 2005;87:99–109.
5. Tanti J-F, Gremeaux T, Van Obberghen E, et al. Serine/threonine phosphorylation of insulin receptor substrate 1 modulates insulin receptor signaling. *J Biol Chem*. 1994;269:6051–6057.

6. Bouzarki K, Roques M, Gual P, et al. Reduced activation of phosphotidylinositol-3 kinase and increased serine 636 phosphorylation of insulin receptor substrate-1 in primary culture of skeletal muscle cells from patients with type 2 diabetes. *Diabetes*. 2003;52:1319–1325.

7. Haruta T, Uno T, Kawahara J, et al. A rapamycin-sensitive pathway down-regulates insulin signaling via phosphorylation and proteasomal degradation of insulin receptor substrate-1. *Mol Endo*. 2000;14:783–794.

8. Danielsson A, Ost A, Nystron FH, et al. Attenuation of insulin-stimulated insulin receptor substrate-1 serine 307 phosphorylation in insulin resistance of type 2 diabetes. *J Biol Chem*. 2005;280:34389–34392.

9. Gao Z, Zuberi A, Quon MJ, Dong Z, Ye J. Aspirin inhibits serine phosphorylation of insulin receptor substrate 1 in tumor necrosis factor-treated cells through targeting multiple serine kinases. *J Biol Chem*. 2003;278:24944–24950.

10. Gao Z, Hwang D, Bataille F, et al. Serine phosphorylation of insulin receptor substrate 1 by inhibitor kB kinase complex. *J Biol Chem*. 2002;277:48115–48121.

11. Jiang G, Dallas-Yang Q, Liu F, et al. Salicylic acid reverses phorbol 12-myristate-13-acetate (PMA)- and tumor necrosis factor α (TNFα)-induced insulin receptor substrate 1 (IRS1) serine 307 phosphorylation and insulin resistance in human embryonic kidney 293 (HEK293) cells. *J Biol Chem*. 2003;278:180–186.

12. Liberman Z, Eldar-Finkelman H. Serine 332 phosphorylation of insulin receptor substrate-1 by glycogen synthase kinase-3 attenuates insulin signaling. *J Biol Chem*. 2005;280:4422–4428.

13. Gual P, Gremeaux T, Gonzalez T, et al. MAP kinases and mTOR mediate insulin-induced phosphorylation of insulin receptor substrate-1 on serine residues 307, 612, and 632. *Diabetologia*. 2003;46:1532–1542.

14. Mothe I, Van Obberghen E. Phosphorylation of insulin receptor substrate-1 on multiple serine residues 612, 632, 662 and 731, modulates insulin action. *J Biol Chem*. 1996;271:11222–11227.

15. Li Y, Soos TJ, Li X, et al. Protein kinase C theta inhibits insulin signaling by phosphorylating IRS1 at Ser1001. *J Biol Chem*. 2004;279:45304–45307.

16. Tremblay F, Brule S, Um SH, et al. Identification of IRS-1 Ser-1101 as a target of S6K1 in nutrient- and obesity-induced insulin resistance. *Proc Natl Acad Sci USA*. 2007;104:14056–14061.

17. Virkamaki A, Ueki K, Kahn CR. Protein–protein interaction in insulin signaling and the molecular mechanisms of insulin resistance. *J Clin Invest*. 1999;103:931–943.

18. Shepherd PR. Mechanisms regulating phosphainositide 3-kinase signalling in insulin-sensitive tissues. *Acta Physiol Scand*. 2005;183:3–12.

19. Myers MG, White MF. Insulin signal transduction and the IRS proteins. *Annu Rev Pharmacol Toxicol*. 1996;36:615–658.

20. Alessi DR, Deak M, Casamayor A, et al. 3-Phosphoinositide-dependent protein kinase-1 (PDK1): structural and functional homology with the Drosophila DSTPK61 kinase. *Curr Biol*. 1997;7:776–789.

21. Farese RV. Insulin-sensitive phospholipid signaling systems and glucose transport. Update II. *Exp Biol Med*. 2001;226:283–295.

22. Valverde AM, Lorenzo M, Navarro P, et al. Okadiac acid inhibits insulin-induced glucose transport in fetal brown adipocytes in an Akt-independent and protein kinase C zeta-dependent manner. *FEBS Lett*. 2000;472:153–158.

23. Sajan MP, Standaert ML, Bandyopadhyay G, et al. Protein kinase C-zeta and phosphoinositide-dependent protein kinase-1 are required for insulin induced activation of ERK in rat adipocytes. *J Biol Chem*. 1999;274:30495–30500.

24. Ravichandran LV, Esposito DL, Chen J, et al. Protein kinase C-zeta phosphorylates insulin receptor substrate-1 and impairs its ability to activate phosphatidylinositol 3-kinase in response to insulin. *J Biol Chem*. 2001;276:3543–3549.

25. Kellerer M, Mushack J, Seffer E, et al. Protein kinase C isoforms alpha, delta and theta require insulin receptor substrate-1 to inhibit the tyrosine kinase activity of the insulin receptor in human kidney embryonic cells (HEK 293 cells). *Diabetologia*. 1998;41:833–838.

26. Farese RV, Sajan MP, Standaert ML. Insulin-sensitive protein kinases (atypical protein kinase C and protein kinase B/Akt: actions and defects in obesity and type II diabetes. *Exp Biol Med (Maywood)*. 2005;230:593–605.

27. Kitamura T, Ogawa W, Sakaue H, et al. Requirement for activation of the serine-threonine kinase Akt (protein kinase B) in insulin stimulation of protein synthesis but not of glucose transport. *Mol Cell Biol*. 1997;18:3708–3717.

28. Cross BAE, Alessi DR, Cohen P, et al. Inhibition of glycogen synthase kinase-3 by insulin mediated by protein kinase B. *Nature*. 1995;378:785–789.

29. Ishikura S, Koshkina A, Klip A. Small G proteins in insulin action: Rab and Rho families at the crossroads of signal transduction and GLUT4 vesicle traffic. *Acta Physiol (Oxf)*. 2008;192:61–74.

30. Musi N, Goodyear LJ. AMP-activated protein kinase and muscle glucose uptake. *Acta Physiol Scand*. 2003;178:337–345.

31. Thong FSL, Bilan PJ, Klip A. The Rab GTPase-activating protein AS160 integrates Akt, protein kinase C, and AMP-activated protein kinase signals regulating GLUT4 traffic. *Diabetes*. 2007;56:414–423.

32. Halse R, Rochford JJ, McCormack JG, et al. Control of glycogen synthesis in cultured human muscle cells. *J Biol Chem*. 1999;274:776–780.

33. Barthel A, Schmoll D, Unterman TG. FoxO proteins in insulin action and metabolism. *Trends Endocrinol Metab*. 2005;16:183–189.

34. Elchebly M, Cheng A, Tremblay ML. Modulation of insulin signaling by protein tyrosine phosphatases. *J Mol Med*. 2000;78:473–482.

35. Hashimoto N, Feener EP, Zhang W-R, et al. Insulin receptor protein-tyrosine phosphatases. *J Biol Chem*. 1992;267:13811–13814.

36. Elchebly M, Payette P, Michaliszyn E, et al. Increased insulin sensitivity and obesity resistance in mice lacking the protein tyrosine phosphatase-1B gene. *Science*. 1999;282:1544–1548.

37. Rocchi S, Tartare-Deckert S, Sawka-Verhelle D, et al. Interaction of SH2-containing protein tyrosine phosphatase 2 with the insulin receptor and the insulin-like growth factor-I receptor: studies of the domains involved using the yeast two-hybrid system. *Endocrinology*. 1996;137:4944–4952.

38. Sugimoto S, Wandless TJ, Sholeson SE, et al. Activation of the SH2-containing protein tyrosine phosphatase, SH-PTP2, by phosphotyrosine-containing peptides derived from insulin receptor substrate-1. *J Biol Chem*. 1994;269:13614–13622.

39. Lazar DF, Saltiel AR. Lipid phosphatases as drug discovery targets for type 2 diabetes. *Nat Rev Drug Disc*. 2006;5:333–342.

40. Brognard J, Sierecki E, Gao T, et al. PHLPP and a second isoform, PHLPP2, differentially attenuate the amplitude of Akt signaling by regulating distinct Akt isoforms. *Mol Cell*. 2007;25:917–931.

41. Avruch J, Khokhlatchev A, Kyriakis JM, et al. Ras activation of the Raf kinase tyrosine kinase recruitment of the MAP kinase cascade. *Rec Prog Horm Res*. 2001;56:127–155.

42. Coffer PJ, van Puijenbroek A, Burgering BM, et al. Insulin activates Stat3 independently of p21ras-ERK and PI-3 K signal transduction. *Oncogene*. 1997;15:2529–2539.

43. Saltiel AR, Pessin JE. Insulin signaling in microdomains of the plasma membrane. *Traffic*. 2003;4:711–716.

44. Michelle Furtado L, Poon V, Klip A. GLUT4 activation: thoughts on possible mechanisms. *Acta Physiol Scand*. 2006;178:287–296.

45. Scheepers A, Joost HG, Schurmann A. The glucose transporter families SGLT and GLUT: molecular basis of normal and aberrant function. *J Parenter Enteral Nutr*. 2004;28:364–371.

46. Hou JC, Pessin JE. Ins (endocytosis) and outs (exocytosis) of GLUT4 trafficking. *Curr Opin Cell Biol*. 2007;19:466–473.

47. Goodyear LG, Kahn BB. Exercise, glucose transport and insulin sensitivity. *Ann Rev Med*. 1998;49:235–261.

48. Lawrence JC, Roach PJ. New insights into the role and mechanism of glycogen synthase activation by insulin. *Diabetes*. 1997;46:541–547.

49. Brady MJ, Saltiel AR. The role of protein phosphatase-1 in insulin action. *Rec Prog Hormone Res*. 2001;56:157–173.

50. Bak J, Jacobsen U, Jorgensen F, et al. Insulin receptor function and glycogen synthase activity in skeletal muscle biopsies from the patients with insulin-dependent diabetes mellitus: Effects of physical training. *J Clin Endocrinol Metab*. 1989;69:158–164.

51. Handberg A, Vaag A, Vinten J, et al. Decreased tyrosine kinase activity in partially purified insulin receptors from muscle of young non-obese first degree relatives of patients with Type 2 (non-insulin-dependent) diabetes mellitus. *Diabetologia*. 1993;36:668–674.

52. Hunter SJ, Garvey WT. Insulin action and insulin resistance: diseases involving defects in insulin receptors, signal transduction and the glucose transport effector system. *Am J Med*. 1998;105:331–345.

53. Obermaier-Kusser B, White MF, Pongrantz DE, et al. A defective intramolecular autoactivation cascade may cause the reduced kinase activity of skeletal muscle insulin receptor from patients with non-insulin-dependent diabetes mellitus. *J Biol Chem*. 1989;264:9497–9504.

54. Freidenberg GR, Henry RR, Klein HH, et al. Decreased kinase activity of insulin receptors from adipocytes of Non-insulin-dependent diabetic subjects. *J Clin Invest*. 1987;79:240–250.

55. Kellerer M, Coghlan M, Capp E, et al. Mechanism of insulin receptor kinase inhibition in non-insulin-dependent diabetes mellitus patients. *J Clin Invest*. 1995;96:6–11.

56. Freidenberg GR, Reichart D, Olefsky JM, et al. Reversibility of defective adipocyte insulin receptor kinase activity in non-insulin-dependent diabetes mellitus. *J Clin Invest*. 1988;82:1398–1406.

57. Lei H-H, Coresh J, Shuldiner AR, et al. Variants of the insulin receptor substrate-1 and fatty acid binding protein 2 genes and the risk of type 2 diabetes, obesity, and hyperinsulinemia in African Americans. *Diabetes*. 1999;48:1868–1872.

58. Yoshimura R, Araki E, Ura S, et al. Impact of IRS-1 mutations on insulin signals. *Diabetes*. 1997;46:929–936.

59. Ura S, Araki E, Kishikawa H, et al. Molecular scanning of the insulin receptor substrate-1 (IRS-1) gene in Japanese patients with NIDDM: identification of five novel polymorphisms. *Diabetologia*. 1996;39:600–608.

60. Bernal D, Almind K, Yenush L, et al. Insulin receptor substrate-2 amino acid polymorphisms are not associated with random type 2 diabetes among caucasians. *Diabetes*. 1998;47:976–979.

61. Bektas A, Warram JH, White MF, et al. Exclusion of insulin receptor substrate 2 (IRS-2) as a major locus for early-onset autosomal dominant type 2 diabetes. *Diabetes*. 1999;48:640–642.

62. Rondinone CM, Wang L-M, Lonnroth P, et al. Insulin receptor substrate (IRS) 1 is reduced and IRS-2 is the main docking protein for phosphatidylinositol 3-kinase in adipocytes from subjects with non-insulin-dependent diabetes mellitus. *Proc Natl Acad Sci USA*. 1997;94:4171–4175.

63. Andreelli F, Laville M, Ducluzeau P-H, et al. Defective regulation of phosphatidylinositol-3-kinase gene expression in skeletal muscle and adipose tissue of non-insulin-dependent diabetes mellitus patients. *Diabetologia*. 1999;42:358–364.

64. Bjornholm M, Kawano Y, Lehtihet M, et al. Insulin receptor substrate-1 phosphorylation and phosphatidylinositol 3-kinase activity in skeletal muscle from NIDDM subjects after in vivo insulin stimulation. *Diabetes*. 1997;46:524–527.

65. Smith U, Axelsen M, Carvalho E, et al. Insulin signaling and action in fat cells: associations with insulin resistance and type 2 diabetes. *Ann NY Acad Sci*. 1999;892:119–126.

66. Krook A, Roth RA, Jiang XJ, et al. Insulin-stimulated Akt kinase activity is reduced in skeletal muscle from NIDDM subjects. *Diabetes*. 1998;47:1281–1286.

67. Kim Y-B, Nikoulina SE, Ciaraldi TP, et al. In vivo activation of Akt/Protein Kinase B (PKB) by insulin is normal in spite of decreased activation of phosphoinositide 3-kinase in skeletal muscle of humans with type 2 diabetes. *J Clin Invest.* 1999;104:733–741.

68. Griffin ME, Marcucci MJ, Cline GW, et al. Free fatty acid-induced insulin resistance is associated with activation of protein kinase C theta and alterations in the insulin signaling cascade. *Diabetes.* 1999;48:1270–1274.

69. Hundal RS, Petersen KF, Mayerson AB, et al. Mechanisms by which high-dose aspirin improves glucose metabolism in type 2 diabetes. *J Clin Invest.* 2002;109:1321–1326.

70. Kossila M, Sinkovic M, Karkkaiinen P, et al. Gene coding for the catalytic subunit p110ß of human phosphatidylinositol 3-kinase. Cloning, genomic structure, and screening for variant in patients with type 2 diabetes. *Diabetes.* 2000;49:1740–1743.

71. Hansen T, Andersen CB, Echwald SM, et al. Identification of a common amino acid polymorphism in the p85alpha regulatory subunit of the phosphatidylinositol 3-kinase: effects on glucose disappearance, glucose effectiveness, and the insulin sensitivity index. *Diabetes.* 1997;46:494–501.

72. Baier LJ, Wiedrich C, Hanson RL, et al. Variant in the regulatory subunit of phosphatidylinositol 3-kinase (p85alpha). *Diabetes.* 1998;47:973–975.

73. Cusi K, Maezono K, Osman A, et al. Insulin resistance differentially affects the PI 3-kinase- and MAP kinase-mediated signaling in human muscle. *J Clin Invest.* 2000;105:311–320.

74. Itani SI, Pories WJ, Macdonald KG, Dohm GL. Increased protein kinase C theta in skeletal muscle of diabetic patients. *Metabolism.* 2001;50:553–557.

75. Ahmad F, Considine RV, Bauer TL, et al. Improved sensitivity to insulin in obese subjects following weight loss is accompanied by reduced protein-tyrosine phosphatases in adipose tissue. *Metabolism.* 1997;46:1140–1145.

76. Cheung A, Kusari J, Jansen D, et al. Marked impairment ofm protein tyrosine phosphatase 1B activity in adipose tissue of obese subjects with and without type 2 diabetes mellitus. *J Lab Clin Med.* 1999;134:115–123.

77. Kusari J, Kenner KA, Suh K-L, et al. Skeletal muscle protein tyrosine phosphatase activity and tyrosine phosphatase 1B protein content are associated with insulin action and resistance. *J Clin Invest.* 1994;93:1156–1162.

78. Worm D, Vinten J, Staehr P, et al. Altered basal and insulin-stimulated phosphotyrosine phosphatase (PTPase) activity in skeletal muscle from NIDDM patients compared with control subjects. *Diabetologia.* 1996;39:1208–1214.

79. Ahmad F, Azevedo JL, Cortright R, et al. Alterations in skeletal muscle protein-tyrosine phosphatase activity and expression in insulin-resistant human obesity and diabetes. *J Clin Invest.* 1997;100:449–458.

80. Palmer ND, Bento JC, Mychaleckyi CD, et al. Associations of protein tyrosine phosphatase 1B gene polymorphisms with measures of glucose homeostasis in Hispanic Americans: the insulin resistance atherosclerosis study (IRAS) family study. *Diabetes.* 2004;53:3013–3019.

81. Florez JC, Agapakis CM, Burtt NP, et al. Association testing of the protein tyrosine phosphatase 1B gene (PTPN1) with type 2 diabetes in 7,883 people. *Diabetes.* 2005;54:1881–1891.

82. Meshkani R, Taghikhani M, Al-Kateb H, et al. Polymorphisms with the protein tyrosine phosphatase 1B (PTPN1) gene and promoter: functional characterization and association with type 2 diabetes and related metabolic traits. *Clin Chem.* 2007;53:1585–1592.

83. Ishihara H, Sasaoka T, Kagawa S, et al. Association of the polymorphisms in the 5′-untranslated region of PTEN gene with type 2 diabetes in a Japanese population. *FEBS Lett.* 2003;20:450–454.

84. Hansen L, Jansen JN, Ekstrom CT, et al. Studies of variability in the PTEN gene among Danish caucasian patients with Type II diabetes mellitus. *Diabetologia.* 2001;44:237–240.

85. Cozzone D, Frojdo S, Disse E, et al. Isoform-specific defects of insulin stimulation of Akt/protein kinase B (PKB) in skeletal muscle cells from type 2 diabetic patients. *Diabetologia.* 2008;51:512–521.

86. Pontiroli AE, Capra F, Vegila F, et al. Genetic contribution of polymorphism of the GLUT1 and GLUT4 genes to the susceptibility to type 2 (non-insulin-dependent) diabetes mellitus in different populations. *Acta Diabetologia.* 1996;33:193–197.

87. Lesage S, Zouali H, Vionnet N, et al. Genetic analyses of glucose transporter genes in French non-insulin-dependent diabetic families. *Diabetes Metab.* 1997;23:137–142.

88. Laybutt DR, Chisholm DJ, Kraegen EW. Specific adaptations in muscle and adipose tissue in response to chronic systemic glucose oversupply in rats. *Am J Physiol.* 1997;273:E1–E9.

89. Garvey WT, Maianu L, Huecksteadt TP, et al. Pretranslational suppression of GLUT4 glucose transporters causes insulin resistance in type II diabetes. *J Clin Invest.* 1991;87:1072–1081.

90. Garvey WT. Glucose transport and NIDDM. *Diabetes Care.* 1992;15:396–417.

91. Ryder JW, Yang J, GAluska D, et al. Use of a novel impermeable biotinylated photolabeling reagent to assess insulin- and hypoxia-stimulated cell surface GLUT4 content in skeletal muscle from type 3 diabetic patients. *Diabetes.* 2000;49:647–654.

92. Garvey WT, Maianu L, Zhu J-H, et al. Evidence for defects in the trafficking and translocation of GLUT4 glucose transporters in skeletal muscle as a cause of human insulin resistance. *J Clin Invest.* 1998;101:2377–2386.

93. Karlsson HKR, Zierath JR, Kane S, et al. Insulin-stimulated phosphorylation of the Akt substrate AS160 is impaired in skeletal muscle of type 2 diabetic subjects. *Diabetes.* 2005;54:1692–1697.

94. Thornburn AW, Gumbiner B, Bulacan F, et al. Intracellular glucose oxidation and glycogen synthase activity are reduced in non-insulin dependent (Type II) diabetes independent of impaired glucose uptake. *J Clin Invest.* 1990;85:522–529.

95. Bjorbaek C, Echwald SM, Hubricht P, et al. Genetic variants in promoters and coding regions of the muscle glycogen synthase and the insulin responsive GLUT4 genes in NIDDM. *Diabetes.* 1994;43:976–983.

96. Vestergaard H, Lund S, Larsen FS, et al. Glycogen synthase and phosphofructokinase protein and mRNA levels in skeletal muscle from insulin-resistant patients with non-insulin-dependent diabetes mellitus. *J Clin Invest*. 1993;91:2342–2350.

97. Bjorbaek C, Vik TA, Echwald SM, et al. Cloning of a human insulin-stimulated protein kinase (ISPK-1) gene and analysis of coding regions and mRNA levels of the ISPK-1 and protein phosphatase-1 genes in muscle from NIDDM patients. *Diabetes*. 1995;44:90–97.

98. Freymond D, Bogardus C, Okubo M, et al. Impaired insulin-stimulated muscle glycogen synthase activation in vivo in man is related to low fasting glycogen synthase phosphatase activity. *J Clin Invest*. 1988;82:1503–1509.

99. Nikoulina SE, Ciaraldi TP, Mudaliar S, et al. Role of glycogen synthase kinase-3 in skeletal muscle insulin resistance of type 2 diabetes. *Diabetes*. 2000;49:263–271.

Chapter 6
The Role of Brain in Glucose Metabolism

Silvana Obici and Paulo José Forcina Martins

Foreword

...Hence we could say that in a diabetic individual the liver secretes too much. The matter which produces sugar cannot be transformed into a product with a more complex organization. The dis-assimilation has become prevalent. Therefore we can consider diabetes as a disease of the nervous system caused by excessive activation of the disassimilator nerve of the liver, which drives the premature disassimilation of [glycogen, translator note] matter that would otherwise be used for nutrition. Hence the treatment of diabetes should address the nervous system. Stimulating the sympathetic nerve could be a valuable tool. But, in order to achieve a treatment with a rationale based on physiology, we should answer many questions, which are still awaiting a solution from the science of physiology.

> Claude Bernard in "Leçons sur les phénomènes de la vie". Cours de physiologies Generale du Museum d'Histoire Naturelle,[1]

Neuroendocrine Control of Glucose Homeostasis

The notion of central nervous system (CNS) control of glucose metabolism has evolved since its initial introduction in the mid-nineteenth century.[2] Claude Bernard first introduced the concept of glucose homeostasis and described a glucoregulatory system involving a brain–liver connection.[1] He observed that blood glucose levels remain surprisingly constant in the face of many physiologic conditions that could affect glucose availability and utilization. Based on his experiments on the puncture of the floor of the fourth cerebral ventricle, he argued that glucose constancy of the "milieu interieur" was regulated by the CNS via two hepatic nerves that would control glucose flux in opposite and physiologically balanced way: the "nerf assimilateur" that stimulates glucose uptake and the "nerf desassimilateur" that stimulates glucose release (Fig. 6.1). The pancreatectomy experiments of Minkwoski in the late nineteenth century and the discovery of the pancreatic hormones insulin and glucagon in the twentieth century shifted the attention to the pancreatic islets as the major site of glucoregulation, substituting neural control of glucose production and utilization to an endocrine control (glucagon and insulin).[2] Work by Shimatzu and colleagues in 1970 underscored the importance of the CNS in the control of glucose homeostasis via innervation of liver and pancreas.[3] In the past few decades, a more complex neuroendocrine model of glucoregulation is emerging (Fig. 6.1c). Several glucoregulatory hormones [including insulin, glucagon-like peptide 1 (GLP1) and some adipokines] initially believed to control glucose homeostasis via their receptors in peripheral organs can affect glucose metabolism via stimulation of their CNS receptors. In addition, circulating nutrients, including glucose and fatty acids, are directly implicated in the regulation of their homeostasis via their ability to stimulate nutrient-sensing pathways in the CNS.

S. Obici (✉)

Department of Psychiatry, Obesity Research Center, University of Cincinnati, Cincinnati, OH, 45237, USA
e-mail: silvana.obici@uc.edu

L. Poretsky (ed.), *Principles of Diabetes Mellitus*, DOI 10.1007/978-0-387-09841-8_6,
© Springer Science+Business Media, LLC 2010

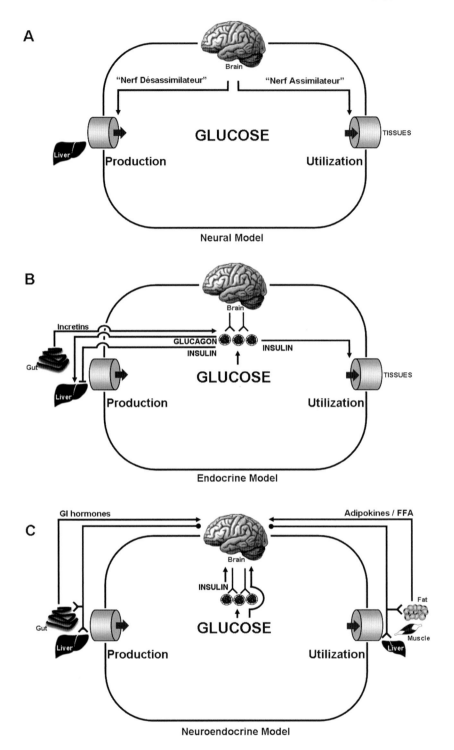

Fig. 6.1 Role of the brain in control of glucose homeostasis: schematic representation of previous and current models. (**a**) Neural model as proposed by Claude Bernard. (**b**) Endocrine (pancreatic) model. (**c**) Neuroendocrine model

This chapter will review the evidence in support of a neuroendocrine model of glucoregulation.

Hypothalamic Insulin Action and Glucose Homeostasis

Although insulin does not appear to influence CNS glucose metabolism, the brain is an insulin-sensitive organ in many respects.[4,5] There is evidence that insulin is promptly transported across the blood–brain barrier via a saturable (receptor-mediated) process and diffusion across the areas of the brain that are outside of the blood–brain barrier.[6] Moreover, insulin levels in the extracellular fluid of hypothalamic nuclei are regulated during meal absorption.[7,8] As in other cell types, the binding of insulin to its receptor triggers a signal transduction cascade initiated by the autophosphorylation of the β-subunit of the insulin receptor (Fig. 6.3) and the phosphorylation and activation of insulin receptor substrate (IRS). Two main downstream pathways of insulin signaling include activation of mitogen-activated protein (MAP) kinases (extracellular signal-regulated kinase 1 and 2 – ERK1, ERK2) and phosphatidylinositol 3-kinase (PI3K). All downstream components of the insulin signaling pathway have been identified in the hypothalamic nuclei.[9–11] The effects of insulin in the CNS include but are not limited to modulation of feeding behavior,[12–14] suppression of neuropeptide Y (NPY) expression,[14–16] hypoglycemia counterregulation,[17] and regulation of autonomic outflow.[5,18,19]

Genetic studies with neural loss of function of the insulin receptor underscore the crucial role of CNS insulin action in the modulation of energy metabolism.[20,21] Ablation of *Insr* gene in nestin-positive neurons results in obesity, hyperinsulinemia, and decreased fertility.[20] In *Caenorhabditis elegans*, the dauer phenotype caused by mutations in the *Insr* ortholog *daf-2* can be rescued by selective re-expression of *daf-2* in the brain.[22]

Hypothalamic Insulin Action Is Sufficient to Modulate Hepatic Glucose Production

Insulin lowers blood glucose by inhibiting endogenous glucose production (EGP) and increasing glucose uptake in insulin-sensitive tissues. Insulin-mediated suppression of EGP occurs via activation of the insulin receptor in hepatocytes (direct effect) and involves the modulation of both glycogen metabolism and gluconeogenesis. The activation of insulin receptors on the surface of hepatocytes leads to the activation of PI3K and serine/threonine-specific protein kinase (Akt) transduction pathway, the phosphorylation of the transcription factor forkhead box O1 (FoxO-1), and the suppression of the expression of gluconeogenic enzymes. Major transcriptional targets of insulin are the promoters of the genes for phosphoenolpyruvate carboxykinase (PEPCK) and glucose-6-phosphatase (G6Pase), rate-limiting enzymes for gluconeogenesis and glucose output, respectively. Insulin controls via direct hepatic action the rate of glycogen synthesis and glycogenolysis. In addition, insulin controls hepatic glucose metabolism by acting in extrahepatic sites (indirect effects, such as insulin-mediated suppression of lipolysis and inhibition of glucagon secretion). Recent evidence has uncovered an additional indirect effect of insulin that regulates hepatic glucose production via hypothalamic insulin action.[23] An infusion of small amounts of insulin into the third cerebral ventricle (ICV) is sufficient to inhibit glucose production, in the presence of basal plasma insulin levels. Furthermore, an infusion of a smaller dose of insulin within the parenchyma of the mediobasal hypothalamus[24] results in lower blood glucose and inhibition of hepatic glucose production. These effects are largely due to a marked inhibition of hepatic gluconeogenesis and are associated with decreases in the hepatic expression of PEPCK and G6Pase. Thus, activation of insulin signaling within the mediobasal hypothalamus is sufficient to decrease blood glucose levels via suppression of glucose production.

ATP-sensitive potassium (K_{ATP}) channels are expressed in the hypothalamus[25] and can be activated by insulin in selective hypothalamic neurons.[26,27] Studies by Pocai and colleagues show that the activation of hypothalamic K_{ATP} channels with diazoxide is sufficient to lower blood glucose levels, decrease glucose production and hepatic gluconeogenesis. In addition, like CNS insulin action, diazoxide decreases liver G6Pase and PEPCK mRNA levels. Thus, direct activation of central K_{ATP} channels is per se sufficient to recapitulate the action of hypothalamic insulin on hepatic glucose production and gluconeogenesis and on hepatic expression of G6Pase and PEPCK. Insulin-mediated activation of hypothalamic K_{ATP} channels is abolished by the K_{ATP} blockers sulfonylureas.[26,27] ICV co-administration of insulin and glibenclamide abolishes the hypothalamic effects of insulin on hepatic glucose metabolism. Thus, modulation of K_{ATP} channel activity within the arcuate nucleus of the hypothalamus can modulate neural output to the liver and control hepatic glucose metabolism.

Some hypothalamic neuronal fibers project to the brain stem and connect with motornuclei of the vagus nerve that innervates the gastrointestinal tract. These areas of the hindbrain are involved in the control of visceral functions including short-term regulation of ingestive behavior[28,29] and the modulation of liver metabolism.[30] Pocai and colleagues have shown that hypothalamic insulin action requires the activation of hepatic efferent vagal fibers because hepatic branch vagotomy abolishes the effects of ICV insulin on EGP and the expression of gluconeogenic enzymes.[24]

Hypothalamic Insulin Action Is Required to Suppress Hepatic Glucose Production

Although these studies establish the existence of a brain–liver neural connection activated by hypothalamic action of insulin, they do not demonstrate that this circuitry is required for the insulin-mediated control of glucose homeostasis. Is hypothalamic insulin action required for the physiologic suppression of glucose production induced by hyperinsulinemia? Obici and colleagues have examined this question by assessing in vivo glucose metabolism during physiologic hyperinsulinemia and simultaneous and selective blockade of insulin action in the hypothalamus.[23] Inhibition of hypothalamic insulin action was achieved in several ways: ICV infusion of anti-insulin antibodies, delivery of antisense oligonucleotides to lower insulin receptor expression, infusion of inhibitors of PI3K. Selective hypothalamic antagonism of insulin action markedly diminishes plasma insulin's ability to inhibit glucose production during hyperinsulinemic clamp procedures.[31] Additionally, ICV or intrahypothalamic infusion of a K_{ATP} blocker markedly impairs the effects of physiologic increases in plasma insulin on glucose production.[24] Similarly, hepatic branch vagotomy impairs the inhibitory effects of systemic insulin on glucose production, gluconeogenesis, and hepatic expression of G6Pase and PEPCK.

The role of K_{ATP} channels in the regulation of hepatic glucose metabolism is supported by the observation that mice with the genetic ablation of the sulfonylurea receptor subunit 1 (SUR1) display a selective impairment of glucose production and gluconeogenesis to insulin-mediated suppression.

The identity of the hypothalamic neurons and circuits responsible for insulin-dependent control of glucose production is still under investigation. Studies using antisense against the insulin receptor indicate that its down-regulation in the medial portion of the arcuate nucleus is sufficient to impair insulin action on glucose production. This area of the arcuate nucleus is enriched with NPY- and AgrP-containing neurons. Indeed, genetic and selective ablation of the insulin receptor in AgrP-positive neurons leads to impaired ability of hyperinsulinemia to suppress glucose production.[32]

Taken together, these results are consistent with a role of hypothalamic insulin action in activating a negative feedback system that controls and restrains the appearance of nutrients in the circulation (Fig. 6.2a). This hypothalamic restraint on glucose output is required for the maintenance of glucose homeostasis and its failure could lead to glucose intolerance. In addition, these experiments imply that impaired hypothalamic insulin signaling is a possible cause of hepatic insulin resistance.

The neuronal circuitry responsive to insulin plays an important role in modulating hepatic gluconeogenesis in response to physiologic elevations of plasma insulin. Since increased gluconeogenesis is a main cause of fasting and postprandial hyperglycemia in type 2 diabetes, impaired hypothalamic insulin signaling might play an important role in the pathogenesis of diabetes.[33]

This novel role of insulin, however, remains to be directly demonstrated in humans.

Hypothalamic Leptin Action

The cloning of leptin, the product of the ob (obese) gene, in the early 1990s has renewed the interest in the relationship between brain and control of energy balance and metabolism. Although the notion that the

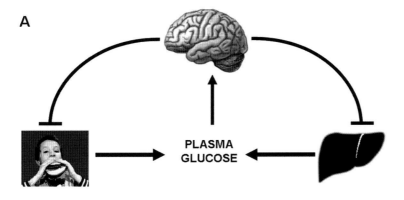

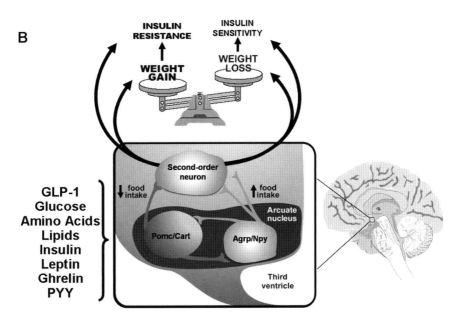

Fig. 6.2 CNS control of the glucose and energy homeostasis. (**a**) The brain senses circulating levels of glucose and nutrients and responds to their fluctuations by modifying the availability of exogenous fuel (feeding behavior) or endogenous fuel (hepatic production). (**b**) Specialized arcuate neurons receive and integrate a variety of peripheral humoral signals that are proportional to fat mass and/or nutritional state. This information is relayed to second-order neurons and used to maintain the homeostasis of energy stores by coordinated changes in food intake and energy expenditure. CNS control of glucose homeostasis may occur through two major mechanisms: (1) alterations in energy balance and body composition occur primarily and result in changes in insulin sensitivity and (2) glucose homeostasis and insulin sensitivity are modulated independently of changes in fat mass or body composition

hypothalamus is a major control center for energy homeostasis was previously well established, the discovery that leptin acts in the hypothalamus to regulate food intake and energy expenditure has greatly advanced our understanding of the neuroendocrine control of energy metabolism.[28] A major target of leptin action in the hypothalamus is the modulation of hypothalamic neuropeptidergic neurons. Leptin can reduce food intake and increase energy expenditure by simultaneously downregulating "orexic" peptides [that promote food intake and energy efficiency, such as neuropeptide Y (NPY), melanocyte-concentrating hormone, MCH, and orexins] and increasing the expression of anorectic peptides (such as the α-melanocyte-stimulating hormone, α-MSH, and corticotrophin releasing hormone, CRH). Two populations of neurons in the arcuate nucleus of the hypothalamus are highly responsive to leptin (Fig. 6.2b). One of these populations responds to leptin by increasing the expression of proopiomelanocortin (POMC), the precursor of α-MSH. The other population of neurons responds to leptin by markedly decreasing the expression of NPY and the agouti-related protein (AgRP). The latter is a natural antagonist of the melanocortin pathway acting on the MC4 (and MC3) receptors.[34,35] The peptide α-MSH is the natural ligand for the CNS melanocortin receptors (MC3 and MC4). The MC4 receptor is expressed in the hypothalamus and has been convincingly implicated in the regulation of energy homeostasis.[36] In particular, genetic knockout of the MC4 receptor gene and ICV administration of agonists and antagonists for this receptor result in dramatic effects on feeding behavior and energy balance.[19-39] Since obesity is tightly associated with insulin resistance, hypothalamic leptin action plays a major role in carbohydrate metabolism and insulin action.[40-43] For example, rodents with a genetic deficiency of leptin function, such as the ob/ob and db/db mice, and the Zucker fa/fa rats, are markedly resistant to insulin action and develop diabetes mellitus later in life. Prolonged leptin administration in leptin-deficient ob/ob mice markedly decreases both plasma insulin and glucose concentration.[44,45] Administration of leptin to ob/ob mice at doses insufficient to induce weight loss rapidly normalizes blood glucose levels, suggesting that leptin has insulin-sensitizing effects independent of its anorectic action.[46] Leptin was also shown to regulate glucose tolerance, insulin signaling/action, and lipid metabolism independently of its anorectic effects.[41,47-52]

Leptin regulates food intake and body adiposity partly via activation of melanocortin receptors in the hypothalamus and in other areas within the central nervous system.[29,45] Bidirectional modulation of central melanocortin action leads to significant changes in peripheral insulin action.[39] On the other hand, the prolonged administration of either leptin or melanocortin agonists or antagonists also impacts on the distribution of body adiposity and on lipid homeostasis.[44,45] The loss of adiposity is likely to influence insulin action, since it is well established that changes in fat mass and/or fat distribution similar to those associated with long-term treatment with either leptin or melanocortin agonists can alter insulin action, particularly in insulin-resistant and obese animals. Thus, short-term administration studies, in the absence of changes in fat mass, might provide a glimpse on the direct role of hypothalamic leptin in the modulation of glucose metabolism.

Leptin appears to exert its pleiotropic behavioral, metabolic, and neuroendocrine actions via multiple neural pathways. What pathways are responsible for the action of CNS leptin on glucose metabolism? Leptin activates central melanocortin receptors mainly via increased biosynthesis of the physiological ligand α-MSH and via decreased biosynthesis of an antagonist agouti-related protein (AgRP) at the level of the hypothalamus.[34] The activation of the central melanocortin pathway mediates in great part leptin action on food intake, energy expenditure, sympathetic nervous system, insulin secretion, and body fat distribution.[40,49,53-55] The acute central activation of melanocortin receptors stimulates the expression of gluconeogenic enzymes within the liver, markedly increases the rate of gluconeogenesis, and decreases the suppressive effect of insulin on glucose production.[43] These rapid metabolic effects of the CNS melanocortin pathway on liver metabolism are completely different from the insulin-sensitizing effects obtained by prolonged stimulation of the CNS melanocortin receptors.[39] In fact, a week-long infusion of α-MSH leads to decreased visceral adiposity and improved insulin action.[39] Similarly, genetic ablation of the MC4 receptor results in hyperphagia, obesity, hyperinsulinemia, glucose intolerance, or diabetes.[38] The contrast between acute and chronic effects of central melanocortin modulation is likely due to the dramatic effects of this pathway on body fat mass and distribution, lipid oxidation and storage, and sympathetic nervous system activity. Acutely, the activation of the melanocortin pathway in the CNS is likely to enhance autonomic outflow to peripheral organs in the absence of changes in visceral adiposity and lipid storage.[38,39] In the liver, an increase in adrenergic tone leads to increased expression of G6Pase and PEPCK and to increased fat oxidation, which in turn can drive up gluconeogenesis.

The effects of leptin on hepatic glucose fluxes appear to be more complex than those of α-MSH. In lean, postabsorptive rats, short-term leptin infusion does not alter systemic insulin action on glucose production or utilization. However, systemic or ICV leptin induces a remarkable redistribution of intrahepatic glucose fluxes, greatly increasing the contribution of gluconeogenesis and simultaneously decreasing the contribution of glycogenolysis to hepatic glucose output.[41,48] Co-administration of a melanocortin receptor antagonist and leptin blunts the stimulatory effect on gluconeogenesis and inhibits the rate of glycogenolysis, consequently enhancing the insulin-mediated inhibition of glucose production.[43] These experiments indicate that hypothalamic leptin action acutely controls gluconeogenic fluxes via the activation of hypothalamic melanocortin receptors. However, when central melanocortin action is blocked, CNS leptin action leads to a marked enhancement of hepatic insulin sensitivity.

The neural mechanisms responsible for leptin amelioration of hepatic insulin sensitivity are still largely unknown. Leptin binding to the long isoform of its receptor activates the Janus kinase-signal transducer–activator of transcription 3 (JAK/STAT3) pathway. This transduction pathway is linked to obesity, because transgenic mice carrying a point mutation of the leptin receptor abolishing JAK2/STAT3 activation are obese and hyperphagic. However, its role in modulating glucose homeostasis is still under investigation. In addition, like insulin, leptin can activate and exert its anorectic action via the PI3K pathway.[56,57] Since the effect of ICV insulin on hepatic glucose production requires central activation of PI3K,[31] the melanocortin-independent action of leptin on hepatic insulin sensitivity might be mediated by its activation of PI3K in neurons.

NPY and insulin action. Neuropeptide Y (NPY) is a potent orexigenic peptide, widely distributed in the mammalian brain and co-expressed in AgRP-positive neurons, whereby it is strongly downregulated by insulin and leptin. Injection of NPY into the hypothalamus or cerebral ventricles has potent and rapid effects on whole body metabolism.[58–60] Leptin and insulin may modulate feeding behavior and glucose homeostasis at least in part by suppressing the release and expression of NPY in the arcuate nucleus. Intracerebroventricular (ICV) injection of NPY decreases hepatic insulin sensitivity.[61] A recent study shows that ICV infusion of NPY impairs hepatic insulin sensitivity via modulation of liver sympathetic innervation.[62]

Hypothalamic Nutrient Sensing

There is a growing body of evidence indicating that circulating nutrients are sensed in the brain and directly participate in the homeostatic control of energy balance and peripheral metabolism. The hypothalamic arcuate nucleus is a regulatory site whereby lipids, glucose, and amino acids levels and their flux are sensed as integrated with other neural and hormonal signals to regulate food intake and energy metabolism. In particular, we will discuss the role of CNS lipid and glucose sensing vis à vis the regulation of hepatic glucose metabolism.

Lipids

The accumulation of lipids in adipose tissue, the site of long-term energy stores, is highly regulated by the brain via the coordinated regulation of feeding behavior (energy intake) and energy expenditure. The "lipostatic hypothesis" maintains that peripheral signals proportional to the size of fat mass communicate energy status to brain centers that in turn regulate energy intake and expenditure.[28,63] Leptin and insulin are classical examples of peripheral signals of energy store size because their plasma levels are proportional to adiposity and they act in the CNS to decrease energy intake.[45,63–65] Recent evidence supports the notion that the lipostatic hypothesis may include CNS control of circulating energy in the form of macronutrients such as fatty acids and glucose. Increased levels of plasma glucose and lipids can stimulate secretion and biosynthesis of insulin and leptin. These signals of adiposity and nutrient availability in turn reach hypothalamic centers and induce rapid shifts in metabolic fluxes of peripheral tissues such as liver and skeletal muscle.[41,52] In addition, hypothalamic neurons are also capable of directly sensing the levels of circulating nutrients.[23,66] The administration of oleic acid in the third cerebral ventricle results in the inhibition of food intake and endogenous glucose production.[31] The CNS effect of oleic acid, a long-chain fatty acid (18 carbons), is not elicited by delivery of medium-chain fatty acids such as octanoic acid (8 carbons). This suggests that the mere availability of macronutrients for oxidation to ATP is not a sufficient signal to the brain for regulation of energy metabolism. Although the brain largely relies on glucose for energy supply, lipids are oxidized in the CNS in small quantities. Studies with radiotracer techniques have shown that, although up to 50% of fatty acids delivered to the whole brain are oxidized to acetate, the bulk of palmitate and oleate incorporated into brain lipids is derived from circulating FAs and not from newly synthesized long-chain fatty acid-coenzyme A (LCFA-CoA).[67] Fatty acids are transported from the circulation to the brain and into cells (Fig. 6.3), converted into LCFA-CoAs, and further metabolized in oxidative (β-oxidation in mitochondria) or biosynthetic pathways (incorporation in phospholipids). Neuronal lipid metabolism has recently been implicated in the control of energy intake and metabolism as a neuronal biochemical sensor of energy flux. Inhibitors of fatty acid synthase have potent anorexic effects mediated via CNS mechanisms.[68] The effect of FAS inhibitors on food intake requires the accumulation of malonyl-CoA, a product of glucose metabolism and potent allosteric inhibitor of carnitine palmitoyltransferase 1 (CPT1). This enzyme is the first committed step for the transport of LCFA-CoAs into mitochondria, where they undergo β-oxidation (Fig. 6.3). In peripheral tissues (liver and muscle), malonyl-CoA has been identified as a fuel sensor that controls the rate of fatty acid oxidation and consequently determines the intracellular levels of LCFA-CoAs.[16,69] Recent evidence suggests that a similar biochemical sensor operates in the brain, and in particular in the hypothalamus.[70] Accumulation of malonyl-CoA by inhibition of fatty acid synthase (FAS) leads to anorexia,[68] whereas lowering malonyl-CoA by overexpression of malonyl-CoA decarboxylase (MCD) causes hyperphagia.[71,72] In addition, MCD overexpression in arcuate prevents the accumulation of arcuate LCFAs and prevents LCFA-mediated inhibition of glucose production.[71] As predicted by the physiologic role of malonyl-CoA as inhibitor of CPT1 and fatty acid oxidation, inhibition of hypothalamic CPT1 increases neuronal levels of LCFA-CoAs and results in anorexia and inhibition of endogenous glucose production.[73] In physiologic conditions, the levels of malonyl-CoA in the hypothalamus vary according to nutritional status, being low in the fasting state and high during refeeding.[74] Taken together, these experiments suggest that peripheral circulating macronutrients (LCFAs and carbohydrates) may represent signals of nutrient availability and activate a neural "lipid-sensing" signal of negative feedback on feeding behavior and glucose production to restrain circulating nutrients from "exogenous" (food) or "endogenous" sources (liver-derived glucose/lipids).

Hypothalamic lipid sensing modulates hepatic glucose fluxes via a neural circuit involving efferent vagal innervation (Fig. 6.3c). The suppression of glucose production elicited by central inhibition of fatty acid oxidation (via CPT1 inhibition) is abolished by selective hepatic vagotomy, whereas vagal deafferentation has no effect.[75]

Hypothalamic sensing of circulating LCFA and hepatic glucose production. CNS delivery of oleic acid results in decreased plasma glucose levels, hepatic glucose production, and expression of hepatic G6Pase.[76,23] These effects are apparently paradoxical because elevated plasma LCFAs are known to increase hepatic glucose production and expression of G6Pase.[77] Indeed, elevated plasma LCFAs in the presence of hyperinsulinemia markedly decrease insulin inhibitory action on glucose production. However, in some circumstances, circulating FFAs do not increase glucose production. In the presence of basal insulin levels, the elevation of plasma LCFA concentration via lipid infusions stimulates gluconeogenesis but does not alter glucose production in nondiabetic humans and animals because of a compensatory decrease in hepatic glycogenolysis.[77] This rapid metabolic adaptation is called hepatic autoregulation. Lam and colleagues have shown that plasma FFA-induced hepatic autoregulation is disrupted when hypothalamic FFA uptake and action are prevented or follow hepatic vagotomy.[78] Thus,

---

Fig. 6.3 (continued) Hypothalamic control of hepatic glucose metabolism. (**a**) Insulin controls hepatic glucose production in part via the activation of its receptors in the arcuate nucleus of the hypothalamus (see text). (**b**) Effects of hypothalamic leptin action on hepatic glucose fluxes. Leptin receptors in the arcuate activate two major distinct signaling pathways: Jak/STAT and IRS/PI3K. Leptin action in the arcuate leads to stimulation of proopiomelanocortin (POMC) neurons and inhibition of NPY/AgRP neurons. The direct and acute effects of CNS leptin action on heptic glucose fluxes can be classified into melanocortin dependent (activation of hepatic gluconeogenesis) and melanocortin independent (decreased glycogenolysis). (**c**) Hypothalamic lipid sensing and brain–liver connection. Circulating LCFAs can alter glucose metabolism by direct action on liver or via an indirect neural circuit. In the hypothalamus, LCFAs are esterified to LCFA-CoAs. Elevation of LCFA-CoAs in the arcuate nucleus results in the opening of K_{ATP} channels and the stimulation of the vagal efferent fibers. These motor neurons originate in the vagal nucleus of the brain stem (NTS/DMX) and innervate the liver. The accumulation of LCFA-CoAs is controlled by the levels of malonyl-CoA, a glucose-derived precursor of fatty acids and potent allosteric inhibitor of CPT1. Increased levels of malonyl-CoA inhibit CPT1 activity, decrease LCFA-CoA oxidation, and increase cytoplasmic LCFA-CoAs levels. This in turn activates a neural hepatic signal for the suppression of glucose production. BBB, blood–brain barrier

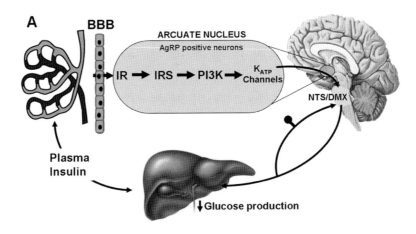

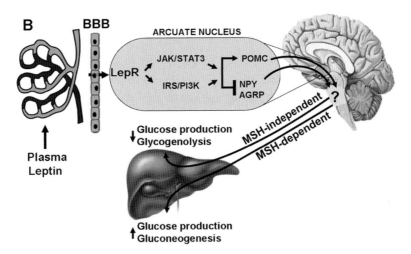

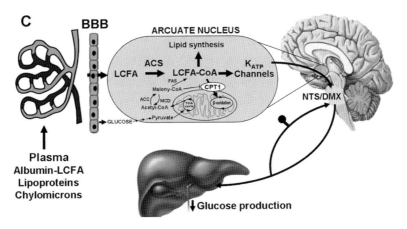

Fig. 6.3 (continued)

circulating LCFAs can alter hepatic glucose production via hepatic and extrahepatic mechanisms. The latter include the stimulation of hypothalamic circuits traveling along the efferent branch of the vagus nerve. Since CNS action of circulating LCFA is required to counteract LCFA-induced stimulation of gluconeogenesis and to prevent an increase in glucose production, FFA-induced hepatic autoregulation might result from the simultaneous activation of hepatic and hypothalamic signals. Interestingly, hypothalamic overexpression of MCD results in the inability to accumulate LCFA-CoA in the arcuate nucleus during peripheral infusion of lipid and in the disruption of FFA-induced hepatic autoregulation.[71] Similarly, hepatic autoregulation is impaired in type 2 diabetes since reciprocal changes in glycogenolysis fail to compensate for changes in gluconeogenesis when the plasma LCFA concentrations are experimentally manipulated.[79]

Glucose

Mayer's "glucostatic" hypothesis postulated the existence of peripheral and neuronal glucose sensors involved in the homeostatic control of energy balance and metabolism.[80] Indeed specialized neurons can alter their firing frequency and membrane potential in response to changes in extracellular glucose levels. Glucose sensing is an essential component of the CNS defense against hypoglycemia and hyperglycemia that triggers counterregulatory responses and attempts to restore normoglycemia. Homeostatic control seemingly operates in the physiologic range of blood glucose ($\sim$5 mM), which is in equilibrium with glucose concentration in the extracellular space in brain ($\sim$2 mM). Lam and colleagues have shown that moderate increases in glucose levels within the hypothalamus lower blood glucose via the inhibition of hepatic glucose production.[81] Furthermore, the restraining effect of CNS glucose on hepatic fluxes requires its conversion to pyruvate and the activation of hypothalamic K_{ATP} channels. In nondiabetic subjects, hyperglycemia is per se sufficient to suppress glucose production. However, hyperglycemia fails to suppress EGP in the presence of hypothalamic blockade of glucose metabolism or K_{ATP} channel activation. Thus, glucose regulation of hepatic glucose production might be mediated in part by extrahepatic, hypothalamic mechanisms. Notably, in diabetic individuals, hyperglycemia fails to decrease glucose production, suggesting a possible impairment of brain glucose sensing.

Other CNS Modulators of Glucose Metabolism

GLP-1

Glucagon-like peptide-1 (GLP-1) is an enteric peptide recently implicated in the neural control of glucose metabolism. GLP-1 is known to stimulate glucose-dependent insulin secretion,[82] reduce glucagon secretion,[83] and inhibit gastric emptying.[84] GLP-1 and its agonists are effective hypoglycemic agents for the treatment of type 2 diabetes.[85] Improved glycemia with GLP-1 is likely due to its multiple actions. GLP-1-induced increase in insulin and decrease in glucagon secretion restrain hepatic glucose production, favor peripheral glucose utilization, and, in concert with delayed gastric emptying, effectively limit postprandial glycemic excursions.[86] Recent evidence suggests that GLP-1 released from intestinal L cells may interact locally with its receptor located on vagal afferent fibers projecting to the nucleus of the solitary tract (NTS) in the brain stem, and ultimately to the arcuate nucleus in the hypothalamus. This would result in the generation of an efferent signal from the arcuate nucleus to increase insulin secretion and decrease hepatic glucose production and muscle glucose utilization.[87] Notably, Sandoval and colleagues have recently shown that direct GLP-1 administration into the arcuate nucleus is sufficient to inhibit hepatic glucose production and glucose uptake. Like insulin, the hypothalamic action of GLP-1 on hepatic glucose metabolism requires the activation of hypothalamic K_{ATP} channels.[88]

Resistin

Resistin is a plasma protein derived from adipose tissue that has been implicated in insulin resistance and inflammation.[89] Acute systemic infusions of resistin result in marked hepatic insulin resistance. ICV or intrahypothalamic infusion of resistin reproduces its systemic effects on hepatic glucose production and inflammation. Of interest, the central administration of resistin markedly and selectively impaired the inhibitory action of insulin on hepatic glycogenolysis with no changes in circulating levels of glucoregulatory hormones or effect on hepatic expression of the key gluconeogenic enzymes. It supports the idea that resistin centrally increased hepatic glucoses fluxes predominantly via glycogenolytic activation.[90] Other studies report that the effects of CNS resistin on glucose production are abrogated in mice lacking NPY or in wild-type mice pretreated with antagonists of the NPY Y1 receptor.[91]

Neurotransmitters

A large body of evidence supports the notion that CNS monoamine neurotransmitters affect energy balance and glucose homeostasis. Hyperphagia and obesity are associated with abnormal hypothalamic dopamine and serotonin tone.[92] Conversely, experiments with streptozotocin-induced diabetic rats show that alterations in insulin and glucose homeostasis can influence mesoaccumbens dopamine and lower striatal concentrations of dopamine.[93] Treatment with dopamine receptor agonists reverts elevated hypothalamic levels of NPY and decreases body weight and hyperglycemia in obese leptin-deficient mice.[94] Agonists of 5-HT receptors are potent anorexic agents. A targeted deletion of the serotonin 5-HT$_{2C}$ receptor gene leads to adult-onset obesity, insulin resistance, and glucose intolerance.[95] Conversely, a selective agonist for 5-HT$_{2C}$ receptors improves glucose tolerance and insulin resistance in diet-induced, insulin-resistant mice, at doses that do not cause changes in fat mass. The beneficial effect of 5-HT$_{2C}$ receptor activation on glucose metabolism requires functional MC4 receptors.[96]

Recent evidence links the use of atypical antipsychotics for the treatment of psychiatry disorders to the onset of obesity, hyperlipidemia, and type 2 diabetes, and underscores the important role of a normal monoaminergic tone in the control of glucose homeostasis. Experiments in dogs show that a short-term treatment with olanzapine causes increased adiposity and markedly reduced hepatic insulin sensitivity.[97] Recent studies in rats show that atypical antipsychotics can acutely impair hepatic insulin sensitivity in the absence of changes in fat mass.[98,99]

A Neural Model of Integration of Peripheral Nutrients and Hormonal Signals

The brain is emerging as an essential regulator of energy metabolism. In particular, the regulation of glucose homeostasis is achieved through complex and still poorly understood neural mechanisms.[100] A major aspect of neural control of glucose metabolism involves the ability of neurons to sense energy flux and glucose availability. As discussed above, nutrients are sensed in neurons either directly or indirectly via the action of nutrient-dependent hormonal signals on neurons. Arcuate neurons are able to alter their firing rate upon changing the extracellular levels of glucose. The presence of K$_{ATP}$ channels in glucose-responsive neurons provides molecular and physiologic mechanism for the ability of neurons to process and integrate nutrients and hormonal signals and translate them into a membrane potential signal (Fig. 6.4). In addition to the postulated role of K$_{ATP}$ channels in the conterregulatory responses to hypoglycemia, these channels have been recently implicated in the neural control of hepatic glucose production.[101] Indeed, several signals converging onto K$_{ATP}$ channels can influence their function and ultimately lead to changes in neuronal electrical activity. As discussed above, glucose, insulin, and LCFA-CoAs can modulate glucose production via activation of K$_{ATP}$ channels in the arcuate nucleus. Nutrients can modulate K$_{ATP}$ channel activity by providing energy for the production of ATP, as demonstrated for glucose-sensing neurons.[102] Parton and colleagues have shown that the selective expression of a mutant K$_{ATP}$ channel unable to bind ATP in POMC neurons results in a mouse with an impaired glucose sensing in POMC neurons

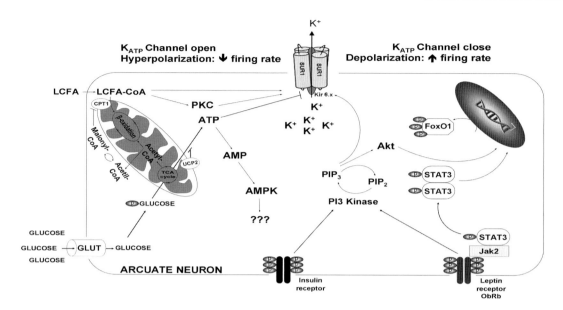

Fig. 6.4 Molecular mechanisms leading to changes in electrical activity in arcuate neurons. A variety of nutrients and hormones can modulate the activity of ATP-sensitive potassium channels (KATP) and rapidly alter neuronal excitability. In addition, modulation of transcriptional activity can alter gene expression for neuropeptides and neurotransmitters

and an impaired systemic tolerance to a glucose load.[103] In addition, LCFA-CoAs can bind directly to the Kir6.2 subunit and modify its sensitivity to ATP. Alternatively, LCFA-CoAs have been shown to activate the channels via activation of PKC.[104] Moreover, insulin and leptin open K_{ATP} channels via PI3K-dependent production of phosphatidylinositol-3,4,5-biphosphate (PIP3).[26,27] Additionally, nutrients and hormonal signals will affect neuronal activity by inducing transcriptional changes that result in the modulation of neuropeptide expression, neurotransmitter metabolism, and synaptic plasticity.

Summary

The concept that brain controls glucose homeostasis goes back to the nineteenth century with the pioneering studies of Claude Bernard, who proposed that the brain controls liver glucose production via its hepatic nerves. The current view is that plasma glucose regulation is under the control of complex neural and endocrine mechanisms. Nonetheless, recent evidence suggests that the CNS is a crucial organ for the control of glucose homeostasis. Circulating nutrients and nutrient-induced hormones (such as insulin and leptin) activate signals of increased energy availability in brain centers that control energy balance and endogenous glucose production. This in turn activates efferent pathways that restrain food intake and excessive endogenous glucose production. This neuroendocrine system of negative feedback ensures the physiologic constancy of plasma glucose levels. The arcuate nucleus of the hypothalamus receives and integrates all peripheral signals of nutrient availability and controls hepatic glucose metabolism via efferent vagal fibers. A major neural mechanism for the integration of metabolic signals is the control of membrane potential through K_{ATP} channels. These channels respond to changes in energy flux (ATP levels) as well as to intracellular changes in second messengers (PIP). Opening of K_{ATP} channels in the arcuate is implicated in the restraint of hepatic glucose production and can occur rapidly in the absence of changes in gene expression. In addition, nutrient and hormones can lead to changes in the expression of neuropeptides (NPY, MSH, AgRP) that have been implicated as CNS modulators of hepatic glucose metabolism. The implication of this recent evidence is that defects in the neural circuitry controlling glucose metabolism can contribute to the pathogenesis of diabetes. There is ample evidence that this occurs in animal models of obesity and type 2 diabetes. An important future challenge is to determine whether these mechanisms play a role in the control of glucose homeostasis in human pathophysiology of glucose metabolism.

References

1. Bernard C. *Leçons sur les phénomènes de la vie. Cours de physiologies generale du Museum d'Histoir Naturelle*. Paris: Librairie Delagrave; 1859.
2. Unger RH. The milieu interieur and the islets of Langerhans. *Diabetologia*. 1981;20:1–11.
3. Shimazu T 1998. *The Hypothalamus and Metabolic Control*. Minatomachi and Matsuyama, eds. Ehime, Japan: Ehime University School of Medicine.
4. Schwartz MW, Porte D Jr. Diabetes, obesity, and the brain. *Science*. 2005;307:375–379.
5. Davis SN, Colburn C, Dobbins R, et al. Evidence that the brain of the conscious dog is insulin sensitive. *J Clin Invest*. 1995;95:593–602.
6. Schwartz MW, Sipols A, Kahn SE, Lattemann DF, Taborsky GJ, Jr., Bergman RN, Woods SC, Porte D, Jr. Kinetics and specificity of insulin uptake from plasma into cerebrospinal fluid. *Am. J. Physiol* 1990;259:E378–E383.
7. Gerozissis K, Rouch C, Nicolaidis S, Orosco M. Brain insulin response to feeding in the rat is both macronutrient and area specific. *Physiol Behav.* 1998;65:271–275.
8. Gerozissis K, Orosco M, Rouch C, Nicolaidis S. Insulin responses to a fat meal in hypothalamic microdialysates and plasma. *Physiol Behav.* 1997;62:767–772.
9. Unger JW, Betz M. Insulin receptors and signal transduction proteins in the hypothalamo-hypophyseal system: a review on morphological findings and functional implications. *Histol. Histopathol.* 1998;13:1215–1224.
10. Marks JL, Porte D, Jr., Stahl WL, Baskin DG. Localization of insulin receptor mRNA in rat brain by in situ hybridization. *Endocrinology* 1990;127:3234–3236.
11. Baskin DG, Gierke EP, Wilcox BJ, Matsumoto AM, Schwartz MW. Food intake and estradiol effects on insulin binding in brain and liver. *Physiol Behav.* 1993;53:757–762.
12. Richardson RD, Ramsay DS, Lernmark A, Scheurink AJ, Baskin DG, Woods SC. Weight loss in rats following intraventricular transplants of pancreatic islets. *Am. J. Physiol* 1994;266:R59–R64.
13. Woods SC, Lotter EC, McKay LD, Porte D, Jr. Chronic intracerebroventricular infusion of insulin reduces food intake and body weight of baboons. *Nature* 1979;282:503–505.
14. Sipols AJ, Baskin DG, Schwartz MW. Effect of intracerebroventricular insulin infusion on diabetic hyperphagia and hypothalamic neuropeptide gene expression. *Diabetes* 1995;44:147–151.
15. Schwartz MW, Marks JL, Sipols AJ, Baskin DG, Woods SC, Kahn SE, Porte D, Jr. Central insulin administration reduces neuropeptide Y mRNA expression in the arcuate nucleus of food-deprived lean (Fa/Fa) but not obese (fa/fa) Zucker rats. *Endocrinology* 1991;128:2645–2647.
16. Sahu A, Dube MG, Phelps CP, Sninsky CA, Kalra PS, Kalra SP. Insulin and insulin-like growth factor II suppress neuropeptide Y release from the nerve terminals in the paraventricular nucleus: a putative hypothalamic site for energy homeostasis. *Endocrinology* 1995;136:5718–5724.
17. Davis SN, Dunham B, Walmsley K, Shavers C, Neal D, Williams P, Cherrington AD. Brain of the conscious dog is sensitive to physiological changes in circulating insulin. *Am. J. Physiol* 1997;272:E567–E575.
18. Liang C, Doherty JU, Faillace R, Maekawa K, Arnold S, Gavras H, Hood WB, Jr. Insulin infusion in conscious dogs. Effects on systemic and coronary hemodynamics, regional blood flows, and plasma catecholamines. *J. Clin. Invest* 1982;69:1321–1336.
19. Rowe JW, YounG JB, Minaker KL, Stevens AL, Pallotta J, Landsberg L. Effect of insulin and glucose infusions on sympathetic nervous system activity in normal man. *Diabetes* 1981;30:219–225.
20. Bruning JC, Gautam D, Burks DJ, et al. Role of brain insulin receptor in control of body weight and reproduction. *Science*. 2000;289:2122–2125.
21. Okamoto H, Obici S, Accili D, Rossetti L. Restoration of liver insulin signaling in Insr knockout mice fails to normalize hepatic insulin action. *J Clin Invest*. 2005;115:1314–1322.
22. Wolkow CA, Kimura KD, Lee MS, Ruvkun G. Regulation of C. elegans life-span by insulinlike signaling in the nervous system. *Science* 2000;290:147–150.
23. Obici S, Zhang BB, Karkanias G, Rossetti L. Hypothalamic insulin signaling is required for inhibition of glucose production. *Nat Med.* 2002;8:1376–1382.
24. Pocai A, Lam TK, Gutierrez-Juarez R, et al. Hypothalamic K(ATP) channels control hepatic glucose production. *Nature*. 2005;434:1026–1031.
25. Karschin C, Ecke C, Ashcroft FM, Karschin A. Overlapping distribution of K(ATP) channel-forming Kir6.2 subunit and the sulfonylurea receptor SUR1 in rodent brain. *FEBS Lett.* 1997;401:59–64.
26. Spanswick D, Smith MA, Groppi VE, Logan SD, Ashford ML. Leptin inhibits hypothalamic neurons by activation of ATP-sensitive potassium channels. *Nature*. 1997;390:521–525.
27. Spanswick D, Smith MA, Mirshamsi S, Routh VH, Ashford ML. Insulin activates ATP-sensitive K+ channels in hypothalamic neurons of lean, but not obese rats. *Nat Neurosci.* 2000;3:757–758.

28. Schwartz MW, Woods SC, Porte D Jr., Seeley RJ, Baskin DG. Central nervous system control of food intake. *Nature.* 2000;404:661–671.

29. Grill HJ, Schwartz MW, Kaplan JM, Foxhall JS, Breininger J, Baskin DG. Evidence that the caudal brainstem is a target for the inhibitory effect of leptin on food intake. *Endocrinology.* 2002;143:239–246.

30. Matsuhisa M, Yamasaki Y, Shiba Y, Nakahara I, Kuroda A, Tomita T, Iida M, Ikeda M, Kajimoto Y, Kubota M, Hori M. Important role of the hepatic vagus nerve in glucose uptake and production by the liver. *Metabolism* 2000;49:11–16.

31. Obici S, Feng Z, Morgan K, Stein D, Karkanias G, Rossetti L. Central administration of oleic acid inhibits glucose production and food intake. *Diabetes.* 2002;51:271–275.

32. Konner AC, Janoschek R, Plum L, et al. Insulin Action in AgRP-Expressing Neurons Is Required for Suppression of Hepatic Glucose Production. *Cell Metab.* 2007;5:438–449.

33. Magnuson MA. Tissue-specific regulation of glucokinase gene expression. *J Cell Biochem.* 1992;48:115–121.

34. Cowley MA, Smart JL, Rubinstein M, et al. Leptin activates anorexigenic POMC neurons through a neural network in the arcuate nucleus. *Nature.* 2001;411:480–484.

35. Cowley MA, Pronchuk N, Fan W, Dinulescu DM, Colmers WF, Cone RD. Integration of NPY, AGRP, and melanocortin signals in the hypothalamic paraventricular nucleus: evidence of a cellular basis for the adipostat. *Neuron* 1999;24: 155–163.

36. Butler AA, Cone RD. Knockout studies defining different roles for melanocortin receptors in energy homeostasis. *Ann.N Y.Acad.Sci.* 2003;994:240–245.

37. Butler AA, Kesterson RA, Khong K, Cullen MJ, Pelleymounter MA, Dekoning J, Baetscher M, Cone RD. A unique metabolic syndrome causes obesity in the melanocortin-3 receptor-deficient mouse. *Endocrinology* 2000;141:3518–3521.

38. Huszar D, Lynch CA, Fairchild-Huntress V, et al. Targeted disruption of the melanocortin-4 receptor results in obesity in mice. *Cell.* 1997;88:131–141.

39. Obici S, Feng ZH, Tan JZ, Liu LS, Karkanias G, Rossetti L. Central melanocortin receptors regulate insulin action. *J Clin Invest.* 2001;108:1079–1085.

40. Barzilai N, She L, Liu L, et al. Decreased visceral adiposity accounts for leptin effect on hepatic but not peripheral insulin action. *Am J Physiol.* 1999;277:E291–E298.

41. Liu L, Karkanias GB, Morales JC, et al. Intracerebroventricular leptin regulates hepatic but not peripheral glucose fluxes. *J Biol Chem.* 1998;273:31160–31167.

42. Fan W, Dinulescu DM, Butler AA, Zhou J, Marks DL, Cone RD. The central melanocortin system can directly regulate serum insulin levels. *Endocrinology* 2000;141:3072–3079.

43. Gutierrez-Juarez R, Obici S, Rossetti L. Melanocortin-independent effects of leptin on hepatic glucose fluxes. *J Biol Chem.* 2004;279:49704–49715.

44. Halaas JL, Gajiwala KS, Maffei M, et al. Weight-reducing effects of the plasma protein encoded by the obese gene. *Science.* 1995;269:543–546.

45. Halaas JL, Boozer C, Blair-West J, Fidahusein N, Denton DA, Friedman JM. Physiological response to long-term peripheral and central leptin infusion in lean and obese mice. *Proc Natl Acad Sci USA.* 1997;94:8878–8883.

46. Pelleymounter MA, Cullen MJ, Baker MB, et al. Effects of the obese gene product on body weight regulation in ob/ob mice. *Science.* 1995;269:540–543.

47. Schwartz MW, Baskin DG, Bukowski TR, Kuijper JL, Foster D, Lasser G, Prunkard DE, Porte D, Jr., Woods SC, Seeley RJ, Weigle DS. Specificity of leptin action on elevated blood glucose levels and hypothalamic neuropeptide Y gene expression in ob/ob mice. *Diabetes* 1996;45:531–535.

48. Rossetti L, Massillon D, Barzilai N, et al. Short term effects of leptin on hepatic gluconeogenesis and in vivo insulin action. *J Biol Chem.* 1997;272:27758–27763.

49. Barzilai N, Wang J, Massilon D, Vuguin P, Hawkins M, Rossetti L. Leptin selectively decreases visceral adiposity and enhances insulin action. *J Clin Invest.* 1997;100:3105–3110.

50. Muoio DM, Dohm GL, Fiedorek FT, Jr., Tapscott EB, Coleman RA, Dohn GL. Leptin directly alters lipid partitioning in skeletal muscle. *Diabetes* 1997;46:1360–1363.

51. Muoio DM, Dohm GL, Tapscott EB, Coleman RA. Leptin opposes insulin's effects on fatty acid partitioning in muscles isolated from obese ob/ob mice. *Am. J. Physiol* 1999;276:E913–E921.

52. Minokoshi Y, Kim YB, Peroni OD, et al. Leptin stimulates fatty-acid oxidation by activating AMP-activated protein kinase. *Nature.* 2002;415:339–343.

53. Balthasar N, Coppari R, McMinn J, et al. Leptin receptor signaling in POMC neurons is required for normal body weight homeostasis. *Neuron.* 2004;42:983–991.

54. da Silva BA, Bjorbaek C, Uotani S, Flier JS. Functional properties of leptin receptor isoforms containing the gln–>pro extracellular domain mutation of the fatty rat. *Endocrinology.* 1998;139:3681–3690.

55. Haynes WG, Morgan DA, Djalali A, Sivitz WI, Mark AL. Interactions between the melanocortin system and leptin in control of sympathetic nerve traffic. *Hypertension.* 1999;33:542–547.

56. Niswender KD, Morton GJ, Stearns WH, Rhodes CJ, Myers MG Jr., Schwartz MW. Intracellular signalling. Key enzyme in leptin-induced anorexia. *Nature.* 2001;413:794–795.

57. Niswender KD, Morrison CD, Clegg DJ, et al. Insulin activation of phosphatidylinositol 3-kinase in the hypothalamic arcuate nucleus: a key mediator of insulin-induced anorexia. *Diabetes.* 2003;52:227–231.

58. Menendez JA, Mcgregor IS, Healey PA, Atrens DM, Leibowitz SF. Metabolic effects of neuropeptide-y injections into the paraventricular nucleus of the hypothalamus. *Brain Res.* 1990;516:8–14.

59. Billington CJ, Briggs JE, Grace M, Levine AS. Effects of intracerebroventricular injection of neuropeptide-y on energy-metabolism. *Am J Physiol.* 1991;260:R321–R327.

60. Marks JL, Waite K. Some acute effects of intracerebroventricular neuropeptide Y on insulin secretion and glucose metabolism in the rat. *J Neuroendocrinol.* 1996;8:507–513.

61. Marks JL, Waite K. Intracerebroventricular neuropeptide Y acutely influences glucose metabolism and insulin sensitivity in the rat. *J Neuroendocrinol.* 1997;9:99–103.

62. van den Hoek AM, van Heijningen C, Schroder-van der Elst JP, et al. Intracerebroventricular administration of neuropeptide Y induces hepatic insulin resistance via sympathetic innervation. *Diabetes.* 2008;57:2304–2310.

63. Baskin DG, Figlewicz LD, Seeley RJ, Woods SC, Porte D Jr., Schwartz MW. Insulin and leptin: dual adiposity signals to the brain for the regulation of food intake and body weight. *Brain Res.* 1999;848:114–123.

64. Schwartz MW, Figlewicz DP, Baskin DG, Woods SC, Porte D Jr. Insulin in the brain: a hormonal regulator of energy balance. *Endocr Rev.* 1992;13:387–414.

65. Seeley RJ, van Dijk G, Campfield LA, et al. Intraventricular leptin reduces food intake and body weight of lean rats but not obese Zucker rats. *Horm Metab Res.* 1996;28:664–668.

66. Levin BE, Dunn-Meynell AA, Routh VH. Brain glucose sensing and body energy homeostasis: role in obesity and diabetes. *Am J Physiol.* 1999;276:R1223–R1231.

67. Miller JC, Gnaedinger JM, Rapaport SI. Utilization of plasma fatty acids in rat brain: distribution of 14C-Palmitate between oxidative and synthetic pathways. *J Neurochem.* 1987;49:1507–1514.

68. Loftus TM, Jaworsky DE, Frehywot GL, et al. Reduced food intake and body weight in mice treated with fatty acid synthase inhibitors. *Science.* 2000;288:2379–2381.

69. McGarry JD, Mannaerts GP, Foster DW. A possible role for malonyl-CoA in the regulation of hepatic fatty acid oxidation and ketogenesis. *J Clin Invest.* 1977;60:265–270.

70. Obici S, Rossetti L. Minireview: nutrient sensing and the regulation of insulin action and energy balance. *Endocrinology.* 2003;144:5172–5178.

71. He W, Lam TKT, Obici S, Rossetti L. Molecular disruption of hypothalamic nutrient sensing induces obesity. *Nat Neurosci.* 2006;9:227–233.

72. Hu Z, Dai Y, Prentki M, Chohnan S, Lane MD. A role for hypothalamic malonyl-CoA in the control of food intake. *J Biol Chem.* 2005;280:39681–39683.

73. Obici S, Feng Z, Arduini A, Conti R, Rossetti L. Inhibition of hypothalamic carnitine palmitoyltransferase-1 decreases food intake and glucose production. *Nat Med.* 2003;9:756–761.

74. Wolfgang MJ, Lane MD. The role of hypothalamic malonyl-CoA in energy homeostasis. *J Biol Chem.* 2006;281:37265–37269.

75. Pocai A, Obici S, Schwartz GJ, Rossetti L. A brain–liver circuit regulates glucose homeostasis. *Cell Metab.* 2005;1:53–61.

76. Morgan K, Obici S, Rossetti L. Hypothalamic responses to long-chain fatty acids are nutritionally regulated. *J Biol Chem.* 2004;279:31139–31148.

77. Lam TK, Carpentier A, Lewis GF, van de WG, Fantus IG, Giacca A. Mechanisms of the free fatty acid-induced increase in hepatic glucose production. *Am J Physiol Endocrinol Metab.* 2003;284:E863–E873.

78. Lam TK, Pocai A, Gutierrez-Juarez R, et al. Hypothalamic sensing of circulating fatty acids is required for glucose homeostasis. *Nat Med.* 2005;11:320–327.

79. Boden G, Chen X, Capulong E, Mozzoli M. Effects of free fatty acids on gluconeogenesis and autoregulation of glucose production in type 2 diabetes. *Diabetes.* 2001;50:810–816.

80. Mayer J. Glucostatic mechanism of regulation of food intake. *N Engl J Med.* 1953;249:13–16.

81. Lam TK, Gutierrez-Juarez R, Pocai A, Rossetti L. Regulation of blood glucose by hypothalamic pyruvate metabolism. *Science.* 2005;309:943–947.

82. Holst JJ, Gromada J. Role of incretin hormones in the regulation of insulin secretion in diabetic and nondiabetic humans. *Am J Physiol Endocrinol Metab.* 2004;287:E199–E206.

83. Schirra J, Nicolaus M, Roggel R, et al. Endogenous glucagon-like peptide 1 controls endocrine pancreatic secretion and antro-pyloro-duodenal motility in humans. *Gut.* 2006;55:243–251.

84. Willms B, Werner J, Holst JJ, Orskov C, Creutzfeldt W, Nauck MA. Gastric emptying glucose responses, insulin secretion after a liquid test meal: effects of exogenous glucagon-like peptide-1 (GLP-1)-(7-36) amide in type 2 (noninsulin-dependent) diabetic patients. *J Clin Endocrinol Metab.* 1996;81:327–332.

85. Zander M, Madsbad S, Madsen JL, Holst JJ. Effect of 6-week course of glucagon-like peptide 1 on glycaemic control, insulin sensitivity, beta-cell function in type 2 diabetes: a parallel-group study. *Lancet.* 2002;359:824–830.

86. Sandoval D. CNS GLP-1 regulation of peripheral glucose homeostasis. *Physiol Behav.* 2008;94:670–674.

87. Knauf C, Cani PD, Perrin C, et al. Brain glucagon-like peptide-1 increases insulin secretion and muscle insulin resistance to favor hepatic glycogen storage. *J Clin Invest.* 2005;115:3554–3563.

88. Sandoval DA, Bagnol D, Woods SC, D'Alessio DA, Seeley RJ. Arcuate glucagon-like peptide 1 receptors regulate glucose homeostasis but not food intake. *Diabetes.* 2008;57:2046–2054.

89. Mojiminiyi OA, Abdella NA. Associations of resistin with inflammation and insulin resistance in patients with type 2 diabetes mellitus. *Scand J Clin Lab Invest.* 2007;67:215–225.

90. Muse ED, Lam TK, Scherer PE, Rossetti L. Hypothalamic resistin induces hepatic insulin resistance. *J Clin Invest.* 2007;117:1670–1678.

91. Singhal NS, Lazar MA, Ahima RS. Central resistin induces hepatic insulin resistance via neuropeptide Y. *J Neurosci.* 2007;27:12924–12932.

92. Meguid MM, Fetissov SO, Varma M, et al. Hypothalamic dopamine and serotonin in the regulation of food intake. *Nutrition.* 2000;16:843–857.

93. Murzi E, Contreras Q, Teneud L, et al. Diabetes decreases limbic extracellular dopamine in rats. *Neurosci Lett.* 1996;202: 141–144.

94. Pijl H. Reduced dopaminergic tone in hypothalamic neural circuits: expression of a "thrifty" genotype underlying the metabolic syndrome?. *Eur J Pharmacol.* 2003;480:125–131.

95. Nonogaki K, Strack AM, Dallman MF, Tecott LH. Leptin-independent hyperphagia and type 2 diabetes in mice with a mutated serotonin 5-HT2C receptor gene. *Nat Med.* 1998;4:1152–1156.

96. Zhou L, Sutton GM, Rochford JJ, et al. Serotonin 2C receptor agonists improve type 2 diabetes via melanocortin-4 receptor signaling pathways. *Cell Metab.* 2007;6:398–405.

97. Ader M, Kim SP, Catalano KJ, et al. Metabolic dysregulation with atypical antipsychotics occurs in the absence of underlying disease: a placebo-controlled study of olanzapine and risperidone in dogs. *Diabetes.* 2005;54:862–871.

98. Houseknecht KL, Robertson AS, Zavadoski W, Gibbs EM, Johnson DE, Rollema H. Acute effects of atypical antipsychotics on whole-body insulin resistance in rats: implications for adverse metabolic effects. *Neuropsychopharmacology.* 2007;32:289–297.

99. Chintoh AF, Mann SW, Lam L, et al. Insulin resistance and decreased glucose-stimulated insulin secretion after acute olanzapine administration. *J Clin Psychopharmacol.* 2008;28:494–499.

100. Rother E, Konner AC, Bruning JC. Neurocircuits integrating hormone and nutrient signaling in control of glucose metabolism. *Am J Physiol Endocrinol Metab.* 2008;294:E810–E816.

101. Prodi E, Obici S. Minireview: the brain as a molecular target for diabetic therapy. *Endocrinology.* 2006;147:2664–2669.

102. Levin BE, Dunn-Meynell AA, Routh VH. Brain glucosensing and the K(ATP) channel. *Nat Neurosci.* 2001;4:459–460.

103. Parton LE, Ye CP, Coppari R, et al. Glucose sensing by POMC neurons regulates glucose homeostasis and is impaired in obesity. *Nature.* 2007;449:228–232.

104. Ross R, Wang PY, Chari M, et al. Hypothalamic protein kinase C regulates glucose production. *Diabetes.* 2008;57:2061–2065.

Part III
Diagnosis and Epidemiology of Diabetes

Chapter 7
Diagnostic Criteria and Classification of Diabetes

James P. Leu and Joel Zonszein

Definition and Nomenclature of Diabetes

Diabetes mellitus is a group of diverse metabolic disorders characterized by hyperglycemia and distinctive complications that include premature atherosclerotic cardiovascular disease and small vessel disease manifested as retinopathy with potential loss of vision; nephropathy leading to renal failure; and peripheral neuropathy with a high risk of foot ulcers and amputations. In the past, the classification of diabetes mellitus was based on clinical findings such as age of onset, so-called juvenile- or adult-onset diabetes, or treatment modalities, such as insulin-dependent versus non-insulin-dependent diabetes. In 1979 the National Diabetes Data Group (NDDG) in conjunction with World Health Organization (WHO) revised and published new and unified criteria for the classification and diagnosis of diabetes mellitus.[1] The NDDG classification was based on the cumulative knowledge of diabetes which consisted of a combination of clinical manifestations, pathogenesis, and treatment. The diagnosis was determined entirely by the degree of hyperglycemia, measured either in the fasting state, randomly, or after a glucose tolerance test. These criteria provided clinicians with a more uniform scale for categorization of patients according to the various degree of glucose intolerance. As more information was accrued on the pathogenesis and etiology of diabetes, the NDDG criteria were modified by the International Expert Committee under the sponsorship of the American Diabetes Association and will be further discussed in this chapter.

Classification

Diabetes mellitus is a complex and heterogeneous disorder with diverse etiologic mechanisms; therefore, any given classification is arbitrary. The current classification includes four main categories.[2] The new criteria are shown in Table 7.1. The terms type 1 and type 2 diabetes mellitus (with Arabic rather than Roman numerals) replaced the previous treatment-based terminology, IDDM and NIDDM. The third group consists of other less common types of diabetes that are caused or associated with certain specific conditions and/or syndromes. The last group includes diabetes diagnosed during pregnancy, called gestational diabetes (GDM). The Expert Committee also identified an intermediate group of individuals whose glucose levels do not meet criteria for diabetes but are too high to be considered normal. These individuals have impaired fasting glucose (IFG) and/or impaired glucose tolerance (IGT). The name "pre-diabetes" has been used again for these entities as progression to diabetes is common, particularly when therapeutic interventions such as lifestyle changes or medications are not provided.[3–7]

J. Zonszein (✉)
Division of Endocrinology and Metabolism, Department of Medicine, Montefiore Medical Center and Albert Einstein College of Medicine, Bronx, NY, USA
e-mail: zonszein@aecom.yu.edu

L. Poretsky (ed.), *Principles of Diabetes Mellitus*, DOI 10.1007/978-0-387-09841-8_7,
© Springer Science+Business Media, LLC 2010

Table 7.1 Etiologic classification of diabetes mellitus

I. Type 1 diabetes
   A. Autoimmune
   B. Idiopathic

II. Type 2 diabetes

III. Others
   A. Genetic defects of β-cell function
   B. Diseases of the exocrine pancreas
   C. Endocrinopathies
   D. Drug or chemical induced
   E. Infections
   F. Other immune-mediated (uncommon)
   G. Other specific genetic syndromes associated with diabetes

IV. Gestational diabetes

Type 1 Diabetes

This form of diabetes accounts for 5–10% of all cases. It results from a progressive cellular-mediated autoimmune destruction of the pancreatic β-cells that leads to complete insulin deficiency.[8] The rate of β-cell destruction is rapid in the majority, particularly in infants and children, but may be insidious in the adults. When β-cell failure is sudden it can cause ketoacidosis, often the first manifestation of the disease. Otherwise, a more indolent onset of disease is common, with severe hyperglycemia and/or ketoacidosis found only in the presence of stress conditions or severe infections. Patients with type 1 diabetes are severely insulin deficient and are dependent on insulin treatment for their survival. Management consists of insulin provided as a replacement hormone. Markers of the immune β-cell destruction include islet cell autoantibodies (ICAs), insulin autoantibodies (IAAs), glutamic acid decarboxylase autoantibodies (GAD$_{65}$), and autoantibodies to the tyrosine phosphatases IA-2 and IA-2α.[9–12] At least one or more of these autoantibodies are present in approximately 90% of the new-onset patients, and therefore can be used clinically to help make the diagnosis. Type 1 diabetes has also a strong HLA association, with linkage to the DQA and B genes. It is influenced by the DRB genes and is associated with other autoimmune disorders.[13] This type of immune-mediated diabetes, while common in childhood and adolescence, can occur at any age, even as late as in the eighth and ninth decades of life. The slow rate of β-cell destruction in adults may mask the presentation making it difficult to distinguish from type 2 diabetes.[14,15] However, positive pancreatic autoantibody establishes the diagnosis and distinguishes type 1 diabetes from the garden variety type 2 diabetes. This type of diabetes is known as Latent Autoimmune Diabetes in Adults, or LADA, an entity that is more common in the Caucasian population. The presence of autoantibodies indicates the need for early insulin treatment.[16]

Idiopathic Diabetes

Some forms of type 1 diabetes are less well understood, and can present with various degrees of β-cell dysfunction. This form of diabetes is inherited, lacks evidence for β-cell autoimmunity, and is not HLA associated. Only a minority of patients fall under this category, which appears to be more common in individuals from African-Caribbean origin. The function of β-cells is variable, and while the disease is often manifested by severe insulinopenia and/or ketoacidosis, β-cell function often recovers, rendering almost normal glucose levels. These patients should be treated initially with insulin, but insulin replacement therapy may not always be necessary after the recovery phase.[17]

Type 2 Diabetes

This type of diabetes consists of heterogeneous conditions responsible for approximately 90% of all individuals with diabetes. It is often associated with central or visceral obesity, as well as other cardiovascular risk factors such as hypertension, and abnormalities of lipoprotein metabolism with the characteristic dyslipidemia of elevated triglycerides and low high-density lipoprotein cholesterol. It is this constellation of cardiovascular risk factors that causes the premature cardiovascular morbidity and mortality, often establishing the diagnosis of type 2 diabetes during hospitalization for a cardiovascular event. Type 2 diabetes is characterized by complex metabolic derangements, with two main abnormalities: insulin resistance and β-cell dysfunction. Circulating insulin levels are higher early in the disease to compensate for insulin resistance, but eventually, insulin production becomes less sufficient and hyperglycemia develops. This is illustrated by the typical progression of the disease that exhibits impaired insulin-mediated glucose utilization with postprandial hyperglycemia in its early stages. Fasting hyperglycemia, the hallmark of type 2 diabetes, ensues at a later stage, secondary to the excessive and inappropriate hepatic glucose production. The capacity of insulin secretion in these patients is often enough to prevent ketosis and ketoacidosis, but still manifest during periods of severe stress or acute medical illness. This disease is closely related to obesity, and it is becoming more common in both developed and developing countries, afflicting younger individuals, and, particularly, ethnic minorities.

Other Specific Types

These numerous conditions are summarized in Table 7.1, but account for only a minor portion of all cases of diabetes. Maturity Onset Diabetes of the Young (MODY) is a group of monogenetic disorders in which a mutation causes hyperglycemia by producing a defect in glucose sensing or insulin secretion with minimal or no defects in insulin action. To date, six genetic loci on different chromosomes have been identified.[18] Patients with MODY usually develop a milder form of hyperglycemia at a young age (before 25 years), have a family history of diabetes, and have fewer chronic complications.

Recently, an example of pharmacogenetics was illustrated by identifying a genetic cause of insulin deficiency and diabetes in neonates. The mutation is in the pancreatic ATP-sensitive potassium (K_{ATP}) channel, a critical regulator of β-cell insulin secretion, and may account for almost 50% of cases of diabetes diagnosed at less than 6 months of age.[19,20] Patients with this disorder suffer from a heterozygous activating mutation of the *KCNJ11* gene, which encodes the Kir6.2 subunit of the K_{ATP} channel. This results in the failure of the channel to close in the presence of glucose, leading to decreased insulin secretion.[21] Sulfonylurea therapy in diabetic patients with this mutation will improve the function of the K_{ATP} channel, and most patients can be successfully switched from insulin therapy to oral sulfonylurea.[22]

Another uncommon but characteristic genetic disorder is a point mutation in mitochondrial DNA manifested as diabetes mellitus and deafness.[23] A similar mutation is found in the MELAS syndrome (mitochondrial myopathy, encephalopathy, lactic acidosis, and stroke-like syndrome); however, diabetes is not part of this syndrome, suggesting different phenotypic expressions. Genetic defects resulting in abnormal insulin production have also been identified including abnormal conversion of proinsulin to insulin,[24] or cases with production of mutant insulin molecules that result in impaired insulin receptor binding.[25] While abnormal circulating insulin is rare, genetic defects of insulin action are more common. These conditions manifest as severe insulin resistance and are found in patients with polycystic ovarian (PCO) syndrome, often presenting with typical skin abnormalities (acanthosis nigricans), obesity, hyperandrogenism, and cystic ovaries.[26–28]

Other causes of diabetes include abnormalities of the exocrine pancreas including pancreatitis, trauma, and cystic fibrosis. Diabetes is also manifested in several endocrinopathies that include Cushing's syndrome and acromegaly, where increased insulin demand results in hyperglycemia when accompanied by inappropriate insulin secretion. Hyperglycemia can also be induced by a number of drugs such as thiazides, dilantin, α-interferon, diazoxide, and glucocorticoids. Finally, viral infections such as coxsackie virus B, cytomegalovirus, adenovirus, and mumps are also associated with β-cell dysfunction resulting in hyperglycemia.[29,30] The high incidence of hepatitis C that is associated with insulin resistance has contributed to the epidemic state of type 2 diabetes.[31,32]

Gestational Diabetes Mellitus (GDM)

Gestational diabetes complicates ~4% of all pregnancies in the United States, but the true prevalence may range from 1 to 14% depending on the population studied. It now represents nearly 90% of all diabetes in pregnancy.[33] Due to its high incidence, the previous recommendation of screening only high-risk patients has now been changed to the early screening of all pregnant women unless they are defined as low risk. This low-risk group includes women who

- are less than 25 years of age
- have a normal body weight
- have no family history (i.e., first-degree relative) of diabetes
- have no history of abnormal glucose metabolism
- have no history of poor obstetric outcome
- are not members of an ethnic/racial group with a high prevalence of diabetes (e.g., Hispanic American, Native American, Asian-American, African-American, and Pacific Islander)

Evaluation for GDM should be done early in pregnancy, particularly in women at high risk (marked obesity, personal history of GDM, glycosuria, or a strong family history of diabetes). If a woman is found not to have GDM at the initial screening, she should be retested between 24 and 28 weeks of gestation. Women of average risk should be tested at 24–28 weeks of gestation. Early screening and diagnosis is crucial as proper monitoring and initiation of therapy reduces perinatal morbidity and mortality.[34,35] The relationship between high blood sugar levels and poor maternal and fetal outcomes was studied in normal (non-gestational diabetes) pregnant women in the Hyperglycemia and Adverse Pregnancy Outcome (HAPO) Study.[36] Preliminary results have shown a direct correlation between high blood sugar and poor outcome for both mother and baby without a glycemic threshold. Women with gestational diabetes mellitus need to be evaluated after delivery, as they may have antecedent diabetes diagnosed at the time of pregnancy. Even with a negative postpartum test these patients need further monitoring as they remain at an increased risk of developing type 2 diabetes and cardiovascular disease.

Diagnostic Criteria

The diagnosis of diabetes is established solely by documentation of abnormal glycemic values. As shown in Table 7.2 there are three criteria used to make a diagnosis of diabetes; elevated fasting glucose, abnormal OGTT, or symptoms of diabetes with hyperglycemia. Glucose tolerance tests are performed by providing either 75 or 100 g of glucose. This test, although more sensitive and specific than fasting glucose alone, is lengthy and cumbersome. Test should be done in the morning after an overnight fast and at least 3 days of unrestricted diet, rich in carbohydrates. The subject should remain seated and not smoking throughout the test. Two or more values must be met or exceeded for a diagnosis. Glycemic values vary greatly, and the degree of hyperglycemia

Table 7.2 Criteria for the diagnosis of diabetes mellitus

- Symptoms of diabetes + random plasma glucose concentration $\geq$ 200 mg/dl (11.1 mmol/l)
- Fasting plasma glucose $\geq$ 126 mg/dl (7.0 mmol/l)
- Two hour plasma glucose $\geq$ 200 mg/dl (11.1 mmol/l) during a 75 g oral glucose tolerance test

or glucose intolerance can improve or worsen according to changes in body weight, food intake, physical activity, stress, pregnancy, use of corticosteroids or other medications, etc.

The use of HbA_{1c} for the diagnosis of diabetes is not currently recommended due to the lack of uniformity in the assays worldwide.[37,38] Studies showing that the frequency distributions for HbA_{1c} are concordant with fasting plasma glucose (FPG) and the 2-h PG determinations have led to the proposal to use HbA_{1c} measurement for diagnostic purposes.[39] There is an ongoing effort for worldwide standardization of HbA_{1c} measurement. A consensus committee organized by the American Diabetes Association (ADA), the European Association for the Study of Diabetes (EASD), the International Federation of Clinical Chemistry and Laboratory Medicine (IFCC), and the International Diabetes Federation (IDF) recently issued a statement stressing the relevance of standardizing the HbA_{1c} test results all over the world, and suggesting using the IFCC reference system as an anchor for standardizing the measurements.[40] At the American Diabetes Association's 69th annual meeting in New Orleans LA, in June 2009, the international committee of experts announced their consensus that the A1C assay is an accurate way to diagnose diabetes in adults and children, but not in pregnant women. The committee is waiting for other major diabetes groups to agree. The international committee advises that anyone with a reading of 6.5% or greater should be considered to have diabetes. While HbA_{1c} levels are not yet approved for diagnosis, it is an excellent marker for cardiovascular morbidity and mortality, even in those without the diagnosis of type 2 diabetes[41] and is the gold standard in monitoring treatment.

While plasma glucose concentrations are distributed over a continuum, the threshold of a fasting plasma glucose (FPG) of ≥ 126 mg/dl has been used for diagnosis based on adverse outcomes related to microvascular complications. In the early stages, particularly in type 2 diabetes, the degree of hyperglycemia is sufficient to cause pathologic changes, but it is not enough to cause clinical symptoms. Thus, a silent phase of the disease can exist for prolonged periods of time before it is diagnosed. Typically the disease progresses from a pre-diabetic condition to overt type 2 diabetes. The criteria for the diagnosis of diabetes, IGT, and IFG are shown in Tables 7.2 and 7.3.

Table 7.3   Criteria for the diagnosis of glucose intolerance and diabetes

	Normal	Impaired fasting glucose (IFG)	Impaired glucose tolerance (IGT)	Diabetes mellitus
Fasting plasma glucose				
mg/dl	<100	100–125	–	≥ 126
mmol/l	<5.6	5.6–6.9	–	≥ 7.0
2-h post OGTT challenge				
mg/dl	<140	–	140–199	≥ 200
mmol/l	<7.8	–	7.8–11.0	≥ 11.1

OGTT, oral glucose tolerance test

To establish the diagnosis, each value must be confirmed on a subsequent day by any one of the three criteria given. The FPG test criteria result in a lower prevalence of diabetes than OGTT (4.35% vs. 6.34%) in individuals without a medical history of diabetes. However, a widespread adoption of OGTT may have a large impact on the number of people diagnosed with diabetes. This is important since presently, a large population of adults with diabetes in the United States remain undiagnosed.[42]

Diagnosis of Pre-diabetes, Impaired Glucose Tolerance (IGT), and Impaired Fasting Glucose (IFG)

Individuals with IGT and/or IFG are currently considered to have "pre-diabetes" as they are at a high risk of progressing to overt diabetes.[37] The threshold to diagnose pre-diabetes has been lowered in parallel to the threshold to diagnose diabetes.[43] The International Expert Committee initially defined normal fasting plasma glucose level as being no higher than 110 mg/dl and introduced the concept of impaired fasting glucose levels with plasma glucose levels between 110 and 125 mg/dl. The recommendation remained controversial because of the discrepancies between fasting plasma glucose and postprandial values. For this reason, the National Diabetes Data Group proposed the use of glycosylated hemoglobin levels for diagnostic purposes.[1] After analysis of data from diverse populations to determine what level of fasting plasma glucose predicted the future outcome of diabetes, the Expert Committee concluded that a level of 110 mg/dl was "inappropriately high" and recommended changing the cutoff point to 100 mg/dl. More recently, in a large cohort of healthy young Israeli military men, higher fasting plasma euglycemic levels (91–99 mg/dl) were found to be predictive of a higher incidence of diabetes, particularly in those with a high body mass index or an increased fasting level of triglycerides.[44] Therefore, fasting plasma glucose levels represent a continuum where the lower the level the better.

Morbidity found in patients with elevated glucose levels is closely influenced by weight, age, sex, and other metabolic substrates. Elevated glucose levels are particularly detrimental when associated with the metabolic syndrome, a constellation of metabolic risk factors such as atherogenic dyslipidemia, elevated blood pressure, a prothrombotic state, and a proinflammatory state.[45,46] When the diagnosis of pre-diabetes is made, patients need to be encouraged to make lifestyle changes and be treated aggressively for other cardiovascular risk factors such as hypertension and dyslipidemia.

Diagnosis of Gestational Diabetes (GDM)

Diabetes in pregnancy (DIP) can be found in individuals with established type 1 diabetes and/or type 2 diabetes. All women diagnosed during pregnancy are defined as GDM, even if the diabetes is suspected to have been present before pregnancy. The definition is independent of treatment use or whether or not it persists after pregnancy. It is likely that unrecognized glucose intolerance or type 2 diabetes may have antedated or begun concomitantly with pregnancy, a common finding in the ethnic/racial minority populations. Prevalence of GDM varies in direct proportion to the prevalence of type 2 diabetes, particularly among different ethnic groups.

The ideal evaluation should be performed before conception; otherwise risk assessment for GDM should be undertaken at the first prenatal visit. Women with low risk should have testing undertaken at 24–28 weeks of gestation, as discussed above, but everyone else should be tested within the first or second visit. There are two approaches to screening for GDM: one-step and two-step approach. The one-step approach is a diagnostic OGTT without prior plasma or serum glucose screening, cost-effective in high-risk patients or populations. The two-step approach is to perform initially a screening test measuring the plasma or serum glucose concentration 1 h after a 50-g oral glucose challenge test (GCT), followed by a diagnostic OGTT on the subset of women exceeding the glucose threshold value on the GCT. When the GCT is employed, approximately 80% of women with GDM are identified with a threshold value of 140 mg/dl. Ninety percent of women with GDM are identified when a cutoff of 130 mg/dl is used. The diagnosis of GDM is made with a 100-g OGTT using the criteria derived from the original work of O'Sullivan and Mahan, modified by Carpenter and Coustan as shown in Table 7.4. If found not to have GDM at the initial screening, women should be retested between 24 and 28 weeks of gestation, as is the recommendation for women of average risk. It is good medical practice to study the patient 6 weeks or more postpartum in order to classify them as normal, pre-diabetes, or diabetes

Table 7.4 Diagnosis of gestational diabetes mellitus with a 100-g glucose challenge

	mg/dl	mmol/l
Fasting	≥95	≥5.3
1 h	≥180	≥10
2 h	≥155	≥8.6
3 h	≥140	≥7.8

Table 7.5 American Diabetes Association criteria to define populations at high risk for diabetes

Age > 45 years
Age < 45 years with the following:
• Member of a minority population
• Obesity (>120% desirable bodyweight or BMI > 27 kg/m^2)
• First relative with diabetes
• Previous history of GDM or delivered a baby weighting >9 lb
• Previous evidence of IGT or IFG
• Hypertension
• Dyslipidemia

Testing for Diabetes in Presumably Healthy Individuals

Undiagnosed type 2 diabetes is common in the United States. The Diabetes Prevention Program Research Group has shown the importance of early detection and lifestyle intervention to prevent future progression to overt diabetes.[3] In order to increase the cost-effectiveness of diagnosing otherwise healthy individuals, testing should be considered in high-risk populations (Table 7.5). Although the OGTT and FPG are both suitable tests, the FPG is preferred for clinical settings as it is easier and more acceptable to the patients.

Summary

Diabetes mellitus is a heterogeneous and complex metabolic disorder characterized by hyperglycemia and complications of premature cardiovascular disease and small vessel disease causing renal failure, eye disease, and neuropathy. Type 2 diabetes is closely associated with obesity and insulin resistance, and its incidence and prevalence has increased dramatically in developed societies; it affects a disproportional number of minority populations and is associated with other cardiovascular risk factors. When not treated, it can result in premature cardiovascular morbidity and mortality. The classification and diagnosis have been continually revised to reflect current knowledge of the disease and the classification is now based on disease etiology. Currently, there is a well-established set of criteria to screen the high-risk population, allowing for an earlier diagnosis and a more focused intervention to prevent future complications.

References

1. National Diabetes Data Group. Classification and diagnosis of diabetes mellitus and other categories of glucose intolerance. *Diabetes*. 1979;28:1039–1057.
2. The Expert Committee on the Diagnosis and Classification of Diabetes Mellitus. Report of the expert committee on the diagnosis and classification of diabetes mellitus. *Diabetes Care*. 2008;31(Suppl 1):S55–S60.
3. Diabetes Prevention Program Research Group. Reduction in the incidence of type 2 diabetes with lifestyle intervention or metformin. *N Engl J Med*. 2002;346:393–403.
4. Tuomilehto J, Lindstrom J, Eriksson JG, et al. Prevention of type 2 diabetes mellitus by changes in lifestyle among subjects with impaired glucose tolerance. *N Engl J Med*. 2001;344:1343–1350.
5. Berkowitz K, Peters R, Kjos SL, et al. Effect of troglitazone on insulin sensitivity and pancreatic beta-cell function in women at high risk for NIDDM. *Diabetes*. 1996;11:1572–1579.
6. Scheen AJ, Ernest P. The xenical in the prevention of diabetes in obese subjects (XENDOS) trial. *Diabetes Metab*. 2002;28: 437–445.
7. DREAM (Diabetes Reduction Assessment with ramipril and rosiglitazone Medication) Trial Investigators. Effect of rosiglitazone on the frequency of diabetes in patients with impaired glucose tolerance or impaired fasting glucose: a randomized controlled trial. *Lancet*. 2006;368:1096–1105.

8. Atkinson MA, Maclaren NK. The pathogenesis of insulin dependent diabetes. *N Engl J Med.* 1994;331:1428–1436.

9. Kaufman D, Erlander M, Clare-Salzler M, Atkinson M, Maclaren N, Tobin A. Autoimmunity to two forms of glutamate decarboxylase in insulin-dependent mellitus. *J Clin Invest.* 1992;89:283–292.

10. Myers MA, Rabin DU, Rowley MJ. Pancreatic islet cell cytoplasmic antibody in diabetes is represented by antibodies to islet cell antigen 512 and glutamic acid decarboxylase. *Diabetes.* 1995;44:1290–1295.

11. Lan MS, Wasserfall C, Maclaren NK, Notkins AL. IA-2, a transmembrane protein of the protein tyrosine phosphatase family, is a major autoantigen in insulin-dependent diabetes mellitus. *Proc Natl Acad Sci USA.* 1996;93:6367–6370.

12. Lu J, Li Q, Xie H, et al. Identification of a second transmembrane protein tyrosine phosphatase, IA-2α, as an autoantigen in insulin-dependent diabetes mellitus: precursor of the 37-kDa tryptic fragment. *Proc Natl Acad Sci USA.* 1996;93:2307–2311.

13. Huang W, Connor E, DelaRosa T, et al. Although DR3-DQB1* may be associated with multiple component diseases of the autoimmune polyglandular syndromes, the human leukocyte antigen DR4-DQB1I0302 haplotype is implicated only in beta cell autoimmunity. *J Clin Endocrinol Metab.* 1996;81:1–5.

14. Landon-Olson M. Latent autoimmune diabetes in adults. *Ann NY Acad Sci.* 2002;958:112–116.

15. Palmer JP, Hampe CS, Chiu H, Goel A, Brooks-Worrell BM. Is latent autoimmune diabetes in adults distinct from type 1 diabetes or just type 1 diabetes at an older age?. *Diabetes.* 2005;54(Suppl 2):S62–S67.

16. Zimmet PZ, Tuomi T, Mackay R, et al. Latent autoimmune diabetes mellitus in adults (LADA): the role of antibodies to glutamic acid decarboxylase in diagnosis and prediction of insulin dependency. *Diabetes Med.* 1994;11:299–303.

17. Banerji M, Lebovitz H. Insulin sensitive and insulin resistant variants in IDDM. *Diabetes.* 1989;38:784–792.

18. Fajans SS, Bell GI, Polonsky KS. Molecular mechanisms and clinical pathophysiology of maturity-onset diabetes of the young. *N Engl J Med.* 2001;345:971–980.

19. Hattersley AT, Ashcroft FM. Activating mutations in Kir6.2 and neonatal diabetes: new clinical syndromes, new scientific insights, and new therapy. *Diabetes.* 2005;54:2503–2513.

20. Flanagan SE, Edghill EL, Gloyn AL, Ellard S, Hattersley AT. Mutations in KCNJ11, which encodes Kir6.2, are a common cause of diabetes diagnosed in the first 6 months of life, with the phenotype determined by genotype. *Diabetologia.* 2006;49: 1190–1197.

21. Gloyn AL, Pearson ER, Antcliff JF, et al. Activating mutations in the gene encoding the ATP-sensitive potassium-channel subunit Kir6.2 and permanent neonatal diabetes. *N Engl J Med.* 2004;350:1838–1849.

22. Pearson ER, Flechtner I, Njolstad PR, et al. Switching from insulin to oral sulfonylureas in patients with diabetes due to Kir6.2 mutations. *N Engl J Med.* 2006;355:467–477.

23. Kadowaki T, Kadowaki H, Mori Y, et al. A subtype of diabetes mellitus associated with a mutation of mitochondrial DNA. *N Engl J Med.* 1994;330:962–968.

24. Gruppuso PA, Gorden P, Kahn CR, Cornblath M, Zeller WP, Schwartz R. Familial hyperproinsulinemia due to a proposed defect in conversion of proinsulin to insulin. *N Engl J Med.* 1984;311:629–634.

25. Given BD, Mako ME, Tager HS, et al. Diabetes due to secretion of an abnormal insulin. *N Engl J Med.* 1980;302:129–135.

26. Taylor SI. Lilly lecture: molecular mechanisms of insulin resistance: lessons from patients with mutations in the insulin-receptor gene. *Diabetes.* 1992;41:1473–1490.

27. Kahn CR, Flier JS, Bar RS, et al. The syndromes of insulin resistance and acanthosis nigricans. *N Engl J Med.* 1976;294: 739–745.

28. Dunaif A, Segal KR, Shelley DR, Green G, Dobrjansky A, Licholai T. Evidence for distinctive and intrinsic defects in insulin action in polycystic ovary syndrome. *Diabetes.* 1992;41:1257–1266.

29. Karjalainen J, Knip M, Hyoty H, et al. Relationship between serum insulin antibodies, islet cell antibodies and Coxsackie-B4 and mumps virus-specific antibodies at the clinical manifestation of type I (insulin-dependent) diabetes. *Diabetologia.* 1988;31:146–152.

30. Pak CY, Eun H, McArthur RG, Yoon J. Association of cytomegalovirus infection with autoimmune type 1 diabetes. *Lancet.* 1988;2:1–4.

31. Hui J, Sud A, Farrell GC, et al. Insulin resistance is associated with chronic hepatitis C and virus infection fibrosis progression. *Gastroenterology.* 2003;125:1695–1704.

32. Mehta S, Brancati F, Sulkowski M, Strathdee S, Szklo M, Thomas D. Prevalence of type 2 diabetes mellitus among persons with hepatitis C virus infection in the United States. *Ann Intern Med.* 2000;133:592–599.

33. Engelgau MM, Herman WH, Smith PJ, German RR, Aubert RE. The epidemiology of diabetes and pregnancy in the U.S., 1988. *Diabetes Care.* 1995;18:1029–1033.

34. Magee MS, Walden CE, Benedetti TJ. Influence of diagnostic criteria on the incidence of gestational diabetes and perinatal morbidity. *JAMA.* 1993;269:609–615.

35. Langer O, Rodriguez DA, Xenakis EMJ, McFarland MB, Berkus MD, Arrendondo F. Intensified versus conventional management of gestational diabetes. *Am J Obstet Gynecol.* 1994;170:1036–1047.

36. HAPO Study Cooperative Research Group. The hyperglycemia and adverse pregnancy outcome (HAPO) study. *Int J Gynaecol Obstet.* 2002;78:69–77.

37. American Diabetes Association. Tests of glycemia in diabetes (Position Statement). *Diabetes Care.* 2001;24(Suppl 1):S80–S82.

38. Engelgau MM, Thompson TJ, Herman WH, et al. Comparison of fasting and 2-hour glucose and HbA$_{1c}$ levels for diagnosing diabetes: diagnostic criteria and performance revisited. *Diabetes Care.* 1997;20:785–791.

39. McCance DR, Hanson RL, Charles MA, et al. Comparison of tests for glycated haemoglobin and fasting and two hour plasma glucose concentrations as diagnostic methods for diabetes. *Brit Med J.* 1994;308:1323–1328.
40. Consensus Committee. Consensus statement on the worldwide standardization of the HbA$_{1c}$ measurement. *Diabetologia.* 2007;50:2042–2043.
41. Barrett-Connor E, Wingard DL. HbA1c levels predict mortality across population ranges. *Brit Med J.* 2001;322:5–6.
42. Harris MI, Hadden WC, Knowler WC, Bennett PH. Prevalence of diabetes and impaired glucose tolerance and plasma glucose levels in the U.S. population aged 20–74 yr. *Diabetes.* 1987;36:523–534.
43. The Expert Committee on the Diagnosis and Classification of Diabetes Mellitus. Report of the expert committee on the diagnosis and classification of diabetes mellitus. *Diabetes Care.* 1997;20:1183–1197.
44. Tirosh A. Normal fasting glucose levels and type 2 diabetes in young men. *N Engl J Med.* 2005;353:1454.
45. Expert Panel on Detection, Evaluation, and Treatment of High Blood Cholesterol in Adults. Executive summary of the third report of the National Cholesterol Education Program (NCEP) expert panel on detection, evaluation, and treatment of high blood cholesterol in adults (Adult Treatment Panel III). *JAMA.* 2001;285:2486–2497.
46. Klein R. Hyperglycemia and microvascular and macrovascular disease in diabetes. *Diabetes Care.* 1995;18:258–268.

Chapter 8
Epidemiology

Shadi Chamany and Bahman P. Tabaei

Introduction

Diabetes is epidemic and its increasing prevalence affects all aspects of society. While some populations are at higher risk for diabetes and may be more prone to the complications of diabetes, this is a disease that has no boundaries and can affect anyone at any point in one's lifetime. The growing burden of diabetes in the United States mirrors that which is occurring around the world and will lead to an increasing financial burden from not only direct costs to society but indirect costs, including overall health status of individuals.

This chapter reviews the concepts of diabetes epidemiology including prevalence and incidence as well as risk factors and determinants of diabetes. Prevalence is defined as the number of persons in a given population affected by a disease at a specific time divided by the number of persons in the given population at that time and is a measure of burden of disease in a population. Incidence is the number of new cases of disease that occur in a given population over a specific period of time and represents the rate at which a population develops disease.

Types of Diabetes

There are two main types of diabetes: type 1, which accounts for 5–10% of cases, and type 2, which accounts for 90–95%. Gestational diabetes and other forms related to pancreatic disease, endocrine disorders, drugs, and genetic mutations make up a small percent of all cases.

Risk Factors

Race, age, family history, environment, and genetics all play a role in type 1 diabetes. The incidence of type 1 diabetes is higher among non-Hispanic whites compared with other racial and ethnic groups.[1] While type 1 diabetes can develop at any age and as many as 40% of people who develop type 1 diabetes are over 30 years of age at diagnosis,[2] the peak incidence is near puberty. The risk of type 1 diabetes in the offspring or a non-twin sibling of an individual with type 1 diabetes is 1–15% and concordance between identical twins is 36%. Environmental factors such as exposure to cow's milk, Coxsackie B virus, human cytomegalovirus, and measles have been considered to increase the risk of type 1 diabetes. Association of HLA class antigens, such as the DR and DQ types, with increased risk of type 1 diabetes has been demonstrated in a variety of populations around the world.[1]

Race, age, and family history are also important risk factors for individuals with type 2 diabetes as are certain lifestyle behaviors and co-morbid conditions (Table 8.1).[3] Certain risk factors, like hypertension, low

S. Chamany (✉)
New York City Department of Health and Mental Hygiene, New York, NY, USA
e-mail: schamany@health.nyc.gov

L. Poretsky (ed.), *Principles of Diabetes Mellitus*, DOI 10.1007/978-0-387-09841-8_8,
© Springer Science+Business Media, LLC 2010

Table 8.1 Risk factors for type 2 diabetes

Age $\geq$ 45 years
Obesity (BMI $\geq$ 25 kg/m^2)^a
Family history of diabetes (i.e., parents or siblings with diabetes)
Habitual physical inactivity
Race/ethnicity (i.e., African-Americans, Hispanic Americans, Native Americans, Asian Americans, and Pacific Islanders)
Previously identified impaired fasting glucose or impaired glucose tolerance
History of gestational diabetes or delivery of a baby weighing > 9 lb
Hypertension ($\geq$ 140/90 mmHg in adults)
HDL cholesterol $\leq$ 35 mg/dl (0.90 mmol/l) and/or a triglyceride level of $\geq$ 250 mg/dl (2.82 mmol/l)
Polycystic ovarian syndrome
History of vascular disease

^{a}May not be correct for all ethnic groups.
Source: Data from American Diabetes Association.[3]

high-density lipoprotein, and high triglycerides, are associated risk factors but not necessarily causal. Increasing prevalence of obesity is one of the most important factors to consider as it is closely linked to increasing prevalence of type 2 diabetes. In the United States, surveys have found that for every 1 kg increase in weight, there is a 4.5–9.0% increase in the risk of incident diabetes.[4,5] Self-reported diabetes was found to be 1.6 times more prevalent among overweight persons [body mass index (BMI) 25–29.9 kg/m^2] compared with normal weight persons (BMI 18.5–24.9 kg/m^2), 3.4 times more prevalent among obese persons (BMI 30–39.9 kg/m^2), and 7.4 times more prevalent among very obese persons (BMI $\geq$ 40 kg/m^2).[6] Several analyses suggest that the relationship between race and ethnicity and diabetes prevalence is not solely based on genetic predisposition but rather a complex web of social factors which are more prevalent in certain racial and ethnic groups like lower income and education level. These factors independently confer a higher risk of obesity and diabetes.[5–10]

Global Burden of Disease

In 2000, the estimated prevalence of diabetes among adults was 2.8%, or 171 million people. The prevalence of diabetes is expected to increase to 4.4%, or 366 million people, by 2030[11,12] (Table 8.2). This estimate is based on the changing demographics of the population over time and assumes that obesity and physical activity prevalence remain constant over time; therefore, it likely underestimates future burden. In absolute numbers, India is and will continue to be the country with the most individuals living with diabetes, projected in 2030 to have nearly 80 million people with diabetes (Table 8.3). The greatest increases in diabetes prevalence will be seen in developing countries where a greater proportion of individuals with diabetes are 45–64 years of age; thus, persons with diabetes will be increasingly younger over time (Fig. 8.1). Overall, diabetes prevalence is higher in men but because diabetes is more prevalent with increasing age and women live longer than men, there are more women with diabetes than men.[11] The estimated number of incident cases of diabetes worldwide was 11.6 million cases in 2002.[13] However, reliable data on global incidence rates of diabetes exist only for those $\leq$ 14 years of age through the World Health Organization's Multinational Project for Childhood Diabetes (DiaMOND) which began in 1990. There is a wide range in incidence rates across countries, as low as 0.1/100,000 in China and as high as 40.9/100,000 in Finland (Fig. 8.2). The average annual increase in incidence between 1990 and 1999 was 2.8%. This increase was seen in most continents except Central America and the West Indies, both of which experienced annual decreases of 3.6%.[14] The prevalence of type 1 diabetes in children $\leq$ 14 years of age worldwide was 0.02% in 2003, or 440,000, with the Southeast Asian region having the highest prevalence followed by the European region.[15]

Table 8.2   Number of individuals with diabetes by World Health Organization (WHO) Region

Region	2000	2030
African region	7,020,000	18,234,000
Eastern Mediterranean	15,188,000	42,600,000
Region of the Americas	33,016,000	66,812,000
European	33,332,000	47,973,000
Southeast Asia	46,903,000	119,541,000
Western Pacific	35,771,000	71,050,100
Total	171,230,000	366,210,100

Source: Data from World Health Organization.[12]

Table 8.3   List of countries with highest numbers of estimated cases of diabetes for 2000 and 2030

	2000		2030	
Ranking	Country	People with diabetes (millions)	Country	People with diabetes (millions)
1	India	31.7	India	79.4
2	China	20.8	China	42.3
3	United States	17.7	United States	30.3
4	Indonesia	8.4	Indonesia	21.3
5	Japan	6.8	Pakistan	13.9
6	Pakistan	5.2	Brazil	11.3
7	Russian Federation	4.6	Bangladesh	11.1
8	Brazil	4.6	Japan	8.9
9	Italy	4.3	Philippines	7.8
10	Bangladesh	3.2	Egypt	6.7

Source: Data from Wild S, Roglic G, Greene A, et al.[11]

Burden of Diabetes in the United States of America

The major sources of information regarding the prevalence and incidence of diabetes in the United States are national surveys. The National Health Interview Survey (NHIS) and the Behavioral Risk Factor Surveillance System (BRFSS) assess diagnosed diabetes, and the National Health and Nutrition Examination Survey (NHANES) assesses diagnosed and undiagnosed diabetes as well as impaired fasting glucose and glucose tolerance. SEARCH for Diabetes in Youth is a multi-center study of diabetes in children and youth which began in 2000.

Prevalence of Self-Reported Diabetes

The prevalence of diabetes has been increasing over the past several decades. In 1980, 2.5% of the entire US population, or 5.6 million, reported having diabetes. In 2006, the prevalence had increased by 132% to 5.8%, or 16.8 million[16] (Fig. 8.3). A small proportion of people with diabetes are less than 20 years of age.[17] A number of factors are suspected to have contributed to this increase: improvements in diabetes care leading to fewer premature deaths, increased screening for diabetes, a shift in the demographic characteristics of the US population with a greater proportion of high-risk racial and ethnic groups, increased prevalence of obesity, the change in the diagnostic threshold from 140 to 126 mg/dl in 1997,[18] and the aging of the population. The latter two factors, while important, are the least likely to be affecting the prevalence since the slope of the increase has remained the same since 1997 and age-adjusted prevalence across these same time periods shows a similar increase.

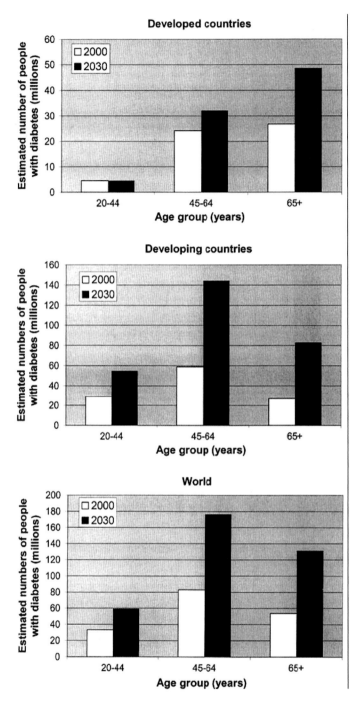

Fig. 8.1 Number of adults with diabetes by age group, year, and country. From Wild S, Roglic G, Greene A, et al. [11] by permission of *Diabetes Care*

In 1995, none of the US states reported having an obesity prevalence of $\geq 20\%$; 10 years later, in 2005, all US states except five reported having an obesity prevalence of $\geq 20\%$ (Fig. 8.4) for an overall prevalence of 24%.[19] The prevalence of measured obesity in NHANES 2005–2006 was 34% as opposed to a lower self-reported obesity from BRFSS.[20] The overall prevalence of obesity among children from birth to 19 years of

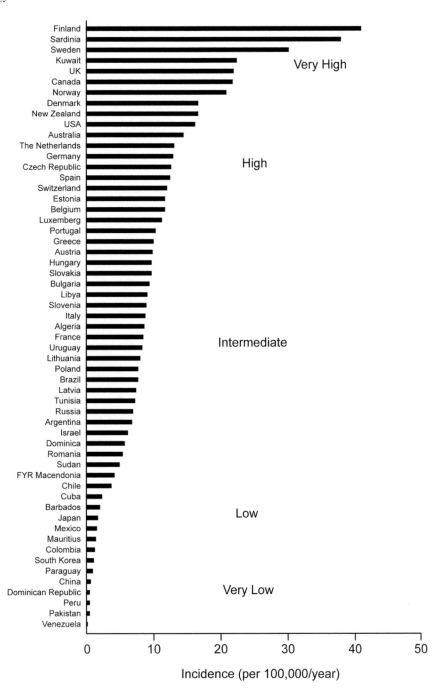

Fig. 8.2 Geographic variation in type 1 diabetes incidence. From DiaMOND Project Group[14] by permission of Diabetic Med.

age was 10–15% in 1999–2000. This had increased since 1988, most prominently among non-Hispanic black and Mexican American adolescents 12–19 years of age, with increases of at least 10% points.[21] Any continuing increases in obesity prevalence will be met with a concomitant increase in diabetes prevalence, including an increased prevalence of type 2 diabetes in children. While the prevalence of diabetes in US children is low in comparison to adults, 0.18%, and is predominately driven by the prevalence of type 1 diabetes, the proportion of type 2 diabetes among cases of newly diagnosed diabetes in children < 20 years of age is not insignificant.

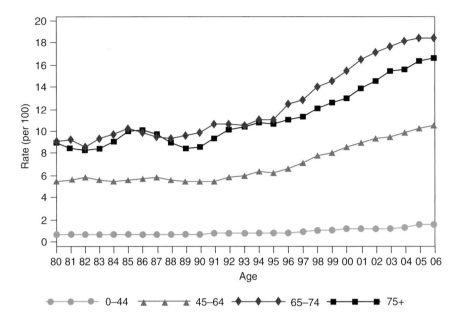

Fig. 8.3 Prevalence of diagnosed diabetes by age, United States, 1980–2006. From Centers for Disease Control and Prevention: National Center for Health Statistics[16]

Overall, type 2 diabetes accounts for 22% of all new cases of diabetes in persons less than 20 years of age, with Asian/Pacific Islanders and American Indian youth 10–19 years of age having much higher proportions, 70 and 86%, respectively.[22] This is consistent with a previous review of population-based case series and clinic-based studies in North American children that found that 8–45% of new cases of diabetes in children are type 2 diabetes.[23]

In addition to varying risk due to weight status, diabetes prevalence differs widely across age and racial/ethnic groups. NHANES 1999–2002 found the overall prevalence of self-reported diabetes to be 6.5%, or 13.5 million adults, with the prevalence being twice as high in non-Hispanic blacks and Mexican Americans compared with non-Hispanic whites.[24] Native Americans are also at high risk for diabetes, particularly the Pima Indians who in 1975 already had a prevalence of diabetes of 13.7%.[25] NHANES prevalence increased with increasing age: the prevalence was 1.7% among 20–39 year old, 6.6% among 40–59 year old, and 15.1% among those 60 years of age and older. The prevalence among men was slightly higher than that among women only in non-Hispanic whites.[24] Lower income and educational status have also been associated with higher prevalence of diabetes, with lower income and lower educational status individuals having 1.5 to 2 times the prevalence of diabetes compared to those with higher income and higher educational status.[5–10]

Prevalence of Undiagnosed Diabetes

This prevalence is ascertained by using a combination of negative self-reported history of diabetes and an elevated fasting plasma glucose ($\geq$ 126 mg/dl) or an abnormal oral glucose tolerance test value ($\geq$ 200 mg/dl at 2 h). Using NHANES 1999–2002, the prevalence of undiagnosed diabetes was 2.8%, or 5.8 million adults. Prevalence of undiagnosed diabetes did not differ by race and ethnicity when age-standardized. As with diagnosed diabetes, the prevalence of undiagnosed diabetes increased with increasing age: the prevalence was 0.7% among 20–39 year old, 3.3% among 40–59 year old, and 5.8% among those 60 years of age and older. Men had a higher prevalence of undiagnosed diabetes compared with women (3.1% vs. 2.1%) but this difference was seen only in the total population and non-Hispanic whites.[24]

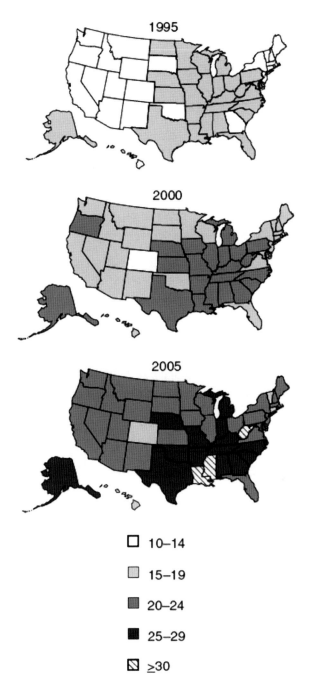

Fig. 8.4 Prevalence of obesity among adults, 1995, 2000, and 2005. From Centers for Disease Control and Prevntion[19]

One major difference between diagnosed and undiagnosed diabetes is that the overall prevalence of undiagnosed diabetes has not increased significantly over time. Between 1976–1980 and 1999–2000, the prevalence of diagnosed diabetes increased significantly from 3.3 to 5.8%, whereas the prevalence of undiagnosed diabetes remained the same between 2.0 and 2.4%. This corresponds to an increase in the proportion of all diabetes cases that are diagnosed from 62.3% in 1976 to 70.7% in 2000, which was most concentrated in persons with a BMI ≥ 35 kg/m^2.[26]

Prevalence of Impaired Fasting Glucose and Impaired Glucose Tolerance

The presence of impaired fasting glucose (IFG) and impaired glucose tolerance (IGT) increases future risk of diabetes.[27] Recent estimates from NHANES 1999–2002 indicate that among adults aged ≥ 20 years, the prevalence of IFG was 26.0%, or 54 million individuals.[24] The overall standardized prevalence in non-Hispanic blacks was lower than the prevalence in non-Hispanic whites and Hispanics (17.7% vs. 26.1% and 31.6%, respectively). As with diagnosed and undiagnosed diabetes, the prevalence of IFG increased with age: the prevalence was 15.9% among 20–39-year old, 29.9% among 40–59-year old, 37.5% among 40–59-year old, and 39.1% among those 60 years of age and older. Men had higher prevalence of IFG compared with women (32.6% vs. 20.0%) and the prevalence differed significantly between racial and ethnic groups. As with undiagnosed diabetes, the overall prevalence of IFG has not increased significantly over time. Between 1988–1994 and 1999–2002, the overall prevalence of IFG was stable (from 25.5 to 26.0%).[24]

Data from NHANES 1988–1994 show that among adults aged 40–74 years, the prevalence of IGT was 15.8%. The prevalence rates were similar for both sexes in each racial and ethnic group. The overall standardized prevalence in non-Hispanic blacks (14.0%) was lower than that in non-Hispanic whites (15.3%) and Hispanics (20.2%). The prevalence of IGT increased with age for all sex and racial and ethnic groups. As with undiagnosed diabetes and IFG, the overall prevalence of IGT has not increased significantly over time. Between 1976–1980 and 1988–1994, the overall prevalence of IGT was stable (15.6%).[28]

Incidence of Diabetes

In 2003, the incidence of diabetes was 6.9 per 1000 adults, or 1,330,000 adults. This was an increase of 41% from 1997 when the incidence was 4.9 per 1000 adults. Incidence varied by age, race/ethnicity, and weight status. The highest incidence was in older age groups: 2.5 per 1000 adults 18–44 year of age; 11.2 per 1000 adults 45–64 years of age; and 16.8 per 1000 adults 65–79 years of age. Non-Hispanic blacks and Hispanics had a higher incidence, 9.9 and 9.1 per 1000, respectively, than whites, 6.6 per 1000. While obesity prevalence increased in all individuals during this time period, incident cases in 2003 were more likely to be obese than incident cases in 1997, with corresponding incidence rates of 17.8 per 1000 among those who were obese compared with 1.9 per 1000 among normal weight individuals.[29]

The incidence of diabetes in children <20 years of age in the United States varies depending on the population studied. In SEARCH, the incidence is 24.3 cases per 100,000, with non-Hispanic whites being disproportionately affected. Females and males have similar incidence and the peak incidence occurs between the ages of 10 and 14.[22] Studies in the United States[30] and worldwide[14] demonstrate increasing incidence among children as well. It is estimated that approximately 15,000 and 65,000 children develop type 1 diabetes per year in the United States and worldwide, respectively.[15]

Gestational Diabetes

Gestational diabetes (GDM) affects 1–14% of pregnancies in the United States each year, resulting in approximately 135,000 cases annually.[31–33] While glucose tolerance in a vast majority of women diagnosed with GDM returns to normal after delivery, 47% of these women go on to develop type 2 diabetes within 5 years,[34] although a systematic review found this range to be from 3 to 70% depending on the population.[35] Risk factors for GDM are previous pregnancy with GDM, older maternal age, family history of diabetes, and obesity.[31,33,36] Non-Hispanic whites have the lowest prevalence of GDM compared with non-Hispanic blacks, Hispanics, and Asians, with Asian women having nearly double the prevalence of non-Hispanic black and Hispanic women.[37,38] Recurrence of GDM is common and ranges from 30 to 84% depending on the type of population studied.[39–41] The incidence of gestational diabetes, like type 1 and type 2, has been increasing over time. Since 1990, several studies have demonstrated a 46–100% increase in incidence, with Asian women experiencing the greatest increases compared with other racial/ethnic groups.[37,38]

Mortality

Diabetes was the sixth leading cause of death in the United States in 2004.[42] Individuals with diabetes have twice the all-cause mortality rate and 2–4 times the cardiovascular disease mortality rate of individuals without diabetes.[43,44] The majority of deaths in individuals with type 1 diabetes occur in middle and late adulthood. In the early years after diagnosis, acute coma is the leading cause of death. Renal disease is the most common cause of death in the middle years, and after 30 years of diagnosis, two-thirds of deaths result from cardiovascular disease.[45] The leading causes of death in individuals with type 2 diabetes are diseases of the heart (55%), diabetes (13%), malignant neoplasms (13%), and cerebrovascular disease (10%).[46] Life expectancy of persons with diabetes aged 55–74 years is on average 4–8 years less than that of persons without diabetes.[43]

Summary

The prevalence and incidence of diabetes is increasing worldwide and in the United States. It is estimated that over 300 million persons will have diabetes by the year 2030. The long-term impact of this growing burden is evidenced in models that estimate that one in three children born in the United States in the year 2000 will develop diabetes in their lifetime.[47] With this growing number of individuals who will develop diabetes, the costs that society will bear in direct medical costs, decreased quality of life, and years of life lost will be immense, disproportionately affecting developing countries and racial and ethnic groups most at risk for diabetes. While managing diabetes and preventing its complications are critical to improving the life of those with diabetes, we must also work to prevent diabetes through individual and community interventions that will support those at risk for obesity and diabetes.

Internet Sites

American Diabetes Association – www.diabetes.org
Centers for Disease Control and Prevention – www.cdc.gov/diabetes; www.cdc.gov/nchs
Juvenile Diabetes Foundation International – www.jdfcure.org
International Diabetes Federation – www.idf.orgorg
National Diabetes Education Program – www.ndep.nih.gov
National Institute of Diabetes and Digestive and Kidney Disease of the National Institutes of Health – www.niddk.nih.gov
SEARCH for Diabetes in Youth – www.searchfordiabetes.org
World Health Organization – www.who.int; www.who.int/diabetes/facts

References

1. Dorman JS, McCarthy BJ, O'Leary LA, et al. Risk factors for insulin-dependent diabetes. In: Harris MO, Cowie CC, Stern MP, Boyko EJ, Reiber GE, Bennett PH eds. *Diabetes in America*. Baltimore, MD: National Institutes of Health; 1995:165–178.
2. Mølbak AC, Christau B, Marner B, et al. Incidence of insulin dependent diabetes mellitus in age groups over 30 years in Denmark. *Diabet Med*. 1994;11:650–655.
3. American Diabetes Association. Screening for type 2 diabetes. *Diabetes Care*. 2004;27:S11–S14.
4. Ford ES, Williamson DF, Simin L. Weight change and diabetes incidence: findings from a national cohort of US adults. *Am J Epidemiol*. 1997;146:214–222.
5. Mokdad AH, Ford ES, Bowman BA, et al. Diabetes trends in the US:1990–1998. *Diabetes Care*. 2000;23:1278–1283.
6. Mokdad AH, Ford ES, Bowman BA, et al. Prevalence of obesity, diabetes, and obesity-related health risk factors, 2001. *J Am Med Assoc*. 2003;289:76–79.
7. Robbins JM, Vaccarino V, Zhang H, et al. Excess type 2 diabetes in African-American women and men aged 40–74 and socioeconomic status: evidence from the Third National Health and Nutrition Examination Survey. *J Epidemiol Community Health*. 2000;54:839–845.

8. Annis AM, Caulder MS, Cook ML, et al. Family history, diabetes, and other demographic and risk factors among participants of the National Health and Nutrition Examination Survey 1999–2002. *Prev Chronic Dis.* 2005;2: 1–12.

9. Signorello LB, Schlundt DG, Cohen SS, et al. Comparing diabetes prevalence between African Americans and whiles of similar socioeconomic status. *AJPH.* 2007;97:2260–2267.

10. Paeratakul S, Lovejoy JC, Ryan DH, et al. The relation of gender, race, and socioeconomic status to obesity and obesity comorbidities in a sample of US adult. *Int J Obesity.* 2002;26:1205–1210.

11. Wild S, Roglic G, Greene A, et al. Global prevalence of diabetes: estimates for the year 2000 and projections for 2030. *Diabetes Care.* 2004;27:1047–1053.

12. World Health Organization. Diabetes Programme Facts and Figures. Available on-line at http://www. who.int/diabetes/facts/world_figures/en/. Accessed December 17, 2007.

13. Revised global burden of disease (GBD) 2002 estimates. Incidence, prevalence, mortality, YLL, YLD, and DALYs by sex, cause and region, estimates for 2002 as reported in the World Health Report 2004. Available online at: http://www.who.int/healthinfo/bodgbd2002revised/en/print.html. Accessed April 16, 2008.

14. DiaMOND Project Group. Incidence and trends in childhood type 1 diabetes worldwide 1990–1999. *Diabet Med.* 2006;23: 857–866.

15. International Diabetes Federation. Diabetes Atlas 3rd Edition: Diabetes in the young. Available at: http://www.eatlas.idf.org/index1599.html. Accessed September 29, 2009.

16. Centers for Disease Control and Prevention: Diabetes Data and Trends. Prevalence of Diabetes. Available online at: http://www.cdc.gov/diabetes/statistics/prevalence_national.htm. Accessed September 29, 2009.

17. Centers for Disease Control and Prevention. National diabetes fact sheet: general information and national estimates on diabetes in the United States, 2007. Atlanta, GA: U.S. Department of Health and Human Services, Center for Disease Control and Prevention, 2008. Available online at: http://www.cdc.gov/diabetes/pubs/ndfs_2007.pdf. Accessed September 29, 2009.

18. Expert Committee on the Diagnosis and Classification of Diabetes Mellitus. Report of the Expert Committee on Diagnosis and Classification of Diabetes Mellitus. *Diabetes Care.* 1997;20:1183–1197.

19. Centers for Disease Control and Prevention. State-specific prevalence of obesity among adults—United States 2005. *MMWR.* 2006;55:985–988.

20. Ogden CL, Carroll MD, McDowell MA, et al. *Obesity Among Adults in the United States— No Change Since 2003–2004.* NCHS data brief no 1. Hyattsville, MD: National Center for Health Statistics; 2007.

21. Ogden CL, Flegal KM, Carroll MD, et al. Prevalence and trends in overweight among US children and adolescents, 1999–2000. *J Am Med Assoc.* 2002;288:1728–1732.

22. The writing group for the SEARCH for diabetes in Youth Study Group. Incidence of diabetes in youth in the United States. *J Am Med Assoc.* 2007;297:2716–2724.

23. Fagot-Campagna A, Pettitt DJ, Engelgau MM, et al. Type 2 diabetes among North American children and adolescents: an epidemiologic review and a public health perspective. *J Pediatr.* 2000;136:664–672.

24. Cowie CC, Rust KF, Byrd-Holt DD, et al. Prevalence of diabetes and impaired fasting glucose in adults in the US population 1999–2002. *Diabetes Care.* 2006;29:1263–1268.

25. Knowler WC, Bennett PH, Hamman RF, et al. Diabetes incidence and prevalence in Pima Indians: a 19-fold greater incidence than in Rochester, Minnesota. *Am J Epidemiol.* 1978;108:497–505.

26. Gregg EW, Cadwell BL, Cheng YJ, et al. Trends in the prevalence and ratio of diagnosed to undiagnosed diabetes according to obesity levels in the U.S. *Diabetes Care.* 2004;27:2806–2812.

27. Nichols GA, Hillier TA, Brown JB. Progression from newly acquired impaired fasting glucose to type 2 diabetes. *Diabetes Care.* 2007;30:228–233.

28. Harris MI, Flegal KM, Cowie CC, et al. Prevalence of diabetes, impaired fasting glucose, and impaired glucose tolerance in U.S. adults. *Diabetes Care.* 1998;21:518–524.

29. Geiss LS, Pan L, Cadwell B, et al. Changes in incidence of diabetes in US adults, 1997–2003. *Am J Prev Med.* 2006;30: 371–377.

30. Pinhas-Hamiel O, Dolan LM, Daniels SR, et al. Increased incidence of non-insulin-dependent diabetes mellitus among adolescents. *J Pediatr.* 1996;128:608–615.

31. Coustan DR. Gestational diabetes. In: Harris MO, Cowie CC, Stern MP, Boyko EJ, Reiber GE, Bennett PH eds. *Diabetes in America.* Baltimore, MD: National Institutes of Health; 1995:703–719.

32. King H. Epidemiology of glucose intolerance and gestational diabetes in women of childbearing age. *Diabetes Care.* 1998;21:B9–B13.

33. Jovanovic L, Pettitt DJ. Gestational diabetes mellitus. *J Am Med Assoc.* 2001;286:2516–2518.

34. Kjos SL, Peters RK, Xiang A, et al. Predicting future diabetes in Latino women with gestational diabetes. Utility of early postpartum glucose tolerance testing. *Diabetes.* 1995;44(5):586–591.

35. Kim C, Newton KM, Knopp RH. Gestational diabetes and the incidence of type 2 diabetes: a systematic review. *Diabetes Care.* 2002;25:1862–1868.

36. American Diabetes Association. Diagnosis and classification of diabetes mellitus. *Diabetes Care.* 2007;30:S42–S47.

37. Dabelea D, Snell-Bergeon JK, Hartsfield CL, et al. Increasing prevalence of gestational diabetes mellitus (GDM) over time and by birth cohort. *Diabetes Care.* 2005;28:579–584.

38. Thorpe LE, Berger D, Ellis JA, et al. Trends and racial/ethnic disparities in gestational diabetes among pregnant women in New York City, 1990-2001. *AJPH*. 2005;95(9):1536–1539.

39. Kim C, Berger DK, Chamany S. Recurrence of gestational diabetes mellitus: a systematic review. *Diabetes Care*. 2007;30: 1314–1319.

40. MacNeill S, Dodds L, Hamilton DC, et al. Rates and risk factors for recurrence of gestational diabetes. *Diabetes Care*. 2001;24:659–662.

41. Lee AJ, Hiscock RJ, Wein P, et al. Gestational diabetes mellitus: clinical predictors and long-term risk of developing type 2 diabetes. *Diabetes Care*. 2007;30:878–883.

42. Kung HC, Hoyert DL, Xu JQ, Murphy SL. Final data for 2005. National vital statistics reports; vol 56 no 10. Hyattsville, MD: National Center for Health Statistics 2008. Available online at: http://www.cdc.gov/nchs/data/nvsr/nvsr56/nvsr56_10.pdf. Accessed May 16, 2008.

43. Gu K, Cowie CC, Harris MI. Mortality in adults with and without diabetes in a national cohort of the US population, 1971–1993. *Diabetes Care*. 1998;21:1138–1145.

44. Gregg EW, Gu Q, Cheng YJ, et al. Mortality trends in men and women with diabetes, 1971 to 2000. *Ann Intern Med*. 2007;147:149–155.

45. Portuese E, Orchard T. Mortality in insulin-dependent diabetes. In: Harris MO, Cowie CC, Stern MP, Boyko EJ, Reiber GE, Bennett PH eds. *Diabetes in America*. Baltimore, MD: National Institutes of Health; 1995:221–232.

46. Geiss LS, Herman WH, Smith PJ. Mortality in non-insulin-dependent diabetes. In: Harris MO, Cowie CC, Stern MP, Boyko EJ, Reiber GE, Bennett PH eds. *Diabetes in America*. Baltimore, MD: National Institutes of Health; 1995:233–257.

47. Narayan KMV, Boyle JP, Thompson TJ, et al. Lifetime risk of diabetes mellitus in the United States. *J Am Med Assoc*. 2003;290:1884–1890.

Chapter 9
Diabetes in Culturally Diverse Populations: From Biology to Culture

A. Enrique Caballero

Introduction

The constantly evolving nature of modern societies has made many health-care professionals around the world face the challenge of providing optimal health care to people from various racial, ethnic, and cultural backgrounds. In the area of diabetes care, this is of particular relevance due to multiple reasons. First of all, racial and ethnic minorities continue to grow in many countries around the globe. In addition, diabetes affects populations at different rates. Furthermore, the quality of diabetes care provided to minority groups often lags behind that provided to the mainstream group.

Whereas it is true that diabetes care encompasses general guidelines and strategies that may be applicable to most patients, there is an increasing need to understand and tailor approaches at an individual level by considering factors such as race, ethnicity, socioeconomics, culture, education, health literacy level, and lifestyle preferences among many others. The lack of routine assessment and integration of these factors into the development and implementation of a comprehensive diabetes care plan may contribute to suboptimal patient outcomes.

Scientific knowledge in the field of diabetes has grown steadily for a long time. Progress in our understanding of the pathophysiology of the disease, its relationship to other comorbidities, the mechanisms that lead to the development of acute and chronic complications, and how to better treat this condition should be seen as a great accomplishment. However, the translation of this great scientific knowledge into effective and sustained patient self-care practices is far from ideal. Real-world clinical practice is full of challenges. In a general sense, a triad of elements participate in this conundrum.

First, the structure of most health-care systems limits the time and quality of clinical encounters between health-care providers and physicians who also have limited resources of all types to integrate a comprehensive diabetes care team. Second, there is a general lack of skills among us as health-care providers on how to effectively assess and integrate this complex level of non-biological factors into an effective treatment plan. In addition, patients are ultimately responsible for improving self-care practices and many personal and social challenges limit their ability to do so.

This chapter aims at providing the reader with general information on the multiple biological, psychological, social, and cultural factors that may influence the development and course of diabetes in culturally diverse populations. Identifying these elements is the first step toward developing effective clinical care and education strategies.

Race and Ethnicity

Race primarily alludes to shared genetically transmitted physical characteristics by large groups, whereas ethnicity relates to people classed according to common racial, national, tribal, religious, linguistic, or cultural origin or

A.E. Caballero (✉)
Harvard Medical School, Joslin Diabetes Center, Boston, MA 02215, USA
e-mail: enrique.caballero@joslin.harvard.edu

L. Poretsky (ed.), *Principles of Diabetes Mellitus*, DOI 10.1007/978-0-387-09841-8_9,
© Springer Science+Business Media, LLC 2010

background.[1] Therefore, ethnicity alludes to a perceived cultural distinctiveness, expressed in language, music, values, art, styles, literature, family life, religion, ritual, food, naming, public life, and material culture.

A good example to distinguish race from ethnicity is the nature of the Latino or the Hispanic population. The term *Latino* or *Hispanic* relates to ethnicity, not race. Racially speaking, Latinos have three possible genetic backgrounds: white, African-American, and/or Native Indians. These genetic backgrounds are seen in any possible combination among Latinos, creating a very heterogeneous group. However, Latinos have multiple shared linguistic, traditional, and cultural values.

Culturally Diverse Populations in the United States

Although white Americans account for three-quarters of the US population, increasing numbers of other racial and ethnic groups contribute to making many cities a true mosaic of heterogeneous cultures. The minority groups with the highest numbers of people in the United States are Latinos/Hispanics, African-Americans, American Indians, Alaska natives, Asian and Pacific Islanders, Southeast Asians, and Arabs. Most of these groups will continue to increase at a higher rate than the non-Hispanic white population. Table 9.1 shows the current and projected increase in the distribution of the US population by race and ethnicity according to the US census data.[2]

Table 9.1 Current and projected percentage of the US population by race and ethnicity from the year 2000 to 2050

Population or percent and race or Hispanic origin	2000	2010	2020	2030	2040	2050
Total	100.0	100.0	100.0	100.0	100.0	100.0
White alone	81.0	79.3	77.6	75.8	73.9	72.1
Black alone	12.7	13.1	13.5	13.9	14.3	14.6
Asian alone	3.8	4.6	5.4	6.2	7.1	8.0
All other races	2.5	3.0	3.5	4.1	4.7	5.3
Hispanic (of any race)	12.6	15.5	17.8	20.1	22.3	24.4
White alone, not Hispanic	69.4	65.1	61.3	57.5	53.7	50.1

Health-Care Disparities

Unfortunately, minority groups have lagged behind in their health care when compared to the predominant group in the United States, as it may happen in other areas around the world. The Institute of Medicine, a private, nonprofit organization that provides health policy advice under a congressional charter granted to the National Academy of Sciences, clearly demonstrated that racial/ethnic minorities have a lower quality of health care than do the mainstream white population. Some of the evaluated outcomes are pertinent to the area of diabetes care.[3] These disparities persist after controlling for level of access to care, socioeconomic status, age, stage of presentation, or existing comorbidities and can be found in multiple health-care settings (e.g., managed care, public, private, teaching, and community centers).[3] This is a complex phenomenon with multiple elements. Two different worlds, that of the patient and that of the health-care provider, usually collide in clinical encounters in a health-care system that is often not conducive to recognize and address cultural differences. Limited cultural awareness on both the health-care provider side and the patient side interferes with an effective clinical encounter. It is highly possible that health-care disparities are not the result of intentional discrimination but due to the lack of effective skills and strategies to interact with people from a different cultural background from our own. In addition, there seem to be some biological differences among culturally diverse populations that may influence the development and course of type 2 diabetes.

The Development of Type 2 Diabetes: Biology and/or Culture?

The prevalence of type 2 diabetes in racial/ethnic minorities has consistently been reported as higher than that in non-Hispanic whites.[4–7] The incidence of type 2 diabetes has also been reported as higher in racial/ethnic minorities in a 20-year follow-up of the Nurses' Health Study.[8] The prevalence of type 1 diabetes is usually about the same or even lower in some of these groups when compared to mainstream groups.

Type 2 diabetes is a heterogeneous disease that results from the combination of genetic predisposition and environmental factors (Fig. 9.1).

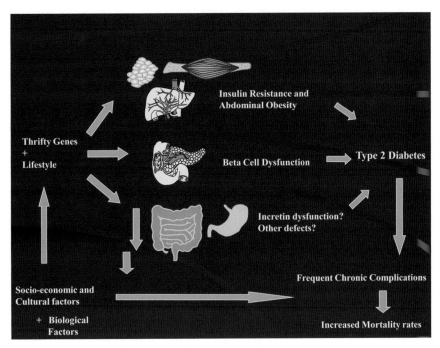

Fig. 9.1 Genes, environment, and social/cultural factors in the development and course of diabetes in culturally diverse populations

The Influence of Biology

Many studies have shown that the minority groups have a strong genetic predisposition for the development of type 2 diabetes. The "thrifty gene" theory has emerged as a possible explanation for this genetic tendency to diabetes. This theory, first proposed by J.V. Neel in 1962, suggests that populations of indigenous people who experienced alternating periods of feast and famine gradually adapted by developing a way to store fat more efficiently during periods of plenty to better survive famine.[9] It is postulated that this genetic adaptation has now become detrimental since food supplies are more constant and abundant, leading to an increased prevalence of obesity and type 2 diabetes in certain populations. Despite the significant amount of research aiming at identifying the precise nature of the "thrifty gene or genes," no uniform genes across ethnic groups have been identified to fully support this theory.[10] It is possible that the genetic basis of the thrifty genotype derives from the multiplicative effects of polymorphisms in multiple pathways such as those involved in insulin signaling, leptin activity, intermediary fat metabolism, and even peroxisome proliferator-activated receptors.[10]

Insulin Resistance/Insulin Secretion

A study in young, healthy Mexican Americans, African-Americans, and Asian-Americans showed that insulin sensitivity was lower in these groups than in whites.[11] None of these people had diabetes and had a similar body weight, reducing the influence of potential factors that could influence the data.[11] In addition, these differences have been shown in youngsters from some of these racial and ethnic minorities, such as Hispanic American and African-American children, even after adjustment for differences in body fat.[12] Furthermore, the associated compensatory responses to increased insulin resistance may differ across these ethnic groups, suggesting that the underlying pathology of diabetes may indeed vary in high-risk ethnic subpopulations.[12] It is postulated that most racial/ethnic minority groups in the United States, such as Latinos or Hispanics, African-Americans, Asian-Americans, South East Asians, American Indian, and Alaska Natives as well as Arab Americans have higher rates of insulin resistance than do the general white population.[13] In addition, it is highly possible that β-cell function in all these groups is more likely to fail over time, which, in conjunction with insulin resistance, leads to type 2 diabetes.[14–18] However, more research is required in this area to identify the precise mechanisms that account for these potential differences.

Obesity/Fat Distribution

Another interesting biological difference among racial/ethnic groups is that related to obesity and in particular, the tendency to accumulate intra-abdominal fat. Abdominal obesity plays a major role in the development of type 2 diabetes and cardiovascular disease. In particular, visceral fat is related to insulin resistance and endothelial dysfunction.[19] Abdominal obesity contributes to insulin resistance and thus to type 2 diabetes and may also impair beta cell function (Fig. 9.1).[20,21]

Obesity continues to be on the rise. The age-adjusted prevalence of obesity was 30.5% in 1999–2000 compared with 22.9% in 1988–1994 in the National Health and Nutrition Examination Survey (NHANES III) ($P < 0.001$). The prevalence of overweight also increased during this period from 55.9 to 64.5% ($P < 0.001$). Extreme obesity (BMI $\geq$ 40) also increased significantly in the population, from 2.9 to 4.7% ($P = 0.002$).[22] An increased rate of obesity was appreciated for non-Hispanic whites, non-Hispanic blacks, and Mexican Americans. Racial/ethnic groups did not differ significantly in the prevalence of obesity or overweight for men. However, among women, the prevalence of obesity and overweight was highest among non-Hispanic black women. More than half of non-Hispanic black women aged 40 years or older were obese and more than 80% were overweight.[22] The proportion of African-Americans and Non-Hispanic whites with abdominal obesity is higher than in whites.[23]

In addition, most minority groups in the United States tend to accumulate more visceral fat than do whites, at any degree of obesity.[13] In African-Americans, there seems to be a reduced content of visceral fat when compared to whites of the same BMI.[24] However, it is still unclear as to whether there is truly a consistent reduction in visceral fat content in this group. In other groups such as South East Asians, visceral fat content has been shown to be higher than that in Caucasians of similar BMI.[25] Therefore, a common clinical picture can be an individual that is not necessarily obese according to usual standards but due to the tendency to accumulate abdominal and visceral fat, insulin resistance and increased risk for type 2 diabetes and cardiovascular disease may exist.[19,20] In fact, the definition of abdominal obesity is race/ethnicity dependent. Different cutoff levels are required in each population around the world.[26]

Furthermore, obesity is also increasing among youngsters in many areas of the world. We recently reported that normoglycemic overweight Hispanic/Latino children have profound endothelial dysfunction and subclinical vascular inflammation in association with body fat and insulin resistance (Table 9.2).[27] Therefore, this high-risk group has not only a significant risk for type 2 diabetes but perhaps for cardiovascular disease as well.

Environmental or Acquired Factors

Environmental factors have undoubtedly contributed to increase in the risk for obesity and diabetes in racial/ethnic minorities (Fig. 9.1). Many of these groups are immigrants to the United States and other countries. Immigrants may have higher rate of type 2 diabetes than do mainstream groups, with multiple lifestyle

Table 9.2 Comparative metabolic and vascular function parameters in overweight vs. lean Hispanic children and adolescents. Constructed from reference[27]

Variable	Controls ($n = 17$)	At risk ($n = 21$)	P value
Age	14.18 ± 2.3	13.33 ± 2.7	0.31
Gender F/M	9/8	10/11	0.746
Percentile BMI	34.8 ± 15.4	97.1 ± 3.5	< 0.0001
Trunk fat	19 ± 5	42 ± 9	< 0.0001
Triglycerides	58.82	108.29	0.004
FPG (mg/dl)	89 ± 4	91 ± 6	0.334
HOMA-IR	2.30 ± 1.1	6.23 ± 3.9	< 0.0001
sICAM (ng/ml)	259.5 ± 60	223.2 ± 47.5	0.047
TNF-α (pg/ml)	2.57 ± 1.1	1.74 ± 0.6	0.008
hs-CRP (mg/l)	2.0	0.13	< 0.0001
PAI-1 (ng/ml)	47 ± 35.7	12 ± 5.2	< 0.0001
tPA (ng/ml)	6.1 ± 1.9	4.1 ± 0.8	0.001
Adiponectin (μg/ml)	8.7 ± 3.3	12.6 ± 5.2	0.022
WBC count ($\times 10^3$)	6.9	5.3	0.031

issues contributing to this phenomenon.[28–31] The common elements of "westernization" that increase the risk for obesity, diabetes, and related diseases include a diet higher in total calories and fat but lower in fiber and a reduced need to expend energy because of labor-saving devices. In addition, particular aspects of preferred foods and lifestyle practices in each of these groups certainly play a role in the development of diabetes and its treatment.[28–31] Cultural factors that influence some of these lifestyle aspects will be discussed in more detail in other sections of this chapter (Table 9.3).

Table 9.3 Main factors to be considered in a culturally oriented clinical encounter and/or education program in patients with diabetes mellitus from diverse racial and ethnic groups

Acculturation
Body image
Cultural awareness
Depression
Educational level
Fears
General family integration and support
Health literacy
Individual and social interaction
Judgment about the disease
Knowledge about the disease
Language
Myths
Nutritional preferences
Other forms of medicine (alternative)
Physical activity preferences
Quality of life
Religion and faith
Socioeconomic status

Diabetes-Related Complications

Unfortunately, minority populations not only develop type 2 diabetes more frequently but also exhibit higher rates of diabetes-related complications than do their white counterparts. Consistent data have emerged from multiple studies showing higher rates of retinopathy, nephropathy, peripheral vascular disease, leg amputations, and cardiovascular disease among many of these groups.[13] For some complications, like chronic kidney disease, some specific factors, such as very high rates of hypertension in African-Americans, partially explain these differences. It is still unclear whether certain biological factors consistently increase the risk of complications in minorities. However, some recent data suggest that glycemic control is particularly poor in some of these groups. The National Health and Nutrition Examination Survey study has shown higher hemoglobin A1c levels among Hispanics, represented by Mexican Americans, and in African-Americans when compared to the white population.[32] Clearly, poor glycemic control contributes to the increased risk of diabetes-related complications.

Social and Cultural Factors

Some of the most relevant social and cultural factors that influence the development and/or the course of type 2 diabetes in culturally diverse populations are listed in Table 9.3. These factors have been arranged in alphabetical order, not in order of importance. Some important factors may therefore be included in another category for simplicity. The primary purpose of the list is to guide the reader as to the multiple factors that may need to be addressed in the day-to-day management of patients with type 2 diabetes.

Acculturation

Culture refers to the behavior patterns, beliefs, arts, and all other products of human work and thought, as expressed in a particular community.[1] *Acculturation* refers to the adoption of some specific elements of one culture by a different cultural group.[1] For immigrants to the United States, it relates to the integration of multiple preferences and behaviors from mainstream culture. No uniform instrument to assess acculturation exists. Self-identification, behavior, and language skills are common elements that may allow classification of individuals into the above categories. Many reports consider language preference as a good estimate of the degree of acculturation of any given individual.[33] Whereas conflicting results exist in the literature as to whether high acculturation translates into better or worse health-care behaviors, some reports point to the fact that groups with low acculturation are more likely to be without a routine place for health care, have no health insurance, and have low levels of education.[34–37] These factors are clearly related to health-care outcomes. At the same time, a high acculturation level can also be associated with higher rates of DM, perhaps through the adoption of a more "diabetogenic" lifestyle, that is, by eating larger portions of foods rich in carbohydrates and fats and by becoming more sedentary.[33–37] It is also true that the acculturation process can lead to the adoption of a healthier lifestyle. Ultimately, individuals choose what behaviors and preferences to adopt. Health-care providers should openly ask patients about behaviors that they have adopted from mainstream culture.

Body Image

The concept of ideal body weight may vary among individuals within and across racial and ethnic groups. Although it would be erroneous to assume that some people prefer to be overweight, the ideal weight that people have conceptualized may be different. In some groups, like Hispanics, African-Americans, some American Indian tribes, and some Arab groups, being robust and slightly overweight has been considered equivalent to being well nourished and financially successful.[13] Children are often encouraged to "eat well" and finish their entire meal. For some groups, achieving a higher socioeconomic status translates into the possibility of eating more, not necessarily eating better. As an example, a study in African-American women with type 2 DM showed that most participants preferred a middle-to-small body size but indicated that a middle-to-large body size was healthier.[38] They also said that a large body size did result in some untoward social consequences. In a recent study in overweight African-American girls, the findings imply that perceptions of weight and healthy lifestyle behaviors are largely determined by environmental and personal influences.[39] When discussing weight-loss strategies, it is therefore crucial that clinicians ask patients about their personal goals.

Cultural Awareness

This element applies to both the patient and the health-care provider. Being aware of how our own culture influences our thoughts, beliefs, and behaviors and respects the fact that others may see the world in a completely different way is the first step toward efficient personal interactions. Cultural competence is defined by the American Medical Association as the knowledge and interpersonal skills that allow health-care providers to understand, appreciate, and work with individuals from cultures other than their own. It involves an awareness and acceptance of cultural differences, self-awareness, knowledge of the patient's culture, and adaptation of skills.

Although no randomized clinical trial has been conducted to demonstrate that diabetes control and/or complication rate are improved by a group of health-care providers with higher cultural competence compared with a group with a lower level, it seems clear that cultural competence can lead to a much more pleasant and productive health-care provider–patient interaction.[40] In the field of DM, it may be particularly relevant because disease control is greatly determined by effective lifestyle and behavior modification. The need to improve the skills of health-care providers in the area of cultural competency has been recognized more than ever before and some interesting studies are starting to emerge.[41] Several states in the United States now require physicians to obtain some annual continuing medical education credits in programs addressing cultural aspects in health care. It is anticipated that more states will join the effort to disseminate accurate information on how to improve the lives of people with DM from various cultures.

Unfortunately, many health-care providers blame the patient for not following a treatment plan. It is disappointing to hear many professionals refer to patients as *noncompliant*. Although it is true that some patients may not adhere to their treatment plan, perhaps it is more helpful to say: "I have not found the best way to interact with my patient so that some specific behavioral changes occur."

It is common to create stereotypes in clinical encounters. However, creating a stereotype about a patient based on his or her racial/ethnic or cultural background is likely to endanger the clinical encounter. It is helpful to be aware of the most common cultural aspects that may influence DM care in any group, but a productive clinical encounter must focus on a particular patient's characteristics and preferences.

On the other hand, patients also need to raise their cultural awareness. In the same way that providers need to understand patients' values and beliefs, so do patients. Although this may be a more challenging task, it may happen naturally as the result of a better and more culturally oriented interaction with health-care providers.

We all have a culture. Therefore, it is important to be able to interact with people within the same and other cultures in a respectful and efficient way. Being aware and sensitive to the impact of culture on diabetes care is the first step. Cultural competence/awareness is highly needed in diabetes care.[42]

Depression

Depression is frequently associated with diabetes. In addition, it is a powerful predictor of poor diabetes-related health outcomes.[43] Multiple factors may account for this association, including low socioeconomic status, lack of family and social support, and sense of isolation, many of which are more common in some ethnic groups, particularly those that have immigrated to the United States.[33–37] In addition, ethnicity is also related to poor glycemic control, which is related to poor clinical outcomes that may exacerbate depression.[32,44] Therefore, a vicious cycle that includes diabetes and depression is very common among patients with diabetes from culturally diverse populations. The presence of depression also influences adherence to any DM treatment plan.[44] Some immigrants to the United States may be more likely to develop stress and depression because of the need to live in, and adapt to, a completely different social and cultural environment. A recent study showed that Puerto Rican elders in Massachusetts are significantly more likely to have physical disability, depression, cognitive impairment, DM, and other chronic health conditions than are non-Hispanic white elders living in the same neighborhoods.[45] Depression is one of the most frequently missed diagnoses in clinical practice.[46] Health-care providers should become familiar with various ways of assessing the presence of depression in their patients.

Although specific scales are useful in assessing depression in specific cultural groups, some general approaches may also be useful in regular clinical encounters.[47] For instance, specific questions such as "Have you felt depressed or sad much of the time this past year?" may provide insight into whether a patient may be depressed.

The evaluation of emotional distress in the patient with diabetes is also crucial for today's effective clinical care.[48]

Educational Level

Some data show that a higher educational level may be related to better diabetes-related outcomes.[49] For instance, the association of educational level with either type 2 DM or CVD was examined in a sample of second-generation Japanese-American men living in King County, Washington. Men with a technical school education showed higher frequencies of both diseases compared with men with any college education or high-school diplomas. The association of educational level with risk of type 2 DM was not explained by other factors, such as occupation, income, diet, physical activity, weight, insulin, lipids, and lipoproteins, whereas the association with CVD was explained in part by the larger average body mass index (BMI), higher total and very-low-density lipoprotein, triglycerides, and lower high-density lipoprotein (HDL) and HDL-2 cholesterol observed in men with technical school educations compared with the other men.[49] Therefore, a low educational level may not be the direct cause of poor outcomes in patients with type 2 DM, but rather a "marker" of multiple socioeconomic and cultural factors that may influence adherence to treatment and the course of the disease.

Another study showed that lower socioeconomic and educational levels are strongly associated with being overweight or obese.[50] However, not all studies have identified educational level as a crucial element to determine responses to lifestyle modification interventions.[51]

It is recommended that health-care providers take into consideration patients' educational level when implementing any educational activity, whether in a regular clinical encounter or through a group DM education program, since it may lead to the identification of other important social and cultural factors that may influence diabetes care.

Fears

Patients may have multiple fears that may influence their adherence to a DM treatment plan. Many patients fear the presence of type 2 DM and its complications. This fear, expressed by a sense of hopelessness, may be due to lack of adequate information about the disease. On the other hand, in some patients, a sense of fear may lead to a more responsible attitude toward the disease and improve self-management behavior.[52]

Another common fear in patients with type 2 DM, particularly in some ethnic groups, is related to the consequences of medications. For instance, insulin use is considered by many as a treatment of last resort that equals the development of severe diabetes-related complications, such as going blind and ultimately dying of the disease. It is perceived as basically a death sentence and reduces patients' likelihood of following a good treatment plan.[53] This concept may be more prevalent in some groups. Our own experience in the Latino Diabetes Initiative at the Joslin Diabetes Center, Boston, Massachusetts, confirms that this fear is common among Latinos. In a recent analysis of our data, approximately, 43% of new patients to our program thought that insulin causes blindness and 25% were not sure whether this was true or not.[54] The basic implication of fear for DM care is quite obvious. Before prescribing medicine, health-care providers should openly ask patients if they have any particular fears about taking insulin or any other diabetes medication. As an anecdotal experience, a few years ago I saw a patient who, according to notes by his primary care physician, had been taking insulin for several years. When referred to us for uncontrolled DM, one of my first questions to him was: "Are you taking your insulin injections?" He openly said to me: "Claro que no, doctor!" (Of course not, doctor!) "No quiero quedarme ciego por usar la insulina" (I don't want to get blind from taking insulin!) Unfortunately, and as happens frequently with many patients, he had already developed severe complications. Both his legs were amputated within

1 year, and he died of a cardiovascular event within 2 years. A very simple question before starting a patient on insulin can be the first step to overcome this common fear to insulin.[55,56] Among Asian-Americans, the effect of substances in the body may be referred as "cold" or "hot." Sometimes, medications that produce "hot" reactions may not be well accepted. For instance, some patients may associate these reactions to those of hypoglycemia, due to the accompanying adrenergic burst. It is then imperative to ask and address these issues with the patients.

General Family Integration and Support

Although family is important for virtually all human beings, the level of closeness and dependence between family members may differ in various populations. In general, some groups such as Latinos, Arabs, Asian Indians, and others often exhibit a collective loyalty to the extended family or the group that supersedes the needs of the individual.[57] This loyalty may provide pros and cons in diabetes care. The benefit is that more members in any given family may provide support to the patient. Some reports suggest that structural togetherness in families is positively related to DM quality of life and satisfaction among patients with DM.[58,59]

The downside is that it is more difficult for some patients to make their own decisions. Nevertheless, openly offering the patient to bring along family members to the clinical encounters may be a good start to address this factor. Inviting relatives to group education activities has been reported as a successful strategy in several groups.[59]

Health Literacy

Health literacy is defined as the degree to which individuals have the capacity to obtain, process, and understand the basic health information and services they need to make appropriate health decisions. Knowing a language is not a guarantee of high health literacy, although it certainly plays a role.

Limited health literacy, common in patients with both type 1 and type 2 DM, has been associated with worse DM outcomes.[60] A particular association that may influence the development of specific DM outcomes is that of health literacy with DM self-management behaviors, as assessed in a population of patients with type 2 DM.[61] Self-management behaviors can be improved in people with low as well as high health literacy.[62] Furthermore, a recent study showed that self-efficacy was associated with self-management behaviors across Asian/Pacific Islanders, African-Americans, Latinos, and white Americans with various degrees of health literacy.[63]

Ideally, specific low-health-literacy patient education programs and materials should be developed for each racial and ethnic group.[64] Health-care providers should evaluate their patients' health literacy levels when implementing a DM education program or even when providing regular patient education materials.[65] There are various ways to evaluate health literacy. A common instrument used for this purpose is the test of functional literacy in adults.[66] The reader may want to become familiar with this instrument as a starting point to formally evaluate patients' health literacy.

Individual and Social Interaction

Every individual has a unique character and personality and different approaches to interacting with other people. There is no right or wrong about how various cultures approach this issue. Each group may just be different. For instance, many Latino patients expect to develop a warm and personal relationship with their physicians.[67] This type of patient–physician relationship would be characterized by interactions that occur at close distances and emphasize physical contact, such as handshakes, a hand on the shoulder, and even hugging under certain circumstances. Some Latino patients with DM may erroneously think that their health-care provider does not care about them if they do not experience this type of interaction. Even though health-care providers cannot easily switch behaviors as they interact with patients with diverse backgrounds and cultures, keeping in mind that certain groups prefer particular approaches may facilitate clinical encounters and help establish a more trusting and effective relationship with patients.

Judgment and Beliefs About the Disease

Every social group shares beliefs about health and illness. Groups and individuals may have a particular DM explanatory model of illness. Knowledge and understanding of these health beliefs and explanatory models are essential for effective clinical encounters and education programs. Some beliefs related to the development of DM include heredity, eating sweets, stress, emotional instability, and, sometimes, even an acute episode of fear or anxiety.

A recent study explored some health-related beliefs and experiences of African-American, Hispanic/Latino, American Indian, and among people with DM.[68] The investigators found that many participants attributed their loss of health to the modern American lifestyle, lack of confidence in the medical system, and the general lack of spirituality in modern life. Interestingly, participants recommended improvements in the areas of health care, DM education, social support, and community action that emphasized respectful and knowledgeable health-care providers, culturally responsive DM education for patients and their families, and broad-based community action as ways to improve DM care and education programs.[68]

Health-care providers should explore beliefs about the development and course of DM with their patients. A simple question to start with is: "Why in your opinion, did you develop DM?" This initial evaluation may guide the clinician on what important factors to address with that patient.[67]

Knowledge About the Disease

Patients' knowledge of DM is usually associated with self-management behaviors but not necessarily or directly associated with DM-related outcomes.[61] However, because improving self-management behaviors is likely to lead to better DM control and, hence, a lower risk of DM complications, general knowledge of DM will continue to be an important aspect of DM education programs.[69-71] Culturally oriented programs should focus on improving patients' knowledge of DM that can specifically help them improve those self-care management behaviors that may be more problematic in specific population groups.[69-71] Specific culturally oriented programs to improve self-management behaviors are necessary.

Language

The most obvious "cultural" barrier in a clinical and educational encounter is the inability to communicate in the same language. It may limit the patient's ability to ask questions, to verbalize important information and concerns, and to establish a natural and spontaneous relationship with the health-care provider. Language has been shown to affect clinical outcomes and may be a serious barrier to effective patient care.[72]

In general, patients prefer health-care providers who have a similar ethnic background. It may improve compliance and follow-up.[72] However, there is currently a pronounced discrepancy between the number of physicians who can communicate in both English and an additional language and the number of non-English-speaking patients. For instance, in 1999, Latino physicians accounted for ~3.3% of practicing physicians in the United States; however, 13.9% of the patient population is of Latino origin.[73] Therefore, the proper use of interpreters is necessary.[74] A word of caution is necessary concerning the common circumstance in which a family member acts as an interpreter during routine clinical encounters. The advantage to this scenario is that the family member may be able to provide additional helpful information to the health-care provider. The disadvantage is that the family member may not be objective about translating all information, may not put aside his or her emotional attachment to the patient, and may communicate only what he or she considers important.

Health-care providers should find the best translating option(s) for their patients. Although speaking the same language facilitates the clinician–patient interaction, other elements (e.g., trust, genuine interest, and honesty) have no language barriers.

Myths

Myths, which are generally not explicit and are usually interwoven with values and beliefs, are common in patients with DM. Such myths include those related to why DM has occurred or why it has taken a specific course. In some groups, a clear link with faith and religion is present.[67] There are many possible myths about the origin of diabetes: – that DM occurs from eating a lot of sweets, is the result of destiny, is caused by lack of faith, or is punishment for a particular action.[75] Certain myths and fears have developed in relation to insulin use, as discussed above.[67,75]

Health-care providers should ask patients about possible myths and be respectful of patients' answers. Understanding what myths patients believe can help clinicians develop specific strategies to dispel them.

Nutritional Preferences

Humans are biologically adapted to their ancestral food environment, in which foods were dispersed and energy expenditure was required to obtain them.[9,10] The modern developed world has a surplus of very accessible, inexpensive food. Unfortunately, this food is usually rich in carbohydrates and saturated fats. Minority populations in the United States have a high risk of developing type 2 DM, partly due to a strong genetic predisposition.[4–8,13] Because more people are incorporating unhealthy foods in their regular meals, eating continuously larger portions, and not engaging in regular physical activity, rates of obesity, type 2 DM, and CVD are rising.[7]

Although similarities between racial and ethnic groups exist, different groups have different food and nutritional preferences. In fact, foods may be so diverse that considerable discrepancies may exist in subgroups in each general racial/ethnic group, such as in Asians (i.e., Japanese, Chinese, Korean, Hawaiian) or Hispanics/Latinos (i.e., Caribbean, Mexican American, Central American, and South American). Food preferences even vary by country or region in each of these subgroups. For instance, food preferences in Venezuela may differ from those in Colombia, and those in the Dominican Republic may differ from those in Puerto Rico.[67]

Food is usually at the core of family and social interaction. It is certainly worthwhile addressing this aspect in detail with the patient with diabetes. Clinicians must identify local educational resources to help their patients receive culturally oriented medical nutrition therapy. Bicultural dieticians are an excellent resource for physicians. In addition, patient education materials in this important area of nutrition may be identified through national organizations such as the American Diabetes Association, the National Institutes of Health, and the National Diabetes Education Program. Some specific programs, such as the Latino Diabetes Initiative and the Asian American Initiative at Joslin Diabetes Center, can also provide some helpful information.

Other Types of Medicines (Alternative)

Many patients with DM combine alternative and traditional medicine. Alternative medicine has long been part of most cultures throughout the world. The most common forms of alternative medicine are herbs, chiropractic care, yoga, relaxation, acupuncture, ayurveda, biofeedback, chelation, energy healing, Reiki therapy, hypnosis, massage, naturopathy, and homeopathy. A recent report showed that of 2472 adults with DM included in the study, 48% used some form of alternative medicine.[76] Interestingly, this study found that the use of alternative medicine was associated with increased likelihood of receiving preventive care services and increased emergency department and primary care visits.[76] This association does not necessarily represent causality. In other words, alternative medicine use may represent a factor that leads to a more proactive health-care behavior and use of conventional medical services in adults with DM; conversely, high use of conventional medical services may lead to increased use of alternative medicine.[77] It is estimated that at least a third of patients with diabetes use some dietary supplements.[78] Information on the effect of alternative medicine on diabetes care is starting to emerge. For instance, a recent study showed that yoga may have a positive influence on BG and lipid levels after a short period of practice in some patients with diabetes.[79] Obviously, more research on alternative medicine use in patients with DM is needed. Health-care providers should not forget to ask patients if they are using any form of alternative medicine. This question should be asked in a sensitive and respectful manner so that patients do not feel threatened or embarrassed.

Physical Activity

The nationwide prevalence of leisure-time physical inactivity for adults in the United States has declined on an average of 0.6% per year during an 11-year period. Many adults continue to have minimal or no physical activity.[80] Among racial/ethnic groups, prevalence of physical inactivity was 18.4% for non-Hispanic white men, 27% for non-Hispanic black men, and 32% in Hispanic men. In women, corresponding figures were 33.9% for non-Hispanic black women, 39.6% in Hispanic women, and 21.6% in white women.[80]

Physical activity preferences may vary among racial and ethnic groups. For instance, older white Americans may prefer jogging or going to the gym; older Latinos may prefer activities such as walking or dancing.[67,81,82] When prescribing an exercise program, physicians and patients should discuss preferred physical activities to enhance continuity.

Further research is needed to identify attitudes toward, and barriers to, physical activity in specific ethnic and racial groups. This type of research may help the development of community culturally oriented programs that, in combination with the availability of accessible facilities and transportation options, may motivate people from certain racial/ethnic populations to engage in regular physical activity.

Quality of Life

Type 2 DM has significant adverse effects on health-related quality of life. The effect of DM on reducing health-related quality of life has also been evaluated and confirmed in multiethnic populations.[83,84] Some factors, such as family structure and support, may improve quality of life in patients with DM, as shown in a study of African-Americans.[59]

Although a patient's quality of life is difficult to routinely assess in clinical practice, health-care providers should try to explore how DM and its complications have affected a patient's quality of life. Quality of life clearly influences patients' behavior, receptiveness to treatment, and adherence to a treatment plan.

Religion and Faith

Religion and faith influence daily life. Religious traditions are expressions of faith in, and reverence for, specific conceptions of ultimate reality. They express one's place in, and relation to, this reality. Ultimate reality may be known as God, Allah, Atman, or Nirvana or by many other names, and it is understood and experienced differently by each religious tradition. The forms of faith and the reverence of a tradition may be expressed and experienced through sacred stories; sacred symbols and objects; sacred music, art, and dance; devotion; meditation; rituals; sacred laws; philosophy; ethics; calls to social transformation; relationship with spirits; and healing.[85]

Some of these expressions may affect the health-care arena. In DM care, a clear example of one important influence is the fasting during the daylight hours that Muslims practice during 1 month each year. This practice requires the health-care provider to show cultural sensitivity and understanding by adjusting any treatment strategies during this time.[86]

For a health-care provider to address the topic of religion and faith, two sets of skills are indispensable. The first involves cultivating self-awareness and reflecting on the components of one's own identity. The second involves learning strategies for talking with patients about this topic and for responding to what patients say.

Socioeconomic Status

Poverty influences not only the development of type 2 DM but also complications of DM.[87–89] A recent study showed that family poverty accounts for differences in diabetic amputation rates of African-Americans, Hispanic Americans, and other persons aged ≥50 years.[88] Place of birth and time in the United States are factors closely related to socioeconomic status, and these two factors may have a direct effect on specific diseases.

For instance, The Multi-Ethnic Study of Atherosclerosis, a population-based study of coronary calcification assessed through a CT scan in a large number of non-Hispanic white Americans, non-Hispanic blacks, Hispanics, and Chinese residing in the United States, found that not being born in the United States was associated with a lower prevalence of calcification in blacks and Hispanics after adjustment for age, sex, income, and education.[89] Years in the United States was positively associated with prevalence of calcification in non-US-born Chinese and non-US-born blacks. Low education was associated with a higher prevalence of calcification in white Americans but a lower prevalence of calcification in Hispanics. US birth and time in the United States were also positively associated with the extent of calcification in persons with detectable calcium.

These differences did not appear to be accounted for by smoking, BMI, LDL and HDL cholesterol, hypertension, and DM.[89] Therefore, multiple socioeconomic and acculturation factors in various racial and ethnic groups seem to be related to the development and progression of various metabolic and vascular conditions. From a practical perspective, health-care providers should always consider their patients' socioeconomic status when understanding the presence of various disease processes and when implementing any treatment plan.

Conclusions/Summary

Many clinicians around the world currently face the challenge of providing care to patients from diverse racial/ethnic populations. The main aspects of diabetes care, including general guidelines and therapeutic approaches, do not need to be distinguished by race and ethnicity. However, as we learn more about biological, medical, social, and cultural differences among patients from different populations, an increasing need to consider them into the development of a comprehensive and culturally oriented treatment plan is evident. Such an approach may result in more effective strategies to improve diabetes care to the most vulnerable populations.

References

1. Merriam-Webster OnLine Dictionary. Available at http://www.m-w.com. Accessed February 13, 2008.
2. US Census Bureau, 2004. US Interim Projections by Age, Sex, Race, and Hispanic Origin. Available at: http://www.census.gov/ipc/www/usinterimproj/. Accessed January 18, 2005.
3. Unequal Treatment Confronting Racial and Ethnic Disparities in Health Care. Institute of Medicine. Available at: www.iom.edu; 2002; Washington, DC: The National Academies Press.
4. National Diabetes Statistics. National Diabetes Information Clearing House; 2005, http://diabetes.niddk.nih.gov/dm/pubs/statistics. Accessed April 15, 2008.
5. National Health and Nutrition Examination Survey (NHANES), 1999–2002. National Center for Health Statistics, Center for Disease Control and Prevention. Available at: http://www.cdc.gov/nhcs/nhanes.htm. Accessed April 15, 2008.
6. McBean AM, Li S, Gilbertson DT, Collins AJ. Differences in diabetes prevalence, incidence and mortality among the elderly of four racial/ethnic groups: whites, blacks. Hispanics and Asians. *Diabetes Care*. 2004;27:2317–2324.
7. Mokdad AH, Ford ES, Bowman BA, et al. Diabetes trends in the US: 1990–1998. *Diabetes Care*. 2000;23:1278–1283.
8. Shai I, Jiang R, Manson JE, et al. Ethnicity, obesity and the risk of type 2 diabetes in women: a 20 year follow-up study. *Diabetes Care*. 2006;29:1585–1590.
9. Neel JV. Diabetes mellitus: a "thrifty" genotype rendered detrimental by "progress"?. *Am J Hum Genet*. 1962;14:353–362.

10. Joffe B, Zimmet P. The thrifty genotype in type 2 diabetes: an unfinished symphony moving to its finale?. *Endocrine*. 1998;9(2):139–141.
11. Chiu KC, Cohan P, Lee NP, Chuang LM. Insulin sensitivity differs among ethnic groups with a compensatory response in beta-cell function. *Diabetes Care*. 2000;23:1353–1358.
12. Goran MI, Bergman RN, Cruz ML, Watanabe R. Insulin resistance and associated compensatory responses in African-American and Hispanic children. *Diabetes Care*. 2002;25:2184–2190.
13. Caballero AE. Diabetes in minority populations. In: Kahn CR, Weir G, King GL, et al., eds. *Joslin's Diabetes Mellitus*. 14th ed. Philadelphia, PA: Lippincott Williams & Wilkins; 2005:505–524.
14. Weiss R, Dziura JD, Burgert TS, Taksali SE, Tamborlane WV, Caprio S. Ethnic differences in beta cell adaptation to insulin resistance in obese children and adolescents. *Diabetologia*. 2006;49(3):571–579.
15. Osei K, Rhinesmith S, Gaillard T, Schuster D. Impaired insulin sensitivity, insulin secretion, and glucose effectiveness predict future development of impaired glucose tolerance and type 2 diabetes in pre-diabetic African-Americans: implications for primary prevention. *Diabetes Care*. 2004;27:1439–1446.
16. Rosouli N, Spencer HJ, Rashidi AA, Elbein SC. Impact of family history of diabetes and ethnicity on beta cell function in obese, glucose-tolerant individuals. *J Clin Endocrinol Metab*. 2007;92(12):4656–4663.
17. Banerji MA. Diabetes in African Americans: unique pathophysiologic features. *Curr Diabetes Rep*. 2004;4(3):219–223.
18. Snehalatha C, Ramachandran A, Sivassankari S, Satyavani K, Vijay V. Insulin secretion and action show differences in impaired fasting glucose and in impaired glucose tolerance in Asian Indians. *Diabetes Metab Res Rev*. 2003;19(4):329–332.
19. Caballero AE. Endothelial dysfunction, inflammation, and insulin resistance: a focus on subjects at risk for type 2 diabetes. *Curr Diabetes Rep*. 2004;4:237–246.
20. Hamdy O, Porramatikul S, Al-Ozairi E. Metabolic obesity: the paradox between visceral and subcutaneous fat. *Curr Diabetes Rev*. 2006;2(4):367–373.
21. Kahn BB, Flier JS. Obesity and Insulin resistance. *J Clin Invest*. 2000;106(4):81.
22. Flegal KM, Carroll MD, Ogden CL, Johnson CL. Prevalence and trends in obesity among US adults, 1999–2000. *JAMA*. 2002;288:1723–1727.
23. Ford ES, Giles WH, Dietz WH. Prevalence of the metabolic syndrome among US adults: findings from the third National Health and Nutrition Examination Survey. *JAMA*. 2002;287:356–359.
24. Bacha F, Saad R, Gungor N, Janosky J, Arslanian SA. Obesity, regional fat distribution and syndrome X in obese black versus white adolescents: race differential in diabetogenic and atherogenic risk factors. *J Clin Endocrinol Metab*. 2003;88:2534–2540.
25. Raji A, Seely EW, Arky RA, Simonson DC. Body fat distribution and insulin resistance in healthy Asian Indians and Caucasians. *J Clin Endocrinol Metab*. 2001;86:5366–5371.
26. ww.idf.org. Ethnic specific values for waist circumference. Accessed June 17, 2007.
27. Caballero AE, Bousquet-Santos K, Robles-Osorio L, et al. Overweight Latino children and adolescents have marked endothelial dysfunction and subclinical vascular inflammation in association with excess body fat and insulin resistance. *Diabetes Care*. 2008;31(3):576–582.
28. Sing GK, Hiatt RA. Trends and disparities in socio-economic and behavioural characteristics, life expectancy, and cause-specific mortality of native-born and foreign-born populations in the United States, 1979–2003. *Int J Epideimol*. 2006;35(4):903–919.
29. Misra A, Ganda OP. Migration and its impact on adiposity and type 2 diabetes. *Nutrition*. 2007;23(9):696–708.
30. Candid LM. Obesity and diabetes in vulnerable populations: reflection on proximal and distal causes. *Ann Fam Med*. 2007;5(6):547–556.
31. Caballero AE. Diabetes in the Hispanic or Latino population: genes, environment, culture and more. *Curr Diabetes Rep*. 2005;5:217–225.
32. Boltri JM, Okosun IS, Davis-Smith M, Vogel RL. Hemoglobin A1c levels in diagnosed and undiagnosed black, Hispanic, and white persons with diabetes: results from NHANES 1999–2000. *Ethn Dis*. 2005;15(4):562–567.
33. Lara M, Gamboa C, Kahramanian MI, Morales L, Hayes Bautista DE. Acculturation and Health in the Unites States: a review of the literature and its sociopolitical context. *Annu Rev Public Health*. 2005;26:367–397.
34. Mainous AG 3rd, Majeed A, Kooopman RJ, et al. Acculturation and diabetes among Hispanics: evidence from the 1999–2002. National Health and Nutrition Examination Survey. *Public Health Rep*. 2006;121(1):60–66.
35. Kandula NR, Diez-Roux AV, Chan C, et al. Association of acculturation levels and prevalence of diabetes mellitus in the multi-ethnic study of atherosclerosis (MESA). *Diabetes Care*. 2008;31(8):1621–1628.
36. Cortes DE, Deres S, Andia J, Colon H, Robles R, Kang SY. Biculturality among Puerto Rican adults in the United States. *Am J Commun Psychol*. 1994 Oct;22(5):707–721.
37. Arcia E, Skinner M, Bailey D, Correa V. Models of acculturation and health behaviors among Latino immigrants to the US. *Soc Sci Med*. 2001;53:41–53.
38. Liburd LC, Anderson LA, Edgar T, Jack L Jr. Body size and body shape: perceptions of black women with diabetes. *Diabetes Educ*. 1999;25(3):382–388.
39. Boyington JE, Carter-Edwards L, Piehl M, Hutson J, Langdon D, McManus S. Cultural attitudes toward weight, diet and physical activity among overweight African American girls. *Prev Chronic Dis*. 2008;5(2):A36.
40. Betancourt JR. Cultural competence – marginal or mainstream movement?. *N Engl J Med*. 2004;351(10):953–955.
41. Reimann JO, Talavera GA, Salmon M, Nunez JA, Velasquez RJ. Cultural competence among physicians treating Mexican Americans who have diabetes: a structural model. *Soc Sci Med*. 2004;59(11):2195–2205.

42. Caballero AE. Cultural competence in diabetes care: an urgent need. *Insulin*. 2007;2:81–90.
43. Black S, Markides K, Ray L. Depression predicts increased incidence of adverse health outcomes in older Mexican Americans with type 2 diabetes. *Diabetes Care*. 2003;10:2822–2828.
44. Lerman I, Lozano L, Villa AR, et al. Psychosocial factors associated with poor diabetes self care management in a specialized center in Mexico city. *Biomed Pharmacother*. 2004;58:566–570.
45. Tucker KL. Stress and nutrition in relation to excess development of chronic disease in Puerto Rican adults living in the Northeast USA. *J Med Invest*. 2005;52(Suppl):252–258.
46. Saver BG, Van-Nguyen V, Keppel G, Doescher MP. A qualitative study of depression in primary care: missed opportunities for diagnosis and education. *J Am Board Fam Med*. 2007;20:28–35.
47. Williams JW, Mulrow CD, Kroenke K, et al. Case-finding for depression in primary care: a randomized trial. *Am J Med*. 1999 Jan;106(1):36–43.
48. Polonsky WH, Fisher L, Earles J, et al. Assessing psychosocial distress in diabetes: development of the diabetes distress scale. *Diabetes Care*. 2005;28(3):626–631.
49. Leonetti DL, Tsunehara CH, Wahl PW, Fujimoto WY. Educational attainment and the risk of non-insulin-dependent diabetes or coronary heart disease in Japanese-American men. *Ethn Dis*. 1992;2(4):326–336.
50. Maty SC, Everson-Rose SA, Haan MN, Raghunathan TE, Kaplan GA. Education, income, occupation and the 34-year incidence (1965–99) of type 2 diabetes in the Alameda County study. *Int J Epidemiol*. 2005;34(6):1274–1281.
51. Gurka MJ, Wolf AM, Conaway MR, et al. Lifestyle intervention in obese patients with type 2 diabetes: impact of the patient's educational background. *Obesity (Silver Spring)*. 2006;14:1085–1092.
52. Glasgow RE, Hampson SE, Strycker LA, Ruggiero L. Personal-model beliefs and social–environmental barriers related to diabetes self-management. *Diabetes Care*. 1997;20:556–561.
53. Hunt LM, Valenzuela MA, Pugh JA. NIDDM patients' fears and hopes about insulin therapy. The basis of patient reluctance. *Diabetes Care*. 1997;20:292–298.
54. Caballero AE, Montagnani V, Ward MA, et al. The assessment of diabetes knowledge, socio-economic and cultural factors for the development of an appropriate education program for Latinos with diabetes. *Diabetes*. 2004;53(Suppl 2):A514.
55. Caballero AE. Building cultural bridges: understanding ethnicity to improve acceptance of insulin therapy in patients with type 2 diabetes. *Ethn Dis*. 2006;16:559–568.
56. Caballero AE. For the patient. Overcoming barriers to using insulin for better diabetes control among Latinos. *Ethn Dis*. 2006;16:591.
57. Wen LK, Parchman ML, Shepherd MD. Family support and diet barriers among older Hispanic adults with type 2 diabetes. *Fam Med*. 2004;36:423–430.
58. Fisher L, Chesla C, Skaff MM, et al. The family and disease management in Hispanic and European-American patients with type 2 diabetes. *Diabetes Care*. 2000;23:267–272.
59. Chesla CA, Fisher L, Mullan JT, et al. Family and disease management in African American patients with type 2 diabetes. *Diabetes Care*. 2004;27:2850–2855.
60. Schillinger D, Grumbach K, Piette J, et al. Association of health literacy with diabetes outcomes. *JAMA*. 2002;288:475–482.
61. Norris SL, Engelgau MM, Narayan KM. Effectiveness of self-management training in type 2 diabetes: a systematic review of randomized controlled trials. *Diabetes Care*. 2001;24:561–587.
62. Kim S, Love F, Quistberg DA, Shea JA. Association of health literacy with self-management behavior in patients with diabetes. *Diabetes Care*. 2004;27:2980–2982.
63. Sarkar U, Fisher L, Schillinger D. Is self-efficacy associated with diabetes self-management across race/ethnicity and health literacy?. *Diabetes Care*. 2006;29:823–829.
64. Rosal MC, Goins KV, Carbone ET, Cortes DE. Views and preferences of low-literate Hispanics regarding diabetes education: results of formative research. *Health Educ Behav*. 2004;31:388–405.
65. Millan-Ferro A, Cortes D, Weinger K, Caballero AE. Development of a culturally oriented educational tool for low health literacy Latino/Hispanic patients with type 2 diabetes and their families. Presented at: The American Diabetes Association Meeting; June 2007; Chicago, IL.
66. Parker RM, Baker DW, Williams MV, Nurss JR. The test of functional health literacy in adults: a new instrument for measuring patients literacy skills. *J Gen Intern Med*. 1995;10:537–541.
67. Caballero AE. Diabetes in Hispanics/Latinos: challenges and opportunities. *Curr Opin Endocrinol Diabetes Obes*. 2007;14:151–157.
68. Devlin H, Roberts M, Okaya A, Xiong YM. Our lives were healthier before: focus groups with African American, American Indian, Hispanic/Latino, and Hmong people with diabetes. *Health Promot Pract*. 2006;7:47–55.
69. Millan-Ferro A, Caballero AE. Cultural approaches to diabetes self-management programs for the Latino community. *Curr Diabetes Rep*. 2007;7(5):391–397.
70. Thackeray R, Merrill RM, Neiger BL. Disparities in diabetes management practice between racial and ethnic groups in the United States. *Diabetes Educ*. 2004;30:665–675.
71. Brown SA, Blozis SA, Kouzekanani K, et al. Dosage effects of diabetes self-management education for Mexican Americans: the Starr county border health initiative. *Diabetes Care*. 2005;28:527–532.
72. Hornberger JC, Gibson CD Jr, Wood W, et al. Eliminating language barriers for non-English-speaking patients. *Med Care*. 1996;34:845–856.

73. Huerta EE, Macario E. Communicating health risk to ethnic groups: reaching Hispanics as a case study. *J Natl Cancer Inst Monogr*. 1999;25:23–26.
74. McCabe M, Gohdes D, Morgan F, Eakin J, Schmitt C. Training effective interpreters for diabetes care and education: a new challenge. *Diabetes Educ*. 2006;32(5):714–720.
75. Meece J. Dispelling myths and removing barriers about insulin in type 2 diabetes. *Diabetes Educ*. 2006;32(Suppl 1):9S–18S.
76. Garrow D, Egede LE. Association between complementary and alternative medicine use, preventive care practices, and use of conventional medical services among adults with diabetes. *Diabetes Care*. 2006;29:15–19.
77. Dham S, Shah V, Hirsch S, Banerji MA. The role of complementary and alternative medicine in diabetes. *Curr Diab Rep*. 2006;6:251–258.
78. Shane-McWhorter L. Botanical dietary supplements and the treatment of diabetes: what is the evidence?. *Curr Diab Rep*. 2005;5:391–398.
79. Bijlani RL, Vempati RP, Yadav RK, et al. A brief but comprehensive lifestyle education program based on yoga reduces risk factors for cardiovascular disease and diabetes mellitus. *J Altern Complement Med*. 2005;11:267–274.
80. Centers for Disease Control and Prevention (CDC). Trends in leisure-time physical inactivity by age, sex, and race/ethnicity – United States, 1994–2004. *MMWR Morb Mortal Wkly Rep*. 2005;54:991–994.
81. Wood FG. Leisure time activity of Mexican Americans with diabetes. *J Adv Nurs*. 2004;45:190–196.
82. Clark DO. Physical activity efficacy and effectiveness among older adults and minorities. *Diabetes Care*. 1997;20:1176–1182.
83. Luscombe FA. Health-related quality of life measurement in type 2 diabetes. *Value Health*. 2000;3(Suppl 1):15–28.
84. Wee HL, Cheung YB, Li SC, et al. The impact of diabetes mellitus and other chronic medical conditions on health related quality of life: is the whole greater than the sum of its parts?. *Health Qual Life Outcomes*. 2005;3:2.
85. Hall DE. Medicine and religion. *N Engl J Med*. 2000;343:1340–1341 author reply 1341–1342.
86. Al-Arouj M, Bouguerra R, Buse J, et al. Recommendations for management of diabetes during Ramadan. *Diabetes Care*. 2005;28:2305–2311.
87. Robbins JM, Vaccarino V, Zhang H, Kasl SV. Socioeconomic status and diagnosed diabetes incidence. *Diabetes Res Clin Pract*. 2005;68:230–236.
88. Wachtel MS. Family poverty accounts for differences in lower-extremity amputation rates of minorities 50 years old or more with diabetes. *J Natl Med Assoc*. 2005;97:334–338.
89. Diez Roux AV, Detrano R, Jackson S, et al. Acculturation and socioeconomic position as predictors of coronary calcification in a multiethnic sample. *Circulation*. 2005;112:1557–1565.

Part IV
Genes and Diabetes

Chapter 10
Genetics of Type 2 Diabetes: From Candidate Genes to Genome-Wide Association Analysis

Kevin Brown and Alan R. Shuldiner

Introduction

Type 2 diabetes mellitus (T2D) is a heterogeneous and complex metabolic disease with a multifactorial etiology under the influence of both the genetic and environmental factors.[1] The most prominent of these environmental factors is excess calorie intake and sedentary lifestyle, leading to obesity, a potent risk factor for T2D. Indeed, the recent epidemic of type 2 diabetes can be accounted for, in large part, to recent changes in these or other environmental factors; our genes have not changed appreciably over the past few decades.[2] Emerging evidence indicates that like other age-related complex diseases, there are many T2D susceptibility gene variants, each relatively common in the population, each contributing a modest effect on disease risk.[3]

There have been rapid advances in our knowledge of variation across the human genome brought about by the Human Genome and HapMap Projects and new high-throughput genome-wide genotyping technologies. These innovations have advanced the field from candidate genes and linkage analysis, which have had limited success in identifying common variants for T2D, to genome-wide association studies in large cohorts of T2D cases and controls.[4] This chapter will review our current state of knowledge regarding the genetic basis of T2D. In addition to the common form(s) of T2D, we include monogenic forms of diabetes, including syndromes in which diabetes is a prominent feature (Fig. 10.1). Although not strictly considered T2D, these monogenic forms of diabetes lie at one end of a spectrum from rare and highly penetrant mutations to common and modest effect penetrant variants characteristic of T2D. They also provide insights into the molecular and cellular basis of glucose homeostasis in humans, especially of the role of beta cell dysfunction. In this chapter, we do not discuss type 1 diabetes or latent autoimmune diabetes in adults (LADA). For excellent recent reviews, see.[5–7]

Genetic Influences of Type 2 Diabetes

The inherited basis of T2D is well documented in twin studies and family studies.[8,9] The concordance of T2D in identical twins is 60–90%.[10,11] Sibling relative risk (λ_s), the risk of having T2D if a sibling has T2D compared to the prevalence in the population, ranges from 2 to 4. For example, the λ_s of T2D in the Amish Family Diabetes Study was estimated to be 3.28.[12] Similarly, traits associated with T2D, e.g., body mass index, blood glucose, and insulin levels, are more similar in family members than the general population.[9,11,12] The heritability (h^2) in the Amish Family Diabetes Study of BMI, glucose, and insulin areas under the curve during an oral glucose tolerance test was 0.42 ($p<0.0001$), 0.15 ($p<0.009$), and 0.42 ($p<0.0001$), respectively.[12] Although shared factors in related individuals other than genes can account for heritability (h^2), shared genes (genetics) is likely a strong component.

A.R. Shuldiner (✉)

Division of Endocrinology, Diabetes and Nutrition, University of Maryland School of Medicine, Geriatric Research and Education Clinical Center, Veterans Administration Medical Center, Baltimore, MD 21201, USA
e-mail: ashuldin@medicine.umaryland.edu

L. Poretsky (ed.), *Principles of Diabetes Mellitus*, DOI 10.1007/978-0-387-09841-8_10,
© Springer Science+Business Media, LLC 2010

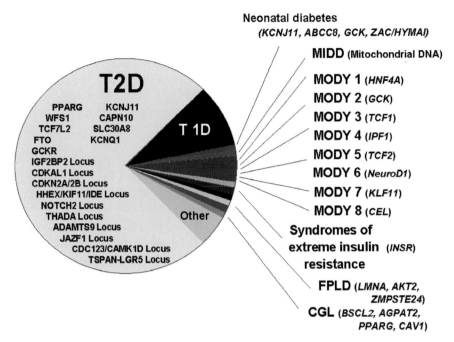

Fig. 10.1 Genetics of diabetes – 2009. Schematic of a pie chart (sectors not drawn to scale) of the multiple genetic causes of diabetes. Rare monogenic causes of diabetes are shown on the right. Common variants in 18 genes or loci each poses a modest increase in risk for type 2 diabetes (T2D). Several genes/loci have been found for type 1 diabetes (T1D), but are not shown in the figure. See text for names of genes depicted and their descriptions

Monogenic Forms of Diabetes

Monogenic forms of diabetes are thought to account for approximately 2–5% of all diabetes cases. They have in common a predictable mode of inheritance and gene mutations that are relatively uncommon in the population, but in which penetrance (the likelihood that someone carrying the mutation will develop diabetes) is high. The identification of these monogenic diabetes genes has provided a unique opportunity to characterize the pathophysiologic mechanisms by which mutations can lead to an increase in the plasma glucose concentration.

Maturity-Onset Diabetes of the Young (MODY)

The classical form of monogenic diabetes is maturity-onset diabetes of the young (MODY). Initially characterized in a large family from Michigan,[13] MODY is a genetically heterogeneous group of clinical disorders. Although they can vary in presentation, common features of all MODYs include nonketotic diabetes mellitus, an autosomal dominant mode of inheritance, typical presentation by the mid-twenties, and a primary defect in pancreatic beta cell function.

MODY can result from mutations in any one of at least eight different genes. The first to be identified was glucokinase (*GCK; MODY2*).[14] Subsequently six other MODY genes encoding different transcription factors pivotal to beta cell development and function were identified, including hepatocyte nuclear factor (HNF)-4α (*HNF4A; MODY1*),[15] HNF-1α (*TCF1; MODY3*),[16] insulin promoter factor-1 (*IPF1; MODY4*),[17] HNF-1β (*TCF2; MODY5*),[18] neurogenic differentiation 1/beta cell E-box *trans*-activator 2 (NEUROD1; *MODY6*),[19] and Kruppel-like factor 11 (*KLF11; MODY 7*).[20] MODY8 encodes the gene for the lipolytic enzyme carboxyl-enterolipase (*CEL*), which is expressed in the pancreas.[21]

MODY Caused by Mutations in Enzymes Involved in Substrate Metabolism

Glucokinase is expressed in the pancreatic beta cell and the liver. It catalyzes the transfer of phosphate from adenosine triphosphate (ATP) to glucose to generate glucose-6-phosphate.[21,22] This reaction is the rate-limiting step in glucose metabolism. Glucokinase functions as the glucose sensor in the beta cell by controlling the rate of entry of glucose into the glycolytic pathway. In the liver glucokinase plays a key role in glycogen synthesis, particularly in the postprandial state. Heterozygous mutations leading to partial deficiency of glucokinase are associated with MODY2,[14] while homozygous mutations resulting in complete deficiency of this enzyme lead to permanent neonatal diabetes mellitus.[23] As predicted by the physiologic functions of glucokinase, the increase in plasma glucose concentrations seen in patients with this form of diabetes is due to a combination of reduced glucose-induced insulin secretion from the pancreatic beta cell and reduced glycogen storage in the liver after glucose ingestion.[24,25] More than 150 different mutations in the glucokinase gene have been described.[14,22] These mutations include missense and nonsense mutations that alter enzyme activity or stability of the protein. Many patients with MODY2 have mild fasting hyperglycemia.[24] Less than half present with overt diabetes, and those with diabetes tend to be controlled with an appropriate diet. These patients also appear to be relatively resistant to microvascular complications in the eyes or kidneys.

Carboxyl-ester lipase (*CEL*) is a lipolytic enzyme that is secreted by the exocrine pancreas. The initial report of MODY8 was of two families with diabetes and exocrine deficiency. Each family was found to have different single base deletions (1686delT and 1785delC) in exon 11 of *CEL* resulting in altered reading frames and truncated proteins.[21] CEL is a major component of pancreatic fluid and it aids in the duodenal hydrolysis of cholesterol esters. Radiological changes in pancreatic architecture are sometimes found in patients with MODY8 and the onset of diabetes tends to occur at a later age than other types of MODY and tends to be mild.[26]

Transcription Factor MODYs

The transcription factors HNF-1α, HNF-1β, and HNF-4α, encoded by *TCF1*, TCF2 and *HNF4A* genes, respectively, play a key role in the tissue-specific regulation of gene expression in the liver and are also expressed in other tissues including pancreatic islets, kidney, and genital tissues. HNF-1α and HNF-1β are members of the homeodomain-containing family of transcription factors, and HNF-4α is an orphan nuclear receptor. HNF-1α, HNF-1β, and HNF-4α make up part of an interacting network that function together to control gene expression during embryonic development and in adult tissues in which they are coexpressed. In the pancreatic beta cell, these transcription factors regulate differentiation and the expression of the insulin gene as well as proteins involved in glucose transport and metabolism: mitochondrial metabolism (linked to insulin secretion) and lipoprotein metabolism. Persons with mutations in these genes have defects in insulin secretory responses to a variety of secretagogues, particularly glucose, that are present before the onset of hyperglycemia, suggesting that they represent the primary functional defect. Reduced glucagon response to arginine has also been observed, suggesting that the pancreatic alpha cell is also involved in a broader pancreatic developmental abnormality. In a large series from the United Kingdom, *TCF1* mutations (MODY3) are the most common cause of MODY, representing approximately 65% of cases, with *HNF4A* (MODY1) and *TCF2* (MODY5) mutations accounting for 5 and 1% of cases, respectively.[26,27] Interestingly, a mutation in *TCF1* (glycine substituted for serine at codon 319 (G319S)), only found in the Canadian Native American Oji-Cree population, is present in 40% of the population and contributes a 1.97-fold (heterozygotes) and 4.00-fold (homozygotes) increased risk of diabetes compared to noncarriers.[28]

IPF-1 is a homeodomain-containing transcription factor that was originally isolated as a transcriptional regulator of the insulin and somatostatin genes.[29] It also plays a central role in the development of the pancreas as well as in regulating expression of a variety of other pancreatic islet genes including glucokinase, islet amyloid polypeptide, and glucose transporter 2 genes.[30] A child born with severe diabetes and pancreatic agenesis was found to be homozygous for an *IPF1* mutation that lacked the homeodomain required for DNA binding and nuclear localization.[30,31] Heterozygous family members developed an early-onset autosomal dominant form of diabetes (i.e., MODY4).[17] Additional *IPF1* mutations have been discovered in pedigrees with pancreatic agenesis/MODY4.[32]

The basic helix-loop-helix transcription factor neurogenic differentiation-1 (NeuroD1/BETA2) (MODY6) was isolated on the basis of its ability to activate transcription of the insulin gene and is also required for normal pancreatic islet development.[32,33] Two patients with heterozygous mutations in *NEUROD1* and diabetes (R111L and 206+C) have been described[19] and a third has been identified in an Icelandic population.[34] Studies in other populations have failed to detect mutations in *NEUROD1* even in subjects with a MODY phenotype. Thus, mutations in *NEUROD1* are a rare cause of MODY.

KLF-11 (MODY7) is a TGF-β inducible transcription factor that regulates exocrine cell growth and exocrine cell fate. TGF-β signaling is crucial for pancreatic development and KLF-11 is a glucose-induced regulator of the insulin gene.[35] Neve[20] identified two rare mutations (A347S and T220M) in *KLF11* in two MODY families. These mutations segregated with diabetes in the families and were shown to cause impaired transcriptional activity in vitro. Although presumed to affect beta cell mass or function, the exact mechanism whereby this gene influences diabetes is not known.

Neonatal Diabetes

Permanent Neonatal Diabetes

The most common cause of permanent neonatal diabetes (PND) is heterozygous activating mutations in the *KCNJ11* gene, which encodes the Kir6.2 subunit of the ATP-sensitive K+ channel of the beta cell.[36,37] Many mutations have been described causing both familial and sporadic (usually because of new mutations) PND. Activating mutations in the Kir6.2 subunit increase the number of open channels on the cell membrane, resulting in hyperpolarization of the beta cell and subsequent prevention of insulin release.[38–40] In addition to diabetes, some patients with mutations in *KCNJ11* have global developmental delay, muscle weakness, epilepsy, and dysmorphic features. Conversely, homozygous inactivating mutations in the *KCNJ11* cause familial persistent hyperinsulinemic hypoglycemia of infancy.[41]

Generally, treatment for PND has been lifelong insulin therapy. Recently, however, it has been shown that some patients with PND caused by mutations in *KCNJ11* respond to high-dose oral sulfonylureas.[42] Sulfonylureas bind to the regulatory subunit (also known as the sulfonylurea receptor) of the ATP-sensitive K+ channel, closing it to stimulate insulin release. Although these findings are still preliminary and long-term follow-up studies are needed, PND caused by *KCNJ11* mutations is an excellent example of molecular diagnosis making a dramatic difference in treatment options.

In addition to mutations in *KCNJ11*, activating mutations in *ABCC8*, encoding the regulatory subunit of the beta cell ATP-sensitive K+ channel, which prevents its closure and hence insulin secretion, and homozygous inactivating mutations in glucokinase (*GCK; MODY2*), which disrupts glucose-stimulated insulin secretion, may also cause PND.[43,44] Other rare syndromic forms of neonatal diabetes are due to mutations in *EIF2AK3* (also known as *PERK*) in Wolcott–Rallison syndrome; *FOXP3*, which is associated with early immune dysregulation;[45] *PTF1A*, also associated with cerebellar agenesis;[46] and *GLIS3*, also associated with congenital hypothyroidism.[47]

Transient Neonatal Diabetes

Transient neonatal diabetes is defined as diabetes beginning by the first 6 weeks of life in term infants with recovery by 18 months of age.[48] Clinically, patients have intrauterine growth retardation, low birth weight, and decreased adipose tissue. Patients may present with dehydration, failure to thrive, hyperglycemia, and mild ketosis. Endogenous insulin production is low with the requirement for exogenous insulin. Approximately 40% of patients go on to develop recurrence of diabetes, most commonly during adolescence and early adulthood. It is usually mild and does not require insulin therapy.

Evidence suggests that transient neonatal diabetes is genetically heterogeneous. There is some overlap in genetic etiologies of transient and permanent neonatal diabetes, with mutations in *ABCC8* and *KCNJ11* also being associated with transient neonatal diabetes.[36,37,49] Another form may be due to overexpression of an imprinted and paternally expressed gene(s) within a critical region of chromosome 6q24.[50,51] Two imprinted genes, *ZAC* (zinc finger protein associated with apoptosis and cell cycle arrest) and *HYMAI* (imprinted in hydatidiform mole), have been identified as potential candidates. Genetic mechanisms shown to result in transient neonatal diabetes include paternal uniparental isodisomy of chromosome 6, paternally inherited duplication of 6q24, and a methylation defect at a CpG island overlapping exon 1 of *ZAC/HYMAI*.[50–52]

Mitochondrial Diabetes

Mitochondria are intracellular organelles that are responsible for generating energy through the process of oxidative phosphorylation. These organelles have their own DNA which is circular about approximately 16 kb in length and maternally inherited. Mutations in mitochondrial DNA have characteristically been associated with neurologic and neuromuscular syndromes, but diabetes can also be a feature. The most common cause of mitochondrial diabetes is the syndrome of maternally inherited diabetes and deafness (MIDD), most often caused by an A3243G point mutation in the gene encoding leucine tRNA.[53–55] The age of diagnosis of MIDD varies widely, generally occurring in the fourth decade of life, although the onset may be earlier. At onset, hyperglycemia is usually mild but many patients go on to require insulin treatment because the insulin deficiency is progressive. Carriers of the A3243G mutation characteristically have sensory neural hearing impairment, the onset of which typically precedes the onset of diabetes by several years. Patients may also develop pigmentary retinal dystrophy and neuromuscular disorder characterized by a cardiomyopathy or muscular weakness.[57]

The mitochondrial DNA mutations impair glucose-induced insulin secretion by the pancreas.[58,59] Patients are typically treated with insulin, diet, or sulfonylureas. Metformin is contraindicated because of its risk of inducing lactic acidosis and the vulnerability of these patients of developing it. The same mutation may result in the less common disease of mitochondrial encephalopathy with lactic acidosis and stroke-like episodes, which is also associated with diabetes. Drastically different phenotypes on the basis of the same mutation may be determined by the degree of heteroplasmy in the mitochondrial DNA. Unlike nuclear DNA, which is restricted to only two copies per somatic cell, mtDNA exists in several hundred copies per cell, any proportion of which can have the mutation while the rest of the copies can be normal; this is referred to as "heteroplasmy." There may be tissue-specific differences in heteroplasmy leading to different clinical manifestations. Two other syndromes, caused by deletions in mitochondrial DNA, tend to be more severe and associated with diabetes. One of these, the Kearns–Sayre syndrome, is characterized by cardiomyopathy, pigmentary degeneration of the retina, chronic progressive external ophthalmoplegia, ataxia, and sensorineural hearing loss. In Pearson's syndrome, patients present with exocrine pancreatic dysfunction, sideroblastic anemia, and lactic acidosis. The onset of diabetes is usually in early infancy and requires treatment with insulin. Patients generally do not survive beyond the first decade of life.

Cystic Fibrosis-Related Diabetes

Cystic fibrosis is a multisystem disorder due to genetic and functional deficiency of the CFTR chloride channel which affects the lungs, pancreas, intestine, and male reproductive tract. In the pancreas, cystic fibrosis initially affects the exocrine pancreas, and later nonimmune destruction of pancreatic islet cells ensues.[60] Increased life span in patients with cystic fibrosis due to improved treatments of the pulmonary manifestations has resulted in a marked increase in cystic fibrosis-related diabetes; up to 50% of cystic fibrosis patients develop diabetes. Due to insulin deficiency, insulin treatment is typically required.[60,61]

Monogenic Forms of Diabetes with Insulin Resistance

Syndromes of Extreme Insulin Resistance

More than 70 mutations have been identified in the insulin receptor (*INSR*) gene in patients with syndromes of extreme insulin resistance.[62–65] There are at least three clinical syndromes caused by homozygous or compound heterozygous mutations in the insulin receptor gene. Type A insulin resistance is defined by the presence of insulin resistance, acanthosis nigricans, and hyperandrogenism. Patients with leprechaunism have multiple abnormalities, including intrauterine growth retardation, fasting hypoglycemia, and death within the first 1–2 years of life. The Rabson–Mendenhall syndrome is associated with short stature, protuberant abdomen, and abnormalities of teeth and nails as well as pineal hyperplasia, which were characteristics in the original description of this syndrome.[66]

In all three syndromes, insulin resistance is extreme. Endogenous insulin levels are high due to compensatory hypersecretion by pancreatic beta cells. The high circulating insulin levels that cross-talk with (functionally normal) IGF-1 receptors are thought to be responsible for the acanthosis nigricans and hyperandrogenism observed in the type A syndrome. Despite endogenous hyperinsulinemia, patients often require very large doses of exogenous insulin for a therapeutic response.

INSR mutations may impair receptor function by a number of different mechanisms, including decreasing the number of receptors expressed on the cell surface, for example, by decreasing the rate of receptor biosynthesis (class 1), accelerating the rate of receptor degradation (class 5), or inhibiting the transport of receptors to the plasma membrane (class 2).[67] Other mutations may alter intrinsic function of the receptor by decreasing affinity of insulin binding (class 3) or if the receptor tyrosine kinase is inactivated (class 4). It is unknown why some insulin receptor mutations result in type A syndrome while others lead to the more severe phenotypes.

Lipoatrophic Diabetes

Another form of monogenic diabetes is lipoatrophic diabetes; this is associated with paucity or absence of adipose tissue, severe insulin resistance, hypertriglyceridemia, fatty liver, and often diabetes. Hypertriglyceridemia may cause recurrent bouts of pancreatitis. As might be expected, the adipose gene product, leptin, is low. There are several genetic forms of this disease (for review, see[68]).

Face-sparing partial lipoatrophy (Dunnigan syndrome or Kobberling–Dunnigan syndrome) is an autosomal dominant form caused by mutations in the lamin A/C (*LMNA*) gene.[69,70] These patients have adequate fat in their face and upper body, with progressively diminishing fat in their trunk and lower extremities. Lamin A/C is a structural protein located in the inner nuclear membrane present in virtually all cells with nuclei. The mechanism whereby *LMNA* mutations cause partial lipoatrophy is unknown. Mutations in v-AKT murine thymoma oncogene homolog 2 (AKT2), involved in insulin signaling, and zinc metalloprotease (ZMPSTE24), involved in processing of lamins, also have been shown to cause partial lipoatrophic diabetes.[71,72]

Another form of lipoatrophic diabetes is congenital generalized lipoatrophy (Berardinelli–Seip syndrome). This syndrome is characterized by lack of fat tissue throughout the body, insulin resistance, hypertriglyceridemia, and often diabetes. It is autosomal recessive and due to mutations in either 1-acyl-sn-glycerol-3-phosphate acyltransferase-2 (*AGPAT2*)[73] or in the Seipin (*BSCL2*)[74] gene product. AGPAT2 is likely to affect triglyceride synthesis in adipose tissue, while Seipin may act by inhibiting lipid droplet formation in adipocytes.[75] Similarly a recently described mutation in caveolin 1 (*CAV1*) may also cause partial congenital generalized lipoatrophy, possibly through altering lipid droplet formation in adipocytes.[76]

Mutations in Peroxisome Proliferator-Activated Receptor-γ

Peroxisome proliferator-activated receptor gamma (PPARγ) is a member of the PPAR subfamily of nuclear receptors. It is an important regulator of lipid and glucose homeostasis and cellular differentiation. It is highly expressed in adipose tissue, but is also expressed in the pancreatic beta cell. Binding of the ligand to the receptor causes it to heterodimerize with the retinoid X receptor, bind specific DNA elements, and induce a transcriptional cascade that leads to adipocyte differentiation and increased insulin sensitivity. PPARγ is the target for the thiazolidinediones.

Mutations in the *PPARG* gene can cause autosomal dominant lipoatrophic syndromes associated with early-onset diabetes. Several mutations have been described.[77–79] For example, Barroso and coworkers reported two dominant negative mutations (P467L and V290M) in three subjects with severe insulin resistance and early-onset diabetes.[77] Located in the ligand-binding domain, both receptor mutants showed decreased transcriptional activation and inhibited the action of wild-type PPARγ. A heterozygous P388L mutation, located in the ligand-binding domain of PPARγ, was found in a Canadian kindred with familial lipodystrophy and was similarly shown to act in a dominant negative fashion.[78] By contrast, a rare activating mutation in *PPARG* in which proline is substituted by glutamine (P115Q) found in a German population was associated with extreme obesity and mild insulin resistance (likely secondary to obesity and not PPARγ activation).[80]

Polygenic Forms of Type 2 Diabetes (T2D)

As described above, there have been significant advances in identifying genes responsible for monogenic diabetes and monogenic syndromes associated with diabetes. However, these forms represent no more than 2–5% of diabetes. Far more common is the polygenic form(s), broadly referred to as T2D, which has complex pathophysiology, with both genetic and environmental factors playing major roles. The phenotypic manifestations include defects in insulin secretory pathways and resistance to the action of insulin in multiple tissue sites, such as liver, muscle, and fat. Insulin resistance from an underlying defect, often compounded by excess body weight, predisposes person to T2D before the onset of hyperglycemia. This association has been interpreted by many to suggest that insulin resistance plays a primary role in the development of T2D. However, pancreatic beta cell dysfunction is also present very early in the course of glucose dysregulation. Indeed, both insulin resistance and beta cell dysfunction have been demonstrated in nondiabetic first-degree relatives of persons with T2D, suggesting a genetic component to each. Since insulin resistance is associated with compensatory changes in insulin secretion, aberrations in insulin secretion can cause insulin resistance, and both insulin resistance and insulin secretion are affected by ambient glucose concentrations, it has been extremely difficult to disentangle these processes at the physiological level. In most patients with T2D, both defects exist, with great interindividual variability in the relative contributions of each to the disease.

There have been intensive efforts to identify gene variants for typical T2D over the past 2–3 decades. Initially, due to limitations in our knowledge of the human genome and technologies to query variation in the genome, identification of these genes was slow and required equal parts of meticulous research and good fortune. Candidate gene studies have been successful in identifying common variants in three genes (*PPARG*, *KCNJ11*, and *WFS1*) that increase risk of T2D. Genome-wide linkage analysis in multiplex T2D families led to the identification of two additional genes (*CAPN10* and *TCF7L2*), as well as several well-replicated chromosomal loci that may harbor additional (yet to be identified) T2D genes. More recently, genome-wide association studies (GWAS), performed by genotyping a very large number (>300,000) of single nucleotide polymorphisms (SNPs) across the genome in DNA samples from large numbers of T2D cases and nondiabetic controls, have successfully identified addition genes or chromosomal loci associated with T2D. At the time of completion of this chapter, 14 T2D genes/loci have been identified by GWAS. A common theme is that sequence variations in these genes/loci are common in the population, and each imposes a modest increase in T2D risk. Interestingly, most of the T2D susceptibility genes identified by GWAS to date likely exert their effect by affecting beta cell function.

T2D Genes Identified by Candidate Gene Approach

Although hundreds of candidate genes have been investigated, few have been studied in enough detail in large enough sample sizes to definitively rule out their role in T2D. Initial reports of association of a candidate gene with T2D are often followed by lack of replication suggesting that many of the initial discoveries are false-positive findings or private to a given population. A detailed review of all candidate gene studies is beyond the scope of this chapter; however, those most highly replicated candidate gene variants are described below.

Potassium Inwardly Rectifying Channel Subfamily J Member 11

The ATP-sensitive K+ channel (K_{ATP}) is expressed in beta cells and is a key regulator of glucose-stimulated insulin secretion. It is composed of Kir6.2, a potassium inwardly rectifying channel, and the sulfonylurea receptor (encoded by *ABCC8*), the regulatory subunit and site of binding of sulfonylureas. Kir6.2 is encoded by the *KCNJ11* gene located on chromosome 11p15.1. As previously discussed, rare activating mutations in *KCNJ11*, and *ABCC8* cause monogenic neonatal diabetes. In polygenic T2D, a common missense mutation where glutamate (E) is and *ABCC8* substituted for lysine (K) at position 23 (E23K) has been consistently associated with T2DM.[81,82] The codon 23 lysine allele is common in Caucasians, with an allele frequency of ~0.37, and less common in African-Americans, with an allele frequency of ~0.08. The increased T2D risk in K23 carriers is modest, with an overall allelic odds ratio (OR) of 1.1–1.2.[83] The K23 allele is associated with decreased insulin secretion, the presumed mechanism for increased diabetes risk.[84,85] Moreover, there is some evidence that patients with the K23 may be have a higher likelihood of secondary failure on sulfonylureas.[86]

Peroxisome Proliferator-Activated Receptor-γ

A common variant in *PPARG* occurs when a proline is substituted for an alanine at codon 12 (P12A) of its gene.[87] The frequency of the alanine allele is highest in Caucasian populations (allele frequency = 0.11–0.19) and lower in African-Americans (allele frequency = 0.02).[88] A12 *PPARG* has been reproducibly associated with a decreased risk for T2D, i.e., the presence of the more common P12 allele confers an approximately 1.25-fold increased risk for T2D.[88–90] The P12 T2D risk allele is also associated with greater insulin resistance, the presumed mechanism whereby this allele confers increased T2D risk.[90]

Other Candidate Genes

Rare mutations in *WFS1* cause Wolfarin's syndrome, which is characterized by diabetes insipidus, diabetes mellitus, optic atrophy, and deafness. In a large pooled case–control study, Sandhu and coworkers[91] identified common intronic variants associated with typical T2D. These variants reside in a large region of linkage disequilibrium across the entire gene, making identification of the functional variant difficult. The risk allele has a frequency of 0.6 and results in a 1.1-fold increase in T2D risk. Several groups have replicated this association with T2D[92] and also demonstrated that subjects with the risk allele have decreased insulin secretion, the likely mechanism whereby this variant increases T2D risk.[93]

As described above, rare mutations in *HNF4A* cause MODY1. Two studies[94,95] reported an association between common SNPs in the islet-specific promoter (P2) of *HNF4A* and T2D. Some, but not all subsequent, reports replicated these findings.[96,97] A recent more detailed study of the P2 promoter suggest that there may be population heterogeneity, in which the genotyped SNP(s) are not causative, but are in linkage disequilibrium with a causative variant in some populations, i.e., Ashkenazi, but not others (UK Caucasians).[97] Further investigation of the P2 region across additional populations will be necessary to better understand the genetic architecture of this region and its contribution to T2D risk.

Type 2 Diabetes Genes Identified by Linkage Analysis Approach

Transcription Factor 7-Like 2 (TCF7L2)

Genome-wide linkage analysis identified a region of linkage to T2D on chromosome 10.[98] Fine mapping localized marker DG10S478 of *TCF7L2* on 10q25 that was strongly associated with T2D.[99] *TCF7L2* (formerly *TCF4*) encodes transcription factor 7-like 2, a member of the T cell transcription factor family. Further analysis identified a common SNP, rs7903146 in intron 3, which is the strongest and most replicated variant studied to date. This variant may be causal, or in linkage disequilibrium with the (yet to be identified) causal variant. The T-allele of rs7903146 imposes an approximately 1.4-fold increased risk for T2D. Many studies have replicated these findings.[100,101] TCF7L2 has an important role in the WNT signaling pathway and in the regulation of cell proliferation and differentiation. In enteroendocrine cells, WNT signaling through TCF7L2 has been shown to influence glucagon-like peptide-1 (GLP-1) secretion. Nondiabetic subjects with the T-allele have decreased meal-induced insulin secretion and increased hepatic glucose output, likely due to alterations in GLP-1 signaling.[102] T2D patients with the T-allele may have decreased response to sulfonylurea therapy.[103] In the Diabetes Prevention Program cohort, those with the T-allele were more likely to progress to diabetes; progression to T2D in those with the risk allele was attenuated in the lifestyle arm, consisting of diet/modest weight loss and exercise.[104]

Calpain 10 (CAPN 10)

Genome-wide linkage analysis identified a region on chromosome 2q that was linked to T2D in Mexican Americans.[105] Further analysis identified three common variants in *CAPN10* that constitute a T2D risk haplotype. *CAPN10* encodes a calcium-regulated cysteine protease, ubiquitously expressed in multiple tissues. Calpains catalyze proteolysis of substrates involved in cytoskeletal remodeling and signal transduction. A number of studies have subsequently confirmed associations between variation in this gene and T2D,[106] while others have not.[107] Some evidence suggests different risk alleles/haplotypes in different populations.[108–110] How *CAPN10* variants influence T2D risk is not known,[111] but may include elements of both insulin resistance[112] and insulin secretion[113] given the ubiquitous expression of this protease.

Type 2 Diabetes Genes Identified by Genome-Wide Association Study (GWAS) Approach

SLC30A8

In a genome-wide case–control association study in a French cohort, Sladek and coworkers first reported association between T2D and a missense mutation (R325W) in the solute carrier family 30 member 8 gene (*SLC30A8*) on chromosome 8q24.11.[114] This finding has subsequently been replicated in other GWAS[115–118] and more targeted replication studies. The risk allele is very common in the population (allele frequency = 0.65) and results in a modest increase in T2D risk (odds ratio = 1.18). *SLC30A8* encodes zinc transporter 8 (ZNT8). ZNT8 is expressed predominantly in pancreatic beta cells and transports zinc from the cytoplasm into insulin secretory vesicles, in which insulin is stored as a hexamer bound with two Zn^{+2} ions. Zinc plays an important role in insulin trafficking, i.e., synthesis, storage, and secretion. It has also been implicated in regulation of pro-inflammatory cytokines and beta cell apoptosis.[119] The missense mutation (R325W) may affect zinc accumulation in insulin granules and hence influence insulin processing, stability and trafficking. Recent data have implicated this variant in autoimmunity in type 1 diabetes.[120]

GCKR

An intronic SNP in the glucokinase regulatory protein *(GCKR)* gene was initially identified in a GWAS of T2D to be associated with fasting serum triglyceride levels.[115] This association was subsequently replicated in several studies and extended to include association with T2D.[121] Subsequently, a nonsynonymous mutation (P336L) in *GCKR* was found to be in high linkage disequilibrium with the initial SNP, and is likely the causative variant. Interestingly, the minor 336L allele is associated with higher triglyceride levels and lower fasting glucose and decreased risk of T2D. GCKR is localized in the nucleus where it sequesters glucokinase and inhibits its activity in the fasting state.[122] Sequestration to the nucleus by GCKR may also protect glucokinase from degradation. Thus altered GCKR activity could have differential effects in the fed and fasted state, perhaps explaining the apparent paradoxical effect on glucose and triglycerides.

FTO

The fat mass- and obesity-associated *(FTO)* gene is located on chromosome 16q12. Initially found to be associated with T2D in the Wellcome Trust Case Control Consortium cohort,[118] the effect on T2D risk was shown to be due to its association with increased BMI/obesity.[123] Association with BMI and obesity has been robustly replicated in several studies.[124,125] The obesity/T2D associated variant is located in intron 2, has an allele frequency of 0.38, and increases T2D risk by approximately 1.3-fold. How FTO affects BMI is not known. FTO protein is ubiquitously expressed, with relatively high expression in adrenal glands and brain, especially in hypothalamus and pituitary. The protein shares sequence homology to 2-oxoglutarate-dependent oxygenases and may play a role in nucleic acid demethylation.[126] A recent study showed that children with the BMI-associated FTO variant have increased food intake.[127]

KCNQ1

Two recent GWAS analyses in Asian populations identified a new T2D susceptibility gene, *KCNQ1* on chromosome 11p15.5.[128,129] The T2D risk allele is located in intron 15 and has an allele frequency of 0.65 in Asians and imposes a 1.3- to 1.4-fold increased risk of T2D. A subsequent study in 3734 Asians replicated association with T2D (odds ratio = 1.48). The risk associated variant has a frequency of 0.94 in Caucasian populations and was also associated with T2D. *KCNQ1* encodes a potassium voltage-gated channel and is expressed in the heart and to a lesser extent in other tissues including pancreas, liver, and adipose tissue. Rare mutations in *KCNQ1* cause long QT syndrome, and *KCNQ1* knockout mice have cardiac dysfunction and abnormalities in gastric parietal cells and gastric acid secretion.[130] Subjects with the T2D risk allele appear to have decreased insulin secretion.[131]

IGF2BP2 Locus

Several GWAS studies identified variants in the insulin-like growth factor 2 mRNA binding protein 2 (*IGF2BP2*) gene on chromosome 3q27 to be associated with T2D.[115,116,118] The frequency of the risk allele is 0.29 and imposes a modest increased risk for T2D (odds ratio = 1.14). Through its ability to bind to IGF2 mRNA, *IGF2BP2* regulates *IGF2* gene expression. It is expressed in oocytes, granulosa cells of small and growing follicles, Leydig cells, spermatogonia, and semen. It is also expressed weakly in heart, placenta, skeletal muscle, bone marrow, colon, kidney, salivary glands, testis, and pancreas. How variants in *IGF2BP2* influence T2D risk is not known. Some studies support a role in insulin sensitivity,[132,133] and others have implicated insulin secretion.[134,135] This locus contains a number of other genes that may play a role in glucose homeostasis including adiponectin (*ADIPOQ*), protein phosphatase 1, regulatory subunit 1 (*PPP1R2*), and alpha-2-HS-glycoprotein (*AHSG*).

CDKAL1 Locus

Initially reported in the GWAS study of Steinthorsdottir and coworkers,[117] and replicated by others, a common noncoding variant in *CDKAL1* on chromosome 6p22.3 was found to be associated with T2D. The risk allele (odds ratio = 1.2) has a frequency of 0.31. *CKDAL1* encodes CDK5 regulatory subunit associated protein 1-like 1, a transmembrane bound regulator of cyclin kinase. Thus it is thought to play a role in regulation of cell cycle. Limited data suggest that the risk allele is associated with decreased insulin secretion.[134,136]

CDKN2A/CDKN2B Locus

Cyclin-dependent kinase inhibitors 2A and 2B (*CDKN2A* and *CDKN2B*) are adjacent genes on chromosome 9p21 that encode cyclin-dependent kinase inhibitor proteins p16^{INK4a}/p14 and p16^{INK4b}. These proteins inhibit cyclin-dependent kinase 4 (CDK4) and thus play a key role in regulating cell division (reviewed in Kim and Sharpless[137]). p16^{INK4a} is a high-risk melanoma gene and has been implicated in pancreatic and other malignancy cancer.[138] p16^{INK4a} and p16^{INK4b} are also regulators of pancreatic beta cell replication. Mice rendered deficient in p16^{INK4a} demonstrate islet proliferation while overexpression results in decreased islet proliferation.[139] SNP rs10811661 (risk allele frequency 0.83) lies in a noncoding region near *CDKN2A/B* and imparts a 1.2-fold risk for T2D[115,116,118] and has been associated with decreased insulin secretion.[140] Interesting, SNPs in the same region, but in a clearly different haplotype block, have been shown to be associated with coronary artery disease as well as abdominal aortic aneurism, intracranial aneurism, and peripheral artery disease.[141,142]

HHEX/KIF11/IDE Locus

Association with T2D to a locus on chromosome 10q23 was shown by Sladek and coworkers[114] with modest evidence for replication in subsequent scans. The T2D risk SNP has an allele frequency of 0.53 and is associated with a 1.13 increase in diabetes risk. Located in a large region of linkage disequilibrium, there are three reasonable candidate genes, hematopoietically expressed homeobox (*HHEX*), insulin degrading enzyme (*IDE*), and kinesin family member 11 (*KIF11*). *HHEX* is involved in WNT signaling. It is expressed during development in several tissues including liver, pancreas, and heart. *IDE* is a neutral metallopeptidase that can degrade insulin as well as other proteins, including beta amyloid. *KIF11* is involved in mitotic spindle assembly and chromosomal segregation. Although which of these three genes harbors the functional variant is not known, the risk allele is associated with decreased insulin secretion.[140]

Other Loci from GWAS Meta-Analysis

A follow-up meta-analysis of three Caucasian genome-wide association studies with a total of 10,000 T2D cases and nondiabetic controls and nearly 54,000 replication samples uncovered several additional genes/loci associated with T2D at the genome-wide significance level.[143] The fact that such a large sample size was required means that these new loci have a very modest effect on phenotype (odds ratios ~1.1). None of these loci contain genes that are obvious biological candidates for diabetes. These include the neurogenic locus notch homolog protein 2 (NOTCH2) on chromosome 1p12, thyroid adenoma-associated gene (THADA) on chromosome 2p21, a disintegrin-like and metalloproteinase with thrombospondin type 1 motif 9 (ADAMTS9) on chromosome 3p14, juxtaposed with another zinc finger gene 1 (JAZF1) on chromosome 7p15, and loci near CDC123-CAMK1D (chromosome 10p13-p14) and TSPAN-LGR5 (chromosome 12q21).

There have been a number of smaller GWA studies in American populations (Amish,[144] Pima Indian,[145,146] Mexican American,[146] Framingham Study[147]). These studies identified variants in a number of potentially interesting genes and loci, e.g., GRB10 in the Amish, that will require additional study.

Concluding Remarks and Future Directions

Since 1993, there have been remarkable advances in our understanding of the genetic basis of diabetes. Several genes that contain mutations that are relatively rare in the population and which have a large effect on the phenotype cause monogenic forms of diabetes. People with these mutations have a high likelihood of developing diabetes; however, they are responsible for only a small percentage of patients with diabetes. Discovery of these genes have uncovered new pathways and mechanisms pivotal to glucose homeostasis.

More recently, advances in our knowledge of common variation across the genome, coupled with high-throughput genotyping methods, have identified more than a dozen genes or chromosomal loci associated with typical T2D. With the possible exception of the R325W nonsynonymous mutation in *SLC30A8* and P336L mutation in *GCKR*, the specific genes and/or their functional variants are not yet known. Additional fine mapping, sequencing, and functional analyses at these chromosomal loci will be necessary. These T2D risk alleles are common in the population, but have a very modest effect on risk (odds ratios 1.1–1.4) and thus are poor predictors of T2D alone and in combination.[148,149] Nonetheless they have the potential to inform us of novel mechanisms and pathways for design of new strategies for prevention and treatment. Moreover, the pharmacogenomic implications of these gene variants are largely unexplored.

Since current GWAS chips do an excellent job at capturing the vast majority of common variation across the genome (at least in Caucasian populations), many wonder why more of the heritable component of T2D was not discovered with this approach. Future studies need to focus on GWAS in other populations as well as a systematic search for other kinds of genetic variation, e.g., copy number variants, inversions, other structural variants, that may not have been captured by current SNP chips. In addition, exome and whole-genome sequencing will be necessary to query the role of rare variants in the etiology of typical T2D. With dramatic advances in throughput and cost of DNA sequence analysis, and availability of DNA samples from large numbers of T2D cases and controls, advances in unraveling the complex genetic architecture of T2D have never been more promising.

References

1. Stumvoll M, Goldstein BJ, van Haeften TW. Type 2 diabetes: pathogenesis and treatment. *Lancet.* 2009;371:2153–2156.
2. Mokdad AH, Ford ES, Bowman BA, et al. Prevalence of obesity, diabetes, and obesity-related health risk factors, 2001. *JAMA.* 2003;289:76–79.
3. McCarthy MI, Abecasis GR, Cardon LR, et al. Genome-wide association studies for complex traits: consensus, uncertainty and challenges. *Nat Rev Genet.* 2008;9:356–369.
4. Manolio TA, Brooks LD, Collins FS. A HapMap harvest of insights into the genetics of common disease. *J Clin Invest.* 2008;118:1590–1605.
5. Cervin C, Lyssenko V, Bakhtadze E, et al. Genetic similarities between latent autoimmune diabetes in adults, type 1 diabetes, and type 2 diabetes. *Diabetes.* 2008;57:1433–1437.
6. Lettre G, Rioux JD. Autoimmune diseases: insights from genome-wide association studies. *Hum Mol Genet.* 2008;17:R116–R121.
7. Ounissi-Benkalha H, Polychronakos C. The molecular genetics of type 1 diabetes: new genes and emerging mechanisms. *Trends Mol Med.* 2008;14:268–275.
8. Adeghate E, Schattner P, Dunn E. An update on the etiology and epidemiology of diabetes mellitus. *Ann NY Acad Sci.* 2006;1084:1–29.
9. Lyssenko V, Almgren P, Anevski D, et al. Predictors of and longitudinal changes in insulin sensitivity and secretion preceding onset of type 2 diabetes. *Diabetes.* 2005;54:166–174.
10. Newman B, Selby JV, King MC, Slemenda C, Fabsitz R, Friedman GD. Concordance for type 2 (non-insulin-dependent) diabetes mellitus in male twins. *Diabetologia.* 1987;30:763–768.
11. Mayer EJ, Newman B, Austin MA, et al. Genetic and environmental influences on insulin levels and the insulin resistance syndrome: an analysis of women twins. *Am J Epidemiol.* 1996;143:323–332.
12. Hsueh WC, Mitchell BD, Aburomia R, et al. Diabetes in the Old Order Amish: characterization and heritability analysis of the Amish Family Diabetes study. *Diabetes Care.* 2000;23:595–601.
13. Fajans SS. Maturity-onset diabetes of the young (MODY). *Diabetes Metab Rev.* 1989;5:579–606.
14. Vionnet N, Stoffel M, Takeda J, et al. Nonsense mutation in the glucokinase gene causes early-onset non-insulin-dependent diabetes mellitus. *Nature.* 1992;356:721–722.

15. Yamagata K, Furuta H, Oda N, et al. Mutations in the hepatocyte nuclear factor-4alpha gene in maturity-onset diabetes of the young (MODY1). *Nature*. 1996;384:458–460.

16. Yamagata K, Oda N, Kaisaki PJ, et al. Mutations in the hepatocyte nuclear factor-1alpha gene in maturity-onset diabetes of the young (MODY3). *Nature*. 1996;384:455–458.

17. Stoffers DA, Ferrer J, Clarke WL, Habener JF. Early-onset type-II diabetes mellitus (MODY4) linked to IPF1. *Nat Genet*. 1997;17:138–139.

18. Horikawa Y, Iwasaki N, Hara M, et al. Mutation in hepatocyte nuclear factor-1 beta gene (TCF2) associated with MODY. *Nat Genet*. 1997;17:384–385.

19. Malecki MT, Jhala US, Antonellis A, et al. Mutations in NEUROD1 are associated with the development of type 2 diabetes mellitus. *Nat Genet*. 1999;23:323–328.

20. Neve B, Fernandez-Zapico ME, Shkenazi-Katalan V, et al. Role of transcription factor KLF11 and its diabetes-associated gene variants in pancreatic beta cell function. *Proc Natl Acad Sci USA*. 2005;102:4807–4812.

21. Raeder H, Johansson S, Holm PI, et al. Mutations in the CEL VNTR cause a syndrome of diabetes and pancreatic exocrine dysfunction. *Nat Genet*. 2006;38:54–62.

22. Iynedjian PB. Molecular physiology of mammalian glucokinase. *Cell Mol Life Sci*. 2009;66:27–42.

23. Gloyn AL, Noordam K, Willemsen MA, et al. Insights into the biochemical and genetic basis of glucokinase activation from naturally occurring hypoglycemia mutations. *Diabetes*. 2003;52:2433–2440.

24. Vaxillaire M, Froguel P. Genetic basis of maturity-onset diabetes of the young. *Endocrinol Metab Clin North Am*. 2006;35:371–384, x.

25. Velho G, Petersen KF, Perseghin G, et al. Impaired hepatic glycogen synthesis in glucokinase-deficient (MODY-2) subjects. *J Clin Invest*. 1996;98:1755–1761.

26. Raeder H, Haldorsen IS, Ersland L, et al. Pancreatic lipomatosis is a structural marker in nondiabetic children with mutations in carboxyl-ester lipase. *Diabetes*. 2007;56:444–449.

27. Frayling TM, Bulamn MP, Ellard S, et al. Mutations in the hepatocyte nuclear factor-1alpha gene are a common cause of maturity-onset diabetes of the young in the U.K. *Diabetes*. 1997;46:720–725.

28. Hegele RA, Cao H, Harris SB, Hanley AJ, Zinman B. The hepatic nuclear factor-1alpha G319S variant is associated with early-onset type 2 diabetes in Canadian Oji-Cree. *J Clin Endocrinol Metab*. 1999;84:1077–1082.

29. Ohlsson H, Karlsson K, Edlund T. IPF1, a homeodomain-containing transactivator of the insulin gene. *EMBO J*. 1993;12:4251–4259.

30. Waeber G, Thompson N, Nicod P, Bonny C. Transcriptional activation of the GLUT2 gene by the IPF-1/STF-1/IDX-1 homeobox factor. *Mol Endocrinol*. 1996;10:1327–1334.

31. Stoffers DA, Zinkin NT, Stanojevic V, Clarke WL, Habener JF. Pancreatic agenesis attributable to a single nucleotide deletion in the human IPF1 gene coding sequence. *Nat Genet*. 1997;15:106–110.

32. Cockburn BN, Bermano G, Boodram LL, et al. Insulin promoter factor-1 mutations and diabetes in Trinidad: identification of a novel diabetes-associated mutation (E224K) in an Indo-Trinidadian family. *J Clin Endocrinol Metab*. 2004;89:971–978.

33. Naya FJ, Stellrecht CM, Tsai MJ. Tissue-specific regulation of the insulin gene by a novel basic helix-loop-helix transcription factor. *Genes Dev*. 1995;9:1009–1019.

34. Kristinsson SY, Thorolfsdottir ET, Talseth B, et al. MODY in Iceland is associated with mutations in HNF-1alpha and a novel mutation in NeuroD1. *Diabetologia*. 2001;44:2098–2103.

35. Fernandez-Zapico ME, Mladek A, Ellenrieder V, Folch-Puy E, Miller L, Urrutia R. An mSin3A interaction domain links the transcriptional activity of KLF11 with its role in growth regulation. *EMBO J*. 2003;22:4748–4758.

36. Barbetti F. Diagnosis of neonatal and infancy-onset diabetes. *Endocr Dev*. 2007;11:83–93.

37. Tammaro P. Neonatal diabetes. *Endocr Dev*. 2007;11:70–82.

38. Edghill EL, Gloyn AL, Gillespie KM, et al. Activating mutations in the KCNJ11 gene encoding the ATP-sensitive K+ channel subunit Kir6.2 are rare in clinically defined type 1 diabetes diagnosed before 2 years. *Diabetes*. 2004;53:2998–3001.

39. Gloyn AL, Pearson ER, Antcliff JF, et al. Activating mutations in the gene encoding the ATP-sensitive potassium-channel subunit Kir6.2 and permanent neonatal diabetes. *N Engl J Med*. 2004;350:1838–1849.

40. Vaxillaire M, Populaire C, Busiah K, et al. Kir6.2 mutations are a common cause of permanent neonatal diabetes in a large cohort of French patients. *Diabetes*. 2004;53:2719–2722.

41. Tornovsky S, Crane A, Cosgrove KE, et al. Hyperinsulinism of infancy: novel ABCC8 and KCNJ11 mutations and evidence for additional locus heterogeneity. *J Clin Endocrinol Metab*. 2004;89:6224–6234.

42. Murphy R, Ellard S, Hattersley AT. Clinical implications of a molecular genetic classification of monogenic beta-cell diabetes. *Nat Clin Pract Endocrinol Metab*. 2008;4:200–213.

43. Babenko AP, Polak M, Cave H, et al. Activating mutations in the ABCC8 gene in neonatal diabetes mellitus. *N Engl J Med*. 2006;355:456–466.

44. Njolstad PR, Sagen JV, Bjorkhaug L, et al. Permanent neonatal diabetes caused by glucokinase deficiency: inborn error of the glucose-insulin signaling pathway. *Diabetes*. 2003;52:2854–2860.

45. Rubio-Cabezas O, Minton JA, Caswell R, et al. Clinical heterogeneity in patients with FOXP3 mutations presenting with permanent neonatal diabetes. *Diabetes Care*. 2009;32:111–116.

46. Sellick GS, Barker KT, Stolte-Dijkstra I, et al. Mutations in PTF1A cause pancreatic and cerebellar agenesis. *Nat Genet.* 2004;36:1301–1305.

47. Senee V, Chelala C, Duchatelet S, et al. Mutations in GLIS3 are responsible for a rare syndrome with neonatal diabetes mellitus and congenital hypothyroidism. *Nat Genet.* 2006;38:682–687.

48. Hamilton-Shield JP. Overview of neonatal diabetes. *Endocr Dev.* 2007;12:12–23.

49. Suzuki S, Makita Y, Mukai T, Matsuo K, Ueda O, Fujieda K. Molecular basis of neonatal diabetes in Japanese patients. *J Clin Endocrinol Metab.* 2007;92:3979–3985.

50. Arima T, Drewell RA, Oshimura M, Wake N, Surani MA. A novel imprinted gene, HYMAI, is located within an imprinted domain on human chromosome 6 containing ZAC. *Genomics.* 2000;67:248–255.

51. Temple IK, Shield JP. Transient neonatal diabetes, a disorder of imprinting. *J Med Genet.* 2002;39:872–875.

52. Arima T, Yamasaki K, John RM, et al. The human HYMAI/PLAGL1 differentially methylated region acts as an imprint control region in mice. *Genomics.* 2006;88:650–658.

53. Reardon W, Ross RJ, Sweeney MG, et al. Diabetes mellitus associated with a pathogenic point mutation in mitochondrial DNA. *Lancet.* 1992;340:1376–1379.

54. van den Ouweland JM, Lemkes HH, Ruitenbeek W, et al. Mutation in mitochondrial tRNA(Leu)(UUR) gene in a large pedigree with maternally transmitted type II diabetes mellitus and deafness. *Nat Genet.* 1992;1:368–371.

55. Velho G, Byrne MM, Clement K, et al. Clinical phenotypes, insulin secretion, and insulin sensitivity in kindreds with maternally inherited diabetes and deafness due to mitochondrial tRNALeu(UUR) gene mutation. *Diabetes.* 1996;45:478–487.

56. Ballinger SW, Shoffner JM, Hedaya EV, et al. Maternally transmitted diabetes and deafness associated with a 10.4 kb mitochondrial DNA deletion. *Nat Genet.* 1992;1:11–15.

57. Smith PR, Bain SC, Good PA, et al. Pigmentary retinal dystrophy and the syndrome of maternally inherited diabetes and deafness caused by the mitochondrial DNA 3243 tRNA(Leu) A to G mutation. *Ophthalmology.* 1999;106:1101–1108.

58. Maassen JA, Janssen GM, 't Hart LM. Molecular mechanisms of mitochondrial diabetes (MIDD). *Ann Med.* 2005;37:213–221.

59. Murphy R, Turnbull DM, Walker M, Hattersley AT. Clinical features, diagnosis and management of maternally inherited diabetes and deafness (MIDD) associated with the 3243A>G mitochondrial point mutation. *Diabet Med.* 2008;25: 383–399.

60. Costa M, Potvin S, Berthiaume Y, et al. Diabetes: a major co-morbidity of cystic fibrosis. *Diabetes Metab.* 2005;31: 221–232.

61. O'Riordan SM, Robinson PD, Donaghue KC, Moran A. Management of cystic fibrosis-related diabetes. *Pediatr Diabetes.* 2008;9:338–344.

62. Kadowaki T, Bevins CL, Cama A, et al. Two mutant alleles of the insulin receptor gene in a patient with extreme insulin resistance. *Science.* 1988;240:787–790.

63. Mercado MM, McLenithan JC, Silver KD, Shuldiner AR. Genetics of insulin resistance. *Curr Diabetes Rep.* 2002;2:83–95.

64. Moller DE, Cohen O, Yamaguchi Y, et al. Prevalence of mutations in the insulin receptor gene in subjects with features of the type A syndrome of insulin resistance. *Diabetes.* 1994;43:247–255.

65. Taylor SI, Cama A, Accili D, et al. Mutations in the insulin receptor gene. *Endocr Rev.* 1992;13:566–595.

66. Taylor SI, Arioglu E. Genetically defined forms of diabetes in children. *J Clin Endocrinol Metab.* 1999;84:4390–4396.

67. Taylor SI. Lilly Lecture: molecular mechanisms of insulin resistance. Lessons from patients with mutations in the insulin-receptor gene. *Diabetes.* 1992;41:1473–1490.

68. Garg A, Agarwal AK. Lipodystrophies: disorders of adipose tissue biology. *Biochim Biophys Acta.* 2009;1791(6):507–513.

69. Cao H, Hegele RA. Nuclear lamin A/C R482Q mutation in canadian kindreds with Dunnigan-type familial partial lipodystrophy. *Hum Mol Genet.* 2000;9:109–112.

70. Shackleton S, Lloyd DJ, Jackson SN, et al. LMNA, encoding lamin A/C, is mutated in partial lipodystrophy. *Nat Genet.* 2000;24:153–156.

71. Agarwal AK, Fryns JP, Auchus RJ, Garg A. Zinc metalloproteinase, ZMPSTE24, is mutated in mandibuloacral dysplasia. *Hum Mol Genet.* 2003;12:1995–2001.

72. George S, Rochford JJ, Wolfrum C, et al. A family with severe insulin resistance and diabetes due to a mutation in AKT2. *Science.* 2004;304:1325–1328.

73. Agarwal AK, Arioglu E, De AS, et al. AGPAT2 is mutated in congenital generalized lipodystrophy linked to chromosome 9q34. *Nat Genet.* 2002;31:21–23.

74. Magre J, Delepine M, Khallouf E, et al. Identification of the gene altered in Berardinelli-Seip congenital lipodystrophy on chromosome 11q13. *Nat Genet.* 2001;28:365–370.

75. Szymanski KM, Binns D, Bartz R, et al. The lipodystrophy protein seipin is found at endoplasmic reticulum lipid droplet junctions and is important for droplet morphology. *Proc Natl Acad Sci USA.* 2007;104:20890–20895.

76. Kim CA, Delepine M, Boutet E, et al. Association of a homozygous nonsense caveolin-1 mutation with Berardinelli-Seip congenital lipodystrophy. *J Clin Endocrinol Metab.* 2008;93:1129–1134.

77. Barroso I, Gurnell M, Crowley VE, et al. Dominant negative mutations in human PPARgamma associated with severe insulin resistance, diabetes mellitus and hypertension. *Nature.* 1999;402:880–883.

78. Hegele RA, Cao H, Frankowski C, Mathews ST, Leff T. PPARG F388L, a transactivation-deficient mutant, in familial partial lipodystrophy. *Diabetes.* 2002;51:3586–3590.

79. Savage DB, Tan GD, Acerini CL, et al. Human metabolic syndrome resulting from dominant-negative mutations in the nuclear receptor peroxisome proliferator-activated receptor-gamma. *Diabetes*. 2003;52:910–917.

80. Ristow M, Muller-Wieland D, Pfeiffer A, Krone W, Kahn CR. Obesity associated with a mutation in a genetic regulator of adipocyte differentiation. *N Engl J Med*. 1998;339:953–959.

81. Hani EH, Boutin P, Durand E, et al. Missense mutations in the pancreatic islet beta cell inwardly rectifying K+ channel gene (KIR6.2/BIR): a meta-analysis suggests a role in the polygenic basis of Type II diabetes mellitus in Caucasians. *Diabetologia*. 1998;41:1511–1515.

82. Barroso I, Luan J, Middelberg RP, et al. Candidate gene association study in type 2 diabetes indicates a role for genes involved in beta-cell function as well as insulin action. *PLoS Biol*. 2003;1:E20.

83. Gloyn AL, Weedon MN, Owen KR, et al. Large-scale association studies of variants in genes encoding the pancreatic beta-cell KATP channel subunits Kir6.2 (KCNJ11) and SUR1 (ABCC8) confirm that the KCNJ11 E23K variant is associated with type 2 diabetes. *Diabetes*. 2003;52:568–572.

84. Nielsen EM, Hansen L, Carstensen B, et al. The E23K variant of Kir6.2 associates with impaired post-OGTT serum insulin response and increased risk of type 2 diabetes. *Diabetes*. 2003;52:573–577.

85. Lyssenko V, Almgren P, Anevski D, et al. Genetic prediction of future type 2 diabetes. *PLoS Med*. 2005;2:e345.

86. Sesti G, Laratta E, Cardellini M, et al. The E23K variant of KCNJ11 encoding the pancreatic beta-cell adenosine 5′-triphosphate-sensitive potassium channel subunit Kir6.2 is associated with an increased risk of secondary failure to sulfonylurea in patients with type 2 diabetes. *J Clin Endocrinol Metab*. 2006;91:2334–2339.

87. Yen CJ, Beamer BA, Negri C, et al. Molecular scanning of the human peroxisome proliferator activated receptor gamma (hPPAR gamma) gene in diabetic Caucasians: identification of a Pro12Ala PPAR gamma 2 missense mutation. *Biochem Biophys Res Commun*. 1997;241:270–274.

88. Celi FS, Shuldiner AR. The role of peroxisome proliferator-activated receptor gamma in diabetes and obesity. *Curr Diabetes Rep*. 2002;2:179–185.

89. Altshuler D, Hirschhorn JN, Klannemark M, et al. The common PPARgamma Pro12Ala polymorphism is associated with decreased risk of type 2 diabetes. *Nat Genet*. 2000;26:76–80.

90. Deeb SS, Fajas L, Nemoto M, et al. A Pro12Ala substitution in PPARgamma2 associated with decreased receptor activity, lower body mass index and improved insulin sensitivity. *Nat Genet*. 1998;20:284–287.

91. Sandhu MS, Weedon MN, Fawcett KA, et al. Common variants in WFS1 confer risk of type 2 diabetes. *Nat Genet*. 2007;39:951–953.

92. Wasson J, Permutt MA. Candidate gene studies reveal that the WFS1 gene joins the expanding list of novel type 2 diabetes genes. *Diabetologia*. 2008;51:391–393.

93. Sparso T, Andersen G, Albrechtsen A, et al. Impact of polymorphisms in WFS1 on prediabetic phenotypes in a population-based sample of middle-aged people with normal and abnormal glucose regulation. *Diabetologia*. 2008;51:1646–1652.

94. Love-Gregory LD, Wasson J, Ma J, et al. A common polymorphism in the upstream promoter region of the hepatocyte nuclear factor-4 alpha gene on chromosome 20q is associated with type 2 diabetes and appears to contribute to the evidence for linkage in an ashkenazi jewish population. *Diabetes*. 2004;53:1134–1140.

95. Silander K, Mohlke KL, Scott LJ, et al. Genetic variation near the hepatocyte nuclear factor-4 alpha gene predicts susceptibility to type 2 diabetes. *Diabetes*. 2004;53:1141–1149.

96. Damcott CM, Hoppman N, Ott SH, et al. Polymorphisms in both promoters of hepatocyte nuclear factor 4-alpha are associated with type 2 diabetes in the Amish. *Diabetes*. 2004;53:3337–3341.

97. Johansson S, Raeder H, Eide SA, et al. Studies in 3,523 Norwegians and meta-analysis in 11,571 subjects indicate that variants in the hepatocyte nuclear factor 4 alpha (HNF4A) P2 region are associated with type 2 diabetes in Scandinavians. *Diabetes*. 2007;56:3112–3117.

98. Reynisdottir I, Thorleifsson G, Benediktsson R, et al. Localization of a susceptibility gene for type 2 diabetes to chromosome 5q34-q35.2. *Am J Hum Genet*. 2003;73:323–335.

99. Grant SF, Thorleifsson G, Reynisdottir I, et al. Variant of transcription factor 7-like 2 (TCF7L2) gene confers risk of type 2 diabetes. *Nat Genet*. 2006;38:320–323.

100. Damcott CM, Pollin TI, Reinhart LJ, et al. Polymorphisms in the transcription factor 7-like 2 (TCF7L2) gene are associated with type 2 diabetes in the Amish: replication and evidence for a role in both insulin secretion and insulin resistance. *Diabetes*. 2006;55:2654–2659.

101. Tong Y, Lin Y, Zhang Y, et al. Association between TCF7L2 gene polymorphisms and susceptibility to type 2 diabetes mellitus: a large Human Genome Epidemiology (HuGE) review and meta-analysis. *BMC Med Genet*. 2009;10:15.

102. Pilgaard K, Jensen CB, Schou JH, et al. The T allele of rs7903146 TCF7L2 is associated with impaired insulinotropic action of incretin hormones, reduced 24 h profiles of plasma insulin and glucagon, and increased hepatic glucose production in young healthy men. *Diabetologia*. 2009;52(7):1227–1230.

103. Pearson ER, Donnelly LA, Kimber C, et al. Variation in TCF7L2 influences therapeutic response to sulfonylureas: a GoDARTs study. *Diabetes*. 2007;56:2178–2182.

104. Florez JC, Jablonski KA, Bayley N, et al. TCF7L2 polymorphisms and progression to diabetes in the Diabetes Prevention Program. *N Engl J Med*. 2006;355:241–250.

105. Hanis CL, Boerwinkle E, Chakraborty R, et al. A genome-wide search for human non-insulin-dependent (type 2) diabetes genes reveals a major susceptibility locus on chromosome 2. *Nat Genet*. 1996;13:161–166.

106. Garant MJ, Kao WH, Brancati F, et al. SNP43 of CAPN10 and the risk of type 2 diabetes in African-Americans: the Atherosclerosis Risk in Communities study. *Diabetes*. 2002;51:231–237.

107. Elbein SC, Chu W, Ren Q, et al. Role of calpain-10 gene variants in familial type 2 diabetes in Caucasians. *J Clin Endocrinol Metab*. 2002;87:650–654.

108. Fullerton SM, Bartoszewicz A, Ybazeta G, et al. Geographic and haplotype structure of candidate type 2 diabetes susceptibility variants at the calpain-10 locus. *Am J Hum Genet*. 2002;70:1096–1106.

109. Song Y, Niu T, Manson JE, Kwiatkowski DJ, Liu S. Are variants in the CAPN10 gene related to risk of type 2 diabetes? A quantitative assessment of population and family-based association studies. *Am J Hum Genet*. 2004;74:208–222.

110. Weedon MN, Schwarz PE, Horikawa Y, et al. Meta-analysis and a large association study confirm a role for calpain-10 variation in type 2 diabetes susceptibility. *Am J Hum Genet*. 2003;73:1208–1212.

111. Jensen DP, Urhammer SA, Eiberg H, et al. Variation in CAPN10 in relation to type 2 diabetes, obesity and quantitative metabolic traits: studies in 6018 whites. *Mol Genet Metab*. 2006;89:360–367.

112. Saez ME, Gonzalez-Sanchez JL, Ramirez-Lorca R, et al. The CAPN10 gene is associated with insulin resistance phenotypes in the Spanish population. *PLoS ONE*. 2008;3:e2953.

113. Turner MD, Fulcher FK, Jones CV, et al. Calpain facilitates actin reorganization during glucose-stimulated insulin secretion. *Biochem Biophys Res Commun*. 2007;352:650–655.

114. Sladek R, Rocheleau G, Rung J, et al. A genome-wide association study identifies novel risk loci for type 2 diabetes. *Nature*. 2007;445:881–885.

115. Saxena R, Voight BF, Lyssenko V, et al. Genome-wide association analysis identifies loci for type 2 diabetes and triglyceride levels. *Science*. 2007;316:1331–1336.

116. Scott LJ, Mohlke KL, Bonnycastle LL, et al. A genome-wide association study of type 2 diabetes in Finns detects multiple susceptibility variants. *Science*. 2007;316:1341–1345.

117. Steinthorsdottir V, Thorleifsson G, Reynisdottir I, et al. A variant in CDKAL1 influences insulin response and risk of type 2 diabetes. *Nat Genet*. 2007;39:770–775.

118. Zeggini E, Weedon MN, Lindgren CM, et al. Replication of genome-wide association signals in UK samples reveals risk loci for type 2 diabetes. *Science*. 2007;316:1336–1341.

119. Egefjord L, Jensen JL, Bang-Berthelsen CH, et al. Zinc transporter gene expression is regulated by pro-inflammatory cytokines: a potential role for zinc transporters in beta-cell apoptosis? *BMC Endocr Disord*. 2009;9:7.

120. Wenzlau JM, Liu Y, Yu L, et al. A common nonsynonymous single nucleotide polymorphism in the SLC30A8 gene determines ZnT8 autoantibody specificity in type 1 diabetes. *Diabetes*. 2008;57:2693–2697.

121. Vaxillaire M, Cavalcanti-Proenca C, Dechaume A, et al. The common P446L polymorphism in GCKR inversely modulates fasting glucose and triglyceride levels and reduces type 2 diabetes risk in the DESIR prospective general French population. *Diabetes*. 2008;57:2253–2257.

122. Farrelly D, Brown KS, Tieman A, et al. Mice mutant for glucokinase regulatory protein exhibit decreased liver glucokinase: a sequestration mechanism in metabolic regulation. *Proc Natl Acad Sci USA*. 1999;96:14511–14516.

123. Frayling TM, Timpson NJ, Weedon MN, et al. A common variant in the FTO gene is associated with body mass index and predisposes to childhood and adult obesity. *Science*. 2007;316:889–894.

124. Rampersaud E, Mitchell BD, Pollin TI, et al. Physical activity and the association of common FTO gene variants with body mass index and obesity. *Arch Intern Med*. 2008;168:1791–1797.

125. Meyre D, Delplanque J, Chevre JC, et al. Genome-wide association study for early-onset and morbid adult obesity identifies three new risk loci in European populations. *Nat Genet*. 2009;41:157–159.

126. Gerken T, Girard CA, Tung YC, et al. The obesity-associated FTO gene encodes a 2-oxoglutarate-dependent nucleic acid demethylase. *Science*. 2007;318:1469–1472.

127. Cecil JE, Tavendale R, Watt P, Hetherington MM, Palmer CN. An obesity-associated FTO gene variant and increased energy intake in children. *N Engl J Med*. 2008;359:2558–2566.

128. Unoki H, Takahashi A, Kawaguchi T, et al. SNPs in KCNQ1 are associated with susceptibility to type 2 diabetes in East Asian and European populations. *Nat Genet*. 2008;40:1098–1102.

129. Yasuda K, Miyake K, Horikawa Y, et al. Variants in KCNQ1 are associated with susceptibility to type 2 diabetes mellitus. *Nat Genet*. 2008;40:1092–1097.

130. Lee MP, Ravenel JD, Hu RJ, et al. Targeted disruption of the Kvlqt1 gene causes deafness and gastric hyperplasia in mice. *J Clin Invest*. 2000;106:1447–1455.

131. Tan JT, Nurbaya S, Gardner D, Sandra Y, Tai ES, Ng DP. Genetic variation in KCNQ1 associates with fasting glucose and beta-cell function: a study of 3734 subjects comprising the ethnicities living in Singapore. *Diabetes*. 2009;58:1445–1449.

132. Li X, Allayee H, Xiang AH, et al. Variation in IGF2BP2 interacts with adiposity to alter insulin sensitivity in Mexican Americans. *Obesity (Silver Spring)*. 2009;17(4):729–736.

133. Ruchat SM, Elks CE, Loos RJ, et al. Association between insulin secretion, insulin sensitivity and type 2 diabetes susceptibility variants identified in genome-wide association studies. *Acta Diabetol*. 2008;46:217–226.

134. Groenewoud MJ, Dekker JM, Fritsche A, et al. Variants of CDKAL1 and IGF2BP2 affect first-phase insulin secretion during hyperglycaemic clamps. *Diabetologia*. 2008;51:1659–1663.

135. Pascoe L, Tura A, Patel SK, et al. Common variants of the novel type 2 diabetes genes CDKAL1 and HHEX/IDE are associated with decreased pancreatic beta-cell function. *Diabetes*. 2007;56:3101–3104.

136. Stancakova A, Pihlajamaki J, Kuusisto J, et al. Single-nucleotide polymorphism rs7754840 of CDKAL1 is associated with impaired insulin secretion in nondiabetic offspring of type 2 diabetic subjects and in a large sample of men with normal glucose tolerance. *J Clin Endocrinol Metab*. 2008;93:1924–1930.

137. Kim WY, Sharpless NE. The regulation of INK4/ARF in cancer and aging. *Cell*. 2006;127:265–275.

138. Kamb A, Gruis NA, Weaver-Feldhaus J, et al. A cell cycle regulator potentially involved in genesis of many tumor types. *Science*. 1994;264:436–440.

139. Krishnamurthy J, Ramsey MR, Ligon KL, et al. p16INK4a induces an age-dependent decline in islet regenerative potential. *Nature*. 2006;443:453–457.

140. Grarup N, Rose CS, Andersson EA, et al. Studies of association of variants near the HHEX, CDKN2A/B, and IGF2BP2 genes with type 2 diabetes and impaired insulin release in 10,705 Danish subjects: validation and extension of genome-wide association studies. *Diabetes*. 2007;56:3105–3111.

141. Helgadottir A, Thorleifsson G, Manolescu A, et al. A common variant on chromosome 9p21 affects the risk of myocardial infarction. *Science*. 2007;316:1491–1493.

142. Samani NJ, Erdmann J, Hall AS, et al. Genomewide association analysis of coronary artery disease. *N Engl J Med*. 2007;357:443–453.

143. Zeggini E, Scott LJ, Saxena R, et al. Meta-analysis of genome-wide association data and large-scale replication identifies additional susceptibility loci for type 2 diabetes. *Nat Genet*. 2008;40:638–645.

144. Rampersaud E, Damcott CM, Fu M, et al. Identification of novel candidate genes for type 2 diabetes from a genome-wide association scan in the Old Order Amish: evidence for replication from diabetes-related quantitative traits and from independent populations. *Diabetes*. 2007;56:3053–3062.

145. Hanson RL, Bogardus C, Duggan D, et al. A search for variants associated with young-onset type 2 diabetes in American Indians in a 100 K genotyping array. *Diabetes*. 2007;56:3045–3052.

146. Hayes MG, Pluzhnikov A, Miyake K, et al. Identification of type 2 diabetes genes in Mexican Americans through genome-wide association studies. *Diabetes*. 2007;56:3033–3044.

147. Florez JC, Manning AK, Dupuis J, et al. A 100 K genome-wide association scan for diabetes and related traits in the Framingham Heart study: replication and integration with other genome-wide datasets. *Diabetes*. 2007;56:3063–3074.

148. Lyssenko V, Jonsson A, Almgren P, et al. Clinical risk factors, DNA variants, and the development of type 2 diabetes. *N Engl J Med*. 2008;359:2220–2232.

149. Meigs JB, Shrader P, Sullivan LM, et al. Genotype score in addition to common risk factors for prediction of type 2 diabetes. *N Engl J Med*. 2008;359:2208–2219.

Chapter 11
Rodent Models of Diabetes

Ronald J. Christopher, Koji Takeuchi, and Bumsup Lee

Introduction

Animal models have been used extensively to study the pathophysiology of type 1 and type 2 diabetes. These models have been invaluable in the development of therapeutic agents to treat the diseases and associated complications. Rodents, primarily mice and rats, are the predominant animals used as models of diabetes. The use of these animals is relatively inexpensive and practical. The importance of mouse models has increased after the introduction of advanced methods for genetic manipulation, such as tissue-specific transgenic expression and targeted gene knockout.

The use of larger animals has been limited by both the expense and the requirement for specialized expertise and facilities. A larger body size, however, can facilitate more frequent blood sampling, longitudinal tissue sampling, and the use of multiple indwelling catheters. Nonhuman primates with insulin resistance and diabetes have been used to study both the disease and therapeutic approaches. However, experimentation with nonhuman primates is more heavily regulated than that with rodents, and the scarcity of the animals and resulting higher costs restrict the application of the nonhuman primate for the study of diabetes.

This chapter focuses on rodent models for studying type 1 and type 2 diabetes including models that develop the disease spontaneously or through induction by chemical agents that alter the function of pancreatic β-cells or by genetic alterations. With transgenic mouse models of type 1 diabetes the researcher is able to probe the molecular mechanisms involving autoimmunity against β-cells as well as genes influenced by the disease. The animal models of type 2 diabetes can be spontaneous or induced (by chemicals or dietary or surgical manipulations and/or by combinations thereof). In recent years many new genetically modified animal models including transgenic, generalized gene knockout, and tissue-specific knockout mice have been engineered for the study of diabetes. In this chapter we describe characteristic features, underlying causes/mechanisms, and advantages/disadvantages of a variety of animal models used in diabetes research.

Models of Type 1 Diabetes

The most widely used animal models of type 1 diabetes are those with selective destruction of pancreatic β-cells. These include both animals that spontaneously develop autoimmune destruction of islets and those that are induced by chemical ablation (Table 11.1). In addition, genetic models have been generated to identify the specific mutations and the transcription factors controlling pancreatic islet organogenesis and β-cell physiology.

R.J. Christopher (✉)
Takeda San Diego, Inc., San Diego, CA 92121, USA
e-mail: ron.christopher@takedasd.com

L. Poretsky (ed.), *Principles of Diabetes Mellitus*, DOI 10.1007/978-0-387-09841-8_11,
© Springer Science+Business Media, LLC 2010

Table 11.1 Animal models of type 1 diabetes

Spontaneous type 1 diabetes	
Mouse	NOD (non-obese diabetic)
Rat	BB (BioBreeding)
	BBDR/Wor and BBdp
	LETL (Long-Evans Tokushima lean)
	KDP (Komeda diabetes prone)
	LEW.1AR1/Ztm-iddm
	LEW.1WR1
Chemicals to induce type 1 diabetes	
	Alloxan
	Streptozotocin
	Vacor
	Dithizone
	8-Hydroxyquinolone

Spontaneous Animal Models of Type 1 Diabetes

The NOD (non-obese diabetic) mouse was developed at the Shionogi Research Laboratories in Osaka, Japan, by selectively breeding offspring and was first used in the study of cataract development (the JcI-ICR mouse).[1] In the NOD mouse, lymphocytic infiltration of the pancreatic islets and insulitis are seen at 4–5 weeks of age followed by subclinical β-cell destruction and decreasing insulin levels. Between 12 and 30 weeks of age the incidence of diabetes in some colonies reaches 90% in females and 60% in males.

BioBreeding (BB) rats were first observed to exhibit spontaneous hyperglycemia and ketoacidosis in the 1970s in a colony of Wistar rats at BioBreeding laboratories in Ottawa, Canada.[2] Affected animals were used to establish other BB rat colonies; BBdp/Wor rats were inbred in Worcester, Massachusetts and BBdp rats were outbred in Ottawa, Canada. Several other immunologically and genetically distinct BB rat substrains have been created. The BB rat refers to all rats derived from the original founder; more specific designations are used to refer to the substrains. The BB rat is one of the best models of type 1 diabetes and has disease onset and pathogenesis closely resembling the human disease. The most obvious immunopathology in BB rats is profound T-cell lymphopenia. The number of CD4+ T cells is severely reduced and the CD8+ T cells are nearly completely absent. The lymphopenia appears to be inherited as a recessive mutation controlled by a single gene, *Gimap5*. The autoimmune rats appear to require at least one gene to develop diabetes, rat major histocompatibility complex (MHC) designated *RT1* that includes two class I loci (designated A and C) and two class II loci (designated B/D). In the BB rat, the *RT1 B/D* region is designated *Iddm1* and expression of diabetes requires the presence of at least one class II *RT1 B/D* allele.

The LETL (Long-Evans Tokushima lean) rat[3] and its substrain, the KDP (Komeda diabetes-prone) rat,[4] were developed in Japan. These animals closely resemble human type 1 diabetes both in the mechanism of induction and in the pathophysiological consequences. They can therefore be used to study disease prevention, early markers of diabetes, and therapeutic approaches.

Evidence to date demonstrates that the MHC class II genes are major contributors to the development of type 1 diabetes in these models and humans. Having the diabetogenic MHC class II genes is a necessary, but not sufficient, condition for development of the phenotype.[5] Identification of non-MHC genes that contribute to type 1 diabetes is underway. For example, a genome-wide scan of the NOD mouse suggests that there are 11 loci contributing to diabetes in this mouse strain and that these loci are widely distributed in the genome.[6] Due to the independent origins of the different autoimmune models, it is likely that some of the contributing genes will vary between the models. Cell types implicated in development of insulitis include CD4+ and CD8+ T lymphocytes, dendritic cells, and monocytes/macrophages. T-lymphocyte infiltration in mice with spontaneous or experimentally induced immune disorders rapidly targets pancreatic islets and leads to insulitis and diabetes. These cells contributing to the development of type 1 diabetes are used for investigating the detailed mechanisms underlying the autoimmune process in pancreatic islet β-cells.[7]

Chemical-Induced Animal Models of Type 1 Diabetes

Streptozotocin and alloxan are the most frequently used chemicals to injure β-cells. A single intravenous dose of alloxan generates highly reactive hydroxyl radicals that damage DNA and increase the cytosolic calcium concentration.[8] This results in β-cell destruction within minutes to hours following the injection. Permanent insulinopenia with hyperglycemia and ketoacidosis typically appears after 12 h and insulin therapy is required to keep the animals alive. Because of the severity of β-cell injury and the inability to titrate the degree of injury following dosing, alloxan is less frequently used than streptozotocin.

Streptozotocin is a nitrosourea derivative isolated from *Streptomyces achromogenes* with broad-spectrum antibiotic and anti-neoplastic activity.[9] It is a powerful alkylating agent that has been shown to interfere with glucose transport and glucokinase function and to induce multiple DNA strand breaks. As a result of streptozotocin exposure, β-cells undergo destruction by necrosis. A single large dose of streptozotocin can produce diabetes in rodents or, alternatively, multiple small doses can be used. The multiple dose technique is valuable to produce animals with sufficient β-cell loss to cause diabetes, while leaving enough residual insulin secretory capacity to avoid ketoacidosis and the need for insulin treatment. This is a major practical advantage of streptozotocin for producing animals that mimic type 1 or type 2 diabetes.

Chemical-induced animal models of type 1 diabetes have virtually the same phenotype as humans with type 1 diabetes although the mechanism of pancreatic β-cell damage is different. Therefore, these models are valuable to study the long-term treatment of diabetes and the prevention and treatment of the complications of diabetes, but not the pathophysiology of the onset of type 1 diabetes.

Genetic Animal Models of Type 1 Diabetes

Transgenic mouse models of type 1 diabetes include T-cell receptor transgenic mice and the rat insulin promoter-driven expression of neo-antigen and the molecules on β-cells that enhance diabetogenic stimuli. Genetic ablation and targeted overexpression of transcription factor genes in mice are used to study pancreas and islet organogenesis and β-cell physiology (some of the transcription factors include: IPF1/PDX1, Isl1, NeuroD1/β2, Pax4, Pax6, Nkx2.2, HNF-1α, HNF-1β, HNF-4α).[10] The human and mouse phenotypes are similar for mutations in some of these genes, although some strains of mice with mutations tend not to develop diabetes, but rather novel autoimmune phenotypes.

Models of Type 2 Diabetes

Animal models of type 2 diabetes have played a significant role both in the advancement of our understanding of the pathophysiology of the disease and in the development of therapeutic agents for its treatment. The most commonly used models are either rat or mouse (Table 11.2) although some work is performed in selected groups of larger animals and nonhuman primates.

The genetic components of obesity and diabetes can be driven by either monogenic or polygenic mutations. A number of monogenic animal models of type 2 diabetes have been used extensively and are very well characterized. These models express phenotypic characteristics that realistically represent the pathophysiology of type 2 diabetes in humans. In humans, however, type 2 diabetes is a heterogeneous polygenic disease and polygenic inheritance is the predominant mode of inheritance. Multiple polygenic animal models are also available. Although numerous genes have been identified that are associated with the development of type 2 diabetes, the target genes implicated in the etiology of the type 2 diabetes are not fully understood. Therefore, as with the animal models of type 1 diabetes, many type 2 diabetes animal models have proven to be valuable tools and are routinely used for studying the pathophysiology of the disease and the prevention or treatment of complications, but not the development of the disease.

Table 11.2 Animal models of type 2 diabetes

Animal models	Application in research and pharmaceutical development
Mice	
ob/ob	Testing the agents of insulin sensitizers, antiobesity, and some other antihyperglycemics
db/db	Investigating type 2 diabetes/diabetic dyslipidemia and testing insulin mimetics and insulin sensitizers
KKA^y	Investigating insulin signaling pathways, including glucose uptake, pentose pathways, and impaired insulin-sensitive phosphodiesterase in fat cells
NZO	Studying relationship between autoimmunity, obesity, and diabetes
NONcNZO10	Investigating diabetes, obesity and testing antidiabetic agents
TSOD	Investigating insulin resistance, adiposity, and diabetic complications of peripheral neuropathy
M16	Studying early-onset polygenic obesity and type 2 diabetes at young ages
NSY	Investigating the pathogenesis and genetic predisposition to type 2 diabetes
Akita	Testing certain chemical diabetogens for islet transplantation studies due to its absence of β-cell autoimmunity
Rats	
Zucker *fa/fa*	Studying obesity and type 2 diabetes associated with increased VLDL and TG levels and hypertension
	Screening insulin sensitizing and antiobesity agents for the testing the potentiators of insulin secretion or incretin mimetic agents
ZDF	Investigating the mechanisms associated with insulin resistance and β-cell dysfunction in type 2 diabetes, as well as for testing insulin sensitizers and insulinotropic agents
Wistar fatty	Pharmacological research testing for insulin secretagogues and sensitizers
OLETF	Pharmacological research testing for antidiabetic and antihypertensive drugs
GK	Studying the relation of changes in β-cell mass and occurrence of type 2 diabetes and diabetic complications (particularly diabetic nephropathy)
SHROB (Koletsky)	Investigating diabetic and hypertensive nephropathies and diabetic retinopathy
SHR/N-*cp*	Investigating obesity-associated type 2 diabetes and the influence of dietary carbohydrate on the development of diabetes in certain genetically predisposed carbohydrate-sensitive individuals
JCR/LA-*cp*	Pharmacological and dietary intervention prior to the onset of cardiovascular lesions or hyperinsulinemia to determine the efficacy for preventing or slowing the occurrence of cardiovascular lesions
SDT	Studying pathogenesis and treatment of diabetic retinopathy

Monogenic Models of Type 2 Diabetes and Obesity

Leptin Receptor or Leptin Mutation

Leptin is a 16 kDa peptide, produced predominantly by adipose tissue, which plays an important role in regulating appetite and energy expenditure, by acting on its receptor in the hypothalamus. Its release by fat cells is proportional to body fat stores and plasma leptin levels correlate with the degree of adiposity. Leptin deficiency results in hyperphagia, decreased energy expenditure, and obesity. Leptin-deficient animals have increased circulating levels of neuropeptide Y (NPY), a potent appetite stimulant, and cortisol, which contributes to muscle insulin resistance. The most widely used models lack either leptin (*ob/ob* mouse) or the leptin receptor (*db/db* mouse and Zucker *fa/fa* rat). The Zucker diabetic fatty (ZDF) rat is a spontaneous variant of the Zucker *fa/fa* rat that is severely diabetic.[11,12]

ob/ob mouse: The *ob/ob* (obese) mouse model originated at The Jackson Laboratory, Bar Harbor, ME,[13] and represents a very popular model to study type 2 diabetes, obesity, and food intake. This monogenic model is the result of an autosomal recessive mutation (C428T) on chromosome 6 in the C57BL/6 J mouse. The mutation in the *ob/ob* mouse is in the coding gene for leptin (referenced as *Lep^ob*) resulting in premature termination of leptin synthesis and the ablation of leptin signaling. The *ob/ob* mice are hyperphagic and show the obese phenotype at 2 weeks of age with the body weight expected to reach approximately 40 and 60 g at 6 and 14 weeks of age, respectively. In normal male C57BL/6 J mice, the body weight reaches approximately 20 and 27 g at 6 and 14 weeks of age, respectively. The *ob/ob* mice also show marked hyperglycemia, mildly impaired glucose tolerance, severe hyperinsulinemia, and impaired fertility and wound healing. Insulin resistance is observed both in peripheral tissues and in the liver. The mice become severely diabetic with ultimate deterioration of pancreatic islets, progressively leading to death. Both hypertrophy and hyperplasia of pancreatic islets are evident prior to the final deterioration.

db/db mouse: The *db/db* (diabetic) mouse also originated at The Jackson Laboratory, Bar Harbor, ME.[13] A single base autosomal recessive mutation (G to T) in the structural gene of the leptin receptor (referenced as *lepr^db*) on chromosome 4 in the C57BL/KsJ mouse eliminates leptin signaling. These mice are spontaneously hyperphagic, obese, hyperglycemic, hyperinsulinemic, and insulin resistant within the first month of age. Increased plasma insulin levels persist until 10 weeks of age followed by a decrease in plasma insulin levels commensurate to the loss of pancreatic β-cells. In this model plasma glucose levels exceed 500 mg/dL at older ages. The mice exhibit ketosis, progressive body weight loss, and diabetic complications (nephropathy) and do not survive beyond 8–10 months. In *db/db* mice, lack of the leptin receptor results in hypothalamic disturbances and NPY abnormalities as seen in *ob/ob* mice. However, leptin is still produced by the adipose tissue and NPY-induced hyperinsulinemia and hypercorticosteronism result in *ob* gene hyperexpression and hyperleptinemia.

Zucker *fa/fa* and ZDF rats: The Zucker *fa/fa* (fatty) rat was discovered in 1961 and is the most popular rat model for studying obesity and the prediabetic state. The model is the result of an autosomal recessive (*fa*) mutation (Gln269Pro) of the structural gene for the leptin receptor (referenced as *Lepr^fa*) on chromosome 5 resulting in reduced, but not eliminated, expression of the leptin receptor on the cell surface with marked intracellular retention and decreased leptin binding. These rats are obese and hyperphagic with increased subcutaneous fat even at 4 weeks of age. They also exhibit mild hyperglycemia, insulin resistance, hyperlipidemia, and hyperinsulinemia. Pancreatic β-cell numbers decrease with age. The hyperphagia in these rats is attributed to the hypothalamic defect in leptin receptor signaling.[12]

The Zucker diabetic fatty (ZDF) rat is a substrain of the Zucker *fa/fa* rat selectively inbred for hyperglycemia and has utility in studying type 2 diabetes. Unlike the Zucker *fa/fa* rat, male ZDF rats progress to frank diabetes due to failure to compensate adequately for insulin resistance. They are less obese but more insulin resistant than Zucker *fa/fa* rats. Males are more prone to the development of diabetes, usually at 7–10 weeks of age. Females are obese and insulin resistant but do not develop diabetes. ZDF rats exhibit an impaired insulin secretory response to glucose while retaining an intact response to non-glucose secretagogues like arginine, a phenomenon similar to that observed in human type 2 diabetic patients. Downregulation of β-cell GLUT-2 transporters coupled with impaired insulin synthesis is also responsible for hyperglycemia in ZDF rats.[14] Significant abnormalities are found in pancreatic function and structure after the onset of diabetes in ZDF rats. Although the β-cell proliferation rate remains high, decreased β-cell mass is observed in the ZDF rats. The lower cell mass is thought to be due to an increase in β-cell apoptosis. These β-cell abnormalities are reduced by treatment with antidiabetic agents such as the insulin sensitizers, thiazolidinediones, suggesting that the β-cell dysfunction in the ZDF rat is derived from glucose toxicity and β-cell exhaustion.[15]

Melanocortin pathway mutations: *agouti yellow* (A^y) and related mice. The agouti protein is a melanocortin antagonist; it competes with melanocortins for binding to the melanocortin receptors (MCRs). The MCRs are involved in controlling the central and peripheral components of the hypothalamo-hypophyseal-adrenal system. Autosomal dominant mutation of the agouti gene (agouti yellow: A^y) in heterozygous A^y/a mice leads to ectopic overexpression of agouti protein and produces a yellow coat color.[16] Increased food intake, obesity, and insulin resistance are attributed to antagonism of α-melanocyte-stimulating hormone (αMSH) at the hypothalamic MC4R, and to a lesser extent, MC3R.

Carboxypeptidase E Mutation

Carboxypeptidase E (CPE) is an enzyme responsible for the final proteolytic processing step of prohormone intermediates in the brain and various neuroendocrine tissues. Mice with a spontaneous homozygous fat mutation of CPE (Cpe^{fat}) lack CPE activity in the islets of Langerhans and the pituitary. The Cpe^{fat} mice arose spontaneously in the HRS/J strain and were backcrossed five generations to C57BLKS/J mice. Cpe^{fat} mice with a C57BLKS/J genetic background have a diabetes phenotype that is primarily restricted to males and is more severe than that seen in the original HRS/J strain. Animals become severely obese, hyperinsulinemic, and hyperglycemic. Cpe^{fat} mice with the HRS/J background exhibit early-onset hyperinsulinemia with subsequent postpubertal moderate obesity without hyperglycemia.[17]

Polygenic Models of Type 2 Diabetes and Obesity

Spontaneous monogenic models for type 2 diabetes have helped to understand the pathogenesis of type 2 diabetes. However, the identified murine diabetogenic genes account for only a small part of human type 2 diabetes and the clinical phenotypes of the monogenic models are extreme: massive obesity and hyperphagia, either extremely high or no leptin in circulation, and extreme hyperinsulinism. Therefore, development of polygenic models of diabetes is necessary to better represent the human disease and to help identify the genes that underlie the disease in man.

Several spontaneous polygenic models of type 2 diabetes, such as the Otsuka Long-Evans Tokushima fatty (OLETF) rat, the KKA^y mouse, the Nagoya–Shibata–Yasuda (NSY) mouse, and the Tsumura Suzuki obese diabetes (TSOD) mouse, develop overt obesity and hyperinsulinemia prior to the onset of diabetes. Notably, Goto–Kakizaki (GK) rats exhibit distinct dysfunction of pancreatic β-cells and develop type 2 diabetes without developing obesity. The NSY mice develop diabetes very late in life without either extreme obesity or severe hyperinsulinemia.

KK and KKA^y mouse: The Kuo Kondo (KK) mouse developed in Japan is a spontaneous diabetes model produced by selective inbreeding for large body size. KK mice are hyperphagic, hyperinsulinemic, insulin resistant and show moderate obesity by 2 months of age. Insulin resistance precedes the onset of obesity. The increase in pancreatic insulin content is associated with an increase in the number and size of pancreatic islets.

The KKA^y mouse (also known as yellow KK obese mouse) was established by transferring the yellow obese (A^y) gene into the KK strain. Unlike KK mice that carry only the diabetes gene, these mice additionally carry the lethal A^y gene. KKA^y mice are heterozygous and show severe obesity, hyperglycemia, hyperinsulinemia, and glucose intolerance by 8 weeks of age indicating that obesity is an important factor for onset of overt diabetes in the KK strain. Hyperphagia and obesity in young animals are more pronounced in males than in females. Pancreatic islets are hypertrophied and β-cells are degranulated. The primary cause of diabetes in these mice is insulin resistance due to defects in both insulin receptor and post-receptor signaling systems, including glucose uptake, pentose pathways, and impaired insulin-sensitive phosphodiesterase activity in fat cells.[18] The characteristics of the KKA^y mice are useful for the evaluation of antidiabetic and antiobesity agents. Pioglitazone, an insulin sensitizer of the thiazolidinedione chemical class, was initially discovered by screening in KKA^y mice.[19]

NZO mouse: The New Zealand obese (NZO) mouse was obtained by selective inbreeding over several generations with the parents selected for their agouti coat color at the University of Otago Medical School in Dunedin, New Zealand. The NZO mouse is a spontaneous model for studies of obese type 2 diabetes. It is a model of spontaneous polygenic obesity and insulin resistance and exhibits hyperphagia, obesity, mild hyperglycemia, hyperinsulinemia, impaired glucose tolerance, and insulin resistance. Hyperglycemia and impaired glucose tolerance increase continuously with advancing age. After initial β-cell hyperplasia, decompensation in males is accompanied by reduced β-cell mass, degranulation, and ultrastructural changes. Reduced liver glycogen synthase activity is considered a primary early defect contributing to the development of diabetes. The mice are shown to have hepatic insulin resistance from an early age with increased gluconeogenesis as a result of abnormal regulation of fructose-1,6-bisphosphatase.[20]

NONcNZO10 mouse: The NONcNZO10 mouse is a new polygenic mouse model of type 2 diabetes with obesity. The mouse is a recombinant congenic mouse model developed at The Jackson Laboratory by introgressing five genomic intervals from the type 2 diabetes-prone and obese NZO/HlLt (NZO) inbred strain into the nominally non-obese nondiabetic (NON/Lt or NON) strain background.[21] Whereas parental NZO males exhibit the unwanted phenotypes of hyperphagia, morbid obesity, poor fertility, and a variable frequency of hyperglycemia, NONcNZO10 males are not hyperphagic, develop more moderate levels of obesity, and reproduce normally. At 8 weeks of age, the mice develop liver and skeletal muscle insulin resistance with modest elevations of plasma insulin levels. The obese and hyperglycemic state is developed by 13 weeks of age with exacerbated insulin resistance in skeletal muscle, liver, and heart associated with increased lipids. The NONcNZO10 mice weigh more than NON males, but significantly less than the NZO males. Pancreatic islets show similar atrophic changes to those seen in diabetic NZO males. Increased serum triglycerides and liver steatosis are observed. Females are resistant to diabetes and can serve as normoglycemic controls. Unlike *ob/ob* and *db/db* mice which are monogenic and exhibit a morbid obesity, these mice are polygenic, not hyperphagic, have a normal leptin/leptin receptor axis, do not exhibit hypercorticism, and show no obvious thermoregulatory defects (i.e., poor heat tolerance, reduced sweating).[12]

TSOD mouse: The Tsumura Suzuki obese diabetes (TSOD) mouse originates from selective inbreeding of the outbred, nondiabetic ddY strain and is a spontaneous mouse model for studies on obese type 2 diabetes. The salient phenotype is obesity and hyperphagia with male mice developing diabetes. A selectively inbred nondiabetic, obese Tsumura Suzuki non-obese (TSNO) mouse was also generated. The male TSOD mice develop polydipsia and polyuria at about 2 months of age followed by the gradual development of obesity, hyperglycemia, and hyperinsulinemia. Body weight reaches more than 60 g at 16 weeks of age while normal C57BL/6 J mice typically weigh 27 g at this same age. Obesity gradually increases until about 12 months of age. Pancreatic islets of male TSOD mice hypertrophy without signs of insulitis or fibrous formation. The reduced insulin sensitivity in diabetic TSOD mice is partly due to impaired insulin-dependent glucose transporter (GLUT4) translocation in both skeletal muscle and adipocytes.[12]

M16 mouse: The M16 mouse is an outbred model of early-onset polygenic obesity and diabetes. The M16 mouse results from long-term selective breeding from an Institute of Cancer Research, London, UK (ICR) base population, with an emphasis on obesity and obesity-induced diabetes. M16 mice exhibit early-onset obesity and are larger than control animals at all ages. They are characterized by increased body fat percentage, fat cell size, fat cell number, and organ weights as compared to control ICR mice. These mice are moderately obese, hyperphagic, hyperglycemic, hyperinsulinemic, hyperleptinemic, and hypercholesterolemic.[12]

NSY mouse: The Nagoya–Shibata–Yasuda (NSY) mouse was developed by selective inbreeding using an outbred Jc1:ICR mouse colony (which is also the ancestral strain from which NOD mice were developed). NSY mice spontaneously develop obesity and type 2 diabetes in an age-dependent manner. The mice show impaired insulin secretion, mild insulin resistance, but normal islet morphology. There is a marked gender difference with almost all males developing hyperglycemia, but less than a third of females being affected.[22]

Akita mouse: This non-obese mutant C57BL/6 Akita (Ins2^{Akita}) mouse was derived from the colony of C57BL/6 in Akita, Japan, and is a model for non-obese type 2 diabetes. This model does not exhibit either obesity or insulitis, but has pancreatic β-cell dysfunction, distinguishing it from other animal models. The Ins2^{Akita} mouse has a spontaneous autosomal dominant mutation in the insulin 2 gene (C96Y). The Ins2^{Akita} mutation impairs normal insulin processing by disrupting a disulfide bond between the A and B chains of the insulin 2 peptide impairing the secretion of mature insulin. The mouse is characterized by hyperglycemia, hypoinsulinemia, polydipsia, and polyuria, beginning around 3–4 weeks of age. Histologically, at 4–35 weeks of age, the density of active pancreatic β-cells is reduced without insulitis and islets release very little mature insulin. Accumulation of mutant proinsulin in the endoplasmic reticulum (ER) results in the increase in ER stress in the pancreatic β-cell and induction of β-cell apoptosis.[22]

Wistar Fatty Rat

The Wistar fatty (WF/Ta-*fa*) rat model of obese type 2 diabetes was established in 1981. This model was developed by transferring the *fa* gene from the genetically obese Zucker *fa/fa* rat to the somewhat carbohydrate-intolerant lean Wistar–Kyoto (WKY) rat. At the fifth generation of backcrossing, the male obese hybrids were found to be hyperglycemic, hyperlipidemic and hyperinsulinemic, and severely obese. The rats are maintained at Takeda Pharmaceuticals Company Limited in Japan. Although both WF/Ta-*fa* and Zucker *fa/fa* rats share the *fa* gene for obesity, their metabolic profiles differ in several respects. Obese male WF/Ta-*fa* rats are more hyperglycemic, glucose intolerant, and insulin resistant, but they are less hyperlipidemic than obese male Zucker *fa/fa* rats. Male, but not female WF/Ta-*fa*, rats show hyperglycemia, glucosuria, and polyuria as early as 8 weeks of age with plasma glucose levels reaching 300–400 mg/dL at this stage. Glucose tolerance and the insulin response to oral glucose are decreased with advancing age in males. The diabetic changes appear to be caused by an interaction between a genetic predisposition to develop diabetes in the WKY rat and *fa*-induced obesity.[23] WKY rats are less sensitive to insulin than Zucker *fa/fa* rats as determined by a glucose tolerance test and steady-state blood glucose measurement.

GK rat: The Goto–Kakizaki (GK) rat represents one of the more popular rat models for non-obese type 2 diabetes with insulin deficiency. The GK rat is one of the best characterized animal models to study the relationship between changes in β-cell mass and the occurrence of type 2 diabetes and diabetic complications, particularly diabetic nephropathy. The GK rat was established by repeated selective inbreeding of Wistar rats with the highest blood glucose over many generations.[24] The rats are characterized by a moderate, but stable fasting hyperglycemia, hypoinsulinemia, normolipidemia, impaired glucose tolerance which appears at 2 weeks of age in all animals, and an early onset of diabetic complications. In the adult GK rats total pancreatic β-cell mass and pancreatic insulin stores decrease by 60%. The reduced β-cell mass and function in the GK rat model may result from inadequate pancreatic growth factors necessary for the growth and development of fetal pancreatic cells during gestation and secondary loss of β-cell differentiation due to chronic exposure to hyperglycemia. As a result, the GK rat at birth has a reduced number of islets. In addition to the defects in β-cells, impaired insulin sensitivity in the liver, skeletal muscle, and adipose tissues has also been reported. Impaired insulin secretion and hepatic glucose overproduction are early events in diabetic GK rats contributing to the development of hyperglycemia rather than the peripheral (muscle and adipose tissue) insulin resistance.

SHROB or Koletsky rat: The genetically obese hypertensive (SHROB or Koletsky) rat was established after a genetic mutation spontaneously appeared in offspring of a cross between a female Kyoto–Wistar spontaneously hypertensive rat (SHR) and a normotensive Sprague–Dawley male. The SHROB is a unique strain with genetic obesity, hypertriglyceridemia, hyperinsulinemia, renal disease with proteinuria, and spontaneous hypertension, characteristic of human metabolic syndrome X (i.e., insulin resistance, hypertension, abnormalities of blood clotting, low HDL and high LDL cholesterol levels, and high triglyceride levels).[25] The phenotype results from a single homozygous recessive trait, originally designated *fa*[k], and is allelic with the Zucker fatty trait (*fa*) but of distinct origin. The *fa*[k] mutation introduces a premature stop codon in the extracellular domain of the leptin receptor, resulting in a natural receptor knockout. The SHROB rats are glucose intolerant compared to heterozygous or wild-type SHR, but retain fasting euglycemia even on a high-sucrose diet. Insulin-stimulated phosphorylation of tyrosine residues on the insulin receptor and on the associated docking protein IRS-1 is reduced in skeletal muscle and liver compared to SHR, due mainly to diminished expression of the insulin receptor and IRS-1 proteins.

SHR/N-cp rat: The spontaneously hypertensive rat/NIH-corpulent (SHR/N-*cp*) rat was established at the National Institutes of Health Animal Genetic Resource as a genetic model of obesity and diabetes.[26] The mutation corpulent *cp* arose spontaneously after several generations of inbreeding in a stock derived from an SHR/N female crossed with a male, normotensive Sprague–Dawley rat. The fully backcrossed SHR/N-*cp* strain differs genetically from its partner SHR/N strain only by the presence of the *cp* mutation. Mating of heterozygotes yields obese to lean rats in a ratio of 1:3. Lean rats consist of two-thirds heterozygotes (*cp/+*) and one-third homozygotes (+/+). Similar to the SHROB rat, male homozygous SHR/N-*cp* rats develop high blood pressure and are hyperphagic, obese, hyperinsulinemic, and hyperleptinemic. The SHR/N-*cp* rat is useful for investigating obesity-associated type 2 diabetes and also for studying the influence of dietary carbohydrate on the development of diabetes in genetically predisposed carbohydrate-sensitive individuals.

JCR/LA-cp rat: JCR/LA-*cp* is a rat model of obesity and insulin resistance with spontaneous cardiovascular disease. Following isolation of the mutant *cp* gene, rats containing this mutation were initially bred into two standard strains: the LA/N and the SHR/N. The progenies were then backcrossed more than 12 times to the parent strains to yield two congenic strains: LA/N-*cp* and SHR/N-*cp*. The JCR (James C Russel): LA-*cp* strain was derived from the LA/N-*cp* at the fifth backcross to the parent LA/N strain. The homozygous dominant (+/+)

and heterozygous (+/*cp*) rats are metabolically unaffected. The rats carrying the autosomal recessive *cp* mutation exhibit an extreme metabolic profile including insulin resistance, hyperinsulinemia, pancreatic β-cell hyperplasia, obesity, glucose intolerance, and severe hyperlipidemia. The *cp* mutation introduces a stop codon in the leptin receptor resulting in the expression of nonfunctional receptor protein. The leptin receptor-deficient state along with hypothalamic dysregulation of peptides contributes to hyperphagia and other metabolic abnormalities in these corpulent rats. The major drawback of this rat as a pure model of diabetes is that it is normoglycemic when fasted. The primary attraction of the JCR/LA-*cp* rat as a research model is its development of atherosclerotic and myocardial lesions in association with the metabolic syndrome X profile. The distinct feature of this animal is that the vasculopathy progresses inherently without any dietary cholesterol and high-fat diet interventions. The cardiovascular disease is strongly correlated with the hyperinsulinemia, which develops as the animals mature from 4 to 8 weeks of age.[12]

OLETF rat: The Otsuka Long-Evans Tokushima fatty (OLETF) rats are a spontaneous rat model for obese type 2 diabetes that originated from an outbred colony of Long-Evans rats discovered in 1984 and bred for glucose intolerance. The rats are maintained at Otsuka Pharmaceutical Company Limited, Japan. They are mildly obese, with males more likely to develop diabetes in adult life than females. OLETF rats carry a null allele for the cholecystokinin A receptor which may be involved in the regulation of food intake; however, whether this is causally related to the phenotype is still unclear. No mutations in the leptin or leptin receptor genes are reported for this strain. At around 18–25 weeks of age predominantly male rats develop diabetes. The rats exhibit innate polyphagia, mild obesity, hyperinsulinemia, hypertriglyceridemia, hypercholesterolemia, chronic hyperglycemia, and impaired glucose tolerance at about 16 weeks of age. Plasma insulin levels are high at 30 and 50 weeks of age accompanied by hyperplasia of pancreatic β-cells, but decrease at 70 weeks of age, probably because of decreased β-cell function over 40 weeks of age. Defects in β-cell proliferation per se are responsible for the development of diabetes in OLETF rats and β-cell function is decreased at 40 weeks of age.[27]

Target-Directed (Knockout) Models

The function and importance of particular genes can be directly tested by creation of genetically modified mice with targeted gene knockouts or overexpression. Conditional or tissue-specific knockouts are also used to increase the specificity and selectivity of the changes. Transgenic animals incorporate modified genes (transgenes) into the host genome. These techniques facilitate the selective perturbation of a single gene in the context of an otherwise undisturbed genome. The effect of transgene expression is strongly modified by the genetic background of the animal, so that results may vary depending on the particular strain employed. Knockout animals are produced using a genetic construct to disrupt the target gene. These constructs contain DNA sequences homologous to the target gene that are constructed to include a disruption or a deletion. They are injected into embryonic stem cells and undergo recombination with the normal gene of the stem cells. Selected embryonic stem cells containing recombinations are then injected into preimplantation mouse embryos, transferred to mice and allowed to develop to term. Using these approaches, a large number of animals have been produced in an attempt to gain insights into the pathogenesis of diabetes. Some of more popular models are listed in Table 11.3.

Insulin Receptor Knockout: Mice lacking the insulin receptor (IR) have severe diabetes with ketoacidosis, markedly increased plasma free fatty acids, triglycerides, and reduced hepatic glycogen content.[28] The phenotype is more severe than that in humans lacking IR and the mice die by a week after birth. Mice selectively lacking IR in muscle display severely reduced insulin-stimulated muscle glucose uptake and elevated fat mass, but their insulin and glucose levels are normal. Pancreatic β-cell-specific IR knockout mice exhibit a selective loss of insulin secretion in response to glucose with progressively impaired glucose tolerance indicating an important functional role of IR in pancreatic β-cell glucose sensing.

IRS-1, IRS-2: Insulin receptor substrate-1 (IRS-1) knockout mice have normal glucose levels and develop mild peripheral (muscle) insulin resistance with compensatory insulin hypersecretion due to an increase in β-cell mass.[29]

Table 11.3 Knockout animal models of diabetes

Gene	Phenotype
IR	Severe hyperglycemia, neonatal death from ketoacidosis
IRS-1	Mild insulin resistance, normoglycemia, increase in β-cell mass
IRS-2	Reduced β-cell mass, progressive glucose intolerance, impaired liver response
GLP-1R	Hyperglycemia, insulin resistance, reduced β-cell mass
GLP-1	Fasting hyperglycemia, abnormal glucose excursion, reduced insulin secretion
GIP-R	Reduced fat mass without reduction of lean mass or food intake, improved insulin sensitivity, improved glucose tolerance, increased plasma adiponectin levels, increased spontaneous physical activity
GIP	Glucose intolerance
CD26/DPP-4	Reduced glycemic excursion, increased glucose-stimulated insulin secretion, decreased degradation of GLP-1 and GIP, failed to become obese on a high-fat diet, reduced food intake together with enhanced metabolic energy expenditure, resistant to diabetogenic doses of streptozotocin
GLUT-2	Reduced β-cell mass, hyperglycemia, glucose intolerance, hypoinsulinemia, die at 3 weeks of age
GLUT-4	Insulin resistance, impaired glucose tolerance, mild hyperinsulinemia, abnormalities in glucose and lipid metabolism, reduced resting glycogen content, enhanced susceptibility to fatigue
PTP1B	Increased sensitivity toward insulin-induced insulin receptor and IRS-1 tyrosine phosphorylation, resistant to diet-induced diabetes and obesity, enhanced leptin-mediated loss of body weight, enhanced growth hormone sensitivity
β3R	Increased body weight and fat stores
PPARγ	Resistant to high-fat diet-induced obesity, decreased insulin sensitivity
GK	Severe hyperglycemia, perinatal death, glucose intolerance
UCP2	Increased circulating insulin levels, resistant to genetic or nutritional diabetes, resistant to lipotoxicity

IR: insulin receptor, IRS: insulin receptor substrate, GLP-1: glucagon-like peptide-1, GLP-1R: glucagon-like peptide-1 receptor, GIP-R: gastric inhibitory polypeptide receptor, DPP-4: dipeptidyl peptidase 4, GLUT: glucose transporter, PTP1B: protein tyrosine phosphatase 1B, β3R: adrenergic receptor β3, PPAR: peroxisome proliferator activator receptors, GK: Goto–Kakizaki, UCP: uncoupling protein.

IRS-2 knockout mice have a limited ability to increase insulin secretion due to reduced β-cell mass resulting in progressive glucose intolerance.[30] Compared to IRS-1, IRS-2 deficiency leads to overt peripheral insulin resistance and diabetes with impaired liver response and progressive β-cell loss. Plasma glucose levels are increased as early as 3 days after birth. The mice show glucose intolerance and fasting hyperglycemia at 6 weeks of age and they are diabetic with polydipsia and polyuria and die of hyperosmolar coma at 10 weeks of age. IRS-2 knockout females tend to have higher food intake and increased body fat mass as well as defects in reproduction.

GLUT-4: GLUT4 knockout mice are insulin resistant, but euglycemic with a reduced amount of white adipose tissue and cardiac hypertrophy.[31] Muscle GLUT4 knockout mice show severe insulin resistance in muscle, liver, and white adipose tissue. Similarly, selective adipose tissue GLUT4 knockout mice exhibit insulin resistance in the adipose tissue and likely secondary insulin resistance in muscle and liver.

GLP-1R: Although glucagon-like peptide-1 (GLP-1) plays a central role in the regulation of glycemia, disruption of GLP-1R signaling in the CNS (by knockout of the receptor) is not associated with perturbation of feeding behavior or obesity in vivo.[32] GLP-1R knockout mice are viable, develop normally but exhibit increased levels of blood glucose following an oral glucose challenge in association with diminished levels of circulating insulin. This knockout mouse exhibits compensatory changes in the enteroinsular axis via increased glucose-dependent insulinotropic polypeptide (GIP) secretion and enhanced GIP action. No significant perturbation in the insulin response to perfused glucagon was detected under conditions of low (4.4 mmol/L) or high (16.6 mmol/L) glucose in GLP-1R knockout mice. Total pancreatic insulin, but not glucagon content, is reduced in GLP-1R knockouts compared to wild-type mice.

DPP-4/CD26: DPP-4 knockout mice appear normal and are resistant to the development of glucose intolerance and diabetes following several months of high-fat feeding. The mice fail to become obese on a high-fat diet, exhibit reduced food intake together with enhanced metabolic energy expenditure, and are comparatively resistant to diabetogenic doses of streptozotocin. Glycemic excursion is significantly reduced in association with increased levels of glucose-stimulated insulin secretion and decreased degradation of GLP-1 and GIP.[33] Despite the putative importance of DPP-4/CD26 for immune function, the knockout mice develop normally with no major immune phenotype reported in the absence of immunological challenge.

Chemical-Induced Models

Alloxan or Streptozotocin

Rats and mice treated with low doses of alloxan show well-characterized symptoms of type 2 diabetes such as hyperglycemia, glucosuria, polyphagia, and polydipsia. They also develop various complications such as neuropathy, cardiomyopathy, and retinopathy. An alloxan-susceptible (ALS) mouse model prone to develop type 2 diabetes was developed by inbreeding outbred CD-1 mice with selection for susceptibility to alloxan.

Streptozotocin is the preferred agent to induce experimental type 2 diabetes. It has some advantages over alloxan for sustained hyperglycemia and the development of well-characterized diabetic complications with a lower incidence of ketosis and mortality.

Nicotinamide and Streptozotocin

An animal model of type 2 diabetes is produced by combining streptozotocin with nicotinamide adenine dinucleotide (NAD) administration.[34] The rats administered NAD followed by streptozotocin develop moderate and stable hyperglycemia without any significant change in their plasma insulin level. NAD is an antioxidant which exerts protective effects on the cytotoxic action of streptozotocin and causes only minor damage to pancreatic β-cell mass. This model provides a useful tool for investigation of insulinotropic agents in the treatment of type 2 diabetes.

n-STZ Rat

Neonatal (n)-STZ rats are generated by administration of streptozotocin on the day of birth to Sherman or Wistar rats. Treated rats exhibit insulin-deficient acute diabetes 3–5 days post-dosing.[35] They have high plasma glucose (345 mg/dL) and their pancreatic insulin store is decreased about 93% with a low incidence of mortality (<30%). By the end of the first week, plasma glucose and insulin levels no longer differ from those of controls. By 8 weeks of age, the rats show mild hyperglycemia (150–180 mg/dL), glucose intolerance, and 50% decrease in pancreatic insulin content without changes in pancreatic glucagon. Variants of this model are produced by changing the day of the streptozotocin injection after birth, such as day 2 (n2-STZ version) or day 5 after birth (n5-STZ version).

These three models show non-insulin-dependent diabetes with graded severity in the adult rat. The n2-STZ rats exhibit characteristics of basal hyperglycemia, basal hypoinsulinemia, glucose intolerance, and decreased pancreatic insulin content which are similar to those seen in the n-STZ rats. The n5-STZ rats, however, show frank basal hyperglycemia with glucose intolerance, increased glycated hemoglobin (HbA1C), a strong reduction of the pancreatic insulin store, a 50% reduction in basal plasma insulin level, and a lack of plasma insulin response to glucose. All three n-STZ rat models have defects in insulin secretion and sensitivity which resemble human type 2 diabetes.

MSG and GTG

Rodents treated postnatally with monosodium glutamate (MSG) develop hypothalamic obesity and become stunted adults. Postnatal MSG treatment produces cell destruction in the arcuate nucleus of the hypothalamus. MSG obese rats show decreased leptin sensitivity, hyperinsulinemia, and tissue insulin resistance.[36]

Type 2 diabetes with obesity is induced in mice using goldthioglucose (GTG) injection.[37] The GTG produces necrosis in the ventromedial hypothalamus with subsequent development of hyperphagia, obesity, hyperinsulinemia, hyperglycemia, and insulin resistance.

Diet-Induced Models

Animals develop some degree of type 2 diabetes when fed specific diets including high-fat diets, diets with varied palatable foods (cafeteria diet), and diets with high energy density (high-fat or high-carbohydrate diets). Insulin resistance in response to diet can differ greatly between strains and species. C57BL/6 J mice fed a high-fat diet show marked obesity, hyperinsulinemia, insulin resistance, and glucose intolerance. These mice have been used to test the ability of various antidiabetic agents, including orally active DPP-4 inhibitors, to normalize glucose tolerance in association with augmented insulin secretion.[38]

The combination of high-fat/carbohydrate diet with low-dose streptozotocin treatment in genetically insulin-resistant rats produces hyperinsulinemia and insulin resistance. Diet-sensitive Cohen diabetic (CDs) rats develop type 2 diabetes only when they are fed a diabetogenic high-sucrose, copper-poor diet. In CDs rats the development of type 2 diabetes is directly attributed to deficient β-cell function and reduced insulin secretion. Compared to genetic models, these type 2 diabetic rats represent a good alternative and are cost-effective.

The sand rat, spiny mouse, and tucotuco are animals that have also been used as models of diet-induced obesity and type 2 diabetes. Although the sand rat (*Psammomys obesus*) remains normal in its natural habitat, when fed on standard laboratory chow in captivity it develops obesity and diabetes. The sensitivity to development of diabetes mellitus increases from weaning to a peak at about 5 months of age and decreases thereafter. The spiny mouse (*Acomys cahirinus*) is a small rodent living in semidesert areas of the Eastern Mediterranean. When placed on high-energy rodent lab chow in captivity they gain weight and develop glucose intolerance with reduced insulin secretion. When fed high-energy rodent diets in captivity the tuco-tuco (*Ctenomys talarum*) exhibits characteristics similar to the sand rat and spiny mouse.

Summary

Animal models have been invaluable tools for identifying candidate diabetes susceptibility genes and environmental factors that contribute to the development of diabetes and for dissecting molecular mechanisms that underlie the pathogenesis of diabetes. This, in turn, has contributed substantially to the development of improved antidiabetic agents and to the understanding of ways to prevent or slow disease progression. The substantial advances in understanding diabetes in recent years and the emergence of the "omics" technologies – transcriptomics (transcriptional profiling), genomics (gene profiling), proteomics (protein profiling), and metabolomics (metabolic profiling) – give researchers confidence that susceptibility genes and other contributing factors to diabetes will be identified at an increasing rate. The animal models of diabetes described in this chapter exhibit various characteristic features of diabetes in humans and have therefore allowed and facilitated experimentation that would have been impossible in humans. However, none of the models can completely represent all aspects of human diabetes. Nevertheless, each model acts as an essential tool for investigating the genetic, endocrine, metabolic, and morphologic changes and underlying mechanisms that potentially contribute to the development and progression of diabetes in humans.

References

1. Makino S, Kunimoto K, Munaoko Y, et al. Breeding of a non-obese diabetic strain of mice. *Exp Anim.* 1980;29:1–13.
2. Colle E, Guttmann RD, Seemayer TA. Spontaneous diabetes mellitus syndrome in the rat. I. Association with the major histocompatibility complex. *J Exp Med.* 1981;154:1237–1242.
3. Kawano K, Hirashima T, Mori S, et al. New inbred strain of Long-Evans Tokushima Lean rats with IDDM without lymphopenia. *Diabetes.* 1991;40:1375–1381.

4. Komeda K, Noda M, Terao K, et al. Establishment of two substrains, diabetes-prone and non-diabetic, from Long-Evans Tokushima Lean (LETL) rats. *Endocr J*. 1998;45:737–744.

5. Todd JA. Genetic analysis of Type 1 diabetes using whole genome approaches. *Proc Natl Acad Sci USA*. 1995;12:8560–8565.

6. Litherland SA, Grebe KM, Belkin NS, et al. Nonobese diabetic mouse congenic analysis reveals chromosome 11 locus contributing to diabetes susceptibility, macrophage STAT5 dysfunction, and granulocyte-macrophage colony-stimulating factor overproduction. *J Immunol*. 2005;175(7):4561–4565.

7. Eizirik DL, Mandrup-Poulsen T. A choice of death – the signal transduction of immune-mediated β-cell apoptosis. *Diabetologia*. 2001;44:2115–2133.

8. Asayama K, Nyfeler F, English D, et al. Alloxan-induced free radical production in isolated cells. Selective effect on islet cells. *Diabetes*. 1984;33(10):1008–1011.

9. Bono VH. Review of mechanism of action studies of the nitrosoureas *Streptomyces achromogenes*. *Cancer Treat Rep*. 1976;60:699–702.

10. Wilson ME, Scheel D, German MS. Gene expression cascades in pancreatic development. *Mech Dev*. 2003;120:65–80.

11. Chua S Jr, Herberg L, Leiter EH. Obesity/diabetes in mice with mutations in leptin or leptin receptor genes. In: Shafrir E, ed. *Animal Models of Diabetes: Frontiers in Research*. Boca Raton, FL: CRC Press; 2007:61–102.

12. Srinivasan K, Ramarao P. Animal models in type 2 diabetes research: an overview. *Indian J Med Res*. 2007;125(3):451–472.

13. Coleman DL. Obese and diabetes: two mutant genes causing diabetes-obesity syndromes in mice. *Diabetologia*. 1978;14(3):141–148.

14. Peterson RG. The Zucker diabetic fatty (ZDF) rats – lessons from a leptin receptor defect diabetic model. In: Shafrir E, ed. *Animal Models of Diabetes: Frontiers in Research*. Boca Raton, FL: CRC Press; 2007:103–118.

15. Pickavance LC, Widdowson PS, Foster JR, et al. Chronic treatment with the thiazolidinedione, MCC-555, is associated with reductions in nitric oxide synthase activity and beta-cell apoptosis in the pancreas of the Zucker Diabetic Fatty rat. *Int J Exp Pathol*. 2003;84(2):83–89.

16. Chiu S, Fisler JS, Espinal GM, et al. The yellow agouti mutation alters some but not all responses to diet and exercise. *Obes Res*. 2004;12(8):1243–1255.

17. Leiter EH. Carboxypeptidase E and obesity in the mouse. *J Endocrinol*. 1997;155(2):211–214.

18. Taketomi S. KK and KKAy mice: models of type 2 diabetes with obesity. In: Shafrir E, ed. *Animal Models of Diabetes: Frontiers in Research*. Boca Raton, FL: CRC Press; 2007:335–348.

19. Sohda T, Kawamatsu Y, Fujita T, et al. Discovery and development of a new insulin sensitizing agent, pioglitazone. *Yakugaku Zasshi*. 2002;122(11):909–918.

20. Fam BC, Andrikopoulos S. The New Zealand obese mouse: polygenic model of obesity, glucose intolerance, and the metabolic syndrome. In: Shafrir E, ed. *Animal Models of Diabetes: Frontiers in Research*. Boca Raton, FL: CRC Press; 2007:139–158.

21. Cho YR, Kim HJ, Park SY, et al. Hyperglycemia, maturity-onset obesity, and insulin resistance in NONcNZO10/LtJ males, a new mouse model of type 2 diabetes. *Am J Physiol Endocrinol Metab*. 2007;293(1):E327–E336.

22. Clee SM, Attie AD. The genetic landscape of type 2 diabetes in mice. *Endocr Rev*. 2007;28(1):48–83.

23. Ikeda H, Sugiyama Y, Matsuo T. Characterization of the Wistar fatty rat. In: Oomura Y, et al., eds. *Progress in Obesity Research*. London, Paris: John Libbey; 1990:435–439.

24. Östenson C. The Goto-Kakizaki rat. In: Shafrir E, ed. *Animal Models of Diabetes: Frontiers in Research*. Boca Raton, FL: CRC Press; 2007:119–138.

25. Koletsky RJ, Velliquette RA, Ernsberger P. The SHROB (Koletsky) rat as a model for metabolic syndrome. In: Shafrir E, ed. *Animal Models of Diabetes: Frontiers in Research*. Boca Raton, FL: CRC Press; 2007:185–208.

26. Michaelis OE 4th, Ellwood KC, Judge JM, et al. Effect of dietary sucrose on the SHR/N-corpulent rat: a new model for insulin-independent diabetes. *Am J Clin Nutr*. 1984;39(4):612–618.

27. Kawano K. OLETF rats: model for the metabolic syndrome and diabetic nephropathy in humans. In: Shafrir E, ed. *Animal Models of Diabetes: Frontiers in Research*. Boca Raton, FL: CRC Press; 2007:209–222.

28. Accili D, Drago J, Lee EJ, et al. Early neonatal death in mice homozygous for a null allele of the insulin receptor gene. *Nat Genet*. 1996;12(1):106–109.

29. Tamemoto H, Tobe K, Yamauchi T, et al. Insulin resistance syndrome in mice deficient in insulin receptor substrate-1. *Ann NY Acad Sci*. 1997;827(1):85–93.

30. Withers DJ, Gutierrez JS, Towery H, et al. Disruption of IRS-2 causes type 2 diabetes in mice. *Nature*. 1998;391:900–904.

31. Wright JR Jr, O'Hali W, Yang H, et al. GLUT-4 Deficiency and severe peripheral resistance to insulin in the teleost fish tilapia. *Gen Comp Endocrinol*. 1998;111(1):20–27.

32. Scrocchi LS, Brown TJ, MacLusky N, et al. Glucose intolerance but normal satiety in mice with a null mutation in the glucagon-like peptide 1 receptor gene. *Nat Med*. 1996;2:1254–1258.

33. Marguet D, Baggio L, Kobayashi T, et al. Enhanced insulin secretion and improved glucose tolerance in mice lacking CD26. *Proc Natl Acad Sci USA*. 2000;97(12):6874–6879.

34. Masiello P, Bergamini E. Nicotinamide and streptozotocin diabetes in the rat. Factors influencing the effectiveness of the protection. *Experientia*. 1977;33(9):1246–1247.

35. Portha B, Movassat J, Cuzin-Tourrel C, et al. Neonatally streptozotocin-induced (n-STZ) diabetic rats: a family of type 2 diabetes models. In: Shafrir E, ed. *Animal Models of Diabetes: Frontiers in Research*. Boca Raton, FL: CRC Press; 2007:223–250.

36. Morrison JF, Shehab S, Sheen R, et al. Sensory and autonomic nerve changes in the MSG-treated rat: a model of type II diabetes. *Exp Physiol*. 2007;93:213–222.

37. Bryson JM, Cooney GJ, Wensley VR, et al. Tissue differences in the response of the pyruvate dehydrogenase complex to a glucose load during the development of obesity in gold-thioglucose-obese mice. *Biochem J*. 1995;305(Pt 3):811–816.

38. Winzell MS, Ahrén B. The high-fat diet-fed mouse: a model for studying mechanisms and treatment of impaired glucose tolerance and type 2 diabetes. *Diabetes*. 2004;53(Suppl 3):S215–S219.

Internet Sites for Additional Relevant Information+

1. Charles River Laboratory (http://www.criver.com/research_models_and_services/research_models/dm_rats3.html)
2. Harlan (http://www.harlan.com/models/usmodels.asp)
3. Jackson Laboratory (http://jaxmice.jax.org/info/index.html)
4. Drucker's lab (http://www.glucagon.com/index.html)
5. National Institute of Health (http://www.nih.gov/index.html)
6. National Institute of Diabetes and Digestive and Kidney Disease (http://www2.niddk.nih.gov/)
7. Juvenile Diabetes Foundation (http://www.jdrf.org/index.cfm?page_id=100686)
8. BRM (http://biomere.com/diabetes_type2.php)

Part V
Diabetes Syndromes

Chapter 12
Type 1 Diabetes Mellitus: Epidemiology, Genetics, Pathogenesis, and Clinical Manifestations

Omar Ali

Type 1 diabetes is characterized by an absolute deficiency of insulin secretion, a generally rapid onset, and dependence on exogenous insulin at the time of diagnosis. These patients are also prone to ketosis.[159]

Insulin deficiency in type 1a diabetes is caused by immune-mediated destruction of beta cells and is associated with evidence of autoimmunity. A smaller group of type 1 diabetic patients exhibit no evidence of autoimmunity and the cause of insulin deficiency remains undefined. These cases are categorized as type 1b diabetes or idiopathic type 1 diabetes and are relatively more common in African and Asian populations.[1] This category is heterogeneous, may be caused by different mechanisms in different populations, and remains poorly understood at this time. This chapter focuses on autoimmune type 1a diabetes unless otherwise specified.

Epidemiology

Type 1 diabetes is the most common form of diabetes among children and adolescents of European origin and is one of the most common chronic diseases of childhood. But this disease is not confined to childhood; cases continue to appear throughout life and approximately half the cases of type 1 diabetes are diagnosed as adults. Highlights of the descriptive epidemiology of type 1 diabetes follow.

Geographic location. One of the most striking characteristics of type 1 diabetes is the large geographic variability in the incidence of the disease (Fig. 12.1, worldwide incidence). Scandinavia and the Mediterranean island of Sardinia have the highest incidence rates in the world while oriental and equatorial populations have the lowest rates. A child in Finland is 400 times more likely to develop diabetes than one in certain regions of China. Even within Scandinavia, with genetically homogenous populations and equally developed societies living at the same latitude, incidence rates vary widely from a high of 45 per 100,000 in Finland (1996) to 28 in Sweden[2] and 20 in Denmark.[3]

The cause of this geographical variation is not immediately apparent. The existence of a strong North–South gradient and the fact that vitamin D is an immune modulator has led to speculation that decreased exposure to ultraviolet light and consequent lack of vitamin D may explain some of this gradient.[4] But there are some areas of increased incidence in sun-drenched regions (Kuwait, Puerto Rico, Sardinia) as well as some areas of very low incidence in the northern latitudes (e.g., Lithuania is only 75 miles from Finland but the incidence of diabetes is dramatically lower). So, while vitamin D levels or sun exposure may play a role, they cannot be the sole explanation of the observed variation.

Another notable feature of this geographical distribution is that great variation can be seen within the same country, even in countries with relatively homogenous populations. Thus, within China the incidence varies from 0.1 per 100,000 per year in Zunyi to 4.5 in Sichuan.[5] In Finland, the incidence is higher in the rural heartland than it is in the urban areas, though this distinction may disappear in the future because the incidence is rising faster

O. Ali (✉)
Medical College of Wisconsin, Milwaukee, WI, USA
e-mail: oali@mcw.edu

L. Poretsky (ed.), *Principles of Diabetes Mellitus*, DOI 10.1007/978-0-387-09841-8_12,
© Springer Science+Business Media, LLC 2010

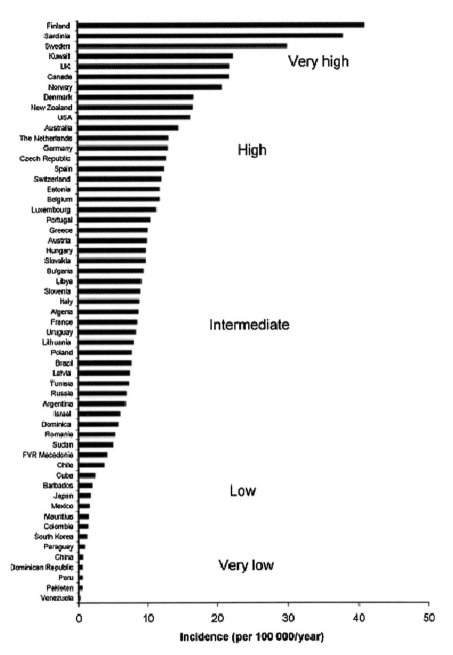

Fig. 12.1 Age-standardized incidence of type 1 diabetes in children under 14 years of age (per 100,000 per year)

in the urban population.[6] A similar trend, with higher incidence in the rural population and lower incidence in the crowded and relatively deprived urban populations, has been found in Sweden,[7] UK,[8] and Northern Ireland,[9] but not in Italy[10] or Lithuania.[11] These differences also remain unexplained at this time.

While incidence rates are much higher in European populations, the absolute number of new cases is almost equal in Asia and Europe because the population base is so much larger in Asia. It is estimated that of the 400,000 total new cases of type 1 diabetes occurring annually in all children under age 14, about half are in Asia even though the incidence rates in that continent are much lower, because the total number of children in Asia is larger.

Increase in incidence. There has been a steady increase in the incidence of type 1 diabetes in most populations studied. For example, the incidence of type 1 diabetes in Austria doubled from 7.3/100,000 in the period 1979–1984 to 14.6/100,000 in the time period 2000–2005.[12] Studies from Croatia,[13] France,[14] Germany,[15] Finland,[16] Newfoundland,[17] and China[18] all show that the incidence of type 1 diabetes is increasing at a rate of 2–5% per year. In addition, most of these studies also show that the rate of increase is greatest in the youngest subgroups (those less than 4 years of age). According to the latest report from Eurodiab,[19] countries in Eastern Europe that historically had a relatively low incidence of type 1 diabetes are the ones now showing the steepest increase. Even the Asian and African countries where the incidence was as low as 0.1/100,000 are now reporting an increase in incidence. Since the genetic composition of these populations has not changed significantly in this short time, the increase is almost certainly due to environmental factors. But in spite of intense speculation and research, the exact nature of the environmental factors that may be causing this increase remains unclear.

It should also be kept in mind that while most population groups are seeing an increase in the incidence of type 1 diabetes, this is not a universal finding. For example, at least one well-documented Swedish rural community saw no increase in the incidence of type 1 (or type 2) diabetes between 1971 and 2001[20] and the Norwegian registry did not detect any increase in incidence between 1989 and 1998.[21]

Effect of migration. In some populations migrants tend to take on the incidence rates of the host countries within one or two generations. For example, a study in Leicestershire in the UK found that type 1 diabetes incidence rates among children of South Asian origin were almost identical with those of local whites and were more than 20-fold higher than the rates reported from their ancestral homelands in South Asia.[22] This suggests that children who move from low-incidence areas to high-incidence areas can acquire the higher risk due to environmental factors. This conclusion is further supported by the observation that as type 1 diabetes has increased in incidence, the proportion of high-risk haplotypes within the diabetic population has decreased.[23] In other words, as the environment becomes more "diabetogenic," relatively lower risk haplotypes also develop diabetes and therefore the contribution of the highest risk haplotypes becomes diluted.

On the other hand, a study in Lazio (mainland Italy) found that the children of Sardinian immigrants had a type 1 diabetes incidence identical with the high incidence in Sardinia and fourfold higher than the incidence among children whose parents were native to Lazio.[24] Children with one Sardinian parent had an incidence about midway between the incidence found in Sardinia and that found in Lazio. This may indicate that in a permissive environment, migrants who carry a higher genetic risk (as Sardinians appear to do) continue to succumb at a higher rate than the rest of the population.

Age. Type 1 diabetes incidence peaks at the ages of 4–6 and 10–14 years.[25] The age distribution of type 1 diabetes onset is similar across different European populations[26] but the average age of presentation tends to be higher in African and Asian (low risk) populations. It has been suggested that these peaks coincide with higher exposure to infectious agents (at entry to school) and higher insulin demand (due to insulin resistance at puberty), but this remains to be conclusively proven. About half of all type 1 diabetics present as adults and new cases continue to present past age 70. Some adults present with evidence of autoimmunity, but with less severe insulin deficiency at presentation than is usually seen in children. These cases, which have some clinical characteristics of type 2 diabetes (relatively preserved insulin secretion, gradual onset, not dependent on exogenous insulin at diagnosis) but also exhibit evidence of autoimmunity, are sometimes said to have "Latent Autoimmune Diabetes of Adults" (LADA) and may or may not be classified as having type 1 diabetes.

Race and ethnicity. There are striking racial differences in type 1 diabetes risk in multiracial populations, although not of the same magnitude as the geographic differences. In the USA, non-Hispanic whites between the ages of 10 and 14 have an incidence rate of 32.9, which is comparable to Scandinavian populations. At the same age, the incidence rate among Hispanics is 17.6 and that in African-Americans is 19.2. Asian-Americans, with an incidence of 8.3 and American-Indians with an incidence of 7.1, have the lowest incidence rates in the American population. Comparable racial disparities have also been found in other countries. For example, in Montreal Canada, children of British descent had about 50% higher risk of type 1 diabetes than children of French descent.[27] And in a study of the incidence of diabetes mellitus in a region in Chile between 1983 and 1993, there was a significant difference between the incidence of type 1 diabetes in native Chileans (0.42/100,000) compared to Caucasian Chileans (1.58/100,000).[28] Some of the observed differences may be due to environmental factors, but others are likely to be genetic in origin. On the other hand, racially and ethnically distinct populations can show convergence of diabetes rates (as in European and South Asian children in the UK and Arab and Jewish children in Israel[29]) and genetically similar populations can show very wide differences in diabetes incidence (for instance, the incidence in Karelians is 7.4 versus an incidence of 41 across the border in Finland[30]), indicating that environmental factors may play an even bigger role than genetic differences between populations.

Seasonality. Pooled data from many different countries show significant seasonality in date of diagnosis for type 1 diabetes in all age groups. These data show a maximum incidence in the winter period around December to January and a minimum in summer around June to July. Data from Australia and New Zealand show similar seasonality (peak incidence in winter, which in the southern hemisphere is in June and July).[31] The amplitudes of these differences are smallest for the youngest age group and largest for the oldest age group.[32,33] Very detailed and accurate records from Denmark also show that this seasonal variation seems to vary by year.[34] For example, in 2004, Denmark saw a peak during summer and it was noted that in that year summer was exceptionally wet and there was less sunshine.

On the other hand, in several populations, seasonality is absent.[35,36] It is possible that some environmental factor (for example, vitamin D, sunshine, or viral exposure) plays a role in the observed seasonality, but its effect may also be overshadowed in some populations by other genetic and environmental factors.

Another aspect of seasonality is the observation that diabetes incidence may also vary by season of birth. Thus, some studies report that the risk is higher in children born in summer (and hence, in children conceived in early winter).[37] This raises the possibility that some factor in early intrauterine life (for example, a viral infection in the mother) increases the diabetes risk in the unborn child.[38] As with so much in type 1 diabetes, this interesting hypothesis is yet to be proven.

Gender. In general, males and females have similar risk of type 1 diabetes,[39] with the pubertal peak of incidence in females preceding that in males by 1–2 years. In lower risk populations, such as Japan, there is a female preponderance with females outnumbering males by 1.4:1.[40]

Genetics of Type 1 Diabetes

While rare monogenic forms of autoimmune type 1 diabetes are known (see below), in most cases, type 1 diabetes is a complex disorder in which multiple genes and environmental factors interact to cause the disease or confer protection against it.[41]

There is a clear familial clustering of type 1 diabetes, with prevalence in siblings approaching 6% while the prevalence in the general population in the USA is only 0.4%. This difference yields a relative risk value of 15 (6/0.4). Risk of diabetes is also increased when a parent has diabetes and this risk differs between the two parents; the risk is 2% if the mother has diabetes, but 7% when the father has diabetes.[42] At this time, we have no explanation for this difference in risk transmission between fathers and mothers. Twin studies show that the heritability of type 1 diabetes is high (0.72 ± 0.21 in one population-based Danish study[43]) but is less than unity, indicating that there is also a non-shared environmental component. In monozygotic twins, the concordance rate ranges from 30 to 65%,[44] whereas dizygotic twins have a concordance rate of 6–10%. Since the concordance rate of dizygotic twins is higher than the sibling risk, factors other than the shared genotypes (for example, the shared intrauterine environment) may play a role in increasing the risk in dizygotic twins (Table 12.1).

Table 12.1 Genetic susceptibility to type 1 diabetes mellitus

European origin general population: 0.4%
Sibling: 6%
Offspring of diabetic mother: 2%
Offspring of diabetic father: 7%
Monozygotic twin: 30–65%
Dizygotic twin: 6–10%
Parents of diabetic child: 3%

It should be kept in mind that although there is a large genetic component in type 1 diabetes, 85% of newly diagnosed type 1 diabetic patients do *not* have a family member with type 1 diabetes. Thus, we cannot rely on family history to identify patients who may be at risk for the future development of type 1 diabetes as most cases will develop in individuals with no such family history.

Monogenic type 1 diabetes. Classic single-gene defects are an extremely rare cause of type 1 diabetes, but they are not unknown. In two rare syndromes (IPEX and APS-1) the genetic susceptibility that leads to diabetes is due to a classic single-gene defect. The IPEX (immune dysfunction, polyendocrinopathy, enteropathy, X-linked) syndrome is caused by mutations of the *FOXP3* gene. These mutations lead to the lack of a major population of regulatory T lymphocytes with resulting overwhelming autoimmunity and development of diabetes (as early as 2 days of age) in approximately 80% of the children with this disorder.

The APS-I syndrome (autoimmune polyendocrinopathy syndrome type 1) is caused by mutations of the *AIRE* (autoimmune regulator) gene, leading to abnormalities in expression of peripheral antigens within the thymus and/or abnormalities of negative selection in the thymus. This results in widespread autoimmunity. Approximately 18% of children with this syndrome develop type 1a diabetes.

Genes altering the risk of autoimmune type 1 diabetes. As noted above, most patients with type 1 diabetes do not have single-gene defects. Instead, their risk of developing type 1 diabetes is modified by the influence of several risk loci. The genomic region with by far the greatest contribution to the risk of type 1 diabetes is the major histocompatibility complex on chromosome 6. One other region which consistently shows up in genetic studies is the promoter region 5′ of the insulin gene on chromosome 11. More recent studies have identified several other risk loci (Fig. 12.2) but except for PTPN22, their contribution is relatively small, thus making them less useful for predicting the genetic risk of type 1 diabetes in a given individual.

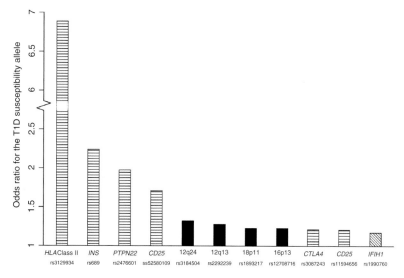

Fig. 12.2 Odds ratios for the susceptibility allele for the ten independent T1D-associated genes or regions

MHC/HLA encoded susceptibility to type 1 diabetes. The major histocompatibility complex (MHC) is a large genomic region or gene family that is found in most vertebrates and that encodes a variety of genes that are involved in immune recognition and response. In humans, the MHC region is usually referred to as the HLA (human leukocyte antigen) region and it is a superlocus that contains a large number of genes related to immune system function in humans (Fig. 12.3). These genes are further divided into HLA class I, II, III, and IV genes. Class I HLA genes encode antigens that are expressed on all body cells and include three major gene types, HLA A, B, and C. HLA class II genes encode antigens that are only expressed on certain immune cells and include HLA DP, DQ, and DR antigens. Class II genes are the ones most strongly associated with risk of type 1 diabetes, but as genetic studies become more detailed, it is becoming apparent that some of the risk associated

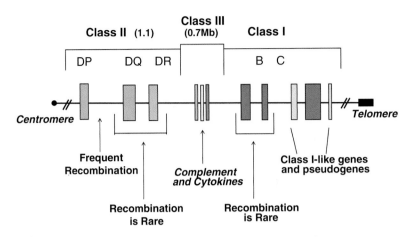

Fig. 12.3 The human leukocyte antigen complex (6p21.31)

with various HLA types is due to variation in genes in HLA classes other than class II. Overall, genetic variation in the HLA region can explain 40–50% of the genetic risk of type 1 diabetes.[45]

Initially, much of the risk associated with diabetes appeared to be linked to DR3 and DR4 alleles, but the genes of the HLA locus display strong linkage disequilibrium and it is now known that some of the earlier identified risk alleles (like DR3/DR4) confer much of their increased risk because of their linkage with other alleles in the DQ region with which they are tightly linked with relatively low recombination rates.

The HLA DR3/4-DQ2/8 is a high-risk genotype which is present in 2.3% of all newborns in Colorado, but is seen in more than 30% of children who develop diabetes. Compared to a population prevalence of type 1 diabetes of approximately 1/300, DR3/4-DQ2/8 newborns from the general population have a 1/20 genetic risk. This risk of development of type 1 diabetes is even higher when the high-risk HLA haplotypes are shared with a sibling or parent with type 1 diabetes. Thus, if one sibling has type 1 diabetes and shares the same high-risk DR3/4-DQ2/8 haplotype with another sibling, then the risk of autoimmunity in the other sibling is 50%. On the other hand, if a subject happens to have the same DR3/4-DQ2/8 haplotype in the general population, he or she has a risk of only 5% (1/20). And this risk approaches 80% when siblings share both HLA haplotypes identical by descent.[46] This is known as the "relative paradox" and points to the existence of other shared genetic risk factors (most likely in the extended HLA haplotype).

With advances in genotyping, further discrimination is now possible and we can identify more specific risk ratios for specific haplotypes. For example, the DRB1*0401-DQA1*0301 g-DQB1*0302 haplotype has an odds ratio (OR) of 8.39 while the DRB1*0401-DQA1*0301 g-DQB1*0301 has an OR of 0.35, implicating the DQB1*0302 allele as a critical susceptibility allele. Risk of diabetes is influenced by both *DRB1*04 variants and DQ alleles on DR4 haplotypes.[47] Thus there is a hierarchy of *DRB1*04 haplotypes, even with the same *DQA1*0301–DQB1*0302 alleles, with higher risk from *DRB1*0405 (OR = 11.4), *DRB1*0401 (OR = 8.4), *DRB1*0402 (OR = 3.6), and *DRB1*0404 (OR = 1.6), while *DRB1*0403 is protective (OR = 0.27). Similarly, for *DRB1*0401, variation of *DQB1* influences risk, as haplotypes with *DQB1*0302 (OR = 8.4) are highly susceptible, while those with *DQB1*0301 (OR = 0.35) are modestly protective.

There are some dramatically protective DR–DQ haplotypes [e.g., DRB1*1501-DQA1*0102-DQB1*0602 (OR = 0.03), DRB1*1401-DQA1*0101-DQB1*0503 (OR = 0.02), and DRB1*0701-DQA1*0201-DQB1*0303 (OR = 0.02)]. The DR2 haplotype (DRB1*1501-DQA1*0102-DQB1*0602) is dominantly protective and is present in 20% of general population but is seen in only 1% of type 1A diabetes patients (Table 12.2).[48]

Role of aspartate at position 57 in DQB1. DQB1*0302 (high risk for diabetes) differs from DQB1*0301 (protective against diabetes) only at position 57, where it lacks an aspartic acid residue.[49] The DQB1*0201 allele (increased risk for diabetes) also lacks aspartic acid at position 57, and it has been proposed that this residue may be involved in the molecular mechanism underlying diabetes susceptibility.[50] It has been proposed that the presence of aspartate at this position alters the protein recognition and protein binding characteristics of this molecule.[51] But while the absence of aspartate at this position appears to be important in most Caucasian

Table 12.2 *HLA-DRB1∗04* and *DQB1* effects on type 1 diabetes risk

HLA-DRB1∗04	HLA-DQB1	Odds ratio
0405	0302	11.4
0401	0302	8.4
0402	0302	3.6
0404	0302	1.6
0403	0302	0.27
0401	0301	0.35

studies, it does not have the same role in Korean[52] and Japanese[53] populations. Moreover, certain low-risk DQB1 genotypes also lack aspartic acid at position 57, including DQB1∗0302/DQB1∗0201 (DR7) and DQB1∗0201 (DR3)/DQB1∗0201 (DR7). Thus the presence of aspartate at this position is usually, but not always, protective in Caucasian populations. In other populations, it may even be associated with increased risk in association with particular haplotypes.

Role of HLA class I. While the alleles of class II HLA genes appear to have the strongest associations with diabetes, recent genotyping studies and analyses of pooled data have identified associations with other elements in the HLA complex, especially HLA-A and HLA-B. The most significant association is with HLA-B39, which confers high risk for type 1A diabetes in three different populations, makes up the majority of the signal from HLA-B, and is associated with a lower age of onset of the disease.[54]

The above-mentioned HLA-risk haplotypes appear to confer increased risk in all populations, but they are not equally distributed in different populations. Part of the reason for the lower incidence of type 1 diabetes in Asian populations is lower prevalence of the highest risk haplotypes in those populations and the existence of unique haplotypes in which the high-risk alleles are associated with protective alleles.[55]

The Insulin Gene Locus, IDDM2. The second locus found to be associated with risk of type 1 diabetes was labeled IDDM2 and has been localized a region upstream of the insulin gene (5′ of the insulin gene). It is estimated that this locus accounts for about 10% of the familial risk of type 1 diabetes.[56] Susceptibility in this region has been primarily mapped to a variable number of tandem repeats (VNTR) about 500 bp upstream of the insulin gene.[57] This highly polymorphic region consists of anywhere from 30 to several hundred repeats of a 14–15 bp unit sequence (ACAGGGGTCTGGGG). The number of repeats tends to cluster into three ranges: class I (short) with 26–63 repeats, class II (intermediate) with an average of 85 repeats, and class III (long) with 140–210 repeats. Caucasians and Asians mostly have class I and class III alleles and class II alleles are relatively rare in these populations, but somewhat more common in Africans (in line with the generally greater diversity of haplotypes in the older African population).[58]

Class I (short) alleles are associated with a higher risk of type 1 diabetes, while class III (longer) alleles appear to be protective. Thus, homozygosity for class I alleles is found in 75–85% of diabetic patients, as compared to a frequency of 50–60% in the general population. It has been hypothesized that this locus alters the risk of type 1 diabetes by altering immune tolerance of insulin and this effect is due to a variation in insulin production in thymic cells, with smaller alleles being associated with lower insulin production.[59] An effect of this locus on IGF-2 transcription was also postulated, but has not been confirmed.[60]

PTPN22 (lymphoid tyrosine phosphatase). In 2004, it was reported that a single-nucleotide polymorphism (SNP) in the *PTPN22* gene on chromosome 1p13 that encodes lymphoid tyrosine phosphatase (Lyp) correlates strongly with the incidence of type 1 diabetes in two independent populations.[61] Since then, this discovery had been replicated in several populations and the gene has been found to have an association with several other autoimmune diseases.[62]

Lyp is an enzyme that has a role in signal transduction downstream of the T-cell receptor and the risk variant may represent a gain of function (increased inhibition of signal transduction), which raises the possibility that an inhibitor of this protein may hold promise as a preventive intervention in type 1 diabetes.[63]

CTLA-4. The cytotoxic T lymphocyte associated-4 (CTLA-4) gene is located on chromosome 2q33 and has been found to be associated with type 1 diabetes risk[64] as well as the risk of other autoimmune disorders[65] in several studies. This gene is a negative regulator of T cell activation and therefore is a good biological candidate for type 1 diabetes risk modification. Because of its role in immune regulation, this gene is another candidate for therapeutic intervention and a fusion protein with human immunoglobulin is already being tested by Diabetes Trial Net as a possible preventive treatment.

IL2-receptor. SNPs in or near the gene for the interleukin-2 receptor have been found to have an association with type 1 diabetes risk.[66] Since IL2-receptor is an important modulator of immunity, it is another obvious candidate for the development of potential therapeutic interventions.

Interferon-induced helicase. Another gene that has recently been identified as having a modest effect on the risk of type 1 diabetes is the interferon-induced helicase (IFIH1) gene.[67] This gene is thought to play a role in protecting the host from viral infections and given the specificity of different helicases for different RNA viruses, it is possible that knowledge of this gene locus will help to narrow down the list of viral pathogens that may have a role in type 1 diabetes.[68]

CYP27B1. Cytochrome P450, subfamily 27, polypeptide 1 gene encodes vitamin D 1alpha hydroxylase. Because of the known role of vitamin D in immune regulation and because of epidemiologic evidence that vitamin D may play a role in type 1 diabetes, this gene was examined as a candidate gene and two SNPS were found to be associated.[69]

Other genes. Several other genes (e.g., PTPN-2) and linkage blocks, including two linkage blocks on chromosome 12 (12q13 and 12q24) and blocks on 16p13, 18p11, and 18q22 have been found to be significant in GWA studies[70,71] and further fine mapping and functional studies of genes in these regions are pending.

In addition, it has been suggested that viral infections (or other environmental factors) may activate dormant retroviruses in the human genome, or may introduce new retroviruses into the genome. A human endogenous retrovirus (IDDMK1, 222) was reported to be expressed in leukocytes from type 1 diabetes patients, but not in controls.[72] This, however, was not confirmed in subsequent studies.[73] At this time, the retroviral hypothesis remains unproven.

Environmental Factors

The fact that 50% or so of monozygotic twins are discordant for type 1 diabetes, the variation seen in urban and rural areas populated by the same ethnic group, the change in incidence that occurs with migration, the increase in incidence that has been seen in almost all populations in the last few decades, and the occurrence of seasonality all provide evidence that environmental factors also play a significant role in the causation of type 1 diabetes. The various factors that have been suggested are discussed below.

Viral infections. There are several mechanisms by which viruses may play a role in triggering or accelerating type 1 diabetes. For instance, some viruses are capable of infecting and destroying beta cells directly. In addition, viral antigens may share sequences with beta-cell antigens (molecular mimicry) or may cause the release of sequestered islet antigens (bystander damage). Repeated viral infections may induce immune dysregulation and trigger autoimmunity or aggravate pre-existing autoimmunity. Evidence for the role of several different viruses in the pathogens of type 1 diabetes is discussed below, but it should be kept in mind that most of the evidence is descriptive or suggestive, not definitive. It is possible that various viruses do play a role in the pathogenesis of type 1 diabetes, but no single virus and no single pathogenic mechanism, stands out in the environmental etiology of type 1 diabetes. Instead, a variety of viruses and mechanisms may contribute to the development of diabetes in genetically susceptible hosts.

Viruses implicated in animal models of diabetes. BBDP (*BioBreeding Diabetes Prone*) rats are prone to insulitis and type 1 diabetes and were discovered in a colony of outbred Wistar rats at the Biobreeding laboratories in Ottawa, Canada, in 1974.[74] BBDR (BioBreeding Diabetes *Resistant*) rats are derived from BBDP rats, but do not develop diabetes spontaneously. It was then discovered that if BBDR rats become infected with Kilham Rat Virus (KRV), a member of the parvovirus family, they develop type 1 diabetes. Another example in which viral infection can cause diabetes is seen in neonatal hamsters, in which rubella infection leads to diabetes.[75] The significance of these examples for humans remains unknown.

Enteroviruses. The viruses most often suspected of playing a role in type 1 diabetes are the small RNA viruses of the picornavirus family.[76] Studies have shown an increase in evidence of enteroviral infection in type 1 diabetics and an increased prevalence of enteroviral RNA in prenatal blood samples from children who subsequently developed type 1 diabetes. In addition, there are case reports[77,78] of association between enteroviral infection and subsequent type 1 diabetes. Molecular mimicry[79] and bystander damage[80] have also been suggested as mechanisms by which enteroviruses may cause type 1 diabetes. It has been proposed that some of the increase in incidence that is being seen in developed countries is due to the fact that childhood enteroviral infections have become rarer and therefore, mothers do not provide antibodies to the fetus or neonate and make them more susceptible to persistent enterovirus infection.[81] While interesting, these speculations are unproven and the true significance of enteroviral infection in type 1 diabetes remains unknown.

Congenital rubella syndrome. The clearest evidence of a role for viral infection in human type 1 diabetes is seen in congenital rubella syndrome (CRS).[82] Prenatal infection with rubella is associated with beta-cell autoimmunity in up to 70%, with development of type 1 diabetes in up to 40% of infected children. The time lag between infection and development of diabetes may be as high as 20 years. Type 1 diabetes after congenital rubella is more likely in patients that carry the higher risk genotypes. Interestingly, there appears to be no increase in risk of diabetes when rubella infection develops after birth, or when live virus rubella immunization is used. Exactly how rubella infection leads to diabetes and why it is pathogenic *only* if infection occurs prenatally, remains unknown.

Mumps virus. It has been observed that mumps infection leads to the development of beta-cell autoimmunity with high frequency, and to type 1 diabetes in some cases.[83] It has also been noted that there is an uptick in the incidence of type 1 diabetes 2–4 years after an epidemic of mumps infection.[84] But a larger European study did not find any association between mumps infection and subsequent development of diabetes. Mumps vaccination, on the other hand, appears to be protective against type 1 diabetes.[85] But while mumps may play a role in some cases of diabetes, the fact that type 1 diabetes incidence has increased steadily in several countries after universal mumps vaccination was introduced, and that incidence is extremely low in several populations where mumps is still prevalent, indicates that mumps is not an important causal factor in diabetes.

Rotavirus. Rotavirus infection in Non-Obese Diabetic (NOD) mice can involve the pancreas[86] and the rotavirus protein VP7 shows sequence homology with the autoantigens tyrosine phosphatase IA-2 and Glutamic Acid Decarboxylase (GAD).[87] But to date, there is no conclusive evidence that rotavirus infections play any role in causing or aggravating beta-cell autoimmunity in humans.

Parvoviruses. As noted above, the parvovirus KRV can induce diabetes in the BBDR rat. One case has been reported in which type 1 diabetes, Graves' disease, and rheumatoid arthritis developed in a woman after acute parvovirus infection,[88] but evidence of any large-scale association with type 1 diabetes in humans is lacking.

Cytomegalovirus (CMV). CMV viruses are capable of infecting beta cells[89] and molecular mimicry[90] is a possibility, but there is no evidence that CMV infection plays any significant role in most cases of type 1 diabetes.

Role of childhood immunizations. Several large-scale, well-designed studies have conclusively shown that routine childhood immunizations do *not* increase the risk of type 1 diabetes.[91–93] On the contrary, immunization against mumps and pertussis may decrease the risk of type 1 diabetes.[85]

The hygiene hypothesis: possible protective role of infections. While some viral infections may increase the risk of type 1 diabetes, infectious agents may also play a protective role *against* diabetes. The hygiene hypothesis states that lack of exposure to childhood infections may somehow increase an individual's chances of developing autoimmune diseases, including type 1 diabetes. Epidemiologic patterns suggest that this *may* indeed be the case. For example, rates of type 1 diabetes and other autoimmune disorders are generally lower in underdeveloped nations with high prevalence of childhood infections, and tend to increase as these countries become more developed. As noted above, the incidence of type 1 diabetes differs almost sixfold between Russian Karelia and Finland even though both are populated by a genetically related population and are located next to each other at the same latitude. The incidence of autoimmunity in the two populations varies inversely with IgE antibody levels and IgE is involved in the response to parasitic infestation. All these observations indicate that decreased exposure to certain parasites and other microbes in early childhood may lead to an increased risk of autoimmunity in later life, including autoimmune diabetes. On the other hand, retrospective case–control studies have been equivocal at best[94–96] and direct evidence of protection by childhood infections is still lacking.

In animal studies, it has been shown that diabetes can be prevented in the NOD mouse model by infecting the mice with mycobacteria, salmonella or helminthes, or even by exposing them to products of these organisms.[97–99] But the NOD mouse is not a perfect model of human type 1 diabetes and a very large number of interventions (some of them apparently trivial) can prevent the development of diabetes in this animal, so the significance of these observations for human type 1 diabetes is open to debate.

DIET. Breast feeding may lower the risk of type 1 diabetes, either directly or by delaying exposure to cow's milk protein.[100,101] Early introduction of cow's milk protein[102] and early exposure to gluten[103] have both been implicated in the development of autoimmunity and it has been suggested that this is due to the "leakiness" of the immature gut to protein antigens. Antigens that have been implicated include beta lactoglobulin,[104] a major lipocalin protein in bovine milk, which is homologous to the human protein glycodelin (PP14), a T-cell modulator. Other studies have focused on bovine serum albumin[105] as the inciting antigen, but the data are contradictory and not yet conclusive.

Other dietary factors that have been suggested at various times as playing a role in diabetes risk include omega-3 fatty acids, vitamin D, ascorbic acid, zinc, and vitamin E. Vitamin D is biologically plausible (it has a role in immune regulation), deficiency is more common in Northern countries like Finland, and there is some epidemiologic evidence that decreased vitamin D levels in pregnancy or early childhood may be associated with diabetes risk; but the evidence is not yet conclusive and it is hoped that ongoing studies like the TEDDY (the Environmental Determinants of Diabetes in the Young) study will help to resolve some of the uncertainties in this area.

Environmental chemicals. Dietary nitrosamines and nitrates can induce beta-cell autoimmunity in animal models[106] and some epidemiologic studies suggested that they may play a role in type 1 diabetes,[107] but other studies contradicted these findings and at least one large prospective study has failed to find any association with chemicals in water supply.[108] At this time, the role of environmental chemicals in type 1 diabetes awaits clarification.

Psychological stress. Several studies[109,110] show an increased prevalence of stressful psychological situations among children who subsequently developed type 1 diabetes. Whether these stresses only aggravate pre-existing autoimmunity or whether they can actually trigger autoimmunity remains unknown.

Role of insulin resistance: the accelerator hypothesis. The accelerator hypothesis proposes that type 1 and type 2 diabetes are the same disorder of insulin resistance, set against different genetic backgrounds.[111] This "strong statement" of the accelerator hypothesis has been criticized[112] as ignoring the abundant genetic and clinical evidence that the two diseases are distinct. Still, the hypothesis has focused attention on the role of insulin resistance and obesity in type 1 diabetes and there is evidence that the incidence of type 1 diabetes is indeed higher in children who exhibit more rapid weight gain.[113] Whether this is simply another factor that stresses the beta cell in the course of a primarily autoimmune disorder, or whether type 1 and type 2 diabetes can really be regarded as the same disease, is still open to question.

Pathogenesis and Natural History of Type 1 Diabetes

In type 1a diabetes mellitus, a genetically susceptible host develops autoimmunity against his or her own beta cells. What triggers this autoimmune response remains unclear at this time. In some (but *not all*) patients, this autoimmune process results in progressive destruction of beta cells until a critical mass of beta cells is lost and insulin deficiency develops. Insulin deficiency in turn leads to the onset of clinical signs and symptoms of type 1 diabetes. At the time of diagnosis, some viable beta cells are still present and these may produce enough insulin to lead to a partial remission of the disease (honeymoon period) but over time, almost all beta cells are destroyed and the patient becomes totally dependent on exogenous insulin for survival. Over time, some of these patients develop secondary complications of diabetes that appear to be related to how well controlled the diabetes has been. Thus, the natural history of type 1 diabetes involves some or all of the following stages (Fig. 12.4):

1. Initiation of autoimmunity
2. Preclinical autoimmunity with progressive loss of beta-cell function

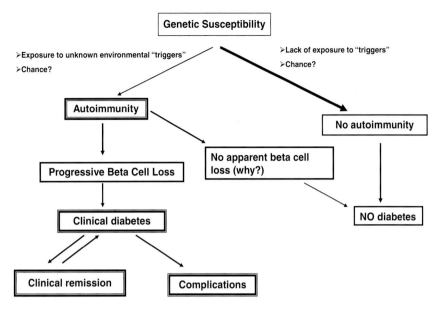

Fig. 12.4 Natural history of type 1 diabetes mellitus

3. Onset of clinical disease
4. Transient remission
5. Established disease
6. Development of complications

1. *Initiation of autoimmunity.* Genetic susceptibility to type 1 diabetes is determined by several genes (see genetics), with the largest contribution coming from variants in the HLA system. But it is important to keep in mind that even with the highest risk haplotypes, most carriers will NOT develop type 1 diabetes. Even in monozygotic twins, the concordance is 30–65%. What determines whether a genetically susceptible person goes on to develop autoimmunity is still unclear. As detailed earlier, a number of factors including prenatal influences, diet in infancy, viral infections, lack of exposure to certain infections, and even psychological stress have been implicated in the pathogenesis of type 1 diabetes, but their exact role and the mechanism by which they trigger or aggravate autoimmunity remains uncertain. What is clear is that markers of autoimmunity are much more prevalent than clinical type 1 diabetes, indicating that initiation of autoimmunity is a necessary but not a sufficient condition for type 1 diabetes.

   Whatever the triggering factor, it seems that in most cases of type 1 diabetes that are diagnosed in childhood, the onset of autoimmunity occurs very early in life. In a majority of the children diagnosed before the age of 10, the first signs of autoimmunity appear before the age of 2.[114] Development of autoimmunity is associated with the appearance of several autoantibodies. Insulin-associated antibodies (IAA) are usually the first to appear in young children, followed by glutamic acid decarboxylase 65 kDa (GAD65) and tyrosine phosphatase insulinoma-associated 2 (IA-2) antibodies. The earliest antibodies are predominantly of the IgG1 subclass. Not only is there "spreading" of autoimmunity to more antigens (IAA, then GAD 65 and IA-2) but there is also epitope spreading within one antigen. For example, initial GAD65 antibodies tend to be against the middle region or the carboxyl-terminal region, while amino-terminal antibodies usually appear later and are less common in children.[115]

2. *Preclinical autoimmunity with progressive loss of beta-cell function.* In some, but not all patients, the appearance of autoimmunity is followed by progressive destruction of beta cells. Antibodies are a marker for the presence of autoimmunity, but the actual damage to the beta cells is primarily T cell mediated.[116] Histologic analysis of the pancreas from patients with recent-onset type 1 diabetes reveals insulitis, with an infiltration of the islets of Langerhans by mononuclear cells, including T and B lymphocytes, monocytes/macrophages,

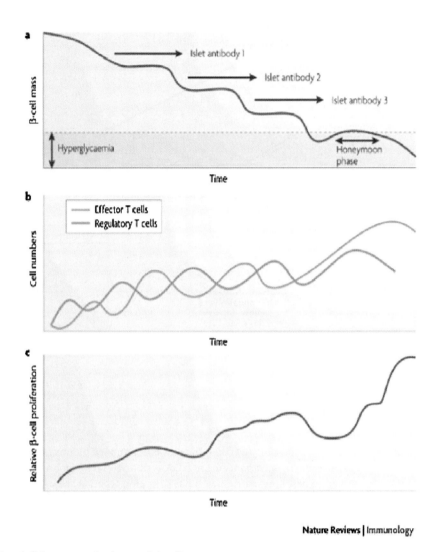

Nature Reviews | Immunology

Fig. 12.5 Type 1 diabetes as a relapsing–remitting disease

and natural killer (NK) cells.[117,118] In the NOD mouse, a similar cellular infiltrate is followed by linear loss of beta cells until they completely disappear. But it appears that the process in human type 1 diabetes is not necessarily linear and there may be an undulating downhill course in the development of type 1 diabetes (Fig. 12.5).[119]

Role of autoantibodies. The risk of developing clinical disease increases dramatically with an increase in the number of antibodies; only 30% of children with one antibody will progress to diabetes, but this risk increases to 70% when two antibodies are present and 90% when three are present.[120] The risk of progression also varies with the intensity of the antibody response and those with higher antibody titers are more likely to progress to clinical disease. Another factor that appears to influence progression of beta-cell damage is the age at which autoimmunity develops; children in whom IAA antibodies appeared within the first 2 years of life rapidly developed anti-islet cell antibodies and progressed to diabetes more frequently than children in whom the first antibodies appeared between ages 5 and 8.[121]

Role of genetics in disease progression. Genetics plays a role in progression to clinical disease. In a large study of healthy children, the appearance of single antibodies is relatively common and usually transient, and does not correlate with the presence of high-risk HLA alleles,[122] but those carrying high-risk HLA alleles are more likely to develop multiple antibodies and progress to disease. Similarly, the appearance of antibodies is more likely to predict diabetes in those with a family history of diabetes versus those with no family history of type 1 diabetes.[123] Thus, it may be the case that environmental factors can induce transient autoimmunity in many children, but those with genetic susceptibility are more likely to see progression of autoimmunity and eventual development of diabetes.

Role of environmental factors. In addition to genetic factors, environmental factors may also act as accelerators of type 1 diabetes after the initial appearance of autoimmunity. This is evident from the fact that the incidence of type 1 diabetes can vary several fold between populations that have the same prevalence of autoimmunity. For instance, the incidence of type 1 diabetes in Finland is almost fourfold higher than in Lithuania, but the incidence of autoimmunity is similar in both countries.[124]

The fact that all children with evidence of autoimmunity do not progress to diabetes indicates that there are "checkpoints" at which the autoimmune process can be halted or reversed before it progresses to full-blown diabetes. This has raised the possibility of preventing type 1 diabetes by intervening in the preclinical stage.

3. *Onset of clinical disease.* Patients with progressive beta-cell destruction will eventually present with clinical type 1 diabetes. It was thought that 90% of the total beta-cell mass is destroyed by the time clinical disease develops, but later studies have revealed that this is not always the case. It now appears that beta-cell destruction is more rapid and more complete in younger children, while in older children and adults the proportion of surviving beta cells is greater (10–20% in autopsy specimens) and some beta cells (about 1% of the normal mass) survive up to 30 years after the onset of diabetes.[125] Since autopsies are usually done on patients who died of diabetic ketoacidosis, these figures may underestimate the actual beta-cell mass present at diagnosis. Functional studies indicate that up to 40% of the insulin secretory capacity may be preserved in adults at the time of presentation of type 1 diabetes.[126] The fact that newly diagnosed diabetic individuals may still have significant surviving beta-cell mass is important because it raises the possibility of secondary prevention of type 1 diabetes. Similarly, the existence of viable beta cells, years or decades after initial presentation, indicates that even long-standing diabetic patients may be able to exhibit some recovery of beta-cell function if the autoimmune destructive process can be halted (Fig. 12.6).

Clinical features at the time of presentation range from asymptomatic (discovered on lab testing), to mild symptoms, to severe life-threatening diabetic ketoacidosis.

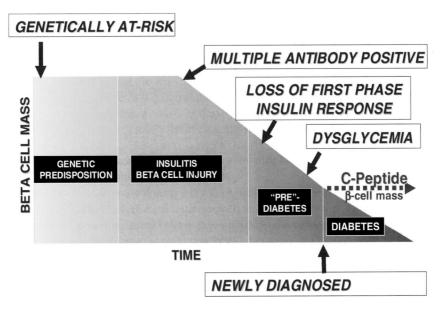

Fig. 12.6 Beta-cell mass at various stages in the natural history of diabetes

A. *Asymptomatic at diagnosis.* A small number of patients with type 1 diabetes are diagnosed before the appearance of any clinical symptoms because blood or urine testing is performed due to an unrelated illness, or in the course of a research study, or by parents who already have one diabetic child and happen to test a sibling. Such patients may need little or no treatment at diagnosis and may exhibit a prolonged "honeymoon period," but eventually almost all of them will progress to more typical type 1 diabetes.

B. *Classic presentation.* The classic presentation of type 1 diabetes is with polyuria, polydipsia, polyphagia, and weight loss.[127] With progressive loss of insulin secretion, fasting and postprandial glucose values become elevated. As blood glucose level rises, it exceeds the renal threshold for glucose (generally around 180 mg/dl) and the patient develops glucosuria. Osmotic diuresis then leads to polyuria and dehydration and this stimulates thirst, leading to polydipsia. At the same time, insulin deficiency leads to a switch from anabolic to catabolic metabolism and this, in combination with glucosuria, leads to weight loss in spite of polyphagia. Nocturnal enuresis due to polyuria is also a very common symptom in children. Other symptoms like fatigue, blurred vision, and muscle cramps may also be seen. Pyogenic skin infection and candidal vaginitis in prepubertal girls, or balanitis in uncircumcised boys, may be the presenting complaint in some cases, but careful history taking will almost invariably reveal that polyuria, polydipsia, or weight loss are also present.

C. *Diabetic ketoacidosis.* Of children with type 1 diabetes, 20–40% present with diabetic ketoacidosis (DKA). Younger patients are more likely to present with DKA, as are patients of lower socioeconomic status, female gender, and lack of family history of type 1 diabetes. Areas with a low prevalence of type 1 diabetes are also more likely to see DKA on presentation as caretakers and medical personnel are unfamiliar with the early symptoms of the disease.[128] Young children are more likely to present with DKA because younger children have lost more of their beta-cell mass at diagnosis and are more likely to have absolute insulin deficiency, and because early symptoms may be missed more frequently in very young children. Incidence of diabetic ketoacidosis at diagnosis has declined in some countries as the general public and medical professionals have become more familiar with early signs and symptoms.[129]

Patients who present with DKA have usually had a period of polyuria and polydipsia that was not recognized as significant. The occurrence of DKA may be precipitated by a stressful event (for example, an acute infection) or may simply reflect the progression of earlier symptoms to the point that homeostatic mechanisms fail and DKA develops. As the patient becomes increasingly dehydrated and lipolysis accelerates due to lack of insulin, increased delivery of fatty acids to the liver and subsequent increase in ketogenesis develop. Increasing ketonemia leads to acidosis, which may be worsened by lactic acidosis due to dehydration. Dehydration also leads to decreased renal function, further compromising acid excretion and worsening acidosis. Acidosis may lead to CNS depression and Kussmaul respirations. Elevated ketones can also cause nausea, abdominal pain, and vomiting. An elevated leukocyte count and nonspecific elevation of serum amylase are frequently seen, but serum lipase is usually not elevated.

The occurrence of cerebral edema may complicate 0.5–1% of cases of DKA. Mortality in patients with DKA ranges from 0.15 to 0.5% in advanced countries and 57–87% of deaths are thought to be due to cerebral edema. Other relatively rare causes of death in DKA include hypokalemia, hyperkalemia, hypoglycemia, thrombosis, septicemia, and multi-organ failure.[130] These complications and their management are discussed in Chapter 18.

D. *Acute fulminant diabetes.* An unusual form of type 1 diabetes characterized by very short history of symptoms (only a few days rather than weeks or months), rapid deterioration, minimal elevation of hemoglobin A1c in spite of severe hyperglycemia (indicating that the pathologic process is of short duration), and frequent history of recent acute illness was initially reported from Japan and Korea,[131,132] It has now been reported in at least three Caucasian adults in France as well. Typical autoimmune type 1 diabetes develops relatively slowly (over months or years) and evidence of autoimmunity is present long before the onset of clinical diabetes. In contrast, acute fulminant diabetes appears to develop in a matter of days in previously euglycemic individuals and is frequently accompanied by signs of exocrine pancreatic damage (acute pancreatitis). The occurrence of recent acute illness and evidence of viral infection are frequently seen. Evidence of autoimmunity may be seen, but the most commonly associated antibodies are directed against amylase rather than against beta-cell antigens.[133] All these facts indicate that acute fulminant diabetes may be the result of acute pancreatitis (including autoimmune pancreatitis) and represents a disease distinct from typical type 1 diabetes.

4. *Transient remission (honeymoon period).* After initial diagnosis of type 1 diabetes, most patients experience a transient decrease in their requirements of exogenous insulin, with a small minority (2–12%) showing total remission for a variable period of time.[134] It is likely that prolonged hyperglycemia and fatty acid excess inhibits the function of otherwise viable beta cells ("glucotoxicity" and "lipotoxicity") and when normoglycemia is reestablished after diagnosis, these cells recover function and thus increase the patient's capacity to secrete endogenous insulin. Unfortunately, this natural remission is almost always temporary and insulin requirements tend to increase gradually or abruptly within a few months in most patients. In extremely rare cases, the remission may last for years.[135] Younger children tend to have a shorter remission as beta-cell destruction is more rapid and more complete in this age group.[136] Less severe initial presentation is associated with longer remission, as are low islet cell antibody and IA-2 antibody levels. Efforts to prolong or accentuate this remission are the basis for various interventions that may be regarded as secondary prevention of diabetes.

5. *Established disease.* In most patients, almost all residual beta-cell function is lost within 1–3 years of diagnosis and the patient is then totally dependent on the administration of exogenous insulin. Management of this stage is discussed in detail in Chapter 43.

6. *Chronic complications of type 1 diabetes.* Patients with type 1 diabetes develop vascular complications (microangiopathy and atherosclerosis) that can lead to cardiovascular disease, retinopathy, nephropathy, neuropathy, peripheral circulatory disease, and other forms of end-organ damage. Poor glycemic control is associated with more rapid development of complications, probably via multiple mechanisms. These are discussed in greater detail in Part VI but a few salient features are highlighted here.

   1. Cardiovascular mortality is very significantly elevated in type 1 diabetes and is 2–20-fold higher in young adults with type 1 diabetes as compared to their peers. In fact, cardiovascular disease has now overtaken nephropathy as a cause of premature death in adults with diabetes.[137–139]

   2. Atherosclerosis begins at an early stage in the disease,[140] therefore all patients with type 1 diabetes should be screened for cardiovascular risk factors like lipid levels and hypertension, and these should be aggressively treated in order to prevent premature cardiovascular disease.[141]

Associated autoimmune disorders. Autoimmune type 1 diabetes is associated with an increased incidence of several other autoimmune disorders, the most prominent of which are celiac disease and autoimmune thyroiditis. The prevalence of thyroid antibodies in children with type 1 diabetes ranges from 7 to 40% in different studies[142–144], while the prevalence of celiac disease ranges from 1 to 16.4%.[145–147] In a recent large study from Germany and Austria, the prevalence of celiac-associated antibodies was approximately 11%, while the prevalence of antithyroid antibodies was 15%.[148]

Primary prevention of type 1 diabetes. While some genetic factors clearly increase the risk of type 1 diabetes, not all high-risk subjects develop autoimmunity, and not all those who develop markers of autoimmunity go on to develop type 1 diabetes. This indicates that there are "checkpoints" on the road to diabetes at which the autoimmune process may be stopped or reversed. Intervening to prevent progression to type 1 diabetes (primary prevention) may therefore be feasible and several trials have attempted to test various interventions in this regard.

A safe, effective, inexpensive, and easily administered intervention could theoretically be targeted at all newborns, but no such universally effective intervention is yet available. Delaying the introduction of cow's milk protein, delaying introduction of cereals, and increasing the duration of breast feeding are all potentially beneficial and trials of these interventions are ongoing.[149,150] But the fact that the disease has continued to increase in incidence in Northern Europe in spite of increase in breast feeding indicates that these interventions may not be sufficient to reverse the epidemic.

Other dietary interventions that are being tested, or may be tested in high-risk subjects, include omega-3 fatty acid supplementation, vitamin D supplementation, and the use of cod liver oil during pregnancy.[151] In all these cases, there are some hints of possible benefit but nothing has been conclusively proven until now.

In high-risk populations (relatives of type 1 diabetic individuals, especially those with high-risk genotypes), it is feasible to test more targeted interventions. One of the first interventions to be tested in a high-risk population was the use of nicotinamide supplementation, but this failed to prevent type 1 diabetes.[152] Parenteral insulin[153] and nasal insulin[154] proved similarly ineffective in preventing diabetes, but oral insulin appeared to delay the incidence of diabetes in some patients.[155] A larger trial of oral insulin is currently ongoing and results are awaited.

Other studies that are ongoing or planned will look at the effect of GAD-alum and anti-CD3 antibodies in subjects at high risk for the development of type 1 diabetes.

Secondary prevention. Depending on age, anywhere from 10–20 to 40% (or more) of a person's beta cells may be intact at the time of diagnosis. In addition, small numbers of beta cells may survive (or develop anew) up to 30 years after diagnosis. This raises the possibility that diabetes can be cured or ameliorated by stopping the autoimmune destructive process *after* initial diagnosis (secondary prevention).

Immunosuppressants like cyclosporine have been tested for this purpose,[156] but while they may prolong the honeymoon period, they are associated with significant side effects and are only effective as long as they are being administered, so their use for this purpose has been abandoned. Trials using CD3 antibodies have been more promising, but some patients did develop flu-like symptoms and reactivation of Epstein–Barr Virus infection.[157] Further trials of this therapy and other therapies targeted at various components of T cells and B cells are planned or ongoing.[158]

The possibility of using glucagon-like peptide (GLP-1) agonists (e.g., exenatide) alone or in combination with immunomodulatory therapies is also being explored as these agents are capable of increasing beta-cell mass in animals (though not necessarily in humans).

Summary

Type 1 diabetes is a heterogenous clinical syndrome, characterized by absolute insulin deficiency. It can present at any age, with about half the cases being diagnosed in childhood. Most cases in children are associated with autoimmune destruction of the pancreatic beta cells. Several genes, especially certain HLA haplotypes, are associated with increased risk of the disease, but environmental factors also play a significant role and their role may be greater in older patients. It is hoped that better understanding of the disease process will lead to more accurate identification of susceptible persons and effective interventions to prevent the disease in susceptible hosts.

References

1. Abiru N, Kawasaki E, Eguch K. Current knowledge of Japanese type 1 diabetic syndrome. *Diabetes Metab Res Rev.* 2002;18:357–366.
2. Pundziute-Lycka A, Dahlquist G, Nystrom L, et al. Type I diabetes in the 0–34 years group in Sweden. *Diabetologia.* 2002;45:783–791.
3. Svensson J, Carstensen B, Molbak A, et al. Increased risk of childhood Type 1 diabetes in children born after 1985. *Diabetes Care.* 2002;25:2197–2201.
4. Mohr SB, Garland CF, Gorham ED, Garland FC. The association between ultraviolet B irradiance, vitamin D status and incidence rates of type 1 diabetes in 51 regions worldwide. *Diabetologia.* 2008 Aug;51(8):1391–1398. Epub 2008 Jun 12.
5. Diamond Project Group. Incidence and trends of childhood type 1 diabetes worldwide 1990–1999. *Diabet Med.* 2006;23: 857–866.
6. Rytkönen M, Moltchanova E, Ranta J, Taskinen O, Tuomilehto J, Karvonen M, SPAT Study Group, Finnish Childhood Diabetes Registry Group. The incidence of type 1 diabetes among children in Finland – rural–urban difference. *Health Place.* 2003 Dec;9(4):315–325.
7. Holmqvist BM, Lofman O, Samuelsson U. A low incidence of Type 1 diabetes between 1977 and 2001 in south-eastern Sweden in areas with high population density and which are more deprived. *Diabet Med.* 2008 Mar;25(3):255–260. Epub 2008 Jan 14.
8. Staines A, Bodansky HJ, McKinney PA, et al. Small area variation in the incidence of childhood insulin-dependent diabetes mellitus in Yorkshire, UK: links with overcrowding and population density. *Int J Epidemiol.* 1997;6:1307–1313.
9. Patterson CC, Carson DJ, Hadden DR. Epidemiology of childhood IDDM in Northern Ireland 1989–1994: low incidence in areas with highest population density and most household crowding. Northern Ireland Diabetes Study Group. *Diabetologia.* 1996;9:1063–1069.

10. Cherubini V, Carle F, Gesuita R, et al. Large incidence variation of Type 1 diabetes in central-southern Italy 1990–1995: lower risk in rural areas. *Diabetologia*. 1999;7:789–792.

11. Pundziute-Lycka A, Urbonaite B, Ostrauskas R, Zalinkevicius R, Dahlquist GG. Incidence of type 1 diabetes in Lithuanians aged 0–39 years varies by the urban-rural setting, and the time change differs for men and women during 1991–2000. *Diabetes Care*. 2003;3:671–676.

12. Schober E, Rami B, Waldhoer T, Austrian Diabetes Incidence Study Group. Steep increase of incidence of childhood diabetes since 1999 in Austria. Time trend analysis 1979–2005. A nationwide study. *Eur J Pediatr*. 2008 Mar;167(3):293–297. Epub 2007 Apr.

13. Stipancic G, La Grasta Sabolic L, Malenica M, Radica A, Skrabic V, Tiljak MK. Incidence and trends of childhood Type 1 diabetes in Croatia from 1995 to 2003. *Diabetes Res Clin Pract*. 2008 Apr;80(1):122–127. Epub 2007 Dec.

14. Barat P, Valade A, Brosselin P, Alberti C, Maurice-Tison S, Lévy-Marchal C. The growing incidence of type 1 diabetes in children: the 17-year French experience in Aquitaine. *Diabet Metab*. 2008 Dec;34(6 Pt 1):601–605. Epub 2008 Oct 25.

15. Ehehalt S, Blumenstock G, Willasch AM, Hub R, Ranke MB, Neu A, DIARY-Study Group Baden-Württemberg. Continuous rise in incidence of childhood Type 1 diabetes in Germany. *Diabet Med*. 2008 Jun;25(6):755–757.

16. Harjutsalo V, Sjöberg L, Tuomilehto J. Time trends in the incidence of type 1 diabetes in Finnish children: a cohort study. *Lancet*. 2008 May 24;371(9626):1777–1782.

17. Newhook LA, Grant M, Sloka S, et al. Very high and increasing incidence of type 1 diabetes mellitus in Newfoundland and Labrador, Canada. *Pediatr Diabetes*. 2008 Jun;9(3 Pt 2):62–68. Epub 2008 Jan.

18. Zhang H, Xia W, Yu Q, et al. Increasing incidence of type 1 diabetes in children aged 0–14 years in Harbin, China (1990–2000). *Prim Care Diabetes*. 2008 Sep;2(3):121–126. Epub 2008 Jul 16.

19. Patterson C, Behalf of the EURODIAB collaboration of childhood type 1 diabetes registers. 15 Year trends in the incidence of Type 1 diabetes in Europe. *Pediatr Diabetes*. 2007;8(Suppl 7):7.

20. Jansson SP, Andersson DK, Svärdsudd K. Prevalence and incidence rate of diabetes mellitus in a Swedish community during 30 years of follow-up. *Diabetologia*. 2007 Apr;50(4):703–710. Epub 2007 Feb 1.

21. Joner G, Stene LC, Søvik O, Norwegian Childhood Diabetes Study Group. Nationwide, prospective registration of type 1 diabetes in children aged <15 years in Norway 1989–1998: no increase but significant regional variation in incidence. *Diabetes Care*. 2004 Jul;27(7):1618–1622.

22. Raymond NT, Jones JR, Swift PG, et al. Comparative incidence of type 1 diabetes in children aged under 15 years from South Asian and white or other ethnic backgrounds in Leicestershire, UK, 1989 to 1998. *Diabetologia*. 2001;44(Suppl 3):B32–B36.

23. Gillespie KM, Bain SC, Barnett AH, et al. The rising incidence of childhood type 1 diabetes and reduced contributions of high-risk HLA haplotypes. *Lancet*. 2004;364:1699–1700.

24. Muntoni S, Fonte MT, Stoduto S, et al. Incidence of insulin-dependent diabetes mellitus among Sardinian-heritage children born in Lazio region, Italy. *Lancet*. 1997 Jan 18;349(9046):160–162.

25. Haller MJ, Atkinson MA, Schatz D. Type 1 diabetes mellitus: etiology, presentation, and management. *Pediatr Clin North Am*. 2005 Dec;52(6):1553–1578.

26. Rewers M, Stone RA, LaPorte RE, et al. Poisson regression modeling of temporal variation in incidence of childhood insulin-dependent diabetes mellitus in Allegheny County, Pennsylvania, and Wielkopolska, Poland, 1970–1985. *Am J Epidemiol*. 1989;129:569–581.

27. Siemiatycki J, Colle E, Campbell S, Dewar RA, Belmonte MM. Case-control study of IDDM. *Diabetes Care*. 1989;12:209–216.

28. Larenas G, Montecinos A, Manosalva M, et al. Incidence of insulin-dependent diabetes mellitus in the IX region of Chile: ethnic differences. *Diabetes Res Clin Pract*. 1996;34:S147–S151.

29. Koton S, Israel IDDM Registry Study Group – IIRSG. Incidence of type 1 diabetes mellitus in the 0- to 17-yr-old Israel population, 1997–2003. *Pediatr Diabetes*. 2007 Apr;8(2):60–66.

30. Kondrashova A, Viskari H, Kulmala P, et al. Signs of beta-cell autoimmunity in nondiabetic schoolchildren: a comparison between Russian Karelia with a low incidence of type 1 diabetes and Finland with a high incidence rate. *Diabetes Care*. 2007 Jan;30(1):95–100.

31. Willis JA, Scott RS, Darlow BA, Lewy H, Ashkenazi I, Laron Z. Seasonality of birth and onset of clinical disease in children and adolescents (0–19 years) with type 1 diabetes mellitus in Canterbury, New Zealand. *J Pediatr Endocrinol Metab*. 2002 May;15(5):645–647.

32. Levy-Marchal C, Patterson C, Green A. Variation by age group and seasonality at diagnosis of childhood IDDM in Europe. The EURODIAB ACE Study Group. *Diabetologia*. 1995;38:823–830.

33. Green A, Patterson CC. Trends in the incidence of childhood-onset diabetes in Europe 1989–1998. *Diabetologia*. 2001;44(Suppl 3):B3–B8.

34. Svensson J, Lyngaae-Jørgensen A, Carstensen B, Simonsen LB, Mortensen HB. Long-term trends in the incidence of type 1 diabetes in Denmark: the seasonal variation changes over time. *Pediatr Diabetes*. 2008 Nov 24;10(4):248–254.

35. Ye J, Chen RG, Ashkenazi I, Laron Z. Lack of seasonality in the month of onset of childhood IDDM (0.7–15 years) in Shanghai, China. *J Pediatr Endocrinol Metab*. 1998;11:461–464.

36. Kida K, Mimura G, Ito T, Murakami K, Ashkenazi I, Laron Z. Incidence of Type 1 diabetes mellitus in children aged 0–14 in Japan, 1986–1990, including an analysis for seasonality of onset and month of birth: JDS study. The Data Committee for Childhood Diabetes of the Japan Diabetes Society (JDS). *Diabet Med*. 2000;17:59–63.

37. Laron Z, Lewy H, Wilderman I, et al. Seasonality of month of birth of children and adolescents with type 1 diabetes mellitus in homogenous and heterogeneous populations. *Isr Med Assoc J.* 2005 Jun;7(6):381–384.

38. Laron Z. Interplay between heredity and environment in the recent explosion of type 1 childhood diabetes mellitus. *Am J Med Genet.* 2002 May 30;115(1):4–7.

39. Gale EA, Gillespie KM. Diabetes and gender. *Diabetologia.* 2001;44:3–15.

40. Kawasaki E, Matsuura N, Eguchi K. Type 1 diabetes in Japan. *Diabetologia.* 2006 May;49(5):828–836. Epub 2006 Mar 28.

41. Risch N. Assessing the role of HLA-linked and unlinked determinants of disease. *Am J Hum Genet.* 1987;40:1–14.

42. Hämäläinen AM, Knip M. Autoimmunity and familial risk of type 1 diabetes. *Curr Diab Rep.* 2002 Aug;2(4):347–353.

43. Kyvik KO, Green A, Beck-Nielsen H. Concordance rates of insulin dependent diabetes mellitus: a population based study of young Danish twins. *BMJ.* 1995 Oct 7;311(7010):913–917.

44. Redondo MJ, Jeffrey J, Fain PR, Eisenbarth GS, Orban T. Concordance for islet autoimmunity among monozygotic twins. *N Engl J Med.* 2008 Dec 25;359(26):2849–2850.

45. Noble JA, Valdes AM, Cook M, Klitz W, Thomson G, Erlich HA. The role of HLA class II genes in insulin-dependent diabetes mellitus: molecular analysis of 180 Caucasian, multiplex families. *Am J Hum Genet.* 1996;59(5):1134–1148.

46. Aly TA, Ide A, Jahromi MM, et al. Extreme genetic risk for type 1A diabetes. *Proc Natl Acad Sci USA.* 2006 Sept 19;103(38):14074–14079. Epub 2006 Sept 11.

47. Erlich H, Valdes AM, Noble J, et al. HLA DR-DQ haplotypes and genotypes and type 1 diabetes risk: analysis of the type 1 diabetes genetics consortium families. *Diabetes.* 2008;57:1084–1092.

48. Redondo MJ, Fain PR, Eisenbarth GS. Genetics of type 1A diabetes. *Recent Prog Horm Res.* 2001;56:69–89.

49. Todd JA, Bell JI, McDevitt HO. HLA-DQβ gene contributes to susceptibility and resistance to insulin-dependent diabetes mellitus. *Nature.* 1987;329:599–604.

50. Morel PA, Dorman JS, Todd JA, McDevitt HO, Trucco M. Aspartic acid at position 57 of the HLA-DQ beta chain protects against type I diabetes: a family study. *Proc Natl Acad Sci USA.* 1988;85(21):8111–8115.

51. Kwok WW, Domeier ME, Johnson ML, Nepom GT, Koelle DM. HLA-DQB1 codon 57 is critical for peptide binding and recognition. *J Exp Med.* 1996;183(3):1253–1258.

52. Lee HC, Ikegami H, Fujisawa T, et al. Role of HLA class II alleles in Korean patients with IDDM. *Diabetes Res Clin Pract.* 1996 Mar;31(1–3):9–15.

53. Awata T, Kuzuya T, Matsuda A, et al. High frequency of aspartic acid at position 57 of HLA-DQ B-chain in Japanese IDDM patients and nondiabetic subjects. *Diabetes.* 1990;39(2):266–269.

54. Nejentsev S, Howson JM, Walker NM, et al. Localization of type 1 diabetes susceptibility to the MHC class I genes HLA-B and HLA-A. *Nature.* 2007 Dec 6;450(7171):887–892. Epub 2007 Nov 14.

55. Park Y. Why is type 1 diabetes uncommon in Asia? *Ann NY Acad Sci.* 2006 Oct;1079:31–40.

56. Bennett ST, Todd JA. Human type 1 diabetes and the insulin gene: principles of mapping polygenes. *Annu Rev Genet.* 1996;30:343–370.

57. Bell GI, Selby MJ, Rutter WJ. The highly polymorphic region near the human insulin gene is composed of simple tandemly repeating sequences. *Nature.* 1982;295(5844):31–35.

58. Stead JD, Hurles ME, Jeffreys AJ. Global haplotype diversity in the human insulin gene region. *Genome Res.* 2003;13: 2101–2111.

59. Pugliese A, Zeller M, Fernandez A Jr, et al. The insulin gene is transcribed in the human thymus and transcription levels correlated with allelic variation at the INS VNTR-IDDM2 susceptibility locus for type 1 diabetes. *Nat Genet.* 1997 Mar;15(3):293–297.

60. Vafiadis P, Grabs R, Goodyer CG, Colle E, Polychronakos C. A functional analysis of the role of IGF2 in IDDM2-encoded susceptibility to type 1 diabetes. *Diabetes.* 1998;47(5):831–836.

61. Bottini N, Musumeci L, Alonso A, et al. A functional variant of lymphoid tyrosine phosphatase is associated with type I diabetes. *Nat Genet.* 2004;36:337–338.

62. Bottini N, Vang T, Cucca F, Mustelin T. Role of PTPN22 in type 1 diabetes and other autoimmune diseases. *Semin Immunol.* 2006 Aug;18(4):207–213. Epub 2006 May 11.

63. Rieck M, Arechiga A, Onengut-Gumuscu S, Greenbaum C, Concannon P, Buckner JH. Genetic variation in PTPN22 corresponds to altered function of T and B lymphocytes. *J Immunol.* 2007;179:4704–4710.

64. Nisticò L, Buzzetti R, Pritchard LE, et al. The CTLA-4 gene region of chromosome 2q33 is linked to, and associated with, type 1 diabetes. Belgian Diabetes Registry. *Hum Mol Genet.* 1996 Jul;5(7):1075–1080.

65. Chistiakov DA, Turakulov RI. CTLA-4 and its role in autoimmune thyroid disease. *J Mol Endocrinol.* 2003 Aug;31(1):21–36. Review.

66. Lowe CE, Cooper JD, Brusko T, et al. Large-scale genetic fine mapping and genotype-phenotype associations implicate polymorphism in the IL2RA region in type 1 diabetes. *Nat Genet.* 2007;39(9):1074–1082.

67. Smyth DJ, Cooper JD, Bailey R, et al. A genome-wide association study of nonsynonymous SNPs identifies a type 1 diabetes locus in the interferon-induced helicase (IFIH1) region. *Nat Genet.* 2006;38(6):617–619.

68. Kato H, Takeuchi O, Sato S, et al. Differential roles of MDA5 and RIG-I helicases in the recognition of RNA viruses. *Nature.* 2006 May 4;441(7089):101–105. Epub 2006 Apr 9.

69. Bailey R, Cooper JD, Zeitels L, et al. Association of the vitamin D metabolism gene CYP27B1 with type 1 diabetes. *Diabetes.* 2007 Oct;56(10):2616–2621. Epub 2007 Jul 2.

70. Todd JA, Walker NM, Cooper JD, et al. Robust associations of four new chromosome regions from genome-wide analyses of type 1 diabetes. *Nat Genet*. 2007 Jul;39(7):857–864. Epub 2007 Jun 6.

71. Wellcome Trust Case Control Consortium. Genome-wide association study of 14,000 cases of seven common diseases and 3,000 shared controls. *Nature*. 2007;447(7145):661–678.

72. Conrad B, Weissmahr RN, Böni J, Arcari R, Schüpbach J, Mach B. A human endogenous retroviral superantigen as candidate autoimmune gene in type 1 diabetes. *Cell*. 1997;90(2):303–313.

73. Knerr I, Repp R, Dotsch J, et al. Quantitation of gene expression by real-time PCR disproves a "retroviral hypothesis" for childhood-onset diabetes mellitus. *Pediatr Res*. 1999;46(1):57–60.

74. Nakhooda AF, Like AA, Chappel CI, et al. The spontaneously diabetic Wistar rat. Metabolic and morphologic studies. *Diabetes*. 1977;26:100–112.

75. Rayfield EJ, Kelly KJ, Yoon JW. Rubella virus-induced diabetes in the hamster. *Diabetes*. 1986;35:1278–1281.

76. Tauriainen S, Salminen K, Hyoty H. Can enteroviruses cause type 1 diabetes? *Ann NY Acad Sci*. 2003;1005:13–22.

77. Yoon JW, Austin M, Onodera T, et al. Isolation of a virus from the pancreas of a child with diabetic ketoacidosis. *N Engl J Med*. 1979;300:1173–1179.

78. Champsaur HF, Bottazzo GF, Bertrams J, et al. Virologic, immunologic, and genetic factors in insulin-dependent diabetes mellitus. *J Pediatr*. 1982;100:15–20.

79. Harkonen T, Lankinen H, Davydova B, et al. Enterovirus infection can induce immune responses that cross-react with beta-cell autoantigen tyrosine phosphatase IA-2/IAR. *J Med Virol*. 2002;66:340–350.

80. Horwitz MS, Bradley LM, Harbertson J, et al. Diabetes induced by Coxsackie virus: initiation by bystander damage and not molecular mimicry. *Nat Med*. 1998;4:781–785.

81. Viskari H, Ludvigsson J, Uibo R, et al. Relationship between the incidence of type 1 diabetes and maternal enterovirus antibodies: time trends and geographical variation. *Diabetologia*. 2005;48:1280–1287.

82. Menser MA, Forrest JM, Bransby RD. Rubella infection and diabetes-mellitus. *Lancet*. 1978;1:57–60.

83. Helmke K, Otten A, Willems W. Islet cell antibodies in children with mumps infection. *Lancet*. 1980;2:211–212.

84. Hyoty H, Leinikki P, Reunanen A, et al. Mumps infections in the etiology of type 1 (insulin-dependent) diabetes. *Diabetes Res*. 1988;9:111–116.

85. Altobelli E, Petrocelli R, Verrotti A, Valenti M. Infections and risk of type I diabetes in childhood: a population-based case-control study. *Eur J Epidemiol*. 2003;18(5):425–430.

86. Coulson BS, Witterick PD, Tan Y, et al. Growth of rotaviruses in primary pancreatic cells. *J Virol*. 2002;76:9537–9544.

87. Honeyman MC, Stone NL, Harrison LC. T-cell epitopes in type 1 diabetes autoantigen tyrosine phosphatase IA-2: potential for mimicry with rotavirus and other environmental agents. *Mol Med*. 1998;4:231–239.

88. Munakata Y, Kodera T, Saito T, et al. Rheumatoid arthritis, type 1 diabetes, and Graves' disease after acute parvovirus B19 infection. *Lancet*. 2005;366:780.

89. Jenson AB, Rosenberg HS, Notkins AL. Pancreatic islet-cell damage in children with fatal viral-infections. *Lancet*. 1980;2:354–358.

90. Pak CY, Cha CY, Rajotte RV, et al. Human pancreatic-islet cell specific 38 kilodalton autoantigen identified by cytomegalovirus-induced monoclonal islet cell autoantibody. *Diabetologia*. 1990;33:569–572.

91. Graves PM, Barriga KJ, Norris JM, et al. Lack of association between early childhood immunizations and beta-cell autoimmunity. *Diabetes Care*. 1999;22:1694–1697.

92. EURODIAB Substudy 2 Study Group. Infections and vaccinations as risk factors for childhood type I (insulin-dependent) diabetes mellitus: a multicentre case-control investigation. *Diabetologia*. 2000;43:47–53.

93. DeStefano F, Mullooly JP, Okoro CA, et al. Childhood vaccinations, vaccination timing, and risk of type 1 diabetes mellitus. *Pediatrics*. 2001;108:E112.

94. Cardwell CR, Carson DJ, Patterson CC. No association between routinely recorded infections in early life and subsequent risk of childhood-onset Type 1 diabetes: a matched case-control study using the UK General Practice Research Database. *Diabet Med*. 2008 Mar;25(3):261–267. Epub 2008 Jan 14.

95. Pundziute-Lyckå A, Urbonaite B, Dahlquist G. Infections and risk of Type I (insulin-dependent) diabetes mellitus in Lithuanian children. *Diabetologia*. 2000 Oct;43(10):1229–1234.

96. Altobelli E, Petrocelli R, Verrotti A, Valenti M. Infections and risk of type I diabetes in childhood: a population-based case-control study. *Eur J Epidemiol*. 2003;18(5):425–430.

97. Cooke A, Tonks P, Jones FM, et al. Infection with Schistosoma mansoni prevents insulin dependent diabetes mellitus in non-obese diabetic mice. *Parasite Immunol*. 1999;21:169–176.

98. Bras A, Aguas AP. Diabetes-prone NOD mice are resistant to Mycobacterium avium and the infection prevents autoimmune disease. *Immunology*. 1996;89:20–25.

99. Saunders KA, Raine T, Cooke A, Lawrence CE. Inhibition of autoimmune type 1 diabetes by gastrointestinal helminth infection. *Infect Immun*. 2007;75:397–407.

100. Sadauskaite-Kuehne V, Ludvigsson J, Padaiga Z, Jasinskiene E, Samuelsson U. Longer breastfeeding is an independent protective factor against development of type 1 diabetes mellitus in childhood. *Diabetes Metab Res Rev*. 2004 Mar–Apr;20(2):150–157.

101. Rosenbauer J, Herzig P, Giani G. Early infant feeding and risk of type 1 diabetes mellitus – a nationwide population-based case-control study in pre-school children. *Diabetes Metab Res Rev*. 2008 Mar–Apr;24(3):211–222.

102. Ziegler AG, Schmid S, Huber D, et al. Early infant feeding and risk of developing type 1 diabetes-associated autoantibodies. *JAMA*. 2003;290:1721–1728.

103. Norris JM, Barriga K, Klingensmith G, et al. Timing of initial cereal exposure in infancy and risk of islet autoimmunity. *JAMA*. 2003;290:1713–1720.

104. Goldfarb MF. Relation of time of introduction of cow milk protein to an infant and risk of type-1 diabetes mellitus. *J Proteome Res*. 2008 May;7(5):2165–2167. Epub 2008 Apr 15.

105. Karjalainen J, Martin JM, Knip M, et al. A bovine albumin peptide as a possible trigger of insulin-dependent diabetes mellitus [see comments]. *N Engl J Med*. 1992;327:302–307.

106. Rayfield EJ, Ishimura K. Environmental factors and insulin dependent diabetes mellitus. *Diabetes Metab Rev*. 1987;3: 925–957.

107. Dahlquist GG, Blom LG, Persson L-Å, Sandström AIM, Wall SGI. Dietary factors and the risk of developing insulin dependent diabetes in childhood. *Br Med J*. 1990;300:1302–1306.

108. Winkler C, Mollenhauer U, Hummel S, Bonifacio E, Ziegler AG. Exposure to environmental factors in drinking water: risk of islet autoimmunity and type 1 diabetes – the BABYDIAB study. *Horm Metab Res*. 2008 Aug;40(8):566–571. Epub 2008 May 21.

109. Hägglöf B, Blom L, Dahlquist G, Lönnberg G, Sahlin B. The Swedish childhood diabetes study: indications of severe psychological stress as a risk factor for type 1 (insulin-dependent) diabetes mellitus in childhood. *Diabetologia*. 1991 Aug;34(8):579–583.

110. Karavanaki K, Tsoka E, Liacopoulou M, et al. Psychological stress as a factor potentially contributing to the pathogenesis of Type 1 diabetes mellitus. *J Endocrinol Invest*. 2008 May;31(5):406–415.

111. Wilkin TJ. The accelerator hypothesis: weight gain as the missing link between Type I and Type II diabetes. *Diabetologia*. 2001;44:914–922.

112. Daneman D. Is the 'Accelerator Hypothesis' worthy of our attention? *Diabet Med*. 2005 Feb;22(2):115–117.

113. Betts PR, Mulligan J, Ward P, Smith B, Wilkin T. Increasing body weight predicts the earlier onset of insulin-dependent diabetes in childhood: testing the 'accelerator hypothesis'. *Diabet Med*. 2005;2:144–151.

114. Ziegler AG, Hummel M, Schenker M, Bonifacio E. Autoantibody appearance and risk for development of childhood diabetes in offspring of parents with type 1 diabetes: the 2-year analysis of the German BABYDIAB Study. *Diabetes*. 1999;48:460–468.

115. Achenbach P, Bonifacio E, Koczwara K, Ziegler AG. Natural history of type 1 diabetes. *Diabetes*. 2005 Dec;54(Suppl 2): S25–S31.

116. Mallone R, van Endert P. T cells in the pathogenesis of type 1 diabetes. *Curr Diabetes Rep*. 2008 Apr;8(2):101–106.

117. Gepts W, Lecompte PM. The pancreatic islets in diabetes. *Am J Med*. 1981;70:105–115.

118. Hanninen A, Jalkanen S, Salmi M, et al. Macrophages, T cell receptor usage, and endothelial cell activation in the pancreas at the onset of insulin-dependent diabetes mellitus. *J Clin Invest*. 1992;90:1901–1910.

119. von Herrath M, Sanda S, Herold K. Type 1 diabetes as a relapsing–remitting disease? *Nat Rev Immunol*. 2007 Dec;7:988–994.

120. Siljander HT, Veijola R, Reunanen A, Virtanen SM, Akerblom HK, Knip M. Prediction of type 1 diabetes among siblings of affected children and in the general population. *Diabetologia*. 2007 Nov;50(11):2272–2275.

121. Hummel M, Bonifacio E, Schmid S, Walter M, Knopff A, Ziegler AG. Brief communication: early appearance of islet autoantibodies predicts childhood type 1 diabetes in offspring of diabetic parents. *Ann Intern Med*. 2004 Jun 1;140(11):882–886.

122. Gullstrand C, Wahlberg J, Ilonen J, Vaarala O, Ludvigsson J. Progression to type 1 diabetes and autoantibody positivity in relation to HLA-risk genotypes in children participating in the ABIS study. *Pediatr Diabetes*. 2008 Jun;9(3 Pt 1):182–190. Epub 2008 Mar 5.

123. Knip M, Karjalainen J, Akerblom HK. Islet cell antibodies are less predictive of IDDM among unaffected children in the general population than in sibs of children with diabetes. The Childhood Diabetes in Finland Study Group. *Diabetes Care*. 1998 Oct;21(10):1670–1673.

124. Samuelsson U, Sadauskaite V, Padaiga Z, Ludvigsson J, DEBS Study Group. A fourfold difference in the incidence of type 1 diabetes between Sweden and Lithuania but similar prevalence of autoimmunity. *Diabetes Res Clin Pract*. 2004 Nov;66(2):173–181.

125. Matveyenko AV, Butler PC. Relationship between beta-cell mass and diabetes onset. *Diabetes Obes Metab*. 2008 Nov;10(Suppl 4):23–31.

126. Sherry NA, Tsai EB, Herold KC. Natural history of beta-cell function in type 1 diabetes. *Diabetes*. 2005;54(Suppl 2):S32–S39.

127. Roche EF, Menon A, Gill D, Hoey H. Clinical presentation of type 1 diabetes. *Pediatr Diabetes*. 2005 Jun;6(2):75–78.

128. Lévy-Marchal C, Patterson CC, Green A, EURODIAB ACE Study Group. Geographical variation of presentation at diagnosis of type I diabetes in children: the EURODIAB study (European and Diabetes). *Diabetologia*. 2001 Oct;44(Suppl 3):B75–B80.

129. Hekkala A, Knip M, Veijola R. Ketoacidosis at diagnosis of type 1 diabetes in children in northern Finland: temporal changes over 20 years. *Diabetes Care*. 2007 Apr;30(4):861–866.

130. Dunger DB, Sperling MA, Acerini CL, et al. ESPE/LWPES consensus statement on diabetic ketoacidosis in children and adolescents. *Arch Dis Child*. 2004 Feb;89(2):188–194.

131. Hanafusa T, Imagawa A. Fulminant type 1 diabetes: a novel clinical entity requiring special attention by all medical practitioners. *Nat Clin Pract Endocrinol Metab*. 2007 Jan;3(1):36–45.

132. Cho YM, Kim JT, Ko KS, et al. Fulminant type 1 diabetes in Korea: high prevalence among patients with adult-onset type 1 diabetes. *Diabetologia*. 2007 Nov;50(11):2276–2279. Epub 2007 Aug 28.

133. Endo T, Takizawa S, Tanaka S, et al. Amylase {alpha}-2A autoantibodies: novel marker of autoimmune pancreatitis and fulminant type 1 diabetes mellitus. *Diabetes.* 2008 Nov 10;58:732–737.

134. Martin S, Pawlowski B, Greulich B, Zieglen A, Mandrup-Poulsen T, Mahan J. Natural course of remission in IDDM during 1st year after diagnosis. *Diabetes Care.* 1992;15:66–74.

135. Wallensteen M, Dahlguiat G, Persson B, et al. Factors influencing the magnitude, duration and rate of fall of β cell function in type 1 (insulin-dependent) diabetic children followed for two years from their clinical diagnosis. *Diabetologia.* 1988;31: 664–669.

136. Dost A, Herbst A, Kintzel K, et al. Shorter remission period in young versus older children with diabetes mellitus type 1. *Exp Clin Endocrinol Diabetes.* 2007 Jan;115(1):33–37.

137. Skrivarhaug T, Bangstad HJ, Stene LC, Sandvik L, Hanssen KF, Joner G. Long-term mortality in a nationwide cohort of childhood-onset type 1 diabetic patients in Norway. *Diabetologia.* 2006;49:298–305.

138. Laing SP, Swerdlow AJ, Slater SD, et al. Mortality from heart disease in a cohort of 23,000 patients with insulin-treated diabetes. *Diabetologia.* 2003;46:760–765.

139. Dahl-Jorgensen K, Larsen JR, Hanssen KF. Atherosclerosis in childhood and adolescent type 1 diabetes: early disease, early treatment? *Diabetologia.* 2005;48:1445–1453.

140. Krantz JS, Mack WJ, Hodis HN, Liu CR, Liu CH, Kaufman FR. Early onset of subclinical atherosclerosis in young persons with type 1 diabetes. *J Pediatr.* 2004;145:452–457.

141. Libby P, Nathan DM, Abraham K, et al. Report of the National Heart, Lung, and Blood Institute-National Institute of Diabetes and Digestive and Kidney Diseases working group on cardiovascular complications of type 1 diabetes mellitus. *Circulation.* 2005;111:3489–3493.

142. Lorini R, D'Annunzio G, Vitali L, Scaramuzza A. IDDM and autoimmune thyroid disease in the pediatric age group. *J Pediatr Endocrinol Metab.* 1996;9:89–94.

143. Kordonouri O, Klinghammer A, Lang EB, Grueters-kieslich A, Grabert M, Holl RW. Thyroid autoimmunity in children and adolescents with type 1 diabetes. *Diabetes Care.* 2002;25:1346–1350.

144. Sumnik Z, Cinek O, Bratanic N, et al. Thyroid autoimmunity in children with coexisting type 1 diabetes mellitus and celiac disease: a multicenter study. *J Pediatr Endocrinol Metab.* 2006;19:517–522.

145. Cronin C, Shanahan F. Insulin-dependent diabetes mellitus and coeliac disease. *Lancet.* 1997;349:1096–1097.

146. Crone J, Rami B, Huber WD, Granditsch G, Schober E. Prevalence of coeliac disease and follow-up of EMA in children and adolescents with type 1 diabetes mellitus. *J Pediatr Gastroenterol Nutr.* 2003;37:67–71.

147. Freemark M, Levitsky LL. Screening for celiac disease in children with type 1 diabetes. *Diabetes Care.* 2003;26:1932–1939.

148. Fröhlich-Reiterer EE, Hofer S, Kaspers S, et al. Screening frequency for celiac disease and autoimmune thyroiditis in children and adolescents with type 1 diabetes mellitus – data from a German/Austrian multicentre survey. *Pediatr Diabetes.* 2008 Dec;9(6):546–553.

149. TRIGR Study Group. Study design of the Trial to Reduce IDDM in the Genetically at Risk (TRIGR). *Pediatr Diabetes.* 2007 Jun;8(3):117–137.

150. Schmid S, Buuck D, Knopff A, Bonifacio E, Ziegler AG. BABYDIET, a feasibility study to prevent the appearance of islet autoantibodies in relatives of patients with Type 1 diabetes by delaying exposure to gluten. *Diabetologia.* 2004 Jun;47(6):1130–1131.

151. Stene LC, Joner G, Norwegian Childhood Diabetes Study Group. Use of cod liver oil during the first year of life is associated with lower risk of childhood-onset type 1 diabetes: a large, population-based, case-control study. *Am J Clin Nutr.* 2003 Dec;78(6):1128–1134.

152. Gale EA, Bingley PJ, Emmett CL, Collier T, European Nicotinamide Diabetes Intervention Trial (ENDIT) Group. European Nicotinamide Diabetes Intervention Trial (ENDIT): a randomised controlled trial of intervention before the onset of type 1 diabetes. *Lancet.* 2004 Mar 20;363(9413):925–931.

153. Diabetes Prevention Trial-Type 1 Study Group. Effects of insulin in relatives of patients with type 1 diabetes mellitus. *N Engl J Med.* 2002;346:1685–1691.

154. Näntö-Salonen K, Kupila A, Simell S, et al. Nasal insulin to prevent type 1 diabetes in children with HLA genotypes and autoantibodies conferring increased risk of disease: a double-blind, randomised controlled trial. *Lancet.* 2008;372:1746–1755.

155. Diabetes Prevention Trial-Type 1 Diabetes Study Group. Effects of oral insulin in relatives of patients with type 1 diabetes mellitus. *Diabetes Care.* 2005;28:1068–1076.

156. Mandrup-Poulsen TR, Mølvig JC, Andersen V, et al. Immunosuppression with cyclosporin induces clinical remission and improved beta cell function in patients with newly diagnosed insulin-dependent diabetes. A national and international multicenter study. *Ugeskr Laeger.* 1990 Jul 2;152(27):1963–1969.

157. Herold KC, Hagopian W, Auger JA, et al. Anti-CD3 monoclonal antibody in new-onset type 1 diabetes mellitus. *N Engl J Med.* 2002 May 30;346(22):1692–1698.

158. Li L, Yi Z, Tisch R, Wang B. Immunotherapy of type 1 diabetes. *Arch Immunol Ther Exp (Warsz).* 2008 Jul–Aug;56(4): 227–236.

159. American Diabetes Association. Diagnosis and classification of diabetes mellitus. *Diabetes Care.* 2008 Jan;31(Suppl 1): S55–S60.

Chapter 13
Type 2 Diabetes Mellitus: Epidemiology, Genetics, Pathogenesis, and Clinical Manifestations

Vivian Fonseca and Jennifer John-Kalarickal

Introduction

Type 2 diabetes mellitus (T2DM) affects about 3% of the population or 100 million people worldwide. The prevalence is higher in the United States, affecting 6–7% of the population and is increasing at an astounding rate. According to the National Institutes of Health (NIH) and Centers for Disease Control (CDC), over 30% of individuals with diabetes are undiagnosed. Furthermore, a third of children born in the United States in the year 2000 will develop diabetes, an estimated 28 million diabetic individuals within the next 50 years.[1]

Although diabetes is a common disease, its pathogenesis remains unclear, probably due to a host of reasons. Perhaps the most important is the heterogeneity of type 2 diabetes because of an interplay between a variety of genetic and environmental factors (see Table 13.1). Although the diagnosis rests on documentation of hyperglycemia, it is important to appreciate that other metabolic abnormalities, such as disorders of lipid metabolism, are also present and may even precede the emergence of hyperglycemia (see Chapter 28).

The syndrome of diabetes, simply put, is due to deficient insulin action. As depicted in Fig. 13.1, this results from inadequate insulin secretion and/or diminished tissue response to insulin at one or more points in the complex pathways of hormone action. These impairments frequently coexist in the same patient, and it is often unclear which abnormality is the primary cause of the hyperglycemia. Furthermore, since insulin resistance and abnormalities of insulin secretion may be associated with other pathologies, such as liver disease, renal disease, glucocorticoid, growth hormone, or thyroid hormone excess, diabetes may be secondary to other conditions (see Chapter 16).

Etiology of Type 2 Diabetes Mellitus

Genetic and Environmental Predictors of Type 2 Diabetes

Twin studies suggest that genetic makeup accounts for 60–90% of the susceptibility to type 2 diabetes. The concordance rate in monozygotic twins is 70–90% compared to only 15–25% in dizygotic twins. Due to the age-dependent penetrance of type 2 diabetes, the concordance rate in the monozygotic twin studies increases with age, approaching 100% with lifelong follow-up. Type 2 diabetes and impaired glucose tolerance (IGT) cluster in families. Thus, most patients have a positive family history, and the lifetime risk for developing type 2 diabetes is increased up to 40% (more than five times the background rate) by having a first-degree relative with the disease. If both parents have type 2 diabetes, the risk to the offspring may be as high as 70%. Available evidence supports a polygenic mode of inheritance with a considerable environmental input [2] (see Tables 13.2 and 13.3).

V. Fonseca (✉)

Section of Endocrinology, Tullis Tulane Alumni Chair in Diabetes and Tulane University Health Sciences Center, New Orleans, LA 70118, USA

e-mail: vfonseca@tulane.edu

Table 13.1 Sites of possible abnormalities/treatment targets in type 2 diabetes mellitus

PPAR-gamma
IRS1
Glucagon synthase
TCF7L2
Glucagon
GLP-1
DPP-IV

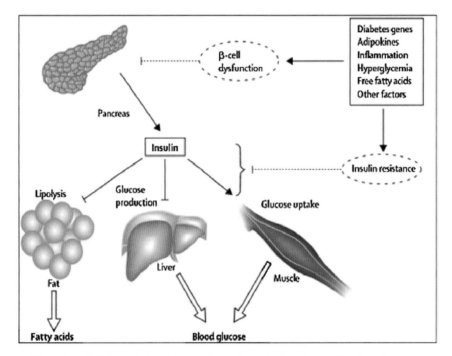

Fig. 13.1 Abnormalities in type 2 diabetes that contribute to hyperglycemia. Insulin secretion from the pancreas normally reduces glucose output by the liver, enhances glucose uptake by skeletal muscle, and suppresses fatty acid release from fat tissue. Decreased insulin secretion will reduce insulin signaling in its target tissues. Insulin resistance affects the action of insulin in each of the major target tissues, leading to increased circulating fatty acids and the hyperglycemia of diabetes. In turn, the raised concentrations of glucose and fatty acids in the bloodstream will feed back to worsen both insulin secretion and insulin resistance (from Stumvoll et al.[86])

The striking ethnic variation in type 2 diabetes prevalence (see Chapter 8) supports the importance of genetic factors: in the United States the prevalence is 2–4% in Caucasians, 4–6% in African-Americans, 10–15% in Mexican-Americans, and 35% in the Pima Indians in Arizona. In adult Pimas, over 75% of whom are obese, a positive family history of type 2 diabetes is a better predictor of the incidence of type 2 diabetes than the combined effects of obesity, gender, and physical fitness.

Environmental influences interact with genetic factors to determine susceptibility to type 2 diabetes by affecting insulin action and/or insulin secretion. The prevalence of type 2 diabetes has increased markedly in populations that have rapidly adopted a Western lifestyle (for example, the Pima Indians) and in many populations that have migrated to regions with a more affluent lifestyle compared to their native country (see Chapter 8). Physical inactivity, obesity, and dietary influences are likely factors that may increase the risk of diabetes in a genetically predisposed individual. Obesity is a strong independent risk factor, and the duration of obesity is also highly predictive of type 2 diabetes.[3] The distribution of the excess fat within the body is important. Thus, truncal obesity is more strongly associated with insulin resistance, and in several prospective studies measures of abdominal obesity such as the waist–hip ratio or the extent of intra-abdominal fat accumulation as measured

Table 13.2 Risk predictors of diabetes

Gender
    female > male
Ethnicity
    Hispanic
    Asians
Genetic defects
    β-Cell function
    Insulin action
Disease of the exocrine pancreas
Excessive weight
Endocrinopathies
    Cushing's syndrome
    Acromegaly
Medications
    Glucocorticoids

Table 13.3 A list of genes implicated in the pathogenesis of diabetes

PPAR-gamma
PPARGC1
KCNJ11
TCF7L2
CDKAL1
HHEX
SLC30A8 and SLC2A1
Chr11
GYS1
IRS1
INS
KCJN11
ABCC8
CAPN10
IGF2BP2
CDKN2A/B
FTO

Adapted from Stumvoll et al.[86] and Narayan et al.[3].

by computerized tomography have been found to be strong predictors of type 2 diabetes.[4,5] Sedentary persons are more likely to develop type 2 diabetes.[6] The antidiabetogenic effect of moderate regular physical activity is likely related to the beneficial effects on insulin action and prevention of obesity: the protective effect appears to be greatest in those at highest risk for type 2 diabetes, such as obese subjects and those with a positive family history.

Type 2 diabetes evolves in stages (Fig. 13.2). Whether insulin resistance or impaired insulin secretion is the primary abnormality or indeed whether both are independent primary defects has been debated. A major difficulty in resolving the issue is due to the fact that insulin resistance can lead to abnormalities of insulin secretion and vice versa. One hypothesis (based on prospective studies in high-risk populations, such as the Pima Indians before they become hyperglycemic and develop secondary defects, and studies of nondiabetic first-degree relatives of type 2 diabetic patients) suggests that in most populations the early defect in type 2 diabetes is insulin resistance which is present when fasting plasma glucose and glucose tolerance are normal.[5–8] Thus, insulin resistance is thought to be an inherited initial defect in most patients and factors such as obesity, sedentary lifestyle, and aging may be additive. At this early stage fasting insulin levels and glucose-stimulated insulin responses are increased and sufficient to maintain normal glucose tolerance. Subjects who develop IGT typically have increased fasting and postprandial insulin levels that do not fully compensate for insulin resistance.

Natural history of type 2 diabetes

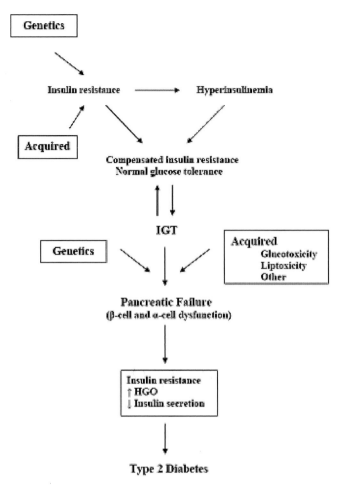

Fig. 13.2 Proposed etiology for the development of type 2 diabetes mellitus

In some this is due to a more marked insulin resistance, but in many it appears to be due to a poor insulin response.[9] Eventually, compensation fails in some subjects, because islet β-cell function declines. The etiology of this decline may be due to a number of factors such as genetic abnormalities affecting β-cell function and/or to acquired defects (such as glucotoxicity and lipotoxicity). One study of insulin-resistant offspring of type 2 diabetic patients found an inherited defect in mitochondrial function.[10] In addition hyperglycemia in itself can worsen insulin resistance due to its effects on β-cells, particularly on insulin gene expression.[11] The development and progression of insulin resistance may also be related to substances released from adipocytes, such as adiponectin, resistin, leptin, and tumor necrosis factor-alpha (TNF-α), as seen in obesity. Other inflammatory markers such as plasminogen activating inhibitor-1(PAI-1) have also been associated with insulin resistance.[12]

Several adipokines are increased in plasma in visceral obesity; however, the concentrations of the adipose-specific protein adiponectin are decreased, reducing its insulin-sensitizing effects in liver and muscle.[13,14] Resistin is thought to mediate liver insulin resistance.[15] Leptin has been implicated in the regulation of adipose mass [16] and is positively correlated to various measures of adiposity.[17] It has been reported to alter both insulin sensitivity[18,19] and insulin secretion.[15] TNF-α enhances adipocyte lipolysis, which further increases nonesterified free fatty acids, and also elicits its own direct negative effects on insulin signaling pathways.[20]

Abnormalities of hepatic glucose metabolism also become apparent during the transition from IGT to overt type 2 diabetes. Subjects with IGT may display hepatic insulin insensitivity but have normal basal rates of hepatic glucose output (HGO): HGO tends to increase at fasting glucose levels above 140 mg/dL. Furthermore, lack of postprandial suppression of HGO and reduced suppression of glucagon contribute to postprandial glucose excursions.[21,22] Thus, excess glucose output by the liver as well as inappropriate glucagon secretion contributes to the pathogenesis of hyperglycemia in type 2 diabetes.

The proportion of insulin-resistant subjects who progress to type 2 diabetes varies between ethnic groups. In most populations the conversion rate from IGT to type 2 diabetes is 2–6% per year over 10 years.[23] In the Diabetes Prevention Program Research Group study conversion rate was as high as 11%.[24] A small percentage of subjects with IGT may revert to normal glucose tolerance while others remain with IGT for many years.

Metabolic Disturbances in Type 2 Diabetes

Hyperglycemia is often accompanied by increased levels of the gluconeogenic precursors, lactate, alanine, pyruvate, and glycerol. Lipolysis is often increased, particularly in obese patients and those with poor insulin secretion resulting in elevated fasting and postprandial plasma free fatty acid (FFA) levels and increased hepatic VLDL production. Under normal circumstances enough insulin is present to prevent unrestrained lipolysis and the development of ketoacidosis, but ketoacidosis may develop during intercurrent illness (trauma, severe infection, myocardial infarction) because of increased counter-regulatory hormone levels. Dyslipidemia in type 2 diabetes, like the abnormalities of glucose metabolism, may be related to a combination of insulin resistance and inadequate insulin secretion as discussed in Chapter 28. Tissue protein metabolism is more sensitive to insulin compared with that of glucose, so tissue wasting is not typical. The remainder of this chapter will focus on the disturbances of glucose metabolism.

Clinical Features of Type 2 Diabetes

The typical patient is an overweight individual often without symptoms. In recent years, type 2 diabetes has started to appear in children in association with increasing rates of obesity. In fact, in some regions the prevalence of type 2 diabetes in children exceeds that of type 1 diabetes. This trend is particularly evident in certain minority groups in the United States, such as Hispanic and African-American children.[25] Figure 13.3 presents the typical mode of presentation of type 2 diabetes. Some present with hyperglycemic symptoms (polydipsia, polyuria, fatigue) but most are diagnosed incidentally by screening or during medical examinations conducted for

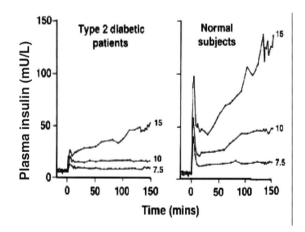

Fig. 13.3 Plasma insulin responses to intravenous glucose in controls and type 2 diabetic patients treated with diet alone. Blood glucose was kept at 7.5 mmol/L (135 mg/dL), 10 mmol/L (180 mg/dL), and 15 mmol/L (270 mg/dL) from 0 until 150 min on three separate days in the two groups of subjects. First-phase insulin secretion is virtually absent and second-phase insulin responses are markedly reduced in the diabetic patients (from Hosker et al.[87])

unrelated reasons. In some, diabetes is diagnosed when they present with infections, especially urinary tract and skin infections and genital candidiasis (particularly, in women). Other patients present with complications of the diabetic condition itself, most commonly, macrovascular disease manifesting as angina, myocardial infarction, stroke, or peripheral vascular disease. A small proportion present with microvascular complications (retinopathy, maculopathy, neuropathy, nephropathy). Because diabetic tissue damage can be detected clinically at the time of diagnosis in a large proportion of patients,[26] it is clear that many patients may have had significant hyperglycemia for 5–10 years before the diagnosis is made.

The age-adjusted life expectancy of a patient with type 2 diabetes is reduced by approximately 5–10 years compared with the general population.[27,28] Overall mortality is increased 2- to 4-fold; over 50% die from ischemic heart disease. Myocardial infarction is more common and carries a worse prognosis. Stroke and peripheral vascular disease are more common. Retinopathy (especially maculopathy), cataracts, and neuropathy are also common, contributing substantially to morbidity. At least one-third of male patients have some degree of impotence. Diabetic nephropathy is increasing in prevalence and type 2 diabetes is now the leading cause of end-stage renal disease in many countries. In several studies, over 10% of patients within 1 year of diagnosis already had gross proteinuria. These patients were probably hyperglycemic for several years prior to diagnosis of diabetes. Microvascular complications and the importance of blood glucose and blood pressure control in their prevention are discussed fully in Part VI.

Type 2 diabetes is associated with a set of cardiovascular risk factors that often precede the development of hyperglycemia, being found in subjects with IGT and in the normoglycemic first-degree relatives of type 2 diabetic patients. These factors include hypertension (>50% of patients), hypertriglyceridemia, smaller denser LDL particles, low HDL cholesterol, and abnormalities of blood coagulation, fibrinolysis, and inflammation. The association of this cluster of abnormalities with insulin resistance, hyperinsulinemia, and often central obesity has been designated as the metabolic syndrome; however, use of this term is controversial.[29] Because these risk factors operate in the pre-hyperglycemic phase it is not surprising that about 10% of patients already have macroangiopathy at diagnosis of their diabetes. Because excess mortality in type 2 diabetes is largely due to ischemic heart disease, effective management requires not only near-normalization of blood glucose levels but also modification of these risk factors through blood pressure control, treatment of dyslipidemia, use of antiplatelet agents, and lifestyle modifications.

Insulin Secretion

In IGT insulin secretion may be normal, increased, or decreased. This variability is partly due to the heterogeneity of this category and partly due to confounding effects of obesity and insulin resistance, which are associated with enhanced insulin secretion in normoglycemic subject.[7] However, compared to normoglycemic subjects matched for degree of insulin resistance and obesity, IGT subjects secrete less insulin at any given glucose level.[9] Islet β-cell function declines on the way from IGT to diabetes and during established type 2 diabetes.[30,31] This progressive deterioration in β-cell function appears to be the main reason why patients who are initially well controlled on a single oral hypoglycemic agent, over the years, require escalation of their therapy (e.g., combined oral agents and/or insulin) to achieve glycemic control. Qualitative secretory abnormalities may also contribute to impaired glucose homeostasis (Table 13.4).

Table 13.4 Insulin secretory defects in type 2 diabetes

Decreased insulin secretory capacity
Decreased β-cell sensitivity to glucose
Loss of first-phase insulin secretion to glucose
Increased release of proinsulin and its split products
Disruption of normal pattern of pulsatile secretion
Morphological changes (decreased β-cell mass; amyloid
  deposits)

Basal and Glucose-Stimulated Insulin Secretion

Basal insulin levels are often increased in type 2 diabetes, especially in obese hyperglycemic patients. However, these elevated insulin levels are maintained only in the presence of fasting hyperglycemia; normal subjects, matched for BMI and rendered similarly hyperglycemic by infusion of glucose, have higher circulating insulin levels. In fact the secretory defect may be more marked than suggested by peripheral insulin levels. This is because in many patients, an increased proportion of proinsulin and its major intermediate conversion product, des-31-32-proinsulin, are released along with insulin. Proinsulin and its intermediates cross-react with insulin in most immunoassays so that the plasma concentration of 'true insulin' is often overestimated in type 2 diabetic patients.[32] Proinsulin and its derivatives may account for as much as 30–50% of total immunoreactive plasma insulin because in addition to increased release from the β-cell their circulating half-life is longer than that of insulin. Basal levels of "true insulin" are either normal or moderately elevated in type 2 diabetes.

Insulin secretion in response to a sustained intravenous glucose stimulus is normally biphasic (Chapter 3). A short-lived surge (first phase) that peaks 1–3 min after a rise in glucose levels and returns to baseline by 6–10 min is followed by a gradual increase (second phase). The first phase is typically lost once fasting plasma glucose exceeds 126 mg/dL and second-phase insulin secretion is markedly reduced at any given glucose level by comparison with age- and BMI-matched normal subjects (Fig. 13.3). In general, the severity of diabetes is inversely related to the second-phase response.

Insulin levels are more variable after oral glucose. The insulin response is usually reduced in patients with obvious fasting hyperglycemia, but may be greater than normal when fasting glucose levels are below 150 mg/dL (Fig. 13.4).

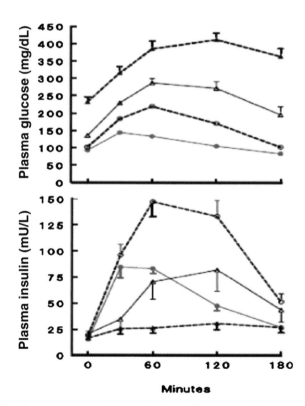

Fig. 13.4 Plasma glucose and insulin responses to oral glucose in four subject groups: (●), normal; (o), impaired glucose tolerance; (Δ), type 2 diabetic individuals with fasting plasma glucose below 150 mg/dL; (▲), type 2 diabetic individuals with fasting plasma glucose above 150 mg/dL (from Reaven et al.[88])

Incretin Effect

In subjects with type 2 diabetes the β-cell secretion of insulin expressed as C-peptide levels is greater after the oral administration of glucose than after the intravenous administration of glucose. This difference in insulin secretion is referred to as the "incretin effect."[33,34] Incretins are peptide hormones that originate in the gastrointestinal tract and play an integral role in glucose homeostasis. The two major incretins in humans are glucagon-like peptide 1 (GLP-1) and glucose-dependent insulinotropic peptide (GIP).[35] These hormones are released during nutrient absorption in the gastrointestinal tract and augment insulin secretion. They are both glucose dependent and increase insulin secretion. However, only GLP-1 suppresses glucagon secretion.[34,36] Both GLP-1 and GIP are rapidly inactivated by the enzyme DPP-IV.[37,38]

Insulin Secretion in Response to Non-glucose Stimuli and Mixed Meals

The β-cell defects in type 2 diabetes are relatively (but not completely) specific for glucose. The insulin response to other stimuli, such as arginine, may be near-normal if measured in patients when their fasting glucose level is high. However, because the ability of hyperglycemia to enhance the response to various non-glucose stimuli is impaired in parallel with the decline in insulin secretion in response to glucose,[39] the insulin response to non-glucose stimuli is usually subnormal when patients and controls are studied at the same glucose level. The relative preservation of insulin responses to certain amino acids and insulinogenic gut peptides (incretins) released during meal absorption may explain why the insulin response to mixed meals is better than that to oral glucose. The patient with mild to moderate hyperglycemia often has an exaggerated insulin response 2–4 h after a meal (even allowing for increased circulating proinsulin).[40] Once fasting plasma glucose exceeds 200–220 mg/dL, decreased insulin levels are more common. The insulin response to meals is often delayed and this may contribute to postprandial hyperglycemia: when insulin is given intravenously to supplement the early response, both postprandial hyperglycemia and the delayed hyperinsulinemia are reduced.[41]

Possible Causes of β-Cell Dysfunction

Possible causes of β-cell dysfunction in type 2 diabetes include a defect in β-cell glucose metabolism and glucose sensing, deficiency of some key stimulatory molecule, reduction in β-cell mass, and deposition of amyloid. Some defects may be hereditary while others are acquired. The number of β-cells may be reduced by 20–50% in patients with long-standing type 2 diabetes.[39] However, in the absence of insulin resistance, more than 80% of β-cells must be lost before insulinopenic diabetes develops, and the function of the remaining β-cells must be impaired. Reduced number of β-cells could be a consequence of long-standing diabetes. Conversely, a decrease in β-cell numbers could lead to decreased function of the remaining β-cells.

Glucotoxicity and Lipotoxicity

The "glucotoxicity" theory holds that some of the β-cell defects are secondary to chronic hyperglycemia. Support for the theory comes from (1) studies showing that prolonged exposure of rat or human islets to high glucose levels can induce a number of defects, and (2) the observation that the absent first-phase insulin response and defective glucose recognition by β-cells in type 2 diabetes may be ameliorated after a period of good glycemic control irrespective of the treatment used (diet, insulin, or oral agents).[42,43] This reversibility suggests that the abnormalities may be secondary, at least in part, to hyperglycemia or some other factor associated with uncontrolled diabetes (e.g., elevated plasma FFAs). According to the "lipotoxicity" theory, chronically increased uptake of FFA by islet β-cells and/or a defect in β-cell FFA metabolism leads to islet lipid deposition which contributes to the decline in insulin secretion in type 2 diabetes (Fig. 13.5).[44,45] Genetic factors may influence islet FFA handling and hence susceptibility to β-cell lipotoxicity.[44] It seems likely that glucotoxicity and lipotoxicity play some role in the impaired β-cell function.

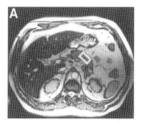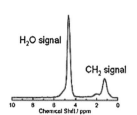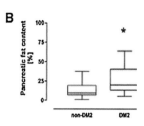

Fig. 13.5 H-magnetic resonance spectra (CH$_2$ peak at 1.3 ppm is main signal of lipids) were obtained from abdominal magnetic resonance imaging scans in the pancreas (**a**). Median (interquartile range) lipid content of the pancreas (**b**) in type 2 diabetic versus nondiabetic men is shown. $^*p < 0.05$. DM2 = type 2 diabetes (from Tushuizen et al.,[45])

Islet Amyloid and Islet Amyloid Polypeptide

Islet amyloid polypeptide (IAPP), also known as amylin, is a 37 amino acid polypeptide which is stored in the insulin secretory granules and co-secreted with insulin from pancreatic β-cells.[46] Subjects with impaired glucose tolerance and more strikingly those with type 2 diabetes have impaired amylin response. Circulating levels of amylin decrease as amyloid deposits accumulate and β-cell function deteriorates. Islet amyloid deposits are composed of insoluble fibrils formed from islet amyloid polypeptide and are found at postmortem examination in up to 90% of type 2 diabetic patients. Amyloid formation could be due to increased IAPP production and/or decreased IAPP clearance. The fibrils are deposited between the capillaries, the endocrine cells, and within invaginations of the β-cell membrane. Even small deposits could pose a physical barrier to the diffusion of nutrients from the circulation and of hormones from the islet cells. The IAPP fibrils might also interfere with membrane function and hence glucose signaling and secretory granule release. Therefore, amyloid deposition may play a role in the reduction of β-cell mass.[39]

Glucagon-Like Peptide-1 (GLP-1)

GLP-1 is a ubiquitous hormone. Its receptors are located within several organs, including the brain, duodenum, kidneys, liver, lungs, pancreas, and stomach (see Fig. 13.6). The receptors for this hormone mediate their action through a G-protein-coupled adenylate cyclase, resulting in an increase in cyclic adenosine monophosphate and activation of protein kinase A. These effects lead to increased insulin secretion.[47]

Endogenous GLP-1 is a gastrointestinal hormone derived from a precursor of glucagons and secreted from the L cells of the distal aspect of the small intestine. It is reduced in the fasting state and increases rapidly after a meal. Its primary action is to stimulate glucose-dependent insulin secretion and also to increase gastrointestinal motility.[36]

The release of GLP-1 is attenuated in patients with T2DM after ingestion of a mixed meal. This attenuation has been demonstrated in patients with T2DM, with a significant reduction of the GLP-1 area under the curve during a period of 240 min after a meal, compared with individuals with normal glucose levels.[48]

GLP-1 action leads to increased insulin secretion in addition to decreased glucagon section. These changes lead to improved glycemic control and a reduction of FFAs, which, in turn, may result in attenuation of both glucotoxicity and lipotoxicity in patients. In addition, GLP-1 stimulation produces direct effects on β-cells, resulting in proliferation of β-cells, increased cell regeneration, and reduced cell apoptosis.[49]

Insulin Resistance

Insulin resistance may be defined as a subnormal biologic response to a given concentration of insulin. The most widely used methods of estimating insulin sensitivity with respect to glucose metabolism are the glucose clamp and the minimal model.[50] With both methods, type 2 diabetic patients and obese nondiabetic subjects are characteristically less insulin sensitive than normal controls.

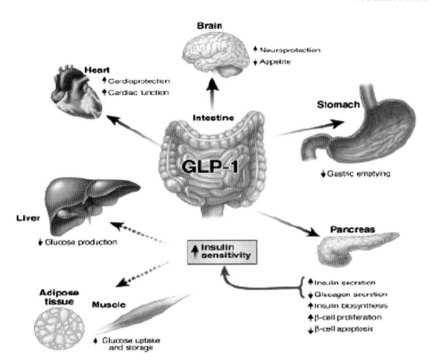

Fig. 13.6 GLP-1 actions in peripheral tissues. The majority of the effects of GLP-1 are mediated by direct interaction with GLP-1Rs on specific tissues. However, the actions of GLP-1 in liver, fat, and muscle most likely occur through indirect mechanisms (from Baggio and Drucker[89])

The glucose clamp technique entails a constant intravenous infusion of insulin for several hours, while blood glucose is kept at a predetermined level by a feedback-controlled infusion of glucose. As the insulin acts to stimulate tissue glucose uptake and suppress HGO, the amount of glucose needed to maintain the target glucose level increases progressively until a steady state is reached at which time the rate of whole body glucose disposal is the sum of the glucose infusion rate and the rate of any residual output of glucose from the liver. The latter can be quantified if a radioactive or stable isotope of glucose is infused during the study. The more sensitive the subject the higher the glucose disposal rate at any given glucose and insulin level. Bergman's minimal model is easier to perform but the analysis is somewhat more complicated: timed blood samples are collected for measurement of plasma glucose and insulin for about 3 h following an intravenous glucose bolus. The glucose and insulin values are entered into a computer model to generate an index of insulin sensitivity.[50]

Figure 13.7 depicts dose–response curves for insulin-stimulated whole body glucose uptake during glucose clamp studies. Type 2 diabetic patients exhibit both a rightward shift (diminished sensitivity) and a marked decrease in the maximal rate (decreased responsiveness). The changes tend to be more pronounced in obese diabetic patients. Obesity is associated with a variable degree of insulin resistance: some subjects are mildly resistant and display only a rightward shift in their dose–response curve while others are more resistant and exhibit both a rightward shift and a decreased maximal response. However, even the latter group tends to be less resistant than equally obese type 2 diabetic patients.

When glucose is infused intravenously (e.g., during a glucose clamp) 80–85% of overall insulin-stimulated glucose uptake is accounted for by skeletal muscle. It follows therefore that muscle is resistant to insulin in type 2 diabetes and obesity. Some glucose is oxidized but most (especially at higher insulin doses) is stored as muscle glycogen. In type 2 diabetes defects in both oxidative and nonoxidative glucose reduction (predominantly glycogen storage) are found, although the defect in the latter is greater.[51] A decreased rate of muscle glycogen synthesis in type 2 diabetes has been directly shown and the magnitude of this defect correlates well with the impairment of whole body glucose uptake.[51]

Studies using nuclear magnetic resonance spectroscopy to examine muscle metabolism strongly suggest that the lower rates of muscle glucose uptake and glycogen synthesis in type 2 diabetic patients are due primarily to

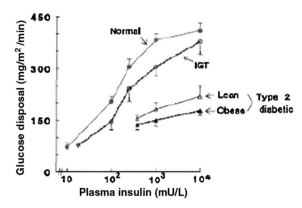

Fig. 13.7 Mean insulin dose–response curves for whole body glucose disposal during glucose clamps at the indicated steady-state plasma insulin levels. The IGT subjects have a rightward shift in the curve but no change in the maximal response. The lean and obese type 2 diabetic patients have both a rightward shift and a reduced maximal response (from Kolterman et al.[90])

a defect in glucose transport.[51] This does not preclude additional defects that may affect glucose metabolism. Indeed, a number of abnormalities are demonstrable in muscle of type 2 diabetic patients. These include impaired synthesis of hexokinase II probably due to decreased hexokinase II gene transcription in response to insulin.[52] Since hexokinase phosphorylates glucose to glucose-6-phosphate it augments glucose uptake by maintaining a glucose gradient across the membrane (lower inside). Thus, an impairment of glucose phosphorylation could contribute to decreased glucose uptake. Activation of glycogen synthase (rate-limiting enzyme for glycogen synthesis from glucose-6-phosphate) and pyruvate dehydrogenase (rate limiting for oxidation of pyruvate produced by glycolysis) is also impaired in diabetes.[53,54]

Insulin-stimulated glucose transport is decreased in adipocytes and skeletal muscle strips from type 2 diabetic patients and obese subjects.[55] Glucose transport activity in these tissues correlates well with whole body insulin sensitivity in both obese and type 2 diabetic subjects. In addition lipids intrahepatic and intrahepatocellular lipid accumulation is associated with obesity and may exacerbate insulin resistance.

Mechanisms of Insulin Resistance

Decreased numbers of insulin receptors can lead to insulin resistance. However, in adipocytes and skeletal muscle only a fraction (10–20%) of surface receptors need to be occupied for maximal stimulation of glucose transport by insulin. With fewer cell surface receptors there is a rightward shift in the insulin dose–response curve, but a normal maximal response. A reduced maximal response in diabetes implies a post-binding defect because the number of receptors is unlikely to be reduced below 10–20% of normal. In obesity and subjects with IGT there are fewer insulin receptors on insulin target tissues, probably because of down-regulation by hyperinsulinemia. This decrease could contribute to their insulin insensitivity (Fig. 13.7). Insulin receptors are also moderately reduced in most obese and non-obese type 2 diabetic patients, but in these patients insulin resistance is primarily due to post-binding defects.

Because resistance is evident in different actions of insulin (e.g., glucose transport, regulation of gene expression) which may involve different signaling elements, it is thought that the primary defect(s) responsible for insulin resistance must involve some early common step in the insulin signaling pathway (see Chapter 5 for a description of normal insulin signaling). The focus of attention has been on three early targets: the insulin receptor itself, the family of insulin receptor substrates (especially IRS-1 and IRS-2), and phosphatidylinositol-3-kinase [PI-3-kinase], a lipid kinase critical for insulin's effects on glucose transport and some other actions of insulin. The insulin receptor gene sequence is normal in >99% of subjects with typical type 2 diabetes indicating that the receptor is not a diabetes susceptibility gene, except in a small fraction of patients. Decreased tyrosine kinase activity of liver, muscle, and adipocyte insulin receptors has been found in type 2 diabetes, but this is probably an acquired defect as it is reversible with weight loss and improved glycemic control in obese type 2 diabetic patients.[56]

The insulin receptor substrates, IRS-1 and IRS-2 (see Chapter 5), play a key role in transmission of the signal from the insulin receptor to downstream proteins. Their function is influenced by their phosphorylation state. In type 2 diabetes the ability of insulin to stimulate IRS-1 phosphorylation on tyrosines is impaired in both adipocytes and skeletal muscle.[56,57] Decreased muscle IRS-2 phosphorylation in response to insulin has also been reported. PI-3-kinase, which is essential for insulin's effects on a glucose transporter isoform (Glut-4) translocation and glycogen synthase activation, is activated by binding to tyrosine phosphorylated IRS-1 and IRS-2. The insulin-induced association of PI-3-kinase with IRS-1 and IRS-2 and hence activation of PI-3-kinase are impaired in muscle of type 2 diabetic patients.[57]

The glucose transport system is a possible site for a post-receptor defect. Skeletal muscle, adipocytes, and cardiac muscle express Glut-4, which in the basal state is primarily in an intracellular vesicular location. Insulin stimulates glucose transport in these tissues by causing the recruitment of Glut-4 proteins from the intracellular pool to the plasma membrane. In the vast majority of type 2 diabetic patients the Glut-4 gene coding sequence and muscle Glut-4 protein levels are normal but insulin-stimulated translocation of Glut-4 to the plasma membrane is impaired.[55,58] The trafficking of Glut-4 to and from the plasma membrane is a complex process: a large number of proteins are involved in the movement of vesicles, membrane fusion, and endocytotic events. Impaired Glut-4 translocation could be due to an abnormality in any of these proteins or it could be due to an impairment of insulin signaling.

Insulin Resistance: Acquired and Genetic Components

A combination of inherited and acquired factors contributes to the insulin resistance in type 2 diabetes. Apart from obesity, dietary influences, and physical inactivity, the development of type 2 diabetes leads to a worsening of insulin resistance.[59,60] Two factors that may contribute to insulin resistance once diabetes has developed are elevated plasma FFA levels and hyperglycemia. Animal and clinical studies suggest that both hyperglycemia and increased FFA availability may play an important role in the acquired component of insulin resistance in type 2 diabetes.[61,62] The component of insulin resistance that appears to be due to the diabetes may be reversible by tight blood glucose control (which also lowers plasma FFA levels). Thus insulin sensitivity is improved (but not normalized) by tight glycemic control; the degree of improvement varies from as little as 10% to as much as 75% in various studies.[4,43,63,64]

Several genes, including the insulin receptor, Glut-4, glycogen synthase, and PI-3-kinase, have been examined as potential candidate genes in insulin resistance and type 2 diabetes (see Table 13.3). An important conceptual advance in our understanding of potential mechanisms of insulin resistance leading to the development of type 2 diabetes has come from transgenic mouse models in which specific genes thought to play a key role in insulin action have been disrupted either in a specific tissue or at the whole body level. Such studies have shown that a major disruption of a single gene (for example, the insulin receptor or IRS-1) may have little phenotypic effect; however, a combination of relatively minor defects, for example, of the insulin receptor and downstream signaling molecules such as IRS-1 and IRS-2, can act synergistically to cause insulin resistance and glucose intolerance.[65] This fits nicely with the polygenic model of type 2 diabetes inheritance and also allows for the synergistic interaction of genetic and acquired defects such as the down-regulation of insulin receptors by high circulating insulin levels or defects induced by hyperglycemia and/or elevated fatty acid levels.

Glucose Metabolism in Type 2 Diabetes

Hyperglycemia is due to a variable combination of overproduction of glucose by the liver and impaired insulin-stimulated tissue glucose uptake. Hyperglycemia, through a mass action effect, results in enhanced non-insulin-mediated glucose uptake by tissues other than brain (including insulin target tissues), thereby compensating to a variable extent for impaired insulin-mediated glucose uptake. The contributions of hepatic glucose overproduction and peripheral tissue insulin resistance to hyperglycemia in type 2 diabetes vary between fasting and postprandial states and are discussed below.

Hepatic Glucose Output (HGO)

After an overnight fast, glucose is produced at about 1.8–2.2 mg/kg/min with about 90% coming from the liver. In type 2 diabetic patients with fasting plasma glucose levels above 140 mg/dL, basal HGO tends to be modestly increased, and fasting glucose levels correlate with HGO.[8] This suggests that in the more severely hyperglycemic patient increased HGO contributes to fasting hyperglycemia. In patients with mildly elevated fasting plasma glucose (<140 mg/dL) who have better insulin secretion, HGO may be normal. One could speculate that in these patients an increase in HGO contributes to the initial rise in plasma glucose but as their fasting glucose level rises they secrete more insulin which restores HGO toward normal with establishment of a new steady state in which fasting glucose and insulin levels are elevated but HGO is within the normal range, albeit not normal for the prevailing insulin and glucose levels. Most studies suggest that gluconeogenesis is increased in diabetic patients with fasting hyperglycemia and that this explains their increased HGO.[66,67] Factors that may augment gluconeogenesis in diabetes include hepatic insulin resistance, relative insulin deficiency, and increased plasma levels of glucagon, gluconeogenic precursors, and FFA. There has been particular interest in the role of FFA. Not only do they supply energy for gluconeogenesis but also they stimulate several gluconeogenic enzymes, and insulin's ability to suppress HGO may be partly indirect and mediated by suppression of fat cell lipolysis and plasma FFA levels.[68] Suppression of HGO after meals is also impaired.[69,70] The effect is to deliver more glucose into the systemic circulation (together with that absorbed from the gut) so that hepatic overproduction of glucose also contributes to postprandial hyperglycemia (Fig. 13.8).

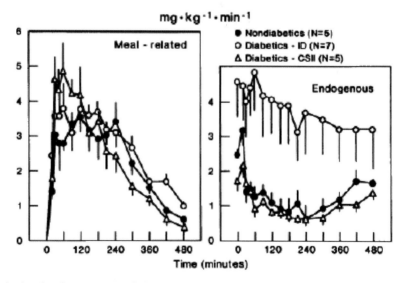

Fig. 13.8 Meal-derived and endogenous rate of glucose appearance in nondiabetic subjects and diabetic subjects when insulin deficient (ID) and while treated with continuous subcutaneous insulin infusion (CSII). Meal was taken at 0 min. There is a lack of appropriate endogenous suppression of glucose production (from Pehling et al.[70])

Glucagon

Glucagon is released from the α-cells of the pancreas. Fasting plasma glucagon levels are elevated in type 2 diabetic patients,[71] and the insulin/glucagon ratio is an important determinant of basal hepatic glucose production.[72,73] After a meal, plasma glucose and insulin levels rise and act together to suppress glucagon secretion by the α-cell.[74] The resultant decline in plasma glucagon concentration contributes to the reduction in hepatic glucose production and plays an important role in maintenance of normal glucose homeostasis.

Despite marked hyperglycemia, type 2 diabetic subjects have high fasting plasma glucagon levels,[75] increased acute glucagon response to an intravenous arginine stimulus,[76] and impaired glucagon suppression after glucose ingestion.[75,77–79] In nondiabetic subjects, an increased glucagon response to arginine predicts worsening of glucose tolerance and progression to type 2 diabetes.[80] Studies employing the pancreatic clamp technique have demonstrated that lack of glucagon suppression after carbohydrate ingestion causes postprandial hyperglycemia in healthy nondiabetic subjects [81] and contributes to postprandial hyperglycemia in type 2 diabetes.[82,83] Studies in humans with IGT suggest that both glucose- and insulin-mediated suppression of glucagon secretion are impaired. One study found that during an oral glucose tolerance test (OGTT) the decrement in the plasma glucagon concentration (area under the curve) was correlated inversely with the fasting plasma glucose (FPG) concentration ($r = -0.35; p < 0.001$). As the fasting glucose level increased, the suppression of plasma glucagon progressively diminished.[84]

The impairment in glucagon suppression after glucose ingestion could result from the inability of the α-cell to respond adequately to the inhibitory effect of either hyperinsulinemia or hyperglycemia. The perturbed glucagon secretion in conjunction with impaired insulin secretion is likely to contribute to the elevated rate of hepatic glucose production [85] and postprandial hyperglycemia [82] in type 2 diabetic patients.

Pathogenesis of Fasting Hyperglycemia

In the fasted state insulin levels are low and 75–85% of glucose uptake is non-insulin mediated. Insulin-independent glucose uptake by the brain accounts for a large part of this basal uptake (50–60%) and is normal in diabetes. Because skeletal muscle accounts for only 15–20% of basal glucose uptake, it follows that insulin resistance causing an impairment of insulin-mediated muscle glucose uptake will have relatively little effect on basal glucose utilization rates or fasting glucose levels; more glucose has to enter the circulation (primarily from the liver) for fasting glucose levels to increase substantially. In the setting of insulin resistance and impaired insulin secretion, insulin-mediated glucose uptake cannot increase appropriately in response to an increase in HGO, and small increases in glucose production cause a proportional increase in glucose levels. As the glucose level rises, the mass action effect of hyperglycemia promotes glucose disposal and the system re-equilibrates. At this point increased glucose entry into the circulation is matched by increased glucose disposal (including urinary glucose loss) in the presence of fasting hyperglycemia.

Pathogenesis of Postprandial Hyperglycemia

Most ingested glucose enters the systemic circulation (<10% is taken up by the liver on first pass) and is then taken up by peripheral tissues (50–60% is taken up by skeletal muscle) and, to a lesser extent, by the liver. Several factors contribute to postprandial hyperglycemia in type 2 diabetes. First, the total amount of glucose entering the systemic circulation is increased because of inadequate suppression of HGO (see above). Second, the efficiency of glucose removal is reduced because of muscle insulin resistance and relative or absolute insulin deficiency. Third, hepatic uptake of glucose (newly absorbed and recirculating) is impaired, although this defect makes a relatively small contribution since the liver normally takes up only 20–35% of a glucose load. The marked increase in plasma glucose levels seen in type 2 diabetes after carbohydrate ingestion promotes glucose uptake by muscle and other tissues by mass action, and this compensates for diminished insulin-mediated glucose uptake. However, the intracellular disposition of the glucose is abnormal. For example, hyperglycemia does not fully compensate for impaired muscle glycogen synthase activation by insulin [53] so less of the glucose taken up by muscle is stored as glycogen and more is metabolized through glycolysis. This in turn leads to increased release of the gluconeogenic precursors, lactate, alanine, and pyruvate which are taken up by the liver and help to sustain the increased rates of gluconeogenesis and HGO.

Summary

The development of type 2 diabetes requires the presence of defects of both insulin action and insulin secretion due to both genetic and environmental factors. Epidemiological and clinical evidence suggests that in most population insulin resistance most commonly initiates the sequence of events leading to type 2 diabetes. As long as the islet β-cells can compensate with a high enough insulin output to overcome the insulin resistance, glucose tolerance remains normal or only mildly impaired. However, a progressive decline in β-cell function in a subset of insulin-resistant subjects eventually leads to overt hyperglycemia. Insulin resistance affects the main insulin target tissues, namely skeletal muscle, the liver, and adipose tissue. Metabolic abnormalities in type 2 diabetes resulting from the effects of insulin resistance and impaired insulin secretion on these target tissues include decreased insulin-stimulated skeletal muscle glucose uptake, overproduction of glucose by the liver, and impaired suppression of adipocyte lipolysis. Impaired insulin-stimulated muscle glucose uptake is the main cause of postprandial hyperglycemia. Overproduction of glucose by the liver and glucagon dysregulation are the main causes of fasting hyperglycemia. These defects also contribute to postprandial hyperglycemia. Impaired suppression of lipolysis results in higher fasting and 24-h circulating plasma FFA levels, which may in turn contribute to both muscle insulin resistance and overproduction of glucose by the liver. Chronically elevated FFA levels may also have adverse effects on islet β-cell function. Further, substances released from adipocytes may further contribute to the insulin resistance. Hyperglycemia, in addition to being the key determinant for the development of microvascular diabetic complications, also has adverse effects on both islet β-cell and α-cell function and may exacerbate the insulin-resistant state (glucotoxicity). Ischemic heart disease is the main cause of the excess mortality in type 2 diabetes. Effective management of type 2 diabetes to ensure immediate well-being and for prevention of both microvascular and macrovascular complications requires near-normalization of blood glucose levels by diet, lifestyle modifications, and glucose lowering agents, as well as attention to other risk factors which involves blood pressure control, use of antiplatelet agents, and treatment of dyslipidemia.

References

1. Narayan KMV, Boyle JP, Thompson TJ, Sorensen SW, Williamson DF. Lifetime risk for diabetes mellitus in the United States. *JAMA*. 2003;290(14):1884–1890.
2. Froguel P, Velho G. Genetic determinants of type 2 diabetes. *Recent Prog Horm Res*. 2001;56:91–105.
3. Narayan KMV, Boyle JP, Thompson TJ, Gregg EW, Williamson DF. Effect of BMI on lifetime risk for diabetes in the U.S. *Diabetes Care*. 2007;30(6):1562–1566.
4. Grundy S. Metabolic complications of obesity. *Endocrine*. 2000;13:155–165.
5. Groop L. Insulin resistance: the fundamental trigger of type 2 diabetes. *Diabetes Obes Metab*. 1999;1(Suppl 1):S1–S7.
6. Clark D. Physical activity efficacy and effectiveness among older adults and minorities. *Diabetes Care*. 1997;20:1176–1182.
7. Cavaghan M, Ehrmann D, Polonsky K. Interactions between insulin resistance and insulin secretion in the development of glucose intolerance. *J Clin Invest*. 2000;106:329–333.
8. Stern M. Strategies and prospects for finding insulin resistance genes. *J Clin Invest*. 2000;106(3):323–327.
9. Polonshy K, Sturis J, Bell G. Non-insulin-dependent diabetes mellitus – a genetically programmed failure of the beta cell to compensate for insulin resistance. *N Engl J Med*. 1996;334:777–783.
10. Peterson K, Dufour S, Befroy D, et al. Impaired mitochondrial activity in the insulin-resistant offspring of patients with type 2 diabetes. *N Engl J Med*. 2004;350:664.
11. Moran A, Zhang H, Olson L, et al. Differentiation of glucose toxicity from beta cell exhaustion during the evolution of defective insulin gene expression in the pancreatic islet cell line, HIT-T15. *J Clin Invest*. 1997;99:534.
12. Festa A, D'Agostino R Jr, Rich SS, Jenny NS, Tracy RP, Haffner SM. Promoter (4G/5G) plasminogen activator inhibitor-1 genotype and plasminogen activator inhibitor-1 levels in Blacks, Hispanics, and Non-Hispanic Whites: the Insulin Resistance Atherosclerosis study. *Circulation*. 2003;107(19):2422–2427.
13. Rajala MW, Scherer PE. Minireview: the adipocyte – at the crossroads of energy homeostasis, inflammation, and atherosclerosis. *Endocrinology*. 2003;144(9):3765–3773.
14. Goldstein BJ, Scalia R. Adiponectin: a novel adipokine linking adipocytes and vascular function. *J Clin Endocrinol Metab*. 2004;89(6):2563–2568.
15. Kieffer T, Habener J. The adipoinsular axis: effects of leptin on pancreatic ß-cells. *Am J Physiol*. 2000;278:E1–E14.
16. Caro J, Sinha M, Kolaczynski J, Zhang P, Considine R. Leptin: the tale of an obesity gene. *Diabetes*. 1996;45:1455–1462.

17. McGregor G, Desaga J, Ehlenz K, et al. Radioimmunological measurement of leptin in plasma of obese and diabetic human subjects. *Endocrinology*. 1996;137:1501–1504.

18. Svitz W, Walsh S, Morgan D, Thomas M, Haynes W. Effects of leptin on insulin sensitivity in normal rats. *Endocrinology*. 1997;138:3395–3401.

19. Oral EA, Simha V, Ruiz E, et al. Leptin-replacement therapy for lipodystrophy. *N Engl J Med*. 2002;346(8):570–578.

20. Hotamisligil G. Molecular mechanisms of insulin resistance and the role of the adipocyte. *J Int Assoc Study Obes*. 2000;24(Suppl 4):S23–S27.

21. Consuli A. Role of liver in pathophysiology of NIDDM. *Diabetes Care*. 1992;15:430–441.

22. Unger R. Glucagon physiology and pathophysiology in the light of new advances. *Diabetologia*. 1985;28:574–578.

23. Alberti K. The clinical significance of impaired glucose tolerance. *Diabetes Metab*. 1996;13:927–937.

24. Diabetes Prevention Program Research Group. Reduction in the incidence of type 2 diabetes with lifestyle intervention or metformin. *N Engl J Med*. 2002;346(6):393–403.

25. Fagot-Campagna A. Emergence of type 2 diabetes mellitus in children: epidemiological evidence. *J Pediatr Endocrinol Metab*. 2000;13(Suppl 6):1395–1402.

26. UK Prospective Diabetes Study Group. Intensive blood-glucose control with sulphonylureas or insulin compared with conventional treatment and risk of complications in patients with type 2 diabetes (UKPDS 33). *Lancet*. 1998;352:837–853.

27. Bale GS, Entmacher PS. Estimated life expectancy of diabetics. *Diabetes*. 1977;26(5):434–438.

28. Gu K, Covie C, Harris M. Mortality in adults with and without diabetes in a national cohort of the U.S. population, 1971–1993. *Diabetes Care*. 1998;21(7):1138–1145.

29. Kahn R, Buse J, Ferrannini E, Stern M. The metabolic syndrome: time for a critical appraisal: joint statement from the American Diabetes Association and the European Association for the Study of Diabetes. *Diabetes Care*. 2005;28:2289.

30. UK Prospective Diabetes Study Group. UK prospective diabetes study 16: overview of 6 years' therapy of type II diabetes: a progressive disease. *Diabetes*. 1995;44:1249–1258.

31. Kahn S. The importance of the beta-cell in the pathogenesis of type 2 diabetes mellitus. *Am J Med*. 2000;108(Suppl 6a):2S–8S.

32. Temple R, Clark P, Nagi D, et al. Radioimmunoassay may overestimate insulin in non-insulin-dependent diabetics. *Clin Endocrinol*. 1990;32:689–693.

33. Nauck M, Stöckmann F, Ebert R, Creutzfeldt W. Reduced incretin effect in type 2 (non-insulin-dependent) diabetes. *Diabetologia*. 1986;29(1):46–52.

34. Nauck MA, Homberger E, Siegel EG, et al. Incretin effects of increasing glucose loads in man calculated from venous insulin and C-peptide responses. *J Clin Endocrinol Metab*. 1986;63(2):492–498.

35. Freeman JS. The pathophysiologic role of incretins. *J Am Osteopath Assoc*. 2007;107(Suppl 3):S6–S9.

36. Drucker DJ. Enhancing incretin action for the treatment of type 2 diabetes. *Diabetes Care*. 2003;26(10):2929–2940.

37. Mentlein R, Gallwitz B, Schmidt WE. Dipeptidyl-peptidase IV hydrolyses gastric inhibitory polypeptide, glucagon-like peptide-1(7-36)amide, peptide histidine methionine and is responsible for their degradation in human serum. *Eur J Biochem*. 1993;214(3):829–835.

38. Kieffer TJ, McIntosh CH, Pederson RA. Degradation of glucose-dependent insulinotropic polypeptide and truncated glucagon-like peptide 1 in vitro and in vivo by dipeptidyl peptidase IV. *Endocrinology*. 1995;136(8):3585–3596.

39. Porte DJ, Kahn S. Beta-cell dysfunction and failure in type 2 diabetes: potential mechanisms. *Diabetes*. 2001;50(Suppl 1): S160–S163.

40. Reaven G, Chen Y, Hollenbeck C, et al. Plasma insulin, C- peptide, and proinsulin concentrations in obese and nonobese individuals with varying degrees of glucose tolerance. *J Clin Endocrinol Metab*. 1993;76:44–48.

41. Bruce D, Chisholm D, Storlien L, Kraegen E. Physiological importance of deficiency in early prandial insulin secretion in noninsulin-dependent diabetes. *Diabetes*. 1998;37:736–744.

42. Garvey W, Olefsky J, Griffin J, et al. The effects of insulin treatment on insulin secretion and action in type II diabetes mellitus. *Diabetes*. 1985;34:222–234.

43. Henry R, Wallace P, Olefsky J. The effects of weight loss on the mechanism of hyperglycemia in obese noninsulin-dependent diabetes mellitus. *Diabetes*. 1986;35:990–998.

44. McGarry J, Dobbins R. Fatty acids, lipotoxicity and insulin secretion. *Diabetologia*. 1999;42:128–138.

45. Tushuizen ME, Bunck MC, Pouwels PJ, et al. Pancreatic fat content and {beta}-cell function in men with and without type 2 diabetes. *Diabetes Care*. 2007;30(11):2916–2921.

46. Cooper G, Day A, Willis A, Roberts A, Reid K, Leighton B. Amylin and the amylin gene: structure, function and relationship to islet amyloid and to diabetes mellitus. *Biochim Biophys Acta*. 1989;1014(3):247–258.

47. Fehmann HC, Goke R, Goke B. Cell and molecular biology of the incretin hormones glucagon-like peptide-I and glucose-dependent insulin releasing polypeptide. *Endocr Rev*. 1995;16(3):390–410.

48. Toft-Nielsen MB, Damholt MB, Madsbad S, et al. Determinants of the impaired secretion of glucagon-like peptide-1 in type 2 diabetic patients. *J Clin Endocrinol Metab*. 2001;86(8):3717–3723.

49. Drucker DJ. Glucagon-like peptide-1 and the Islet {beta}-cell: augmentation of cell proliferation and inhibition of apoptosis. *Endocrinology*. 2003;144(12):5145–5148.

50. Ferrannini E, Mari A. How to measure insulin sensitivity. *J Hypertens*. 1998;16:895–906.

51. Cline G, Petersen K, Krssak M, et al. Impaired glucose transport as a cause of decreased insulin-stimulated muscle glycogen synthesis in type 2 diabetes. *N Engl J Med*. 1999;341:240–246.

52. Kruszynska Y, Mulford M, Baloga J, Yu J, Olefsky J. Regulation of skeletal muscle hexokinase II by insulin in nondiabetic and NIDDM subjects. *Diabetes*. 1998;47:1107–1113.

53. Thorburn A, Gumbiner B, Bulacan F, et al. Multiple defects in muscle glycogen synthase activity contribute to reduced glycogen synthesis in non-insulin dependent diabetes mellitus. *J Clin Invest*. 1991;87:489–495.

54. DeFronza R, Bonadonna R, Ferrannini E. Pathogenesis of NIDDM. A balanced overview. *Diabetes Care*. 1992;15:318–368.

55. Kruszynska Y, Olefsky J. Cellular and molecular mechanisms of non-insulin dependent diabetes mellitus. *J Invest Med*. 1996;44:413–428.

56. Thies R, Molina J, Ciaraldi T, et al. Insulin receptor autophosphorylation and endogenous substrate phosphorylation in human adipocytes from control, obese and non-insulin dependent diabetic subjects. *Diabetes*. 1990;39:250–259.

57. Cusi K, Katsumi M, Osman A, et al. Insulin resistance differentially affects the PI-3-kinase- and MAP kinase-mediated signaling in human muscle. *J Clin Invest*. 2000;105:311–320.

58. Kelley D, Mintun M, Watkins S, et al. The effect of non-Insulin dependent diabetes mellitus and obesity on glucose transport and phosphorylation in skeletal muscle. *J Clin Invest*. 1996;97:2705–2713.

59. Vaag A, Henriksen J, Madsbad S, Holm N, Beck-Nielsen H. Insulin secretion, insulin action, and hepatic glucose production in identical twins discordant for non-insulin-dependent diabetes mellitus. *J Clin Invest*. 1995;95:690–698.

60. Eriksson J, Franssila-Kallunki A, Ekstrand A, et al. Early metabolic defects in persons at increased risk for non-insulin dependent diabetes mellitus. *N Engl J Med*. 1989;321:337–343.

61. Yki-Jarvinen H. Glucose toxicity. *Endocr Rev*. 1992;13:415–431.

62. Shulman G. Cellular mechanisms of insulin resistance in humans. *Am J Cardiol*. 1999;83:3 J–10 J.

63. Henry R, Gumbiner B, Ditzler T, Wallace P, Lyon R, Glauber H. Intensive conventional insulin therapy for type II diabetes. Metabolic effects during a 6-mo outpatient trial. *Diabetes Care*. 1993;16:21–31.

64. Hollenbeck C, Reaven G. Treatment of patients with non-insulin dependent diabetes mellitus: diabetic control and insulin secretion and action after different treatment modalities. *Diabetic Med*. 1987;4:311–316.

65. Kadowaki T. Insights into insulin resistance and type 2 diabetes from knockout mouse models. *J Clin Invest*. 2000;106:459–465.

66. Gastaldelli A, Baldi S, Pettiti M, et al. Influence of obesity and type 2 diabetes on gluconeogenesis and glucose output in humans: a quantitative study. *Diabetes*. 2000;49:1367–1373.

67. Wajngot A, Chandramouli V, Schumann W, et al. Quantitative contributions of gluconeogenesis to glucose production during fasting in type 2 diabetes mellitus. *Metabolism*. 2001;50:47–52.

68. Bergman R. Non-esterified fatty acids and the liver: why is insulin secreted into the portal vein? *Diabetologia*. 2000;43:946–952.

69. Mitrakou A, Kelley D, Veneman T, et al. Contribution of abnormal muscle and liver glucose metabolism to postprandial hyperglycemia in NIDDM. *Diabetes*. 1990;39(11):1381–1390.

70. Pehling G, Tessari P, Gerich J, Haymond M, Service F, Rizza R. Abnormal meal carbohydrate disposition in insulin-dependent diabetes. Relative contributions of endogenous glucose production and initial splanchnic uptake and effect of intensive insulin therapy. *J Clin Invest*. 1984;74:985–991.

71. Matsuda M, DeFronzo R. Insulin sensitivity indices obtained from oral glucose tolerance testing: comparison with the euglycemic insulin clamp. *Diabetes Care*. 1999;22:1462–1470.

72. Jiang G, Zhang B. Glucagon and regulation of glucose metabolism. *AJP Endocrinol Metab*. 2003;284:E671–E678.

73. Cherrington A. Banting Lecture 1997. Control of glucose uptake and release by the liver in vivo. *Diabetes*. 1999;48:1198–1214.

74. Gerich J, Charles M, Grodsky G. Regulation of pancreatic insulin and glucagon secretion. *Annu Rev Physiol*. 1976;38:353–388.

75. Reaven G, Chen Y, Godlay A, Swislocki A, Jaspan J. Documentation of hyperglucagonemia throughout the day in nonobese and obese patients with noninsulin-dependent diabetes mellitus. *J Clin Endocrinol Metab*. 1987;64:106–110.

76. Larsson H, Ahren B. Islet dysfunction in insulin resistance involves impaired insulin secretion and increased glucagon secretion in postmenopausal women with impaired glucose tolerance. *Diabetes Care*. 2000;23:650–657.

77. Muller W, Faloona G, Aguilar-Parada E, Unger R. Abnormal α-cell function in diabetes. Response to carbohydrate and protein ingestion. *N Engl J Med*. 1970;283:109–115.

78. Dimitriadis G, Pehling G, Gerich J. Abnormal glucose modulation of islet alpha- and â-cell responses to arginine in non-insulin-dependent diabetes mellitus. *Diabetes*. 1985;34:541–547.

79. Baron A, Schaeffer L, Shragg P, Kolterman O. Role of hyperglucagonemia in maintenance of increased rates of hepatic glucose output in type II diabetics. *Diabetes*. 1897;36:274–283.

80. Larsson H, Ahrn B. Glucose intolerance is predicted by low insulin secretion and high glucagon secretion: outcome of a prospective study in postmenopausal Caucasian women. *Diabetologia*. 2000;43:194–202.

81. Shah P, Basu A, Basu R, Rizza R. Impact of lack of suppression of glucagon on glucose tolerance in humans. *Am J Physiol*. 1999;277:E283–E290.

82. Shah P, Vella A, Basu A, Basu R, Schwenk W, Rizza R. Lack of suppression of glucagon contributes to postprandial hyperglycemia in subjects with type 2 diabetes mellitus. *J Clin Endocrinol Metab*. 2000;85:4053–4059.

83. Ahren B, Larsson H. Impaired glucose tolerance (IGT) is associated with reduced insulin-induced suppression of glucagon concentrations. *Diabetologia*. 2001;44:1998–2003.

84. Abdul-Ghani M, DeFronzo RA. Fasting hyperglycemia impairs glucose- but not insulin-mediated suppression of glucagon secretion. *J Clin Endocrinol Metab*. 2007;92(5):1778–1784.

85. DeFronzo R, Ferrannini E, Simonson D. Fasting hyperglycemia in non-insulin-dependent diabetes mellitus: contributions of excessive hepatic glucose production and impaired tissue glucose uptake. *Metabolism*. 1989;38:387–395.

86. Stumvoll M, Goldstein BJ, van Haeften TW. Type 2 diabetes: principles of pathogenesis and therapy. *Lancet.* 2005;365: 1333–1346.
87. Hosker JP, Rudenski AS, Burnett MA, Matthew DR, Turner RC. *Metabolism.* 1988;38:767–772.
88. Reaven GM, Bernstein R, Davis B, Olefsky JM. Nonketotic diabetes mellitus: insulin deficiency or insulin resistance? *Am J Med.* 1976;60:80–88.
89. Baggio LL, Drucker DJ. *Gastroenterology.* 2007;132(6):2131–2157.
90. Kolterman OG, Gray RS, Griffin J, Burstein P, Insel J. Receptor and postreceptor defects contribute to the insulin resistance in noninsulin-dependent diabetes mellitus. *J Clin Invest.* 1981;68(4):957–969.

Chapter 14
Maturity-Onset Diabetes of the Young: Molecular Genetics, Clinical Manifestations, and Therapy

Markus Stoffel

Definition and Genetic Classification of Monogenic Diabetes

Type 2 diabetes accounts for the majority ($\geq$90%) of all diabetes. It ranks among the top 10 causes of death in western nations and afflicts about 5% of populations in industrialized countries. Type 2 diabetes is a heterogeneous, complex metabolic syndrome in which hyperglycemia results from decreased insulin effectiveness (insulin resistance) and an impaired insulin secretory response to glucose. Genetic and lifestyle factors (e.g., weight, physical activity) predispose to the development of these defects; however, the genetic mechanisms that underlie the pathophysiology of most forms of type 2 diabetes are incompletely understood.

Although most forms of type 2 diabetes appear to be polygenic, monogenic forms have also been identified. Two broad categories of monogenic diabetes can be defined, neonatal diabetes and maturity-onset diabetes of the young (MODY). Neonatal diabetes is a rare condition and is defined as a disease onset before 6 months of age. Clinically, neonatal diabetes has two subdivisions, termed transient (TNDM) and permanent (PNDM) forms. Over 10 distinct genetic anomalies or mutations have been identified causing the disease (Table 14.1). The majority of cases of transient neonatal diabetes have a mutation that maps to a locus on the long arm of chromosome 6, and mutations in two overlapping genes, ZAC and HYMA1, have been identified as the predominant cause of transient neonatal diabetes.[1] Mutations in the genes encoding the β-cell ATP-sensitive potassium channel, a key regulator of nutrient-induced insulin secretion in pancreatic β-cells, have been shown to cause TNDM. Activating mutations in the two ATP-sensitive K^- channel (KATP channel) subunits Kir6.2 and SUR1, which prevent closure of the KATP channel and thus inhibit insulin secretion, are now known to be the predominant cause of permanent neonatal diabetes.[2–4] Permanent neonatal diabetes can be caused by mutations in β-cell transcription factors leading to abnormal pancreatic development and are often associated with other significant developmental anomalies, defects in the glucose sensing, insulin secretory defects, and accelerated β-cell decompensation. Approximately 30% of cases of permanent diabetes have yet to have a genetic cause identified. About 10% of neonatal diabetes is caused by syndromes that frequently are associated with pancreatic aplasia and that can be caused by mutations in several transcription factors (Table 14.1).

Maturity-onset diabetes of the young (MODY) describes a subgroup of autosomal dominantly inherited diabetes that, despite having a young age of onset (at least one family member diagnosed before 25 years of age), is noninsulin dependent. Patients with MODY can be distinguished from patients with type 1 diabetes by a lack of autoantibodies against pancreatic antigens (e.g., glutamic acid decarboxylase, GAD-Ab) and detection of measurable C-peptide in the presence of measurable hyperglycemia outside of the honeymoon period (the period of up to 5 years after diagnosis). The phenotype of patients with MODY is variable, underlining that this disorder is genetically heterogeneous. The term "maturity onset" implies a resemblance to type 2 diabetes; however, it should be noted that all MODY subtypes exhibit very different clinical and etiological features from type 2 diabetes. At least seven discrete genetic etiologies of diabetes have been described, and these account for much of

M. Stoffel (✉)

Institute of Molecular Systems Biology, Swiss Federal Institute of Technology, Zurich 8093, Switzerland

e-mail: stoffel@imsb.biol.ethz.ch

L. Poretsky (ed.), *Principles of Diabetes Mellitus*, DOI 10.1007/978-0-387-09841-8_14,

© Springer Science+Business Media, LLC 2010

Table 14.1 Genetic forms of neonatal diabetes

- Transient (TNDM)
  - 6q ZAC
  - KCNJ11
  - ABC C8
- Permanent (PNDM)
  - KCNJ11
  - ABC C8
  - INS
  - GCK
- Syndromes (pancreatic aplasia)
  - PDX1, HNF1b, PTF1A, FOXP3, EIF2AK3

the clinical heterogeneity apparent among patients receiving a diagnosis of MODY on the basis of this clinical definition (Table 14.2). The different genetic subtypes differ in age of onset, pattern of hyperglycemia, response to treatment, and associated extrapancreatic manifestations. It therefore may not be appropriate to group them all into a single category.

Table 14.2 Definition of MODY

- Impaired glucose tolerance
- Age of onset <25 years
- Autosomal dominant inheritance

Using genetic linkage and candidate gene approaches, mutations in genes on chromosomes 2, 7, 12, 13, 19, and 20 have been linked to MODY and collectively may represent up to 3% of all patients with type 2 diabetes (Table 14.3). The gene on chromosome 7 (MODY2) encodes the glycolytic enzyme glucokinase which plays a key role in generating the metabolic signal for insulin secretion and integrating hepatic glucose uptake.[5] The genes on chromosomes 20 (*MODY1*), 12 (*MODY3*), 19 (*MODY5*), and 13 (*MODY4*) contain mutations in transcription factors, hepatocyte nuclear factor (HNF)-4α, HNF-1α, HNF-1β, and PDX-1, respectively.[6–10] Mutations in NEURO-D1/BETA-2 (MODY6) are responsible for an autosomal dominant form of diabetes that may have a more variable age of onset.[11,12] Rare mutations in the insulin gene have also been shown to give rise to a MODY-like phenotype in humans.[13]

Table 14.3 Genetic classification of MODY

MODY1: Hepatocyte nuclear factor 4α	(HNF-4α)
MODY2: Glucokinase	(GCK)
MODY3: Hepatocyte nuclear factor 1α	(HNF-1α)
MODY4: Insulin promoter factor	(IPF-1/PDX-1)
MODY5: Hepatocyte nuclear factor 1β	(HNF-1β)
MODY6: Neurogenic differentiation-1	(NEURO-D1/BETA-2)
Insulin gene mutations	(INS)
Carboxyl ester lipase gene mutations	(CEL)

Biochemical and genetic studies have shown that MODY genes are functionally related and form a transcriptional network that is critical for formal pancreatic islet development, differentiation, and metabolism. This chapter will discuss the function and molecular defects of different MODY genes and the clinical manifestations of the various subtypes.

MODY Genes and Phenotypes

Hepatocyte Nuclear Factor-4α (MODY1)

HNF-4α is an orphan member of the superfamily of ligand-dependent transcription factors. It contains a zinc finger region (amino acids 48–128) and binds DNA as a homodimer. Two transcriptional activation domains, designated AF-1 and AF-2, flank the DNA-binding domain. AF-1 consists of the first 24 amino acids and functions as a constitutive autonomous activator of transcription. The AF2 transactivation domain of HNF-4α, spanning amino acid residues 128–366, includes the dimerization interface and ligand-binding domain.

The HNF-4α gene is located on chromosome 20q (20q12-q13.1) and plays a critical role in the normal function of liver, intestine, kidney, and pancreatic islets.[14,15] Clinical studies demonstrated that loss-of-function mutations in HNF-4α (Fig. 14.1) cause diabetes by compromising β-cell function. Prediabetic subjects with HNF-4α mutations have normal sensitivity to insulin and first-phase insulin responses to intravenous glucose.[16] However, compared with normal subjects, MODY1 patients exhibit a decrease in plasma C-peptide concentration, decrease in absolute amplitude of insulin secretory oscillations, and reduced insulin secretion rates in response to intravenous glucose infusions as blood glucose levels increase above 7 mmol/l.[16] Furthermore, HNF-4α haploinsufficiency leads to diminished glucagon secretory responses to arginine, suggesting a role of the MODY1 gene in α-cell function.[17]

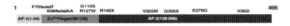

Fig. 14.1 Functional domains and mutations in HNF-4α

Clinically, MODY1 patients frequently develop severe diabetes and complications, including micro- and macrovascular angiopathy and peripheral neuropathy (Table 14.4). About 30% of cases with MODY1 require insulin therapy and the majority of the remainder are treated with oral antidiabetic drugs. Molecular studies indicate that the mechanism by which HNF-4α deficiency results in an impairment of insulin secretion involves abnormal pancreatic islet gene expression. Several genes of the glucose-stimulated insulin secretion pathway in pancreatic β-cells are regulated by HNF-4α. They include the glucose transporter-2 (GLUT-2) and enzymes of glycolysis, including aldolase B, glyceraldehyde-3-phosphate dehydrogenase, and L-pyruvate kinase.[15] HNF-4α also regulates the expression of other transcription factors, such as HNF-1α (the MODY3 gene), which itself is a transcriptional activator of the insulin gene.[15] Together, these observations suggest that diminished HNF-4α activity can impair glucose-stimulated insulin secretion by decreasing the expression of genes involved in glucose entry and metabolism in pancreatic β-cells as well as insulin gene transcription.[15] Since HNF-4α proteins are not only expressed in pancreatic β-cells but also played a key role in hepatocyte differentiation, mutations in this gene could be expected to result in pleiotropic phenotypes. Indeed, subjects with HNF-4α haploinsufficiency have diminished serum apolipoprotein (Apo)A2, apoC3, Lp(a), and triglyceride levels compared to normal controls or patients with other forms of early-onset diabetes.[18]

Table 14.4 Clinical features of HNF-4α mutations

- Decreased insulin secretion
- Decreased glucagon response to arginine
- Variable phenotype: low/normal plasma C-peptide, insulin levels
- Low/normal serum APOAII, CIII, triglyceride levels
- Tendency to develop diabetic complications
- Transient neonatal hyperinsulinemic hypoglycemia and macrosomia

The first HNF-4α/MODY1 mutation was found in R-W pedigree, a family of German ancestry. The affected members of the R-W family have a nonsense mutation, Q268X, in the HNF-4α gene.[6] This mutation generates a truncated protein that contains an intact DNA-binding domain but lacks part of the AF2 region. Functional studies of this mutation revealed that the mutant protein lacks transcriptional activity and does not interact with the wild-type HNF-4α in a dominant-negative fashion.[15]

Additional HNF-4α variants associated with MODY1 have since then been identified and include F75fsdelT, K99fsdelAA, R154X, R127W, V255M, E276Q, V393I, and G115S.[19,20] F75fsdelT and K99fsdelAA are frameshift mutations that lead to truncated HNF-4α proteins. HNF-4α(R154X) produces a truncated protein containing only the DNA-binding domain and the AF1 transactivation domain. This mutant protein lacks transactivation potential and may exert a mild dominant-negative effect on the activity of wild-type HNF-4α in β-cells. In contrast to the frameshift or nonsense mutants, the functional properties of HNF-4α missense mutants are more varied. HNF-4α(V393I), located in the AF2 domain, leads to a two-fold decrease in transactivation potential.[21] Other sequence variants, such as HNF-4α(R127W) and HNF-4α (V255M), have a modest reduction in transcriptional activation.[22] Only one missense mutation that is located in the DNA-binding domain of HNF-4α has been reported. This mutation, HNF-4α(G115S), leads to an impairment in the ability of the mutant protein to bind to HNF4 consensus binding sites, thereby reducing its transactivation activity.

Heterozygous *HNF-4α* mutations may also cause transient or persistent hyperinsulinemic hypoglycemia and are associated with macrosomia. This marked increase in birth weight reflects increased insulin secretion in the fetus, with some neonates exhibiting transient or prolonged hypoglycemia. The most likely explanation is that increased insulin secretion in the fetus progresses to reduced insulin secretion and diabetes in adolescence or early adulthood.

Glucokinase (MODY2)

The phosphorylation of glucose at the sixth carbon position is the first step in glycolysis and is catalyzed by a family of enzymes called hexokinases. Glucokinase (GCK) is expressed mainly in the liver and endocrine pancreas and is a unique member of this family. In contrast to hexokinases 1, 2, and 3, glucokinase (hexokinase 4) is characterized by a high substrate specificity for glucose, a high K_M of about 10 mM (versus 0.1–0.001 mM for the other hexokinases), and a lack of inhibition by metabolites, such as glucose 6-phospahate or glucose 1,6 bisphosphate. These unique biochemical properties allow glucokinase to serve as the glucose sensor of the pancreatic β-cell by integrating glucose metabolism and insulin secretion.[5]

Genetic linkage between DNA polymorphisms in the glucokinase gene (Fig. 14.2) on the short arm of chromosome 7 (7p15-p14) and MODY was initially reported in families of French origin. More than 80 different GCK mutations have been identified since then and, depending on the population, may represent from 11 to 63% of all MODY. Impairment in the enzymatic activity of mutant GCK leads to decreased glycolytic flux in pancreatic β-cells.[23] This translates in vivo into a rightward shift in the dose–response curve relating blood glucose and insulin secretion rates (ISR) obtained during a graded intravenous glucose infusion. Average ISRs over a glucose range between 5 and 9 mM are 61% lower in MODY2 subjects than in control subjects.[23] The release of insulin in response to arginine in MODY2 is preserved, indicating that the insulin secretion defect in MODY2 patients is due to abnormal glucose sensing. Complete loss of glucokinase activity in subjects with homozygous

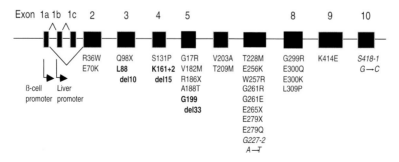

Fig. 14.2 Mutations in the glucokinase gene

mutations in the GCK gene (T228M and M210K) causes neonatal diabetes, a rare form of diabetes that requires insulin therapy within the first weeks of life.[24] In contrast, individuals with activating glucokinase mutations (e.g., HNF-4αV455M) develop an autosomal dominant form of familial hyperinsulinism due to a leftward shift of the dose–response curve relating blood glucose and insulin secretion rates.[25] These genetic findings highlight the importance of glucokinase as a glucose sensor and critical regulator for insulin secretion in pancreatic β-cells.

Glucokinase-deficient mice have been shown to be an excellent animal model for the genetic defect in humans. Mice that lack glucokinase activity die perinatally with severe hyperglycemia and phenotypically resemble rare forms of neonatal diabetes. Heterozygous mice have elevated blood glucose levels and reduced insulin secretion. Expression of GCK in β-cells in the absence of expression in the liver can prevent perinatal death of GCK null mice, providing strong evidence for the need of β-cell GCK in glucose sensing and for maintaining normal glucose levels.[26]

[13]C nuclear magnetic spectroscopy studies have revealed that a hepatic glucose cycling defect also contributes to the molecular etiologies of MODY2 phenotype. MODY2 patients have decreased net accumulation of hepatic glycogen and augmented hepatic gluconeogenesis after a meal.[27] These results suggest that, in addition to β-cell dysfunction, abnormalities in liver glycogen metabolism contribute to the hyperglycemia in patients with glucokinase-deficient diabetes.[27]

Fetal insulin secretion in response to maternal glycemia is an important determinant for intrauterine growth. Glucose-sensing defects in pancreatic β-cells, caused by a heterozygous mutation in the glucokinase gene, can reduce fetal growth and birth weight in addition to causing hyperglycemia after birth.[28] Fetuses that have inherited a glucokinase mutation from the mother or father have a reduced birth weight of 521 g ($p = 0.0002$) compared to unaffected siblings.[28] It is likely that these changes in birth weight reflect changes in fetal insulin secretion that are influenced directly by the fetal genotype and indirectly, through maternal hyperglycemia, by the maternal GCK genotype.[28]

In contrast to MODY1 and MODY3 patients, who frequently develop diabetes at the time of puberty, hyperglycemia in subjects with GCK mutations frequently manifests in the neonatal period and invariably develops before adolescence.[28,29] Glucokinase deficiency is not associated with an increased incidence of diabetic complications, including proliferative retinopathy, neuropathy, or proteinuria, and other manifestations of the metabolic syndrome such as hypertension, obesity, or dyslipidemia.[29,30] This finding is also consistent with the low frequency of coronary heart disease in MODY2 patients. Hypoglycemic medication is not appropriate for most patients with heterozygous GCK mutations because their hyperglycemia is invariable mild, their glycemic regulation is maintained, and medication has a minimal effect. Pregnancy is the one exception in which hypoglycemic therapy might be considered, in particular when excess fetal growth can be documented. Clinical features of MODY2 are summarized in Table 14.5.

Table 14.5 Clinical features of GCK mutations

- Mild defect in insulin secretion
- Mild fasting and postprandial hyperglycemia
- Low/normal plasma C-peptide, insulin levels
- Little tendency for disease progression
- Age of onset: perinatal
- Low birth weight of affected newborns
- Homozygous GCK mutation: neonatal (insulin-dependent) diabetes
- Activating GCK mutations: autosomal dominant familial hyperinsulinism

Hepatocyte Nuclear Factor-1α (MODY3)

HNF-1α is a homeodomain transcription factor composed of an N-terminal dimerization domain, a POU-homeobox DNA-binding domain, and a C-terminal transactivation domain. HNF-1α is expressed in liver, kidney, intestine, and pancreatic islets where it directs tissue-specific gene expression. The gene encoding HNF-1α is located on the long arm of chromosome 12 (12q24.2) and was identified as the MODY3 gene through a combination of genetic linkage analysis and positional cloning.[9] Depending on the population, MODY3 accounts for 21–73% of all MODY. More than 60 different HNF-1α mutations have been found to co-segregate with diabetes in UK, German, French, Danish, Italian, Finnish, North American, and Japanese families (Fig. 14.3). They include missense, nonsense, deletion, insertion, and frame shift mutations. Most HNF-1α mutations can be predicted to result in loss of function. However, mutant HNF-1α proteins with an intact dimerization domain may impair pancreatic β-cell function by forming nonproductive dimers with wild-type protein, thereby exhibiting dominant-negative activity. This mechanism has been shown for frameshift mutation HNF-1α-P291fsinsC. Overexpression of HNF-1α-P291fsinsC in MIN6 cells, a murine β-cell line, resulted in 40% inhibition of the endogenous HNF-1α activity in a dose-dependent manner.[31] Furthermore, the formation of heterodimers between wild-type and HNF-1α-P291fsinsC mutant proteins has been observed, indicating that this mutant protein has dominant-negative activity.[31] Codon 291, in the poly-C tract of exon 4, is a frequent site for mutations in the HNF-1α gene. This is likely due to slipped mispairing during DNA replication, thereby causing this region to be a mutation hotspot.[32]

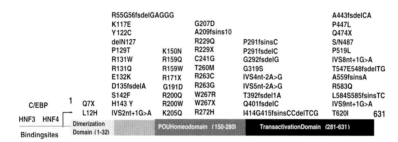

Fig. 14.3 Functional domains and mutations in HNF-1α

Hypomorphic HNF-1α mutations may also contribute to the development of type 2 diabetes in some populations. The HNF-1α(G319S) variant is associated with type 2 diabetes in the Canadian Oji-Cree population with odd ratios of 4.0 and 1.97 in individuals with homozygous and heterozygous G319S mutations, respectively.[33] This mutation is located in the proline-rich transactivation domain and substitutes a conserved glycine residue. Clinical studies indicate that the G319S variant in the Canadian Oji-Cree population is associated with earlier onset of diabetes in women, lower body mass index, and higher plasma glucose after oral glucose challenge.[33]

HNF-1α mutations lead to β-cell dysfunction and result in elevated fasting glycemia and impaired glucose-stimulated insulin secretion.[34] Other clinical features of MODY3 (Table 14.6) include increased proinsulin-to-insulin ratios, increased responsiveness to sulfonylureas, and lower body mass index (BMI).[29,34,35] HNF-1α mutations are highly penetrant, with 63% of MODY3 diagnosed by the age of 25 years, 78.6% by 35 years, and 95.5% by 55 years.[36] Subjects with HNF-1α mutations have a more rapid deterioration in β-cell function than MODY2 subjects.[29] Heterozygous HNF-1α patients frequently require treatment with oral hypoglycemic agents or insulin.[29]

Table 14.6 Clinical features of HNF-1α mutations

- Defect in insulin secretion
- Fasting and postprandial hyperglycemia
- Low plasma C-peptide, insulin levels
- Tendency for disease progression
- Increased sensitivity to sulfonylurea therapy

Mice lacking HNf-1α develop diabetes within the first month of life due to defects in insulin secretion. Pancreatic islets from HNf-1α null mice have impaired β-cell glycolytic signaling due to decreased expression of glucose transporter-2 and glycolytic enzymes, such as L-pyruvate kinase and glucokinase.[37,38] Mutant HNf-1α mice also exhibit dwarfism, renal Fanconi-like syndrome, glycogen storage disease 1b, and defects in bile acid and plasma HDL-cholesterol metabolism.[39–42] However, the hepatic and renal manifestations develop only in the absence of HNF-1α but are not a feature of heterozygous mice.

Insulin Promoter Factor-1 (MODY4)

Insulin promoter factor-1 or pancreatic and duodenal homeobox gene-1 (IPF-1, PDX-1) (Fig. 14.4) is a homeodomain transcription factor that is required for endocrine and exocrine pancreas development as well as insulin gene expression in the adult islet. PDX-1 binds to promoters of target genes as a heterodimer with the ubiquitously expressed homeodomain protein PBX.[43] PDX-1 is an essential gene for early pancreas development. During development in mice, PDX-1 is initially expressed at 8.5 days postcoitum (dpc) in the dorsal and ventral gut epithelia that will later develop into a pancreas. At 9.5 dpc, PDX-1 expression marks the dorsal and ventral pancreatic buds of the gut and later is restricted to differentiating insulin-producing β-cells and somatostatin-producing δ-cell.[44] Targeted disruption of the PDX-1 gene results in a failure of the pancreas to develop.[45] Furthermore, β-cell-specific inactivation of the mouse PDX-1 gene leads to β-cell dedifferentiation, loss of proper glucose sensing, insulin processing, and the development of diabetes.[46] Thus, PDX-1 appears to be a key regulator in early pancreas formation and later in maintaining islet pattern of hormone expression and normoglycemia.

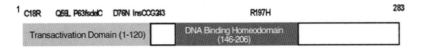

Fig. 14.4   Functional domains and mutations in PDX-1

The PDX-1 gene maps to human chromosome 13 (13q12.1) and is involved in several human disorders including pancreatic agenesis and diabetes.[7,8] A single nucleotide deletion within codon 63 (Pro63fsdelC) of the human PDX-1 gene has been reported to cause pancreatic agenesis. This patient inherited the mutant allele from his parents who were heterozygous for the same mutation.[7] Heterozygous family members have early-onset diabetes (range 17–67 years) (Table 14.7).[8] The point deletion leads to an out-of-frame protein downstream of the PDX-1 transactivation domain, resulting in a nonfunctional protein lacking the homeodomain that is essential for DNA binding.[7] Expression studies of the mutant PDX1(Pro63fsdelC) protein in eukaryotic cells revealed a second PDX-1 isoform that resulted from an internal translation initiating at an out-of-frame AUG.[46] The reading frame crosses over to the wild-type IPF1 reading frame at the site of the point deletion just carboxy-proximal to the transactivation domain, resulting in a second PDX1 isoform that contains the COOH-terminal DNA-binding domain but lacks the amino-terminal transactivation domain.[46] This terminal domain PDX-1 isoform may inhibit the transactivation functions of wild-type PDX-1, suggesting that a dominant-negative mechanism may contribute to the development of diabetes in individuals with this mutation. Six of eight affected heterozygotes in this pedigree were treated with diet or oral hypoglycemic agents. None of the family members carrying the PDX-1(Pro63fsdelC) mutation showed ketosis or other indications of severe insulin deficiency.[8]

Table 14.7   Clinical features of PDX-1/IPF-1 mutations

- Defect in insulin secretion
- Fasting and postprandial hyperglycemia
- Low plasma C-peptide, insulin levels
- Tendency for disease progression
- Homozygous PDX-1 mutation: pancreatic agenesis

Other PDX-1 mutations that predispose carriers to diabetes include D76N, C18R, R197H, Q59L, and InsCCG243.[47,48,49] The PDX-1(InsCCG243) mutation is linked in two French families with a late-onset form of type 2 diabetes and autosomal inheritance, in which insulin secretion becomes progressively impaired over time. The nondiabetic carriers have lower than normal insulin levels at high glucose levels.[48] The InsCCG243 mutation occurs at the COOH-terminal border of PDX-1 homeodomain required for transactivation. Three PDX-1 missense mutations (C18R, D76N, and R197H) were found in diabetic subjects from Great Britain. Functional analysis of these mutations suggests that they exhibit decreased binding activity to the human insulin gene promoter and reduced activation of the insulin gene in response to hyperglycemia.[49] These mutations are estimated to have a frequency of 1% in the English population and may predispose to type 2 diabetes (relative risk of 3.0).[48] The PDX-1 mutations (D76N) and (Q59L) were also found in French, late-onset type 2 diabetic families with a relative risk of 12.6 for diabetes and with decreased glucose-stimulated insulin secretion in nondiabetic individuals.[48] These mutations are located in the amino-terminal transactivation region that mediates insulin transcription. In summary, hypomorphic PDX-1 variants may lead to a progressive impairment of β-cell function and glucose homeostasis in concert with other inherited metabolic abnormalities and risk factors such as age, obesity-related insulin resistance, and physical inactivity. Therefore, PDX-1 mutations may also be involved in the polygenic basis of late-onset type 2 diabetes.[48,49]

Hepatocyte Nuclear Factor-1β (MODY5)

HNF-1α and -1β are homologous proteins belonging to a large superfamily of homeodomain-containing transcription factors. As such, HNF-1β is structurally similar to HNF-1α with an N-terminal dimerization domain, a POU-homeobox DNA-binding domain, and a C-terminal transactivation domain. HNF-1α and -1β bind to DNA as homo- and/or heterodimers. The HNF-1 genes have an overlapping tissue distribution but HNF-1α/HNF1β ratios differ from one organ to another with HNF-1α being the predominant form in the liver and HNF-1β the major form in the kidney. Inactivation of the HNF-1β gene in mice results in early embryonic lethality by day 7.5 of development. HNF-1β-deficient embryos exhibit an abnormal extraembryonic region, poorly organized ectoderm, and no discernible visceral endoderm.[50,51]

The gene encoding HNF-1β (Fig. 14.5) maps to chromosome 17q (17cen-q21.3) and genetic variation in this gene is responsible for several human disorders including MODY5 (Table 14.8), familial hypoplastic glomerulocystic kidney disease, and Müllerian aplasia.[10,52–54] HNF-1β mutations are rare causes of MODY and only a few MODY5 families have been identified and studied. MODY5 develops early in life (10–25 years) and ultimately requires insulin replacement therapy to control hyperglycemia. The first HNF-1β mutation found to be associated with MODY was HNF-1β(R177X).[10] Nephropathy, in addition to diabetes, was found in this pedigree suggesting that decreased expression levels of HNF-1β in the kidney contribute to renal dysfunction.[10] This loss-of-function mutation generated a truncated protein lacking the C-terminal transactivation domain.[10]

Diabetes, renal dysfunction progressing to end-stage renal disease, and Müllerian aplasia were found in a Norwegian family.[52] This syndrome was caused by a 75-bp deletion in exon 2 of the HNF-1β gene. The deletion

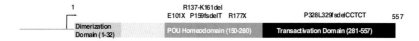

Fig. 14.5 Functional domains and mutations in HNF-1β

Table 14.8 Clinical features of HNF-1β mutations

- Renal dysfunction and early-onset diabetes
- Decreased insulin sensitivity
- Variable renal phenotype: nephron agenesis, cysts, familial hypoplastic glomerulocystic kidney disease, Müllerian aplasia
- Low plasma C-peptide, insulin levels
- Pancreas atrophy
- Tendency for disease progression, progressive hypoplastic glomerulocystic nephropathy
- Increased risk for prostate cancer

is located in the POU DNA-binding homeodomain and functional studies revealed that the HNF1β (R137-K161del) mutant lost its DNA-binding property and could not activate a reporter gene, indicating that this mutant is functionally inactive.[52]

In contrast to other MODY types, patients with mutations in the HNF-1β gene have early and rapidly progressing familial hypoplastic glomerulocystic kidney disease that is distinct from the diabetic nephropathy in type 1 or type 2 diabetes. In addition, they may have increased risk to develop prostate cancer.[55] They may also exhibit other clinical features such as uterine and genital abnormalities, gout, hyperuricemia, exocrine pancreatic dysfunction, abnormal liver function tests, and insulin resistance.[56]

Three other HNF-1β mutations, P328L329fsdelCCTCT, P159fsdelT, and E101X, were found in families with a history of renal dysfunction and early-onset diabetes.[53,54] Both, frameshift P159fsdelT and nonsense E101X, mutations lack the POU DNA-binding domain and result in inactive protein.[53] HNF-1β(P328L329fsdelCCTCT) is a 5-bp deletion resulting in a truncated protein that retains the DNA-binding domain. This mutation is associated with nephron agenesis and exhibits gain-of-function activity with increased transcriptional activation potential in vitro.[54] In summary, there is increasing evidence that normal expression levels and activity of HNF-1β are critical for β-cell function and pancreas and kidney development and that both loss-of-function and gain-of-function mutations can lead to disease in these organs.

Neurogenic Differentiation Factor 1 (MODY6)

NEURO-D1/Beta-2 (Fig. 14.6) belongs to the basic helix-loop-helix (bHLH) family of transcription factors that is involved in determining cell type during development. NEURO-D1 is composed of a bHLH DNA-binding domain and a C-terminal transactivation domain that interacts with the cellular co-activator p300 and CBP. NEURO-D1 is expressed in pancreatic islets, intestine, and the brain.[57] Mice deficient for NEURO-D1 function have abnormal islet morphology, overt diabetes, and die after birth.[57]

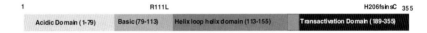

Fig. 14.6 Functional domains and mutations in NEURO-D1/BETA-2

Mutations in the NEURO-D1 gene have recently been reported as being associated with diabetes in two families with autosomal dominant inheritance.[11] One of the families had a G to T substitution in codon 111, causing a substitution of Arg to Leu (R111L) in the proximal bHLH domain. In vitro studies suggest that Neuro-D1(R111L) has lost its DNA-binding activity and is less effective in transactivating the insulin promoter. Clinical features of subjects with this mutation are similar to type 2 diabetes with high fasting serum insulin levels, elevated levels of insulin 2 h after oral glucose, and an average age of diagnosis of 40 (range 30–59 years).[11]

The second mutation in the NEURO-D1 gene consists of an insertion of a cytosine residue in a poly-C tract in codon 206 (206+C).[11] NeuroD (H206fsinsC) gives rise to a truncated polypeptide lacking the C-terminal transactivation domain, a region that associates with the co-activators CBP and p300. This mutant retains its ability to bind to DNA; however, it has lost its ability to activate transcription through the deletion of the protein domain that interacts with co-activator p300.[11] The clinical profile of patients with this truncated protein is more severe and shares clinical features of MODY such as low endogenous insulin secretion and early age of onset (range 17–56 years).[11]

Insulin Gene Mutations

Insulin is synthesized in β-cells of the islets of Langerhans and is a central hormone that maintains glucose homeostasis. Insulin-deficient mice die shortly after birth due to severe hyperglycemia.[58] All cell types of the endocrine pancreas are present in insulin-deficient mice suggesting that insulin is not required for development and differentiation of the endocrine pancreas.[58]

Naturally occurring mutations in the insulin gene that result in the synthesis of abnormal insulin proteins have been found in humans to result in a MODY-like phenotype.[13] These abnormal insulin proteins have altered metabolic properties and usually present with inappropriately high serum insulin levels and high insulin/C-peptide ratios due to abnormal posttranslational processing and an increased half-life. In many cases, diabetes develops only in individuals with underlying insulin resistance or other risk factors for diabetes. Some mutations in the insulin gene have been reported to segregate with early-onset diabetes with incomplete penetrance and are inherited in an autosomal dominant manner.[13]

Carboxyl Ester Lipase Gene Mutations

Mutations in the variable number of tandem repeats (VNTR) of the carboxyl ester lipase gene (*CEL*) can cause β-cell dysfunction and early-onset diabetes (mean age of diagnosis 36 years). *CEL* is expressed in the exocrine acinar cells. Affected individuals have phenotypes consistent with reduced CEL activity. Furthermore, they develop glucose intolerance and often exhibit asymptomatic exocrine failure and altered serum lipids.[59] The mechanism by which carboxyl ester lipase deficiency in the acinar cells causes progressive failure of the β-cells is unknown. The pancreas of subjects with CEL mutations shows atrophy and possible fat infiltration on imaging and marked fibrosis at autopsy.[60]

Summary

Maturity-onset diabetes of the young (MODY) is a group of monogenic forms of type 2 diabetes that are characterized by an early disease onset, autosomal dominant inheritance, and defects in insulin secretion. Genetic studies have identified mutations in at least eight genes associated with different forms of MODY. The majority of the MODY subtypes are caused by mutations in transcription factors that include hepatocyte nuclear factor (HNF)-4α, HNF-1α, PDX-1, HNF-1β, and NEURO-D1/BETA-2. In addition, genetic defects in the glucokinase gene, the glucose sensor of the pancreatic β-cells, and the insulin gene also lead to impaired glucose tolerance. The genetic heterogeneity of MODY is reflected in the phenotypic spectrum of the disease. MODY is caused by impaired glucose-stimulated insulin secretion due to defects in pancreatic β-cells and can be discriminated from type 1 diabetes by lack of glutamic acid decarboxylase antibodies. Insulin sensitivity in MODY is normal or increased and insulin resistance is generally not associated with MODY. Glucokinase-deficient diabetes (MODY2) has little tendency to progress, whereas all other forms can develop severe diabetic complications. Patients with familial mild hyperglycemia that does not deteriorate with age should be tested for GCK mutations. Molecular diagnostic testing is now available in many countries and can improve the management of monogenic forms of diabetes. Restoration of normoglycemia should be attempted with diet and exercise (to maximize insulin sensitivity), oral antidiabetic therapy (insulin secretagogues such as sulfonylureas), and/or insulin.

References

1. Gloyn AL, et al. Assessment of the role of a common genetic variation in the transient neonatal diabetes mellitus region in type 2 diabetes: a comparative genomic and tagging single nucleotide polymorphism approach. *Diabetes*. 2006;55:2272–2276.
2. Gloyn AL, et al. Activating mutations in the gene encoding the ATP-sensitive potassium-channel subunit Kir6.2 and permanent neonatal diabetes. *N Engl J Med*. 2004;350:1838–1849.
3. Flanaghan SE, et al. Mutations in ATP sensitive K+ channel genes cause transient neonatal diabetes and permanent diabetes in childhood or adulthood. *Diabetes*. 2007;56:1930–1937.
4. Babenko AP, et al. Activating mutations in the ABC C8 gene in neonatal diabetes mellitus. *N Engl J Med*. 2006;355:456–466.
5. Matschinsky FM. Glucokinase as glucose sensor and metabolic signal generator in pancreatic beta-cells and hepatocytes. *Diabetes*. 1990;39:647–652.
6. Yamagata K, Furuta H, Oda N, et al. Mutations in the hepatocyte nuclear factor-4alpha gene in maturity-onset diabetes of the young (MODY1). [see comments]. *Nature*. 1996;384:458–460.
7. Stoffers DA, Zinkin NT, Stanojevic V, Clarke WL, Habener JF. Pancreatic agenesis attributable to a single nucleotide deletion in the human IPF1 gene coding sequence. *Nat Genet*. 1997;15:106–110.

8. Stoffers DA, Ferrer J, Clarke WL, Habener JF. Early-onset type-II diabetes mellitus (MODY4) linked to IPF1. *Nat Genet.* 1997;17:138–139.

9. Yamagata K, Oda N, Kaisaki PJ, et al. Mutations in the hepatocyte nuclear factor-1alpha gene in maturity-onset diabetes of the young (MODY3). [see comments]. *Nature.* 1996;384:455–458.

10. Horikawa Y, Iwasaki N, Hara M, et al. Mutation in hepatocyte nuclear factor-1 beta gene (TCF2) associated with MODY. *Nat Genet.* 1997;17:384–385.

11. Malecki MT, Jhala US, Antonellis A, et al. Mutations in NEUROD1 are associated with the development of type 2 diabetes mellitus. *Nat Genet.* 1999;23:323–328.

12. Waeber G, Delplanque J, Bonny C, et al. The gene MAPK8IP1, encoding islet-brain-1, is a candidate for type 2 diabetes. *Nat Genet.* 2000;24:291–295.

13. Vinik A, Bell G. Mutant insulin syndromes. [erratum appears in Horm Metab Res 1988 Mar;20(3):191]. *Hormone Metab Res.* 1988;20:1–10.

14. Chen WS, Manova K, Weinstein DC, et al. Disruption of the HNF-4 gene, expressed in visceral endoderm, leads to cell death in embryonic ectoderm and impaired gastrulation of mouse embryos. *Genes Dev.* 1994;8:2466–2477.

15. Stoffel M, Duncan SA. The maturity-onset diabetes of the young (MODY1) transcription factor HNF4alpha regulates expression of genes required for glucose transport and metabolism. *Proc Natl Acad Sci USA.* 1997;94:13209–13214.

16. Byrne MM, Sturis J, Fajans SS, et al. Altered insulin secretory responses to glucose in subjects with a mutation in the MODY1 gene on chromosome 20. *Diabetes.* 1995;44:699–704.

17. Herman WH, Fajans SS, Smith MJ, Polonsky KS, Bell GI, Halter JB. Diminished insulin and glucagon secretory responses to arginine in nondiabetic subjects with a mutation in the hepatocyte nuclear factor-4alpha/MODY1 gene. *Diabetes.* 1997;46:1749–1754.

18. Shih DQ, Dansky HM, Fleisher M, Assmann G, Fajans SS, Stoffel M. Genotype/phenotype relationships in HNF-4alpha/MODY1: haploinsufficiency is associated with reduced apolipoprotein (AII), apolipoprotein (CIII), lipoprotein(a), and triglyceride levels. *Diabetes.* 2000;49:832–837.

19. Moller AM, Urhammer SA, Dalgaard LT, et al. Studies of the genetic variability of the coding region of the hepatocyte nuclear factor-4alpha in Caucasians with maturity onset NIDDM. *Diabetologia.* 1997;40:980–983.

20. Malecki MT, Yang Y, Antonellis A, Curtis S, Warram JH, Krolewski AS. Identification of new mutations in the hepatocyte nuclear factor 4alpha gene among families with early onset Type 2 diabetes mellitus. *Diabet Med.* 1999;16:193–200.

21. Hani EH, Suaud L, Boutin P, et al. A missense mutation in hepatocyte nuclear factor-4 alpha, resulting in a reduced transactivation activity, in human late-onset non-insulin-dependent diabetes mellitus. *J Clin Invest.* 1998;101:521–526.

22. Navas MA, Munoz-Elias EJ, Kim J, Shih D, Stoffel M. Functional characterization of the MODY1 gene mutations HNF4(R127W), HNF4(V255M), and HNF4(E276Q). *Diabetes.* 1999;48:1459–1465.

23. Byrne MM, Sturis J, Clement K, et al. Insulin secretory abnormalities in subjects with hyperglycemia due to glucokinase mutations. *J Clin Invest.* 1994;93:1120–1130.

24. Njolstad PR, Sovik O, Cuesta-Munoz A, et al. Neonatal diabetes mellitus due to complete glucokinase deficiency. *N Engl J Med.* 2001;344:1588–1592.

25. Glaser B, Kesavan P, Heyman M, et al. Familial hyperinsulinism caused by an activating glucokinase mutation. *N Engl J Med.* 1998;338:226–230.

26. Grupe A, Hultgren B, Ryan A, Ma YH, Bauer M, Stewart TA. Transgenic knockouts reveal a critical requirement for pancreatic beta cell glucokinase in maintaining glucose homeostasis. *Cell.* 1995;83:69–78.

27. Velho G, Petersen KF, Perseghin G, et al. Impaired hepatic glycogen synthesis in glucokinase-deficient (MODY-2) subjects. *J Clin Invest.* 1996;98:1755–1761.

28. Hattersley AT, Beards F, Ballantyne E, Appleton M, Harvey R, Ellard S. Mutations in the glucokinase gene of the fetus result in reduced birth weight. [see comments]. *Nat Genet.* 1998;19:268–270.

29. Pearson ER, Velho G, Clark P, et al. Beta-cell genes and diabetes: quantitative and qualitative differences in the pathophysiology of hepatic nuclear factor-1alpha and glucokinase mutations. *Diabetes.* 2001;50(Suppl 1):S101–S107.

30. Froguel P, Zouali H, Vionnet N, et al. Familial hyperglycemia due to mutations in glucokinase. Definition of a subtype of diabetes mellitus. [see comments]. *N Engl J Med.* 1993;328:697–702.

31. Yamagata K, Yang Q, Yamamoto K, et al. Mutation P291fsinsC in the transcription factor hepatocyte nuclear factor-1alpha is dominant negative. *Diabetes.* 1998;47:1231–1235.

32. Kaisaki PJ, Menzel S, Lindner T, et al. Mutations in the hepatocyte nuclear factor-1alpha gene in MODY and early-onset NIDDM: evidence for a mutational hotspot in exon 4. [erratum appears in Diabetes 1997 Jul;46(7):1239]. *Diabetes.* 1997;46:528–535.

33. Hegele RA, Cao H, Harris SB, Hanley AJ, Zinman B. The hepatic nuclear factor-1alpha G319S variant is associated with early-onset type 2 diabetes in Canadian Oji-Cree. *J Clin Endocrinol Metab.* 1999;84:1077–1082.

34. Lehto M, Tuomi T, Mahtani MM, et al. Characterization of the MODY3 phenotype. Early-onset diabetes caused by an insulin secretion defect. *J Clin Invest.* 1997;99:582–591.

35. Hansen T, Eiberg H, Rouard M, et al. Novel MODY3 mutations in the hepatocyte nuclear factor-1alpha gene: evidence for a hyperexcitability of pancreatic beta-cells to intravenous secretagogues in a glucose-tolerant carrier of a P447L mutation. *Diabetes.* 1997;46:726–730.

36. Frayling TM, Evans JC, Bulman MP, et al. Beta-cell genes and diabetes: molecular and clinical characterization of mutations in transcription factors. *Diabetes*. 2001;50(Suppl 1):S94–S100.

37. Dukes ID, Sreenan S, Roe MW, et al. Defective pancreatic beta-cell glycolytic signaling in hepatocyte nuclear factor-1alpha-deficient mice. *J Biol Chem*. 1998;273:24457–24464.

38. Shih DQ, Screenan S, Munoz KN, et al. Loss of HNF-1a function in mice leads to abnormal expression of genes involved in pancreatic islet development and metabolism. *Diabetes*. 2001;50:2472–2480.

39. Pontoglio M, Barra J, Hadchouel M, et al. Hepatocyte nuclear factor 1 inactivation results in hepatic dysfunction, phenylketonuria, and renal Fanconi syndrome. *Cell*. 1996;84:575–585.

40. Lee YH, Sauer B, Gonzalez FJ. Laron dwarfism and non-insulin-dependent diabetes mellitus in the Hnf-1alpha knockout mouse. *Mol Cell Biol*. 1998;18:3059–3068.

41. Hiraiwa H, Pan C-J, Lin B, Akiyama TE, Gonzalez FJ, Chou JY. A molecular link between the common phenotypes of type 1 glycogen storage disease and HNF1-alpha-null mice. *J Biol Chem*. 2001;276:7963–7967.

42. Shih DQ, Bussen M, Sehayek E, et al. Hepatocyte nuclear factor-1alpha is an essential regulator of bile acid and plasma cholesterol metabolism. *Nat Genet*. 2001;27:375–382.

43. Dutta S, Gannon M, Peers B, Wright C, Bonner-Weir S, Montminy M. PDX:PBX complexes are required for normal proliferation of pancreatic cells during development. *Proc Natl Acad Sci USA*. 2001;98:1065–1070.

44. Ohlsson H, Karlsson K, Edlund T. IPF1, a homeodomain-containing transactivator of the insulin gene. *EMBO J*. 1993;12:4251–4259.

45. Jonsson J, Carlsson L, Edlund T, Edlund H. Insulin-promoter-factor 1 is required for pancreas development in mice. *Nature*. 1994;371:606–609.

46. Ahlgren U, Jonsson J, Jonsson L, Simu K, Edlund H. Beta-cell-specific inactivation of the mouse Ipf1/Pdx1 gene results in loss of the beta-cell phenotype and maturity onset diabetes. *Genes Dev*. 1998;12:1763–1768.

47. Stoffers DA, Stanojevic V, Habener JF. Insulin promoter factor-1 gene mutation linked to early-onset type 2 diabetes mellitus directs expression of a dominant negative isoprotein. *J Clin Invest*.1998;102:232–241.

48. Hani EH, Stoffers DA, Chevre JC, et al. Defective mutations in the insulin promoter factor-1 (IPF-1) gene in late-onset type 2 diabetes mellitus. *J Clin Invest*. 1999;104:R41–R48.

49. Macfarlane WM, Frayling TM, Ellard S, et al. Missense mutations in the insulin promoter factor-1 gene predispose to type 2 diabetes. *J Clin Invest*. 1999;104:R33–R39.

50. Coffinier C, Thepot D, Babinet C, Yaniv M, Barra J. Essential role for the homeoprotein vHNF1/HNF1beta in visceral endoderm differentiation. *Development*. 1999;126:4785–4794.

51. Barbacci E, Reber M, Ott MO, Breillat C, Huetz F, Cereghini S. Variant hepatocyte nuclear factor 1 is required for visceral endoderm specification. *Development*. 1999;126:4795–4805.

52. Lindner TH, Njolstad PR, Horikawa Y, Bostad L, Bell GI, Sovik O. A novel syndrome of diabetes mellitus, renal dysfunction and genital malformation associated with a partial deletion of the pseudo-POU domain of hepatocyte nuclear factor-1beta. *Hum Mol Genet*. 1999;8:2001–2008.

53. Bingham C, Bulman MP, Ellard S, et al. Mutations in the hepatocyte nuclear factor-1beta gene are associated with familial hypoplastic glomerulocystic kidney disease. *Am J Hum Gen*. 2001;68:219–224.

54. Bingham C, Ellard S, Allen L, et al. Abnormal nephron development associated with a frameshift mutation in the transcription factor hepatocyte nuclear factor-1 beta. [see comments]. *Kid Intl*. 2000;57:898–907.

55. Gudmundsson J, et al. Two variants on chromosome 17 confer prostate cancer risk, and the one in TCF2 protects against type 2 diabetes. *Nat Genet*. 2007;39:977–983.

56. Pearson ER, et al. Contrasting diabetes phenotypes associated with hepatocyte nuclear factor 1a and -1b mutations. *Diabetes Care*. 2004;27:1102–1107.

57. Naya FJ, Huang HP, Qiu Y, et al. Diabetes, defective pancreatic morphogenesis, and abnormal enteroendocrine differentiation in BETA2/neuroD-deficient mice. *Genes Dev*. 1997;11:2323–2334.

58. Duvillie B, Cordonnier N, Deltour L, et al. Phenotypic alterations in insulin-deficient mutant mice. *Proc Natl Acad Sci USA*. 1997;94:5137–5140.

59. Raeder H, Johansson S, Holm PI, et al. Mutations in the CEL VNTR cause a syndrome of diabetes and pancreatic exocrine dysfunction. *Nat Genet*. 2006;38:54–62.

60. Raeder H, et al. Pancreatic lipomatosis is a structural marker in nondiabetic children with mutations in carboxyl-ester lipase. *Diabetes*. 2007;56:444–449.

Chapter 15
Diabetes in Pregnancy

Adina E. Schneider, Elliot J. Rayfield, Agustin Busta, and Yuriy Gurevich

Introduction

Based on the 2002 birth data in the United States,[1] maternal diabetes affects more than 321,760 of the 4,022,000 pregnancies that result in birth, and is a significant cause of maternal and fetal morbidity.[2] Gestational diabetes mellitus (GDM) makes up approximately 50% of maternal diabetes.[3] The remaining cases are due to type 1 diabetes and diagnosed or undiagnosed type 2 diabetes, collectively referred to as pregestational diabetes. GDM affects up to 14% of pregnant women, depending on the population.[4] In North America, the prevalence of GDM is higher in Asians, African-Americans, Native North Americans from Canada, and Hispanics than in non-Hispanic whites.[5]

A subset of women with gestational diabetes has circulating islet cell antibodies. They might have a latent form of type 1 diabetes.[6] Majority of complications arise in patients with gestational and undiagnosed type 2 diabetes. Patients with gestational diabetes usually develop hyperglycemia during the second half of pregnancy. Hyperglycemia at this stage of gestation clearly causes fetal macrosomia and neonatal hypoglycemia. Patients with pregestational diabetes are at risk for hyperglycemia early in pregnancy; this hyperglycemia is associated with significantly increased rates of fetal loss and fetal malformations.

The evidence that has accrued over the past 20 years reveals that tight glycemic control can prevent most of the maternal and fetal complications of diabetes. The neonatal death rate in pregnancies complicated by diabetes was 50% prior to the introduction of insulin, 10% in 1939 after the introduction of insulin, and approached that in nondiabetic pregnancies by the 1980s.[7]

Pathophysiology of Pregnancy

The first trimester of pregnancy is associated with increased insulin sensitivity, which may be due to increased adipocyte binding of insulin in the presence of increased estradiol levels.[8] In addition, insulin secretion in response to glucose appears to be enhanced during the first 20 weeks of pregnancy.[9] During normal pregnancy fasting and postprandial glucose levels are lower than that in the nonpregnant state and HBA1C falls approximately 20%. This fact is also due in part to the fetal utilization of glucose, which occurs predominantly through a glucose transporter (GLUT)-1 isoform on the trophoblast.[10]

However, as the levels of cortisol, progesterone, estrogen, prolactin, and human placental lactogen raise later in pregnancy, a state of insulin resistance ensues (Fig. 15.1). Fasting insulin levels rise and C-peptide peaks at about 28–32 weeks gestation. Human placental lactogen (hPL), which is homologous to growth hormone, causes reduction in phosphorylation of insulin receptor substrate (IRS)-1. It is likely responsible for most of the observed insulin resistance.[8] The reduction in insulin sensitivity in pregnancy can approach 80%.[11] It might represent an

A. Busta (✉)
Division of Endocrinology and Metabolism, Albert Einstein College of Medicine, Beth Israel Medical Center, New York, NY, USA
e-mail: abusta@chpnet.org

L. Poretsky (ed.), *Principles of Diabetes Mellitus*, DOI 10.1007/978-0-387-09841-8_15,
© Springer Science+Business Media, LLC 2010

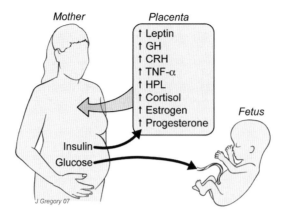

Fig. 15.1 Movement of hormones and glucose across the placental barrier

adaptive mechanism leading to an ample supply of glucose to the fetus by altering maternal metabolism from carbohydrates to lipids.[11] Moreover, it has been demonstrated that women with GDM have a 67% decline in β-cell compensation for insulin resistance in comparison with normal pregnant women.[12] It is interesting to mention, however, that a study of pregnant women living at high altitude in Peru demonstrated lower maternal fasting plasma glucose levels than that at sea level in the presence of similar insulin secretion, indicating higher peripheral insulin sensitivity.[13]

Several other changes which take place in GDM might impact insulin resistance. Elevated leptin concentrations have been observed in GDM.[14] It has been demonstrated that levels of tumor necrosis factor-alpha (TNF-α) increase from early to late pregnancy.[15] Some investigators suggested that TNF-α is the most important contributor to insulin resistance in pregnancy.[16]

Hypothalamic hormone concentrations that are undetectable in the systemic circulation of nonpregnant women increase during pregnancy. In response to cortisol, corticotropin-releasing hormone (CRH) is liberated by placenta throughout pregnancy, enhancing maternal and fetal pituitary functions. The placenta also produces somatostatin which inhibits hPL. Reduction in the secretion of somatostatin in later part of pregnancy may contribute to insulin resistance.

Secretion of pituitary GH is diminished by 20 weeks and supplanted by placental GH. Human placental growth hormone has been shown to cause insulin resistance in transgenic animals.[17] ACTH levels increase during pregnancy, probably secondary to placental CRH, leading to an increase in plasma cortisol levels.

According to the data presented at the Fifth International Workshop-Conference on GDM, post-receptor mechanism of insulin resistance in GDM involves β-subunit of insulin receptor as well as IRS-1 in the skeletal muscle.[18]

Gestational Diabetes

Gestational diabetes (GDM) is defined as glucose intolerance of varying severity with onset or first recognition during pregnancy. As discussed above, insulin resistance is a normal consequence of pregnancy. Women with GDM, in contrast to normal pregnant women, have an impaired ability to secrete insulin.[19] Perhaps the first reference to GDM in the literature was made in 1946, when Miller observed an 8% neonatal mortality among infants born to mothers who subsequently developed diabetes. [20]

Diagnosis

The diagnosis of GDM is determined by the results of an oral glucose tolerance test (OGTT). The currently used values for the 100-g test are based on the calculations of O'Sullivan and Mahan who performed the 100-g

OGTT on 752 pregnant women and set the diagnostic threshold at greater than 2 standard deviations above the mean.[21] This cutoff was based on a retrospective evaluation of 1013 subjects; 22% of the women who had a glucose tolerance test of greater than 2 SD above the mean developed diabetes in the next 7–8 years. In 1978 ACOG (American Congress of Obstetricians and Gynecologists) recommended the use of the O'Sullivan–Mahan criteria for the diagnosis of gestational diabetes. Coustan and Carpenter revised these criteria in 1982 to account for the shift from venous to plasma blood glucose levels and for changes in technology.[22]

Table 15.1 shows the criteria for diagnosis of GDM after a 100- or 75-g oral glucose load. The 75-g load is advocated by the World Health Organization (WHO) and is more sensitive and less specific than the 100-g load, which is advocated by the American Diabetes Association (ADA). An observational study conducted in Brazil in approximately 5000 women reported a prevalence of GDM of 2.4% based on ADA criteria using the 2-h 75-g OGTT diagnostic criteria, and 7.2% based on WHO criteria.[23] Either test should be performed in the morning with the patient seated after an overnight fast of 8–14 h. Over the preceding 3 days the patient should have unrestricted carbohydrate intake and unrestricted physical activity. Two or more positive values are necessary for the diagnosis of GDM.

Table 15.1 Diagnostic criteria for GDM

	ADA	ADA	WHO
Glucose load	100 g	75 g	75 g
Fasting plasma glucose (mg/dl)	95	95	126
1 h	180	180	–
2 h	155	155	140
3 h	140		–

To deal with disparity in diagnostic testing used throughout the world and its impact on estimation of prevalence of GDM and pregnancy outcomes, a *Hyperglycemia and Adverse Pregnancy Outcome* (HAPO) prospective observational study was undertaken.[24] Investigators analyzed several pregnancy outcomes in over 23,000 women with impaired glycemic control as determined by 75-g oral glucose tolerance test at 24–32 weeks gestation. Average fasting, 1-, and 2-h plasma glucose levels were 80.9 mg/dl, 134.1 mg/dl, and 111.0 mg/dl, respectively. The study demonstrated that primary outcomes (umbilical cord-blood C-peptide level, birth weight, neonatal hypoglycemia, and rate of cesarean delivery) were directly related to the levels of fasting, plasma glucose and 1-, and 2-h post-challenge glucose.

Despite the aforementioned criteria for diagnosis of GDM, there is evidence to suggest that one abnormal glucose tolerance test value is associated with increased risk of macrosomia, preeclampsia, and eclampsia.[25] It has also been demonstrated that treatment of women with one abnormal OGTT value results in reduction of such complications.[26]

Screening

It is essential that all women presenting for the first prenatal visit be assessed for their risk of developing gestational diabetes. A fasting plasma glucose level ≥126 mg/dl (7.0 mmol/l) or a casual plasma glucose ≥200 mg/dl (11.1 mmol/l) meets the threshold for the diagnosis of diabetes, if confirmed on a subsequent day, and precludes the need for any glucose challenge.

The ADA and ACOG advocate a two-step approach to screening. A 50-g glucose challenge test is performed on all average risk patients at 24–28 weeks. If the threshold level (>140 mg/dl at 1 h) is met, the above 100-g oral glucose tolerance test is performed.[27] Cutoff of 140 mg/dl at 1 h has been traditionally used, identifying 80% of patients with gestational diabetes. The cutoff of 130 mg/dl, however, identifies approximately 90%, but has a higher false-positive rate.[28] Both ADA and American College of Obstetricians and Gynecologists (ACOG) consider either cutoff as abnormal.[28]

Women who are deemed to be at high risk should undergo blood glucose testing as early as possible in the pregnancy using the one- or two-step procedure. If they do not meet the diagnostic threshold the testing should be repeated at 24–28 weeks. High-risk characteristics include: obesity, family history of type 2 DM, personal history of prior GDM, glucose intolerance, or glucosuria.[27] Polycystic ovary syndrome could be a risk factor for GDM as well.[29]

An area of continued controversy is whether low-risk women should undergo screening. Low-risk characteristics include: age <25, normal weight before pregnancy, no known diabetes in first-degree relatives, no history of poor obstetric outcome, no history of abnormal glucose metabolism, and member of an ethnic group with a low prevalence of GDM. The ADA does not recommend screening women who meet all of the aforementioned criteria. In a study of 573 low-risk pregnant women, a 2.8% prevalence of GDM was found using the 75-g glucose tolerance test. There was no difference in pregnancy outcomes in this group when compared to other patients with GDM. Ten percent of all cases of GDM would have been missed if low-risk patients had not been screened.[30] Thus, many experts advocate continued screening of all pregnant women.[31] While American College of Obstetrics and Gynecology (ACOG) recommends that all pregnant patients should be screened for GDM, United States Preventive Services Task Force (USPSTF) proposed that there was insufficient evidence to recommend for or against universal screening for GDM.[32]

One-step approach involves a diagnostic oral glucose tolerance test (OGTT) without prior plasma or serum glucose screening. The one-step approach may be cost-effective in high-risk patients or populations (e.g., some Native American groups).

Morbidity

The consequences of untreated gestational diabetes have been well described. Maternal glucose crosses the placenta, while insulin does not. Thus, maternal hyperglycemia leads to fetal hyperinsulinemia, which results in macrosomia (typically defined as birth weight more than 4000 g) and neonatal hypoglycemia. Maternal consequences of gestational diabetes include: preeclampsia, polyhydramnios, operative delivery, and future development of overt diabetes. Fetal and infant consequences include: macrosomia, shoulder dystocia, polycythemia, hyperbilirubinemia, and increased risk of developing obesity and diabetes in later life (Table 15.2).[33]

Table 15.2 Morbidity of gestational diabetes

Maternal	Fetal and newborn
Preeclampsia	Neonatal hypoglycemia
C-section	Macrosomia
Polyhydramnios	Shoulder dystocia
	Polycythemia
	Hypocalcemia
	Hyperbilirubinemia
	Future DM, obesity

There is now ample evidence that identification and treatment of women who meet the above diagnostic criteria are associated with decreased perinatal morbidity. It appears that strict metabolic control is necessary to reduce macrosomia and mortality. A reduction in macrosomia has been shown to occur only in patients who achieve a FBG of <95 mg/dl.[34] A prospective controlled trial compared the pregnancy outcomes of 102 women with gestational diabetes who were under strict control with 102 nondiabetic controls. The women with gestational diabetes were treated with diet or diet and insulin to achieve a BG < 130 mg/dl 1 h after breakfast. The perinatal outcomes in the pregnancies complicated by gestational diabetes were equal to the control pregnancies.[35] An important study showed that postprandial, rather than preprandial, blood glucose monitoring resulted in improved glycemic control and decreased the risk of macrosomia (12% vs. 42%, $p = 0.010$), cesarean delivery (12% vs. 36%, $p = 0.04$), and neonatal hypoglycemia (3% vs. 25%, $p = 0.05$).[36]

Target Glucose Levels

Noting that there is considerable variation in peak glucose excursion after initiation of a meal (45–120 min), the Fifth International Workshop-Conference on Gestational Diabetes Mellitus proposed the following recommendations for glycemic goals in GDM (plasma glucose):[18]

Fasting	<96 mg/dl
1-h postprandial	<140 mg/dl
2-h postprandial	<120 mg/dl

However, the goals put forward by other investigators are more stringent[37]:

Fasting	<90 mg/dl
1-h postprandial	<120 mg/dl

Fifth International Workshop-Conference also pointed out that overtreatment of glycemia (meal capillary glucose levels <87 mg/dl) can result in increased risk of intrauterine growth retardation (IUGR).[18]

In order to meet the above goals for normoglycemia in pregnancy, self-monitoring of blood glucose is essential. Weekly monitoring of blood glucose levels is unlikely to identify women at risk for perinatal complications. Self-monitoring of blood glucose levels is necessary even in patients treated with diet therapy alone so that those failing to meet euglycemic goals can be identified as early as possible. Blood glucose testing should preferably be performed before meals, after meals, and at bedtime to ensure attainment of ideal glycemic control.

Diet Therapy and Exercise

A nutritionist or other professional should provide dietary advice to women with gestational diabetes. Limiting carbohydrate intake to 35–45% of total calories is the cornerstone of this therapy.[38] The avoidance of simple carbohydrates is advocated as they lead to high postprandial glucose values. In addition caloric restriction should be imposed on obese patients. A weight gain of only 7 kg is permitted for patients with a pre-pregnancy BMI of >29 kg/m^2, while patients with a pre-pregnancy BMI of <19 kg/m^2 should gain up to 18 kg.[39] Excessive weight gain can be associated with macrosomia. Physical exercise has been shown to improve maternal glucose control and is advocated by the ADA for patients with gestational diabetes.[40] Fifth International Workshop-Conference recommends 30 min of physical activity a day if possible. This can consist of brisk walking or seated arm exercises for 10 min after each meal.[18]

Insulin

Women who fail to meet the above stated glycemic goals or who show signs of excess fetal growth should be started on insulin therapy. Since pregnancy is an insulin-resistant state, high doses of insulin are often required to maintain euglycemia. An initial starting dose of insulin can be estimated as 0.7 units/kg/day up to 18th week of gestation, 0.8 units/kg/day for weeks 18–26, 0.9 units/kg/day for weeks 26–36, and 1.0 units/kg/day from week 36 to delivery.[2] Women who are obese might require doses of up to 2 units/kg/day. Most patients will require at least three injections (prebreakfast, predinner, bedtime) to achieve the described goals.

The new synthetic human insulin analogs, lispro and aspart, are now in common use during pregnancy. Their rapid onset of action has been shown to improve postprandial blood glucose levels, which is particularly important in pregnant diabetics. They are considered to be category B for pregnancy by the Food and Drug Administration. There have been no reports of another short-acting analog glulisine use in pregnancy. There is not much available experience with long-acting insulin analogs such as insulin glargine. Its use is not currently recommended. Of interest, a recent case–control study (use of glargine during pregnancy) demonstrated no difference in neonatal morbidity or fetal macrosomia in a group of women treated with insulin glargine vs. intermediate-acting human insulin.[41] NPH is a preferred intermediate agent of choice.

Oral agents are not approved for use in pregnancy. Nevertheless, studies have shown similar outcomes in a group of 201 patients with gestational diabetes treated with glyburide compared with a group of 203 insulin-treated patients.[42] Larger studies that address the effect of glyburide on postpartum progression of the woman with GDM toward glucose intolerance/diabetes, GDM recurrence, and long-term impact on the offspring are needed before the use of sulfonylureas can be recommended during pregnancy.[18]

Metformin crosses the placenta and, at present, the FDA does not recommend it for the treatment for GDM. However, a recent randomized open-label trial assigned 751 women with GDM at 20–33 weeks gestation to receive either metformin or insulin.[43] This study demonstrated that the rate of primary composite outcome (neonatal hypoglycemia, respiratory distress, need for phototherapy, birth trauma, 5-min Apgar score <7, or prematurity) was comparable in both groups. Nevertheless, 46.3% of patients in the metformin group required supplemental insulin. The rate of c-section was not reported.

Labor and Delivery

It is very important to prevent maternal hyperglycemia late in gestation as it can result in fetal hyperinsulinemia and neonatal hypoglycemia. Blood glucose should be maintained in the range of 70–90 mg/dl.[2] As the delivery of placenta occurs, there is a considerable reduction in pregnancy-related insulin resistance. Most women with GDM will not require insulin once active labor begins and rarely require insulin after delivery. Blood glucose needs to be obtained on the day after delivery to make sure hyperglycemia is resolved.

There are no data to support delivery of women with GDM before 38 weeks gestation if evidence of maternal or fetal compromise is absent. There is a lack of information on the risk of perinatal morbidity/mortality in the infants of women with well-controlled GDM if pregnancy proceeds beyond 40 weeks gestation. However, it is prudent to intensify fetal surveillance when pregnancy continues beyond 40 weeks gestation.[18]

Postpartum

According to the Fifth International Workshop, there is evidence to suggest that breastfeeding might have a beneficial effect on the development of postpartum diabetes in women with GDM. Therefore, breastfeeding should be encouraged.[18]

Since insulin is degraded in the GI tract of an infant, women who are breastfeeding can safely use any type of insulin. Glyburide and glipizide may also be utilized.[44] There are some data to suggest that metformin is excreted into breast milk in small amounts. However, this seems not to have any deleterious effects on the infant.[45] At present, larger studies are needed to determine safety of metformin in breastfeeding mothers.

Fetal Surveillance

The intensity of fetal monitoring is determined by the severity of GDM. At a minimum, patients treated with diet alone should be taught to measure fetal movements during the last 8–10 weeks of pregnancy. Patients who are being treated with insulin should undergo non-stress testing beginning at 32 weeks gestation. Fetal ultrasound may be used to assess fetal size at 29–33 weeks and should be used for detection of fetal anomalies in patients who had GDM diagnosed during the first trimester or who have fasting plasma glucose of >120 mg/dl.[39] Recent evidence suggested use of fetal ultrasound rather than strict glycemic parameters as a guide for initiation of insulin therapy. This approach would minimize glucose testing and insulin utilization in low-risk pregnancies.[46]

Long-Term Consequences to Mother and Offspring

Women who have had GDM are at high risk for developing type 2 diabetes. Approximately 35–60% of these women develop type 2 diabetes within 10 years.[18] Risk factors for development of diabetes in these women are the following: gestational age at diagnosis, severity of GDM, level of glycemia at the first postpartum visit, obesity, and further pregnancy.[40] Women with GDM should be evaluated for glucose intolerance using a 75-g oral glucose tolerance test 6–12 weeks postpartum and annually thereafter. Measuring fasting glucose only does not carry adequate sensitivity.[18] Counseling women on the risks of glucose intolerance and future diabetes is essential.

The children of women who have had GDM have increased risk of developing obesity and abnormal glucose tolerance by the time of puberty. The health-care providers of these children should be aware of this risk so that they can encourage their patients to make appropriate lifestyle changes.[39]

Pregestational Diabetes

When treating patients with type 1 and type 2 diabetes, it is essential to assess not only the effect the diabetes has on the pregnancy but also the impact the pregnancy has on diabetic complications, such as retinopathy and nephropathy.[7]

Unlike most patients with gestational diabetes who develop hyperglycemia during the second half of pregnancy, patients with pregestational diabetes may be hyperglycemic from conception. The presence of poor glycemic control during the first 7 weeks of fetal development results in significant rates of congenital malformations and fetal mortality.[47] It cannot be overemphasized that women with pregestational diabetes should receive intensive preconception counseling and achieve tight glycemic control before becoming pregnant. If no such counseling took place, and a woman presents at the beginning of her pregnancy, it is imperative that glucose control is achieved in 24–48 h only after a consultation with an ophthalmologist (see diabetic retinopathy).[2]

Congenital Malformations

Before the introduction of insulin diabetic women were rarely able to produce viable offspring. The introduction of insulin and improvement in glycemic control have led to decreased rates of fetal death and congenital malformations. Malformations appear to be a result of metabolic derangements, predominantly hyperglycemia, early in organogenesis. The exact mechanism by which hyperglycemia causes anomalies remains undetermined, but likely involves generation of oxygen free radicals and the disruption of the embryonic yolk sac.[48] Alterations in other metabolites such as myo-inositol,[49] arachidonic acid,[50] prostaglandins[48] have also been postulated to play a role in the dysmorphogenesis. These data are largely derived from animal studies and further work will need to be done to fully understand the pathogenesis of the malformations.

The level of glycemic control early in organogenesis has been shown to impact rates of malformations. Miller et al. showed that a HBA1C in the first trimester of >8.5% was associated with a malformation rate of 22.4%, a HBA1C 7–8.4% was associated with a rate of 5%, while a HBA1C <6.9% was associated with no excessive malformations.[51] The duration of diabetes and the presence of vasculopathy have also been shown to be associated with an increased risk of anomalies.[52]

Clinical trials have clearly shown that attainment of euglycemia before conception eliminates the excessive risk of congenital malformations. The incidence of major malformations in women with careful preconception care has been reported to be 0.8–1.6%, which is similar to nondiabetic mothers, compared with 6.5–8.2% in women who did not receive preconception care.[53–55]

Preconception Care

Pregnancy must be a planned event for women with type 1 and type 2 diabetes. It had been pointed out that women with type 2 diabetes are less likely to receive preconception care because the disease has often gone undiagnosed.[47] In addition, type 2 diabetes is also more prevalent in minority groups who may have limited access to care.

The goals of preconception care are to achieve a HBA1C as low as possible without the development of hypoglycemia.[56] Patients with type 2 diabetes who are being treated with oral agents must be switched to insulin, as there are currently no oral agents approved for use in pregnancy in the United States. Patients should become facile with frequent blood glucose monitoring and self-adjustment of insulin. Conception should be deferred until the patient is normoglycemic:

Fasting plasma glucose (PG) <95 mg/dl
1-h postprandial PG <140 mg/dl
2-h postprandial PG <120 mg/dl

Another important aspect of preconception care is the identification of diabetic complications that might be aggravated by pregnancy. A dilated retinal exam, blood pressure measurement, and cardiovascular exam are suggested.[66] Evaluation of renal function, via a 24-h urine collection for microalbumin/creatinine, and thyroid function, via TSH, are essential components of the initial visit. Hypertensive women should be treated with agents such as aldomet, which have been shown to be safe in pregnancy; ACE inhibitors, diuretics, and beta blockers should be avoided because of the associated risk of congenital malformations (Table 15.3).[56]

Table 15.3 Preconception care – initial visit

HbA1C
Blood glucose record
24-h urine microalbumin/creat
TSH
Blood pressure
Retinal exam
Cardiovascular evaluation
Neurological exam
Nutritional evaluation
Counseling on risks of pregnancy

Diabetic Retinopathy

Progression of diabetic retinopathy is a risk of tightened metabolic control in early pregnancy. A prospective study of 140 diabetic women without proliferative retinopathy revealed progression of retinopathy in 10.3% of patients with no retinopathy, 21.1% of patients with microaneurysms, 54.8% of patients with moderate to severe nonproliferative retinopathy. Proliferative retinopathy developed in 6.3% of patients with mild and 29% of patients with moderate to severe retinopathy. The odds ratio of developing proliferative disease in patients with HBA1C >6 SD above the mean vs. 2 SD above the mean was 2.7.[57] Risk factors for progression to proliferative retinopathy are the following: baseline retinopathy, elevated HBA1C at conception, rapid normalization of blood glucose, duration of diabetes greater than 6 years, and proteinuria.[47] One of the proposed mechanisms of retinopathy that occurs with rapid normalization of blood sugar is retinal deterioration due to increased growth-promoting factors and retinal extravasation of serum proteins.[2]

Diabetic Nephropathy

Careful assessment of renal function is mandatory in all diabetic women planning a pregnancy. The increased glomerular filtration rate seen in pregnancy often results in increased proteinuria; thus, a 24-h urine for microalbumin and creatinine should be collected prior to conception. Although pregnancy is associated with a transient decline in renal function, it does not appear to hasten the onset of end-stage renal disease in women with nephropathy.[58] The ideal medical therapy for diabetic nephropathy, ACE inhibitors, is contraindicated during pregnancy. Alpha methyl-dopa is considered safe during early pregnancy. Diltiazem, which is a more effective agent in preventing progression of nephropathy, can be used at the end of the first trimester.[59] Preeclampsia is the most common complication in patients with overt nephropathy; other maternal complications include anemia and nephrotic syndrome. Fetal complications include fetal distress, intrauterine growth retardation, preterm delivery, and stillbirth. Diabetic nephropathy, in the absence of HTN, impacts fetal outcome when renal function is impaired by at least 50%.[47] With improved preconception and perinatal glycemic and blood pressure control, perinatal mortality has decreased to 5%.[47]

Treatment

Close follow-up by a diabetic team is required throughout gestation to assure maintenance of strict glycemic control. Office visits every 2–3 weeks are usually necessary with more frequent telephone contact as needed (Table 15.4).

Table 15.4 Plan of care in diabetic pregnancy

Five to nine blood glucose measurements/day
HBA1C every 4–6 weeks
Office visits every 2–3 weeks
Telephone contact (as needed)
Fetal surveillance

Multiple blood glucose measurements and insulin injections are often required to achieve tight glycemic control. As noted previously, postprandial monitoring seems to result in improved fetal outcome. Indeed, postprandial blood glucose levels are the most important predictor of fetal macrosomia.[60] HBA1C should be monitored to confirm the level of control. The usual insulin requirements in type 1 diabetes are similar to those used in GDM as outlined above. Insulin pump therapy can achieve glucose control and perinatal outcomes equal to multiple injection regimens.[61]

As discussed for women with gestational diabetes, women with type 2 diabetes must be treated with insulin during pregnancy. Again, insulin requirements in these patients are often high due to obesity and insulin resistance.

Diet and Exercise

As discussed for women with gestational diabetes, a nutritionist or other professional should follow pregnant patients with type 1 or type 2 diabetes closely. Recommended caloric intake should be determined by pregestational weight. A total of 24 kcal/kg/day is recommended for women at ideal body weight. About 40–50% of calories should be from carbohydrate, 20% from protein, and 30–40% from fat. Calories are distributed over the course of the day as follows: 10% for breakfast, 30% for lunch, 30% for dinner, and 30% for snacks.[47] Like for women with gestational diabetes, exercise may be beneficial for pregnant patients with type 2 diabetes. Exercise in pregnant women with type 1 diabetes may lead to increased hypoglycemic episodes and is only permitted in women who participated in an exercise program prior to becoming pregnant.[47]

Hypoglycemia

Hypoglycemia is an important complication of tight glucose control during pregnancy. Early pregnancy is associated with decreased fasting glucose levels due to increased glucose uptake by the placental fetal unit and decreased hepatic glucose production. Thirty-three percent of all pregnant women treated with insulin have at least one episode of hypoglycemia during pregnancy.[62] The majority of these episodes occur during the first trimester. Recurrent episodes of hypoglycemia may be associated with small for gestational age infants[39] and severe prolonged episodes of hypoglycemia can result in intrauterine fetal demise.[63]

Diabetic Ketoacidosis (DKA)

Although its frequency has decreased markedly, diabetic ketoacidosis remains a serious emergency in the pregnant woman with type 1 diabetes and is associated with increased fetal morbidity and mortality. Ketogenesis appears to be accelerated during the third trimester. The mechanism by which DKA results in poor fetal outcome is not clear but is hypothesized to involve fetal hypoxia. Another possibility is that the fetus develops acidosis and hypokalemia with subsequent cardiac arrest.[64] The fetal heart rate should be continuously monitored while the mother is undergoing intensive treatment for DKA. It is also prudent to alert a neonatologist.

Labor and Delivery

The maintenance of maternal euglycemia at delivery is necessary in order to prevent neonatal hypoglycemia. The goal of insulin therapy is to keep the blood glucose between 70 and 90 mg/dl.[47] This can be best accomplished via a continuous intravenous insulin infusion. When active labor begins the maternal insulin requirements usually decline and drop even further as the placenta is expelled. Thus, intravenous glucose should be started once active labor begins. After the delivery the mother may not require any insulin therapy for 24–72 h. The cause of this clinical observation remains speculative but may be attributed to a state of functional hypopituitarism after delivery of the placenta (Lois Jovanovic, September 2001, personal communication) or recovery of β-cells.[65]

Fetal Surveillance

Fetal surveillance may be deferred until the 35th week in patients with pregestational diabetes who have been under strict metabolic control. Those patients with poor control, nephropathy, hypertension, or vascular disease should begin surveillance at week 26. The best method of surveillance is via fetal ultrasound, which can estimate gestational age, screen for anomalies, determine amniotic fluid volume, and assess fetus status through Doppler and biophysical profiles.[47]

Summary

The presence of diabetes in a pregnant woman can result in serious maternal and neonatal morbidity and mortality if not treated appropriately. Screening pregnant women for gestational diabetes and attainment of euglycemia, either by diet or insulin therapy, clearly prevents potentially catastrophic maternal and fetal events. Pregnancies that suffer from hyperglycemia early in gestation are at high risk for fetal loss and malformations. Thus, preconception care is essential for all type 1 and type 2 diabetic women. Diabetic women of reproductive age must be continually reminded of the need to plan their pregnancies. Maintenance of strict glycemic control requires tremendous effort on the part of the patient and the health-care team. This should be considered an achievable goal in all pregnant women with diabetes.

References

1. Martin JA, Hamilton BE, Sutton PD, et al. Births: final data for 2002. *Natl Vital Stat Rep*. 2003;52:1.
2. Jovanovic L, Nakai Y. Successful pregnancy in women with type 1 diabetes: from preconception through postpartum care. *Endocrinol Metab Clin North Am*. 2006;35:79–97.

3. American Diabetes Association. Gestational diabetes. Available at: http://www.diabetes.org/gestational-diabetes.jsp. Accessed June 12, 2008.
4. Coustan DR. Gestational diabetes. In: Harris MI, Cowie CC, Stern MP, Boyko EJ, Reiber GE, Bennett PH, eds. *Diabetes in America*. 2nd ed. Baltimore, MD: National Institutes of Health; 1995:703–717.
5. Hunt KJ, Schuller KL. The increasing prevalence of diabetes in pregnancy. *Obstet Gynecol Clin North Am*. 2007;34(2):173–199.
6. Mauricio D, Balsells M, Morales J, Corcoy R, Puig-Domingo M, de Leiva A. Islet cell autoimmunity in women with gestational diabetes and risk of progression to insulin-dependent diabetes mellitus. *Diabetes Metab Rev*. 1996;12(4):275–285.
7. Ryan EA. Prevention and treatment of diabetes and its complications: pregnancy and diabetes. *Medical Clinics of North America*. 1998;82:823–845.
8. Boden G. Fuel metabolism in pregnancy and gestational diabetes mellitus. *Obstet Gynecol Clin*. 1996;23:1–10.
9. Kuhl C. Etiology and pathogenesis of gestational diabetes. *Diabetes Care*. 1998;21(Suppl 2):B19.
10. Desoye G, Hauguel-de Mouzon S, Shafrir E. The Placenta in diabetic pregnancy. In: Hod M, Jovanovic L, Di Renzo G, de Leiva A, Langer O, eds. *Textbook of Diabetes and Pregnancy*. New York: Martin Dunitz; 2003:126–149.
11. Setji T, Brown A, Feinglos M. Gestational diabetes mellitus. *Clin Diabetes*. 2005;23:17–22.
12. Xiang AH, Peters RK, Trigo E, Kjos SL, Lee WP, Buchanan TA. Multiple metabolic defects during late pregnancy in women at high risk for type 2 diabetes. *Diabetes*. 1999;48:848–854.
13. Krampl E, Kametas NA, Nowotny P, Roden M, Nicolaides KH. Glucose metabolism in pregnancy at high altitude. *Diabetes Care*. 2001;24(5):817–822.
14. Yogev Y, Ben-Haroush A, Hod M. Pathogenesis of gestational diabetes mellitus. In: Hod M, Jovanovic L, Di Renzo G, de Leiva A, Langer O, eds. *Textbook of Diabetes and Pregnancy*. New York: Martin Dunitz; 2003:39–49
15. Lain K, Catalano P. Metabolic changes in pregnancy. *Clin Obstet Gynecol*. 2007;50(4):938–948.
16. Kirwan JP, Haugel-De Mouzon S, Lepercq J, et al. TNF-alpha is a predictor of insulin resistance in human pregnancy. *Diabetes*. 2002;51:2207–2213.
17. Barbour LA, Shao J, Qiao L, et al. Human placental growth hormone causes severe insulin resistance in transgenic mice. *Am J Obstet Gynecol*. 2002;186:512–517.
18. Metzger B, Buchanan T, Coustan D, et al. Summary and recommendations of the fifth international workshop-conference on gestational diabetes mellitus. *Diabetes Care*. 2007;30(Suppl 2):S251–S260.
19. Buchanan TA. Pancreatic B cell defects in gestational diabetes: implications for pathogenesis and prevention of type 2 diabetes. *J Clin Endocrinol Metab*. 2001;86:989–993.
20. Miller HC. The effect of diabetic and prediabetic pregnancies on the fetus and newborn infant. *J Pediatr*. 1946;26:455–461.
21. O'Sullivan JB, Mahan CM. Criteria for the oral glucose tolerance test in pregnancy. *Diabetes*. 1964;13:285.
22. Coustan DR, Carpenter MW. The diagnosis of gestational diabetes. *Diabetes Care*. 1998;21:B5–B8.
23. Schmidt MI, Duncan BD, Reichelt AJ, Branchtein L, Matos MC, et al. Gestational diabetes mellitus diagnosed with a 2-h 75-g oral glucose tolerance test and adverse pregnancy outcomes. *Diabetes Care*. 2001;24:1151–1155.
24. The HAPO Study Cooperative Research Group. Hyperglycemia and adverse pregnancy outcomes. *N Engl J Med*. 2008;358:1991–2001.
25. Lindsay MK, Graves W, Klein L. The relationship of one abnormal glucose tolerance test value and pregnancy complications. *Obstet Gynecol*. 1989;73(1):103–106.
26. Langer O, Anyaegbunam A, Brustman L, Divon M. Management of women with one abnormal oral glucose tolerance test value reduces adverse outcome in pregnancy. *Am J Obstet Gynecol*. 1989;161(3):593–599.
27. American Diabetes Association. ADA position statement. *Diabetes Care*. 2001;24(Suppl 1):S77–S79.
28. Brody SC, Harris R, Lohr K. Screening for gestational diabetes: a summary of the evidence for the U.S. Preventive Services Task Force. *Obstet Gynecol*. 2003;101(2):380–392.
29. Mikola M, Hiilesmaa V, Halttunen M, Suhonen L, Tiitinen A. Obstetric outcome in women with polycystic ovarian syndrome. *Hum Reprod*. 2001;16:226–229.
30. Moses R, Moses J, Davis W. Gestational diabetes: Do lean young caucasian women need to be tested?. *Diabetes Care*. 1998;21:1803–1807.
31. Pettitt D. GDM: Who to test, how to test. *Diabetes Care*. 1998;21:1789–1790.
32. U.S. Preventive Services Task Force. Screening for gestational diabetes mellitus: recommendations and rationale. *Obstet Gynecol*. 2003;101(2):393–395.
33. Jovanovic L. American Diabetes Association's fourth international workshop – conference on gestational diabetes mellitus: summary and discussion. Therapeutic interventions. *Diabetes Care*. 1998;21(Suppl 2):B131-B137.
34. Oppermann W, Gugliucci C, O'Sullivan MJ, et al. Gestation diabetes and macrosomia. In: Camerini-Davalos RA, Cole HS, eds. *Early Control in Early Life*. New York: NY Academic; 1975:455–468.
35. Drexel H, Alefred B, Sigurd S, et al. Prevention of perinatal morbidity by tight metabolic control in gestational diabetes. *Diabetes Care*. 1988;11:761–776.
36. De Veciana M, Major C, Morgan M, Asrat T, et al. Postprandial versus preprandial blood glucose monitoring in women with gestational diabetes mellitus requiring insulin therapy. *N Engl J Med*. 1995;333:1237–1241.
37. Jovanovic-Peterson L, Bevier W, Peterson CM. The Santa Barbara County Health Care Services Program: birth weight change concomitant with screening for and treatment of glucose-intolerance of pregnancy: a potential cost-effective intervention?. *Am J Perinat*. 1997;14:221–227.

38. Major CA, Henry MH, De Veciana M, Morgan MA. The effects of carbohydrate restriction in patients with diet controlled gestational diabetes. *Obstet Gynecol*. 1998;91:600–604.

39. Metzger B, Coustan D. Summary and recommendations of the fourth international workshop – conference on gestational diabetes mellitus. *Diabetes Care*. 1998;21(Suppl 2):B161.

40. Jovanovic-Peterson L. *Medical Management of Pregnancy Complicated by Diabetes*. Alexandria, VA: American Diabetes Association; 1995.

41. Price N, Bartlett C, Gillmer MD. Use of insulin glargine during pregnancy: a case-control pilot study. *BJOG*. 2007;114:453–457.

42. Langer O, Conway DL, Berkus MD, et al. A comparison of glyburide and insulin in women with gestational diabetes mellitus. *N Engl J Med*. 2000;343:1134–1138.

43. Rowan JA, Hague WM, Gao W, Battin MR, Moore MP. Metformin versus insulin for the treatment of gestational diabetes. *N Engl J Med*. 2008;358:2003–2015.

44. Feig DS, Briggs GG, Kraemer JM, et al. Transfer of glyburide and glipizide into breast milk. *Diabetes Care*. 2005;28:1851–1855.

45. Hale TW, Kristensin JH, Hackett LP, et al. Transfer of metformin into human milk. *Diabetologia*. 2004;45:1509–1514.

46. Schaefer-Graf UM, Kjos SL, Fauzan OH, et al. A randomized trial evaluating a predominately fetal growth-based strategy to guide management of gestational diabetes in Caucasian women. *Diabetes Care*. 2004;27:297–302.

47. Jovanovic L. Medical emergencies in the patient with diabetes during pregnancy. *Endocrinol Metab Clin North Am*. 2000;29(4):771–787.

48. Reece EA, Eriksson UJ. The pathogenesis of diabetes associated congenital malformations. *Obstet Gynecol Clin*. 1996;23:29–45.

49. Hod M, Star S, Passoneau J, et al. Effect of hyperglycemia on sorbitol and myo-inositol content of cultured rat conceptus: failure of aldose reductase inhibitors to modify myo-inositol and dysmorphogeneis. *Biochem Biophys Res Commun*. 1986;140:974–980.

50. Pinter E, Reece EA, Ogbum P, et al. Relative essential fatty acid deficiency in hyperglycemia – induced embryopathy. *Am J Obstet Gynecol*. 1988;159:1484–1490.

51. Miller E, Hare JW, Cloherty JP, et al. Elevated maternal HBA1c and major congenital anomalies in infants of diabetic mothers. *N Engl J Med*. 1998;304:1331–1334.

52. Karlsson K, Kjeller I. The outcome of diabetic pregnancies in relation to the mother's blood glucose level. *Am J Obstet Gynecol*. 1972;112:213–220.

53. Fuhrmann K, Reiker H, Semmler K, et al. The effect of intensified conventional insulin therapy before and during pregnancy on the malformation rate in offspring of diabetic mothers. *Exp Clin Endocrinol*. 1984;83:173–177.

54. Damm P, Molsted-Pederson L. Significant decrease in congenital malformations in newborn infants of an unselected population of diabetic women. *Am J Obstet Gynecol*. 1989;161:1163–1167.

55. Willhoite MB, Benvert HW, Palomaki GE, et al. The impact of preconception counseling on pregnancy outcomes: the experience of the Maine Diabetes in Pregnancy Program. *Diabetes Care*. 1993;16:450–455.

56. American Diabetes Association. ADA position statement: preconception care of women with diabetes. *Diabetes Care*. 2001;24(Suppl 1):S66–S68.

57. Chew E, et al. Metabolic control and progression of retinopathy, the diabetes in early pregnancy study. *Diabetes Care*. 1995;18:631–637.

58. Leguizamon G, Reece EA. Effect of medical therapy on progressive nephropathy: influence of pregnancy, diabetes, and hypertension. *J Maternal Fetal Med*. 2000;9:70–78.

59. Kitzmiller JL, Combs CA. Diabetic nephropathy and pregnancy. *Obstet Gynecol Clin*. 1996;23:173.

60. Jovanovic-Peterson L, Peterson CM, Reed GF, et al. Maternal postprandial glucose levels predict birth weight: the diabetes in early pregnancy study. *Am J Obstet Gynecol*. 1991;164:103–111.

61. Gabbe S. New concepts and applications in the use of the insulin pump during pregnancy. *J Maternal Fetal Med*. 2000;9:42–45.

62. Coustan DR, Reece RA, Sherwin RS, et al. A randomized trial of the insulin pump vs. intensive conventional therapy in diabetic pregnancies. *JAMA*. 1986;255:631–636.

63. Whiteman VE, Homko CJ, Reece EA. Management of hypoglycemia and diabetic ketoacidosis in pregnancy. *Obstet Gynecol Clin*. 1996;23:87–107.

64. Kitzmiller JL. Diabetic ketoacidosis and pregnancy. *Contemp Obstet Gynecol*. 1982;20:141–148.

65. AACE Guidelines. AACE medical guidelines for clinical practice for the management of diabetes mellitus. *Endocr Pract*. 2007;13(Suppl 1):59–63.

Chapter 16
Secondary Causes of Diabetes Mellitus

Yana B. Garger, Prajesh M. Joshi, Ashutosh S. Pareek, Carla M. Romero, Amit K. Seth, and Adrienne M. Fleckman

Introduction

The diabetic syndromes include type 1 diabetes with immune destruction of the pancreatic islets, type 2 diabetes with a complex pathophysiology of insulin resistance combined with insulin secretory failure, distinct monogenetic abnormalities (maturity onset diabetes of the young – MODY), and extreme insulin resistance of several different etiologies. In addition, secondary causes of diabetes mellitus refer to a category in which diabetes is associated with other diseases or conditions. Presumably, the diabetes is caused by those conditions and could be reversed if those conditions were cured.

Secondary causes constitute less than 2% of total cases of diabetes mellitus. Mechanistically they can be considered in the broad categories of decreased insulin secretion, insulin resistance, and increased counter-regulation, although classification schemes are typically anatomical and pathophysiological (Table 16.1).

Decreased insulin secretion is generally seen in pancreatic diabetes following destruction of the endocrine pancreas with loss or impairment of insulin secretion and in somatostatinoma. Liver disease causes insulin resistance via unknown mechanisms. Counter-regulatory hormones balance the glucose-lowering action of insulin. Excess levels of the counter-regulatory hormones glucagon, catecholamines, cortisol, and growth hormone seen with exogenous administration or excess secretion by their respective tumors can elevate the blood glucose level. The pathogenesis of secondary diabetes is sometimes defined to include autoimmune mechanisms and antagonism of insulin action (discussed in other chapters). There are also a variety of infections (congenital rubella, cytomegalovirus) and rare genetic syndromes that are associated with insulin resistance or diabetes mellitus through unknown mechanisms.[1]

Diseases of the Exocrine Pancreas

Acute Pancreatitis

Acute inflammation of the pancreas can cause transient glucose elevation.[2] The incidence of abnormal carbohydrate metabolism in acute pancreatitis varies from 8 to 83%.[3] The wide range can be related to the cause of acute inflammation, with alcohol having a more damaging effect on pancreatic tissue and a higher incidence of glucose intolerance.[4] Hyperglycemia has also been correlated with tissue necrosis and a higher mortality.[2,5] The plasma insulin concentration is lower in patients with acute pancreatitis than in healthy control subjects and is associated with impaired insulin secretion in response to glucose or glucagon. Glucagon concentration is usually elevated and tends to remain high for at least 1 week.[6,7] Hyperglycemia usually subsides within weeks of the

A.M. Fleckman (✉)
Department of Medicine, Albert Einstein College of Medicine, Beth Israel Medical Center, New York, NY, USA
e-mail: fleckman@chpnet.org

L. Poretsky (ed.), *Principles of Diabetes Mellitus*, DOI 10.1007/978-0-387-09841-8_16,
© Springer Science+Business Media, LLC 2010

Table 16.1 Classification of secondary causes of diabetes mellitus

Diseases of the exocrine pancreas	*Endocrinopathies*
Pancreatectomy	Acromegaly
Acute pancreatitis	Cushing's syndrome
Chronic pancreatitis	Pheochromocytoma
Hemochromatosis	Hyperthyroidism
Carcinoma	Hyperparathyroidism
Cystic fibrosis	Hyperaldosteronism
Abnormalities of the endocrine pancreas and the endocrine gut	*Genetic syndromes*
Glucagonoma	Klinefelter's syndrome
Somatostatinoma	Turner's syndrome
Gastrinoma	Wolfram's syndrome
VIPoma (vasoactive intestinal peptide tumor)	Friedreich's syndrome
Carcinoid syndrome	Huntington's chorea
	Lawrence–Moon–Biedl syndrome
	Myotonic dystrophy
	Porphyria
	Prader–Willi syndrome
Liver disease	
Chronic liver disease and cirrhosis	
Hepatitis C	
Acute hepatitis	

acute attack. However, 24–35% of patients have glucose intolerance and 12% have diabetes mellitus following a single bout of acute pancreatitis.[8]

Chronic Pancreatitis

Chronic pancreatitis is an inflammatory condition that influences both digestive and endocrine function of the pancreas.[9] Although glucose intolerance is frequent in patients with chronic pancreatitis, overt diabetes mellitus usually occurs late in the course of the disease. Patients with chronic calcifying pancreatitis are at higher risk (60–70%) of developing diabetes and glucose intolerance than are patients with non-calcifying disease (15–30%),[10] with both insulin and glucagon secretion disturbed more strongly in calcific than in noncalcific pancreatitis.[11] Diabetes caused by chronic pancreatitis requires insulin therapy because of β-cell destruction, although lack of immunologic destruction may contribute to a slower destruction of the β-cells in chronic pancreatitis than in type 1 diabetes with greater preservation of β-cell function. Concomitant damage to the glucagon-secreting alpha cells results in a high incidence of hypoglycemia, with residual counter-regulation attributable to catecholamine secretion.[12] Despite the requirement for insulin in diabetes mellitus secondary to chronic pancreatitis, glucagon-like peptide 1(7–36) amide (GLP-1), an intestinally derived insulinotropic hormone, may be considered in select patients with preservation of α- and β-cell secretory capacity.[13] Neuropathy and retinopathy occur in increased frequency in these patients, while nephropathy and diabetic ketoacidosis are rare.[14]

Pancreatic Cancer

Impaired glucose tolerance, an early manifestation of pancreatic cancer in over 40%, may occur before the tumor becomes apparent.[15] Pancreatic cancer may be associated with abnormal islet cell function by primary alteration of islet cells by carcinogen, secondary damage by cancer cells,[16] or stimulation of the secretion of islet amyloid polypeptide (IAPP) through an unknown mechanism. IAPP causes cytotoxicity and apoptosis.[17,18] It was found that pancreatectomy in pancreatic cancer with diabetes mellitus and high level of IAPP is associated with the cure of diabetes and the disappearance of IAPP.[19]

Pancreatectomy

Total pancreatectomy, primarily used for the treatment of pancreatic cancer with large lesions in the head of the pancreas, is associated with a high incidence of glucose intolerance. Pancreatic resections that spare the duodenum, such as distal pancreatectomy, are associated with a lower incidence of new or worsened diabetes than is the standard or pylorus-preserving pancreaticoduodenectomy (Whipple procedure) or total pancreatectomy.

In addition to insulin deficiency, the endocrine abnormalities that accompany pancreatic resection can include pancreatic polypeptide (PP) deficiency with preservation of glucagon production if the resection is proximal or glucagon deficiency if the resection is distal. Glucagon deficiency increases susceptibility to hypoglycemia through loss of counter-regulation, and PP deficiency is considered to impair hepatic insulin action, thereby contributing to hyperglycemia. The resulting hepatic insulin resistance with persistent endogenous glucose production and enhanced peripheral insulin sensitivity results in a brittle form of diabetes, which can be difficult to manage.[20]

Cystic Fibrosis-Related Diabetes (CFRD)

Cystic fibrosis (CF) comprises a clinical triad of abnormalities involving the sweat glands, the exocrine pancreas, and the respiratory epithelium. CFRD, the principal extra-pulmonary complication of cystic fibrosis, occurs in 15–30% of adults with mean age of onset of 18–21 years[21,22] and up to 1% of children with the disease.[23] CFRD is primarily an insulinopenic condition. Early in the course of the disease, the β-cells appear normal. As the disease progresses, insulin secretion is impaired and delayed as a result of β-cell failure secondary to fibrosis, fatty infiltration, and amyloid deposition. Insulin resistance plays only a minor role. CFRD is associated with worsening of nutritional status, increased morbidity, decreased survival, and decrease in pulmonary function in patients with CF.[24] Early treatment with insulin may decrease morbidity.[25]

Pancreatic Infiltrative Diseases

Primary/Secondary Hemochromatosis

Hemochromatosis (bronze diabetes) is a state of iron overload due to either hereditary or secondary (acquired) causes. The acquired causes include transfusional iron overload anemias (thalassemia major, sideroblastic anemia, and chronic hemolytic anemia), chronic liver diseases (hepatitis C, alcoholic liver disease, nonalcoholic fatty liver),[26] and dietary or parenteral iron overload. Deposition of iron in the pancreas causes fibrosis and secondary diabetes in 30–60% of patients with advanced disease. Contributing factors include an inherited predisposition for diabetes mellitus, cirrhosis, and direct damage to the pancreas by deposition of iron.[27]

Although the exact mechanism of iron-induced diabetes is uncertain, iron excess seems to contribute initially to insulin resistance and subsequently to decreased insulin secretion as well as hepatic dysfunction.[28] Pancreatic islets have an extreme susceptibility to oxidative damage from iron-derived free radicals, perhaps because of the reliance on mitochondrial metabolism of glucose for glucose-induced insulin secretion, and low expression of the antioxidant defense system (Table 16.2).[29]

Abnormalities of the Endocrine Pancreas and the Endocrine Gut

β-Cells of the pancreas are responsible for insulin secretion and glucose homeostasis. Abnormalities in the non-β-cells of the pancreas can also be associated with abnormalities in glucose metabolism and cause glucose

Table 16.2 Frequency of diabetes mellitus in pancreatic diseases

Disease	Frequency (%)	Disease	Frequency (%)
Acute pancreatitis	8–83	Partial pancreatectomy	20
Chronic pancreatitis	15	Total pancreatectomy	100
Chronic calcific pancreatitis	60–70	Cystic fibrosis	13
Pancreatic cancer	40	Hemochromatosis	30–60

intolerance or secondary diabetes. Endocrine tumors of the non-β-cells of the pancreas and/or the gut that cause glucose intolerance include the following:

1. Hypersecretion of glucagon (glucagonoma)
2. Hypersecretion of somatostatin (somatostatinoma)
3. VIPoma (vasoactive intestinal peptide tumor)
4. Hypersecretion of gastrin (gastrinoma)
5. Carcinoid syndrome

Glucagonoma

The glucagonoma syndrome is a rare disorder of a glucagon-secreting tumor, with an annual incidence of 0.1 cases per million.[30,31] Presentation is usually in the fifth decade of life, with an even distribution between females and males. The tumors arise almost exclusively in the pancreas and are malignant in behavior, with 50% having metastasized to liver or lymph nodes at the time of diagnosis. Patients develop the "4D syndrome" of *d*iabetes, *d*ermatitis (necrolytic migratory erythema), *d*eep-vein thrombosis, and *d*epression. Hypersecretion of glucagon also produces glucose intolerance in 80% of patients, with or without frank diabetes mellitus.[32] Glucagon is one of the "counter-regulatory" hormones that balance the glucose-lowering action of insulin with actions to raise the circulating glucose levels. Glucagon increases hepatic glucose output via glycogenolysis and gluconeogenesis[33] causing hyperglycemia in the glucagonoma syndrome.

Somatostatinoma

Somatostatinomas are neuroendocrine tumors that usually originate in the pancreas or the intestine. The release of large amounts of somatostatin causes a distinct clinical syndrome characterized by diabetes mellitus, gallbladder disease, diarrhea, and weight loss. The development of diabetes mellitus is likely secondary to the inhibitory action of somatostatin on insulin release as well as replacement of functional pancreatic tissue.[34,35]

VIPoma Syndrome

The VIPoma syndrome is due to a rare pancreatic endocrine tumor that secretes excessive amounts of vasoactive intestinal peptide (VIP). This causes a distinct syndrome of fasting large volume diarrhea, hypokalemia, and hypochlorhydria (due to gastric acid suppression). Hyperglycemia is noted in 25–50% of patients with VIPomas. It has been attributed to the glycogenolytic effects of VIP on the liver.[36]

Gastrinoma (Zollinger–Ellison) Syndrome

Zollinger–Ellison (ZE) syndrome is characterized by gastrin-producing tumors (gastrinoma), hypersecretion of gastric acid, and recurrent peptic ulcers. The tumors usually originate from the pancreas and less frequently from the duodenum. Glucose intolerance and diabetes have been reported in patients with ZE syndrome.[37] It is unclear if gastrin overproduction is the cause of glucose intolerance. Twenty to sixty percent of patients with ZE syndrome have gastrinoma as part of the genetic multiple endocrine neoplasia (MEN) syndrome.

Carcinoid Syndrome

One report focuses on the link between diabetes mellitus and carcinoid tumors, relating a 50–80% incidence of diabetes or glucose intolerance to active secretion of serotonin.[38] It is more probable that diabetes seen with carcinoid syndrome is related to tumor secretory products such as somatostatin, glucagon, or ACTH causing Cushing's syndrome.[39]

Liver Disease as a Cause of Secondary Diabetes Mellitus

The liver plays a major role in glucose homeostasis.[40] It produces glucose by both glycogenolysis (breakdown of glycogen) and gluconeogenesis (newly synthesized glucose). It is a major organ in glucose storage in the form of glycogen.

Insulin increases hepatic glucose uptake and suppresses hepatic glucose production. This results in increase in glycogen synthesis and deposition in the liver. Opposing this action, glucagon decreases hepatic glucose uptake from the portal system.

Nonalcoholic Fatty Liver Disease (NAFLD), Chronic Hepatitis, and Cirrhosis

The incidence of impaired glucose tolerance and diabetes is increased in chronic liver disease.[41,42] Insulin resistance is a characteristic feature of patients with liver cirrhosis.[43] Even in the absence of cirrhosis, portal hypertension is associated with insulin resistance,[44] manifested as insulin resistance in 80% of cirrhotic patients, with 20–60% developing overt diabetes mellitus.[45] In total, an astounding 95% of patients with cirrhosis have diabetes or glucose intolerance.[46] Both insulin resistance and inadequate insulin secretion by the β-cells contribute to glucose intolerance in patients with cirrhosis.[43] Inflammatory pathways are invoked as a link between liver disease and glucose intolerance, especially in NAFLD.[47,48] Hyperglycemia in chronic liver disease may also occur as a result of the therapeutic administration of various medications including interferons and corticosteroids. Cirrhotic patients with overt diabetes have a high mortality rate, with an increased risk of liver cell failure. Thus, the presence of diabetes in cirrhotic patients is a risk factor for long-term survival.[46,49,50]

Hepatitis C

Overt diabetes mellitus is more prevalent in patients with chronic hepatitis C than in patients with other liver diseases.[51–57] Risk factors for the development of glucose intolerance in patients with hepatitis C include hepatitis C viremia, male gender, hypertension, BMI, and age.[58] The mechanism by which hepatitis C virus (HCV) infection induces glucose intolerance and diabetes is unknown. Many theories, including cytopathic and immunological mechanisms, have been proposed for the effect of HCV on extrahepatic tissues.[59,60] One possible mechanism is the upregulation of TNF-α by HCV. TNF-α has been shown to block tyrosine phosphorylation of insulin receptor substrate (IRS)-1, disrupting an important step in the insulin signaling cascade, with restoration of insulin sensitivity following administration of antibodies against TNF-α.[61] The HCV core protein upregulates the suppressor of cytokine signaling (SOCS)3 and downregulates, via ubiquitination, insulin receptor substrates (IRS) 1 and 2.[61–64] Thus, via these two mechanisms, the HCV core protein is thought to lead to insulin resistance. Insulin resistance impairs sustained response to antiviral therapy and is associated with increased severity of fibrosis in patients with chronic HCV.[65–68]

Acute Hepatitis

Acute hepatitis is associated with transient glucose intolerance or hypoglycemia,[69,70] with rare persistence of diabetes.[71,72]

For more detailed discussion of the relationship between liver disease and diabetes, please see Chapter 35.

Drug-Induced or Chemical-Induced Diabetes

Many drugs are known to cause glucose intolerance or diabetes mellitus (Table 16.3).[73]

Table 16.3 Some drugs causing impaired glucose tolerance and diabetes

Alcohol	Atypical antipsychotics
Nicotinic acid (Niacin)	Steroids, particularly glucocorticoids
Thiazides	Thyroid hormone
β-Blockers	β-Interferon
Calcium channel blockers	Cyclosporin
Clonidine	Diazoxide
Dilantin	Pentamidine
HIV* protease inhibitors	Megestrol acetate
Oral contraceptive pills	Vacor

*Human immunodeficiency virus.

Alcohol, when ingested acutely, has been associated with hypoglycemia due to its inhibitory effect on gluconeogenesis. This effect is mostly seen in fasted individuals with depleted glycogen stores who are dependent on gluconeogenesis to maintain hepatic glucose production. Acute large alcohol intake can cause insulin resistance in peripheral tissues, particularly in the muscles. When ingested on chronic basis, excessive alcohol intake has been associated with moderate to severe insulin resistance and glucose intolerance.

β-Adrenergic blockers are widely used in clinical practice. They are considered, along with diuretics, the first line of therapy for hypertension. They are known to promote hypoglycemia both by inhibiting hepatic glucose production directly and by blocking the counter-regulatory hormonal response to hypoglycemia. Studies have shown that non-diabetic patients on β-blockers (particularly the non-selective) may exhibit disturbance in their glucose homeostasis in the form of worsening glucose tolerance. This might be due to worsening insulin secretion or insulin action.

Pentamidine has multiphasic effect on the β-cell of the pancreas. Initially, pentamidine causes β-cell degranulation with the release of insulin, which results in hypoglycemia. Later, it causes β-cell destruction and impaired insulin secretion, resulting in hyperglycemia and even diabetic ketoacidosis.[74] Intravenous pentamidine can permanently destroy pancreatic β-cells and has been incriminated in the development of secondary diabetes in multiple cases.[75,76] These reactions, however, are considered rare. Impairment of insulin action can result from the administration of multiple drugs and hormones, such as nicotinic acid and steroids.[77,78]

Patients on α-interferon treatment for chronic hepatitis C are reported to develop diabetes with islet cell antibodies and, in some cases, insulin deficiency.[79] Vacor (pyriminil, synthetic organic rodenticide) can cause hyperglycemia, ketoacidosis, and irreversible diabetes, in addition to its toxic effect on the central and peripheral nervous system.[80]

Protease Inhibitors, Human Immunodeficiency Virus (HIV), and Glucose Intolerance

Undesirable physical and metabolic changes associated with HIV infection and therapy assume greater importance as life expectancy improves.[81] An acquired lipodystrophy syndrome occurs in a high proportion of chronically HIV-infected individuals and variably includes central obesity, dorsal fat pad, facial wasting, and wasting of the extremities. Insulin resistance, frank diabetes, and hyperlipidemia are associated with this lipodystrophy and presumably carry an increased risk of premature cardiovascular mortality.[82] The metabolic syndrome can occur in HIV-infected individuals in the absence of HIV-specific medications, increases in incidence with the use of some classes of drugs including reverse transcriptase inhibitors, and is greatest in those patients on protease inhibitors.[83] Investigation into mechanisms has included the role of mitochondrial toxicity in producing the syndrome, protection of lipid particles from degradation,[84] increased fatty acid and cholesterol biosynthesis,[85] inhibition of fat cell differentiation,[86] and inhibition of glucose transport into fat and muscle.[87] There is no accepted or proven safe therapy.

For detailed discussion of the relationship between HIV infection and diabetes, see Chapter 38.

Endocrinopathies

Acromegaly, a State of Growth Hormone Excess, Is Associated with Hyperglycemia and Insulin Resistance

The major players in the growth hormone (GH) system are GH and IGF-1 (insulin-like growth factor-1). GH and IGF-1 affect glucose and fat metabolism, as well as growth. They have opposing effects on carbohydrate metabolism (Fig. 16.1). A family of IGF-binding proteins (IGF-BPs) affects tissue delivery, availability of IGF-1, and gene transcription, thereby altering the balance between growth hormone and IGF-1. In some tissues, the IGF effects cooperate with the GH effects (for example, growth of long bones) and in other tissues, they are antagonistic (the metabolic effects).

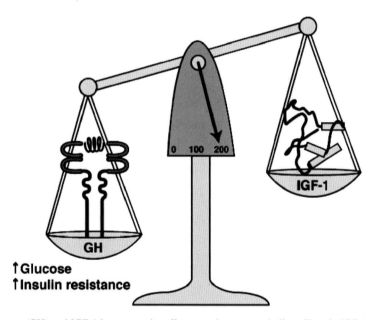

Fig. 16.1 Growth hormone (GH) and IGF-1 have opposite effects on glucose metabolism. Hepatic IGF-1 appears to be an insulin sensitizer and can lower blood glucose levels, while elevated GH raises blood glucose and is associated with insulin resistance[93]

Growth, mediated by IGF-1, is an anabolic process that requires cellular uptake of building components, such as amino acids and glucose. Administered separately from growth hormone, IGF-1 lowers elevated blood glucose levels and can cause hypoglycemia. In fact, IGF-1 has been used to treat diabetic ketoacidosis in insulin-resistant individuals.[88]

Growth hormone can be regarded as the metabolic partner of IGF-1 because growth hormone provides substrate for the effects of IGF-1. GH-stimulated fat mobilization and new glucose formation (gluconeogenesis) are required to make building components (substrate) available. Growth hormone acts on the fat cell to stimulate the hormone-sensitive lipase, causing lipolysis (breakdown of fat) with the release of glycerol and free fatty acids (FFAs). Glycerol is a precursor of hepatic gluconeogenesis. FFAs stimulate gluconeogenesis and are the precursors of ketogenesis.[89] FFA elevation also increases output of the lipoprotein VLDL, thereby elevating triglyceride levels.[90] FFAs become the preferred substrate for muscle uptake and oxidation. GH also causes inhibition of muscle uptake and oxidation of glucose, even though insulin concentrations are increased because of insulin resistance secondary to GH action.[91] GH excess in children and adolescents prior to closure of the growth plate of the long bones results in continued growth (gigantism). In adults, GH excess causes acromegaly (acral overgrowth). Acromegaly occurs with GH-secreting pituitary tumors and rarely with ectopic production of growth hormone-releasing hormone, usually by bronchial carcinoids or pancreatic neuroendocrine tumors. Even though GH stimulates IGF-1 secretion and IGF-1 levels are elevated in acromegaly, GH excess is potentially diabetogenic. The actions of GH to mobilize FFAs, stimulate gluconeogenesis, and inhibit insulin action may lead to impaired fasting glucose (30%) and frank diabetes mellitus (16%) in acromegaly.[92]

Cushing's Syndrome, Glucocorticoids, and 11-β-Hydroxysteroid Dehydrogenase

Glucocorticoids were named for their ability to raise blood glucose.[94] Excess glucocorticoid secretion or administration can lead to diabetes mellitus. Cushing's syndrome results from excess endogenous glucocorticoid (cortisol) secretion from adrenal gland tumors; from pituitary or other tumors secreting excessive amounts of ACTH, which stimulates adrenal cortisol production; or from exogenously administered glucocorticoids used in the treatment of asthma or autoimmune disorders. Glucose intolerance and diabetes mellitus are common in Cushing's syndrome, with frank diabetes or impaired glucose tolerance occurring in 50–90% of affected individuals. Cortisol is one of the counter-regulatory hormones and acts at many steps. One action is to increase the appetite, thereby increasing energy intake with an initial rise in blood glucose level. The lipogenic action of cortisol, to store nutrients in visceral fat tissue, contributes to insulin resistance. The major actions of cortisol, like those of growth hormone, lead to extrahepatic substrate mobilization. The lipolytic action of cortisol mobilizes energy from adipose tissue, providing precursors for increased hepatic glucose production.[95] Cortisol antagonizes the effects of insulin in muscle, preventing protein synthesis and inhibiting glucose utilization; further, its catabolic actions include muscle breakdown,[96] with the effect of delivering gluconeogenic precursors to the liver. In the liver, cortisol stimulates both gluconeogenesis and glycogen breakdown.

The pivotal role that cortisol may play in insulin resistance and type 2 diabetes mellitus is highlighted by observations that increased cortisol production in visceral fat can be shown in a transgenic mouse model to recreate the metabolic syndrome of insulin resistance, diabetes, and hypertension (Fig. 16.2).[97,98]

Pheochromocytoma

Pheochromocytomas, a general term applied to tumors of the adrenal medulla and the extra-adrenal chromaffin tissue, secrete catecholamines, especially norepinephrine. Headache related to extreme elevations of blood pressure (α_1-adrenergic stimulation), palpitations (β_1-adrenergic stimulation), anxiety, and diaphoresis dominates the clinical presentation. Diabetes occurs in up to 65% of pheochromocytomas, may mirror the paroxysmal rises in blood pressure, and has been demonstrated to resolve following tumor resection.[100] Pheochromocytomas whose major secretory product is epinephrine are much more likely than norepinephrine-secreting tumors to present with arrhythmias, non-cardiac pulmonary edema, hypotension, and hyperglycemia. This distinct presentation reflects the combined α- and β-adrenergic stimulation of epinephrine (Fig. 16.3). The more common norepinephrine-secreting tumors may also cause hyperglycemia since norepinephrine is also a mixed agonist, although with less β activity than does epinephrine.[101]

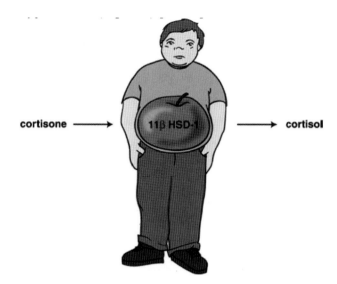

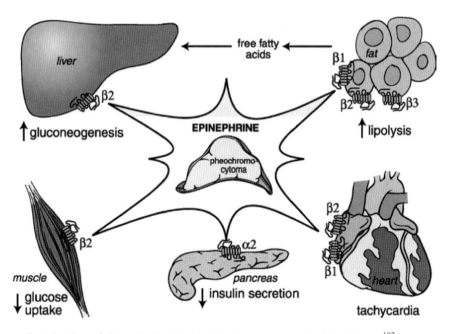

Fig. 16.2 Increased activity of 11-β-hydroxysteroid dehydrogenase type 1 in transgenic mice increases cortisol production in visceral fat and causes abdominal obesity and the metabolic syndrome resembling that seen in "apple-shaped" people[99]

Fig. 16.3 The coordinated actions of elevated epinephrine in pheochromocytoma raise blood glucose[102]

Hyperthyroidism

Thyroid hormone increases glucose transporters 4 (GLUT-4) in fat tissue and muscle, thereby enhancing the stimulatory effect of insulin.[103] Given the increase in metabolic rate caused by thyroid hormones, it is logical that increased fuel would be made available to tissues. It is paradoxical then that hyperthyroidism is sometimes associated with deterioration of glucose control or with onset of frank diabetes mellitus. Partial explanations implicate increased growth hormone secretion[104]; a hepatic gene expression profile that promotes gluconeogenesis and glycogenolysis, and decreases insulin action[105]; and increased hepatic GLUT-2 transporters, through which glucose effluxes out of the liver.[106]

Hyperaldosteronism

Primary hyperaldosteronism, the elevated secretion of the mineralocorticoid aldosterone resulting from adrenal cortical tumors, genetic mutations, or idiopathic hyperaldosteronism, is classified with the endocrinopathies that cause "other specific types" of diabetes mellitus.[1] Yet, little is known about the occurrence, the mechanism, or the resolution of the glucose intolerance seen with hypersecretion of aldosterone. One retrospective study found a prevalence of diabetes of 5–24% in hyperaldosteronism.[107] Physiologic potassium levels play a fundamental role in insulin secretion. Potassium stimulates glucose-induced insulin secretion, and insulin lowers serum potassium by driving the cation intracellularly.[108] The hypokalemia that occurs with renal potassium wasting in primary aldosteronism presumably has a restraining or inhibiting effect on insulin secretion and leads to glucose intolerance and diabetes in susceptible individuals. In addition, insulin resistance may occur.[109] The diabetes that occurs with hyperaldosteronism may (personal observation) or may not[110] resolve with cure of hyperaldosteronism.

Conclusion

Diverse organs and drugs are implicated in secondary diabetes mellitus. Pancreatic destruction is treatable only with insulin replacement. The link between liver disease and diabetes is poorly understood. The lipodystrophy and metabolic consequences of HIV infection and its therapies are under active investigation. Sometimes medications that cause diabetes may be discontinued, but others are life saving and lack appropriate substitutions. Cure of the endocrinopathies that cause diabetes may ameliorate or cure the associated diabetes. Ultimately, the explanation for the mechanisms that cause secondary diabetes mellitus can be sought in the basic physiology and pathophysiology of the secretion of insulin and its action on target tissues.

References

1. American Diabetes Association. Diagnosis and classification of diabetes mellitus. *Diabetes Care.* 2008;31(Suppl 1):S55–S60.
2. Pitchumoni CS, Patel NM, Shah P. Factors influencing mortality in acute pancreatitis. *J Clin Gastroenterol.* 2005;39:798–814.
3. Thow J, Semad A, Alberti KGMM. Epidemiology and general aspects of diabetes secondary to pancreatopathy. In: Tiengo A, Alberti KGMM, Del Prato S, Vranic M, eds. *Diabetes Secondary to Pancreatopathy.* Amsterdam: Excerpta Medica; 1988: 7–20.
4. Del Prato S, Tiengo A. Diabetes secondary to acquired disease of the pancreas. In: Alberti KGMM, DeFronzo RA, Keen H, Zimmet P, eds. *International Textbook of Diabetes Mellitus.* New York: John Wiley & Sons, Inc.; 1992:199.
5. Ueda T, Takeyama Y, Yasuda T, et al. Simple scoring system for the prediction of the prognosis of severe acute pancreatitis. *Surgery.* 2007;141:51–58.
6. Drew SI, Joffe B, Vinik AI, et al. The first 24 hours of acute pancreatitis. Changes in biochemical and endocrine homeostasis inpatients with pancreatitis compared to those in control subjects undergoing stress for reasons other than pancreatitis. *Am J Med.* 1978;64:795–803.
7. Donowitz M, Hendeler R, Spiro HM, et al. Glucagon secretion in acute and chronic pancreatitis. *J Intern Med.* 1975;83: 778–781.
8. Kaya E, Dervisoglu A, Polat C. Evaluation of diagnostic findings and scoring systems in outcome prediction in acute pancreatitis. *World J Gastroenterol.* 2007;13(22):3090–3094.
9. Andersen DK. Mechanisms and emerging treatments of the metabolic complications of chronic pancreatitis. *Pancreas.* 2007;35(1):1–15.
10. Mlka D, Hammel P, Sauvanet A, et al. Risk factors for diabetes mellitus in chronic pancreatitis. *Gastroenterology.* 2000;119:1324–1332.
11. Angelopoulos N, Dervenis C, Goula A, et al. Endocrine pancreatic insufficiency in chronic pancreatitis. *Pancreatology.* 2005;5:122–131.

12. Larsen S. Diabetes mellitus secondary to chronic pancreatitis. *Dan Med Bull*. 1993;40(2):153–162.
13. Hedetoft C, Sheikh SP, Larsen S, Holst JJ. Effect of glucagons-like peptide 1(7-36)amide in insulin-treated patients with diabetes mellitus secondary to chronic pancreatitis. *Pancreas*. 2000;20(1):25–31.
14. Mergener K, Baillie J. Chronic pancreatitis. *Lancet*. 1997;350:1379–1385.
15. Chari ST, Leibson CL, Rabe KG, et al. Pancreatic cancer-associated diabetes mellitus: prevalence and temporal association with diagnosis of cancer. *Gastroenterology*. 2008;134:95–101.
16. Murat S, Parviz PM. Diabetes and its relationship to pancreatic carcinoma. *Pancreas*. 2003;26(4):381–387.
17. Hull RL, Westermark GT, Westermark P, Kahn SE. Islet amyloid: a critical entity in the pathogenesis of type 2 diabetes. *J Clin Endocrinol Metab*. 2004;89:3629–3643.
18. Casas S, Gomis R, Gribble FM, et al. Impairment of the ubiquitin–proteasome pathway is a downstream endoplasmic reticulum stress response induced by extracellular human islet amyloid polypeptide and contributes to pancreatic β-cell apoptosis. *Diabetes*. 2007;56:2284–2294.
19. Permert J, Larsson J, Fruin AB, et al. Islet hormone secretion in pancreatic cancer patients with diabetes. *Pancreas*. 1997;15:60–68.
20. Slezak LA, Andersen DK. Pancreatic resection: effects on glucose metabolism. *World J Surg*. 2001;25:452–460.
21. Brennan AL, Geddes DM, Gyi KM, Baker EH. Clinical importance of cystic fibrosis-related diabetes. *J Cyst Fibros*. 2004;3(4):209–222.
22. Dobson L, Stride A, Bingham C, et al. Microalbuminuria as a screening tool in cystic fibrosis-related diabetes. *Pediatr Pulmonol*. 2005;39(2):103–107.
23. Shwachman H, Kowalski M, Khaw KT. Cystic fibrosis: a new outlook, 70 patients above 25 years of age. *Medicine*. 1977;56:24–49.
24. Alves Cde A, Aguiar RA, Alves AC, Santana MA. Diabetes mellitus in patients with cystic fibrosis. *J Bras Pneumol*. 2007;33(2):213–221.
25. Bizzarri C, Lucidi V, Ciampalini P, et al. Clinical effects of early treatment with insulin glargine in patients with cystic fibrosis and impaired glucose tolerance. *J Endocrinol Invest*. 2006;29(3):RC1–RC4.
26. Williams R, Williams HS, Scheuer PJ, et al. Iron absorption and siderosis in chronic liver disease. *Quart J Med*. 1967;35:151–166.
27. Powell LW, Yapp TR. Hemochromatosis. *Clin Liver Dis*. 2000;4(1):211–228.
28. Wilson J, Lindquist J, Grambow S, et al. Potential role of increased iron stores in diabetes. *Am J Med Sci*. 2003;325(6):332–339.
29. Swaminathan S, Fonseca V, Alam M, Shah S. The role of iron in diabetes and its complications. *Diabetes Care*. 2007;30(7):1926–1933.
30. Wermers RA, Fatourechi V, Wynne AG, et al. The glucagonoma syndrome. *Medicine*. 1996;75:53.
31. Warner R. Enteroendocrine tumors other than carcinoid: a review of clinically significant advances. *Gastroenterol*. 2005;128:1668–1684.
32. Beek AP, de Haas ERM, van Vloten WA, et al. The glucagonoma syndrome and necrolytic migratory erythema: a clinical review. *Eur J Endocrinol*. 2004;151:531–537.
33. Lefgbvre PJ. Glucagon and its family revisited. *Diabetes Care*. 1995;18:715–730.
34. Vinik AI, Strodel WE, Eckhauser FE, et al. Somatostatinomas, PPomas, neurotensinomas. *Semin Oncol*. 1987;14:263–281.
35. Sassolas G, Chayvialle JA. GRFomas, somatostatinomas: clinical presentation, diagnosis, and advances in management. In: Mignon M, Jensen RT, eds. *Endocrine Tumors of the Pancreas: Recent Advances in Research and Management*. Frontiers of Gastrointestinal Research, Vol. 23. Basel, Switzerland: S. Karger; 1995:194.
36. Matuchansky C, Rambuaud JC. VIPomas and endocrine cholera: clinical presentation, diagnosis, and advances in management. In: Mignon M, Jensen RT, eds. *Endocrine Tumors of the Pancreas: Recent Advances in Research and Management*. Frontiers of Gastrointestinal Research, Vol. 23. Basel, Switzerland: S. Karger; 1995:166.
37. McCallum RW, Parameswaran V, Burgess JR. Multiple endocrine neoplasia type 1 (MEN 1) is associated with an increased prevalence of diabetes mellitus and impaired fasting glucose. *Clin Endocrinol*. 2006;65:163–168.
38. Feldman JM, Plonk JW, Bivens CH, Levobitz HE. Glucose intolerance in the carcinoid syndrome. *Diabetes*. 1975;24:664–671.
39. Mitzner LD, Nohria A, Chacho M, Inzucchi SE. Sequential hypoglycemia, hyperglycemia, and the carcinoid syndrome arising from a plurihormonal neuroendocrine neoplasm. *Endocr Pract*. 2000;6:370–374.
40. DeFronzo RA, Ferrannini E. Regulation of hepatic glucose metabolism in humans. *Diabetes Metab Rev*. 1987;3:415–459.
41. Zein NN. Prevalence of diabetes mellitus in patients with end-stage liver cirrhosis due to hepatitis C, alcohol, or cholestatic disease. *J Hepatol*. 2000;32:209–217.
42. Tolman KG, Fonseca V, Dalpiaz A, Tan MH. Spectrum of liver disease in type 2 diabetes and management of patients with diabetes and liver disease. *Diabetes Care*. 2007;30(3):734–743.
43. Albright ES, Bell DSH. The liver, liver disease, and diabetes mellitus. *Endocrinol*. 2003;13(1):58–66.
44. Cavallo-Perin P, Cassader M, Bozzo C, et al. Mechanism of insulin resistance in human liver cirrhosis: evidence of combined receptor and postreceptor defect. *J Clin Invest*. 1985;75:1659–1665.
45. Harrison SA. Liver disease in patients with diabetes mellitus. *J Clin Gastroenterol*. 2006;40:68–76.
46. Holstein A, Hinze S, Thiessen E, et al. Clinical implications of hepatogenous diabetes in liver cirrhosis. *J Gastroenterol Hepatol*. 2002;17(6):677–681.

47. Shoelson SE, Lee J, Goldfine AB. Inflammation and insulin resistance. *J Clin Invest*. 2006;116:1793–1801.
48. Samuel VT, Liu ZX, Wang A, et al. Inhibition of protein kinase Cε prevents hepatic insulin resistance in nonalcoholic fatty liver disease. *J Clin Invest*. 2007;117:739–745.
49. Fartoux L, Poujol-Robert A, Guéchot J, et al. Insulin resistance is a cause of steatosis and fibrosis progression in chronic hepatitis C. *Gut*. 2005;54(7):1003–1008.
50. Hickman IJ, Macdonald GA. Impact of diabetes on the severity of liver disease. *Am J Med*. 2007;120(10):829–834.
51. Fraser GM, Harman I, Meller N, et al. Diabetes mellitus is associated with chronic hepatitis C but not chronic hepatitis B infection. *Isr J Med Sci*. 1996;32:526–530.
52. Knobler H, Schihmanter R, Zifroni A, et al. Increased risk of type 2 diabetes in noncirrhotic patients with chronic hepatitis C virus infection. *Mayo Clin Proc*. 2000;75:355–359.
53. Huang JF, Dai CY, Hwang SJ, et al. Hepatitis C viremia increases the association with type 2 diabetes mellitus in a hepatitis B and C endemic area: an epidemiological link with virological implication. *Am J Gastroenterol*. 2007;102(6):1237–1243.
54. Mehta SH, Brancati FL, Strathdee SA, et al. Hepatitis C virus infection and incident type 2 diabetes. *Hepatology*. 2003;38(1):50–56.
55. Zein CO, Levy C, Basu A, Zein NN. Chronic hepatitis C and type II diabetes mellitus: a prospective cross-sectional study. *Am J Gastroenterol*. 2005;100(1):48–55.
56. Lecube A, Hernández C, Genescà J, Simó R. Glucose abnormalities in patients with hepatitis C virus infection: epidemiology and pathogenesis. *Diabetes Care*. 2006;29(5):1140–1149.
57. Mehta SH, Brancati FL, Sulkowski MS, et al. Prevalence of type 2 diabetes mellitus among persons with hepatitis C virus infection in the United States. *Hepatology*. 2001;33(6):1554.
58. Huang JF, Dai CY, Hwang SJ, et al. Hepatitis C viremia increases the association with type 2 diabetes mellitus in a hepatitis B and C endemic area: an epidemiological link with virological implication. *Am J Gastroenterol*. 2007;102(6):1237–1243.
59. Hadziyannis SJ. The spectrum of extrahepatic manifestations in hepatitis C virus infection. *J Vir Hepat*. 1997;4:9–28.
60. Oben JA, Paulon E. Fatty liver in chronic hepatitis C infection: unraveling the mechanisms. *Gut*. 2007;56:1186–1188.
61. Knobler H, Schattner A. TNF-alpha, chronic hepatitis C and diabetes: a novel triad. *QJM*. 2005;98(1):1–6.
62. Chen LK, Chou YC, Tsai ST, et al. Hepatitis C virus infection-related type 1 diabetes mellitus. *Diabetes Med*. 2005;22(3):340–343.
63. Kawaguchi T, Yoshida T, Harada M, et al. Hepatitis C virus down-regulates insulin receptor substrates 1 and 2 through up-regulation of suppressor of cytokine signaling 3. *Am J Pathol*. 2004;165(5):1499–1508.
64. Aytug S, Reich D, Sapiro LE, et al. Impaired IRS-1/PI3-kinase signaling in patients with HCV: a mechanism for increased prevalence of type 2 diabetes. *Hepatology*. 2003;38(6):1384–1392.
65. Romero-Gómez M, Del Mar Viloria M, Andrade RJ, et al. Insulin resistance impairs sustained response rate to peginterferon plus ribavirin in chronic hepatitis C patients. *Gastroenterology*. 2005;128(3):636–641.
66. Hickman IJ, Powell EE, Prins JB, et al. In overweight patients with chronic hepatitis C, circulating insulin is associated with hepatic fibrosis: implications for therapy. *J Hepatol*. 2003;39(6):1042–1048.
67. Taura N, Ichikawa T, Hamasaki K, et al. Association between liver fibrosis and insulin sensitivity in chronic hepatitis C patients. *Am J Gastroenterol*. 2006;101(12):2752–2759.
68. Trombetta M, Spiazzi G, Zoppini G, Muggeo M. Review article: type 2 diabetes and chronic liver disease in the Verona diabetes study. *Aliment Pharmacol Ther*. 2005;22(Suppl 2):24–27.
69. Record CO, Alberti KG, Williamson DH, Wright R. Glucose tolerance and metabolic changes in human viral hepatitis. *Clin Sci Mol Med*. 1973;45:677–690.
70. Bianchi G, Marchesini G, Zoli M, et al. Prognostic significance of diabetes in patients with cirrhosis. *Hepatology*. 1994;20:119–125.
71. Vesely DL, Dilley RW, Duckworth WC, Paustian FF. Hepatitis A-induced diabetes mellitus, acute renal failure, and liver failure. *Am J Med Sci*. 1999;317(6):419–425.
72. Masuda H, Atsumi T, Fujisaku A, et al. Acute onset of type 1 diabetes accompanied by acute hepatitis C: the potential role of proinflammatory cytokine in the pathogenesis of autoimmune diabetes. *Diabetes Res Clin Pract*. 2007;75(3):357–361.
73. Luna B, Feinglos MN. Drug-induced hyperglycemia. *JAMA*. 2001;286(16):1945–1948.
74. Lambertus MW, Murthy AR, Nagami P, et al. Diabetic ketoacidosis following pentamidine therapy in a patient with the acquired immunodeficiency syndrome. *West J Med*. 1988;149:602–604.
75. Bouchard P, Sai P, Reach G, et al. Diabetes mellitus following pentamidine-induced hypoglycemia in humans. *Diabetes*. 1982;31:40–45.
76. Assan R, Perronne C, Assan D, et al. Pentamidine-induced derangements of glucose homeostasis. *Diabetes Care*. 1995;18:47–55.
77. Pandit MK, Burke J, Gustafson AB, et al. Drug-induced disorders of glucose tolerance. *Ann Intern Med*. 1993;118:529–540.
78. O'Byrne S, Feely J. Effects of drugs on glucose tolerance in non-insulin-dependent diabetes (parts I and II). *Drugs*. 1990;40:203–219.
79. Shiba T, Morino Y, Tagawa K, et al. Onset of diabetes with high titer anti-GAD antibody after IFN therapy for chronic hepatitis. *Diabetes Res Clin Pract*. 1996;30:237–241.
80. Gallanosa AG, Spyker DA, Curnow RT. Diabetes mellitus associated with autonomic and peripheral neuropathy after Vacor poisoning: a review. *Clin Toxicol*. 1981;18:441–449.

81. Florescu D, Kotler DP. Insulin resistance, glucose intolerance and diabetes mellitus in HIV-infected patients. *Antivir Ther.* 2007;12:149–162.

82. Moyle G. Metabolic issues associated with protease inhibitors. *J Acquir Immune Defic Syndr.* 2007;45:S19–S26.

83. Martinez E, Mocroft A, Garcia-Viejo MA, et al. Risk of lipodystrophy in HIV-1-infected patients treated with protease inhibitors: a prospective cohort study. *Lancet.* 2001;357:592–598.

84. Liang J, Distler O, Cooper DA, et al. HIV protease inhibitors protect apolipoprotein B from degradation by the proteasome: a potential mechanism for protease inhibitor-induced hyperlipidemia. *Nat Med.* 2001;7:1327–1331.

85. Riddle TM, Kuhel DG, Woollett LA, et al. HIV protease inhibitor induces fatty acid and sterol biosynthesis in liver and adipose tissues due to the accumulation of activated sterol regulatory element-binding proteins in the nucleus. *J Biol Chem.* 2001;276:37514–37519.

86. Martine C, Auclair M, Vigouroux C, et al. The HIV protease inhibitor indinavir impairs sterol regulatory element-binding protein-1 intranuclear localization, inhibits preadipocyte differentiation, and induces insulin resistance. *Diabetes.* 2001;50:1378–1388.

87. Murata H, Hruz PW, Mueckler M. The mechanism of insulin resistance caused by HIV protease inhibitor therapy. *J Biol Chem.* 2000;275:20251–20254.

88. Usala AL, Madigan T, Burguera B, et al. Treatment of insulin-resistant diabetic ketoacidosis with insulin-like growth factor I in an adolescent with insulin-dependent diabetes [Brief report]. *N Engl J Med.* 1992;327:853–857.

89. Boden G. Role of fatty acids in the pathogenesis of insulin resistance and NIDDM. *Diabetes.* 1997;46:3–10.

90. Leung KC, Ho KKY. Stimulation of mitochondrial fatty acid oxidation by growth hormone in human fibroblasts. *J Clin Endocrinol Metab.* 1997;82:4208–4213.

91. Goodman HN. The metabolic actions of growth hormone. In: Jefferson LS, Cherrington AD, Goodman HM, eds. *Handbook of Physiology*, Section, 7; The Endocrine System, Vol. 2. The Endocrine Pancreas and Regulation of Metabolism. New York: Oxford University Press, Inc.; 2001:849–906.

92. Vilar L, Naves LA, Costa SS, et al. Increase of classic and nonclassic cardiovascular risk factors in patients with acromegaly. *Endocr Pract.* 2007;13:363–372.

93. Butler AA, LeRoith D. Minireview: tissue-specific versus generalized gene targeting of the igf1 and igf1r genes and their roles in insulin-like growth factor physiology. *Endocrinol.* 2001;142:1685–1688.

94. Munck A, Naray-Fejes-Toth A. Glucocorticoid physiology. In: DeGroot LJ, Jameson LJ, eds. *Endocrinology.* 5th ed. Philadelphia, PA: Elsevier Saunders; 2006:2287–2309.

95. Salati LM. Regulation of fatty acid biosynthesis and lipolysis. In: Jefferson LS, Cherrington AD, Goodman HM, eds. *Handbook of Physiology*, Section, 7; The Endocrine System, Vol. 2. The Endocrine Pancreas and Regulation of Metabolism. New York: Oxford University Press, Inc.; 2001:495–527.

96. Jefferson LS, Vary TC, Kimball SR. Regulation of protein metabolism in muscle. In: Jefferson LS, Cherrington AD, Goodman HM, eds. *Handbook of Physiology*, Section, 7; The Endocrine System, Vol. 2. The Endocrine Pancreas and Regulation of Metabolism. New York: Oxford University Press, Inc.; 2001:536.

97. Masuzaki H, Paterson J, Shinyama H, et al. A transgenic model of visceral obesity and the metabolic syndrome. *Science.* 2001;294:2166–2170.

98. Qatanani M, Lazar MA. Mechanisms of obesity-associated insulin resistance: many choices on the menu. *Genes Dev.* 2007;21:1443–1455.

99. Gura T. Pot-bellied mice point to obesity enzyme [News of the Week]. *Science.* 2001;294:2071–2072.

100. Manger WM, Gifford RW. *Clinical and Experimental Pheochromocytoma.* 2nd ed. Cambridge: Blackwell Science, Inc.; 1996:209.

101. Pacak K. Preoperative management of the pheochromocytoma patient. *J Clin Endocrinol Metab.* 2007;92(11):4069–4079.

102. Cryer PE. Catecholamines, pheochromocytoma and diabetes. *Diabetes Rev.* 1993;1:309–317.

103. Romero R, Casanova B, Pulido N, et al. Stimulation of glucose transport by thyroid hormone in 3T3-L1 adipocytes: increased abundance of GLUT1 and GLUT4 glucose transporter proteins. *J Endocrinol.* 2000;164:187–195.

104. Tosi F, Moghetti P, Castello R, et al. Early changes in plasma glucagon and growth hormone response to oral glucose in experimental hyperthyroidism. *Metab Clin Exp.* 1996;45:1029–1033.

105. Feng X, Jiang Y, Meltzer P, Yen PM. Thyroid hormone regulation of hepatic genes in vivo detected by complementary DNA microarray. *Mol Endocrinol.* 2000 July;14(7):947–955.

106. Mokuno T, Uchimura K, Hayashi R, et al. Glucose transporter 2 concentrations in hyper- and hypothyroid rat livers. *J Endocrinol.* 1999;160:285–289.

107. Kreze A Sr., Kreze-Spirova E, Mikulecky M. Diabetes mellitus in primary aldosteronism. *Bratisl Lek Listy.* 2000;101:187–190.

108. Ferrannini E, Galvan AQ, Santoro D, Natali A. Potassium as a link between insulin and the rennin–angiotensin–aldosterone system. *J Hypertension.* 1992;10(Suppl 1):S5–S10.

109. Hitomi H, Kiyomoto H, Nishiyama A, et al. Aldosterone suppresses insulin signaling via the downregulation of insulin receptor substrate-1 in vascular smooth muscle cells. *Hypertension.* 2007;50:750–755.

110. Strauch B, Widimsky J, Sindelka G, Skrha J. Does the treatment of primary hyperaldosteronism influence glucose tolerance? *Physiol Res.* 2003;52(4):503–506.

Useful Websites

Endotext.org   http://www.endotext.org/index.htm – This is a complete textbook of endocrinology on the web that is available free.

http://www.endocrineweb.com/index.html – This is a site designed for patients and their families.

http://digestive.niddk.nih.gov/ddiseases/a-z.asp – Diseases of the pancreas can be found at this site.

http://digestive.niddk.nih.gov/ddiseases/pubs/hemochromatosis/index.htm

http://www.cancer.gov/ – This is a wonderful site to look up all of the endocrine tumors by system, body location, or type.

Mayo   Clinic   Staff.   "Primary   Aldosteronism."   http://www.mayoclinic.com/health/primary-aldosteronism/DS00563. January 5, 2007. Accessed February 16, 2008.

Chapter 17
Syndromes of Extreme Insulin Resistance

George Grunberger and Bianca Alfonso

Introduction

This group of syndromes shares severe insulin resistance and hyperinsulinemia with variable clinical manifestations.[1,2] Attention has been paid to these rare disorders because they provide insight into several aspects of insulin action at the molecular level and advance our understanding of the more common insulin-resistant disorders, such as polycystic ovarian syndrome[3] and type 2 diabetes mellitus.[4]

Insulin resistance is defined as a state of suboptimal biological response to a given concentration of insulin.[2] It is possible, therefore, to overcome the resistance by increasing the quantity of insulin secreted. Mild to moderate insulin resistance is seen in such clinical conditions as obesity, hypertension, and type 2 diabetes. These are discussed in detail in other chapters.

In *extreme* insulin resistance syndromes, hereditary and/or acquired defects in insulin action at different molecular levels result in the diseases described below. In this chapter we review the pathogenesis and classification of syndromes of extreme insulin resistance and then follow by describing the general and specific features of these conditions.

Laboratory Assessment of Insulin Resistance

Various tests can be used to assess the presence and/or the level of insulin resistance.

1. *Fasting serum/plasma glucose* may be normal or elevated. This is primarily determined by the magnitude of the basal insulin response.
2. *Glucose tolerance test* may be normal or severely impaired. This is primarily determined by the magnitude of insulin response to carbohydrate or other secretagogue stimuli. The fasted patient is given a 75 g dose of oral glucose, after which plasma insulin and serum glucose levels are obtained over the next 2 h. Multiple parameters can then be calculated based on these two values. The index of whole-body insulin sensitivity, ISI (composite), takes into account hepatic and peripheral insulin sensitivity. This index is calculated based on the following formula:

$$10,000/\sqrt{\dfrac{[\text{fasting glucose (mg/dL)} \times \text{fasting insulin (}\mu\text{U/mL)]}}{\times[\text{mean glucose} \times \text{mean insulin}]}}$$

The insulin sensitivity index-glycemia (ISI-gly) reflects peripheral insulin sensitivity (the lower the ISI-gly, the lower the sensitivity). Another formula is used to calculate ISI-gly:

G. Grunberger (✉)
Grunberger Diabetes Institute, Wayne State University School of Medicine, Detroit, MI, USA
e-mail: g.grunberger@gdi-pc.com

L. Poretsky (ed.), *Principles of Diabetes Mellitus*, DOI 10.1007/978-0-387-09841-8_17,
© Springer Science+Business Media, LLC 2010

$$ISI - gly = 2/[(insulin_p \times glucose_p) + 1]$$

Insulin$_p$ and glucose$_p$ represent the sum of measurements of insulin and glucose obtained before and after a 75-g oral glucose dose divided by their respective normal values.

Both of these indices have been reported to correlate well with insulin measurements obtained from the euglycemic hyperinsulinemic clamp. These results are affected by individual gastric emptying rates.[5]

3. *Serum insulin* level, in conjunction with serum glucose, in fasting state or after oral glucose tolerance. Fasting insulin levels > 50–70 μU/mL or insulin levels more than 350 μU/mL post-OGTT suggest severe insulin resistance (normal insulin levels: fasting insulin < 20 μU/mL and post-OGTT insulin <150 μU/mL).[6] These markers have some important limitations. Insulin levels depend on the β-cell reserve and insulin degradation. There is no standard method for insulin measurement and reference ranges are not available for all of the assays. Also, proinsulin cross-reacts with some of the assays used.[5] The fasting glucose/insulin ratio could be more useful than insulin values alone. This ratio has been compared to the insulin sensitivity values obtained with the frequently sampled intravenous glucose tolerance test (FSIVGTT) (see below) and suggested to be used as a screening tool for insulin resistance.[7]

4. *Quantitative insulin sensitivity check index (QUICKI)*. This is a marker of insulin sensitivity calculated based on the following formula:

$$QUICKI = 1/[\log insulin\,(\mu U/mL) + \log glucose\,(mg/dL)]$$

Both insulin and glucose values are obtained in a fasting state.

The insulin sensitivity is directly proportional to QUICKI – the lower this index, the lower the sensitivity. This index showed a powerful correlation with the values obtained from FSIVGTT (see below). Compared to HOMA (see below), QUICKI is more accurate when used in calculations over a larger range of insulin sensitivities.[5] Used in large population studies, QUICKI was better than fasting insulin alone in predicting the future development of type 2 diabetes.[8] In another study, it was used in diagnosing metabolic syndrome.[9] QUICKI does not take post-glucose load insulin and glucose values into account and it cannot be applied as easily to subjects that have uncontrolled diabetes or patients with no endogenous insulin production.

In patients with mild insulin resistance, a revised QUICKI formula correlates better with the gold standard than does the original QUICKI:[10]

$$Revised\,QUICKI = 1/[\log insulin\,(\mu U/mL) + \log glucose\,(mg/dL) + \log$$
$$nonesterified\,fatty\,acids\,(NEFA)\,(mmol/L)].$$

5. The *homeostasis model assessment (HOMA) index*, which is calculated using the formula described by Matthews and associates: fasting serum insulin (μU/mL) multiplied by fasting plasma glucose (mmol/L) and then divided by 22.5. The higher the HOMA index, the lower the insulin sensitivity (i.e., more severe insulin resistance). This method is an inexpensive and validated way for evaluating insulin resistance.

6. Assessment of sequential plasma glucose levels after intravenous administration of insulin (*insulin tolerance test*) showing decreased response to exogenous insulin. This test was first described in 1929. It estimates the net effects of insulin on liver and peripheral tissues. The patient receives an intravenous bolus of insulin (0.1 U/kg), and blood glucose is measured at 15 and 5 min before the insulin injection and then at 3, 6, 9, 12, 15, 20, and 30 min thereafter. Exogenous glucose is given to the patient at 30 min to prevent a continuous fall in blood glucose. The rate of glucose disappearance constant (k_{ITT}) represents the slope of the decline in blood glucose plotted logarithmically, and it is correlated with the insulin sensitivity parameters obtained with the euglycemic hyperinsulinemic clamp. This test comes with its own drawbacks: it could cause hypoglycemia and it does not determine the site of insulin action defect. Also, the results of this test are difficult to interpret,

given the fact that insulin's effects are opposed by the physiological release of catecholamines, glucagon, cortisol, and growth hormone.[5]

7. Estimation of the insulin sensitivity index from the frequently sampled intravenous glucose tolerance test (FSIVGTT). Different protocols are described for the FSIVGTT. In the standard FSIVGTT, four baseline insulin levels and blood glucose levels are drawn after placement of an intravenous cannula. The patient is then administered a fixed dose of intravenous glucose, after which 25 blood samples are obtained over the next 180 min. Indices of insulin sensitivity and glucose effectiveness are calculated using a computer software. This test provides information about the insulin sensitivity and the β-cell function. The limitations of this test include long duration, dependence on the computer software, and its unsuitability for subjects with reduced endogenous insulin response.[5]

8. Measurement of in vivo insulin-mediated glucose disposal by the euglycemic hyperinsulinemic clamp. This test is the gold standard for investigating insulin sensitivity in vivo but it is mainly performed in research settings. The patient is given an intravenous infusion of insulin at a constant rate, along with glucose at a variable rate to maintain the blood glucose at 5–5.5 mmol/L. The hepatic glucose output is inhibited by the infused insulin so that, when a steady state is reached, the rate of glucose infusion is the same as the peripheral glucose disposal rate (metabolic clearance rate or M value). If the patient is very sensitive to insulin, it will require high amounts of exogenous glucose to maintain euglycemia, whereas patients with insulin resistance require small amounts of exogenous glucose. A high M value (> 7.5 mg/kg/min) indicates that the individual is insulin sensitive, and a low M value (< 4.0 mg/kg/min) indicates a relative insulin-resistant state[5]; M < 2.0 mg/kg/min suggests severe insulin resistance.[6] This test is a lengthy test and has a potential for hypoglycemia. The person performing the test needs to be experienced with this technique.[5]

Pathogenesis and Classification

Significant progress has been made in our understanding of the molecular basis underlying the syndromes of extreme insulin resistance. Some of these diseases are due to genetic defects or mutations in the insulin receptor gene, as seen in the type A syndrome, leprechaunism as well as in the Rabson–Mendenhall syndrome, while circulating antibodies against the insulin receptor are detected in the type B syndrome. The etiology of some of the extreme insulin resistance syndromes is still a mystery, as is the case in many lipodystrophic syndromes.

It is important to mention that some conditions should not be mistakenly categorized under extreme insulin resistance syndromes. These conditions are discussed below.

Conditions that Mimic Insulin Resistance

Although hyperinsulinemia is seen in these genetic diseases, insulin resistance is not present. In fact individuals with these disorders respond appropriately to exogenous insulin.

(1) Familial hyperproinsulinemia

   This trait is inherited as an autosomal dominant pattern and leads to the inability to convert proinsulin to insulin.[11,12]

(2) Mutant insulin molecules

   These molecules may act as weak insulin agonists with lower affinity for the insulin receptors.

(3) Increased insulin degradation

   This phenomenon has been observed in insulin-treated diabetic patients. They respond to exogenous insulin given intravenously but are resistant to subcutaneous insulin.[13] It seems that insulin may be degraded in, or prevented from getting absorbed from, the subcutaneous tissue.

Syndromes of Extreme Insulin Resistance

In this chapter we classify the extreme insulin resistance syndromes according to the underlying etiology.

(1) Anti-insulin antibodies

Anti-insulin antibodies have been reported in patients with diabetes who were on poorly purified or animal intermittent insulin.[14] This complication was remarkably minimized after the introduction of human or highly purified insulin. In diabetic patients using human insulin, only few develop very high capacity immunoglobulins that might lead to extreme insulin resistance.

(2) Autoantibodies against insulin receptors

This condition is characterized by spontaneous development of antibodies against insulin receptors. These antibodies can interfere with the ability of insulin to bind to its receptors, resulting in insulin resistance. However, hypoglycemia due to direct activation of insulin receptors by these antibodies has also been described.[15]

(3) Mutation in insulin receptor genes

Insulin receptor is composed of two α- and two β-subunits. Insulin activates, by binding to its α-subunit, the intrinsic tyrosine kinase of the receptor's transmembrane β-subunit. Subsequently, activation of several downstream signaling pathways takes place. The end results of this activation and signal transduction are the well-known biological effects of insulin on its target cells, including glucose and amino acid uptake, glycogenesis, antilipolysis, and others.[16]

The abovementioned cascade of molecular events can be interrupted at various steps, resulting in an impaired insulin action and a potential development of extreme insulin-resistant clinical conditions. Many mutations have been identified in the insulin receptor gene. These mutations may lead to the following:

- Decreased insulin receptor biosynthesis
- Premature chain termination in extracellular or intracellular domain
- Accelerated receptor degradation
- Defect in the receptor transport to plasma membranes
- Decreased insulin-binding affinity
- Impaired tyrosine kinase activity
- Impaired binding interactions with signaling molecules

(4) Defects in target cell

When adequate amounts of insulin are synthesized, secreted into the extracellular space, and gain access to the target tissues, abnormal function is then attributed to the target cell. Since the first step in insulin action is binding to specific cell surface receptors, we must first consider the receptor as a potential site of dysfunction. Studies in the past have revealed a number of general principles regarding the insulin receptor:

(a) Using direct binding techniques, estimates can be obtained of both the affinity and the concentration of cell surface receptors.

(b) Affinity is a complex function and is determined both by multiplicity of binding sites and by negatively cooperative interactions (which are interactions among the receptor sites so that the affinity of the receptors for the hormone progressively decreases as more sites are occupied by insulin).

(c) The receptor is highly regulated. Temperature, pH, and ligand concentration are among the various factors that regulate the receptor.

(d) At physiologic temperatures, both the ligand and the receptor are internalized by the cell. This receptor-mediated process provides a mechanism to remove the ligand from the cell surface and terminate its signal and a mechanism that may regulate the concentration of receptors on the cell surface.[17]

Interestingly, in target and nontarget tissues, insulin is processed in a similar manner.[18] This suggests that biologic activity and receptor regulation are separate functions; however, when target and nontarget cells are exposed to a similar environment, their cell surface receptors are regulated in a similar fashion.

(5) Decreased insulin clearance

Insulin clearance from the circulation may become impaired in some conditions due to certain insulin receptor defects.[19] So, hyperinsulinemia seen in patients with extreme insulin resistance may result both from increased β-cell secretion and from decreased insulin clearance.

(6) Other causes of extreme insulin resistance

Some hormonal or metabolic abnormalities may lead, occasionally, to extreme insulin resistance. These abnormalities include excess of glucocorticoids, growth hormone, catecholamines, glucagon, and free fatty acids.

Specific syndromes of insulin resistance are summarized in Table 17.1 and discussed below.

Table 17.1 Specific syndromes of extreme insulin resistance

A. Familial lipodystrophy syndromes
  1. Familial generalized lipodystrophy
  2. Familial partial lipodystrophy
    • Kobberling variety
    • Dunnigan variety
    • Mandibuloacral dysplasia variety
    • Familial partial lipodystrophy associated with PPAR gamma (peroxisome proliferator-activated receptor-γ) gene mutations
    • Familial partial lipodystrophy due to v-AKT murine thymoma oncogene homolog 2 (*AKT2*) gene mutations

B. Acquired lipodystrophy syndromes
  1. Acquired generalized lipodystrophy
  2. Acquired partial lipodystrophy
  3. Lipodystrophy in HIV patients
  4. Localized lipodystrophies
    • Drug-induced
    • Pressure-induced
    • Panniculitis variety
    • Centrifugal variety
    • Idiopathic

C. Insulin receptor defects
  1. Type A insulin resistance syndrome
  2. Leprechaunism
  3. Rabson-Mendenhall syndrome

D. Type B insulin resistance syndrome

General Clinical Features of Extreme Insulin Resistance

General clinical manifestations of these syndromes can be classified into two main categories: features related to deficiency of insulin action and those secondary to the effects of high levels of insulin in some relatively insulin-sensitive tissues (Table 17.2).

(1) Features related to deficiency of insulin action

In extreme insulin-resistant states, the effect of insulin at the target tissue is diminished. Therefore, pancreatic β-cells try to compensate by producing more insulin. If the pancreatic islets are unable to keep up with the increased demand, pathologies will occur including impaired glucose homeostasis and possibly lipodystrophy.

Table 17.2 Common features of extreme insulin resistance syndromes

Glucose homeostasis	Impaired glucose tolerance, diabetes, hypoglycemia
Lipid metabolism	Hypertriglyceridemia
Reproductive	Hirsutism, virilization, PCO, amenorrhea
Adipose tissue	Lipoatrophy, lipohypertrophy, obesity
Developmental	Decreased or increased linear growth, mental retardation
Musculoskeletal	Muscle hypertrophy, acromegalic features, muscle cramps
Dermatologic	Acanthosis nigricans, eruptive xanthoma
Abdominal	Fatty liver, cirrhosis, pancreatitis
Cardiac	Cardiomegaly, hypertension

- Glucose homeostasis

Hyperinsulinemia is the hallmark of extreme insulin resistance. The consequences of extreme insulin resistance on glucose homeostasis can range from normal fasting glucose with impaired glucose tolerance to frank type 2-like diabetes mellitus. Diabetes mellitus can sometimes be the presenting complaint in patients with extreme insulin resistance. Tens of thousands of units of insulin administered each day may have only a small or no effect on glucose lowering in some diabetic patients affected by these devastating syndromes. Lastly, hypoglycemia may rarely result from insulin receptor activation by insulin receptor autoantibodies as mentioned above.[15]

- Lipoatrophy

Lipoatrophy is manifested by an adipose tissue loss. It is seen in some of the extreme insulin resistance syndromes as is detailed below. It is thought that the lack of the lipogenic effect of insulin may be contributing to the loss of adipose tissue.

(2) Features directly related to high circulating insulin

Although many tissues are resistant to insulin action in the extreme insulin resistance syndromes, some tissues that remain relatively sensitive to insulin may show the characteristic features of hyperinsulinemia.

- Acanthosis nigricans

Acanthosis nigricans is a hyperpigmented velvety lesion found usually in the neck and the axillary areas (Fig. 17.1a), and occasionally elsewhere. The palms and soles are typically not involved. Pathologically, it is characterized by an increased number of melanocytes associated with hyperkeratotic epidermal papillomatosis. Acanthosis nigricans is strongly associated with insulin resistance. However, the condition is nonspecific, also occurring in obesity, endocrine diseases (such as Cushing's syndrome and acromegaly) as well as in association with malignant tumors.

Acanthosis nigricans is present in all patients with congenital syndromes of extreme insulin resistance[20] and in many patients with acquired forms. The severity of acanthosis nigricans correlates with the degree of insulin resistance and the level of serum insulin. Thus, the condition ranges from mild and limited lesions to diffuse skin involvement (Fig. 17.1b). The exact mechanism leading to acanthosis nigricans in extreme insulin resistance syndromes is still unclear. It is speculated that the related IGF-1 receptors in the skin are activated by the ambient hyperinsulinemia[21] through receptor "specificity spillover."[22] The presence of acanthosis nigricans may warrant an evaluation for an insulin-resistant state.

- Ovarian hyperandrogenism

Increased androgen level in females with extreme insulin resistance syndromes is not an uncommon feature. This abnormality may cause amenorrhea, hirsutism, or frank virilization along with polycystic changes in the ovaries. However, these abnormalities are not specific and can be seen in other conditions. The high levels of insulin in extreme insulin resistance syndromes stimulate androgen-producing cells in the ovary[3] where receptors for both insulin and IGF-1 are present. Fasting insulin correlates significantly with mean ovarian volume[23].

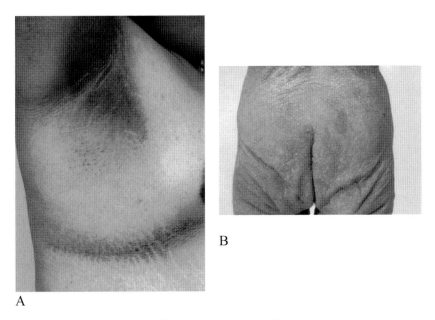

Fig. 17.1 Acanthosis nigricans severity correlates with insulin resistance level

Specific Syndromes of Insulin Resistance

Lipodystrophic Syndromes

Lipodystrophic syndromes are a heterogeneous group of disorders characterized by the absence of an adipose tissue as well as an extreme insulin-resistant state in most cases. The clinical diagnosis can be made based on the physical exam, certain metabolic abnormalities (fasting insulin level over 30 μU/mL, fasting triglycerides level >200 mg/dL, presence of diabetes mellitus), and genetic abnormalities in some types of lipodystrophic syndrome.[24] The adipose tissue loss can be familial or acquired, generalized or focal. Several modalities used to evaluate the adipose tissue status include CT scan, MRI, or dual-energy X-ray absorptiometry. The etiology of the fat loss is still incompletely understood. The absence of fat and leptin deficiency may contribute to the insulin resistance in these syndromes as will be discussed later.

A. Familial lipodystrophy syndromes

1. Familial generalized lipodystrophy (Berardinelli–Seip syndrome)
    Berardinelli and Seip have separately initially described this autosomal recessive syndrome. This is a rare disease, reported in about 250 patients only. Males and females are affected equally, but the metabolic abnormalities appear to be more severe in females.[24]
    Proposed criteria for the diagnosis of congenital generalized lipoatrophy (presence of two of the three major criteria and at least three supportive criteria needed for diagnosis) [24]

    (a) Major criteria

    o Autosomal recessive inheritance
    o Paucity of fat apparent at birth or within the first year of life
    o Emergence of at least one of the following metabolic abnormalities within the first decade of life:

    – Fasting insulin levels of more than 30 mU/mL
    – Fasting triglycerides levels of 200 mg/dL

– Presence of diabetes as defined by American Diabetes Association criteria (fasting blood sugar >126 mg/dL on two consecutive tests or 2-h oral glucose tolerance test glucose level >200 mg/dL on two consecutive tests)
– Enlarged liver with evidence of fatty infiltration and no other genetic disease present

(b) Supporting criteria

○ Acromegalic features
○ Cardiomegaly
○ Increased body hair during childhood
○ Evidence of hyperandrogenism in girls
○ Preservation of supportive fat in temporal fossa, palms, and soles of the feet; presence of glandular breast tissue in girls
○ Evidence of hypogonadotropic hypogonadism
○ Long bones with multiple sclerotic and lytic lesions
○ MR images that reveal complete absence of fat in abdomen and extremities as well as absence of bone marrow fat
○ Early heavy proteinuria with no other features of nephrotic syndrome
○ Leptin levels of less than 2 ng/mL
○ Decreased IQ or attention deficit, particularly in boys

Clinical manifestations: The loss of adipose tissue is diffuse and affects visceral as well as subcutaneous tissue. The lack of fat is seen at birth or within 2 years of life. Although extreme insulin resistance state is apparent in the first decade of life, diabetes is usually manifested in the second decade. The characteristic muscular phenotype observed in many patients with this syndrome is attributed to the adipose tissue loss, high muscular glycogen stores, and possible hyperinsulinemia-mediated changes as described earlier. Various complications have been described, including acute pancreatitis associated with profound hypertriglyceridemia, fatty liver and cirrhosis which may recur after liver transplant,[25] hyperandrogenic state with PCOS, accelerated early growth in children with final short stature, different degrees of mental retardation, cardiac hypertrophy, and arterial hypertension (Fig. 17.2).

Etiology: Two genetic abnormalities that translate into two different forms of familial generalized lipodystrophy (type 1 and type 2) have been identified.[26] Besides these, there are patients that do not express these two aberrant genes. Familial generalized type 1 has an abnormal gene on chromosome 9q34 *([1-acylglycerol-3-phosphate O-acyltransferase 2 (AGPAT2)]*.[27] AGPAT2 enzyme is involved in the synthesis of triglycerides and phospholipids. Parental consanguinity is found to be high in this syndrome. The exact mechanism of adipose tissue loss is unclear and different suggestions are available including impaired lipogenesis, increased lipolysis, underdevelopment of adipocytes, decreased synthesis of triglycerides in adipose tissue, and reduced bioavailability of phosphatidic acid and other phospholipids.[26] Finally, the pathogenesis of insulin resistance is also unknown and the available data suggest insulin-binding defects, insulin receptor defects, and post-receptor defect. Elevated free fatty acids seen in this syndrome may contribute to the severe insulin resistance.

Familial generalized lipodystrophy type 2 has an abnormal *seipin* gene linked to chromosome 11q13. Even though the function of the protein encoded by this gene is unknown and the underlying process causing the lipodystrophy is unclear, there are suggestions that the central nervous system is involved.[28]

2. Familial partial lipodystrophy syndromes

• Kobberling variety

The adipose tissue loss is limited to the extremities with normal or even remarkable accumulation of adipose tissue in other subcutaneous as well as visceral areas. The face is spared in this syndrome.

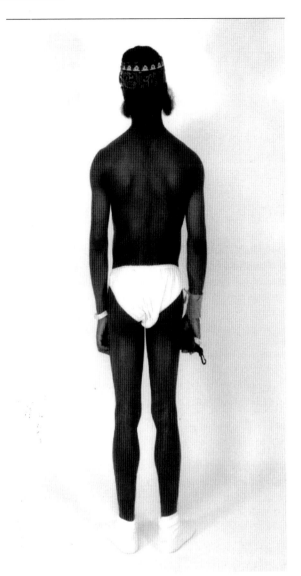

Fig. 17.2 The muscular appearance of a patient with familial generalized lipodystrophy

- Dunnigan variety

An autosomal dominant disease was mapped to chromosome 1q21-22[29,30] which harbors the *LMNA* gene encoding nuclear lamins A and C. Nuclear lamin A/C R482Q mutation is found in this variety.[31] It appears that abnormal lamin A/C causes premature death of adipocytes in the extremities. The site of the mutation influences the phenotype.[32] Patients are born with normal fat distribution but after puberty the fat loss involves the extremities and the trunk and spares the face and the neck (Fig. 17.3). Patients have high triglycerides, low HDL, diabetes, and atherosclerosis, all of which are worse in females.[26]

Proposed criteria for the diagnosis of familial partial lipodystrophy or Dunnigan–Kobberling syndrome (presence of two major criteria or of one major and two supporting criteria needed for diagnosis).[24]

(a) Major criteria

- Autosomal dominant inheritance in pedigree (male patients are easy to miss; therefore, at least one affected first-degree female relative required to substantiate the diagnosis)

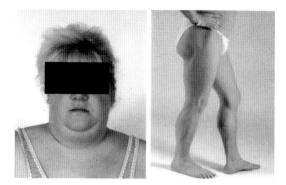

Fig. 17.3 Some phenotypic features of a patient with Dunnigan variety

    ○ Change in body habitus at or after puberty (clear increase of fat deposits around face and neck)
    ○ Presence of mutations on *lamin A* gene (if the test is available)
    ○ Clear absence of subcutaneous fat in the extremities and trunk with increased fat around face and neck or viscera (suspected on the basis of physical examination and supported by MR imaging findings)
    ○ At least one of the following metabolic abnormalities:

        – Fasting insulin level of more than 30 mU/mL
        – Fasting triglycerides level of more than 200 mg/mL
        – Presence of diabetes as defined by American Diabetes Association criteria
        – Evidence of fatty infiltration of the liver

(b) Supporting criteria

    ○ Presence of "buffalo hump"
    ○ High-density lipoprotein level of less than 35 mg/dL
    ○ Evidence of premature coronary artery disease
    ○ Evidence of hyperandrogenism or menstrual abnormalities in female patients

• Mandibuloacral dysplasia variety

This is an autosomal recessive condition with stiff joints, mandibuloacral dysplasia, dental and dermal abnormalities, along with lipodystrophy. It is rare, described in approximately 40 patients. Some of the patients have high lipid levels, diabetes, and insulin resistance. A mutation in the *LMNA* gene has been reported in 12 patients with this lipodystrophic syndrome.[33,34]

• Familial partial lipodystrophy associated with *PPAR gamma* (peroxisome proliferator-activated receptor-γ) gene mutations

A different variant of familial partial lipodystrophy has been reported recently, in which the patients have a mutation of the peroxisome proliferator-activated receptor-γ (*PPAR gamma*) gene. These patients have diabetes, high triglycerides, hypertension, and insulin resistance. The fat is lost more from the forearms and calves, and the truncal region is spared.[4,35,36] Since PPAR gamma protein has a crucial role in adipogenesis, it is thought that mutations in this gene cause lipodystrophy.

• Familial partial lipodystrophy due to v-AKT murine thymoma oncogene homolog 2 (*AKT2*) gene mutations

Another form of partial lipodystrophy was described in four members of a family, all carrying a mutation in the *AKT2* gene. These patients had insulin resistance and hypertension. Some of them developed diabetes in the fourth decade of life. One member had reduced body fat and lipodystrophy affecting her extremities. It appears that *AKT2* mutations lead to decreased adipocyte differentiation and also impaired insulin action at cellular level.[37]

B. Acquired lipodystrophy syndromes

  1. Acquired generalized lipodystrophy (Lawrence syndrome)

     This syndrome has been described in approximately 80 patients. The male-to-female ratio is 1:3.[38] The disease is usually manifested in the first or the second decade of life with insulin resistance syndrome. No similar family history is found and adipose tissue is healthy at birth. The fat is lost during childhood and adolescence, especially from face and extremities.[38] Low levels of leptin and adiponectin have been found in the majority of these patients.[39] Some of these patients have associated autoimmune diseases.[38] Viral infection preceded the relatively rapid appearance of the syndrome in other cases. Inflammatory cells and panniculitis[40] are seen on skin biopsy. Therefore, inflammatory destructive process involving the adipose tissue may play a role in the pathogenesis of this syndrome. In fact, antibodies against adipocyte membranes have been found in one study.[41]

  2. Acquired partial lipodystrophy (Barraquer–Simons syndrome or cephalothoracic lipodystrophy)

     Although this is one of the most common forms of acquired lipodystrophies, this is a rare disease, reported in approximately 250 patients.[42] The male-to-female ratio is 1:4.

The characteristic feature of this disorder is fat loss in the trunk and the face, with excessive fat accumulation immediately below the waist (Fig. 17.4).

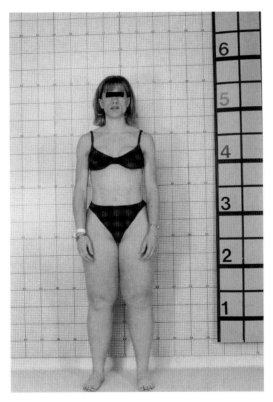

Fig. 17.4 The fat accumulation below the waist is associated with fat loss in other locations in a patient with cephalothoracic lipodystrophy

It is seen mainly in women and may follow a viral infection. The etiology is still unknown. However, an association between cephalothoracic lipodystrophy and the nephritic factor, low complement in type II mesangioproliferative glomerulonephritis, has been documented. Rarely patients develop insulin resistance with its manifestations or dyslipidemia. Other autoimmune syndromes can be seen (association with systemic lupus erythematosus or juvenile dermatomyositis have been reported in a few cases).[43,44] Majority of patients have C3 nephritic factor immunoglobulin, which is suggested to cause lysis of adipose tissue.[45]

3. Lipodystrophy in HIV patients

This is the most common form of lipodystrophy, occurring in approximately 40% of the HIV patients treated with a protease inhibitor for more than 1 year.[46]

This increasingly recognized serious condition is characterized by lipoatrophy in the face and limbs, dorsocervical and visceral adiposity,[47] associated with hypertriglyceridemia, low high-density lipoprotein cholesterol, and severe insulin resistance with potentially increased risk of cardiovascular disease. No clear explanation for the syndrome has been confirmed, but emergence of this syndrome has been correlated with the widespread introduction of protease inhibitors to the highly active antiretroviral therapy (HAART) regimens. The risk is also increased if nucleoside analogue reverse transcriptase inhibitors are combined with protease inhibitors.[48] The lipodystrophic changes could be reversed upon stopping protease inhibitors.[49] The precise molecular mechanism of fat redistribution is still unknown. It is suggested that protease inhibitors impair preadipocyte differentiation[50,51] and promote apoptosis[51] via inhibition of glucose transport,[52] thereby rendering the adipose tissue resistant to insulin. Altered insulin signaling at the level of phosphatidylinositol 3-kinase is suggested to be causing or contributing to insulin resistance state.[53] Adipose tissue in these patients has altered messenger RNA expression of sterol regulatory element-binding protein 1c (SREBP1c) and peroxisome proliferator-activated receptor gamma (PPAR-γ), resulting in the overexpression of SREBP1c and the decreased expression of PPAR-γ.[54] In mice, overexpression of SREBP1c results in lipodystrophy,[55] and in humans, reduced PPAR-γ is associated with familial partial lipodystrophy.

4. Localized lipodystrophies

This group of lipodystrophies includes patients that have loss of subcutaneous fat from small areas of the body but do not have insulin resistance or metabolic abnormalities.

This loss of fat can be caused by injected drugs (insulin, glucocorticoids, antibiotics), recurrent pressure, and panniculitis. Some cases have unknown causes. A rare localized lipodystrophic syndrome (lipodystrophia centrifugalis abdominalis infantilis) has been described in Japan, Korea, and Singapore. These patients are young children who present with fat loss in a centrifugal pattern, usually before 3 years of age. Approximately half of the patients recover later in life.[42]

C. Insulin receptor defects

1. Type A insulin resistance syndrome

The transmission of type A syndrome is found to follow autosomal dominant or autosomal recessive pattern with variable penetrance.[1,2]

Clinical manifestations: This syndrome was originally described in young nonobese women with extreme hyperinsulinemia, variable resistance to exogenous insulin, hirsutism, polycystic ovaries, and android habitus.[1] Now it includes females and males that have severe insulin resistance and acanthosis nigricans and do not have autoantibodies to the insulin receptor. Postpubertal females have signs of androgen excess of ovarian origin (hirsutism, acne, oligomenorrhea, infertility, or frank virilism with increased testosterone levels).[56] Only about a third of these patients, however, have had fasting hyperglycemia. Most have glucose intolerance, but some patients have normal glucose tolerance, and these patients demonstrate the greatest degree of basal- and glucose-stimulated hyperinsulinemia. All of these patients have had elevated plasma testosterone values usually associated with normal concentration of gonadotropins and all have had PCOS. Acromegalic features have been reported in some patients with type A extreme insulin resistance syndrome.[57] Although both GH and IGF-1 levels are normal, IGF-1 receptor activation by the high levels of insulin has been speculated to contribute to "pseudoacromegaly." Weight reduction may help to reduce the insulin levels and some of its manifestations to some extent.

The remarkable muscular pattern seen in these patients may be related to the hyperandrogenic state and/or to insulin-mediated IGF-1 stimulation. In one study, type A syndrome was associated with increased intraocular pressure and retinal vascular permeability, which improved by IGF-1 administration.[58]

Etiology: Several types of insulin receptor defects have been described. Typically, insulin binding to freshly obtained circulating monocytes and erythrocytes has been decreased. Less commonly, insulin binding has been completely normal. Thus, insulin resistance is a fixed feature of the type A syndrome but insulin binding is either low or normal. Studies of the function of the β-subunit of the monocyte insulin receptors showed concomitant decrease in the receptor autophosphorylation and tyrosine kinase activity with the binding activity in patients with low insulin binding. Interestingly, in one of the patients with normal insulin binding, insulin receptor autophosphorylation and tyrosine kinase activity from circulating monocytes and erythrocytes as well as cultured fibroblasts were greatly decreased.[59] Uncoupling of the receptor binding and phosphorylation thus exist in cells of some patients with type A syndrome. A variant of this syndrome has been seen in a brother and sister who also exhibited muscle cramps, and another family with features of this syndrome has also been described. A case with a lamina A mutation was described in a 24-year-old nonobese woman who had insulin resistance, acanthosis nigricans, and no lipodystrophy.[60] Another variation of this syndrome seen with precocious puberty, pineal tumors, and developmental defects is referred to as the *Rabson–Mendenhall syndrome (see below)*. It has been reported that PC-1 transmembrane glycoprotein inhibits insulin receptor function by interacting with the α-subunit of the insulin receptor in patients with type A syndrome.[61]

2. Leprechaunism (Donohue syndrome)

   Leprechaunism is a complex congenital insulin resistance syndrome.

   Clinical manifestations: These infants are small for gestational age and continue to grow slowly in extrauterine life. They have a characteristically abnormal appearance (Fig. 17.5) with such features as low-set ears, saddle nose deformity, hypertrichosis, decreased subcutaneous fat, and, occasionally, acanthosis nigricans. Curiously, in these infants a tendency to fasting hypoglycemia coexists with extreme resistance to insulin. Typically, the patients die within the first year of life, although an occasional child may live significantly longer.

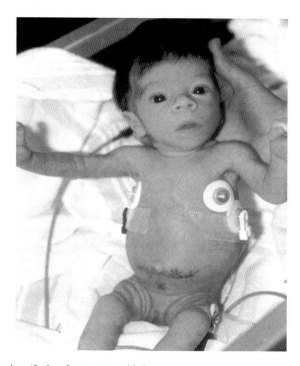

Fig. 17.5 Features of leprechaunism (fat loss is apparent at birth)

Etiology: Insulin-binding studies have revealed significant heterogeneity. Leprechaunism appears to be caused by defects in the insulin receptor. Over 20 kinds of mutations in the insulin receptor gene have been reported in patients with leprechaunism thus far. Frequent small feeding may help in reducing the risk of hypoglycemia and the postprandial hyperglycemia.

3. Rabson–Mendenhall syndrome

This autosomal recessive syndrome was described in 1956 in a family with hyperplasia of pineal gland and diabetes mellitus. Further characteristic features are low birth weight, thickened nails, hirsutism, acanthosis nigricans, dental precocity and dysplasia, polycystic ovaries, abdominal protuberance, and phallic enlargement. Most affected children die of ketoacidosis and intercurrent infections associated with extreme insulin resistance. Rabson–Mendenhall syndrome appears to lie between type A syndrome and leprechaunism on the spectrum of severity of insulin receptor dysfunction.

D. Type B insulin resistance syndrome

This syndrome was initially described in three female patients and shown to be associated with a plasma inhibitor of insulin binding.[62] Subsequently, about 20 patients have been studied. Most have been women of variable age; only two are male patients in the sixth decade of life.

Clinical manifestations: Patients exhibit acanthosis nigricans, and in one patient this disorder involved the entire body. Almost all patients have fasting hyperglycemia, and in these patients, up to 100,000 units of insulin/day may be required to normalize the blood glucose. Some patients may have fasting hypoglycemia.[56] All of these patients have features typical of autoimmune diseases, such as pancytopenia and increased erythrocyte sedimentation rate. In some, a lupus or Sjögren-like syndrome is present with arthralgias, proteinuria, parotid enlargement, and positive antinuclear antibody. About half the patients have anti-DNA antibodies but positive lupus preparations are uncommon. The symptoms may wax and wane reflecting the levels of antibodies, and in some cases, spontaneous remission has been described.[63,64]

Etiology: In patients with suggestive clinical features, the diagnosis is confirmed by demonstrating an inhibitor of insulin binding. The circulating inhibitor has been shown to be a polyclonal immunoglobulin behaving as an antibody to the insulin receptor.

These antireceptor autoantibodies can mimic insulin action in vitro. We have studied one patient who manifested only hypoglycemia.[15] Administration of corticosteroids resulted in a prompt increase in plasma glucose levels in all of similar patients reported to date. Thus, autoantibodies to the insulin receptor must be considered in the differential diagnosis of hypoglycemia. Most patients, however, demonstrate hyperglycemia and insulin resistance. Insulin binding is qualitatively abnormal in circulating cells from these patients. Abnormal insulin binding results from antibody binding on or near the insulin receptor. This yields a competition curve that has decreased specific tracer binding but also a marked increase in the amount of insulin necessary for 50% competition of binding. The net outcome is a major alteration in the affinity of the receptor for insulin. This abnormality can be reversed by the removal of the circulating antibody by plasma exchange or by an acid wash procedure, indicating that the underlying receptor is normal. Furthermore, insulin receptors in cultured cells from these patients exhibit normal binding. Analysis of the function of the β-subunit of the receptor from cells of patients with type B syndrome revealed a generally proportional decrease in the receptor kinase activity and insulin binding. Therefore, the phosphorylating activity expressed per receptor appears to be normal.

A variant of type B syndrome is seen is some ataxia telangiectasia patients with the antireceptor antibodies of IgM subtype.[65]

Although initially the type A and B syndromes were described as distinctly different, we now know that patients with typical clinical and laboratory features of the type B syndrome may manifest the major features of the type A syndrome, including polycystic ovaries, elevated plasma testosterone, and hirsutism. Thus, it is apparent that the type A and B syndromes have overlapping phenotypic features. Furthermore, it is clear that all of the syndromes of severe insulin resistance and acanthosis nigricans have many common clinical features.

Therapeutic Modalities

Many patients with extreme insulin resistance are refractory to therapeutic maneuvers and various agents produce variable results. Common modalities include treating the individual manifestations of different diseases such as dyslipidemia (drugs or plasmapheresis), PCOS and hyperandrogenemia, diabetes (including diet, exercise, and weight reduction if appropriate), cosmetic surgery (such as liposuction of lipohypertrophic lesions), and so forth.

1. Thiazolidinediones and metformin

   Thiazolidinediones act by activating PPAR-γ and inducing adipocyte differentiation,[66] so they are especially effective in treating familial partial lipodystrophy that results from PPAR-γ mutations.[36] Thiazolidinediones may improve insulin resistance, diabetes, hyperlipidemia, and lipodystrophy.[66,67] Metformin acts in early steps of insulin signal transduction and decreases ovarian and adrenal cytochrome P450c17 activity. Metformin may improve insulin resistance and lipodystrophy[68,69] and decrease hyperandrogenemia.[70] Metformin treatment may result in weight loss by reducing the appetite.

2. Insulin

   Often, very high doses of insulin may be needed in extreme insulin resistance syndromes. Highly concentrated insulin can be used in these cases (500 units/mL). Lifestyle modifications and insulin sensitizers may help to decrease the insulin requirements.

3. Growth hormone and IGF-1

   IGF-1 shares homology with insulin and has the ability to bind to insulin receptors. IGF-1 has been used in some patients with leprechaunism and found to be effective in preventing the growth retardation as well as in improving hyperglycemia in some cases.[71] IGF-1 has also been used in other types of insulin resistance syndrome.[72–74] In HIV lipodystrophy, recombinant human growth hormone has been reported to reverse the buffalo hump and truncal adiposity but not the peripheral lipoatrophy.[75] Even though treatment with recombinant human growth hormone leads to an improved lipid profile with a significant increase in HDL cholesterol and significant decreases in total and LDL cholesterol and triglyceride levels, it also induces hyperglycemia and insulin resistance.[76]

4. Immunomodulation

   This modality has been used in antibody-mediated extreme insulin resistance syndromes. Steroids, cyclosporine, and cyclophosphamide and plasmapheresis have been used.[63,77,78] A combination of a short-term suppression of autoantibodies with plasmapheresis and cyclophosphamide, followed by a chronic maintenance approach with cyclosporin A and azathioprine offers a promise of prevention of relapses. However, immunosuppressive therapy may not have an impact on the natural history of the disease.[63]

5. Leptin replacement and adipose tissue implant

   In animal studies, it was shown that fat transplantation reversed the hyperglycemia and lowered insulin levels in animal models of lipodystrophy.[79,80] Additionally, leptin replacement improved insulin resistance and hyperlipidemia,[80] which was not seen in another study.[81] In one study that included nine women with lipodystrophies and hypoleptinemia, subcutaneous recombinant leptin was shown to improve hyperglycemia and decrease triglyceride levels. Some of these patients were actually able to maintain normoglycemia after discontinuation of hypoglycemic treatments.[82] Leptin has also been reported to improve hepatic steatosis, insulin sensitivity, and decrease intramyocellular lipid levels.[82–84]

6. Insulin receptor activators

   Insulin mimetics, such as L-783,281 and vanadate, seem to act by stimulating insulin receptor activity. Thus, they may potentially have beneficial effect in some types of extreme insulin resistance syndromes.[85]

7. Lifestyle modifications

   Extremely low-fat diet is recommended for the patients that have hypertriglyceridemia, in addition to regular exercise that improves insulin sensitivity and dyslipidemia. Alcohol should be avoided in patients with hepatic steatosis and hypertriglyceridemia.[26]

Summary

Recent explosion of our knowledge of insulin signal transduction at the molecular level gathered from studies of patients with extreme insulin resistance syndromes has allowed us to rapidly translate the findings to the therapeutic area dealing with the much more common insulin-resistant conditions. Because of the rapid progress in this area, it is expected that students of these conditions get into the habit of frequently updating their knowledge from reviewing general science (such as *Nature, Cell, Science*) and specific diabetes/metabolism journals (*Diabetes, Diabetes Care, Diabetologia, Molecular Endocrinology, Endocrinology, Journal of Clinical Endocrinology and Metabolism, Journal of Clinical Investigation*, etc.). Additionally, several professional organizations maintain excellent websites with useful web links on the Internet, allowing a quick search for the updated information. These websites are listed at the end of this chapter.

References

1. Kahn CR, Flier JS, Bar RS, et al. The syndrome of insulin resistance and acanthosis nigricans: insulin receptor disorders in man. *N Engl J Med*. 1976;294:739–745.
2. Moller DE, Flier JS. Insulin resistance: mechanisms, syndromes, and implications. *N Engl J Med*. 1991;325:938–948.
3. Barbieri RL, Smith S, Ryan KJ, et al. The role of hyperinsulinemia in the pathogenesis of ovarian hyperandrogenism. *Fertil Steril*. 1988;50:197–202.
4. Barroso I, Curnell M, Crowley VE, et al. Dominant negative mutation in human PPAR gamma associated with severe insulin resistance, diabetes mellitus, and hypertension. *Nature*. 1999;402:880–883.
5. Borai A, Livingstone C, Ferns GA. The biochemical assessment of insulin resistance. *Ann Clin Biochem*. 2007;44:324–342.
6. Tritos NA, Mantzoros CS. Syndromes of severe insulin resistance. *J Clin Endocrinol Metab*. 1998;83(9):3025–3030.
7. Legro RS, Finegood D, Dunaif A. A fasting glucose to insulin ratio is a useful measure of insulin sensitivity in women with polycystic ovary syndrome. *J Clin Endocrinol Metab*. 1998;83:2694–2698.
8. Vanhala P, Vanhala M, Kumpusalo E, et al. The quantitative insulin sensitivity check index QUICKI predicts the onset of type 2 diabetes better than fasting plasma insulin in obese subjects: a 5 year follow up study. *J Clin Endocrinol Metab*. 2002;87: 5834–5837.
9. Lee S, Choi S, Kim HJ, et al. Cut-off measures of surrogate measures of insulin resistance for metabolic syndrome in Korean non-diabetic adults. *J Korean Med Sci*. 2006;21:695–700.
10. Rabasa-Lhoret R, Bastard JP, Jan V, et al. Modified quantitative insulin sensitivity check index is better correlated to hyperinsulinemic glucose clamp than other fasting-based index of insulin sensitivity in different insulin resistant states. *J Clin Endocrinol Metab*. 2003;88:4917–4923.
11. Collinet M, Berthelon M, Benit P, et al. Familial hyperinsulinemia due to a mutation substituting histidine for arginine at position 65 in proinsulin: identification of the mutation by restriction enzyme mapping. *Eur J Pediatr*. 1998;157:450–460.
12. Haned M, Polonsky KS, Bergenstal RM, et al. Familial hyperinsulinaemia due to a structurally abnormal insulin. Definition of an emerging new clinical syndrome. *N Engl J Med*. 1984;310:1288–1294.
13. Duckworth WC, Bennit RG, Hamel FG. Insulin degradation: progress and potential. *Endo Rev*. 1998;19:608–624.
14. Francis A, Hanning I, Alberti KG. The influence of insulin antibody levels on the plasma profile and action of subcutaneously injected human and bovine short acting insulins. *Diabetologia*. 1985;28:330–334.
15. Taylor SI, Grunberger G, Marcus-Samuels B, et al. Hypoglycemia associated with antibodies to the insulin receptor. *N Engl J Med*. 1982;307:1422–1426.
16. Virkamaki A, Ueki K, Kahn CR. Protein–protein interaction in insulin signaling and the molecular mechanisms of insulin resistance. *J Clin Invest*. 1999;103:931–943.
17. Gorden P, Carpentier JL, Frechet PO, et al. Internalization of polypeptide hormones: mechanism, intracellular localization and significance. *Diabetologia*. 1980;18:263–274.
18. Grunberger G, Robert A, Carpentier JL, et al. Human circulating monocytes internalize 125I-insulin in a similar fashion to rat hepatocytes: relevance to receptor regulation in target and non-target tissue. *J Lab Clin Med*. 1985;106:211–217.
19. Flier JS, Minaker KL, Landsburg L, et al. Impaired in vivo insulin clearance in patients with target cell resistance to insulin. *Diabetes*. 1982;31:132–135.
20. Flier JS. Metabolic importance of acanthosis nigricans. *Arch Derm*. 1985;121:193–194.
21. Cruz PD, Hud JA. Excess insulin binding to insulin-like growth factor receptors: proposed mechanism for acanthosis nigricans. *J Invest Dermatol*. 1992;98(Suppl):82S–85S.
22. Fradkin JE, Eastman RC, Lesniak MA, et al. Specificity spillover at the hormone receptor: exploring its role in human disease. *N Engl J Med*. 1989;320:640–645.
23. Rotman-Pikielny P, Andewelt A, Ozyavuzligil A, et al. Polycystic ovarian syndrome (PCOS): lessons from patients with severe insulin resistance syndromes. The Endocrine Society's 83rd Annual Meeting; 2001:80.

24. Premkumar A, Chow C, Bhandarkar P, et al. Lipoatrophic lipodystrophic syndromes – the spectrum of findings on MR imaging. *AJR*. 2002;178:311–318.
25. Cauble MS, Gilroy R, Sorrel MF, et al. Lipoatrophic diabetes and end-stage liver disease secondary to nonalcoholic steatohepatitis with recurrence after liver transplantation. *Transplantation*. 2001;71:892–895.
26. Garg A. Acquired and inherited lipodystrophies. *N Engl J Med*. 2004;350(12):1220–1234.
27. Garg A, Wilson R, Barnes R, et al. A gene for congenital generalized lipodystrophy maps to human chromosome 9q34. *J Clin Endocrinol Metab*. 1999;84:3390–3394.
28. Magre J, Delepine M, Khallouf E, et al. Identification of the gene altered in Berardinelli-Seip congenital lipodystrophy on chromosome 11q13. *Nat Genet*. 2001;28:365–370.
29. Peters JM, Barnes R, Bennet L, et al. Localization the gene for familial partial lipodystrophy (Dunnigan Variety) to chromosome 1q21-22. *Nat Genet*. 1998;18:292–295.
30. Jackson SN, Pinkey J, Bargiotta A, et al. A defect in the regional deposition of adipose tissue (partial lipodystrophy) is encoded by a gene at chromosome 1q. *Am J Hum Genet*. 1998;63:534–540.
31. Cao H, Hegele RA. Nuclear lamin A/C R482Q mutations in Canadian kindreds with Dunnigan type familial partial lipodystrophy. *Hum Molec Genet*. 2000;9:109–112.
32. Garg A, Vinaitheerthan M, Weatherall PT, et al. Phenotypic heterogeneity in patients with familial partial lipodystrophy (Dunnigan variety) related to the site of missense mutations in lamin A/C gene. *J Clin Endocrinol Metab*. 2001;86:59–65.
33. Simha V, Garg A. Body fat distribution and metabolic derangements in patients with familial partial lipodystrophy associated with mandibuloacral dysplasia. *J Clin Endocrinol Metab*. 2002;87:776–785.
34. Simha V, Agarwal AK, Oral EA, Fryns J-P, Garg A, et al. Genetic and phenotypic heterogeneity in patients with mandibuloacral dysplasia-associated lipodystrophy. *J Clin Endocrinol Metab*. 2003;88:2821–2824.
35. Agarwal AK, Garg A. A novel heterozygous mutation in peroxisome proliferator-activated receptor-gamma gene in a patient with familial partial lipodystrophy. *J Clin Endocrinol Metab*. 2002;87:408–411.
36. Savage DB, Tan GD, Acerini CL, et al. Human metabolic syndrome resulting from dominant-negative mutations in the nuclear receptor peroxisome proliferator-activated receptor-gamma. *Diabetes*. 2003;52:910–917.
37. George S, Rochford JJ, Wolfrum C, et al. A family with severe insulin resistance and diabetes due to a mutation in AKT2. *Science*. 2004;304:1325–1328.
38. Misra A, Garg A. Clinical features and metabolic derangements in acquired generalized lipodystrophy: case reports and review of the literature. *Medicine (Baltimore)*. 2003;82:129–146.
39. Haque WA, Shimomura I, Matsuzawa Y, Garg A. Serum adiponectin and leptin levels in patients with lipodystrophies. *J Clin Endocrinol Metab*. 2002;87:2395–2398.
40. Billings JK, Milgraum SS, Gupta AK, et al. Lipoatrophic panniculitis: a possible autoimmune inflammatory disease of fat report of three cases. *Arch Dermatol*. 1987;123:1662–1666.
41. Hubler A, Abendroth K, Keiner T, et al. Dysregulation of insulin-like growth factors in a case of generalized acquired lipoatrophic diabetes mellitus (Lawrence syndrome) connected with autoantibodies against adipocytes membranes. *Exp Clin Endocrinol Diabetes*. 1998;106:79–84.
42. Garg A. Lipodystrophies. *Am J Med*. 2000;108:143–152.
43. Jasin HE. Systemic lupus erythematosus, partial lipodystrophy and hypocomplementemia. *J Rheumatol*. 1979;6:43–50.
44. Torrelo A, Espana A, Boixeda P, Ledo A. Partial lipodystrophy and dermatomyositis. *Arch Dermatol*. 1991;127:1846–1847.
45. Mathieson PW, Wurzner R, Oliveria DB, et al. Complement mediated adipocytes lysis by nephritic factor sera. *J Exp Med*. 1993;177:1827–1831.
46. Chen D, Misra A, Garg A. Lipodystrophy in human immunodeficiency virus-infected patients. *J Clin Endocrinol Metab*. 2002;87:4845–4856.
47. Tsiodras S, Mantzoros C, Hammer S, et al. Effects of protease inhibitors on hyperglycemia, hyperlipidemia and lipodystrophy. A five-year cohort study. *Arch Int Med*. 2000;160:2050–2056.
48. Van Der Valk M, Gisolf EH, Reiss P, et al. Increased risk of lipodystrophy when nucleoside analogue reverse transcriptase inhibitors are included with protease inhibitors in the treatment of HIV infection. *AIDS*. 2001;15:847–855.
49. Panse I, Vasseur E, Raffin-Manson ML, et al. Lipodystrophy associated with protease inhibitors. *Br J Dermatol*. 2000;142:496–500.
50. Caron M, Auclair M, Vigouroux C, et al. The HIV protease inhibitor indinavir impairs sterol regulatory element-binding protein-1 intranuclear localization, inhibits preadipocyte differentiation, and induces insulin resistance. *Diabetes*. 2001;50:1378–1388.
51. Dowell P, Flexner C, Kwiterovich PO, et al. Suppression of preadipocyte differentiation and promotion of adipocytes death by HIV protease inhibitors. *J Biol Chem*. 2000;275:41325–41332.
52. Murata H, Hruz PW, Mueckler M. The mechanism of insulin resistance caused by HIV protease inhibitor therapy. *J Biol Chem*. 2000;275:20251–20254.
53. Meyer MM, Schuett M, Jost P, et al. Indinavir decreases insulin-stimulated phosphatidylinositol 3-kinase activity and stimulates leptin secretion in human adipocytes. *Diabetes*. 2001;50(Suppl 2):A414.
54. Bastard JP, Caron M, Vidal H, et al. Association between altered expression of adipogenic factor SREBP1 in lipoatrophic adipose tissue from HIV-1-infected patients and abnormal adipocyte differentiation and insulin resistance. *Lancet*. 2002;359:1026–1031.

55. Shimomura I, Hammer RE, Richardson JA, et al. Insulin resistance and diabetes mellitus in transgenic mice expressing nuclear SREBP-1c in adipose tissue: model for congenital generalized lipodystrophy. *Genes Dev*. 1998;12:3182–3194.

56. Tritos NA, Mantzoros CS. Syndromes of severe insulin resistance. *J Clin Endocrinol Metab*. 1998;83:3025–3030.

57. Flier JS, Moller DE, Moses AC, et al. Insulin-mediated pseudoacromegaly: clinical and biochemical characterization of a syndrome of selective insulin resistance. *J Clin Endocrinol Metab*. 1993;76:1533–1541.

58. Martin XD, Zenobi PD. Type A syndrome of insulin resistance: anterior chamber anomalies of the eye and effects of insulin-like growth factor-1 on the retina. *Ophthalmologica*. 2001;215:117–123.

59. Grunberger G, Zick Y, Gorden P. Defect in phosphorylation of insulin receptors in cells from an insulin-resistant patient with normal insulin binding. *Science*. 1984;223:832–934.

60. Young J, morbois-Trabut L, Couzinet B, et al. Type A insulin resistance syndrome revealing a novel lamin A mutation. *Diabetes*. 2005;54:1873–1878.

61. Maddux BA, Goldfine ID. Membrane glycoprotein PC-1 inhibition of insulin receptor function occurs via direct interaction with receptor alpha subunit. *Diabetes*. 2000;49:13–19.

62. Flier JS, Kahn CR, Roth J, et al. Antibodies that impair insulin receptor binding in an unusual diabetic syndrome with severe insulin resistance. *Science*. 1975;190:63–65.

63. Arioglu E, Andewelt A, Diabo C, et al. Clinical course of autoantibody to the insulin receptor syndrome. The Endocrine Society's 83rd Annual Meeting; 2001:113.

64. Flier JS, Bar RS, Muggeo M, et al. The evolving clinical course of patients with insulin receptor autoantibodies: spontaneous remission or receptor proliferation with hypoglycemia. *J Clin Endocrinol Metab*. 1978;47:985–995.

65. Bar RS, Levis WR, Rechler MM, et al. Extreme insulin resistance in ataxia telangiectasia: defect in affinity of insulin receptors. *N Engl J Med*. 1978;298:1164–1171.

66. Burant CF, Sreenan S, Hirano K, et al. Troglitazone action is independent of adipose tissue. *J Clin Invest*. 1997;100:2900–2908.

67. Arioglu E, Duncan-Morin J, Sebring N, et al. Efficacy and safety of troglitazone in the treatment of lipodystrophy syndrome. *Ann Int Med*. 2000;133:263–274.

68. Hadigan C, Corcoran C, Basgoz N, et al. Metformin in the treatment of HIV lipodystrophy syndrome. *JAMA*. 2000;284: 472–477.

69. Di Paolo S. Metformin ameliorates extreme insulin resistance in a patient with anti-insulin receptor antibodies: description of insulin receptor and postreceptor effects in vivo and vitro. *Acta Endocrinol*. 1992;126:117–123.

70. Rique S, Ibanez L, Marcos MV, et al. Effect of metformin on androgen and insulin concentration in type A insulin resistance syndrome. *Diabetologia*. 2000;43:385–386.

71. Nakae J, Kato M, Murashita M, et al. Long-term effect of recombinant human insulin-like growth factor1 on metabolic and growth control in a patient with leprechaunism. *J Clin Endocrinol Metab*. 1998;83:542–549.

72. Morrow LA, O'Brien MB, Moller DE, et al. Recombinant human insulin like growth factor-1 therapy improves glycemic control and insulin action in type A syndrome insulin resistance. *J Clin Endocrinol Metabol*. 1994;79:205–210.

73. Quin JD, Fisher BM, Paterson KR, et al. Acute response to recombinant insulin-like growth factor 1 in a patient with Mendenhall's syndrome. *N Engl J Med*. 1990;323:1425–1426.

74. Yamamoto T, Sato T, Mori T, et al. Clinical efficacy of insulin like growth factor 1 in a patient with auto-antibodies to insulin receptors: a case report. *Diabetes Res Clin Pract*. 2000;49:65–69.

75. Torres RA, Unger KW, Cadman JA, et al. Recombinant human growth hormone improves truncal adiposity and buffalo humps in HIV positive patients on HAART. *AIDS*. 1999;13:2479–2481.

76. Schwarz JM, Mulligan K, Lee J, et al. Effects of recombinant human growth hormone on hepatic lipid and carbohydrate metabolism in HIV-infected patients with fat accumulation. *J Clin Endocrinol Metab*. 2002;87:942–945.

77. Kramer N, Rosenstien ED, Schneider G. Refractory hyperglycemia complicating an evolving connective tissue disease: response to cyclosporin. *J Rheumatol*. 1998;25:816–818.

78. Eriksson JW, Bremell T, Eliasson B, et al. Successful treatment with plasmapheresis, cyclophosphamide, and cyclosporin A in type B syndrome of insulin resistance. Case report. *Diabetes Care*. 1998;21:1217–1220.

79. Gavrilova O, Marcus-Samuels B, Graham D, et al. Surgical implantation of adipose tissue reverses diabetes in lipotropic mice. *J Clin Invest*. 2000;105:271–278.

80. Shimomura I, Hammer RE, Ikemoto S, et al. Leptin reverses insulin resistance and diabetes mellitus in mice with congenital lipodystrophy. *Nature*. 1999;401:73–76.

81. Reitman ML, Gavrilova O. A-ZIP/F-1 mice lacking white fat: a model for understanding lipoatrophic diabetes. *Int J Obes Relat Metab Disord*. 2000;24(Suppl 4):S11–S14.

82. Oral EA, Simha V, Ruiz E, et al. Leptin-replacement therapy for lipodystrophy. *N Engl J Med*. 2002;346:570–578.

83. Petersen KF, Oral EA, Dufour S, et al. Leptin reverses insulin resistance and hepatic steatosis in patients with severe lipodystrophy. *J Clin Invest*. 2002;109:1345–1350.

84. Simha V, Szczepaniak LS, Wagner AJ, et al. Effect of leptin replacement on intrahepatic and intramyocellular lipid content in patients with generalized lipodystrophy. *Diabetes Care*. 2003;26:30–35.

85. Zhang B, Salituro G, Szalkowski D, et al. Discovery of a small molecule insulin mimetic with antidiabetic activity in mice. *Science*. 1999;284:974–977.

Helpful Internet Sources for Additional Information on Insulin Resistance

www.diabetes.org
www.acponline.org
www.asim.org
www.endo-society.org

Part VI
Complications of Diabetes

Chapter 18
Acute Hyperglycemic Syndromes: Diabetic Ketoacidosis and the Hyperosmolar State

Yun Feng and Adrienne M. Fleckman

Diabetic Ketoacidosis: Clinical Presentation

A typical patient with diabetic ketoacidosis (DKA) becomes severely ill over one to several days and represents a medical emergency.

The patient, often a "repeat offender" who stops taking insulin, presents with increasing urination and thirst along with nausea, vomiting, abdominal pain, dehydration, weakness, and dizziness. The patient may become confused and slip into coma. The respiratory compensation that accompanies acidemia causes deep rapid (Kussmaul) breathing. The sweet smell of the volatile ketone body acetone signals the possibility of ketoacidosis.

Diabetes is a heterogeneous disease,[1] and patients with DKA reflect this heterogeneity.[2] The majority of patients with DKA have type 1 diabetes[3] (Fig. 18.1a). Consistent with this type 1 predominance, patients are likely to be young, slender, Caucasian (type 1 diabetes is 2–7 times more common in whites than blacks[4]), and lack a family history of diabetes. Nevertheless, many patients with DKA have type 2 diabetes,[5] particularly those whose diabetes first presents with DKA (Fig. 18.1a and b).

The Differential Diagnosis

The most severe scenario for patients with DKA is the diabetic coma. Stupor and coma have many potential causes (Table 18.1). Alcoholic intoxication causing coma can be assessed by a history of alcohol intake and blood alcohol levels. Decreased level of consciousness without focal findings suggests encephalopathy (unilateral weakness suggests a stroke). The patient may have taken an overdose; toxicology "screen" is helpful to exclude drugs that can cause coma and acidosis. Renal failure with uremic encephalopathy can be detected with blood urea nitrogen (BUN) and creatinine measurements. Evidence of trauma should be sought. Fever and confusion may indicate central nervous system infection. A history of emotional instability may suggest psychosis or a patient who is feigning illness. Witnesses can be questioned about seizure activity, which is often followed by a decreased level of alertness. The mnemonic given in Table 18.1 is not comprehensive; for example, the electrocardiogram may show a cardiac arrhythmia or a myocardial infarction that can cause a drop in blood pressure and change in mental status. While reviewing the differential diagnosis, the physician simultaneously obtains the finger stick (capillary) glucose measurement to exclude hypoglycemia (low blood sugar) or hyperglycemia as a cause of coma. An elevated glucose supports a diagnosis of diabetic ketoacidosis or hyperglycemic hyperosmolar coma.

A.M. Fleckman (✉)

Department of Medicine, Albert Einstein College of Medicine, Beth Israel Medical Center, New York, NY, USA

e-mail: fleckman@chpnet.org

L. Poretsky (ed.), *Principles of Diabetes Mellitus*, DOI 10.1007/978-0-387-09841-8_18,
© Springer Science+Business Media, LLC 2010

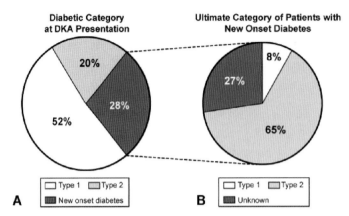

Fig. 18.1 Categories of diabetes in patients with DKA. Diabetic ketoacidosis is predominantly, but not exclusively, a complication of type 1 diabetes[3]

Table 18.1 Differential diagnosis of diabetic coma

A-E-I-O-U	TIPSI
Alcohol	Trauma
Encephalopathy	Infection
Infectious	Meningitis
Neurologic	Sepsis
Insulin	Psychosis
Hypoglycemia, DKA, hyperosmolar, alcoholic ketoacidosis	Seizure
Overdose, Opiates	Post-ictal state
Uremia	

Definition

Diabetic ketoacidosis (DKA) is a state of metabolic decompensation in which insulin deficiency (relative or absolute) causes both hyperglycemia and excess production of ketoacids, resulting in metabolic acidosis.[6]

DKA, the first manifestation of diabetes in a minority of patients, most often occurs in known diabetic individuals taking insufficient insulin. Patients may run out of insulin or not accept the necessity for insulin. Adolescents sometimes discontinue insulin as an act of rebellion. Ill patients, who are not eating well, may reduce or omit insulin doses not realizing that stress, which is accompanied by elevation of "counter-regulatory" hormones, may require *more* than usual insulin.

No absolute numbers separate uncontrolled diabetes from DKA, although there is agreement on a somewhat arbitrary definition: a glucose level >250 mg/dL (13.9 mmol/L), acidemia reflected by a pH lower than 7.30, a serum bicarbonate less than 18 mEq/L, a positive test for serum ketones, and an increase in the anion gap.[7] Reasons for exceptions to this definition are discussed below.

Pathophysiology

The fed state is an insulin-sufficient state. Insulin affects the internal machinery of cells in the liver, fat (adipose tissue), and muscles to promote energy production and storage.

Cellular work requires massive amounts of energy. Intermediary metabolism (named for the *intermediate* compounds that are generated prior to the final metabolic products), largely through the production of ATP (adenosine tri-phosphate), provides this energy and the energy for synthesizing macromolecules.[5,8–10]

Glucose, the major cellular nutrient, is transported into cells where it is metabolized in the glycolytic pathway. Enzymes in this pathway are regulated by insulin (whose action is antagonized by glucagon). At the end of this pathway, the three-carbon glucose metabolite pyruvate is further broken down into small molecules that are used to produce complex cellular components or can be converted into chemical energy (the nucleotide ATP) when transported into the energy generator of the cell (the mitochondria).

When insulin levels are adequate, energy is stored in small quantities as glycogen for immediate use or in large quantities as triglycerides for long-term use.

Inside the hepatocyte, glucose molecules can be linked in a tightly packed branching structure to form glycogen, the polysaccharide that stores glucose. Alternatively, the two-carbon compound acetylcoenzyme A (acetyl-CoA), which is formed from glucose breakdown, can be used to manufacture larger molecules, including fatty acids for energy storage in a large fat depot (adipose tissue). Insulin acts to stimulate and maintain these storage processes.

In DKA, insulin action is inadequate to promote glucose entry into cells. The decreased flux of glucose into cells simulates fasting.

With the fall in intracellular glucose, intermediary metabolism of carbohydrates and lipids shifts away from glucose breakdown and storage to an exaggerated imitation of the fasting state. Metabolism shifts away from the utilization of glucose toward gluconeogenesis, which is the production of glucose from pyruvate (Fig. 18.2). Precursors for gluconeogenesis are obtained from fat, which is melted down into fatty acids and glycerol, and from proteins following breakdown into constituent amino acids. Glycerol, amino acids (particularly alanine), and lactate (derived from red cell metabolism) are converted into glucose.

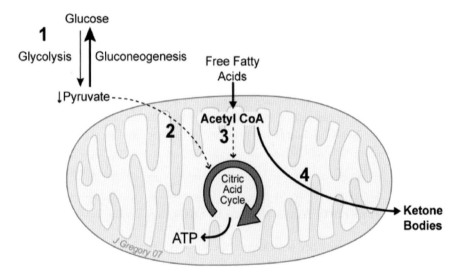

Fig. 18.2 The formation of ketone bodies is linked to increased gluconeogenesis. **1** When insulin levels fall, glycolysis decreases and gluconeogenesis increases, reducing pyruvate levels. **2** Pyruvate is not available for conversion into oxaloacetate. **3** Without oxaloacetate, acetyl-CoA cannot enter the TCA cycle. **4** Free fatty acids, converted into acetyl-CoA, are therefore diverted to mitochondrial ketone body formation

The counter-regulatory hormones glucagon and epinephrine, along with growth hormone and cortisol, stimulated by fasting and by stress, antagonize the effects of insulin.

Counter-regulatory hormones antagonize the glucose-lowering action of insulin and act to raise the blood glucose level. Glucagon, a potent counter-regulatory hormone inhibited by insulin, is secreted from pancreatic alpha cells when cells perceive low glucose. In diabetes, pancreatic insulin levels are reduced and glucagon is chronically elevated. In DKA, in addition to low insulin action, there is the cellular perception of low glucose, which further stimulates glucagon secretion. The excessive glucagon levels of DKA dominate hepatic metabolism, promoting breakdown of glycogen to glucose, stimulating gluconeogenesis, inhibiting fatty acid synthesis, and directing long-chain fatty acids into the mitochondria where they are dedicated to ketoacid formation (Fig. 18.3).

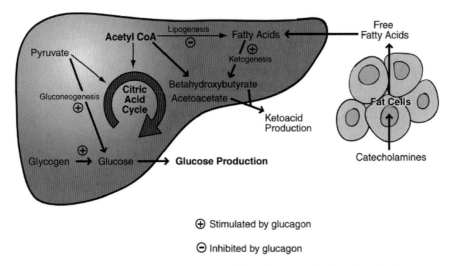

Fig. 18.3 Glucagon plays a central role in DKA. Glucagon stimulates glucose production through gluconeogenesis and glycogen breakdown. Lipogenesis is inhibited by glucagon. Free fatty acids derived from lipolysis in fat cells are transported into the mitochondria. Acetyl-CoA from fatty acid breakdown is diverted to ketoacid production

Catecholamines, acting on β-adrenergic receptors, are the most potent stimulators of lipolysis (breakdown of adipose tissue triglycerides with release of free fatty acids and glycerol). Growth hormone also stimulates lipolysis and liberates free fatty acids.[11] Cortisol contributes to elevations of blood glucose by increasing lipolysis in certain fat depots, increasing the transcription of genes that increase protein catabolism (providing precursors for gluconeogenesis), and upregulating the expression of the rate-limiting enzyme for gluconeogenesis, phosphoenolpyruvate carboxykinase (PEPCK).[12]

The Central Role of Free Fatty Acids (FFAs) in DKA

Free fatty acids leave the fat cell and are transported to the liver.

Without fatty acids there cannot be any ketoacids; without ketoacids there is no diabetic ketoacidosis.[13] Under the influence of insulin, free fatty acids are transported to and imprisoned inside a fat cell (adipocyte) bound as three chains to a glycerol molecule (triglyceride). The catecholamines are ready to "spring" FFAs out of "jail," but they are unable to do so while there is adequate insulin. During starvation, when insulin levels drop, lipids stored in adipose tissue as triglycerides are released from the fat cell as the hydrocarbon long-chain fatty acids. These fatty acids are transported to the liver bound to albumin. From the viewpoint of the FFA, the scene in the liver is chaotic. The liver does not have adequate insulin levels. Glycolysis, the most ancient metabolic pathway, is at a standstill. FFAs further inhibit insulin action and stimulate gluconeogenesis and hepatic production of lipoproteins, contributing to hyperglycemia and to the marked elevation of triglycerides seen in some patients. Under fasting conditions with adequate insulin present, this process (coupled with the release of glycerol) provides sufficient calories to serve as the glucose and energy "grocery store." In DKA, this process leads to uncontrolled glucose elevations.

Malonylcoenzyme A (CoA) levels control free fatty acid transport into the mitochondria, thereby acting as the key control of the rate of hepatic ketoacid production.

Malonyl-CoA is a precursor molecule whose levels rise during the insulin-stimulated process of triglyceride synthesis in the cytoplasm. Malonyl-CoA then inhibits the transport of fatty acids into mitochondria, by inhibiting the fatty acid transporter carnitine palmitoyltransferase 1 (CPT1). During DKA, since insulin levels fall, malonyl-CoA levels decline, permitting a rise in fatty acid transport into mitochondria (Fig. 18.4).

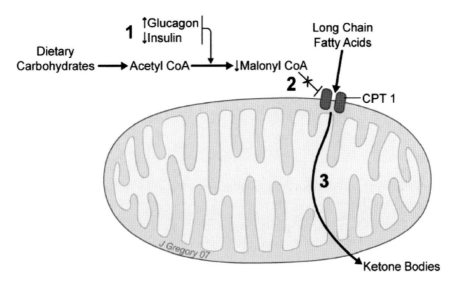

Fig. 18.4 Malonyl-CoA plays a pivotal role in the regulation of ketogenesis. In DKA, the *high* glucagon and the *low* insulin decrease malonyl-CoA production from acetyl-CoA. **1**. The fall in malonyl-CoA releases the inhibition of the transport protein (CPT1) that shuttles long-chain fatty acids into the mitochondria. **2**. Increased long-chain fatty acids are thus available for ketone body formation

The fate of free fatty acids in the hepatic mitochondria is determined by the activity of the glycolytic pathway, because pyruvate is required for FFA derivatives to enter the TCA cycle (Fig. 18.2).

Pyruvate formed during glycolysis is the glucose-derived metabolite that enters the TCA (tricarboxylic acid, also called the Krebs or citric acid) cycle. This pathway is oxygen requiring (oxidative) and generates large amounts of ATP. In DKA, pyruvate is diverted to gluconeogenesis, less is available to enter the TCA cycle, and the rate of oxidative metabolism of glucose declines. In addition, the fall in pyruvate alters fat metabolism in the liver. Under normal conditions of energy generation, fatty acid metabolites can enter the TCA cycle in a process that requires pyruvate. Since pyruvate is necessary for fat to enter the TCA pathway, it is said that fat burns in the flame of carbohydrate. In DKA, this energy-generating "flame" is extinguished (Fig. 18.2).

Some pyruvate is converted to lactate in a process that restores cytoplasmic NAD^+ (nicotinamide adenine dinucleotide), necessary for minimal cellular metabolism. This can cause a lactic acidosis superimposed on top of ketoacidosis[14] (Fig. 18.5).

When fatty acids cannot enter the TCA cycle in hepatic mitochondria, they are diverted to ketone body (ketoacid) formation.

Fatty acids are broken down in the mitochondrial matrix into the two-carbon compound acetyl-CoA. Unable to enter the TCA cycle during intracellular glucose privation, acetyl-CoA in hepatic mitochondria is diverted to the production of the ketoacids β-hydroxybutyrate and acetoacetate.[15]

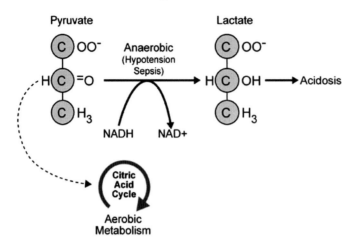

Fig. 18.5 Lactate formed from pyruvate can contribute to acidosis

The "redox" (reduction–oxidation) status of the mitochondria, set by the NADH/NAD⁺ ratio, determines the predominant species of ketoacid.

Coenzymes co-operate with enzymes to catalyze reactions. In these reactions, the coenzymes are reversibly altered and can be cycled back and forth between two forms, creating a "pair." The coenzyme pair NAD⁺ and NADH functions to carry electrons in oxidation–reduction reactions. An increased NADH/NAD⁺ ratio develops in DKA during β-oxidation of fatty acids and also in states of low tissue oxygenation (such as those that occur if the patient has severe fluid loss and is hypotensive from dehydration or sepsis). NADH drives the conversion of the ketoacid acetoacetate to β-hydroxybutyrate. As will be discussed later, laboratories use the nitroprusside reaction, which does not measure β-hydroxybutyrate, to test for ketones. When β-hydroxybutyrate is the major ketoacid, a misleadingly low nitroprusside test can sway the unsuspecting physician away from the correct diagnosis.

Since glucose is not available in DKA, alternative energy-releasing compounds must be utilized. The ketoacids function as an alternate fuel.

Tissues are not able to utilize glucose because of inadequate insulin action. Without insulin (or without *enough* insulin) cells are left without nutrients. The ketone bodies, or ketoacids, do not require insulin for uptake into cells. If glucose is the electric power that drives the body, ketone bodies are the batteries of the brain and the heart. When the electricity fails, hepatic mitochondria produce and export this alternate power. In the heart, skeletal muscle, brain, and kidney, ketone bodies can be converted back to acetyl-CoA, which enters the TCA cycle and provides metabolic energy through generation of ATP[16] (Fig. 18.6).

Assessment of a Patient with DKA

Among the long list of potential precipitating factors for DKA are serious conditions that require diagnosis and specific treatment.

Although diabetic ketoacidosis often occurs in patients who run out of insulin or stop taking insulin, there is frequently an inciting event that must be discovered. The physician's challenge is to find what went wrong, reverse the process, return the patient to health, and prevent the next episode. In considering the possibilities, it is important to remember that common things occur commonly. The patient may have stopped taking insulin

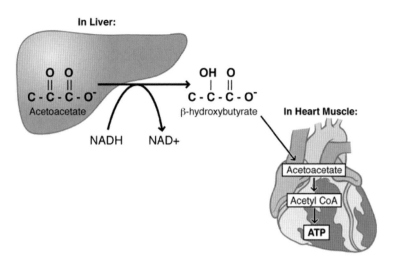

Fig. 18.6 Ketone bodies formed in the liver provide an alternate fuel for the heart, skeletal muscle, and brain

or the pancreas may have gradually lost insulin secretory capacity. Counter-regulatory mechanisms may be activated during any stress and may render antecedent insulin levels insufficient. Particular attention must be given to infections (with elevations of the counter-regulatory hormones cortisol and catecholamines), stroke or heart attacks (extremely high epinephrine production), or pregnancy (placental lactogen or cortisol). Dehydration during gastrointestinal illness accompanied by vomiting or diarrhea may hasten the development of DKA. An alcohol binge may cause rapid "decompensation" in the patient with limited insulin reserve.

Very unusual causes of counter-regulatory hormone elevation precipitating DKA are growth hormone elevations from acromegaly, glucocorticoid excess in Cushing's syndrome, and glucagon in the rare glucagonoma syndrome. Obscure causes of DKA, such as changing to more active pancreatic enzymes to treat chronic pancreatitis with increased absorption of nutrients or somatostatin inhibition of insulin secretion in a somatostatinoma, have been described. In teenagers, eating disorders are a consideration, especially in recurrent DKA. Medications – the anti-psychotic drugs clozapine and olanzapine – are reported to cause DKA.[17,18] An unusual fulminant non-immune form of type 1 diabetes can present with a rapid onset.[19] Rare cases of DKA have occurred following pancreatic destruction by a virus.[20,21]

Infection is the most common precipitating cause of diabetic ketoacidosis; sites that hide infections should be examined carefully.

Elevated glucose levels impair the ability to fight infection, potentially leading to aggressive tissue destruction. Thus it is critical to control the blood glucose and to discover and treat all infections. The physician must be particularly suspicious in patients who are more likely to harbor infections. Infection is twice as likely in women as in men, three times as likely in patients who present with neurologic abnormalities, and two to nine times as likely in patients who fail to clear ketonuria within 12 h. Hidden sites of infection include the teeth, sinuses, gallbladder, abscesses in the peri-rectal area, and pelvis (in women), and must be examined and re-examined. The nose should be carefully inspected for eschar (black necrotic tissue), which might indicate the fungus mucormycosis, classically but rarely seen in DKA.

Measurements, tests, and calculations are used to determine the severity of acidosis, magnitude of ketonemia, and fluid and electrolyte balance.

In order to treat DKA, the physician must measure the degree of acidosis (pH), the ability of the patient to compensate by lowering pCO_2, the elevation of the blood glucose level, and the serum potassium (K^+). Initially, an arterial sample is taken for measuring the pH, pO_2, and pCO_2 in order to know if the patient has low oxygenation (hypoxemia), a primary respiratory acidosis (indicating pulmonary disease or central hypoventilation), or a primary respiratory alkalosis (suggestive of sepsis). After the baseline arterial measurement, the calculated anion gap from chemistries (using measured – not corrected – serum sodium, chloride, and bicarbonate) and the venous pH can be used to evaluate the acid–base status (Table 18.2).[22] To document or follow ketoacid production, serum ketones are typically measured. They are cleared rapidly and may be detected with greater sensitivity in urine, even when low or absent in the serum. Although it is the dominant "ketoacid" in DKA with a ratio as high as 20:1 compared to acetoacetate, β-hydroxybutyrate is not measured in the nitroprusside test for ketoacids because β-hydroxybutyrate is really an acid-alcohol. In the "redox" environment of DKA, an excess ratio of β-hydroxybutyrate to acetoacetate may result in spuriously low ketone body measurements. The astute clinician knows that DKA may occur without a markedly elevated nitroprusside reaction and is guided by the clinical presentation, pH, anion gap, and bicarbonate level.[23]

Table 18.2 Measurements useful in assessing a patient with DKA

Corrected serum $[Na^+]$ = measured serum $[Na^+]$ + 2 * (glucose in mg/dL – 100)/100[24,25]
The anion gap = $[Na^+]$ – ($[Cl^-]$ + $[HCO_3^-]$)
The normal anion gap = 8–12
In pure metabolic acidosis the last two digits of the pH = pCO_2
e.g., if the pH = 7.32, the pCO_2 should be 32
In pure metabolic acidosis the blood gas pCO_2 = (serum HCO_3^- * 1.5) + 8
The calculated effective serum osmolality = 2 (Na^+ + K^+) + (glucose in mg/dL/18)
Normal total body water (TBW) = lean body mass in kg * 60%
Current TBW = (normal serum osmolality * normal TBW)/current osmolality
Water deficit = normal TBW – current TBW

Treatment of Diabetic Ketoacidosis

Introduction

The treating physician seeks to re-establish normal physiology and restore the patient to normal function. Treatment is remarkably straightforward and involves intravenous fluid, insulin, potassium, and vigilance.

The osmotic diuresis of hyperglycemia causes dehydration, which exacerbates the metabolic acidosis.[9] **The severity of dehydration determines initial rates of fluid administration.**

In the hypotensive patient, fluid resuscitation takes precedence over other concerns. A fluid "challenge" is performed with isotonic fluid given in short blocks of time (in adults, at a rate of 10–30 mL/min checking the patient every 10 min; in children at a rate of 10–20 mL/kg over 30 min to 2 h[26,27]). If intravascular fluid depletion is the cause of hypotension, the blood pressure responds rapidly. Failure to respond to a fluid challenge within 30 min suggests another cause for low blood pressure such as cardiac pump failure or peripheral vasodilatation in sepsis. In adults with severe dehydration, initial fluid rates of 1–2 L/h may be required. If the patient is not hypotensive, or once blood pressure is restored, a more balanced approach to fluid administration using 250–500 mL/h is desirable. These slower rates of administration avoid fluid overload with potential for pulmonary edema and hypoxemia, or diuresis of potassium with resultant hypokalemia.[28] Hydration per se decreases counter-regulatory hormone levels, enhances renal perfusion, and establishes a glucose diuresis, lowering the blood sugar toward the renal threshold of 180 mg/dL.[29] It is customary to choose isotonic fluid in the hypotensive, dehydrated patient; half-normal saline as the patient recovers; and dextrose-containing fluid as the blood glucose drops below 200–250 mg/dL. Fluids containing 5% or even 10% dextrose prevent the hypoglycemia that would otherwise occur with continued administration of insulin essential to restrain ketogenesis and prevent recurrence of acidosis.

Medical situations requiring special fluid adjustments include myocardial infarction, congestive heart failure, and acute or chronic renal failure. These situations require individualized fluid management following initial volume resuscitation.[30]

Fluid administration should be slower in pediatric patients than adults.[26,31]

In children, the physician must be concerned about cerebral edema, which occurs in 1% of DKA episodes in children[32] and is responsible for 70% of diabetic deaths occurring before 12 years of age.[33] The assumption that cerebral edema is caused by organic osmoles that accumulate in the brain to balance the cellular dehydrating effect of the hyperosmolar extracellular fluid, and then cause excess fluid movement into cells with hydration, is unproven.[32] The risk factors identified for cerebral edema are more severe acidemia (lower pCO_2), greater dehydration (higher blood urea nitrogen), and the use of bicarbonate.[34] The ketone bodies themselves may increase brain microvascular permeability.[35] Even though the role of rapid fluid administration (greater than 50 mL/kg during the first 4 h of therapy) in causing brain herniation[36] is debated, fluid overload is avoided.

Insulin is administered by continuous infusion in doses that range from 0.5 to 4.0 units of regular insulin or rapid acting insulin analog (lispro or aspart) per hour.[37]

Insulin doses are adjusted against two parameters – restoring a near-normal blood glucose and reversing ketoacidosis. A loading bolus of 10 units regular insulin is commonly administered intravenously while simultaneously beginning continuous infusion at 0.1 units/kg/h. The glucose should fall by 50–75 mg/dL each hour. If the glucose does not fall as expected, the insulin infusion rate should be doubled. Since prevention of ketoacidosis requires less insulin action than prevention of hyperglycemia, it is a paradox in the therapy of DKA that it is more difficult to stop ketone body generation than to lower serum glucose. Therefore, it is essential that the physician maintains constant insulin infusion, if only at physiologic levels of 0.5 to 1 unit/h, to restrain lipolysis (release of FFA from adipose tissue). The continued administration of insulin without causing hypoglycemia often requires concomitant administration of glucose-containing infusions (usually 5% or, if necessary, 10% dextrose in water at approximately 100 mL/h), which should be started when the serum glucose has fallen to 200–250 mg/dL (11–14 mmol/L).

Potassium repletion is necessary because K^+ is lost during the osmotic diuresis of DKA as the K^+ salt of ketoacids.

The serum potassium level reflects both total body stores and the distribution between the intracellular (98% of total body K^+) and extracellular spaces. The osmotic diuresis of DKA causes huge urinary K^+ losses. Yet, the serum K^+ can be low, normal, or high at the time of presentation. Redistribution of K^+ out of the intracellular compartment and into the intravascular space causes a normal or high serum K^+ in the face of total body depletion.

Physiologic insulin levels drive K^+ into cells.[38] With the decreased insulin action of DKA, potassium moves out of cells into the serum. This redistribution may raise serum K^+. Further elevation of serum K^+ may occur because of redistribution related to acidosis (K^+ moving out of cells in exchange for H^+ moving in). Insulin administration during treatment moves potassium back into the cells, halts the generation of ketoacids, and reverses acidosis. Dangerous degrees of hypokalemia may then occur and are postulated to be the cause of the 30–50% DKA mortality in the 1950s.[39] The treating physician must anticipate and prevent this hypokalemia. Typically, 20–40 mEq K^+ is administered with each liter of fluid. If the fluid is administered more rapidly, the patient will (appropriately) receive more K^+ per unit time. Two caveats against K^+ administration are renal impairment, which prevents normal excretion of excess K^+, and dangerous hyperkalemia at the time of presentation. The physician may administer potassium as soon as urine flow is established. In addition, the physician must order an electrocardiogram (EKG) on presentation. If signs of hyperkalemia are present (tall-peaked T waves, followed by low-amplitude P wave and widening QRS complex) (Fig. 18.7), no potassium is given until the "stat" K^+ levels are back from the laboratory. In the absence of signs of hypokalemia on the EKG (low-amplitude T waves with rising amplitude U waves), some physicians do not administer K^+ until the laboratory measurement is available.

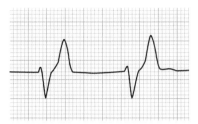

Fig. 18.7 The electrocardiogram in hyperkalemia progressively shows tall-peaked T waves followed by low-amplitude "P" wave (not even discernible in this example) and widening of the QRS

More and more evidence shows that bicarbonate administration plays no role in the therapy of DKA.

When insulin therapy reverses ketoacid formation, bicarbonate is rapidly regenerated from retained ketone body anions. To the extent that these anions were lost in the urine, the kidney takes several days to fully reclaim bicarbonate. In the past, bicarbonate was administered out of concern that severe acidosis would impair cardiac function and precipitate congestive heart failure or vascular collapse. On the other hand, administration of bicarbonate may cause fluid retention, brain edema, and unfavorable pH shifts. Current data suggest that bicarbonate administration does not favorably influence patient outcome down to a pH of 6.90.[40] Below this level, there is a consensus to administer bicarbonate even if its value is unproven.

Complications of DKA include death, brain edema, pancreatitis, hyperlipidemia, hypophosphatemia, and pulmonary edema.

Mortality in DKA is 2–10%, striking mostly the very young and the elderly. Almost 2 out of 1000 episodes of DKA in children will result in death from cerebral edema, the major cause of death and disability for children with diabetic ketoacidosis. Multiple organ failure (cardiac, renal, hepatic, and pulmonary) portends a high mortality in adult patients. Elevated pancreatic enzymes, such as amylase and lipase, are correlated with the degree of hyperglycemia, acidemia, and dehydration. Although not usually clinically important,[41] dehydration with hypoperfusion of the pancreas and elevations of triglycerides may precipitate acute pancreatitis.[42,43] Elevated triglycerides occur because insulin stimulation of endothelial lipoprotein lipase is necessary to remove lipids from the circulation, and insulin inhibition of adipose tissue lipase prevents mobilization of lipids out of the fat cell. Hypertriglyceridemia resolves following DKA unless there is an underlying defect but may contribute to pancreatitis.[44] Mild hypophosphatemia commonly occurs in DKA; there is evidence that treatment is not required unless clearly symptomatic.[45–47] Pulmonary symptoms may indicate pneumonia but may also occur with a "capillary leak" or interstitial edema associated with DKA.[48]

DKA costs lives and dollars; the epidemiology of DKA targets educational and preventive solutions.

In developing countries, mortality rates for type 1 diabetic patients are high, with DKA as the leading cause of death.[49] In US children and young adults with type 1 diabetes mellitus, DKA is also the most common cause of mortality and appears to affect non-whites with greatly increased frequency compared to whites.[50] DKA, with 100,000 admissions annually in the United States,[51] is estimated to represent ~25% of the direct medical care dollars of treating type 1 diabetes mellitus.[52]

Educational programs may decrease the incidence of DKA,[53] although the emotional and psychological factors that stimulate knowledgeable patients to discontinue insulin are not easily addressed. Studies have shown that patients can be safely discharged following care in the emergency room if DKA is mild (pH > 7.20, HCO_3 > 10).[54] Admission to a general hospital bed rather than a more expensive intensive care unit bed is also possible for less severely ill patients.[55] Specialty care may provide significant cost savings: endocrinologists treat and discharge their patients with DKA more rapidly, with fewer tests and fewer readmissions than do general internists.[51]

Patients may present with DKA with exceptions to the definition including lower glucose, higher pH, and negative nitroprusside test for ketones.

The glucose at presentation in DKA varies widely from less than 180 to 1000 mg/dL. If a patient is not eating well prior to the onset of DKA, the glucose may be lower than with a prior good food intake. Young people with good kidney function or pregnant patients with increased glomerular filtration rate (GFR) and lowered glucose threshold can develop DKA with normal blood sugars since they have a greater capacity to excrete glucose.[56] Patients who treat their finger stick glucose elevations with small doses of insulin may develop diabetic ketoacidosis with normal glucose levels if the stress hormones during illness stimulate sufficient lipolysis. DKA may develop unusually rapidly during fasting or dehydration because these conditions increase the counter-regulatory hormone glucagon and increase the pace at which acidosis occurs when insulin is withdrawn. Patients on the insulin pump do not have long-acting insulin on board when the pump malfunctions and may develop DKA within hours.

Patients who have excessive vomiting and develop DKA may have pH levels above the definition for DKA (pH < 7.35) because H^+ lost in emesis fluid superimposes metabolic alkalosis on the metabolic acidosis of DKA. Other states that cause metabolic alkalosis can have the same effect, such as DKA with Cushing's syndrome.

Patients with low tissue oxygenation, sepsis, and hypotension can present with a large predominance of β-hydroxybutyrate over acetoacetate. The test for ketoacids in these patients may be negative at presentation and become positive as the patient improves and converts β-hydroxybutyrate to acetoacetate.

The patient with atypical diabetes mellitus is exceptional in the ability to recover normal pancreatic function.[57–59]

In the United States, perhaps 10% of black Americans who present with DKA will have a subsequent course characterized by long-term remission of diabetes mellitus. This course has been labeled "atypical diabetes mellitus," "type 1.5" diabetes, and "Flatbush" diabetes for the area of Brooklyn, New York, where it has been best characterized. Relapses occurred over a time period of months to longer than 5 years; 20% of patients were in remission beyond 6 years. Patients may have a family history of similar remissions of diabetes mellitus. This pattern is seen in younger, less obese, and more insulin-sensitive patients than the typical patient with type 2 diabetes, and in Japanese and Chinese patients with atypical diabetes mellitus who often do not require insulin after the episode. Unlike in type 1 diabetes, antibodies against glutamic acid decarboxylase (GAD) and islet cell antibodies are negative.

Hyperosmolar Hyperglycemic Syndrome (HHS)

Hyperosmolar hyperglycemic syndrome differs from DKA in the more dramatic degree of dehydration, higher serum glucose, lack of acidosis, advanced patient age, and much higher mortality (Fig. 18.8).[60]

Hyperosmolar hyperglycemic syndrome (HHS) connotes severe hyperglycemia without (or with mild) acidemia or ketoacidosis. The pathophysiologic assumption is that patients with HHS have a greater insulin reserve and, unlike patients with DKA, are able to inhibit lipolysis and avoid ketoacid formation. Typically, serum glucose is higher than in diabetic ketoacidosis, patients are remarkably more dehydrated, older, and with more prominent underlying illnesses. The severe dehydration and hyperglycemia often results in effective serum osmolality (Table 18.2) greater than 320 mOsm/L, a level at which depression of consciousness or coma can be attributed to the hyperosmolar state.[61,62] Patients commonly have type 2 diabetes mellitus, with poor antecedent glucose control. Thrombotic complications, which may occur in DKA,[63] are a feared complication of HHS. Coronary arteries may clot, and arterial clots may propagate from the periphery to include the large central vessels. Presumably, the severe dehydration results in hemoconcentration and a hypercoagulable state. Because of the advanced patient age and the hypercoagulability and decreased perfusion accompanying severe dehydration, myocardial infarction must be specifically excluded as a precipitating or a complicating event [small doses of intravenous heparin (500–1000 units/h) are appropriate unless contraindicated]. Abdominal pain in HHS should

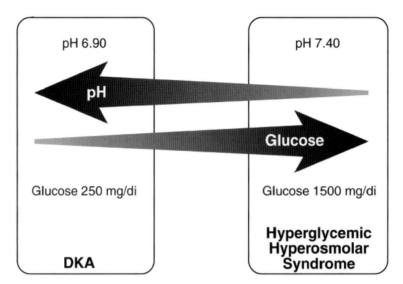

Fig. 18.8 There is no clear separation of DKA and hyperglycemic hyperosmolar syndrome (HHS). The less extreme glucose elevations and more extreme acidosis can be labeled DKA. The more extreme glucose elevations with no or minimal acidosis can be labeled HHS. In between, there is overlap and the clinician tailors therapy accordingly

be evaluated as a medical emergency, with consideration of perforated viscus, acute cholecystitis, and ischemic bowel.

Patients should be treated in an intensive care setting. Fluid management with aggressive rehydration is the critical aspect of treatment of hyperosmolar syndrome. An immediate fluid challenge should be given to guarantee continued renal perfusion and urine output. One or two liters of fluid in the first hour of therapy followed by 1 l/h for the next 4 h are commonly recommended. The water deficit can be calculated from the serum osmolality (the serum sodium can be substituted for osmolality in the equation). Half the water deficit should be replaced in the first 8–12 h. Exceptions include patients with renal or congestive heart failure, who require highly individualized fluid management.

The "corrected" serum sodium (Table 18.2) indicates the degree of free water loss – the higher the corrected sodium, the greater the water loss. In spite of marked free water loss, initial fluid replacement is with isotonic solutions, usually normal saline (NS), to establish blood pressure and perfusion. Hypotonic fluids (1/2 NS) are then administered, followed again by isotonic fluids when the glucose falls significantly (for example, to levels of 300–500 mg/dL). The rationale is that hypotonic fluids distribute more evenly between the intravascular and the extravascular space, whereas isotonic fluids remain in the intravascular space. As hyperglycemia resolves, fluid leaves the intravascular space and moves intracellularly. The movement of fluid out of the intravascular space in a severely dehydrated patient may result in vascular "collapse" (hypotension and irreversible shock).

Insulin plays only a minor role in the treatment of HHS, since these patients are not "ketosis prone," are not acidotic, and do not require restraint of free fatty acid release. The glucose osmotic diuresis that occurs with fluid administration is the most important factor in lowering the blood glucose toward the renal threshold of 180 mg/dL. Small doses of insulin may be useful, but rapid blood lowering of the serum glucose with insulin is not desirable, because the osmotic pull of glucose helps to maintain intravascular volume and to prevent cerebral edema.

When it is over, the physician must educate the patient not to omit insulin at times of stress.

Patients with type 1 diabetes must always take insulin; patients with type 2 diabetes must understand when insulin doses need to be increased. Common misconceptions have to be corrected. The patient must take insulin even when not able to eat. Ordinarily, the diabetic patient will have long-acting depot insulin or continued pump therapy between meals and during overnight fasting. Patients get confused, however, when they are not eating because of illness, such as gastrointestinal "upset." At these times, counter-regulatory hormones may rise and the patient must know that he or she needs to treat both the finger stick glucose and urine ketone elevations measured by "ketostik" or other convenient methods.

Conclusions

The next patient will be different ... but the witnesses – glucose, free fatty acids, serum electrolytes and pH, ketoacids – will always tell their stories. The fingerprint of relative insulin deficiency permitting substrates (free fatty acids, amino acids and glycerol) to reach the liver and counter-regulatory excesses driving hepatic gluconeogenesis and ketogenesis will be clear to your experienced eye. The reversal of controlled storage and synthetic processes resulting in hyperglycemia, systemic acidosis, osmotic diuresis, and dehydration will be familiar. Therapy is straightforward, requiring insulin, fluid, and electrolyte administration. Key to a successful clinical outcome is careful monitoring of the patient, anticipation of responses, and investigation of potential precipitating factors.

Recommended Websites

1. Mayo Clinic Staff. "Diabetic Ketoacidosis." February 8, 2008. http://www.mayoclinic.com/health/diabetic-ketoacidosis/DS00674.
2. Medline Plus. "Diabetic Ketoacidosis." August 8, 2006. Accessed February 16, 2008. http://www.nlm.nih.gov/medlineplus/ency/article/000320.htm.
3. eMedicine from WebMD. "Diabetic Ketoacidosis." February 12, 2008. http://www.emedicine.com/emerg/topic135.htm.

References

1. Pietropaolo M, Barinas-Mitchell E, Kuller LH. The heterogeneity of diabetes: unraveling a dispute: is systemic inflammation related to islet autoimmunity? *Diabetes*. 2007;56:1189–1197.
2. Balasubramanyam A, Garza G, Rodriguez L, et al. Accuracy and predictive value of classification schemes for ketosis-prone diabetes. *Diabetes Care*. 2006;29:2575–2579.
3. Balasubramanyam A, Zern JW, Hyman DJ, et al. New profiles of diabetic ketoacidosis: type 1 vs type 2 diabetes and the effect of ethnicity. *Arch Intern Med*. 1999;159:2317–2322.
4. Umpierrez GE, Woo W, Hagopian WA, et al. Immunogenetic analysis suggests different pathogenesis for obese and lean African-Americans with diabetic ketoacidosis. *Diabetes Care*. 1999;22:1517–1523.
5. Davis SN, Umpierrez GE. Diabetic ketoacidosis in type 2 diabetes mellitus – pathophysiology and clinical presentation. *Nat Clin Pract Endocr Metab*. 2007;3(11):730–731.
6. Fleckman AM. Diabetic ketoacidosis. *Endocrinol Metab Clin N Amer*. 1993;22:181–207.
7. Kitabchi AE, Umpierrez GE, Murphy MB, et al. Hyperglycemic crises in adult patients with diabetes: a consensus statement from the American Diabetes Association. *Diabetes Care*. 2006;29(12):2739–2748.
8. Cooper GM, Hausman RE. *The Cell: A Molecular Approach*. 4th Ed. Washington, D.C., ASM Press, pp. 73–102, 433–471, 2007.
9. Nelson DL, Cox MM. *Lehninger Principles of Biochemistry*, 4th Ed. New York, W.H. Freeman and Co., Chapter 14-1, Glycolysis; Chapter 17, Fatty acid catabolism; Chapter 23.2 Tissue-specific metabolism; 2005.
10. DeFronzo RA, Matsuda M, Barrett EJ. Diabetic ketoacidosis. *Diabetes Rev*. 1994;2:209–238.
11. Ottosson M, Lönnroth P, Björntorp P, et al. Effects of cortisol and growth hormone on lipolysis in human adipose tissue. *J Clin Endocrinol Metab*. 2000;85:799–803.
12. Seckl JR, Walker BR. Minireview: 11beta-hydroxysteroid dehydrogenase type 1 – a tissue-specific amplifier of glucocorticoid action. *Endocrinol*. 2001;142:1371–1376.
13. Zammit VA. Regulation of ketone body metabolism. *Diabetes Rev*. 1994;2:132–155.
14. Kreisberg RA. Lactate homeostasis and lactic acidosis. *Ann Intern Med*. 1980;92(2 Pt 1):227–237.
15. Laffel L. Ketone bodies: a review of physiology, pathophysiology and application of monitoring to diabetes. *Diabetes/Metab Res Rev*. 1999;15:412–426.
16. Berg JM, Tymoczko JL, Stryer L. *Biochemistry*, 6th Ed. New York, W.H. Freeman and Co., Chapter 22, Fatty acid metabolism: Ketone bodies are a major fuel in some tissues, pp. 632–633, 2007.

17. Jin H, Meyer JM, Jeste DV. Phenomenology of and risk factors for new-onset diabetes mellitus and diabetic ketoacidosis associated with atypical antipsychotics: an analysis of 45 published cases. *Ann Clin Psychiatry*. 2002;14(1):59–64.

18. Ramaswamy K, Masand PS, Nasrallah HA. Do certain atypical antipsychotics increase the risk of diabetes? A critical review of 17 pharmacoepidemiologic studies. *Annals Clinical Psychiatry*. 2006;18(3):183–194.

19. Imagawa A, Hanafusa T, Miyagawa JI, et al. A novel subtype of type 1 diabetes mellitus characterized by a rapid onset and an absence of diabetes-related antibodies. *N Engl J Med*. 2000;342:301–307.

20. Yoon JW, Austin M, Onodera T, et al. Isolation of a virus from the pancreas of a child with diabetic ketoacidosis. *N Engl J Med*. 1979;300(21):1173–1179.

21. Chen LK, Chou YC, Tsai ST, et al. Hepatitis C virus infection-related Type 1 diabetes mellitus. *Diabetic Med*. 2005;22(3): 340–343.

22. Brandenburg MA, Dire DJ. Comparison of arterial and venous blood gas values in the initial emergency department evaluation of patients with diabetic ketoacidosis. *Ann Emerg Med*. 1998;31:459–465.

23. Fulop M, Murthy V, Michili A, et al. Serum beta-hydroxybutyrate measurement in patients with uncontrolled diabetes mellitus. *Arch Intern Med*. 1999;159:381–384.

24. Katz MA. Hyperglycemia-induced hyponatremia – calculation of expected serum sodium depression. *N Engl J Med*. 1973;289(16):843–844.

25. Hillier TA, Abbott RD, Barrett EJ. Hyponatremia: evaluating the correction factor for hyperglycemia. *Amer J Med*. 1999;106:399–403.

26. White NH. Diabetic ketoacidosis in children. *Endocrinol Metab Clin*. 2000;29:657–682.

27. Wolfsdorf J, Glaser N, Sperling MA. Diabetic ketoacidosis in infants, children, and adolescents. *Diabetes Care*. 2006;29: 1150–1159.

28. Adrogue' HJ, Barrero J, Eknoyan G. Salutary effects of modest fluid replacement in the treatment of adults with diabetic ketoacidosis. *J Am Med Assoc*. 1989;262:2108–2113.

29. Rave K, Nosek L, Posner J, et al. Renal glucose excretion as a function of blood glucose concentration in subjects with type 2 diabetes – results of a hyperglycaemic glucose clamp study. *Nephrol Dial Transplant*. 2006;21:2166–2171.

30. Kawata H, Inui D, Ohto J, et al. The use of continuous hemodiafiltration in a patient with diabetic ketoacidosis. *J Anesth*. 2006;20(2):129–131.

31. Kaufman FR. Diabetes in children and adolescents: areas of controversy. *Med Clin No Amer*. 1998;82:721–738.

32. Muir A. Cerebral edema in diabetic ketoacidosis: a look beyond rehydration. *J Clin Endocrinol Metab*. 2000;85:509–513.

33. Edge JA, Ford-Adams ME, Dunger DB. Causes of death in children with insulin dependent diabetes 1990–96. *Arch Disease Child*. 1999;81:318–323.

34. Glaser N, Barnett P, McCaslin I, et al. Risk factors for cerebral edema in children with diabetic ketoacidosis. *N Engl J Med*. 2001;344:264–269.

35. Isales CM, Min L, Hoffman WH. Acetoacetate and beta-hydroxybutyrate differentially regulate endothelin-1 and vascular endothelial growth factor in mouse brain microvascular endothelial cells. *J Diabetes Complic*. 1999;13:91–97.

36. Mahoney CP, Vlcek BW, DelAguila M. Risk factors for developing brain herniation during diabetic ketoacidosis. *Pediatr Neurol*. 1999;21:721–727.

37. Wagner A, Risse A, Brill HL, et al. Therapy of severe diabetic ketoacidosis: zero-mortality under very-low-dose insulin application. *Diabetes Care*. 1999;22:674–677.

38. Weiner ID, Wingo CS. Hypokalemia – consequences, causes, and correction. *J Amer Soc Neph*. 1997;8:1179–1188.

39. Tattersall RB. A paper which changed clinical practice (slowly). Jacob Holler on potassium deficiency in diabetic acidosis (1946). *Diabetic Med*. 1999;16:978–984.

40. Viallon A, Zeni F, Lafond P, et al. Does bicarbonate therapy improve the management of severe diabetic ketoacidosis? *Crit Care Med*. 1999;27:2690–2693.

41. Vantyghem MC, Haye S, Balduyck M, et al. Changes in serum amylase, lipase and leukocyte elastase during diabetic ketoacidosis and poorly controlled diabetes. *Acta Diabetol*. 1999;36:39–44.

42. Nair S, Pitchumoni CS. Diabetic ketoacidosis, hyperlipidemia, and acute pancreatitis: the enigmatic triangle. *Amer J Gastro*. 1997;92:1560–1561.

43. Nair S, Yadav D, Pitchumoni CS. Association of diabetic ketoacidosis and acute pancreatitis: observations in 100 consecutive episodes of DKA. *Amer J Gastro*. 2000;95:2795–2800.

44. Fulop M, Eder H. Severe hypertriglyceridemia in diabetic ketosis. *Amer J Med Sci*. 1990;300:361–365.

45. Fisher JN, Kitabchi AE. A randomized study of phosphate therapy in the treatment of diabetic ketoacidosis. *J Clin Endocrinol Metab*. 1983;57:177–180.

46. Gaasbeek A, Meinders AE. Hypophosphatemia: an update on its etiology and treatment. *Amer J Med*. 2005;118: 1094–1101.

47. Megárbane B, Guerrier G, Blancher A, et al. A possible hypophosphatemia-induced, life-threatening encephalopathy in diabetic ketoacidosis: a case report. *Am J Med Sci*. 2007;333(6):384–386.

48. Hoffman WH, Locksmith JP, Burton EM, et al. Interstitial pulmonary edema in children and adolescents with diabetic ketoacidosis. *J Diabetes Comp*. 1998;12:314–320.

49. Podar T, Solntsev A, Reunanen A, et al. Mortality in patients with childhood-onset type 1 diabetes in Finland, Estonia, and Lithuania: follow-up of nationwide cohorts. *Diabetes Care*. 2000;23:290–294.

50. Lipton R, Good G, Mikhailov T, et al. Ethnic differences in mortality from insulin-dependent diabetes mellitus among people less than 25 years of age. *Pediatrics*. 1999;103:952–956.
51. Levetan CS, Passaro MD, Jablonski KA, et al. Effect of physician specialty on outcomes in diabetic ketoacidosis. *Diabetes Care*. 1999;22:1790–1795.
52. Javor KA, Kotsanos JG, McDonald RC, et al. Diabetic ketoacidosis charges relative to medical charges of adult patients with type 1 diabetes. *Diabetes Care*. 1997;20:349–354.
53. Vanelli M, Chiari G, Ghizzoni L, et al. Effectiveness of a prevention program for diabetic ketoacidosis in children: an 8-year study in schools and private practices. *Diabetes Care*. 1999;22:7–9.
54. Bonadio WA, Gutzeit MF, Losek JD, et al. Outpatient management of diabetic ketoacidosis. *Amer J Dis Child*. 1988;142: 448–450.
55. Marinac JS, Jesa L. Using a severity of illness scoring system to assess intensive care unit admissions for diabetic ketoacidosis. *Crit Care Med*. 2000;28:2238–2241.
56. Cullen MT, Reece EA, Homko CJ, et al. The changing presentations of diabetic ketoacidosis during pregnancy. *Am J Perinatol*. 1996;13(7):449–451.
57. Winter WE, Maclaren NK, Riley WJ, et al. Maturity-onset diabetes of youth in black Americans. *N Engl J Med*. 1987;316: 285–291.
58. Banerji MA, Chaiken RL, Huey H, et al. GAD antibody negative NIDDM in adult black subjects with diabetic ketoacidosis and increased frequency of human leukocyte antigen DR3 and DR4. Flatbush diabetes. *Diabetes*. 1994;43:741–745.
59. Banerji MA, Chaiken RL, Lebovitz HE. Long-term normoglycemic remission in black newly diagnosed NIDDM subjects. *Diabetes*. 1996;45:337–341.
60. Matz R. Management of the hyperosmolar hyperglycemic syndrome. *Am Fam Physician*. 1999;60:1468–1476.
61. Fulop M, Tannenbaum H, Dreyer N. Ketotic hyperosmolar coma. *Lancet*. 1973;2:635–639.
62. Daugirdas JT, Kronfol NO, Tzamaloukas AH, et al. Hyperosmolar coma: cellular dehydration and the serum sodium concentration. *Ann Intern Med*. 1989;110:855–857.
63. Ileri NS, Buyukasik Y, Karaahmetoglu S, et al. Evaluation of the haemostatic system during ketoacidotic deterioration of diabetes mellitus. *Haemostasis*. 1999;29:318–325.

Chapter 19
Hypoglycemia in Diabetes Mellitus

Mazen Alsahli and John E. Gerich

General Considerations

As indicated earlier in Chapter 2, human plasma glucose concentrations are maintained within a relatively narrow range throughout the day (usually between 55 and 165 mg/dl, ~3.0 and 9.0 mM/L) despite wide fluctuations in the delivery (e.g., meals) and removal (e.g., exercise) of glucose from the circulation. This is accomplished by a tightly linked balance between glucose production and glucose utilization regulated by complex mechanisms.

Hypoglycemia is to be avoided to protect the brain and prevent cognitive dysfunction. Because of limited availability of ketone bodies and amino acids and the limited transport of free fatty acids across the blood–brain barrier, glucose can be considered to be the sole source of energy for the brain except under conditions of prolonged fasting. In the latter situation, ketone bodies increase several fold so that these may be used as an alternative fuel.[1]

It is generally thought that the brain cannot store or produce glucose and therefore requires a continuous supply of glucose from the circulation. Recent studies in animals, however, suggest that the brain may not contain negligible quantities of glycogen.[2] At physiological plasma glucose levels, phosphorylation of glucose is rate limiting for its utilization. However, because of the kinetics of glucose transfer across the blood–brain barrier, uptake becomes rate limiting as plasma glucose concentrations decrease below the normal range. Consequently, maintenance of the plasma glucose concentration above some critical level is essential to the survival of the brain and thus the organism. It is therefore not surprising that a complex physiological mechanism has evolved to prevent or correct hypoglycemia (vide infra). Nevertheless for many patients with type 1 or type 2 diabetes, hypoglycemia is a frequent complication. Because of its possible detrimental effects on the central nervous system, hypoglycemia is considered to be the main limiting factor for achieving near-normal glycemic control.[3]

Epidemiology of Hypoglycemia

Type 1 Diabetes

The reported incidence of hypoglycemia varies considerably among studies. In general, patients with type 1 diabetes practicing conventional insulin therapy have an average of ~1 episode of symptomatic hypoglycemia per week, whereas those practicing intensive insulin therapy have ~2 such episodes per week.[4] Thus, over 40 years of type 1 diabetes, the average patient can be projected to experience 2000–4000 episodes of symptomatic hypoglycemia. The complete detection of chemical hypoglycemia (commonly defined as a capillary blood glucose concentration < 50 mg/dl[5]) would require continuous blood glucose measurements over prolonged periods.

J.E. Gerich (✉)
University of Rochester School of Medicine, Rochester, NY, USA
e-mail: johngerich@compuserve.com

L. Poretsky (ed.), *Principles of Diabetes Mellitus*, DOI 10.1007/978-0-387-09841-8_19,
© Springer Science+Business Media, LLC 2010

The few studies using this approach have generally found that the frequency and duration of hypoglycemia, especially the nocturnal hypoglycemia, is greater than what was previously thought.[6,7]

For the purpose of reporting hypoglycemia in clinical trials, the American Diabetes Association has developed five categories as outlined in Table 19.1.[8] The incidence of severe hypoglycemia has been determined more precisely since it is defined as that associated with unconsciousness or requiring external assistance. It occurs more often during intensified insulin therapy than during conventional insulin therapy. For example, during the 6.5-year follow-up in the Diabetes Control and Complication Trial (DCCT),[9] 35% of patients in the conventional treatment group and 65% of patients in the intensive treatment group had at least one episode of severe hypoglycemia. This corresponds to about 60 episodes per 100 patient-years in patients being managed to achieve optimal glycemic control by intensive insulin therapy and to about 20 episodes per 100 patient-years in conventionally treated patients.[9] In a recent meta-analysis of 14 studies, which included 1028 patients on intensified insulin therapy and 1039 patients on conventional insulin therapy, the median incidence of severe hypoglycemia was 7.9 and 4.6 episodes per 100 patient-years in the two treatment groups, respectively; the combined odds ratio was 2.99 ($p < 0.0001$).[10] However the increased incidence of severe hypoglycemia in the intensified treatment group was no longer evident as soon as glycosylated hemoglobin was included in a multivariate regression analysis.[10]

Table 19.1 Hypoglycemia categories as defined by the American Diabetes Association[8]

Category	Definition
Documented symptomatic	An event during which typical symptoms of hypoglycemia are associated with a measured plasma glucose concentration ≤70 mg/dl[a]
Severe	An event requiring assistance of another person to actively administer carbohydrate, glucagon, or other resuscitative actions[b]
Asymptomatic	An event not accompanied by typical symptoms of hypoglycemia but by a measured plasma glucose concentration ≤70 mg/dl[a]
Probable symptomatic	An event during which symptoms of hypoglycemia are not accompanied by a plasma glucose determination but that was presumably caused by a plasma glucose concentration ≤70 mg/dl[a]
Relative	An event during which the person with diabetes reports any of the typical symptoms of hypoglycemia and interprets those as indicative of hypoglycemia, but with a measured plasma glucose concentration >70 mg/dl

[a]70 mg/dl equals 3.9 mmol/l
[b]If plasma glucose measurements are not available during such an event, the neurological recovery attributable to the restoration of plasma glucose to normal is considered a sufficient evidence that the event was induced by hypoglycemia

Type 2 Diabetes

Patients with type 2 diabetes generally experience less frequent severe hypoglycemia than those with type 1 diabetes. Both the UKPDS[11] and the Kumamoto study[12] demonstrated a much lower incidence of severe hypoglycemia in insulin-treated patients with type 2 diabetes than what was reported in the DCCT[9] for patients with type 1 diabetes despite similar glycemic control. In the UKPDS, which followed 676 patients with type 2 diabetes on insulin therapy for 3 years, the incidence was 0.83 episodes per 100 patient-years. In the Kumamoto study, which followed 52 type 2 diabetic patients on intensive insulin therapy for over 6 years, no severe hypoglycemic episode was reported. However, one retrospective study, which directly compared the incidence of severe hypoglycemia in 104 insulin-treated patients with type 2 diabetes with that in 104 equally well-controlled type 1 diabetic patients, found a similar incidence of severe hypoglycemia.[13] A later study also found that hypoglycemia requiring emergency assistance was as common in patients with insulin-treated type 2 diabetes as in patients with type 1 diabetes.[14]

In patients with type 2 diabetes treated with sulfonylureas, the incidence of severe hypoglycemia has been reported to be approximately 1.5 episodes per 100 patient-years.[15] Its frequency increases with the potency and duration of action of the sulfonylurea, being greatest for second-generation sulfonylureas, glimepiride, glyburide, and glipizide averaging ∼4–6%.[16]

Risk Factors for Hypoglycemia

Conventional risk factors for hypoglycemia relate to absolute or relative insulin excess. These include insulin doses that are excessive or ill timed, missed meals or snacks, lack of compensation for increased exercise, alcohol ingestion, or mistaken insulin administration. However, a thorough analysis of a large number of episodes of severe hypoglycemia in the DCCT has indicated that such conventional risk factors explained only a minority of the episodes[17,18]; indeed, mathematical models incorporating many of these factors were found to have little predictive power.[17] Instead it is now well established that impaired glucose counterregulation and hypoglycemia unawareness (vide infra) are the major risk factors for severe hypoglycemia in type 1 diabetes.[3,19] These defects are particularly common in patients with a long diabetes duration,[20,21] tight glycemic control,[20,22,23] antecedent hypoglycemia,[24,25] and autonomic neuropathy.[26–28] Hypoglycemia awareness may also be compromised by the use of β-blockers.[29] The risk of severe hypoglycemia is increased 25-fold in patients with impaired hypoglycemia counterregulation[30] and increased sixfold in those with hypoglycemia unawareness.[31] Other risk factors for severe hypoglycemia due to diabetes complications include renal insufficiency, gastroparesis which causes unpredictable and delayed food absorption, poor vision, and (rarely) insulin antibodies. In the latter condition, hypoglycemia occurs via dissociation of insulin from antibodies causing prolonged hyperinsulinemia.[21]

Despite the fact that most episodes of severe hypoglycemia in type 1 diabetes are related to impaired glucose counterregulation and hypoglycemia unawareness, one should also keep in mind that hypoglycemia can be multifactorial and could be due to several unrelated diseases. These include liver disease, malnutrition, sepsis, burns, total parenteral nutrition, malignancy, and administration of certain medications known to reduce plasma glucose concentrations (Table 19.2).[32]

Table 19.2 Drug-induced hypoglycemia

Drugs capable of causing hypoglycemia by themselves		Drugs probably causing hypoglycemia only in combination with insulin/sulfonylurea/meglitinides	
Antidiabetic drugs	Other	Antidiabetic drugs	Other
Insulin	Alcohol	Biguanides	ACE inhibitors
Sulfonylureas	Salicylates	Thiazolidinediones	Phenylbutazone
Meglitinides	Propranolol	α-Glucosidase inhibitors	Lidocaine
	Pentamidine	Exenatide[a]	Coumadin
	Sulfamethoxazole	Sitagliptin	Ranitidine, cimetidine
	Vacor	Pramlintide	Doxepin
	Quinine		Danazol
	Propoxyphene		Azapropazone
	para-Aminobenzoic acid		Oxytetracycline
	Perhexiline		Clofibrate, benzofibrate
			Colchicine
			Ketoconozole
			Chloramphenicol
			Haloperidol
			Monoamine oxidase inhibitors
			Thalidomide
			Orphenadrine
			Selegiline

[a]Combination of exenatide and a thiazolidinedione increased the incidence of hypoglycemia to 11% compared with 7% in placebo in a randomized controlled trial[161]

In principle, the same risk factors for hypoglycemia apply to patients with type 2 diabetes as to patients with type 1 diabetes, although the importance of each has been less well defined.

Gastric bypass surgery is becoming more common as a treatment for morbid obesity. Many of the patients have type 2 diabetes. Hypoglycemia has been reported to occur in some patients usually in the second or third hour postprandially.[33-37] The exact mechanism is currently being investigated but is likely to be multifactorial and related to the changes that follow the surgery such as decreased caloric intake, weight loss, and a change in the nutrient composition and transit time in the gastrointestinal tract.[38-40] Studies have also shown decreased ghrelin secretion, exaggerated release of glucagon-like peptide 1 (GLP-1), and possibly other gastrointestinal hormone changes.[41-45] These hormonal changes should enhance the release of insulin and inhibit the release of pancreatic glucagon. Additionally, several severe cases of hyperinsulinemic hypoglycemia presenting as postprandial hypoglycemia after Roux-en-Y gastric bypass surgery have been published.[46-48] The mechanism by which this occurs is not entirely clear. Examination of pancreatic specimens obtained following partial pancreatectomy performed to treat these cases implicated nesidioblastosis or islet cell hyperplasia as a possible cause.[46,47] A subsequent report, however, found no evidence of increased islet cell mass or neogenesis when some of these specimens were reexamined and compared with those of well-matched subjects.[49] The report suggests that hypoglycemia in these patients is related to a combination of gastric dumping and inappropriately increased insulin secretion due to either failure of beta cells to adapt to changes in post-gastric bypass or an acquired phenomenon. It is also not clear whether patients with diabetes are more or less likely to suffer from post-gastric bypass hypoglycemia when compared to other patients.

Hypoglycemia Counterregulation

Normal Hypoglycemia Counterregulation and Hypoglycemia Awareness

Because of the importance of intact hypoglycemia counterregulation and awareness for the prevention or the correction of hypoglycemia, this shall be briefly reviewed. Glucose counterregulation refers to the sum of the body's defense mechanisms which prevent hypoglycemia from occurring and those which restore euglycemia. Hypoglycemia awareness refers to the symptomatic responses of hypoglycemia which alert the patient of declining blood glucose levels. Our knowledge of counterregulation has accumulated over the past 35 years from studies in which pharmacologic blockade of the secretion or action of individual counterregulatory hormones has been produced during standardized insulin-induced hypoglycemia.[50]

Counterregulatory mechanisms in acute hypoglycemia, i.e., induced by an intravenous insulin injection, differ markedly from those in prolonged hypoglycemia. Clinical hypoglycemia that occurs in patients with diabetes after subcutaneous insulin injection usually develops gradually and is more prolonged.[51] Therefore, in the following discussion, mainly counterregulation of prolonged hypoglycemia will be considered.

In normal postabsorptive humans, i.e., after an overnight fast, the sum of glucose release by liver and kidney nearly equals systemic glucose utilization so that plasma glucose concentrations remain relatively stable. Since insulin suppresses both hepatic and renal glucose release[52,53] and stimulates glucose uptake, exogenous insulin administration causes systemic glucose utilization to exceed systemic glucose release so that plasma glucose concentrations decrease.

As the plasma glucose levels decrease, there is a characteristic hierarchy of responses[54] (Fig. 19.1). Reduction of insulin secretion, the first in the cascade of hypoglycemia counterregulation,[3] derepresses glucose production and reduces glucose utilization. When plasma glucose levels decline to approximately 70 mg/dl, there is an increase in the secretion of counterregulatory hormones (glucagon, epinephrine, growth hormone, cortisol).[26,54-56] Glucagon and epinephrine have immediate effects on glucose kinetics, whereas the effects of growth hormone and cortisol are delayed by several hours.[57,58]

Glucagon exclusively increases hepatic glucose release, initially via glycogenolysis, later mainly via gluconeogenesis,[59] and does not affect renal glucose release or glucose utilization.[60] In contrast, catecholamines have multiorgan effects, including stimulation of hepatic and renal glucose production,[61,62] inhibition of glucose

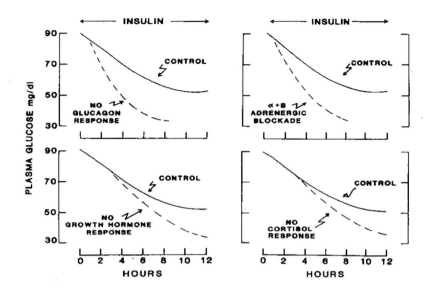

Fig. 19.1 Effect of lack of glucagon, catecholamine (α- and β-adrenergic blockade), growth hormone, and cortisol responses on insulin-induced hypoglycemia in nondiabetic volunteers studied with pituitary–adrenal–pancreatic clamp. From Gerich[50] Copyright © 1988 The American Diabetes Association. Used with permission

utilization,[63,64] stimulation of gluconeogenic substrate supply,[61,62,65] suppression of endogenous insulin secretion,[66] and stimulation of lipolysis.[66] Growth hormone and cortisol suppress insulin-mediated tissue glucose uptake and augment glucose release into the circulation.[67,68]

Under normal physiologic conditions, these responses prevent a further decrease in plasma glucose concentrations and restore normoglycemia. Decreases to ~60 mg/dl (3.4 mM/L) usually evoke the so-called autonomic warning symptoms [69,70] (hunger, anxiety, palpitations, sweating, warmth, nausea) which if interpreted correctly lead a person to eat and prevent more serious hypoglycemia. However, clues of hypoglycemia may vary considerably from person to person.[71] If, for some reason, plasma glucose levels decrease to about 55 mg/dl (~3.0 mM/L), neuroglycopenic signs/symptoms of brain dysfunction (blurred vision, slurred speech, glassy-eyed appearance, confusion, difficulty in concentrating) would occur.[69,70] Further decreases can produce coma, and values below 30 mg/dl (~1.6 mM/L), if prolonged, can cause seizures, permanent neurologic deficits, and death. However, it should be pointed out that in otherwise healthy/young (<45 years) individuals, glucose levels averaging 35 mg/dl (~2.0 mM/L) have been maintained for as long as 8 h without any long-term adverse effects[72] and chronic levels as low as 24 mg/dl (1.3 mM/L) in insulinoma patients have been observed in association with apparently normal cerebral function.[73]

Regarding the importance of each of these responses, the exact role of insulin dissipation for hypoglycemia counterregulation is controversial. Heller et al.[74] reported that dissipation of insulin is important but not critical for recovery from hypoglycemia. In contrast, De Feo et al.[75] and Sacca et al.[76] observed that no recovery from hypoglycemia occurs despite increases in counterregulatory hormones when hypoglycemia is induced by continuous low-dose insulin infusion, resulting in insulin levels lower (~25 μU/ml)[75] or similar (~40 μU/ml)[76] to those observed postprandially. On the other hand, plasma glucose concentrations stabilized and did not decrease further.

Roles of individual counterregulatory hormone responses have been delineated using the pituitary–adrenal–pancreatic (PAP) clamp technique.[77] With this technique, the spontaneous responses of counterregulatory hormones are simulated by infusions of the hormones during blockade of their secretion so that an isolated lack of response of each hormone can be examined. Studies using this technique have demonstrated that glucagon and epinephrine are the predominant counterregulatory hormones and that cortisol and growth hormone also have major roles in glucose counterregulation (Fig. 19.1).[57,58,78] The consequences of lack of glucagon or epinephrine were quantitatively similar.[50]

These studies have also delineated the time course of action and the relative effects of each hormone on glucose production and glucose utilization.[50] As shown in Fig. 19.2, counterregulation initially involves only changes in glucose production predominantly due to glucagon and, to a lesser extent, catecholamines. Later on, changes in glucose utilization become as important as those of glucose production. At this time, cortisol and growth hormone, through their delayed effects on glucose production and glucose utilization become major hormonal factors and may be more important than catecholamines and glucagon.

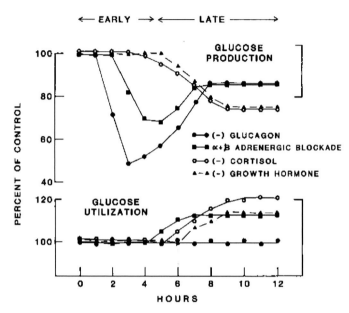

Fig. 19.2 Effect of lack of glucagon, catecholamine (α- and β-adrenergic blockade), growth hormone, and cortisol responses on counterregulatory changes in glucose production and glucose utilization in nondiabetic volunteers studied with pituitary–adrenal–pancreatic clamp. From Gerich[50] Copyright © 1988 The American Diabetes Association. Used with permission

Hypoglycemia Counterregulation and Hypoglycemia Awareness in Type 1 Diabetes

In type 1 diabetes, the physiology of the defense against hypoglycemia is seriously deranged (Fig. 19.3). First, as endogenous insulin secretion becomes totally deficient over the first few years of type 1 diabetes, the appearance of insulin in the circulation becomes unregulated since it relies on absorption from subcutaneous injection sites. Consequently, as plasma glucose levels are falling, insulin levels do not decrease. Second, glucagon responses to hypoglycemia are lost early in the course of type 1 diabetes.[21,79] This defect coincides with the loss of insulin secretion and is therefore the rule in people with type 1 diabetes.[80] Nonetheless, glucose counterregulation appears to be adequate in such patients probably due to compensatory counterregulation by epinephrine.[81] After a few more years, epinephrine responses to hypoglycemia are also commonly reduced.[21,82,83] When compared to patients with a defective glucagon response but normal epinephrine responses, patients with a combined defect in glucagon and epinephrine responses have at least a 25-fold increased risk for severe iatrogenic hypoglycemia.[30,84] The combined defect in glucagon and epinephrine responses is therefore considered as the syndrome of impaired hypoglycemia counterregulation.[3] This is now known to be associated with impaired glucose production in both liver and kidney.[85] Pathophysiologic mechanisms might be different when only glucagon responses are impaired and epinephrine responses are intact. Since glucagon affects exclusively the

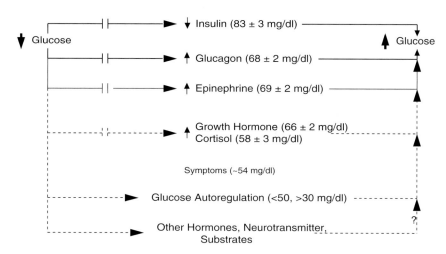

Fig. 19.3 Schematic representation of physiology of glucose counterregulation in normal humans (*arrows*) and defects in type 1 diabetes (*interrupted lines*). Mean ± SE arterialized venous glycemic thresholds for the various responses to falling blood glucose concentrations in normal humans are from Schwartz et al.[54] and Mitrakou et al.[55]

liver whereas epinephrine has a temporary effect on the liver but a sustained effect on the kidney, only hepatic glucose production might be decreased under these conditions.

In addition to impaired glucose counterregulation, people with type 1 diabetes often suffer from hypoglycemia unawareness. These patients no longer have autonomic warning symptoms of developing hypoglycemia which previously prompted them to take appropriate action (i.e., food intake before severe hypoglycemia with neuroglycopenia occurs). Hypoglycemia unawareness has been reported to occur in about 50% of patients with long-standing diabetes and estimated to affect 25% overall.[19,31,86,87] Hypoglycemia unawareness is associated with sixfold increased risk for severe hypoglycemia.[31]

The mechanisms of impaired hypoglycemia counterregulation and hypoglycemia unawareness are not entirely clear but several factors have been proposed. These include altered intra-islet structure and altered cell–cell interaction (reduced glucagon responses),[88,89] autonomic neuropathy (reduced catecholamine responses),[26–28] upregulation of glucose transporters in the central nervous system by antecedent hypoglycemia which prevents central hypoglycemia during subsequent hypoglycemia (reduced hormone and symptom responses),[90] and impaired β-adrenergic sensitivity to catecholamines which reduce autonomic warning symptoms of hypoglycemia.[91] Studies in animals have shown that the ventromedial hypothalamus (VMH) plays a major role in controlling the counterregulatory responses to hypoglycemia and that AMP-activated protein kinase plays a key role in the glucose sensing mechanism used by VMH neurons.[92] These studies also suggest that increased urocortin I, an endogenous type 2 corticotropin-releasing factor receptor (CRFR2) agonist in the VMH during antecedent hypoglycemia, could explain a decreased sympathoadrenal response to subsequent hypoglycemia.[93]

Hypoglycemia Counterregulation and Hypoglycemia Awareness in Type 2 Diabetes

The hormonal glucose counterregulation is usually less impaired in type 2 diabetes than in type 1 diabetes.[94–96] Nevertheless defects can be seen when patients become markedly insulin deficient.[97] One important factor for the nearly intact hormonal glucose counterregulation in type 2 diabetes may be some residual albeit abnormal, insulin secretion. Normally insulin directly suppresses glucagon secretion. There is now experimental evidence to suggest that the glucagon response to hypoglycemia may depend on the decrease in insulin secretion because the latter would derepress glucagon secretion.[89] Since insulin secretion is absent in type 1 diabetes, no decrease in insulin secretion occurs during hypoglycemia. However, in type 2 diabetes, insulin secretion is usually present and decreases appropriately during hypoglycemia, which may explain the intact glucagon response to hypoglycemia until the patient with type 2 diabetes becomes markedly insulin deficient. Since antecedent hypoglycemia is one of the main factors for impaired epinephrine responses to hypoglycemia and since hypoglycemia rarely occurs in people with type 2 diabetes because of their intact glucagon response, epinephrine responses also usually remain intact.

Once patients with type 2 diabetes become markedly insulin deficient, glucagon responses are commonly impaired. However, in contrast to patients with type 1 diabetes, the epinephrine responses usually remain intact and in fact may partially compensate for the reduced glucagon responses to hypoglycemia.[96,98] This may explain the reduced risk for severe hypoglycemia in patients with type 2 diabetes compared to patients with type 1 diabetes. Nevertheless, some studies reported that despite their increased catecholamine responses, patients with type 2 diabetes have impaired endogenous glucose production during hypoglycemia.[98,99] Recently this has been shown to be due to diminished glucose release by the liver which is partially compensated for by an increased glucose release by the kidney.[99] Factors involved in the reduced hepatic glucose release in type 2 diabetes may be diminished hepatic glycogen stores[100] and reduced glucagon activation of hepatic membrane adenylate cyclase.[101] These changes would be expected to impair hepatic glycogenolytic and gluconeogenic responses to glucagon.

Complications of Hypoglycemia

Organ Complications

As mentioned above, an episode of severe hypoglycemia can be detrimental or even fatal mostly due to its effects on the central nervous system. At a plasma glucose concentration of ~55 mg/dl (~3 mM/L), cognitive impairment and EEG changes are demonstrable. Decreases below 40 mg/dl (~2.5 mM/L) result in sleepiness and gross behavioral (e.g., combativeness) abnormalities. Further decreases can produce coma and values below 30 mg/dl (~1.6 mM/L) if prolonged can cause seizures, permanent neurologic deficits, and death.

In individuals with underlying cardiovascular disease, life-threatening arrhythmias, myocardial infarction, and strokes may be precipitated.[102–110] Moreover, in patients with underlying eye disease, hypoglycemia has been shown to trigger retinal hemorrhages.[111] It has been suggested that repeated episodes of severe hypoglycemia may lead to subtle permanent cognitive dysfunction.[112] In addition to its physical morbidity and mortality, recurrent hypoglycemia may also be associated with psychosocial morbidity.[86] In fact many patients with diabetes are as much afraid of severe hypoglycemia as they are of blindness or renal failure.[86]

Severe hypoglycemia has been reported to be at least a contributing factor to the cause of death in 3–13% of patients with type 1 diabetes, which includes motor vehicle accidents, injuries at work.[113,114] Severe hypoglycemia due to sulfonylureas has been shown to have a mortality between 4 and 7%.[16,115,116]

Somogyi Phenomenon

More than 60 years ago, Somogyi postulated that secretion of counterregulatory hormones provoked by insulin-induced hypoglycemia could lead to hyperglycemia. This sequence has become known as rebound hyperglycemia or the Somogyi phenomenon. It is the result of persistent catecholamine action initially and growth hormone and cortisol action later despite return of the plasma glucose concentration to normal. These posthypoglycemia counterregulatory effects, coupled with the dissipation of insulin injected earlier to produce hypoglycemia, result in posthypoglycemic hyperglycemia in patients with type 1 diabetes. In support of this concept, Mintz et al.[117] and Frier et al.[118] have shown that hypoglycemia, even in nondiabetic individuals, could cause subsequent glucose intolerance, and several studies demonstrated that prolonged insulin resistance lasting 4–8 h occurs after hypoglycemia in type 1 diabetes.[119–121]

Despite the evidence cited above, the literature is confounded with studies that have been interpreted to question the mechanism,[122] the frequency,[123] and even the existence[124] of the Somogyi phenomenon. However, to a large extent, study design and selection of patients (inclusion of those with impaired counterregulation[124] or type 2 diabetes[123]) can explain this controversy. It is nevertheless possible that the magnitude of the Somogyi phenomenon has been overestimated in the past. Furthermore, it is of note that the posthypoglycemia hyperglycemia in most patients is probably due to the combination of overtreatment of hypoglycemia with carbohydrate ingestion and the increase in counterregulatory hormones.

Management of Hypoglycemia

Treatment

Treatment is aimed at restoring euglycemia, preventing recurrences, and, if possible, alleviating the underlying cause. In an insulin-taking diabetic patient with mild hypoglycemia due to a skipped meal, 12–18 g oral carbohydrate every 30 min until the blood glucose is above 80 constitutes adequate treatment.[125,126] In a patient with more severe hypoglycemia resulting in obtundation, where oral administration of carbohydrate might result in aspiration, 1 mg glucagon administered subcutaneously or intramuscularly might be sufficient to raise the blood glucose and revive the patient so that oral carbohydrate may be given. Comatose patients should receive intravenous glucose (25 g bolus, followed by an infusion at an initial rate of 2 mg/kg/min, roughly 10 g/hr) for as long as necessary for the insulin or sulfonylurea to wear off. Sulfonylurea overdose can result in prolonged hypoglycemia requiring sustained intravenous glucose infusion aimed at keeping the blood glucose at ∼80 mg/dl (∼4.5 mM/L) to avoid hyperglycemia which would cause further stimulation of insulin secretion, thus setting in motion a vicious cycle. Blood glucose levels should be monitored initially every 30 min and subsequently at 1–2 h intervals. Rarely diazoxide or a somatostatin analogue may be needed to inhibit insulin secretion.[127] Where other drugs may be involved, they should be discontinued if possible (i.e., sulfonamides in a patient with renal insufficiency). In other conditions, the underlying disorder should be treated (e.g., sepsis, heart failure, endocrine deficiency) and the blood glucose supported.

Prevention of Recurrences

Conventional Measures

For prevention of recurrences, it is important to determine whether hypoglycemia was an isolated event or whether it has occurred before. If so, how frequently? Is there any pattern to occurrences, i.e., always at night? For how long have the hypoglycemic episodes been occurring? Are they associated with hypoglycemic warning symptoms? If so, usually at what level of glycemia is hypoglycemia recognized? Are there any precipitating factors, i.e., exercise, skipped meal, erroneous insulin injection, alcohol ingestion, recent weight loss, or other precipitating factors (see above)? Did the patient spontaneously recover? What did the patient do to prevent recurrences or relieve symptoms? What is the patient's occupation?

Obviously, if these questions reveal precipitating factors for hypoglycemia, these should be eliminated. However, if careful testing does not reveal any apparent precipitating factors but reveals hypoglycemia unawareness instead, chances are relatively high that there is also impaired hypoglycemia counterregulation, especially in a patient with frequent hypoglycemic episodes. Consequently the question arises as to how to treat the affected patients.

The principles of intensive therapy – patient education, blood glucose self-monitoring, and an insulin regimen that provides basal insulin levels with prandial increments – still apply to the majority of patients who require insulin to control their diabetes. However, glycemic goals must be individualized according to the frequency of hypoglycemia. Since the prevention or correction of hypoglycemia normally involves dissipation of insulin and activation of counterregulatory hormones as discussed above, it follows that patients with impaired glucose counterregulation are extremely sensitive to very little insulin in excess of its requirement, resulting in hypoglycemia. It is therefore generally accepted that normoglycemia is not a reasonable goal for such patients.[128,129]

Although therapy of type 1 and type 2 diabetes is discussed in detail in other chapters, several suggestions for prevention of hypoglycemia may be useful.

In patients treated with insulin, hypoglycemia can be most successfully prevented by continuous subcutaneous insulin infusion (CSII) by means of a minipump. This has been reported to reduce the frequency of severe hypoglycemia by 50–75% [130,131] despite the fact that glycemic control actually improved. If CSII is not feasible, substitution of preprandial short-acting (regular) insulin for rapid insulin (e.g., lispro or aspart) may reduce the frequency of hypoglycemic episodes by reducing prolonged postprandial hyperinsulinemia. In a recent meta-analysis of eight studies comparing 2327 patients treated with insulin lispro with 2339 patients treated with regular insulin, the frequency of hypoglycemia was approximately 20% less in those who received lispro despite virtually identical glycemic control.[132] Furthermore, substitution of intermediate-acting insulin (NPH) for long-acting insulin analogue (glargine or detemir) has been shown to reduce the frequency of hypoglycemia in patients with type 1 or type 2 diabetes.[133–138]

In patients with type 2 diabetes on oral hypoglycemic agents, substitution of a long-acting sulfonylurea for a short-acting sulfonylurea or a meglitinide (nateglinide, repaglinide) may be useful, especially in patients with chronic renal insufficiency since most of these agents are cleared by the kidney.[139,140]

If these measures result in strict avoidance of hypoglycemia, hypoglycemia awareness may be restored.[141] This might be due to an improvement in β-adrenergic sensitivity.[142] Although strict avoidance of hypoglycemia does not improve glucagon responses to hypoglycemia in type 1 diabetes,[141,143–146] it does increase epinephrine responses.[143,146] This however seems to be limited to patients with a diabetes duration of less than ~15 years. In patients with type 1 diabetes of more than 15 years duration, epinephrine responses may remain markedly impaired.[141,144] Thus there is unfortunately no conventional therapy available to reverse impaired hypoglycemia counterregulation in such patients. Although the effects of avoidance of hypoglycemia have not been studied in patients with type 2 diabetes, it seems likely that these are similar to those in type 1 diabetes.

Pancreas/Islet Transplantation

Because of the irreversibly impaired hypoglycemia counterregulation in long-standing type 1 diabetes, pancreas or islet transplantation has been proposed as a possible treatment in patients who suffer from recurrent severe hypoglycemia despite all conventional measures.[147–149] Pancreatic transplantation is usually reserved for patients undergoing simultaneous kidney transplantation. It has been found to improve glucagon responses to hypoglycemia in most studies[150–156] and to improve or normalize epinephrine responses.[152–154,156–158] Furthermore, it has been reported to improve hypoglycemia awareness in type 1 diabetes.[156]

Experience in the effects of islet transplantation on hypoglycemia counterregulation and awareness is limited and inconsistent. It seems that glucagon responses remain impaired after islet transplantation[147,148,159] possibly because of the transplantation site.[160] However, in one study, epinephrine responses and hypoglycemia awareness were reported to improve in long-standing type 1 diabetes,[148] whereas a later larger study found no evidence of improvement in epinephrine or hypoglycemia awareness despite prolonged insulin independence and near-normal glycemic control in seven islet transplantation patients.[159]

Although pancreas transplantation and islet transplantation may be promising alternatives for some patients with recurrent severe hypoglycemia, risk benefits ratios should be very carefully analyzed because of the invasive nature of these forms of therapy and the necessity for potent long-term immunosuppression.

Summary and Conclusions

In summary, severe hypoglycemia is a relatively common, potentially life-threatening complication of diabetic treatment more often affecting patients with type 1 than those with type 2 diabetes. Major risk factors for severe hypoglycemia are impaired hypoglycemia counterregulation and hypoglycemia unawareness, whereas conventional risk factors explain only a minority of the hypoglycemic episodes. Treatment is to be aimed at acute restoration of normoglycemia and prevention of recurrences. The latter can be accomplished by temporary loosening of glycemic control and changes in types and times of administration of insulin in addition to education, frequent blood glucose monitoring, and ongoing professional guidance. This may restore hypoglycemia counterregulation and hypoglycemia awareness, which subsequently may allow tightening of glycemic control.

Suggested Sites for the Readers

- www.cadre-diabetes.org
- http://professional.diabetes.org

References

1. Owen O, Morgan A, Kemp H, Sullivan J, Herrera M, Cahill G. Brain metabolism during fasting. *J Clin Invest*. 1967;46: 1589–1595.
2. Choi IY, Seaquist ER, Gruetter R. Effect of hypoglycemia on brain glycogen metabolism in vivo. *J Neurosci Res*. 2003;72: 25–32.
3. Cryer P. Banting lecture: hypoglycemia, the limiting factor in the management of IDDM. *Diabetes*. 1994;43:1378–1389.
4. Cryer P, Binder C, Bolli G, et al. Hypoglycemia in IDDM. *Diabetes*. 1989;38:1193–1199.
5. Foster D, Rubenstein A. Hypoglycemia. In: Wilson J, Braunwald E, Isselbacher K, eds. *Harrison's Principles of Internal Medicine*. New York: McGraw-Hill; 1991:1759.
6. Guillod L, Comte-Perret S, Monbaron D, Gaillard RC, Ruiz J. Nocturnal hypoglycaemias in type 1 diabetic patients: what can we learn with continuous glucose monitoring? *Diabetes Metab*. 2007;33:360–365.
7. Wentholt IM, Maran A, Masurel N, Heine RJ, Hoekstra JB, DeVries JH. Nocturnal hypoglycaemia in type 1 diabetic patients, assessed with continuous glucose monitoring: frequency, duration and associations. *Diabet Med*. 2007;24:527–532.
8. Defining and reporting hypoglycemia in diabetes: a report from the American Diabetes Association Workgroup on Hypoglycemia. *Diabetes Care*. 2005;28:1245–1249.
9. DCCT Research Group. The effect of intensive treatment of diabetes on the development and progression of long-term complications in insulin dependent diabetes mellitus. *N Engl J Med*. 1993;329:977–986.
10. Egger M, Smith GD, Stettler C, Diem P. Risk of adverse effects of intensified treatment in insulin-dependent diabetes mellitus: a meta-analysis. *Diabet Med*. 1997;14:919–928.
11. UK Prospective Diabetes. Study (UKPDS) Group. Intensive blood-glucose control with sulphonylureas or insulin compared with conventional treatment and risk of complications in patients with type 2 diabetes (UKPDS 33). *Lancet*. 1998;352: 837–853.
12. Ohkubo Y, Kishikawa H, Araki E, et al. Intensive insulin therapy prevents the progression of diabetic microvascular complications in Japanese patients with non-insulin- dependent diabetes mellitus: a randomized prospective 6-year study. *Diabetes Res Clin Pract*. 1995;28:103–117.
13. Hepburn D, MacLeod K, Pell A, Scougal I, Frier B. Frequency and symptoms of hypoglycemia experienced by patients with type 2 diabetes treated with insulin. *Diabet Med*. 1993;10:231–237.
14. Leese GP, Wang J, Broomhall J, et al. Frequency of severe hypoglycemia requiring emergency treatment in type 1 and type 2 diabetes: a population-based study of health service resource use. *Diabetes Care*. 2003;26:1176–1180.
15. van Staa T, Abenhaim L, Monette J. Rates of hypoglycemia in users of sulfonylureas. *J Clin Epidemiol*. 1997;50:735–741.
16. Gerich J. Sulfonylureas in the treatment of diabetes mellitus. *Mayo Clin Proc*. 1985;60:439–443.
17. DCCT Research Group. Epidemiology of severe hypoglycemia in the diabetes control and complications trial. *Am J Med*. 1991;90:450–459.
18. Nilsson A, Tideholm B, Kalen J, Katzman P. Incidence of severe hypoglycemia and its causes in insulin-treated diabetics. *Acta Med Scand*. 1988;224:257–262.
19. Amiel S. R.D. Lawrence Lecture 1994. Limits of normality: the mechanisms of hypoglycemia unawareness. *Diabetic Med*. 1994;11:918–924.
20. Mokan M, Mitrakou M, Veneman T, et al. Hypoglycemia unawareness in IDDM. *Diabetes Care*. 1994;17:1397–1403.
21. Bolli G, DeFeo P, Compagnucci P, et al. Abnormal glucose counterregulation in insulin-dependent diabetes mellitus: interaction of anti-insulin antibodies and impaired glucagon and epinephrine secretion. *Diabetes*. 1983;32:134–141.
22. Amiel S, Tamborlane W, Simonson D, Sherwin R. Defective glucose counterregulation after strict control of insulin-dependent diabetes mellitus. *N Engl J Med*. 1987;316:1376–1383.
23. Simonson D, Tamborlane W, DeFronzo R, Sherwin R. Intensive insulin therapy reduces counterregulatory responses to hypoglycemia in type I diabetes. *Ann Int Med*. 1985;103:184–188.
24. Davis M, Mellman M, Shamoon H. Further defects in counterregulatory responses induced by recurrent hypoglycemia in IDDM. *Diabetes*. 1992;41:1335–1340.

25. Lingenfelser T, Renn W, Sommerwerck U, et al. Compromised hormonal counterregulation, symptom awareness, and neurophysiologic function after recurrent short-term episodes of insulin-induced hypoglycemia in IDDM patients. *Diabetes.* 1993;42:610–618.
26. Meyer C, Großmann R, Mitrakou A, et al. Effects of autonomic neuropathy on counterregulation and awareness of hypoglycemia in type 1 diabetic patients. *Diabetes Care.* 1998;21:1960–1966.
27. Horie H, Hanafusa T, Matsuyama T, et al. Decreased response of epinephrine and norepinephrine to insulin-induced hypoglycemia in diabetic autonomic neuropathy. *Horm Metab Res.* 1984;16:398–401.
28. Hoeldtke R, Boden G, Shuman C, Owen C. Reduced epinephrine secretion and hypoglycemic unawareness in diabetic autonomic neuropathy. *Ann Int Med.* 1982;96:459–462.
29. Hirsch I, Boyle P, Craft S, Cryer P. Higher glycemic thresholds for symptoms during β-adrenergic blockade in IDDM. *Diabetes.* 1991;40:1177–1186.
30. White N, Skor D, Cryer P, Bier D, Levandoski L, Santiago J. Identification of type I diabetic patients at increased risk for hypoglycemia during intensive therapy. *N Engl J Med.* 1983;308:485–491.
31. Gold A, MacLeod K, Frier B. Frequency of severe hypoglycemia in patients with type 1 diabetes with impaired awareness of hypoglycemia. *Diabetes Care.* 1994;17:697–703.
32. Gerich J. Hypoglycemia. In: DeGroot L, ed. *Endocrinology*. Philadelphia: W.B. Saunders; 2001:921–940.
33. Andreasen J, Orskov C, Holst J. Secretion of glucagon-like peptide-1 and reactive hypoglycemia after partial gastrectomy. *Digestion.* 1994;55:221–228.
34. Miholic J, Orskov C, Holst J, Kotzerke J, Meyer H. Emptying of the gastric substitute, glucagon-like peptide-1 (GLP-1), and reactive hypoglycemia after total gastrectomy. *Dig Dis Sci.* 1991;36:1361–1370.
35. Wapnick S, Jones JJ. Changes in glucose tolerance and serum insulin following partial gastrectomy and intestinal resection. *Gut.* 1972;13:871–873.
36. Leichter S, Permutt M. Effect of adrenergic agents on postgastrectomy hypoglycemia. *Diabetes.* 1975;24:1005–1010.
37. Shultz KT, Neelon FA, Nilsen LB, Lebovitz HE. Mechanism of postgastrectomy hypoglycemia. *Arch Intern Med.* 1971;128:240–246.
38. Guidone C, Manco M, Valera-Mora E, et al. Mechanisms of recovery from type 2 diabetes after malabsorptive bariatric surgery. *Diabetes.* 2006;55:2025–2031.
39. Gumbs AA, Modlin IM, Ballantyne GH. Changes in insulin resistance following bariatric surgery: role of caloric restriction and weight loss. *Obes Surg.* 2005;15:462–473.
40. Maggard MA, Shugarman LR, Suttorp M, et al. Meta-analysis: surgical treatment of obesity. *Ann Intern Med.* 2005;142:547–559.
41. Gebhard B, Holst JJ, Biegelmayer C, Miholic J. Postprandial GLP-1, norepinephrine, and reactive hypoglycemia in dumping syndrome. *Dig Dis Sci.* 2001;46:1915–1923.
42. Lawaetz O, Blackburn AM, Bloom SR, Aritas Y, Ralphs DN. Gut hormone profile and gastric emptying in the dumping syndrome. A hypothesis concerning the pathogenesis. *Scand J Gastroenterol.* 1983;18:73–80.
43. Dube PE, Brubaker PL. Nutrient, neural and endocrine control of glucagon-like peptide secretion. *Horm Metab Res.* 2004;36:755–760.
44. Kellum JM, Kuemmerle JF, O'Dorisio TM, et al. Gastrointestinal hormone responses to meals before and after gastric bypass and vertical banded gastroplasty. *Ann Surg.* 1990;211:763–770.
45. Cummings DE, Weigle DS, Frayo RS, et al. Plasma ghrelin levels after diet-induced weight loss or gastric bypass surgery. *N Engl J Med.* 2002;346:1623–1630.
46. Patti ME, McMahon G, Mun EC, et al. Severe hypoglycaemia post-gastric bypass requiring partial pancreatectomy: evidence for inappropriate insulin secretion and pancreatic islet hyperplasia. *Diabetologia.* 2005;48:2236–2240.
47. Service GJ, Thompson GB, Service FJ, Andrews JC, Collazo-Clavell ML, Lloyd RV. Hyperinsulinemic hypoglycemia with nesidioblastosis after gastric-bypass surgery. *N Engl J Med.* 2005;353:249–254.
48. Won JG, Tseng HS, Yang AH, et al. Clinical features and morphological characterization of 10 patients with noninsulinoma pancreatogenous hypoglycaemia syndrome (NIPHS). *Clin Endocrinol (Oxf).* 2006;65:566–578.
49. Meier JJ, Butler AE, Galasso R, Butler PC. Hyperinsulinemic hypoglycemia after gastric bypass surgery is not accompanied by islet hyperplasia or increased beta-cell turnover. *Diabetes Care.* 2006;29:1554–1559.
50. Gerich J. Glucose counterregulation and its impact on diabetes mellitus. *Diabetes.* 1988;37:1608–1617.
51. Bolli G, Dimitriadis G, Pehling G, et al. Abnormal glucose counterregulation after subcutaneous insulin in insulin-dependent diabetes mellitus. *N Engl J Med.* 1984;310:1706–1711.
52. Cersosimo E, Garlick P, Ferretti J. Renal glucose production during insulin-induced hypoglycemia in humans. *Diabetes.* 1999;48:261–266.
53. Meyer C, Dostou J, Gerich J. Role of the human kidney in glucose counterregulation. *Diabetes.* 1999;48:943–948.
54. Schwartz N, Clutter W, Shah S, Cryer P. The glycemic thresholds for activation of glucose counterregulatory systems are higher than the threshold for symptoms. *J Clin Invest.* 1987;79:777–781.
55. Mitrakou A, Ryan C, Veneman T, et al. Hierarchy of glycemic thresholds for counterregulatory hormone secretion, symptoms, and cerebral dysfunction. *Am J Physiol.* 1991;260:E67–E74.
56. Fanelli C, Pampanelli S, Epifano L, et al. Relative roles of insulin and hypoglycemia on induction of neuroendocrine responses to, symptoms of, and deterioration of cognitive function in hypoglycemia in male and female humans. *Diabetologia.* 1994;37:797–807.

57. DeFeo P, Perriello G, Torlone E, et al. Demonstration of a role of growth hormone in glucose counterregulation. *Am J Physiol.* 1989;256:E835–E843.

58. DeFeo P, Perriello G, Torlone E, et al. Contribution of cortisol to glucose counterregulation in humans. *Am J Physiol.* 1989;257:E35–E42.

59. Lecavalier L, Bolli G, Cryer P, Gerich J. Contributions of gluconeogenesis and glycogenolysis during glucose counterregulation in normal humans. *Am J Physiol.* 1989;256:E844–E851.

60. Stumvoll M, Meyer C, Kreider M, Perriello G, Gerich J. Effects of glucagon on renal and hepatic glutamine gluconeogenesis in normal postabsorptive humans. *Metabolism.* 1998;47:1227–1232.

61. Stumvoll M, Meyer C, Perriello G, Kreider M, Welle S, Gerich J. Human kidney and liver gluconeogenesis: evidence for organ substrate selectivity. *Am J Physiol.* 1998;274:E817–E826.

62. Meyer C, Stumvoll M, Welle S, Nair S, Haymond M, Gerich J. Sites, substrates and mechanisms of epinephrine stimulated glucose production in humans. *Diabetes.* 1998;47(Suppl 1):A305.

63. Rizza R, Haymond M, Cryer P, Gerich J. Differential effects of physiologic concentrations of epinephrine on glucose production and disposal in man. *Am J Physiol.* 1979;237:356–362.

64. Sacca L, Morrone G, Cicala M, Corso G, Ungaro B. Influence of epinephrine, norepinephrine and isoproterenol on glucose homeostasis in normal man. *J Clin Endo Metab.* 1980;50:680–684.

65. Sacca L, Vigorito C, Cicala M, Corso G, Sherwin R. Role of gluconeogenesis in epinephrine-stimulated hepatic glucose production in humans. *Am J Physiol.* 1983;245:E294–E302.

66. Clutter W, Bier D, Shah S, Cryer P. Epinephrine plasma metabolic clearance rates and physiologic thresholds for metabolic and hemodynamic actions in man. *J Clin Invest.* 1980;66:94–101.

67. Gerich J, Campbell P. Overview of counterregulation and its abnormalities in diabetes mellitus and other conditions. *Diabetes Metab Rev.* 1988;4:93–111.

68. McMahon M, Gerich J, Rizza R. Effects of glucocorticoids on carbohydrate metabolism. *Diabetes Metab Rev.* 1988;4:17–30.

69. Hepburn D, Deary I, Frier B, Patrick A, Quinn J, Fisher B. Symptoms of acute insulin-induced hypoglycemia in humans with and without IDDM. Factor-analysis approach. *Diabetes Care.* 1991;14:949–957.

70. Towler D, Havlin C, Craft S, Cryer P. Mechanism of awareness of hypoglycemia: perception of neurogenic (predominantly cholinergic) rather than neuroglycopenic symptoms. *Diabetes.* 1993;42:1791–1798.

71. Cox D, Gonder-Frederick L, Antoun B, Cryer P, Clarke W. Perceived symptoms in the recognition of hypoglycemia. *Diabetes Care.* 1993;16:519–527.

72. Bolli G, DeFeo P, Perriello G, et al. Role of hepatic autoregulation in defense against hypoglycemia in humans. *J Clin Invest.* 1985;75:1623–1631.

73. Mitrakou A, Fanelli C, Veneman T, et al. Reversibility of unawareness of hypoglycemia in patients with insulinomas. *N Engl J Med.* 1993;329:834–839.

74. Heller S, Cryer P. Hypoinsulinemia is not critical to glucose recovery from hypoglycemia in humans. *Am J Physiol.* 1991;261:E41–E48.

75. DeFeo P, Perriello G, DeCosmo S, et al. Comparison of glucose counterregulation during short-term and prolonged hypoglycemia in normal humans. *Diabetes.* 1986;35:563–569.

76. Sacca L, Sherwin R, Hendler R, Felig P. Influence of continuous physiologic hyperinsulinemia on glucose kinetics and counterregulatory hormones in normal and diabetic humans. *J Clin Invest.* 1979;63:849–857.

77. DeFeo P, Perriello G, Ventura M, et al. The pancreatic–adrenocortical–pituitary clamp technique for study of counterregulation in humans. *Am J Physiol.* 1987;252:E565–E570.

78. DeFeo P, Perriello G, Torlone E, et al. Contribution of adrenergic mechanisms to glucose counterregulation in humans. *Am J Physiol.* 1991;261:E725–E736.

79. Gerich J, Langlois M, Noacco C, Karam J, Forsham P. Lack of glucagon response to hypoglycemia in diabetes: evidence for an intrinsic pancreatic alpha-cell defect. *Science.* 1973;182:171–173.

80. Fukuda M, Tanaka A, Tahara Y, et al. Correlation between minimal secretory capacity of pancreatic ß-cells and stability of diabetic control. *Diabetes.* 1988;37:81–88.

81. Rizza R, Cryer P, Gerich J. Role of glucagon, epinephrine and growth hormone in glucose counterregulation. *J Clin Invest.* 1979;64:62–71.

82. Hirsch B, Shamoon H. Defective epinephrine and growth hormone responses in type I diabetes are stimulus specific. *Diabetes.* 1987;36:20–26.

83. Dagogo-Jack S, Craft S, Cryer P. Hypoglycemia-associated autonomic failure in insulin dependent diabetes mellitus. *J Clin Invest.* 1993;91:819–828.

84. Bolli G, DeFeo P, DeCosmo S, et al. A reliable and reproducible test for adequate glucose counterregulation in type I diabetes mellitus. *Diabetes.* 1984;33:732–737.

85. Cersosimo E, Ferretti J, Sasvary D, Garlick P. Adrenergic stimulation of renal glucose release is impaired in type 1 diabetes. *Diabetes.* 2001;50(Suppl 2):A54.

86. Pramming S, Thorsteinsson B, Bendtson I, Binder C. Symptomatic hypoglycemia in 411 type I diabetic patients. *Diabetic Med.* 1991;8:217–222.

87. Hepburn D, Patrick A, Eadington D, Ewing D, Frier B. Unawareness of hypoglycemia in insulin-treated diabetic patients: prevalence and relationship to autonomic neuropathy. *Diabetic Med.* 1990;7:711–717.

88. Raju B, Cryer PE. Loss of the decrement in intraislet insulin plausibly explains loss of the glucagon response to hypoglycemia in insulin-deficient diabetes: documentation of the intraislet insulin hypothesis in humans. *Diabetes*. 2005;54:757–764.

89. Unger R. Insulin–glucagon relationships in the defense against hypoglycemia. *Diabetes*. 1983;32:575–583.

90. Boyle P, Kempers S, O'Connor A, Nagy R. Brain glucose uptake and unawareness of hypoglycemia in patients with insulin-dependent diabetes mellitus. *N Engl J Med*. 1995;333:1726–1731.

91. Fritsche A, Stumvoll M, Grüb M, et al. Effect of hypoglycemia on -adrenergic sensitivity in normal and type 1 diabetic subjects. *Diabetes Care*. 1998;21:1505–1510.

92. McCrimmon RJ, Shaw M, Fan X, et al. Key role for AMP-activated protein kinase in the ventromedial hypothalamus in regulating counterregulatory hormone responses to acute hypoglycemia. *Diabetes*. 2008;57:444–450.

93. McCrimmon RJ, Song Z, Cheng H, et al. Corticotrophin-releasing factor receptors within the ventromedial hypothalamus regulate hypoglycemia-induced hormonal counterregulation. *J Clin Invest*. 2006;116:1723–1730.

94. Heller S, MacDonald I, Tattersall R. Counterregulation in type 2 (noninsulin-dependent) diabetes mellitus: normal endocrine and glycemic responses, up to 10 years after diagnosis. *Diabetologia*. 1987;30:924–929.

95. Levy C, Kinsley B, Bajaj M, Simonson D. Effect of glycemic control on glucose counterregulation during hypoglycemia in NIDDM. *Diabetes Care*. 1998;21:1330–1338.

96. Shamoon H, Friedman S, Canton C, Zacharowicz L, Hu M, Rossetti L. Increased epinephrine and skeletal muscle responses to hypoglycemia in non-insulin-dependent diabetes mellitus. *J Clin Invest*. 1994;93:2562–2571.

97. Segel S, Paramore D, Cryer P. Hypoglycemia-associated autonomic failure in advanced type 2 diabetes. *Diabetes*. 2002;51:724–733.

98. Bolli G, Tsalikian E, Haymond M, Cryer P, Gerich J. Defective glucose counterregulation after subcutaneous insulin in noninsulin-dependent diabetes mellitus. *J Clin Invest*. 1984;73:1532–1541.

99. Woerle HJ, Meyer C, Popa E, Cryer P, Gerich J. Renal compensation for impaired hepatic glucose release during hypoglycemia in type 2 diabetes: further evidence for hepatorenal reciprocity. *Diabetes*. 2003;52:1386–1392.

100. Magnusson I, Rothman D, Katz L, Shulman R, Shulman G. Increased rate of gluconeogenesis in type II diabetes. A 13C nuclear magnetic resonance study. *J Clin Invest*. 1992;90:1323–1327.

101. Arner P, Einarsson K, Ewerth S, Livingston J. Altered action of glucagon on human liver in Type 2 (noninsulin- dependent) diabetes mellitus. *Diabetologia*. 1987;30:323–326.

102. Krahn D, Mackenzie T. Organic personality syndrome caused by insulin-related nocturnal hypoglycemia. *Psychosomatics*. 1984;25:711–712.

103. Silas J, Grant D, Maddocks J. Transient hemiparetic attacks due to unrecognised nocturnal hypoglycaemia. *BMJ*. 1981;282:132–133.

104. Chalmers J, Risk M, Kean D, Grant R, Ashworth B, Campbell I. Severe amnesia after hypoglycemia. Clinical, psychometric, and magnetic resonance imaging correlations. *Diabetes Care*. 1991;14:922–925.

105. Fisher B, Quin J, Rumley A, et al. Effects of acute insulin-induced hypoglycaemia on haemostasis, fibrinolysis and haemorheology in insulin-dependent diabetic patients and control subjects. *Clin Sci*. 1991;80:525–531.

106. Wredling R, Levander S, Adamson U, Lins P. Permanent neuropsychological impairment after recurrent episodes of severe hypoglycaemia in man. *Diabetologia*. 1990;33:152–157.

107. Patrick A, Campbell I. Fatal hypoglycaemia in insulin-treated diabetes mellitus: clinical features and neuropathological changes. *Diabetic Med*. 1990;7:349–354.

108. Pladziewicz D, Nesto R. Hypoglycemia-induced silent myocardial ischemia. *Am J Cardiol*. 1989;63:1531–1532.

109. Duh E, Feinglos M. Hypoglycemia-induced angina pectoris in a patient with diabetes mellitus. *Ann Intern Med*. 1994;121:945–946.

110. Perros P, Frier B. The long-term sequelae of severe hypoglycemia on the brain in insulin-dependent diabetes mellitus. *Horm Metab Res*. 1997;29:197–202.

111. Kohner E, McLeod D, Marshall J. *Complications of Diabetes*. London: Edward Arnold; 1982.

112. Deary I, Crawford J, Hepburn D, Langan S, Blackmore L, Frier B. Severe hypoglycemia and intelligence in adult patients with insulin-treated diabetes. *Diabetes*. 1993;42:341–344.

113. Paz-Guevara A, Hsu T-H, White P. Juvenile diabetes mellitus after forty years. *Diabetes*. 1975;24:559–565.

114. Nabarro J, Mustaffa B, Morris D, Walport M, Kurtz A. Insulin deficient diabetes. Contrasts with other endocrine deficiencies. *Diabetologia*. 1979;16:5–12.

115. Seltzer H. Severe drug-induced hypoglycemia: a review. *Compr Ther*. 1979;5:21–29.

116. Berger W, Caduff F, Pasquel M, Rump A. Die relative haufigkeit der schweren Sulfonylharnstoff- hypoglykamie in den letzten 25 Jahren in der Schweiz. *Schwerz Med Wschr*. 1986;116:145–151.

117. Mintz D, Finster J, Taylor A, Fefea A. Hormonal genesis of glucose intolerance following hypoglycemia. *Am J Med*. 1968;45:187–197.

118. Frier B, Corrall R, Ashby J, Baird J. Attenuation of the pancreatic beta-cell response to a meal following hypoglycemia in man. *Diabetologia*. 1980;18:297–300.

119. Attvall S, Fowelin J, von Schenck H, Smith U. Insulin resistance in type I (insulin-dependent) diabetes following hypoglycemia-evidence for the importance of B-adrenergic stimulation. *Diabetologia*. 1987;30:691–697.

120. Kollind M, Adamson U, Lins P. Insulin resistance following nocturnal hypoglycemia in insulin- dependent diabetes mellitus. *Acta Endocrinol*. 1987;116:314–320.

121. Clore J, Brennan J, Gebhart S, Newsome H, Nestler J, Blackard W. Prolonged insulin resistance following insulin-induced hypoglycemia. *Diabetologia.* 1987;30:851–858.
122. Gale E, Kurtz A, Tattersall R. In search of the Somogyi effect. *Lancet.* 1980;2:279–282.
123. Havlin C, Cryer P. Nocturnal hypoglycemia does not commonly result in major morning hyperglycemia in patients with diabetes mellitus. *Diabetes Care.* 1987;10:141–147.
124. Tordjman K, Havlin C, Levandoski L, White N, Santiago J, Cryer P. Failure of nocturnal hypoglycemia to cause fasting hyperglycemia in patients with insulin-dependent diabetes mellitus. *N Engl J Med.* 1987;317:1552–1559.
125. Gaston S. Outcomes of hypoglycemia treated by standardized protocol in a community hospital. *Diabetes Educ.* 1992;18: 491–494.
126. Slama G, Traynard P, Desplanque N, et al. The search for an optimized treatment of hypoglycemia. Carbohydrates in tablets, solution, or gel for the correction of insulin reactions. *Arch Intern Med.* 1990;150:589–593.
127. Palatnick W, Meatherall R, Tenenbein M. Clinical spectrum of sulfonylurea overdose and experience with diazoxide therapy. *Arch Intern Med.* 1991;151:1859–1862.
128. Cryer P, Gerich J. Glucose counterregulation, hypoglycemia, and intensive insulin therapy in diabetes mellitus. *N Engl J Med.* 1985;313:232–241.
129. Bolli G. How to ameliorate the problem of hypoglycemia in intensive as well as nonintensive treatment of type 1 diabetes. *Diabetes Care.* 1999;22(Suppl 2):B43–B52.
130. Boland E, Grey M, Oesterle A, Fredrickson L, Tamborlane W. Continuous subcutaneous insulin infusion. A new way to lower risk of severe hypoglycemia, improve metabolic control, and enhance coping in adolescents with type 1 diabetes. *Diabetes Care.* 1999;22:1779–1784.
131. Bode B, Steed RD, Davidson P. Reduction in severe hypoglycemia with long-term continuous subcutaneous insulin infusion in type 1 diabetes. *Diabetes Care.* 1996;19:324–327.
132. Brunelle R, Llewelyn J, Anderson J, Gale E, Koivisto V. Meta-analysis of the effect of insulin lispro on severe hypoglycemia in patients with type 1 diabetes. *Diabetes Care.* 1998;21:1726–1731.
133. Pieber T, Eugene-Jolchine I, Derobert E. The European Study Group of HOE 901 in type 1 diabetes. Efficacy and safety of HOE 901 versus NPH insulin in patients with type 1 diabetes. *Diabetes Care.* 2000;23:157–162.
134. Ratner R, Hirsch I, Neifing J, Garg S, Mecca T, Wilson C. Less hypoglycemia with insulin glargine in intensive insulin therapy for type I diabetes. *Diabetes Care.* 2000;23:639–643.
135. Home P, Bartley P, Russell-Jones D, et al. Insulin detemir offers improved glycemic control compared with NPH insulin in people with type 1 diabetes: a randomized clinical trial. *Diabetes Care.* 2004;27:1081–1087.
136. Rosenstock J, Dailey G, Massi-Benedetti M, Fritsche A, Lin Z, Salzman A. Reduced hypoglycemia risk with insulin glargine: a meta-analysis comparing insulin glargine with human NPH insulin in type 2 diabetes. *Diabetes Care.* 2005;28:950–955.
137. Hermansen K, Davies M, Derezinski T, Martinez RG, Clauson P, Home P. A 26-week, randomized, parallel, treat-to-target trial comparing insulin detemir with NPH insulin as add-on therapy to oral glucose-lowering drugs in insulin-naive people with type 2 diabetes. *Diabetes Care.* 2006;29:1269–1274.
138. Garber AJ, Clauson P, Pedersen CB, Kolendorf K. Lower risk of hypoglycemia with insulin detemir than with neutral protamine Hagedorn insulin in older persons with type 2 diabetes: a pooled analysis of phase III trials. *J Am Geriatr Soc.* 2007;55:1735–1740.
139. Nattrass M, Lauritzen T. Review of prandial glucose regulation with repaglinide: a solution to the problem of hypoglycaemia in the treatment of Type 2 diabetes? *Int J Obes Relat Metab Disord.* 2000;24(Suppl 3):S21–S31.
140. Levien TL, Baker DE, Campbell RK, White JR Jr. Nateglinide therapy for type 2 diabetes mellitus. *Ann Pharmacother.* 2001;35:1426–1434.
141. Dagogo-Jack S, Rattarason C, Cryer P. Reversal of hypoglycemia unawareness, but not defective glucose counterregulation in IDDM. *Diabetes.* 1994;43:1426–1434.
142. Fritsche A, Stumvoll M, Haring H, Gerich J. Reversal of hypoglycemia unawareness in a long-term type 1 diabetic patient by improvement of beta-adrenergic sensitivity after prevention of hypoglycemia. *J Clin Endocrinol Metab.* 2000;85:523–525.
143. Fanelli C, Epifano L, Rambotti A, et al. Meticulous prevention of hypoglycemia normalizes the glycemic thresholds and magnitude of most of neuroendocrine responses to, symptoms of, and cognitive function during hypoglycemia in intensively treated patients with short-term IDDM. *Diabetes.* 1993;42:1683–1689.
144. Fanelli C, Pampanelli S, Epifano L, et al. Long-term recovery from unawareness, deficient counterregulation and lack of cognitive dysfunction during hypoglycemia, following institution of rational, intensive insulin therapy in IDDM. *Diabetologia.* 1994;37:1265–1276.
145. Cranston I, Lomas J, Maran A, MacDonald I, Amiel S. Restoration of hypoglycemia unawareness in patients with long-duration insulin-dependent diabetes. *Lancet.* 1994;344:283–287.
146. Davis M, Mellman M, Friedman S, Chang C, Shamoon H. Recovery of epinephrine response but not hypoglycemic symptom threshold after intensive therapy in type 1 diabetes. *Am J Med.* 1994;97:535–542.
147. Kendall D, Teuscher A, Robertson R. Defective glucagon secretion during sustained hypoglycemia following successful islet allo- and autotransplantation in humans. *Diabetes.* 1997;46:23–27.
148. Meyer C, Hering B, Großmann R, et al. Improved glucose counterregulation and autonomic symptoms after intraportal islet transplants alone in patients with long-standing type I diabetes mellitus. *Transplantation.* 1998;66:233–240.

149. Federlin K, Pozza G. Indications for clinical islet transplantation today and in the foreseeable future – The diabetologist's point of view. *J Mol Med*. 1999;77:148–152.

150. Bosi E, Piatti P, Secchi A, et al. Response of glucagon and insulin secretion to insulin-induced hypoglycemia in diabetic patients after pancreatic transplantation. *Diab Nutr Metab*. 1988;1:21–27.

151. Diem P, Redman J, Abid M, et al. Glucagon, catecholamine, and pancreatic polypeptide secretion in type I diabetic recipients of pancreas allografts. *J Clin Invest*. 1990;86:2008–2013.

152. Bolinder J, Wahrenberg H, Persson A, et al. Effect of pancreas transplantation on glucose counterregulation in insulin-dependent diabetic patients prone to severe hypoglycaemia. *J Intern Med*. 1991;230:527–533.

153. Bolinder J, Wahrenberg H, Linde B, Tyden G, Groth C, Ostman J. Improved glucose counterregulation after pancreas transplantation in diabetic patients with unawareness of hypoglycemia. *Transplant Proc*. 1991;23:1667–1669.

154. Landgraf R, Nusser J, Riepl R, et al. Metabolic and hormonal studies of type 1 (insulin-dependent) diabetic patients after successful pancreas and kidney transplantation. *Diabetologia*. 1991;34(Suppl 1):S61–S67.

155. Barrou Z, Seaquist E, Robertson R. Pancreas transplantation in diabetic humans normalizes hepatic glucose production during hypoglycemia. *Diabetes*. 1994;43:661–666.

156. Kendall D, Rooney D, Smets Y, Bolding L, Robertson R. Pancreas transplantation restores epinephrine response and symptom recognition during hypoglycemia in patients with long-standing type 1 diabetes and autonomic neuropathy. *Diabetes*. 1997;46:249–257.

157. Luzi L, Battezzati A, Perseghin G, et al. Lack of feedback inhibition of insulin secretion in denervated human pancreas. *Diabetes*. 1992;41:1632–1639.

158. Battezzati A, Luzi L, Perseghin G, et al. Persistence of counter-regulatory abnormalities in insulin-dependent diabetes mellitus after pancreas transplantation. *Eur J Clin Invest*. 1994;24:751–758.

159. Paty BW, Ryan EA, Shapiro AM, Lakey JR, Robertson RP. Intrahepatic islet transplantation in type 1 diabetic patients does not restore hypoglycemic hormonal counterregulation or symptom recognition after insulin independence. *Diabetes*. 2002;51:3428–3434.

160. Gupta V, Wahoff D, Rooney D, et al. The defective glucagon response from transplanted intrahepatic pancreatic islets during hypoglycemia is transplantation site-determined. *Diabetes*. 1997;46:28–33.

161. Zinman B, Hoogwerf BJ, Duran GS, et al. The effect of adding exenatide to a thiazolidinedione in suboptimally controlled type 2 diabetes: a randomized trial. *Ann Intern Med*. 2007;146:477–485.

Chapter 20
Intake of Advanced Glycation Endproducts: Role in the Development of Diabetic Complications

Helen Vlassara and Gary E. Striker

Introduction

Diabetes is a very common cause of hospitalization and is listed as a diagnosis in 12% of hospital discharges. This diagnosis has a substantial impact on medical costs since hospital stay for diabetic patients is 1–3 days longer than non-diabetics. Cardiovascular complications are a common cause of hospitalizations for diabetic patients, and diabetes is a listed diagnosis in 29% of cardiac surgery patients.[1–4]

The underlying pathogenesis of cardiovascular disease in diabetes includes increased oxidant stress (OS) and inflammation. The manifestations of the diabetic state include metabolic abnormalities, increased OS, and a chronic inflammatory state, which serve to accentuate each other and result in a cycle of increasing organ damage. Since data obtained over the past few years support the new and novel concept that the inflammatory response seen in diabetes results from the cumulative and sustained pressure from oxidant stress, it is important to decrease OS from all potential sources.[4–9] The origin of oxidants in diabetes was initially considered to be entirely endogenous, but there is now an agreement that the environment, especially the diet, is a substantial source of oxidants.[10] This being the case it is important to understand the significant contribution of the diet to OS in diabetics and seek to reduce this input.

Advanced glycation endproducts (AGEs) are among the most commonly encountered oxidants in food.[10] They belong to a class of toxic oxidant molecules, also called glycoxidants. High levels of toxic oxidant AGEs are thought to underlie many of the complications of diabetes.[11,12] One of the ways by which AGEs induce these changes is by generating reactive oxidant species (ROS), which promote the formation of more AGEs, in a vicious action/reaction cycle, which progressively increases oxidative stress (OS) and the risk for both micro- and macrovascular disease (Fig. 20.1). Activation of receptors which recognize AGEs results in activation of downstream signaling pathways (including NFκB) which induce the production of pro-inflammatory cytokines and pro-angiogenic factors, leading to increased OS.[9]

AGE deposition in aging blood vessels and other tissues is well documented, and its role in the pathogenesis of cardiovascular disease and diabetic nephropathy is supported by the fact that structurally unrelated inhibitors of AGE formation provide protection against these diseases.[13–33] The number and breadth of these studies are an indication of the importance of blocking the formation and actions of AGEs. Understanding how AGEs interact with cells and tissues (Fig. 20.2), and how they can be prevented or treated, is an important challenge in the management of diabetes and its complications, across all medical disciplines. This chapter focuses on a non-pharmacological approach to the management of OS in diabetic patients.

H. Vlassara (✉)

Division of Experimental Diabetes and Aging, Division of Geriatrics, Mount Sinai School of Medicine, New York, NY, USA
e-mail: helen.vlassara@mssm.edu

L. Poretsky (ed.), *Principles of Diabetes Mellitus*, DOI 10.1007/978-0-387-09841-8_20,
© Springer Science+Business Media, LLC 2010

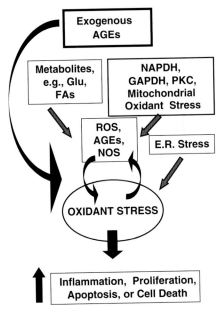

Fig. 20.1 Cellular/tissue injury in chronic disease is due to increased oxidant stress from exogenous and endogenous sources

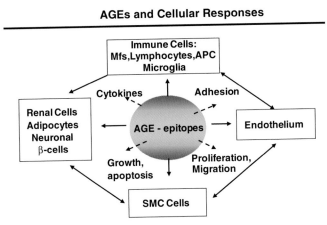

Fig. 20.2 AGEs interact with most cell types in the body, eliciting a variety of responses, depending on cell type and underlying state of OS

Toxic Oxidants (AGEs) and Cellular Responses

The glycoxidation pathway makes a fundamental contribution to OS, which underlies aging-mediated vascular disease and diabetes-related vascular and renal complications.[3,7,8,11,12,21,34–39] There are two sources of AGEs, *endogenous* and *exogenous* (*diet and smoking*[34]). It was previously thought that most AGEs are generated *endogenously* in diabetics by spontaneous reactions between the carbonyl groups of reducing sugars, ascorbate, and other carbohydrates and amino acids (lysine, arginine) or cystine-containing amino-peptides, nucleic acids, and lipids.[39,40–46] However, regular foods are now known to be a major source of AGEs in diabetics, as well as in non-diabetics.[47,48] The term AGEs, while often referring to non-reactive terminal products, such as $^\epsilon N$-carboxymethyllysine (CML) or pentosidine, also includes a broad range of reactive precursors, including 1- or

3-deoxyglucosone as well as methylglyoxal (MG) and their derivatives, a common one being hydroimidazolone, MG-H1. The latter are formed largely by non-oxidative mechanisms from triose phosphate intermediates during anaerobic glycolysis and are elevated in diabetes and aging.[49,50] Amine-containing lipids also form advanced lipoxidation endproducts (ALE), such as 4-hydroxy-nonenal or CML, and other lipid analogues.[11,30,40,41,49–53] Glycoxidation products of proteins and lipids (AGE/ALE) can accelerate the generation of reactive oxygen species (ROS), leading to oxidative and "carbonyl" stress.[38] Autoxidation of glucose is also accompanied by the generation of reactive oxygen species (ROS), such as superoxide radicals.[4,54] ROS enhance glycation and both mechanisms can promote atherogenesis and other complications related to diabetes or aging.[4] In fact, the direct cellular and tissue toxicity of certain AGEs, such as 1- or 3-deoxyglucosone or methylglyoxal derivatives, is now well established.[54]

Other non-glucose dependent AGE pathways involve activated white blood cells, i.e., neutrophils, monocytes, and macrophages. Activated white blood cells produce enzymes, including myeloperoxidase and nicotinamide adenine dinucleotide phosphate (NADPH) oxidase, causing AGE formation by oxidation of amino acids.[4,26,44,55–59] Cell activation by AGEs, i.e. via binding to the AGE receptor RAGE can also promote ROS and AGE formation via the NADPH oxidase pathway, the myeloperoxidase pathway or possibly through the nuclear protein amphoterin (also termed High Mobility Group Box 1) which can activate RAGE and toll-like receptor 4, and thus amplify AGE formation.[11,25,60–63]

Another mechanism of AGE formation is the aldose reductase-mediated polyol pathway. Glucose entering the polyol pathway may directly form AGEs via reactive intermediates, i.e., glyoxal, methyl-glyoxal, or 3-deoxyglucosone, as well as via depletion of NADPH or glutathione, which result in raised intracellular ROS.[56] These changes indirectly result in the further formation of AGEs.[61] Since these two mutually enhancing processes are tightly linked, interventions targeting one will inevitably have an impact on the other.

Sources of Toxic Oxidants (AGEs) in Diabetic Patients

Endogenous Sources: Hyperglycemia promotes metabolic activity and is the best known endogenous pathway by which the levels of AGEs and OS are increased in cells.[9,24,27,44,48,52,60,64–68] However, increased OS leads to the oxidation of other sugars and/or lipids, which create dicarbonyl compounds that use highly reactive carbonyl groups to bind amino acids and form AGEs.[24,52] While hyperglycemia may be one cause of increased OS in diabetic patients, as noted above, other pathways may increase the levels and activity of enzymes, such as NADPH oxidase, which induce AGE formation by oxidizing amino acids in both inflammatory and parenchymal cells.[27,59,64] MG may be formed as an intracellular toxic product of glycolysis. It is metabolized to lactate by enzymes (glyoxylase I and II) that require the non-enzymatic conjugation of glutathione with MG.[49,69] Thus, MG is neutralized when the levels of glutathione are normal, a state that may be compromised in the presence of high OS, such as diabetes.

AGE-modified moieties, especially long-lived proteins and lipids, as well as nucleic acids may be removed by proteolytic digestion, degraded to inactive molecules, and then excreted by the kidneys. However, AGE-derived cross-links are particularly resistant to degradation.[70–72] AGE crosslinks may contribute to the increased levels and delayed clearance of oxidized lipoproteins, the inactivation of immune components, and increased sensitivity of diabetic patients to drug toxicity, infection, and ischemia.[1–4,8,22,58,73–77] In particular, the toxic effects of AGEs on tissue structure and function may include the formation of chemical cross-links within and between connective tissue components or between these elements and plasma constituents, which can impair vasodilation or LDL removal (due to the retention of molecules trapped in the sub-endothelium and/or by impairing recognition and uptake of AGE-modified LDL by the LDL receptor).[20,26,29,52,53,67,78,79] Since AGE-LDL is a particular form of glycoxidized lipoprotein which is cross linked and is thus retained in the aortic wall, it recruits macrophages and promotes their conversion to foam cells and/or the accumulation of smooth muscle cells. As such it is thought to be an efficient pro-atherogenic substance.[5,12,13,25,26,28,40,45,46,49,58,63,80–87]

By creating cross-links between components of the extracellular matrix, and thereby changing their physical properties, AGEs affect both their distensibility and elasticity of arteries. Both type 1 diabetes and type 2 diabetes subjects have increased arterial disease, which is associated with increased cardiovascular mortality based on diastolic dysfunction,[73,88] increased pulse-wave velocity, decreased arterial compliance, and formation of aneurysms. Decreased vascular elasticity due to cross-links, which are resistant to degradation and the normal turnover of collagen and elastin, may play a larger role than previously appreciated.[5,28,38,72,89] This interpretation is reinforced by the observation that AGE inhibition restores these properties in rodents.[13,26,28]

Exogenous Sources: Many studies suggest that the modern diet is also a significant source of toxic oxidants (AGEs) in both man and experimental animals and contribute to the development of diabetes and diabetic complications.[65,90] While it has long been appreciated that AGEs are present in food,[67,68] they were not considered to be an important contaminant, since bioavailability studies showed that "only a small amount" of AGEs was taken into the body.[32,66,86,87,91] This point of view now has to be revised for two reasons. First, the cumulative oxidant properties of AGEs are well known. Second, the amount of oxidants in the modern diet has dramatically increased, particularly the amount of AGEs, as documented throughout this review. In part, this can be traced to the widespread consumption of red meat, processed foods, and soft drinks, as well as the near universal use of pasteurization and other forms of food preservation using heat.[86,87,9] Thus, the amount of toxic oxidants, including AGEs, that is present in the diet is now cause for concern, even if "only" a fraction is absorbed. This fact led to several recent studies of the bioavailability, kinetics, and renal elimination of dietary-derived AGE in healthy adults[90] and diabetic patients, with or without impaired renal function[66], as well as in animals.[32] We found that ~10% of the AGEs in the diet are absorbed, of which 2/3 is incorporated into tissues and turn over very slowly; the other ~1/3 is excreted via the kidneys.[32,66] Since the amount of AGEs in food in the last 50 years has increased, and the lifespan of the population has increased, this amount of absorption assumes greater importance clinically.

While increasedOS and the propensity to develop cardiovascular diseases have been in part attributed to excess fat in the diet, it is now recognized that even diets with a modest amount of lipids may contain high levels of oxidants, generated when proteins or lipids are mixed with reducing sugars and processed under elevated temperatures, as in standard cooking (Table 20.1).[65,92,93] Prime examples of the resultant dietary oxidants include reactive carbonyl compounds, advanced glycation (AGE), and lipoxidation endproducts (ALE), containing CML and MG derivatives in large concentrations.[44,51,94,95] The compounds formed in food are identical to those formed endogenously. Together with the exogenous AGEs the endogenous AGEs contribute to the chronic inflammatory response associated with the complications of aging and diabetes.[8,41,49,52,54,86,91,96]

Table 20.1 Thermally modulated AGE content in common foods

Regular diet (U/mg)		Low-AGE diet	
Beef: *broiled*	5367	*BOILED*	2000
Chicken: *broiled*	5245	*BOILED*	1011
Salmon: *broiled*	1348	*RAW*	502
Potato: *fried*	*1522*	*BOILED*	17

The levels of AGEs in most foods, not only red meats, depend largely on the method of cooking (see potato). Data are shown as CML immunoreactivity based on ELISA.

The data on the effect of cooking temperature on the formation of AGEs, and perhaps other toxic oxidants, are based on direct measurements of CML, MG, and MDA (a lipid peroxide product) in food prepared by different methods.[65,96] Grilling or frying meat increases the amounts of toxic oxidants significantly more than meat prepared by boiling. Frying results in a vast increase in AGEs, compared to boiling. For instance, so-called French fries contain 100-fold more AGEs, compared to boiled potatoes. This results from the addition of lipids to carbohydrates and proteins under conditions of dry heat. The amount of AGEs in the diet largely depends on the temperature during cooking and the degree of hydration (i.e., the amount of water present). For instance, cooking fish or chicken in water results in 4–6 times less AGEs, compared to cooking these foods in the absence of water. In addition, the amount of AGEs in cooked food is directly proportional to the fat content.

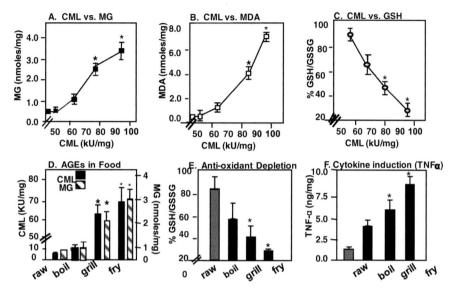

Fig. 20.3 Pro-oxidant and pro-inflammatory activity of food AGEs. (**a**) Correlation between food-derived protein AGEs (CML and MG-derivatives); (**b**) between CML and malondialdehyde (MDA, a lipid oxidation product); (**c**) addition of different amounts of food extracts to human endothelial cell (EC) cultures. CML levels inversely correlate with intracellular levels of glutathione, indicating that food AGEs induce cellular oxidant stress; (**d**) the amount of AGEs (CML and MG) in food (red meat) varies with method of cooking; (**e**) endothelial cell levels of anti-oxidant GSH vary, following the addition of food extracts prepared by different methods; (**f**) levels of the inflammatory cytokine, TNFα in EC, also vary with method of cooking following the addition of identical amounts of food extracts

The question is often raised as to the levels of specific AGEs in food. Therefore, we extracted red meat, prepared by different cooking methods and found that the amount of CML correlated with MG (Fig. 20.3a), that the amount of CML and MG correlated with the levels of MDA (an oxidized lipid) (Fig. 20.3b). In addition, both grilled and fried meat contained increased amount of both CML and MG, compared to either raw or boiled meat (Fig. 20.3c). While a relationship between the AGE content of foods, OS, and diabetic complications had previously been found, we directly tested whether food AGEs have biological activity, by preparing soluble extracts of these meat preparations, and then adding them to endothelial cells in vitro. The amount of intracellular anti-oxidants (i.e., glutathione) negatively correlated with the amount of AGEs in the preparations (Fig. 20.3d). The extracts also caused a decrease in anti-oxidant levels (GSH/GSSG ratio) (Fig. 20.3e), and promoted the release of TNFα (Fig. 20.3f). These data are of particular importance because they clearly show that AGEs are present in the food, and that their levels depend on the method of preparation. In addition, the data show that the AGEs present in the food are biologically active, since they directly cause increased OS and depletion of anti-oxidant defenses. Thus, both the type of food and the means by which it is prepared is critical in determining the total amount of oxidant AGEs present in food. We recently obtained direct proof that AGEs in the diet cause increased OS and raise the levels of circulating AGEs in mice. This was accomplished by adding a well-characterized AGE (MG) to a diet prepared with low heat, so that the initial content of AGEs in the food was reduced and that any changes observed would be directly related to the added AGEs. Examination of the mice from birth to 6 months of age revealed a linear rise in serum AGEs and increased OS levels in the mice fed the diet supplemented with MG (Fig. 20.4).[11] This critical finding provided direct proof of the ability of AGEs ingested via the diet to raise AGEs in the blood and lead to increased OS.

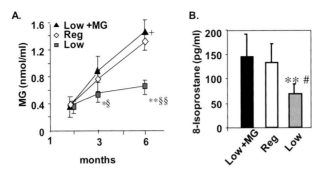

Fig. 20.4 Methyl-glyoxal (MG) derivatives in diet increase serum AGEs and OS. Pups from dams fed a low-AGE diet during gestation and nursing were pair-fed a low diet, a Low+MG, or a regular (Reg) diet at weaning. **(a)** Serum MG levels from weaning to 6 months of age. Low vs. Reg, *$p<0.05$, **$p<0.001$; Low vs. Low+MG, §$p<0.01$, §§$p<0.001$; Low+MG vs. Reg, + $p<0.05$. **(b)** 8-Isoprostane levels. Low vs. Low+MG, **$p<0.01$; Low vs. Reg, #$p<0.01$

Reduction of Toxic Oxidants (AGEs) in Mice

Recent evidence indicates that the cycle of increased levels of AGEs and elevated OS can be interrupted by reducing glycation, either in the body (endogenous) or in the food (exogenous). While anti-oxidant or anti-AGE agents may prevent the formation of AGEs, a non-pharmaceutical intervention such as reducing the amount of AGEs in the food by simply reducing the heat applied may be the most cost-efficient, effective, and widely applicable way of decreasing exposure to oxidants. The reduction of dietary oxidants (AGEs) prevents many of the diabetic complications in several animal models and reinforces the need to continue the search for optimal interventions in the clinical setting.

We have previously shown that sustained parenteral administration of AGEs, or feeding a high-AGE diet, reproduces many of the complications associated with diabetes.[48,66,68,78,97–100] The accumulation of advanced glycation endproducts (AGEs) begins in early life and progressively increases with time.[101] In this context, avoidance of early exposure to AGEs may determine susceptibility to certain diseases, including type 1 and type 2 diabetes. This concept was examined in non-obese diabetic (NOD) mice which have a high propensity to develop type 1 DM (~80% of young NOD females develop diabetes), which is attributed to an autoimmune process (Fig. 20.5, left upper panel).[98] We found that when these mice were exposed to a low-AGE diet the structure of their islets remained normal (Fig. 20.5, right upper panel), and the propensity to develop diabetes was sharply reduced. In fact, this "loss of susceptibility" could be traced to the maternal diet, since offspring of dams maintained on a low-AGE diet during gestation had a greatly reduced incidence of diabetes in the F1 generation, and diabetes was nearly absent in the F2 progeny.[98] The absence of diabetes resulted from preservation of intact pancreatic islets, the loss of several abnormalities in T lymphocytes, and the maintenance of low levels of OS (Fig. 20.6). This phenomenon was epigenetic in nature, since the progeny became diabetic, if they were returned to regular mouse chow, which has a high AGE content, similar to that of the modern human diet.[10,102]

We also tested other models of Type 2 DM, including db/db+/+ and high fat diet-induced type 2 DM in normal C57B6 mice, and found that both diabetes and complications were reduced.[22,28,48,97] Thus, the development of diabetes was blocked in both genetic and non-genetic models by reducing the intake of AGEs in the diet. A conclusion reached from these genetically and pathogenetically diverse models of diabetes was that the maintenance of lower levels of OS, by reducing the intake of AGEs (oxidants) in the diet may be a critical factor in the preservation of normal beta-cell function. Furthermore, the prevention of diabetes was effective in both those with a genetic background prone to the development of diabetes (type 1 and type 2), and the prevention of diabetes by diabetogenic interventions in otherwise normal strains. Furthermore, the data show that the levels of OS may be partly driven by the levels of toxic oxidants in the diet, and showed that the maternal diet was also an important source of oxidant AGEs in the fetus. Finally, the data show that these changes may be entirely preventable by

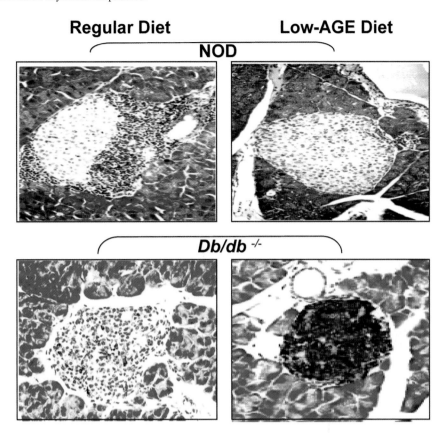

Fig. 20.5 Effect of dietary AGEs on islet morphology. (**a**) Non-diabetic F1 NOD mice, and (**b**) db/db +/+ mice were exposed to either regular (*left*) or low-AGE diet (*right panels*). NOD mouse pancreatic tissues stained by H&E (**a**) showed absence of the severe mononuclear cell infiltration after a low-AGE diet (for >12 mos). Islets of age-matched db/db+/+ mice (**b**), after L-AGE (×5 mos), stained for insulin showed intact insulin production compared to those on regular diet. Mag. ×400

modifying the preparation of the diet, without altering either the calorie content or particular nutrients. The latter point may be critical to normal fetal and post-natal development of diabetic mothers, and possibly even those with gestational diabetes. It also raises the question as to whether this may be important to the prevention of diabetes itself. Nonetheless, the conclusions from these initial studies are that consumption of diets that contain high amounts of AGEs can promote OS in apparently normal adults and that this can begin in the unborn fetus or in childhood. For instance, we and others found that infant formulae contain 28–389 fold (median=70) higher levels of toxic oxidant AGEs than maternal milk.[65,103] The CML in the infant formulae was absorbed and appeared in the urine.[103] Finally, the effect of oxidants in the diet may have other untoward effects as they may neutralize anti-oxidants in normal food, or anti-oxidants added for nutritional or pharmacologic purposes, and many vitamins are altered by oxidants or heat.[96]

Reduction of these toxic dietary AGE oxidants in diabetic mice attenuated diabetic vascular and kidney disease, acute vascular injury, and promoted wound healing.[48,67,68,75,76,104] Diabetic mice fed with standard laboratory diets (which have a high content of AGEs) developed vascular and renal lesions.[105] However, their age-matched cohorts fed with low-AGE isocaloric diets remain largely free of these changes, despite persistence of hyperlipidemia and diabetes.[47,54,67,68,75,76,97,106] A low-AGE diet also led to significant suppression of atherosclerotic plaque formation at the aortic root of diabetic/hyperlipidemic (ApoE[−/−]) mice (Fig. 20.7).[67] In addition, a low-AGE diet provided protection of post-injury arterial inflammation and re-stenosis in ApoE[−/−] mice despite sustained hyperlipidemia.[78] As noted above, feeding diabetic mice a diet with lower levels of toxic

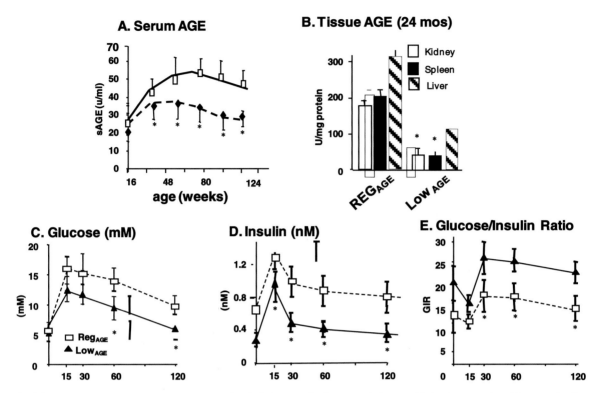

Fig. 20.6 A low-AGE diet suppresses age-associated diabetes. **a, b**: Serum and tissue AGE levels are reduced in normal mice pair-fed a low-AGE diet for life. Reg-AGE (*open symbols*), low-AGE diet (*closed symbols*). (**b**) Kidney, spleen, and liver AGE at 24 mos of age (*n*=8/group). **c–e**: Changes in glucose, insulin response to IGTT and GIR at 4 and 24 mos (*n*=6/group). Note: none of the low-AGE fed mice became diabetic by 3 years of age. All Reg-fed mice were diabetic at various age points before death (*n*=20/group)

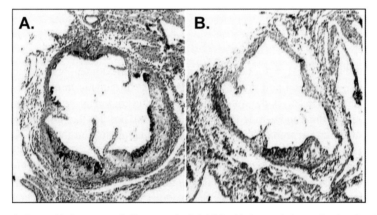

Fig. 20.7 Atheromatous lesion and inflammatory infiltrate are both inhibited in hypercholesterolemic mice (ApoE–/–) after feeding on a low-AGE diet for 5 mos. Aortic root sections from ApoE–/– mice fed a regular diet (**a**) or an AGE-restricted diet (**b**) are stained by a macrophage surface antigen-specific antibody (MOMA). Note the markedly decreased inflammatory cell infiltrate (Mag. ×200)

oxidants (AGEs) prevented the structural and functional changes of diabetic nephropathy in genetic models of type 1 and type 2 diabetes.[77,107] These studies support the proposed synergism between the levels of toxic oxidants in exogenous (diet) and the endogenously derived OS burden in diabetes. In addition, AGEs are antigenic, a property which may contribute to inflammation and atherosclerosis.[77,101]

In normally aging mice, long-term reduction in the intake of exogenous oxidants, without altering caloric intake, ameliorated OS, insulin resistance, and the incidence of diabetes, as well as significantly extending lifespan.[108] These diverse positive effects were attributed to the functional preservation of AGER1, anti-oxidant reserves, and the amelioration of aging-induced OS-response genes, including p66[Shc] and FOXO-1.[57,108,109]

Interventions which reduce the formation of ROS, such as calorie restriction, have long been known to promote lifespan extension.[43,110–112] Since calorie restriction is accomplished by reducing food intake, this effectively reduces the intake of AGEs as an obligate concomitant. We recently found that the well-known beneficial effects of a calorie-restricted diet could be due to the 40% reduction in food intake, primarily because it also restricts the intake of AGEs. In fact, when the AGE content of a calorie-restricted diet was increased, the benefits of calorie restriction on reducing OS, CVD, and CKD were lost.[12] We have shown that a long-term reduction of the intake of toxic AGEs decreases ROS, the expression of OS-response genes, cardiovascular and renal disease, and leads to an increased life span.[76,80,83,102,108,113] Furthermore, these effects were independent of calorie intake.

These experimental studies suggest that while factors such as heredity or nutrient intake play a large role in diabetes, the level of oxidants in the diet may be a key link to both the induction of diabetes and diabetic complications. AGEs may be a major contributor to these lesions, since they cause a wide spectrum of vascular abnormalities, including basement membrane thickening and endothelial injury, resulting in increased vascular permeability, a pro-thrombotic state, and decreased blood flow; all of which are traits of microvascular disease affecting the retina, kidneys, and peripheral nerves.[9,114–119] The specific role that AGEs play in causing microvascular disease is well documented in the kidney glomeruli.[100] However, the role of exogenous AGEs in retinopathy or neuropathy is not yet defined.

Elevated AGEs are also associated with macrovascular abnormalities in diabetic subjects, including coronary atherosclerosis.[14,27,73,120] AGEs decrease both endothelial cell nitric oxide levels and activity, by inhibiting endothelial nitric oxide synthase and prostacyclin or by quenching NO^-.[38,80,120] These changes, in conjunction with the effects attributed to protein kinase C activation, can further increase vasoconstriction.[117,118,121,122] AGEs increase expression of angiotensin II and endothelin in vascular smooth muscle cells, which also contribute to vasoconstriction, enhancing pro-inflammatory processes, and mitogenesis.[121,122] Activation of NFκB and activator protein-1 (AP-1) and other transcription factors by AGEs may lead to increased expression of adhesion molecules (e.g., ICAM-1, VCAM-1) and plasminogen activator inhibitor 1 (PAI-1), and contribute to chronic vascular dysfunction.[117]

In summary, these studies on diabetes and its complications introduce the view that the accumulation of advanced glycation endproducts (AGEs) may begin in utero (during the fetal period), continue in childhood, and progressively increases with normal aging. If the intake of AGEs is high, i.e., similar to that in the average modern diet, the baseline level of OS may be higher than "normal" and the rate of rise would be accelerated. This would reduce anti-oxidant defenses and result in an inflammatory state that may significantly alter innate immune responses to inflammatory processes. The end result could be the earlier onset of obesity and type 1 or type 2 diabetes, accompanied by macrovascular (atherosclerosis) and microvascular (kidney, retinal) diseases.[4,117,118]

Cellular Receptors that Recognize Toxic AGE Oxidants

Among the receptors that bind AGEs, AGER1 is the most extensively studied receptor involved in AGE endocytosis and processing (Fig. 20.8).[52,55,123,124] AGER1 is the principal receptor mediating the removal of excess extracellular AGEs, from both endogenous and exogenous origin. AGER1 is a ã50 kDa integral surface membrane protein that inhibits AGE-induced OS (as depicted in Fig. 20.9), via inhibition of RAGE, MAPK and Ras activation and phosphorylation of EGFR and ERK;[26] inhibition of phosphorylation of ser-36 of p66[Shc], a key pro-apoptotic adaptor protein involved in the phosphorylation and inactivation of members of the FOXO pathway,[109] which normally enhances anti-oxidants such as MnSOD and increases resistance to OS; and also via reduction of AGE-induced mitochondrial OS and mitochondrial injury in endothelial cells. Increased expression of the AGER1 transgene blocks ROS in vitro[55,57] and prevents vascular and kidney injury in mice.[137] These

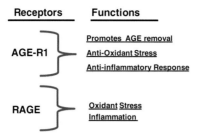

Fig. 20.8 Major AGE receptors and functions: AGER1 is localized on cell surface, mitochondria, and ER. RAGE is principally a cell surface receptor

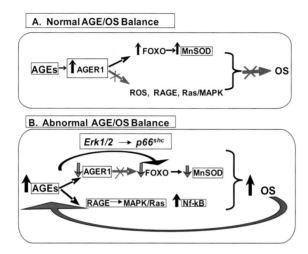

Fig. 20.9 Schematic representation of putative AGE-receptor interactions and their contribution to oxidant balance. (**a**) In the normal state AGER1 can suppress AGE- and ROS-dependent increased RAGE/Ras/MAPK and NFκB activity, as well as p66shc-dependent inactivation of FOXO. These oppose the formation of excess ROS from AGEs. (**b**) Chronic, poorly controlled diabetes, and/or sustained influxes of exogenous oxidants can reduce levels of AGER1 and its anti-OS actions, which will further increase ROS/AGEs

observations point to AGER1 as a potentially important multifunctional component of the anti-OS defense system. The levels of AGER1 are directly correlated with the levels of circulating AGEs in healthy adults, but they are reduced in those with chronically high levels of AGEs, such as found in patients with diabetes.[123,125] Our studies in both human subjects and experimental models show that AGEs and AGE receptors are a part of normal homeostasis.[10,62,102,125] When the levels of AGEs exceed the capacity of the body to detoxify them, they accumulate and raise the levels of OS. If the levels of AGER1 are sufficient, AGER1 actively counteracts this increase and maintains the normal oxidant balance. Elevated levels of AGEs, combined with low AGER1 expression, are a signal that the capacity for removal of AGEs has been exceeded, i.e., in diabetes and chronic kidney disease.[123] The sustained nature of the responses induced by AGEs, coupled with the continued intake of excess dietary oxidants in the Western diet, may constitute the basis for the progressive depletion of innate defenses in diabetes. These changes may include, or be due to, reduced levels of AGER1 (Fig. 20.9). Decreased AGER1 function, allowing AGEs to accumulate, can result in depletion of anti-oxidants and promote high OS. Thus, the maintenance of normal AGER1 levels may be critical to redox homeostasis.

Among the AGE receptors that trigger an inflammatory response, the best known is a multi-ligand protein, RAGE and its variants.[66,81] HMGB1 (amphoterin) has recently been identified as a major RAGE ligand.[60] Activated RAGE leads to the induction of ROS and an inflammatory response.[126–128] RAGE does not participate in AGE removal, but its extracellular domain (sRAGE) is present in circulation. Since, blood levels of sRAGE inversely correlate with the OS state, it has been suggested that sRAGE may bind and assist in clearing AGEs and other oxidants.[129–132] While sRAGE levels have generally been found to be low in diabetic individuals, some have found that they are increased in diabetic patients with coronary vascular disease.[23,82]

Other entities that bind AGEs include AGER2, which is an 80–90 kDa protein possibly involved in early AGE signaling, and AGER3, a 30–35 kDa protein, which may make a contribution to both AGE removal and cell activation.[52,107] AGEs are also bound by ScR-II, CD36, lysozyme and other defensins.[133] While several AGE-receptor gene polymorphisms have been identified, none have been strongly linked to diabetes.[134] Toll-like receptor 4 also binds RAGE ligands (HMGB-1), although it is not known if it also binds AGEs.[60]

Reduction of Exposure to Toxic Oxidants (AGEs) in Humans

Several epidemiologic studies show that a rise in OS among clinically normal subjects may be important in the pathogenesis of insulin resistance and other metabolic diseases.[4,6,7,39,135] We found that the AGE content of regular meals or meals with a low AGE content given to normal subjects is readily reflected in the serum levels of AGEs and in the amount of AGEs excreted in the urine.[66,86,87] In addition, we recently found that serum AGEs correlated with oxidant stress in a cross-sectional study in normal non-diabetic adults of different ages (Fig. 20.10a).[88,125] Those who ate a diet with a low AGE content, had lower levels of markers of inflammation and oxidant stress, i.e., hsCRP, TNFα, and fibrinogen, whereas these levels were much higher in those consuming a diet with a higher AGE content. Of interest, a significant association was noted between serum AGE and HOMA, an indicator of insulin resistance.[88,125,136] The associations between serum AGEs, 8-isoprostane, and HOMA suggest that sAGE may be an important contributor to OS, prior to the onset of diabetes. Hyperglycemia has been assumed to be the source of the increased AGE levels found in diabetes, a condition associated with systemic OS.[3,64] None of the normal subjects in this study were hyperglycemic in the fasting state. Therefore, their higher fasting levels of serum AGE could not be explained on the basis of glycemia. This data provided strong additional evidence that the intake of AGEs in the diet very likely contributes to the increased levels of serum AGEs, and the subsequent increased systemic OS.

These data are consistent with previous observations in patients with diabetes and chronic kidney disease.[47,106] The use of CML-like AGEs as surrogates for other oxidants or carbonyl-rich products in the diet seems justified by the correspondence between the levels of CML-like AGEs in the diet and CML or MG in the circulation, as well as the highly significant correlation ($r=0.7$, $p=0.0001$) between sAGEs and the endogenous lipid peroxidation derivatives, 8-isoprostanes.[125]

Thus, the intake of AGEs contained in the usual adult diet may deliver excessive amounts of AGE oxidants to the body, which may promote cumulative changes in oxidant homeostasis with time. These changes may presage the emergence of metabolic and cardiovascular disturbances, heretofore believed to be part of the normal aging

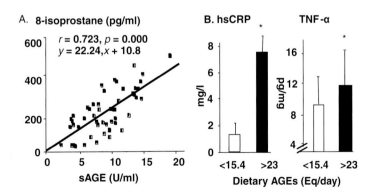

Fig. 20.10   a. Serum AGEs (CML) correlate with plasma lipid peroxidation products (8-isoprostanes) in non-diabetic subjects. **b.** Levels of inflammatory factors, hsCRP and TNFα, are elevated in healthy subjects consuming AGE-rich diets (>23 Eq/d), but not in those consuming a low-AGE diets (<15.4 Eq/d), *$p=0.025$. Note: high-AGE consumers had a BMI >33

process.[4,6–8,35,37,88,137,138] The above data suggest that reduction of the intake of AGEs via the diet may inhibit the accumulation of toxic AGEs, increased oxidant stress, and slow or reduce the emergence of the diabetes and diabetes-related complications. Indeed, a reduced intake of AGEs via the diet in diabetic persons was associated with lowered serum AGEs, OS, and inflammatory markers, e.g., TNFα, hsCRP, and VCAM-1.[see references in 90,102] These findings led to the hypothesis that dietary AGEs, together with those made endogenously, could promote an excessive systemic glycoxidant burden, oxidant stress, and cell activation, all of which would enhance the "vulnerability" of tissues to injury. This is especially true of diabetic patients, since they have elevated levels of AGEs and OS, accompanied by decreased anti-oxidant reserves, at baseline. It is imperative that studies be undertaken in diabetic patients to determine if this approach would also improve diabetic complications.

The Link Between Toxic AGEs and Oxidant Stress (OS)

For the last few decades, the focus has been on the oxidation and glycoxidation products generated by hyperglycemia. Extended studies, including those in type 1 and type 2 diabetes, have lent support to this view, at least in part.[89] However, very recently two other long-term trials raised serious doubts about the utility of strict normalization of glycemic levels in reducing diabetic complications.[1,2] These studies may redirect our thinking to embrace a more diverse realm of controls of risk factors in diabetic patients, perhaps with a focus on OS. It may include prospective on oxidants generated by other mechanisms, including the contribution of dietary AGEs as toxic oxidants. The evidence is increasing that the generation of OS is the basis of many diabetes complications and that it can be lowered by reducing the levels of toxic oxidants from either exogenous or endogenous sources.[64,66,106] The fact that reduction of AGE intake prevents type 1 and type 2 diabetes, as well as diabetic complications in different animal models, noted above corroborates the importance of external sources of AGEs in their pathogenesis and provides a strong impetus for novel clinical interventions.

Diabetes increases the incidence of large vessel diseases such as strokes, myocardial infarction, aortic atherosclerosis, aneurysms, and limb ischemia requiring amputation.[1–4,73] These complications often have catastrophic effects in the short term. Based on the studies in animals discussed above, it is reasonable to postulate that a high dietary intake of toxic AGEs in the usual Western diet may be a major contributor to atherosclerotic lesion severity in the presence of high circulating glucose levels in diabetic patients, an effect that may be preventable by reducing the amount of toxic oxidant AGEs in the diet. Clinical studies to examine this point are now in progress.

Acute Effects of Dietary AGEs in Normal and Diabetic Subjects

After normal subjects are given an AGE-rich meal, the levels of serum AGEs peak within 4–6 h, and return to baseline within 12 h (Fig. 20.11a, solid lines, right panel) and the urinary levels follow.[66] In these individuals, ∼70% of the absorbed oxidants in the diet remain in cells and tissues, and 30% is excreted in the urine.[66] These data point to the unrecognized potential for toxic oxidants from the diet to progressively accumulate over time, particularly in persons consuming a high-AGE diet. As discussed above, even persons who are "normal" in all other aspects can develop high levels of serum AGEs. Importantly, this suggests that the tissue levels of toxic oxidants may progress with time, if the intake remains high.

Since diabetic patients often have long-term elevation of OS and a concomitant decrease in anti-oxidant reserves, it is logical that they would have a decreased ability to deal with a high dietary load of oxidant AGEs. In fact, this is the case as shown by a study of diabetics with either microalbuminuria or overt proteinuria. Long before any clinical or laboratory signs of renal disease are apparent, diabetic patients with microalbuminuria have an impaired ability to excrete the increased load of toxic AGEs presented within the normal diet. Namely, after a high-AGE meal, diabetic patients with microalbuminuria and an estimated GFR in the normal range (Fig. 20.11b, broken line) had sharply increased levels of serum AGEs, and that these levels remained elevated for more than 30 hours. The far smaller peak of AGEs in the urine fell only when the serum AGE levels returned

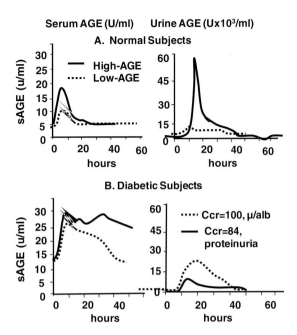

Fig. 20.11 (**a**) Serum and urine AGE kinetics in normal adults after a regular meal (high AGE) or a meal with 50% lower AGEs (low-AGE). (**b**) Diabetic patients with different degrees of diabetic nephropathy were fed the same amount of diet AGEs (regular meal): higher baseline and prolonged elevation of serum AGE levels corresponded to significantly reduced urine AGE levels in those with a lower GFR (*solid lines*). Note, neither group had severe disease but AGE excretion was markedly reduced in both groups

to baseline levels. On the other hand, patients with overt proteinuria, but with only a modestly decreased GFR (20%) (Fig. 20.11b, solid line), had a marked prolongation of the high levels of serum AGEs, while the amount excreted in the urine was significantly decreased. Note that since serum creatinine levels were in the normal range at this level of GFR, these patients would have been considered to have normal renal function by most physicians. Thus, diabetic patients with kidney lesions, as evidenced by albuminuria of any level, appear to have a marked impairment in their ability to handle oxidants presented in the diet. Importantly, this occurs long before physicians generally consider them to have "kidney damage." In addition, these data suggest that the kidney is a major site for the handling of toxic oxidants, and current clinical measures of kidney damage do not accurately measure critical abnormalities in this aspect of kidney function. Since toxic AGEs within the diet directly contribute to elevated OS, and to diabetic complications, the data provided by the studies presented above suggest that it is critical to lower the exposure of patients with diabetes to AGEs within the diet prior to the time they develop clinical evidence of renal disease. This intervention should be in addition to inhibiting the further increase of endogenous AGEs in the body due to elevated OS.

Conclusions

Oxidant stress (OS) is now recognized to be one of the major factors predisposing to diabetic complications. The sources of OS include both the intake of toxic oxidants (AGEs) and their formation intracellularly as part of the hypermetabolic state and other sources of OS. This chapter emphasizes the fact that the intake of toxic oxidants contained in food is a major factor in the pathogenesis of diabetic complications. Furthermore, we show that the amount of toxic oxidants present within the food can be very simply modified by changing the methods by which meals are prepared. The results of decreasing the intake of toxic oxidants by diabetic patients include a decrease in markers of inflammation, vascular injury, and OS. In animals, this is associated with a sharp reduction in the severity of established diabetic complications, the presence of an inflammatory state, vascular injury, insulin resistance, and diabetes. Since reducing the level of toxic oxidants within the diet does not add to health care costs, does not change nutrient intake, and promises to substantially reduce diabetic complications, this intervention should be strongly considered by both physicians and patients in the day-to-day management of diabetic complications.

References

1. Patel A, MacMahon S, Chalmers J, et al. Intensive blood glucose control and vascular outcomes in patients with type 2 diabetes. *N Engl J Med*. 2008;358:2560–2572.
2. Gerstein HC, Miller ME, Byington RP, et al. Effects of intensive glucose lowering in type 2 diabetes. *N Engl J Med*. 2008;358:2545–2559.
3. Abbatecola AM, Ferrucci L, Grella R, et al. Diverse effect of inflammatory markers on insulin resistance and insulin-resistance syndrome in the elderly. *J Am Geriatr Soc*. 2004;52:399–404.
4. de Rekeneire N, Peila R, Ding J, et al. Diabetes, hyperglycemia, and inflammation in older individuals: the health, aging and body composition study. *Diabetes Care*. 2006;29:1902–1908.
5. Zhang L, Zalewski A, Liu Y, et al. Diabetes-induced oxidative stress and low-grade inflammation in porcine coronary arteries. *Circulation*. 2003;108:472–478.
6. Reuben DB, Cheh AI, Harris TB, et al. Peripheral blood markers of inflammation predict mortality and functional decline in high-functioning community-dwelling older persons. *J Am Geriatr Soc*. 2002;50:638–644.
7. Harris TB, Ferrucci L, Tracy RP, et al. Associations of elevated interleukin-6 and C-reactive protein levels with mortality in the elderly. *Am J Med*. 1999;106:506–512.
8. Ershler WB, Ferrucci L, Finch C, et al. Inflammation, inflammatory mediators and aging. In: Sherman RFS, Carrington J, Miller M, Monjan A, eds. *NIA Inflammation and Aging Workshop*. Bethesda, MD: NIH; 2004.
9. Vlassara H, Cai W, Crandall J, et al. Inflammatory mediators are induced by dietary glycotoxins, a major risk factor for diabetic angiopathy. *Proc Natl Acad Sci USA*. 2002;99:15596–15601.
10. Vlassara H, Uribarri J, Cai W, Striker G. Advanced glycation end product homeostasis: exogenous oxidants and innate defenses. *Ann N Y Acad Sci*. 2008;1126:46–52.
11. Cai W, He JC, Zhu L, et al. Oral glycotoxins determine the effects of calorie restriction on oxidant stress, age-related diseases, and lifespan. *Am J Pathol*. 2008;173:327–336.
12. Cai W, He JC, Zhu L, et al. High levels of dietary advanced glycation end products transform low-density lipoprotein into a potent redox-sensitive mitogen-activated protein kinase stimulant in diabetic patients. *Circulation*. 2004;110:285–291.
13. Wolffenbuttel BH, Boulanger CM, Crijns FR, et al. Breakers of advanced glycation end products restore large artery properties in experimental diabetes. *Proc Natl Acad Sci USA*. 1998;95:4630–4634.
14. Williams SB, Cusco JA, Roddy MA, Johnstone MT, Creager MA. Impaired nitric oxide-mediated vasodilation in patients with non-insulin-dependent diabetes mellitus. *J Am Coll Cardiol*. 1996;27:567–574.
15. Williams ME, Bolton WK, Khalifah RG, Degenhardt TP, Schotzinger RJ, McGill JB. Effects of pyridoxamine in combined phase 2 studies of patients with type 1 and type 2 diabetes and overt nephropathy. *Am J Nephrol*. 2007;27:605–614.
16. Waanders F, van den Berg E, Nagai R, van Veen I, Navis G, van Goor H. Renoprotective effects of the AGE-inhibitor pyridoxamine in experimental chronic allograft nephropathy in rats. *Nephrol Dial Transplant*. 2008;23:518–524.
17. Voziyan PA, Hudson BG. Pyridoxamine as a multifunctional pharmaceutical: targeting pathogenic glycation and oxidative damage. *Cell Mol Life Sci*. 2005;62:1671–1681.
18. Thornalley PJ. Use of aminoguanidine (Pimagedine) to prevent the formation of advanced glycation endproducts. *Arch Biochem Biophys*. 2003;419:31–40.
19. Stracke H, Hammes HP, Werkmann D, et al. Efficacy of benfotiamine versus thiamine on function and glycation products of peripheral nerves in diabetic rats. *Exp Clin Endocrinol Diabetes*. 2001;109:330–336.
20. Onorato JM, Jenkins AJ, Thorpe SR, Baynes JW. Pyridoxamine, an inhibitor of advanced glycation reactions, also inhibits advanced lipoxidation reactions. Mechanism of action of pyridoxamine. *J Biol Chem*. 2000;275:21177–21184.
21. Zheng F, Zeng YJ, Plati AR, et al. Combined AGE inhibition and ACEi decreases the progression of established diabetic nephropathy in B6 db/db mice. *Kidney Int*. 2006;70:507–514.
22. Jain SK, Lim G. Pyridoxine and pyridoxamine inhibits superoxide radicals and prevents lipid peroxidation, protein glycosylation, and (Na+ + K+)-ATPase activity reduction in high glucose-treated human erythrocytes. *Free Radic Biol Med*. 2001;30:232–237.
23. Nakamura S, Li H, Adijiang A, Pischetsrieder M, Niwa T. Pyridoxal phosphate prevents progression of diabetic nephropathy. *Nephrol Dial Transplant*. 2007;22:2165–2174.
24. Nagaraj RH, Sarkar P, Mally A, Biemel KM, Lederer MO, Padayatti PS. Effect of pyridoxamine on chemical modification of proteins by carbonyls in diabetic rats: characterization of a major product from the reaction of pyridoxamine and methylglyoxal. *Arch Biochem Biophys*. 2002;402:110–119.

25. Liu H, Zheng F, Uribarri J, et al. Reduced acute vascular injury and atherosclerosis in hyperlipidemic mice transgenic for lysozyme. *Am J Pathol*. 2006;169:303–313.

26. Li YM, Steffes M, Donnelly T, et al. Prevention of cardiovascular and renal pathology of aging by the advanced glycation inhibitor aminoguanidine. *Proc Natl Acad Sci USA*. 1996;93:3902–3907.

27. Kang Z, Li H, Li G, Yin D. Reaction of pyridoxamine with malondialdehyde: mechanism of inhibition of formation of advanced lipoxidation end-products. *Amino Acids*. 2006;30:55–61.

28. Huijberts MS, Wolffenbuttel BH, Boudier HA, et al. Aminoguanidine treatment increases elasticity and decreases fluid filtration of large arteries from diabetic rats. *J Clin Invest*. 1993;92:1407–1411.

29. Degenhardt TP, Alderson NL, Arrington DD, et al. Pyridoxamine inhibits early renal disease and dyslipidemia in the streptozotocin-diabetic rat. *Kidney Int*. 2002;61:939–950.

30. Davies SS, Brantley EJ, Voziyan PA, et al. Pyridoxamine analogues scavenge lipid-derived gamma-ketoaldehydes and protect against H2O2-mediated cytotoxicity. *Biochemistry*. 2006;45:15756–15767.

31. Chetyrkin SV, Zhang W, Hudson BG, Serianni AS, Voziyan PA. Pyridoxamine protects proteins from functional damage by 3-deoxyglucosone: mechanism of action of pyridoxamine. *Biochemistry*. 2008;47:997–1006.

32. He C, Sabol J, Mitsuhashi T, Vlassara H. Dietary glycotoxins: inhibition of reactive products by aminoguanidine facilitates renal clearance and reduces tissue sequestration. *Diabetes*. 1999;48:1308–1315.

33. Booth AA, Khalifah RG, Hudson BG. Thiamine pyrophosphate and pyridoxamine inhibit the formation of antigenic advanced glycation end-products: comparison with aminoguanidine. *Biochem Biophys Res Commun*. 1996;220:113–119.

34. Cerami C, Founds H, Nicholl I, et al. Tobacco smoke is a source of toxic reactive glycation products. *Proc Natl Acad Sci USA*. 1997;94:13915–13920.

35. Stadtman ER. Protein oxidation and aging. *Science*. 1992;257:1220–1224.

36. Smith CD, Carney JM, Tatsumo T, Stadtman ER, Floyd RA, Markesbery WR. Protein oxidation in aging brain. *Ann N Y Acad Sci*. 1992;663:110–119.

37. Martindale JL, Holbrook NJ. Cellular response to oxidative stress: signaling for suicide and survival. *J Cell Physiol*. 2002;192:1–15.

38. Finkel TH, Holbrook NJ. Oxidants, oxidative stress and the biology of ageing. *Nature*. 2000;408:239–247.

39. Cappola AR, Xue QL, Ferrucci L, Guralnik JM, Volpato S, Fried LP. Insulin-like growth factor I and interleukin-6 contribute synergistically to disability and mortality in older women. *J Clin Endocrinol Metab*. 2003;88:2019–2025.

40. Sobenin IA, Tertov VV, Koschinsky T, et al. Modified low density lipoprotein from diabetic patients causes cholesterol accumulation in human intimal aortic cells. *Atherosclerosis*. 1993;100:41–54.

41. Requena JR, Ahmed MU, Fountain CW, et al. Carboxymethylethanolamine, a biomarker of phospholipid modification during the maillard reaction in vivo. *J Biol Chem*. 1997;272:17473–17479.

42. Menini S, Amadio L, Oddi G, et al. Deletion of p66Shc longevity gene protects against experimental diabetic glomerulopathy by preventing diabetes-induced oxidative stress. *Diabetes*. 2006;55:1642–1650.

43. Masoro EJ. Overview of caloric restriction and ageing. *Mech Ageing Dev*. 2005;126:913–922.

44. Cai W, Gao QD, Zhu L, Peppa M, He C, Vlassara H. Oxidative stress-inducing carbonyl compounds from common foods: novel mediators of cellular dysfunction. *Mol Med*. 2002;8:337–346.

45. Bucala R, Makita Z, Vega G, et al. Modification of low density lipoprotein by advanced glycation end products contributes to the dyslipidemia of diabetes and renal insufficiency. *Proc Natl Acad Sci USA*. 1994;91:9441–9445.

46. Bucala R, Makita Z, Koschinsky T, Cerami A, Vlassara H. Lipid advanced glycosylation: pathway for lipid oxidation in vivo. *Proc Natl Acad Sci USA*. 1993;90:6434–6438.

47. Uribarri J, Peppa M, Cai W, et al. Dietary glycotoxins correlate with circulating advanced glycation end product levels in renal failure patients. *Am J Kidney Dis*. 2003;42:532–538.

48. Sandu O, Song K, Cai W, Zheng F, Uribarri J, Vlassara H. Insulin resistance and type 2 diabetes in high-fat-fed mice are linked to high glycotoxin intake. *Diabetes*. 2005;54:2314–2319.

49. Bechmann J. Extensive nitration of protein tyrosines in human atherosclerosis detected by immunohistochemistry. *Biol Chem Hoppe Seyler*. 1994;375:81–88.

50. Hamada Y, Araki N, Koh N, Nakamura J, Horiuchi S, Hotta N. Rapid formation of advanced glycation end products by intermediate metabolites of glycolytic pathway and polyol pathway. *Biochem Biophys Res Commun*. 1996;228:539–543.

51. Henle T. A food chemists view of advanced glycation end-products. *Perit Dial Int*. 2001;21:S125–S130.

52. Li YM, Mitsuhashi T, Wojciechowicz D, et al. Molecular identity and cellular distribution of advanced glycation endproduct receptors: relationship of p60 to OST-48 and p90 to 80 K-H membrane proteins. *Proc Natl Acad Sci USA*. 1996;93:11047–11052.

53. Thornalley PJ. Pharmacology of methylglyoxal: formation, modification of proteins and nucleic acids, and enzymatic detoxification--a role in pathogenesis and antiproliferative chemotherapy. *Gen Pharmacol*. 1996;27:565–573.

54. Requena JR, Baynes JW. Studies in animal models on the role of glycation and advanced glycation end-products (AGEs) in the pathogenesis of diabetic complications: pitfalls and limitations. In: Sima AAF, ed. *Lessons From Animal Models of Diabetes*. Vol VII. Boston, MA: Birkhauser; 2001.

55. Lu C, He JC, Cai W, Liu H, Zhu L, Vlassara H. Advanced glycation endproduct (AGE) receptor 1 is a negative regulator of the inflammatory response to AGE in mesangial cells. *Proc Natl Acad Sci USA*. 2004;101:11767–11772.

56. Inoguchi T, Li P, Umeda F, et al. High glucose level and free fatty acid stimulate reactive oxygen species production through protein kinase C – dependent activation of NAD(P)H oxidase in cultured vascular cells. *Diabetes*. 2000;49: 1939–1945.

57. Cai W, He JC, Zhu L, Lu C, Vlassara H. Advanced glycation end product (AGE) receptor 1 suppresses cell oxidant stress and activation signaling via EGF receptor. *Proc Natl Acad Sci USA*. 2006;103:13801–13806.

58. Black PH. The inflammatory response is an integral part of the stress response: Implications for atherosclerosis, insulin resistance, type II diabetes and metabolic syndrome X. *Brain Behav Immun*. 2003;17:350–364.

59. Anderson MM, Heinecke JW. Production of N(epsilon)-(carboxymethyl)lysine is impaired in mice deficient in NADPH oxidase: a role for phagocyte-derived oxidants in the formation of advanced glycation end products during inflammation. *Diabetes*. 2003;52:2137–2143.

60. van Beijnum JR, Buurman WA, Griffioen AW. Convergence and amplification of toll-like receptor (TLR) and receptor for advanced glycation end products (RAGE) signaling pathways via high mobility group B1 (HMGB1). *Angiogenesis*. 2008;11:91–99.

61. Kagan JC, Su T, Horng T, Chow A, Akira S, Medzhitov R. TRAM couples endocytosis of Toll-like receptor 4 to the induction of interferon-beta. *Nat Immunol*. 2008;9:361–368.

62. Dougan M, Dranoff G. Inciting inflammation: the RAGE about tumor promotion. *J Exp Med*. 2008;205:267–270.

63. Negrean M, Stirban A, Stratmann B, et al. Effects of low- and high-advanced glycation endproduct meals on macro- and microvascular endothelial function and oxidative stress in patients with type 2 diabetes mellitus. *Am J Clin Nutr*. 2007;85:1236–1243.

64. Brownlee M. Biochemistry and molecular cell biology of diabetic complications. *Nature*. 2001;414:813–820.

65. Goldberg T, Cai W, Peppa M, et al. Advanced glycoxidation end products in commonly consumed foods. *J Am Diet Assoc*. 2004;104:1287–1291.

66. Koschinsky T, He CJ, Mitsuhashi T, et al. Orally absorbed reactive glycation products (glycotoxins): an environmental risk factor in diabetic nephropathy. *Proc Natl Acad Sci USA*. 1997;94:6474–6479.

67. Lin RY, Choudhury RP, Cai W, et al. Dietary glycotoxins promote diabetic atherosclerosis in apolipoprotein E-deficient mice. *Atherosclerosis*. 2003;168:213–220.

68. Zheng F, He C, Cai W, Hattori M, Steffes M, Vlassara H. Prevention of diabetic nephropathy in mice by a diet low in glycoxidation products. *Diabetes Metab Res Rev*. 2002;18:224–237.

69. Shinohara M, Thornalley PJ, Giardino I, et al. Overexpression of glyoxalase-I in bovine endothelial cells inhibits intracellular advanced glycation endproduct formation and prevents hyperglycemia-induced increases in macromolecular endocytosis. *J Clin Invest*. 1998;101:1142–1147.

70. Basta G, Schmidt AM, De Caterina R. Advanced glycation end products and vascular inflammation: implications for accelerated atherosclerosis in diabetes. *Cardiovasc Res*. 2004;63:582–592.

71. Monnier VM, Sell DR, Nagaraj RH, et al. Maillard reaction-mediated molecular damage to extracellular matrix and other tissue proteins in diabetes, aging, and uremia. *Diabetes*. 1992;41(Suppl 2):36–41.

72. Sell DR, Monnier VM. End-stage renal disease and diabetes catalyze the formation of a pentose-derived crosslink from aging human collagen. *J Clin Invest*. 1990;85:380–384.

73. Berg TJ, Snorgaard O, Faber J, et al. Serum levels of advanced glycation end products are associated with left ventricular diastolic function in patients with type 1 diabetes. *Diabetes Care*. 1999;22:1186–1190.

74. McCance DR, Dyer DG, Dunn JA, et al. Maillard reaction products and their relation to complications in insulin-dependent diabetes mellitus. *J Clin Invest*. 1993;91:2470–2478.

75. Peppa M, Brem H, Ehrlich P, et al. Adverse effects of dietary glycotoxins on wound healing in genetically diabetic mice. *Diabetes*. 2003;52:2805–2813.

76. Peppa M, Uribarri J, Vlassara H:. Advanced glycoxidation. A new risk factor for cardiovascular disease?. *Cardiovasc Toxicol*. 2002;2:275–287.

77. Shamshi FA, Partal A, Sady C, Glomb MA, Nagaraj RH. Immunological evidence for methylglyoxal-derived modifications in vivo: determination of antigenic epitopes. *J Biol Chem*. 1998;273:6928–6936.

78. Lin RY, Reis ED, Dore AT, et al. Lowering of dietary advanced glycation endproducts (AGE) reduces neointimal formation after arterial injury in genetically hypercholesterolemic mice. *Atherosclerosis*. 2002;163:303–311.

79. Klein RL, Laimins M, Lopes-Virella MF. Isolation, characterization, and metabolism of the glycated and nonglycated subfractions of low-density lipoproteins isolated from type I diabetic patients and nondiabetic subjects. *Diabetes*. 1995;44: 1093–1098.

80. Linden E, Cai W, He JC, et al. Endothelial dysfunction in patients with chronic kidney disease results from advanced glycation end products (AGE)-mediated inhibition of endothelial nitric oxide synthase through RAGE activation. *Clin J Am Soc Nephrol*. 2008;3:691–698.

81. Gao X, Zhang H, Schmidt AM, Zhang C. AGE/RAGE Produces Endothelial Dysfunction in Coronary Arterioles in Type II Diabetic Mice. *Am J Physiol Heart Circ Physiol*. 2008;295:H491–H498.

82. Nakamura K, Yamagishi S, Adachi H, et al. Elevation of soluble form of receptor for advanced glycation end products (sRAGE) in diabetic subjects with coronary artery disease. *Diabetes Metab Res Rev*. 2007;23:368–371.

83. Peppa M, Uribarri J, Vlassara H. The role of advanced glycation end products in the development of atherosclerosis. *Curr Diab Rep*. 2004;4:31–36.

84. Stirban A, Negrean M, Stratmann B, et al. Benfotiamine prevents macro- and microvascular endothelial dysfunction and oxidative stress following a meal rich in advanced glycation end products in individuals with type 2 diabetes. *Diabetes Care.* 2006;29:2064–2071.

85. Stirban A, Negrean M, Gotting C, et al. Dietary advanced glycation endproducts and oxidative stress: in vivo effects on endothelial function and adipokines. *Ann N Y Acad Sci.* 2008;1126:276–279.

86. Thorpe SR, Baynes JW. Role of the Maillard reaction in diabetes mellitus and diseases of aging. *Drugs Aging.* 1996;9: 69–77.

87. Uribarri J, Stirban A, Sander D, et al. Single oral challenge by advanced glycation end products acutely impairs endothelial function in diabetic and nondiabetic subjects. *Diabetes Care.* 2007;30:2579–2582.

88. Vlassara H, Cai W, Goodman S, et al. Protection against loss of innate defenses in adulthood by low AGE intake; role of a new anti-inflammatory AGE-Receptor-1. *J Clin Endocrinol Metab.* 2009;94:4483–4491.

89. Sell DR, Lapolla A, Odetti P, Fogarty J, Monnier VM. Pentosidine formation in skin correlates with severity of complications in individuals with long-standing IDDM. *Diabetes.* 1992;41:1286–1292.

90. Huebschmann AG, Regensteiner JG, Vlassara H, Reusch JE. Diabetes and advanced glycoxidation end products. *Diabetes Care.* 2006;29:1420–1432.

91. Tan D, Wang Y, Lo CY, Sang S, Ho CT. Methylglyoxal: its presence in beverages and potential scavengers. *Ann N Y Acad Sci.* 2008;1126:72–75.

92. Baynes JW. Role of oxidative stress in development of complications in diabetes. *Diabetes.* 1991;40:405–412.

93. Baynes JW, Thorpe SR. Role of oxidative stress in diabetic complications: a new perspective on an old paradigm. *Diabetes.* 1999;48:1–9.

94. O'Brien J. Nutritional and toxicological aspects of the Maillard browning reaction in foods. *Crit Rev Food Sci Nutr.* 1989;28:211–248.

95. Lee TC, Kimiagar M, Pintauro SJ, Chichester CO. Physiological and safety aspects of Maillard browning of foods. *Prog Food Nutr Sci.* 1981;5:243–256.

96. Pouillart P, Mauprivez H, Ait-Ameur L, et al. Strategy for the study of the health impact of dietary Maillard products in clinical studies: the example of the ICARE clinical study on healthy adults. *Ann N Y Acad Sci.* 2008;1126:173–176.

97. Yang CW, Vlassara H, Peten EP, He CJ, Striker GE, Striker LJ. Advanced glycation end products up-regulate gene expression found in diabetic glomerular disease. *Proc Natl Acad Sci USA.* 1994;91:9436–9440.

98. Peppa M, He C, Hattori M, McEvoy R, Zheng F, Vlassara H. Fetal or neonatal low-glycotoxin environment prevents autoimmune diabetes in NOD mice. *Diabetes.* 2003;52:1441–1448.

99. Vlassara H, Striker LJ, Teichberg S, Fuh H, Li YM, Steffes M. Advanced glycation end products induce glomerular sclerosis and albuminuria in normal rats. *Proc Natl Acad Sci USA.* 1994;91:11704–11708.

100. Vlassara H, Bucala R, Striker L. Pathogenic effects of advanced glycosylation: biochemical, biologic, and clinical implications for diabetes and aging. *Lab Invest.* 1994;70:138–151.

101. Booth AA, Khalifah RG, Todd P, Hudson BG. In vitro kinetic studies of formation of antigenic advanced glycation end products (AGEs). Novel inhibition of post-Amadori glycation pathways. *J Biol Chem.* 1997;272:5430–5437.

102. Vlassara H, Striker G. Glycotoxins in the diet promote diabetes and diabetic complications. *Curr Diab Rep.* 2007;7:235–241.

103. Birlouez-Aragon I, Pischetsrieder M, Leclere J, et al. Assessment of protein glycation markers in infant formulas. *Food Chem.* 2004;87:253–259.

104. Sugiyama S, Miyata T, Horie K, et al. Advanced glycation end-products in diabetic nephropathy. *Nephrol Dial Transplant.* 1996;11(Suppl 5):91–94.

105. Sebekova K, Faist V, Hofmann T, Schinzel R, Heidland A. Effects of a diet rich in advanced glycation end products in the rat remnant kidney model. *Am J Kidney Dis.* 2003;41:S48–S51.

106. Uribarri J, Peppa M, Cai W, et al. Restriction of dietary glycotoxins reduces excessive advanced glycation end products in renal failure patients. *J Am Soc Nephrol.* 2003;14:728–731.

107. He C, Zheng F, Sabol J, et al. Differential expression of renal AGE-receptor genes in NOD mouse kidneys: possible role in non-obese diabetic renal disease. *Kidney Int.* 2000;58:1931–1940.

108. Cai W, He JC, Zhu L, et al. Reduced oxidant stress and extended lifespan in mice exposed to a low glycotoxin diet: association with increased AGER1 expression. *Am J Pathol.* 2007;170:1893–1902.

109. Cai W, He JC, Zhu L, Chen X, Striker GE, Vlassara H. AGE-receptor-1 counteracts cellular oxidant stress induced by AGEs via negative regulation of p66shc-dependent FKHRL1 phosphorylation. *Am J Physiol Cell Physiol.* 2008;294: C145–C152.

110. Mattson MP, Wan R. Beneficial effects of intermittent fasting and caloric restriction on the cardiovascular and cerebrovascular systems. *Nutr Biochem.* 2005;16:129–137.

111. Spindler SR, Dhahbi JM. Conserved and tissue-specific genic and physiologic responses to caloric restriction and altered IGFI signaling in mitotic and postmitotic tissues. *Annu Rev Nutr.* 2007;27:193–217.

112. Zimmerman JA, Malloy V, Krajcik R, Orentreich N. Nutritional control of aging. *Exp Gerontol.* 2003;38:47–52.

113. Peppa M, Uribarri J, Vlassara H. Aging and glycoxidant stress. *Hormones (Athens).* 2008;7:123–132.

114. Chou SM, Han CY, Wang HS, Vlassara H, Bucala R. A receptor for advanced glycosylation endproducts (AGEs) is colocalized with neurofilament-bound AGEs and SOD1 in motoneurons of ALS: immunohistochemical study. *J Neurosci.* 1999;169: 87–92.

115. Fosmark DS, Torjesen PA, Kilhovd BK, et al. Increased serum levels of the specific advanced glycation end product methylglyoxal-derived hydroimidazolone are associated with retinopathy in patients with type 2 diabetes mellitus. *Metabolism*. 2006;55:232–236.

116. Makita Z, Radoff S, Rayfield EJ, et al. Advanced glycosylation end products in patients with diabetic nephropathy. *N Engl J Med*. 1991;325:836–842.

117. Murata T, Nagai R, Ishibashi T, Inomuta H, Ikeda K, Horiuchi S. The relationship between accumulation of advanced glycation end products and expression of vascular endothelial growth factor in human diabetic retinas. *Diabetologia*. 1997;40:764–769.

118. Stitt AW, Moore JE, Sharkey JA, et al. Advanced glycation end products in vitreous: Structural and functional implications for diabetic vitreopathy. *Invest Ophthalmol Vis Sci*. 1998;39:2517–2523.

119. Boehm BO, Schilling S, Rosinger S, et al. Elevated serum levels of N(epsilon)-carboxymethyl-lysine, an advanced glycation end product, are associated with proliferative diabetic retinopathy and macular oedema. *Diabetologia*. 2004;47:1376–1379.

120. Zeiher AM, Fisslthaler B, Schray-Utz B, Busse R. Nitric oxide modulates the expression of monocyte chemoattractant protein 1 in cultured human endothelial cells. *Circ Res*. 1995;76:980–986.

121. Yao D, Taguchi T, Matsumura T, et al. High glucose increases angiopoietin-2 transcription in microvascular endothelial cells through methylglyoxal modification of mSin3A. *J Biol Chem*. 2007;282:31038–31045.

122. Quehenberger P, Bierhaus A, Fasching P, et al. Endothelin 1 transcription is controlled by nuclear factor-kappaB in AGE-stimulated cultured endothelial cells. *Diabetes*. 2000;49:1561–1570.

123. He CJ, Koschinsky T, Buenting C, Vlassara H. Presence of diabetic complications in type 1 diabetic patients correlates with low expression of mononuclear cell AGE-receptor-1 and elevated serum AGE. *Mol Med*. 2001;7:159–168.

124. Skolnik EY, Yang Z, Makita Z, Radoff S, Kirstein M, Vlassara H. Human and rat mesangial cell receptors for glucose-modified proteins: potential role in kidney tissue remodelling and diabetic nephropathy. *J Exp Med*. 1991;174:931–939.

125. Uribarri J, Cai W, Peppa M, et al. Circulating glycotoxins and dietary advanced glycation endproducts: two links to inflammatory response, oxidative stress, and aging. *J Gerontol A Biol Sci Med Sci*. 2007;62:427–433.

126. Galichet A, Weibel M, Heizmann CW. Calcium-regulated intramembrane proteolysis of the RAGE receptor. *Biochem Biophys Res Commun*. 2008;370:1–5.

127. Schmidt AM, Hori O, Brett J, Yan SD, Wautier JL, Stern D. Cellular receptors for advanced glycation end products. Implications for induction of oxidant stress and cellular dysfunction in the pathogenesis of vascular lesions. *Arterioscler Thromb*. 1994;14:1521–1528.

128. Schmidt AM, Yan SD, Yan SF, Stern DM. The biology of the receptor for advanced glycation end products and its ligands. *Biochim Biophys Acta*. 2000;1498:99–111.

129. Nakamura K, Yamagishi S, Adachi H, et al. Serum levels of soluble form of receptor for advanced glycation end products (sRAGE) are positively associated with circulating AGEs and soluble form of VCAM-1 in patients with type 2 diabetes. *Microvasc Res*. 2008;76:52–56.

130. Basta G, Sironi AM, Lazzerini G, et al. Circulating soluble receptor for advanced glycation end products is inversely associated with glycemic control and S100A12 protein. *J Clin Endocrinol Metab*. 2006;91:4628–4634.

131. Emanuele E, D'Angelo A, Tomaino C, et al. Circulating levels of soluble receptor for advanced glycation end products in Alzheimer disease and vascular dementia. *Arch Neurol*. 2005;62:1734–1736.

132. Gohda T, Tanimoto M, Moon JY, et al. Increased serum endogenous secretory receptor for advanced glycation end-product (esRAGE) levels in type 2 diabetic patients with decreased renal function. *Diabetes Res Clin Pract*. 2008;81:196–201.

133. Li YM, Tan AX, Vlassara H. Antibacterial activity of lysozyme and lactoferrin is inhibited by binding of advanced glycation-modified proteins to a conserved motif. *Nat Med*. 1995;1:1057–1061.

134. Poirier O, Nicaud V, Vionnet N, et al. Polymorphism screening of four genes encoding advanced glycation end-product putative receptors. Association study with nephropathy in type 1 diabetic patients. *Diabetes*. 2001;50:1214–1218.

135. Ershler WB. Biological interactions of aging and anemia: a focus on cytokines. *J Am Geriatr Soc*. 2003;51:S18–S21.

136. Matthews DR, Hosker JP, Rudenski AS, Naylor BA, Treacher DF, Turner RC. Homeostasis model assessment: insulin resistance and beta-cell function from fasting plasma glucose and insulin concentrations in man. *Diabetologia*. 1985;28:412–419.

137. Bokov A, Chaudhuri A, Richardson A. The role of oxidative damage and stress in aging. *Mech Ageing Dev*. 2004;125:811–826.

138. Peppa M, Uribarri J, Cai W, Lu M, Vlassara H. Glycoxidation and inflammation in renal failure patients. *Am J Kidney Dis*. 2004;43:690–695.

Chapter 21
Diabetic Retinopathy

Ketan Laud and Uri Shabto

Epidemiology

Diabetes mellitus (DM) is a major medical problem in the United States and worldwide. The disease has tremendous social and economic impact as it affects individuals in their economic productive years. It is estimated that societal costs related to the disease exceed a 100 billion dollars per year.[1] Diabetes remains a leading cause of newly diagnosed blindness in the United States and worldwide today.

The prevalence of diabetes in the United States and worldwide is clearly increasing due to various environmental and behavioral factors.[2,3] Ten to fifteen percent of patients with diabetes have type 1 diabetes mellitus and are typically diagnosed prior to 40 years of age. The vast majority of patients are diagnosed after the age of 40 and have type 2 diabetes. Both type 1 and type 2 diabetes patients can develop ocular complications of diabetes, although patients with type 2 diabetes make up the majority of cases due to the larger patient population. The ocular manifestations for both groups are similar however, over a long-term follow-up period.

Roy et al. utilized prevalence data to estimate the prevalence of diabetic retinopathy by age, gender, and race among persons of 18 years and older having type 1 DM diagnosed before 30 years of age.[4] It was determined that among 209 million Americans of 18 years and older, an estimated 889,000 have type 1 diabetes mellitus diagnosed before age 30 years. Among persons with type 1 diabetes mellitus, the crude prevalences of diabetic retinopathy of any level (74.9% vs. 82.3% in black and white persons, respectively) and of vision-threatening retinopathy (30.0% vs. 32.2%, respectively) are high.[4] In another study,[5] pooled analysis of data from eight population-based eye surveys was used to estimate the prevalence of diabetic retinopathy among adults 40 years of age and older in the United States. Among an estimated 10.2 million adults of 40 years and older included in the study, the estimated crude prevalence rates for retinopathy and vision-threatening retinopathy were 40.3 and 8.2%, respectively. The estimated US general population prevalence rates for retinopathy and vision-threatening retinopathy were 3.4% (4.1 million persons) and 0.75% (899,000 persons).[5]

It is important to note that the prevalence of diabetic retinopathy in the general population has been increasing and is related to the increase in patients' life expectancy due to better overall health care and treatment of comorbidities. Fortunately, advances in the treatment of diabetic retinopathy have allowed for improved prognosis and maintenance of visual potential in these patients.

Risk Factors of Diabetic Retinopathy

Duration of Diabetes

The single best predictor of diabetic retinopathy is the duration of the disease.[21–28] Among younger-onset patients with diabetes, the prevalence of any retinopathy was 8% at 3 years, 25% at 5 years, 60% at 10 years,

U. Shabto (✉)

Department of Ophthalmology, The New York Eye and Ear Infirmary, New York, NY, USA

e-mail: redvit@aol.com

L. Poretsky (ed.), *Principles of Diabetes Mellitus*, DOI 10.1007/978-0-387-09841-8_21,
© Springer Science+Business Media, LLC 2010

and 80% at 15 years. The prevalence of proliferative diabetic retinopathy (PDR) was 0% at 3 years and increased to 25% at 15 years.[2] The incidence of retinopathy also increased with increasing duration. The incidence of developing proliferative retinopathy in the younger-onset group increased from 0% in the first 5 years to 27.9% in 13–14 years of diabetes.[2]

Determining the role of duration of diabetes as a predictor of retinopathy in type 2 diabetes mellitus is more challenging because of the uncertainty of the time of onset and therefore duration in many patients. In a well-established study, Yanko et al.[6] found that the prevalence of nonproliferative retinopathy was 23% after 11–13 years of the onset of disease and increased to 60% after 16 or more years. Klein found that 10 years after the diagnosis of type 2 diabetes, 67% of patients had retinopathy and 10% had PDR. The risk was determined to be lowest in patients not requiring insulin.[7]

Glycemic Control

The effect of intensive glycemic control on the development of diabetic retinopathy was addressed by the Diabetes Control and Complications Trial (DCCT),[7,8] involving 1,441 patients with type 1 diabetes across 29 medical centers in the United States and Canada. The DCCT enrolled patients with insulin-dependent diabetes mellitus with minimal (secondary progression cohort) or no (primary prevention cohort) evidence of diabetic retinopathy. Patients were assigned either to conventional treatment (one or two daily injections of insulin) or to intensive diabetes management with three or more daily insulin injections or a continuous subcutaneous insulin infusion.

The DCCT demonstrated that intensive therapy reduced clinically relevant diabetic retinopathy. In the primary-prevention cohort, intensive therapy reduced the adjusted mean risk for the development of retinopathy by 76% as compared with conventional therapy. In the secondary-intervention cohort, intensive therapy slowed the progression of retinopathy by 54% and reduced the development of proliferative or severe nonproliferative retinopathy by 47%. In addition, intensive therapy reduced the occurrence of microalbuminuria, albuminuria, and that of clinical neuropathy in both cohorts.[7,8]

The United Kingdom Prospective Diabetes Study (UKPDS)[9] was a randomized, controlled clinical trial investigating the protective effects of glycemic control in newly diagnosed type 2 diabetics. Patients were randomly assigned to intensive glycemic control with oral agents or insulin or to conventional control with diet. The study demonstrated that improved blood glucose control reduced the risk of developing retinopathy, nephropathy, and possibly neuropathy. The overall rate of microvascular complications was decreased by 25% in patients receiving intensive therapy versus conventional therapy.[10]

Systemic Hypertension

The UKPDS also evaluated the effect of blood pressure control on the progression of diabetic retinopathy. With a median follow-up of 8.4 years, patients assigned to tight blood pressure control had a 34% reduction in progression of retinopathy and a 47% reduced risk of deterioration in visual acuity of three lines associated with a 10 mmHg reduction in systolic blood pressure.[11]

The EURODIAB Controlled Trial of Lisinopril in insulin-dependent diabetes (EUCLID) study group investigated the effect of lisinopril on retinopathy in type 1 diabetes. The study showed a statistically significant 50% reduction in the progression of retinopathy in those taking lisinopril over a 2-year period compared to those not on blood pressure medication, after the adjustment of glycemic control. The results of this study, however, are tempered by the small sample size of the study.

Currently the utility of specific antihypertensive agents in preventing the incidence and progression of diabetic retinopathy cannot be addressed and further investigation will be required.

Dyslipidemia

Elevated serum lipids have been associated with the occurrence and progression of diabetic ocular disease. According to the Early Treatment Diabetic Retinopathy Study (ETDRS), elevated triglycerides, low-density lipoproteins, and very low-density lipoproteins are related to an increased risk for the macular hard exudates that are associated with macular edema.[12] Independent of this association with macular edema, these exudates are associated with an increased risk for vision loss. Increased triglycerides also carry an increased risk for progression of retinopathy.

Pregnancy

Pregnancy is considered a risk factor for the progression of retinopathy. In one study of type 1 diabetes, 7.3% of pregnant women compared with only 3.7% of woman who were not pregnant progressed to proliferative retinopathy.[13] The risk of progression, however, is low for pregnant women who have had type 1 diabetes for less than 10 years or who have mild retinopathy.[14]

Pathophysiology of Diabetic Retinopathy

The precise mechanism resulting in diabetic retinopathy remains unknown. Several metabolic pathways have been implicated in the pathogenesis of diabetic retinopathy including protein kinase C activation, polyol accumulation, and vasoproliferative factors. The net result of these pathways is compromise of the retinal capillaries resulting in their functional incompetence.

Polyol Pathway

Polyol accumulation is linked to the pathogenesis of diabetic retinopathy. Polyol pathway is a two-step pathway in which glucose is initially converted to sorbitol and then to fructose. Experimental animal models have demonstrated that the accumulation of polyol has been associated with the development of basement membrane thickening, pericyte loss, and microaneurysm formation.[15,16] Hyperglycemia leads to an elevation of intracellular sorbitol concentrations by utilization of aldose reductase, the first and rate-limiting enzyme in the polyol pathway. Accumulation of sorbitol causes an osmotic shift, drawing water into lens epithelial cells and producing cataracts in children.[17] Retinal capillary pericytes contain the enzyme aldose reductase, and the accumulation of excess sugar alcohol, catalyzed by aldose reductase in pericytes, has been linked to their degeneration and selective death.[18,19] The efficacy of aldose reductase inhibitors (ARIs) has been evaluated for the prevention of retinal damage in diabetes. The results of several clinical trials, however, have not shown this class of medications to be useful in the management of the development or progression of diabetic retinopathy.[20,21]

Protein Kinase C Activation

Protein kinase C (PKC) is a family of related enzymes that function as signaling components for a variety of growth factors, hormones, neurotransmitters, and cytokines. PKC activation, specifically of the PKC β2-isoform, has been implicated in causing hyperglycemia-related microvascular damage.[22] Changes in endothelial permeability, blood flow, and formation of angiogenic growth factors have been shown to be PKC mediated in experimental models of diabetic retinopathy and result in retinal leakage, ischemia, and neovascularization.[23,24] PKC-β has been shown to be an integral component of cellular signaling by vascular endothelial growth factor (VEGF), an important mediator of retinal neovascularization and vascular permeability.[25,26,27]

PKC activation occurs with its binding to diacylglycerol (DAG) in the presence of calcium. Studies have demonstrated that the hyperglycemia of diabetes induces an early activation of PKC through de novo synthesis of DAG. Other factors including reactive oxygen species, advanced glycation end products, and oxidative stress are associated with DAG-independent activation of PKC.[28] Theoretically, PKC inactivation should suppress the stimuli for the inception and progression of diabetic retinopathy and macular edema. Clinical studies have shown that ruboxistaurin, a PKC-beta isoform selective inhibitor, normalized endothelial dysfunction, renal glomerular filtration rate, and prevented loss of visual acuity in diabetic patients.[29,30] Thus, PKC activation involving several isoforms is likely to be responsible for some aspects of the pathogenesis of diabetic retinopathy, nephropathy, and cardiovascular disease. Ongoing prospective clinical trials investigate whether the treatment with the specific PKC-beta inhibitor can prevent the progression of diabetic retinopathy and diabetic macular edema.

Growth Factors

PKC activation results in increased production of vasoconstrictive, angiogenic, and chemotactic growth factors including TGF-beta, vascular endothelial growth factor (VEGF), growth hormone, insulin-like growth factor I (IGF-I), transforming growth factor-β (TGF-β), and pigment epithelium-derived growth factor (PEDF).

Vascular endothelial growth factor (VEGF) is an important signaling protein involved in vasculogenesis and angiogenesis. In vitro VEGF stimulates endothelial cell mitogenesis and cell migration. In addition, VEGF functions as a vasodilator and increases microvascular permeability. Its expression has been shown to be induced by hypoxia in both retinal pigment epithelial cells and retinal pericytes.[31,32,33] In an animal model, retinal neovascularization was suppressed utilizing soluble VEGF-neutralizing VEGF receptor chimera.

Aiello et al.[34] demonstrated the role of VEGF in the ocular ischemic neovascular response in proliferative diabetic retinopathy, ischemic central retinal vein occlusion, and retinopathy of prematurity. The authors measured intraocular VEGF concentrations of 164 patients undergoing intraocular surgery. They compared VEGF levels in patients with active neovascularization, quiescent neovascularization, and those without any underlying neovascular disorder. VEGF concentrations were highest in the subset of patients with active neovascularization. In addition, comparison of VEGF levels in vitreous humor to that found in the aqueous humor led them to suggest a gradient-driven diffusion of angiogenic factors from the posterior to the anterior segment of the eye in patients with ischemic retinal diseases. They also determined that treatment with panretinal photocoagulation caused regression of retinal neovascularization which coincided with lower VEGF levels.[34] The reduction in retinal ischemia after laser therapy, therefore reduces the production of angiogenic factors, suppressing neovascularization through suppression of VEGF.

Growth hormone and IGF-I have been associated with the development of diabetic retinopathy since retinal neovascularization was found to regress following pituitary infarction.[35] IGF-I was one of the first growth factors to be directly associated with diabetic retinopathy because increased serum levels of IGF-I preceded the onset of proliferative diabetic retinopathy in animal models.[36,37] Since then, increased IGF-I levels were measured in the vitreous of patients with PDR indicating that IGF-I may play a role in retinal neovascularization.[38] Clinical trials are underway to determine the significance of IGF-I in the development of diabetic retinopathy.

TGF-β is a multifunctional growth factor that can cause an accumulation of extracellular matrix. There are three known isoforms of TGF-β (TGF-β_1, TGF-β_2, and TGF-β_3) in the human eye although TGF-β_2 is the predominant isoform in the vitreous humor. There have been several reports of the action of TGF-β_2 in the vitreous. Connor et al.[39] found that TGF-β_2 levels were increased in proliferative vitreoretinopathy. Levels of TGF-β_2 in the vitreous were correlated with the severity of fibrosis suggesting that TGF-β_2 had a role in the formation of proliferating membranes in this disorder. Hirase et al.[40] determined that levels of TGF-β_2 were increased in the vitreous of patients with PDR. In addition, there was also a direct correlation between intraocular fibrosis and TGF-β_2 levels, suggesting that TGF-β_2 plays a role in the pathogenesis of PDR by inducing the formation of proliferating membranes via its interaction with the extracellular matrix.

PEDF is produced by the retinal pigment epithelium and serves as a major inhibitor of intraocular angiogenesis. The vitreous humor which is antiangiogenic and generally devoid of vessels, contains high concentrations of PEDF.[41] Dawson et al.[42] found that removal of PEDF from vitreous fluid abrogated its antiangiogenic activity and revealed an underlying angiogenic stimulatory activity. PEDF regulates blood vessel growth in the eye by altering its levels to the oxygen needs of the eye thereby creating a permissive or inhibitory environment for angiogenesis. This process presumably occurs with regulation of VEGF levels.

Breakdown of Blood–Retinal Barrier

The blood–retinal barrier plays an important part in the pathophysiology of diabetic retinopathy. The blood–retinal barrier is composed of an inner and an outer component. The inner blood–retinal barrier is comprised of the tight junctions between endothelial cells of the retinal blood vessels. A competent inner blood–retinal barrier normally blocks the movement of macromolecules from the vessel lumen to the interstitial space. The outer blood–retinal barrier is comprised of the tight junctions of the retinal pigment epithelial cells (RPE) preventing leakage of fluid from the choroid into the retina.

The incipient stages of diabetic retinopathy are associated with an early breakdown of the blood–retinal barrier resulting in enhanced vascular permeability and macular edema. The breaching of the blood–retinal barrier is believed to represent the earliest known change in diabetic retinopathy occurring prior to the development of microaneurysms and capillary occlusion.[43] Although both the inner and outer components exhibit increased permeability in diabetes, the inner monolayer is the predominant site of leakage in diabetic retinopathy. Interestingly, the retinal vasculature comprising the inner blood–retinal barrier contains VEGF receptors and early blood–retinal barrier breakdown in experimental diabetes is VEGF dependent.[44]

Clinical Trials in Diabetic Retinopathy

Diabetic Retinopathy Study (DRS)

The diabetic retinopathy study (DRS) was undertaken in 1971 to determine whether photocoagulation helps prevent severe visual loss from proliferative diabetic retinopathy and if there was a clinically significant difference in the efficacy and safety of argon versus xenon photocoagulation for proliferative diabetic retinopathy.[45]

This randomized, controlled clinical trial involved more than 1,700 patients enrolled at 15 medical centers.[45] Eligibility criteria included patients younger than 70 years of age with best corrected visual acuity of 20/100 or better in each eye in the presence of PDR in at least one eye or severe nonproliferative diabetic retinopathy in both eyes. Patients were excluded if they had prior treatment with photocoagulation or pituitary ablation, and both eyes had to be suitable for photocoagulation.[45]

In the trial, one eye of each patient was randomly assigned to receive immediate photocoagulation with either argon laser or xenon arc photocoagulation. The fellow eye was observed without treatment.[45] Patients were subsequently monitored at 4-month intervals. Treatment with photocoagulation was carried out in a panretinal or scatter technique extending to or beyond the vortex veins. Argon photocoagulation treatment specified 800–1,600 burns, 500-μm in size with 0.1 s duration.[45] Direct treatment of retinal neovascularization was applied on or within one disc diameter of the optic disc (NVD) or beyond this zone (NVE). Photocoagulation with xenon was carried out in a similar manner with fewer burns of longer duration. Treatment with xenon photocoagulation was directed at NVE. Supplemental focal laser photocoagulation in the argon treatment group was applied when clinically necessary to treat macular edema.

The DRS demonstrated that both argon and xenon photocoagulation reduced the risk of severe visual loss (best corrected visual acuity < 5/200) by more than 50% during a follow-up of over 5 years.[46] Adverse effects of laser photocoagulation included a modest reduction of visual acuity of one line and constriction of the peripheral visual field. The results indicated that these effects were more pronounced in the xenon arc treated group. The study concluded that the risks of severe visual loss outweighed the adverse effect of treatment for two groups of patients: eyes with retinal neovascularization and preretinal or vitreous hemorrhage; and eyes with new vessels on or within one disc diameter of the optic disc (NVD) equaling or exceeding 1/4–1/3 disc area in extent even in the absence of preretinal or vitreous hemorrhage.[46] These eyes were considered at high risk for PDR and required prompt treatment as they had the highest risk of severe visual loss.

Early Treatment Diabetic Retinopathy Study (ETDRS)

The ETDRS was a multicenter, randomized clinical trial involving 3711 participants designed to evaluate the effectiveness of both argon laser photocoagulation and aspirin therapy in the management of patients with non-proliferative diabetic retinopathy and early PDR.[47] In addition, it was designed to determine the best time to initiate photocoagulation treatment in diabetic retinopathy.

The eligibility criteria for the ETDRS were broad, enrolling patients with a mild nonproliferative diabetic retinopathy through early PDR with visual acuity 20/200 or better in each eye.[47] Patients were randomly assigned to receive photocoagulation in one eye with the fellow eye observed. Follow-up examinations were scheduled at least every 4 months and photocoagulation was initiated in eyes assigned to deferral as soon as high-risk proliferative retinopathy was detected.[47] Furthermore, patients were randomly assigned to receive 650 mg per day of aspirin or a placebo. The primary outcome measured in the ETDRS was moderate visual loss (MVL) defined as a doubling of the visual angle, a drop of 15 or more letters on ETDRS visual acuity, or a drop of 3 or more lines of Snellen visual acuity.[47]

The ETDRS defined clinically significant macular edema (CSME) as:

1. Retinal edema located at or within 500 μm of the center of the macula.
2. Hard exudates at or within 500 μm of the center if associated with thickening of the adjacent retina.
3. A zone of thickening larger than one disc area if located within one disc diameter of the center of the macula.

The ETDRS determined that focal laser photocoagulation reduced the risk of MVL by 50%. Treatment increased the chance of visual improvement and was associated in minor losses of visual field. Treatment consisted of argon laser photocoagulation of individual-leaking microaneurysms and grid treatment to areas of diffuse leakage and capillary nonperfusion.[48]

The ETDRS also concluded that early panretinal photocoagulation with or without focal photocoagulation compared with deferral of photocoagulation was associated with a small reduction in the incidence of severe visual loss (visual acuity less than 5/200 at two consecutive visits), but 5-year rates were low in both the early treatment and deferral groups (2.6 and 3.7%, respectively).[49] It was determined that scatter photocoagulation is not recommended for eyes with mild or moderate nonproliferative diabetic retinopathy provided appropriate follow-up care can be maintained. Patients with severe nonproliferative diabetic retinopathy or high-risk PDR should receive prompt photocoagulation. The ETDRS defined severe nonproliferative diabetic retinopathy as:

1. Diffuse intraretinal hemorrhages and microaneurysms in four quadrants.
2. Venous beading in two quadrants.
3. Intraretinal microvascular abnormalities (IRMA) in one quadrant.

Aspirin treatment did not alter the course of diabetic retinopathy in patients enrolled in ETDRS. Aspirin did not prevent the development of high-risk proliferative retinopathy and did not reduce the risk of visual loss, nor did it increase the risk of vitreous hemorrhage in both eyes assigned for laser photocoagulation and deferral of treatment. Furthermore, it was determined that aspirin had no deleterious effects for diabetic patients with retinopathy.[50]

Diabetic Retinopathy Vitrectomy Study (DRVS)

The DRVS was a randomized, multicenter clinical trial designed to compare two therapies, early vitrectomy and conventional management, for recent severe vitreous hemorrhage secondary to diabetic retinopathy.[51] The early vitrectomy group had vitrectomy within 6 months of the onset of vitreous hemorrhage. The conventional management group underwent vitrectomy if hemorrhage failed to clear during a waiting period of 6–12 months or if retinal detachment involving the center of the macula developed at any time.[51]

The results of the DRVS clearly demonstrated the benefit of early vitrectomy for patients with severe PDR. After 2 years of follow-up, 25% of the early vitrectomy group had visual acuity of 10/20 or better compared with 15% in the deferral group.[52] This benefit was most evident for patients with type 1 diabetes, as they represented a younger subset of patients with a relatively more severe PDR. This trend continued at the 4-year follow-up, with 44% of patients in the early vitrectomy group achieving 10/20 visual acuity versus 28% for the conventional management group.[53]

Clinical and Fundus Findings

Nonproliferative Diabetic Retinopathy (NPDR)

Diabetic retinopathy is a retinal vascular disorder characterized by typical microvascular funduscopic changes. These typical funduscopic lesions can be broadly characterized as either nonproliferative or proliferative retinopathy with varying degrees of severity in each subset. They can either precede or follow alterations in retinal function thereby highlighting the importance of timely examinations to detect incipient changes.

The characteristic fundus lesions associated with nonproliferative diabetic retinopathy include cotton wool spots, microaneurysms, dot and blot hemorrhages, retinal vascular caliber changes, hard exudate formation, retinal capillary closure, and macular edema.

Microaneurysms represent saccular outpouchings of the retinal capillary bed. They can present as concentrated lesions in the posterior pole or with widespread distribution throughout the fundus. Their formation is nonspecific to diabetes and can occur in a variety of disorders including hypertension and sickle cell disease. Although their precise pathogenesis remains unknown, they are attributed to pericyte degeneration, endothelial cell proliferation, and retinal capillary closure. They represent the earliest clinical changes of the retinal vasculature in NRDR detectable with ophthalmoscopy. They are best detected with fluorescein angiography in which they typically surround areas of capillary nonperfusion. In the earliest stages, the increase or decrease in microaneurysm formation can be used as an indicator for progression or regression of disease. The microaneurysm count at baseline examination can be used as an important predictor of progression of diabetic retinopathy.[54] They become visually significant when there is an associated leakage of serous contents leading to macular edema.

Cotton wool spots represent retinal nerve fiber layer infarcts associated with stasis of axoplasmic flow. They occur early in the course of NPDR and may be evident prior to the development of microaneurysms and retinal hemorrhages. They are evanescent in nature, usually resolving in several months though they may persist much longer. Their effect on visual acuity and the visual field is dependent on their size and location. Although most commonly seen in diabetic retinopathy, they are also seen in a variety of retinal vascular disorders including hypertensive retinopathy, central retinal vein occlusion, and drug toxicities such as with interferon retinopathy.

The presence of intraretinal microvascular abnormalities and capillary permeability may lead to the formation of retinal hemorrhages. The morphology of the hemorrhages is related to the topography of the anatomical retinal layer from which they are derived. Superficial hemorrhages assume a flame-shaped appearance due to the parallel arrangement of the nerve fiber layer to the retinal surface. Deeper hemorrhages assume a dot-and-blot appearance due to the perpendicular arrangement of cells in the deeper retinal tissue. Occasionally, these hemorrhages may attain a white center, representing fibrin deposition. White-centered hemorrhages are more commonly seen in other conditions such as subacute bacterial endocarditis and acute leukemia. Intraretinal hemorrhages are significant in that they generally parallel the severity of NPDR. Intraretinal hemorrhages are not typically visually significant unless they assume a subfoveal location.

Intraretinal microvascular abnormalities or IRMA are evident in NPDR. They represent dilated vascular segments in a partially occluded capillary bed and represent intraretinal neovascularization or the formation of shunts in areas on nonperfusion. They are clinically significant in that they may leak and cause macular edema and impart a greater risk for the development of PDR.

The venous caliber abnormalities in NPDR include vascular dilation, beading, and the formation of loops. They are indicative of retinal ischemia, and may be associated with central or branch retinal venous occlusions, which are both seen more commonly in the diabetic population.

The primary mechanism of visual loss in nonproliferative retinopathy is through macular edema. The edema can be a result of focal vascular leakage from microaneurysms in the macular, or via diffuse vascular leakage. The edema may be associated with hard exudates or cystoid changes in the macula. If the edema is classified as clinically significant macular edema (CSME), as outlined by the ETDRS, focal laser photocoagulation is performed to avoid precipitous vision loss. Laser photocoagulation is directed at microaneurysms for focal leakage and is applied in a grid pattern for diffuse leakage. Concomitant cardiovascular and renal disease leading to fluid retention and hypertension can further exacerbate the edema. Treatment, therefore, of systemic abnormalities using a multidisciplinary approach should be included in the care of the patient with macular edema.

NPDR can be classified into mild, moderate, and severe forms, with each imparting its own degree of severity and progression to proliferative retinopathy. *Mild* NPDR is characterized by microaneurysms only and impart a 5% risk of developing PDR in 1 year (Fig. 21.1(1)).[55] *Moderate* NPDR is characterized by less than four quadrants of scattered microaneurysms and hemorrhages along with cotton wool spots, venous beading, or IRMA (Fig. 21.1(2)). The risk of progression to PDR within 1 year is between 12 and 27%.[55] Patients with mild and moderate NPDR are treated by medically optimizing glycemic control and any associated hypertension or dyslipidemia. Patients with clinically significant macular edema are treated with focal laser therapy. These patients are not candidates for scatter laser photocoagulation. *Severe* NPDR is characterized by the "4-2-1" rule of four quadrants of hemorrhages and microaneurysms, two quadrants of venous caliber abnormalities, or one quadrant of IRMA (Fig. 21.1(3)). These patients are at high risk for developing PDR with a 52% risk within 1

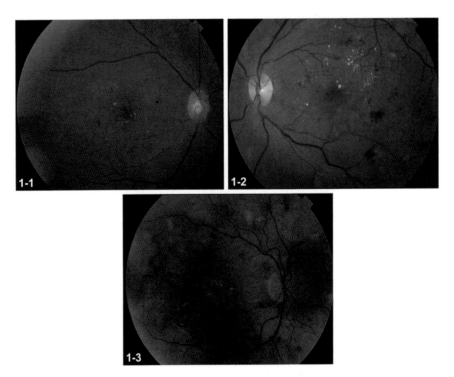

Fig. 21.1 Stages of nonproliferative diabetic retinopathy. Mild NPDR (1) with few dot-blot hemorrhages and intraretinal lipid. Red-free photograph of moderate NPDR (2) depicting a greater number of dot-blot hemorrhages and microaneurysms with associated lipid exudation. Severe NPDR (3) characterized by extensive four quadrant distribution of intraretinal hemorrhages and lipid along with infarctions of the nerve fiber layer (cotton wool spots)

year.[55] These patients are candidates for panretinal photocoagulation (PRP) the timing of which is determined at the discretion of the retinal specialist.

Proliferative Diabetic Retinopathy (PDR)

Proliferative diabetic retinopathy is an advanced form of diabetic retinopathy characterized by the growth of abnormal blood vessels, which extend over the surface of the retina and along the "scaffold" provided by the posterior vitreous hyaloid. These new blood vessels may present as neovascularization of the optic disc (NVD) or anywhere along the retinal periphery (NVE), vitreous hemorrhage, and fibrous proliferation. Active neovascularization commonly occurs at the border of perfused and nonperfused retina and is most severe in eyes with extensive nonperfusion. The newly formed vessels are fragile commonly resulting in vitreous hemorrhage and precipitous vision loss.

The formation of new blood vessels in PDR occurs as a consequence of progressive damage to the retinal blood vessels in NPDR. Eventually, with cumulative damage, there is capillary occlusion resulting in a relative oxygen deficient or ischemic environment. This results in the release of various angiogenic growth factors, the most significant of which is believed to be vascular endothelial growth factor or VEGF. VEGF release serves as the stimulus for the proliferation of new vessels resulting in NVD, NVE, and potential neovascularization within the anterior chamber along the surface of the iris. Neovascularization along the iris surface most commonly occurs at the pupillary margin and is significant in that these fine arborizing vessels can progress along the iris margin and into the trabecular meshwork accompanied by a fibrous membrane. Subsequent contracture of the fibrous membrane leads to synechiae within the trabecular meshwork and secondary angle closure glaucoma.

Clinicians treating PDR assess for the presence of new vessels, their location, and severity when determining the timing of panretinal photocoagulation. Early PDR is that which does not meet the criteria for high-risk PDR. Patients with early PDR have a 75% risk of developing high-risk PDR within a 5-year period. Patients with early PDR and severe NPDR may require treatment with early PRP. Initiation of PRP should be considered for patients with severe NPDR with any new vessels or early PDR with elevated new vessels or NVD.

High-risk PDR is characterized by any of the following:

1. NVD 1/4–1/3 disc area or more in size (Fig. 21.2(1))
2. NVD less than 1/4 disc area in size with concurrent vitreous hemorrhage
3. NVE greater than or equal to 1/2 disc area in size with concurrent vitreous hemorrhage (Fig. 21.2(2))

Patients with high-risk characteristics require prompt treatment with laser photocoagulation to prevent further progression of retinopathy.

Patients with advanced PDR may require vitrectomy surgery to clear an otherwise non-clearing vitreous hemorrhage. Vitreous hemorrhage may occur as a result of vitreous traction on new vessels (Fig. 21.2(3)). Contracture of the vitreous or fibrovascular proliferation can result in the shearing of a new vessel, and subsequent vitreous hemorrhage.

In time, retinal neovascularization may become fibrotic, contract, and lead to tractional retinal detachment (Fig. 21.2(4)). The fibrovascular proliferation in PDR typically occurs along the temporal vascular arcades and on the optic disc and may exhibit tractional forces resulting in macular striae and edema. The tractional retinal detachments that result can involve or spare the macula. They may be associated with both atrophic and tractional retinal breaks resulting in a combined rhegmatogenous-tractional retinal detachment. Patients with posterior tractional retinal detachments not involving the macula may be observed without vitrectomy surgery and can be stable for years. Upon encroachment of the macula, however, tractional retinal detachments can result in profound visual compromise and are therefore an indication for prompt vitrectomy. These tractional forces may be relieved with pars plana vitrectomy utilizing segmentation and delamination techniques.

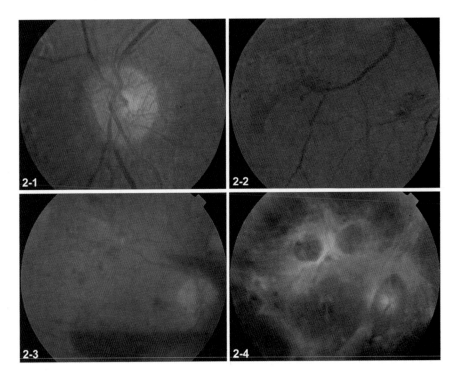

Fig. 21.2 Sequelae of proliferative diabetic retinopathy. Color photographs depicting neovascularization of the optic disc or NVD (1) and neovascularization elsewhere in the retinal periphery or NVE (2). Note the development of preretinal hemorrhage in the subhyaloidal space with progression of PDR (3). Severe proliferation of tractional membranes resulting in detachment of the macula; tractional retinal detachment (4)

Fluorescein Angiography

Fluorescein angiography is a technique for examining the integrity of the retinal circulation using the dye-tracing method. Sodium fluorescein dye is injected into an antecubital vein and then an angiogram is obtained with multiple sequential photographs to monitor dye transit. Sodium fluorescein is a yellow-red dye with a molecular weight of 376.67 Daltons with a spectrum of absorption at 465–490 nm (blue wavelength) and excitation at 520–530 nm (yellow-green wavelength). The angiogram is performed with a camera with exciter and barrier filters that allow for the illumination of the retina with blue light because only yellow-green light (from the fluorescence) can reach the camera. The dye is metabolized within the liver and kidney within 24–36 h turning the patient's urine a yellow-green color. The most common adverse reactions to fluorescein dye are mild including nausea, vomiting, and pruritus and are typically transient. However, severe reactions requiring immediate intervention such as bronchospasm and anaphylaxis can occur and must be monitored. Although there are no adverse effects reported during pregnancy, all efforts are undertaken to avoid fluorescein angiography unless deemed critical in directing diagnosis and management.

Fluorescein angiography is an invaluable tool that aids in the diagnosis and directs management in diabetic retinopathy. By allowing the clinician to identify the spectrum of funduscopic changes prevalent in diabetic retinopathy, fluorescein angiography can be used to monitor the severity of retinopathy and identify risk factors for progression. Various angiographic risk factors have been identified including fluorescein leakage, capillary dilation, and capillary loss.[56,57]

Diabetic retinopathy can result in both hyper- and hypofluorescent patterns of angiography and their distinction and interpretation are essential in identifying treatable lesions. In the setting of clinically significant macular edema (CSME), angiography is utilized to better identify leaking microaneurysms, which may appear as either focal or diffuse areas of permeability (Fig. 21.3(1)). Treatment with laser photocoagulation then can

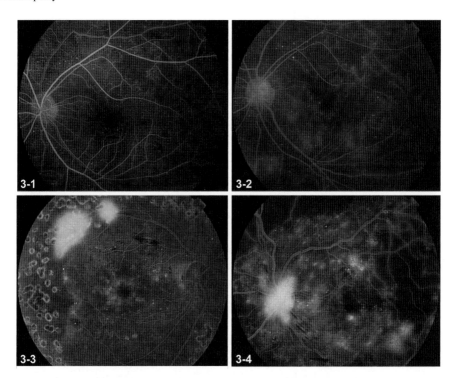

Fig. 21.3 Fluorescein angiographic characteristics. Early frame of fluorescein angiography (1) highlighting multiple areas of hyper-fluorescence corresponding to microaneurysms which demonstrate prominent leakage in the late frame (2). Late frame fluorescein angiogram showing an area of hyperfluorescence along the supero-temporal arcade corresponding to retinal neovascularization and within the macula representing pronounced leakage from the perifoveal capillaries (3). Multiple areas of hyperfluorescence in the late frame angiogram (4) representing fronds of active retinal neovascularization. Hypofluorescent areas (4) seen temporally and superiorly represent ischemic zones of capillary non-perfusion

be directed to the selected microaneurysms or to a cluster of microaneurysms in a grid pattern with diffuse permeability alterations (Fig. 21.3(2)). Marked ischemia can result in areas of capillary closure within the macula potentially limiting vision or further peripherally. These vascular filling defects are well delineated on angiography as hypofluorescent patches representing nonperfused segments (Fig. 21.3(4)). Furthermore, angiography can be used to identify and monitor leaf-like formation of new blood vessels referred to as fronds of neovascularization along the optic disc or elsewhere in the retinal periphery. Areas of neovascularization are easily identified in the early frames of the angiogram and exhibit late hyperfluorescence signaling leakage of dye from these newly formed, incompetent vessels (Fig. 21.3(3)). Other high-risk vascular abnormalities such as *IRMA* are clearly demonstrated with angiography. The use of fluorescein angiography is essential as an adjunct to clinical ophthalmoscopy in the diagnosis and management of diabetic retinopathy.

Optical Coherence Tomography (OCT)

Optical coherence tomography (OCT) captures reflected light from retinal structures to create a cross-sectional image of the retina. Optical coherence tomography (OCT) greatly enhances the ability to detect macular thickening and has brought new insights into the efficacy of various treatments. Use of this imaging modality allows for the quantitative measurement of macular thickness and objective analysis of the foveal architecture. OCT has gained widespread acceptance as an additional modality to help identify and evaluate macular pathology and allows for a reproducible way to monitor macular edema.

The use of OCT with micrometer resolution was first devised by Huang et al. in 1991.[58] The ability to obtain cross-sectional retinal images with micrometer resolution has allowed for better morphological tissue imaging and analysis compared to other imaging modalities. OCT utilizes the principle of low-coherence interferometry where distance information concerning various ocular structures is extracted from time delays of reflected signals. The interference pattern of light is measured over a distance of micrometers in OCT using broadband light sources. In OCT, interferometry is utilized in a noninvasive, noncontact manner to produce high-resolution cross-sectional images of the retina. It is particularly useful in evaluating the extent of diabetic macular edema and in monitoring the efficacy of a given treatment (Fig. 21.4(1–4)). Topographic mapping protocol can be utilized for longitudinally monitoring and objectively quantifying the development of macular edema and for following the resolution of edema after laser treatment.

Novel Therapeutic Approaches

Various novel medical approaches in conjunction with laser photocoagulation are currently being explored for the treatment of diabetic retinopathy and diabetic macular edema. One such treatment is with ruboxistaurin, a selective PKC-b inhibitor. Hyperglycemia activates protein kinase C, and the beta-isoform of protein kinase C mediates early diabetes-induced microvascular complications, including diabetic macular edema. Animal models have suggested that ruboxistaurin ameliorates hyperglycemia-induced complications. Initial results of the 30-month data of the randomized Protein Kinase C-b Inhibitor Diabetic Macular Edema Study (PKC-DMES) indicated that treatment with 32 mg of ruboxistaurin daily did not reduce the risk of progression to sight-threatening diabetic macular edema or focal/grid photocoagulation in diabetic patients.[59] However, subgroup analysis of the data revealed that those treated with ruboxistaurin daily appeared to have slower progression to sight-threatening diabetic macular edema than those taking placebo when the endpoint excluded photocoagulation, as different practitioners had different thresholds for initiating photocoagulation.[59] Thus, the results of this clinical trial demonstrated that daily treatment with ruboxistaurin is an effective therapy for diabetic macular edema and diabetic retinopathy.

Pharmacologic inhibition of VEGF appears to be a promising strategy for diabetic retinopathy, in which breakdown of the blood–retina barrier and neovascularization play a prominent pathogenetic role. Introduction of VEGF into normal primate eyes induces the same pathologic processes as those seen in diabetic retinopathy, including microaneurysm formation and increased vascular permeability.[60] Furthermore, elevated VEGF levels have been found from the analysis of vitreous samples from patients with diabetic macular edema.[61] Therefore VEGF inhibition has garnered interest in ameliorating diabetic retinopathy and diabetic macular edema.

Bevacizumab and ranibizumab (Genentech, Inc., South San Francisco, CA) have emerged as therapeutic options for age-related macular degeneration, with promising functional results. The rationale for evaluating their use is sound in treating patients with diabetic retinopathy and diabetic macular edema. Ranibizumab is a recombinant, humanized Fab fragment of mouse monoclonal antibody directed toward all isoforms of VEGF. Ranibizumab has been shown to significantly reduce foveal thickness and improve visual acuity in patients with diabetic macular edema.[62,63] Bevacizumab is a humanized monoclonal antibody that inhibits all active isoforms of VEGF. Intravitreal bevacizumab is a new treatment modality which is currently being tried out for use in macular edema following central retinal vein occlusion (CRVO), wet age-related macular degeneration (ARMD), rubeosis irides, proliferative diabetic retinopathy (PDR), and retinopathy of prematurity. The short-term results of various investigations demonstrate that bevacizumab is effective in improving visual acuity, reducing retinal thickness, and in causing regression of retinal and iris neovascularization in diabetic patients.[64,65,66] Although these preliminary results are promising, the long-term outcomes from treatment with these agents remain unknown. Randomized, controlled, double-masked trials are needed to test whether intraocular injections of anti-VEGF agents provide long-term benefit to patients with DME.

Further study will determine the long-term effects of pharmacologic therapies for DME and their potential utility as preventive treatments for this condition. The use of combination therapies may offer treatment advantages, particularly when the therapies approach the disease through different pathways. These novel therapeutic approaches will likely be incorporated as adjuncts to laser photocoagulation in the future treatment of diabetic macular edema.

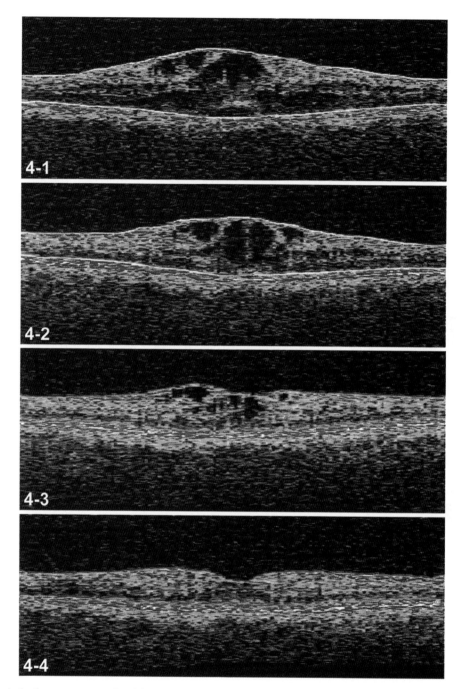

Fig. 21.4 Optical coherence tomography (OCT). OCT demonstrating persistent macular edema in a patient with diabetic retinopathy (1). Note the collection of cystic spaces throughout the retina. Following treatment with intravitreal bevacizumab at monthly intervals there is progressive resolution of the macular edema at 1 month (2), and 2 months (3) from baseline with ultimate restitution of the normal foveal architecture at the 3-month interval (4)

References

1. Bell RA. *Diabetes 2001 Vital Statistics*. Alexandria, VA: American Diabetes Association; 2003.
2. National Health and Nutrition Examination Survey 1999–2002. Prevalence of diabetes and impaired fasting glucose in adults in the U.S. population. *Diabetes Care*. 2006;29:1263–1268.

3. Zimmet P, Alberti KG, Shaw J. Global and societal implications of the diabetes epidemic. *Nature*. 2001;414:782–787.
4. Roy MS, Klein R, O'Colmain BJ, et al. The prevalence of diabetic retinopathy among adults in the United States. *Arch Ophthalmol*. 2004;122:552–563.
5. The Eye Diseases Prevalence Research Group. The prevalence of diabetic retinopathy among adults in the United States. *Arch Ophthalmol*. 2004;122:552–563.
6. Yanko L, Goldbourt U, Michaelson IC, et al. Prevalence and 15-year incidence of retinopathy and associated characteristics in middle-aged and elderly diabetic men. *Br J Ophthalmol*. 1983;67:759.
7. Diabetes Control and Complications Trial Research Group: The effect of intensive diabetes treatment on the progression of diabetic retinopathy in insulin-dependent diabetes mellitus. *Arch Ophthalmol*. 1995;113:36.
8. Diabetes Control and Complications Trial Research Group. The effect of intensive treatment of diabetes on the development and progression of long-term complications in insulin-dependent diabetes mellitus. *N Engl J Med*. 1993;329:977.
9. United Kingdom Prospective Diabetes Study Group: Intensive blood-glucose control with sulphonylureas or insulin compared with conventional treatment and risk of complications in patients with type 2 diabetes (UKPDS 33). *Lancet*. 1998;352:837.
10. Gray A, Raikou M, McGuire A, et al. Cost effectiveness of an intensive blood glucose control policy in patients with type 2 diabetes: economic analysis alongside randomised controlled trial (UKPDS 41). United Kingdom Prospective Diabetes Study Group. *BMJ*. 2000;320:1373.
11. United Kingdom Prospective Diabetes Study Group: Efficacy of atenolol and captopril in reducing risk of lacrovascular and microvascular complications in type 2 diabetes: UKPDS 39. *BMJ*. 1998;317:713.
12. Chew EY, Klein ML, Ferris FL 3rd, et al. Association of elevated serum lipid levels with retinal hard exudate in diabetic retinopathy. Early Treatment Diabetic Retinopathy Study (ETDRS) Report 22. *Arch Ophthalmol*. 1996;114:1079–1084.
13. Klein BE, Moss SE, Klein R. Effect of pregnancy on progression of diabetic retinopathy. *Diabetes Care*. 1990;13:34–40.
14. Temple RC, Aldridge VA, Sampson MJ, Greenwood RH, Heyburn PJ, Glenn A. Impact of pregnancy on the progression of diabetic retinopathy in type 1 diabetes. *Diabet Med*. 2001;18:573–577.
15. Frank RN, Keirn RJ, Kennedy RA, Frank KW. Galactose induced retinal basement membrane thickening: prevention by sorbinil. *Invest Ophthalmol Vis Sci*. 1983;24:1519–1524.
16. Engerman RL, Kern TS. Experimental galactosemia produces diabetic-like retinopathy. *Diabetes*. 1984;33:97–100.
17. Varma SD. Aldose reductase and the etiology of diabetic cataracts. *Curr Top Eye Res*. 1980;3:91.
18. Akagi Y, Kador PF, Kuwabara T, et al. Aldose reductase localization in human retinal mural cells. *Invest Ophthalmol Vis Sci*. 1983;24:1516–1519.
19. Akagi Y, Yajima Y, Kador PF, et al. Localization of aldose reductase in the human eye. *Diabetes*. 1984;33:562–566.
20. Arauz-Pacheco C, Ramirez LC, Pruneda L, Sanborn GE, Rosenstock J, Raskin P. The effect of the aldose reductase inhibitor, ponalrestat, on the progression of diabetic retinopathy. *J Diabetes Complications*. 1992;6:131–137.
21. A randomized trial of sorbinil, an aldose reductase inhibitor, in diabetic retinopathy: the Sorbinil Retinopathy Trial Research Group. *Arch Ophthalmol*. 1990;108:1234–1244.
22. Ishii KD, King GL. Protein kinase C activation and its role in the development of vascular complications in diabetes mellitus. *J Mol Med*. 1998;76:21–31.
23. Lynch JJ, Ferro TJ, Blumenstock FA, Brockenauer AM, Malik AM. Increased endothelial albumin permeability mediated by protein kinase C activation. *J Clin Invest*. 1990;85:1991–1998.
24. Wolf BA, Williamson JR, Easom RA, Chang K, Sherman WR, Turk J. Diacylglycerol accumulation and microvascular abnormalities induced by elevated glucose levels. *J Clin Invest*. 1991;87:31–38.
25. Xia P, Aiello LP, Ishii H, et al. Characterization of vascular endothelial growth factor's effect on the activation of protein kinase C, its isoforms, and endothelial cell growth. *J Clin Invest*. 1996;98:2018–2026.
26. Miller JW, Adamis AP, Aiello LP. Vascular endothelial growth factor in ocular neovascularization and proliferative diabetic retinopathy. *Diabete Metab Rev*. 1997;13:37–50.
27. Aiello LP, Avery RL, Arrigg PG, et al. Vascular endothelial growth factor in ocular fluid of patients with diabetic retinopathy and other retinal disorders. *N Engl J Med*. 1994;331:1480–1487.
28. Das Evcimen N, King GL. The role of protein kinase C activation and the vascular complications of diabetes. *Pharmacol Res*. 2007;55(6):498–510.
29. Joy SV, Scates AC, Bearelly S, et al. Ruboxistaurin, a protein kinase C beta inhibitor, as an emerging treatment for diabetes microvascular complications. *Ann Pharmacother*. 2005;39(10):1693–1699.
30. PKC-DRS2 Group, Aiello LP, Davis MD, et al. Effect of ruboxistaurin on visual loss in patients with diabetic retinopathy. *Ophthalmology*. 2006;113(12):2221–2230.
31. Adamis AP, Shima DT, Yeo KT, et al. Synthesis and secretion of vascular permeability factor/vascular endothelial growth factor by human retinal pigment epithelial cells. *Biochem Biophys Res Commun*. 1993;193:631–638.
32. Plouet J, Chollet P, Moro F, Malecaze F. Secretion of VAS/VEGF by retinal pericytes: a paracrine stimulation of endothelial cell proliferation. *Invest Ophthalmol Vis Sci*. 1993;34:900–900.
33. Aiello LP, Ferrara N, King GL. Hypoxic regulation and bioactivity of vascular endothelial growth factor: characterization in retinal microvascular pericytes and pigment epithelial cells. *Invest Ophthalmol Vis Sci*. 1994;35:1868–1868.

34. Aiello LP, Avery RL, Arrigg PG, et al. Vascular endothelial growth factor in ocular fluid of patients with diabetic retinopathy and other retinal disorders. *N Engl J Med*. 1994;331(22):1519–1520.

35. Poulsen JE. Recovery from retinopathy in a case of diabetes with Simmond's disease. *Diabetes*. 1953;2:7–12.

36. Hyer SL, Sharp PS, Brooks RA, Burrin JM, Kohner EM. Serum IGF-1 concentration in diabetic retinopathy. *Diabet Med*. 1988;5:356–360.

37. Grant MB, Mames RN, Fitzgerald C, Ellis EA, Aboufriekha M, Guy J. Insulin-like growth factor I acts as an angiogenic agent in rabbit cornea and retina: comparative studies with basic fibroblast growth factor. *Diabetologia*. 1993;36: 282–291.

38. Lee HC, Lee KW, Chung CH, et al. IGF-I of serum and vitreous fluid in patients with diabetic proliferative retinopathy. *Diabetes Res Clin Pract*. 1994;24:85–88.

39. Connor TB Jr, Roberts AB, Sporn MB, et al. Correlation of fibrosis and transforming growth factor-beta type 2 levels in the eye. *J Clin Invest*. 1989;83(5):1661–1666.

40. Hirase K, Ikeda T, Sotozono C, et al. Transforming growth factor beta2 in the vitreous in proliferative diabetic retinopathy. *Arch Ophthalmol*. 1998;116(6):738–741.

41. Wu YQ, Becerra SP. Proteolytic activity directed toward pigment epithelium-derived factor in vitreous of bovine eyes. Implications of proteolytic processing. *Invest Ophthalmol Vis Sci*. 1996;37(10):1984–1993.

42. Dawson DW, Volpert OV, Gillis P, et al. Pigment epithelium-derived growth factor: a potent inhibitor of angiogenesis. *Science*. 1999;285:245–248.

43. Cunha-Vaz J, Faria de Abreu JR, Campos AJ. Early breakdown of the blood-retinal barrier in diabetes. *Br J Ophthalmol*. 1975;59(11):649–656.

44. Qaum T, Xu Q, Joussen AM, et al. VEGF-initiated blood-retinal barrier breakdown in early diabetes. *Invest Ophthalmol Vis Sci*. 2001;42(10):2408–2413.

45. The Diabetic Retinopathy Study Research Group: Design, methods, and baseline results. Diabetic Retinopathy Study (DRS) Report Number 6. *Invest Ophthalmol Vis Sci*. 1981;2:210–226.

46. The Diabetic Retinopathy Study Research Group: Photocoagulation treatment of proliferative diabetic retinopathy. Clinical application of Diabetic Retinopathy Study (DRS) findings, DRS Report Number 8. *Ophthalmology*. 1981;88(7): 583–600.

47. Early Treatment Diabetic Retinopathy Study Research Group: Early Treatment Diabetic Retinopathy Study design and baseline patient characteristics. ETDRS Report Number 7. *Ophthalmology*. 1991;98:741–756.

48. Early Treatment Diabetic Retinopathy Study Research Group: Photocoagulation for diabetic macular edema. Early Treatment Diabetic Retinopathy Study Report Number 1. *Arch Ophthalmol*. 1985;103(12):1796–1806.

49. Early Treatment Diabetic Retinopathy Study Research Group: Early photocoagulation for diabetic retinopathy. ETDRS Report Number 9. *Ophthalmology*. 1991;98(5 Suppl):766–785.

50. Early Treatment Diabetic Retinopathy Study Research Group: Effects of aspirin treatment on diabetic retinopathy. ETDRS Report Number 8. *Ophthalmology*. 1991;98(5 Suppl):757–765.

51. The Diabetic Retinopathy Vitrectomy Study Research Group: Two-year course of visual acuity in severe proliferative diabetic retinopathy with conventional management. Diabetic Retinopathy Vitrectomy Study (DRVS) Report 1. *Ophthalmology*. 1985;92(4):492–502.

52. The Diabetic Retinopathy Vitrectomy Study Research Group: Early vitrectomy for severe vitreous hemorrhage in diabetic retinopathy. Two-year results of a randomized trial. Diabetic Retinopathy Vitrectomy Study Report 2. *Arch Ophthalmol*. 1985;103(11):1644–1652.

53. The Diabetic Retinopathy Vitrectomy Study Research Group: Early vitrectomy for severe proliferative diabetic retinopathy in eyes with useful vision. Results of a randomized trial – Diabetic Retinopathy Vitrectomy Study Report 3. *Ophthalmology*. 1988;95(10):1307–1320.

54. Klein R, Meuer SM, Moss SE, Klein BE. The relationship of retinal microaneurysm counts to the 4-year progression of diabetic retinopathy. *Arch Ophthalmol*. 1989;107(12):1780–1785.

55. Early Treatment Diabetic Retinopathy Study Research Group: Fundus photographic risk factors for progression of diabetic retinopathy. ETDRS Report Number 12. *Ophthalmology*. 1991;98(5 Suppl):823–833.

56. Early Treatment Diabetic Retinopathy Study Research Group: Classification of diabetic retinopathy from fluorescein angiograms. ETDRS Report Number 11. *Ophthalmology*. 1991;98:807–822.

57. Early Treatment Diabetic Retinopathy Study Research Group: Fluorescein angiographic risk factors for progression of diabetic retinopathy. ETDRS Report Number 13. *Ophthalmology*. 1991;98:834–840.

58. Huang D, Swanson EA, Lin CP, et al. Optical coherence tomography. *Science*. 1991;254(5035):1178–1181.

59. PKC-DMES Study Group. Effect of ruboxistaurin in patients with diabetic macular edema: thirty-month results of the randomized PKC-DMES clinical trial. *Arch Ophthalmol*. 2007;125(3):318–324.

60. Tolentino MJ, Miller JW, Gragoudas ES, et al. Intravitreous injections of vascular endothelial growth factor produce retinal ischemia and microangiopathy in an adult primate. *Ophthalmology*. 1996;103:1820–1828.

61. Funatsu H, Yamashita H, Noma H, et al. Increased levels of vascular endothelial growth factor and interleukin-6 in the aqueous humor of diabetics with macular edema. *Am J Ophthalmol*. 2002;133:70–77.

62. Nguyen QD, Tatlipinar S, Shah SM, et al. Vascular endothelial growth factor is a critical stimulus for diabetic macular edema. *Am J Ophthalmol*. 2006;142(6):961–969.

63. Chun DW, Heier JS, Topping TM, Duker JS, Bankert JM. A pilot study of multiple intravitreal injections of ranibizumab in patients with center-involving clinically significant diabetic macular edema. *Ophthalmology*. 2006;113(10):1706–1712.
64. Diabetic Retinopathy Clinical Research Network, Scott IU, Edwards AR, et al. A phase II randomized clinical trial of intravitreal bevacizumab for diabetic macular edema. *Ophthalmology*. 2007;114(10):1860–1867.
65. Arevalo JF, Fromow-Guerra J, Quiroz-Mercado H, et al. Pan-American Collaborative Retina Study Group. *Ophthalmology*. 2007;114(4):743–750.
66. Avery RL, Pearlman J, Pieramici DJ, et al. *Ophthalmology*. 2006;113(10):1695.e1–15.

Chapter 22
Diabetic Nephropathy

James F. Winchester, Donald A. Feinfeld, Nikolas B. Harbord, and Alan Dubrow

The Impact of Diabetic Renal Disease

Diabetes mellitus (DM) remains the most common primary cause of incident and prevalent chronic kidney disease (CKD) requiring renal replacement therapy in the United States[1] and the emerging world.[2] In the United States, more than 43% of the new CKD diagnoses in 2004 were attributable to diabetes: a total of 45,871 patients, a rate of 149 per million/population. Although the absolute number of new CKD patients each year is increasing due to population growth, the rate of incident CKD from diabetes has decreased since the year 2000. This trend is reassuring, although CKD attributable to DM remains unacceptably high among blacks, Hispanics, and Native Americans; and continues to increase in the elderly and younger (age 30–39) black adults. The economic impact of advanced kidney disease from diabetes is enormous – total CKD expenditure in 2004 was $32.5 billion, and diabetic patients incur the highest per-person per-year cost. Patients with diabetes have the highest hospitalization rates and mortality (cardiovascular, infectious, and all-cause) among all dialysis patients. They are also less likely to be wait listed for or to receive a kidney transplant. Diabetic individuals fare worse than nondiabetic patients after transplantation, with higher mortality and morbidity from infection.[3] Furthermore, new onset diabetes mellitus (NODM) following kidney transplantation and the use of tacrolimus therapy as the immunosuppressive agent is often associated with obesity and accelerated complications.[4] Advances in vascular biology will likely improve management of cardiovascular disease in the diabetic population. Efforts to attenuate the progression of diabetic nephropathy in the vast pre-CKD-5 population[5] represent the greatest opportunity to improve these adverse circumstances.

Pathophysiology of Diabetic Nephropathy

While the pathophysiology of diabetic nephropathy is understood incompletely, several cardinal etiologic features have emerged. Glycosylation of circulating proteins as well as renal parenchymal proteins, systemic hypertension (including a family history of hypertension), abnormal alteration of intrarenal hemodynamics, as well as smoking play major roles. Since diabetic nephropathy does not develop in every diabetic patient, genetic factors also play a role. Early physiologic abnormalities include increased transglomerular pressure leading to hyperfiltration, manifesting initially with increased glomerular filtration rate (GFR) and small quantities of albumin in the urine (microalbuminuria). Detection of microalbuminuria is essential in diagnosis and follow-up of the disease, since the onset of macroalbuminuria (>300 mg/day) heralds the progression to renal failure. Factors contributing to the renal lesions in both type 1 and type 2 diabetic nephropathy are shown in Table 22.1.

J.F. Winchester (✉)
Division of Nephrology and Hypertension, Department of Medicine, Beth Israel Medical Center,
Albert Einstein College of Medicine, New York, NY, USA
e-mail: jwinches@bethisraelny.org

Table 22.1 Factors contributing to development of diabetic nephropathy

- Sustained hyperglycemia (HbA1c >7.5–8%)
- Familial hypertension (in a parent or sibling)
  - o Abnormalities in red blood cell Na/Li countertransport
  - o Genetic polymorphism for the DD genotype of the
     angiotensin-converting enzyme in type I diabetes
- Familial diabetic nephropathy
  - o Twins
- Ethnic diversity
  - o Native Americans
  - o African-Americans
  - o Mexican
  - o Hispanic Americans
  - o Japanese
- Metabolic syndrome

Appearance of urine albumin of glomerular origin is caused by increased intraglomerular pressure, loss of negatively charged glycosaminoglycans in the basement membrane, and eventually, increased basement membrane pore size. Microscopically, there is a thickening of the glomerular basement membrane, an increased mesangial matrix, and an increased population of mesangial cells.[6] Mesangial expansion is associated with a decrease in capillary filtration surface area, which also correlates with (decreased) glomerular filtration rate. Tubulo-interstitial disease develops probably as a result of a "phlogistic" or inflammatory response to albumin accumulation in proximal convoluted tubule cells[7]; this results in thickening of the tubular basement membrane, tubular atrophy, interstitial fibrosis, and arteriosclerosis. The podocyte also has a role in progression of diabetic nephropathy. Podocyte foot processes (pedicels) interdigitate upon and support the glomerular basement membrane, preventing protein escape. Normally negatively charged, the podocytes repel negatively charged molecules such as albumin. The loss of charge demonstrated in diabetic nephropathy (and other glomerular diseases) explains the passage of proteins into the urinary space. One of the mechanisms by which this occurs is the loss of nephrin and other podocyte proteins (podocin). Eventually the podocytes fuse (or efface) and their slit diaphragms disappear. These changes result in proteinuria and the podocyte-controlled pressure-sensitive maintenance of intraglomerular pressure.

Biochemical mechanisms involved in the pathogenesis of diabetic nephropathy (Fig. 22.1) include direct glucose toxicity, glycation of proteins, formation of advanced glycation end products (AGEs), and increased flux through the polyol and hexosamine metabolic pathways, resulting in overproduction of reactive oxygen species (ROS) molecules which stimulate each of the above pathways.[8] Glucose itself stimulates some signaling molecules (see below), as does the raised intraglomerular pressure. Several isoforms of protein kinase C, diacyl glycerol, mitogenic kinases, and transcription factors may also be activated in diabetic nephropathy.

In addition, a large number of growth factors may be implicated.[9] Transforming growth factor β1 and connective tissue growth factor may result in mesangial and interstitial fibrosis. Growth hormone and insulin-like growth factor-1 are associated with glomerular hyperfiltration and hypertrophy. Circulating and intraglomerular vascular endothelial growth factor (VEGF) increases are evident,[10] while inhibition of VEGF has been associated with improved diabetic retinopathy.[11] Angiotensin II has several important pathophysiologic roles: by its pressor effect it causes preferential constriction of the efferent glomerular arteriole;[12] it increases glomerular capillary permeability to proteins; and its growth effects stimulate mesangial cell proliferation and accumulation of mesangial matrix. Via stretch receptors stimulated by increased efferent glomerular pressure, the mesangial cell induces transforming growth factor β1 and fibronectin expression.[13] Highlighting the importance of growth factors is the recent demonstration that imatinib (an inhibitor of tyrosine kinase) ameliorates the effect of PDGF (platelet-derived growth factor) in promoting collagen formation, interstitial macrophage infiltrates, and glomerular injury in a mouse model of accelerated diabetic nephropathy.[14]

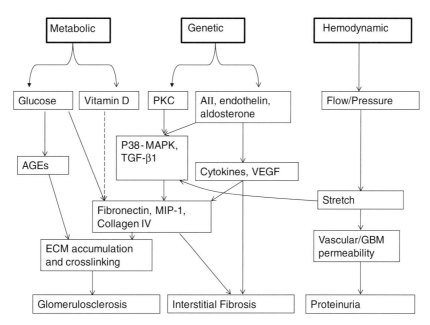

Fig. 22.1 Schematic of pathogenesis of diabetic nephropathy. Abbreviations: PKC – phosphokinase C, AII – angiotensin 2, P38-MAPK – P38-mitogen activated protein kinase, TGF-β1 – transforming growth factor β1, AGEs – advanced glycosylation end-products, VEGF – vascular endolthelial growth factor, MIP-1 – macrophage-inhibitory protein – 1, ECM – extracellular matrix, - - - - - - = inhibitory

   Parathyroid hormone (PTH) is known to have a mitogenic effect in the kidney, and there is upregulation of parathyroid hormone-related protein (PTHrP) in diabetic nephropathy as well as the PTH1 receptor, probably as a result of hyperglycemia, and also through stimulation by angiotensin II.[15] Of more recent interest is the relevance of vitamin D deficiency in the pathogenesis of diabetic nephropathy. Cultured glomerular podocytes have mRNA for 1,25-dihydroxy vitamin D3, vitamin D receptor, and calbindin D28K; in the presence of high glucose these mRNA concentrations increase.[16] High glucose concentrations also result in production of fibronectin and collagen IV protein, a process which is blocked by 1,25-dihydroxy vitamin D3. Additionally, 1,25-dihydroxy vitamin D3 blocks the high glucose-induced macrophage-inhibitory protein-1 (MIP-1),[17] the renin–angiotensin system and TGF-β in mesangial and juxtaglomerular cells.[18] Thus, there seems to be an emerging role for vitamin D in the suppression of diabetic nephropathy; clinical trials are underway in diabetes and other glomerular diseases.

   Genetic influences also play a role as evidenced by twin and family studies in type 1 and type 2 diabetes. There is an excess of hypertension, dyslipidemia, insulin resistance, and premature cardiovascular disease in relatives of individuals with proteinuric diabetic nephropathy compared with diabetic individuals with normal albumin excretion.[19] Familial clustering of patients with nephropathy has been observed and may result from environmental influences (poor glycemic or blood pressure control) or from independent genetic influences.[20,21] Diabetic siblings of patients with combined diabetes and renal disease are five times more likely to develop nephropathy than are diabetic siblings of diabetic patients without renal disease. There is a strong concordance of both nephropathy and renal histopathology in twins with type 1 diabetes.[22] In Brazilian families with two or more diabetic members, the presence of diabetic nephropathy in the propositi is associated with a 3.75-fold increased risk of diabetic nephropathy in the diabetic siblings.[23]

   In some studies, gene polymorphisms have been reported in the renin–angiotensin pathway, peroxisome proliferator activated receptor gamma, endothelial nitric oxide, glucose transporter 1, aldose reductase, and apolipoprotein E.[24] Diabetic nephropathy has been linked to cardiovascular disease and hypertension with inherited abnormalities of sodium–lithium countertransport.[25,26] In a study of 89 patients with type 1 diabetes, the presence of increased maximal velocity of sodium–lithium countertransport and a parent with hypertension significantly increased the risk of nephropathy.[25] Additionally, parents of patients with type 1 diabetes complicated by nephropathy have decreased survival due to a fourfold increased risk of stroke.[27] Familial clustering and the benefits of angiotensin-converting enzyme (ACE) inhibition on diabetic nephropathy have stimulated investigation into the genetics of the renin–angiotensin system. Increased levels of ACE have been found in patients with type 1 diabetes and nephropathy, particularly carriers of certain abnormal alleles of the ACE gene.[28] In a study of type 1 patients with CKD compared with type 1 patients with diabetes for at least 15 years without microalbuminuria, the presence of the double deletion (DD) genotype at the ACE locus increased twofold the risk of severe renal failure (CKD-5).[29] There are also non-genomic and environmental influences on gene polymorphism and physiology which may explain divergent findings of gene polymorphism in diabetic nephropathy.[30] No single gene defect is likely to identify those at risk of nephropathy.

Since CKD is known to be more prevalent in certain ethnic groups – Native Americans, Mexican-Americans, and African-Americans – than in Caucasian-Americans, there should be an increased awareness and increased vigilance of these high-risk populations.

The typical histological picture is diffuse sclerosis of the mesangium and thickening of the basement membrane. Nodular glomerulosclerosis (Kimmelstiel–Wilson kidney) is common and often co-exists with global glomerular sclerosis on the same biopsy or autopsy specimen.

Clinical Picture and Spectrum of Diabetic Nephropathy

Diabetic nephropathy tends to be a progressive disease that often leads to end-stage renal failure (CKD-5). A succession of stages of nephropathy is well described (Table 22.2). The clinical problem is that once the disease has become overt, a great deal of renal damage has already occurred, and the opportunity for intervention is limited.

Table 22.2 Classification of chronic kidney disease (CKD) based on glomerular filtration rate (GFR)[a]

Stage 1: GFR >90 ml/min/1.73 m^2
Stage 2: GFR 60–90 ml/min/1.73 m^2
Stage 3: GFR 30–59 ml/min/1.73 m^2
Stage 4: GFR 15–29 ml/min/1.73 m^2
Stage 5: GFR <15 ml/min/1.73 m^2

[a]Modification of diet in renal disease (MDRD) equation for calculation of GFR (calculators found on many internet sites)
GFR (mL/min/1.73 m^2) = $175 \times (S_{cr})^{-1.154} \times (Age)^{-0.203} \times (0.742$ if female) $\times$ (1.210 if African-American) (conventional units)
Note: S_{cr} stands for serum creatinine

Ironically, the earliest clinically demonstrable effect of diabetes on the kidney is an increase in glomerular filtration rate, reported in both type 1[31] and type 2[32] diabetes. Such hyperfiltration is a harbinger of subsequent deterioration of renal function. It is felt that the increase in glomerular pressure, coupled with hypertrophy, is a stimulus to the processes that ultimately cause glomerular sclerosis. This hypothesis provides a rationale for treatment modalities that lower glomerular capillary pressure (see below). Following the onset of hyperfiltration there is usually a latency period of 5–20 years, during which the basement membranes gradually become damaged, setting off the sequence of events that leads to end-stage renal failure.

Injury to basement membranes ultimately leads to an increase in glomerular permeability to albumin (vide supra). Normal urinary albumin loss is <10 mg/day. Patients with early diabetic nephropathy develop urinary albumin excretion rates of 30–300 mg/day, which has been termed "microalbuminuria" and may be detected on a 24-hour urine specimen or by a "spot" urine albumin:creatinine ratio > 0.3 on a random urine specimen. At this stage a regular urinalysis will be negative for protein. Testing for microalbuminuria should be performed when the patient is feeling well and is at rest, as exercise, fever, acute illness, congestive heart failure, and severe hyperglycemia or hypertension may transiently elevate urinary albumin. Screening for microalbuminuria should be done annually in all patients with type 2 or type 1 diabetes after 5 years or at puberty since urinary albumin excretion increases in all individuals with diabetes at about 20% per year.

Microalbuminuria has been shown to be a good predictor of progressive diabetic nephropathy.[33] About 75–80% of type 1 and 34–42% of type 2 diabetes patients with microalbuminuria will go on to develop renal dysfunction. The next stage is overt proteinuria (macroalbuminuria), which is detectable on standard urinalysis. Overt proteinuria presages an inexorable decline in GFR in 75% of type 1 and 20% of type 2 diabetes patients. The rate of decline is variable from patient to patient (up to 20 ml/min of GFR/year), but the development and severity of hypertension are major influences.[34] Since both diabetes and hypertension can cause endothelial injury, there may be a synergistic effect of these processes on glomerular capillaries.[35] Other risk factors for progression of the renal dysfunction are listed in Table 22.1.

Up to this point the renal dysfunction is usually asymptomatic. However, in the next stage the proteinuria increases to nephrotic levels (above 3 g/day or a urine protein:creatinine ratio $\geq$ 3:1). The full-blown nephrotic syndrome usually ensues, with clinical edema and laboratory evidence of hypoalbuminemia and hyperlipidemia. The latter may, of course, worsen the systemic vascular disease. The nephrotic patient is also at risk for hypercoagulability, which can lead to coronary or cerebral arterial occlusion, peripheral ischemia, or renal vein thrombosis with its risk of pulmonary embolism. By this time diabetic retinopathy is also usually manifested.

Normal kidneys remove around 1/3 of circulating insulin from the blood.[36] Once GFR falls to around 30 ml/min or less (late Stage 3–Stage 4 CKD), the half-life of insulin is increased by as much as 2.5-fold,[37] so small doses of insulin can have a profound and prolonged hypoglycemic effect. In type 2 diabetes the temporal rhythms of insulin secretion often become abnormal.[31]

Patients with diabetic renal disease whose GFR is < 60 ml/min/1.73 m^2 (i.e., Stages 3–4) are at risk to develop hyporeninemic hypoaldosteronism. This complication is caused by impaired renin release due to atrophy of the juxtaglomerular apparatus, with low aldosterone levels. The atrophy of renin-secreting cells has been variously attributed to concomitant autonomic neuropathy,[38] β-adrenergic stimulation-induced renin secretion, volume expansion inhibiting renin production,[39] and suppression of renin by retained potassium.[40] The response to endogenous and exogenous mineralocorticoid is impaired by the tubulo-interstitial nephritis that usually accompanies chronic diabetic glomerulosclerosis. Clinically, both hyperkalemia and hyperchloremic metabolic acidosis are seen, due to the failure of mineralocorticoid stimulation of K$^+$ and H$^+$ secretion in the distal nephron. Drugs that block the renin–angiotensin–aldosterone axis, which are commonly used in the treatment of diabetic nephropathy, may exacerbate these electrolyte disorders, especially the high K$^+$. Treatment usually involves a low-potassium diet coupled with a diuretic,[33] pharmacologic doses of mineralocorticoid,[41] or sodium bicarbonate.

Risk of Other Complications

Patients with types 1 and 2 diabetes mellitus are at risk for vascular complications and investigators have typically separated macroangiopathy (coronary syndromes, stroke, and peripheral vascular disease) from microangiopathy (retinopathy and nephropathy). The distinction is largely anatomic, as vascular disease involves a common pathophysiology of endothelial injury, activation of the renin–angiotensin–aldosterone (RAA) system, oxidative stress, inflammation and cytokine dysregulation, and disordered repair/remodeling. While there is evidence of simultaneous damage to the microcirculation of the retina and glomerulus, the clinical presentation may be variably represented in the triopathy of diabetes – retinopathy, nephropathy, and neuropathy. Recently, a link between insulin and cardiovascular disease has been described in type 2 diabetes,[42] while a reduced cardiovascular risk was associated with pioglitazone[43] with equivalent glucose control. On the other hand, rosiglitazone has been shown to increase cardiovascular risk.[44]

Treatment of Diabetic Nephropathy

Kidney biopsy is not typically performed to diagnose diabetic glomerulosclerosis, particularly if diabetic retinopathy is present. Detection of microalbuminuria indicates incipient nephropathy. Quantification of proteinuria allows surveillance and identifies progression, with clinical albuminuria suggesting established nephropathy. Interventional clinical trials have demonstrated proteinuria to be a surrogate end point for treatment and subsequent reduction of renal and cardiovascular disease risk.

Tight glycemic control is effective in the prevention and treatment of established nephropathy. In type 1 diabetes, intensive insulin therapy – decreasing mean glycated hemogloblin A1c to <7% – reduces the risk of development of microalbuminuria, progression to clinical albuminuria, and the rate of urinary albumin excretion (UAE).[45,46] Decreased hyperfiltration and hypertrophy are evident within 3 weeks of intensive insulin therapy.[47] Tight glycemic control with an intensive insulin regimen appears to provide sustained benefit in incident microalbuminuria, albuminuria, and creatinine elevation for nearly a decade, even with later recidivism in the degree of glycemic control.[48] Improved glycemic control also reduces microvascular disease in type 2 diabetes. In the UKPDS, intensive blood glucose control with sulfonylureas, metformin, and insulin reduced the risk of microvascular disease by 25% in older, obese patients, when compared with dietary control.[49] The UKPDS investigators demonstrated a strong association between treatment of hyperglycemia and reduction in diabetic complications, with a 37% microvascular risk reduction for every 1% decrease in mean hemoglobin A1c.[50] This study has come under scrutiny recently, and others have shown no clear benefit in terms of outcomes. [51] In a trial of younger, non-obese type 2 diabetes patients, intensive insulin therapy also reduced development and progression of nephropathy, as defined by proteinuria.[52] There is some debate as to the optimal target hemoglobin A1c and glycemia threshold for microvascular risk.

Blood pressure (BP) management is another well-established intervention for diabetic nephropathy, although an optimal target range is uncertain. In type 1 diabetic patients with normotension (<120/80 mmHg), there may be an association between progression to microalbuminuria and higher mean 24-h ambulatory BP; particularly higher night-time diastolic BP blunting night/day circadian variation.[53] However, the EUCLID Study Group reported no significant reduction in proteinuria among normotensive (<120/80 mmHg), normoalbuminuric type 1 patients with additional diastolic BP reduction over 2 years.[54] In normoalbuminuric type 2 patients, additional proteinuria reduction is possible with BP reduction within the category designated as pre-hypertension (<140/80 mmHg).[55] Finally, UKPDS data suggest that systolic BP reduction to less than 120 mmHg confers the lowest risk of microvascular complications, with a more than 13% risk reduction observed for each 10 mmHg decrease in systolic BP.[56] In summary, diabetic individuals with and without proteinuria may well benefit from measures to reduce SBPs below 140 mmHg and at least to 120 mmHg.

Renin–angiotensin–aldosterone system blockers are the preferred first-line agents for diabetic patients with hypertension or nephropathy in many guideline statements.[57,58] This makes sense in view of the pathophysiologic activation of the RAAS system. Decreased risk of doubling of serum creatinine, death, dialysis, and transplant as well as progression to clinical proteinuria have been demonstrated with angiotensin-converting enzyme inhibitors (ACEI's) in the Collaborative Study Group[59] and Micro-Hope[60] trials, respectively. Angiotensin receptor blockers (ARBs) also decreased progression to clinical albuminuria in IRMA-II,[61] and to doubling of serum creatinine, progression to CKD, and death in both the RENAAL[62] and IDNT[63] trials. Claims of specific renoprotective benefit in all of these trials are confounded by insufficient BP data[59] and unequal blood pressure reduction as compared with a placebo.[60–62] Furthermore, in trials where equivalent blood pressure reduction was achieved, ACEI's were not superior to a β-blocker[64] nor a dihydropyridine calcium-channel blocker[65] in reducing proteinuria. A meta-analysis[66] has also concluded that when compared with other active intervention providing equal BP reduction, ACEIs and ARBs provide no specific renoprotection in diabetic patients with regard to creatinine, GFR, or progression to CKD, although they improved proteinuria. The preponderance of evidence suggests that achievement of sufficient blood pressure reduction appears to be more beneficial than use of any particular class of antihypertensive agent.

Aldosterone and angiotensin II (AII) likely contribute to glomerulosclerosis and proteinuria in experimental nephropathy;[67] and aldosterone breakthrough in diabetic patients on ACEI monotherapy is associated with refractory proteinuria[68] and declining GFR.[69] Aldosterone breakthrough is likely the result of AII breakthrough due to either inadequate ACE inhibition[70] or non-ACE-dependent generation of AII.[71] Therapeutic methods to antagonize breakthrough with high-dose ARB therapy,[72] combination of ACEI and ARB,[73] and use of ARB or ACEI with aldosterone antagonists[74] have all been demonstrated to reduce proteinuria in diabetic nephropathy with surprisingly infrequent hyperkalemia. These measures may reduce diabetic proteinuria in short term studies solely through blood pressure reduction. A well-powered study[75] involving eplerenone (a non-gynecomastia producing aldosterone antagonist) (with ACEI) suggests epleronone is well tolerated, and provides proteinuria reduction at 50 mg, independent of blood pressure. There are currently no studies of combination therapy involving endpoints other than proteinuria and such measures are not advised in greatly advanced CKD without potassium monitoring. Renin antagonists such as aliskerin have not yet been sufficiently studied in diabetic patients with nephropathy.

Other measures may be of potential benefit to attenuate development and progression of diabetic nephropathy. The use of HMG-CoA reductase inhibitors (statins) may have a modest effect on preservation of GFR and proteinuria reduction in patients with established cardiovascular disease. This observation is the result of meta-analyses[76, 77] of cardiovascular trial data as no large controlled trials with specified renal endpoints have been conducted. Given the strong correlation between cardiovascular and renal risk factors, statins should be included in comprehensive diabetic treatment regimens. Future therapies may include metalloprotease inhibitors, glycosaminoglycans (GAG), cross-link breakers, AGE receptor inhibitors, and endothelin-converting enzyme inhibitors.

Internet Sites Pertaining to Diabetic Nephropathy

1. http://care.diabetesjournals.org/cgi/content/full/27/suppl_1/s79
2. http://kidney.niddk.nih.gov/kudiseases/pubs/kdd/
3. http://clinicaltrials.gov
4. http://www.kidney.org

References

1. *United States Renal Data System: 2006 Annual Data Report*. Bethesda: US Department of Health and Human Services, Public Health Service, National Institutes of Health; 2006.
2. Hossain P, Kawar B, El Nahas M. Obesity and diabetes in the developing world – a growing challenge. *N Eng J Med*. 2007;356:213–215.
3. Ramezani M, Ghoddousi K, Hashemi M, et al. Diabetes as the cause of end-stage renal disease affects the pattern of post kidney transplant rehospitalizations. *Transplant Proc*. 2007;39:966–969.
4. Burroughs TE, Swindle J, Takemoto S, et al. Diabetic complications associated with new-onset diabetes mellitus in renal transplant recipients. *Transplantation*. 2007;83:1027–1034.
5. Centers for Disease Control and Prevention (CDC). Prevalence of chronic kidney disease and associated risk factors – United States, 1999–2004. *MMWR Morb Mortal Wkly Rep*. 2007;56:161–165.
6. Osterby R, Parving HH, Hommel E, et al. Glomerular structure and function in diabetic nephropathy. Early to advanced stages. *Diabetes*. 1990;39:1057–1063.
7. Gilbert RE, Cooper ME. The tubulointerstitium in progressive diabetic kidney disease: more than an aftermath of glomerular injury? *Kidney Int*. 1999;56:1627–1637.
8. Brownlee M. Biochemistry and molecular cell biology of diabetic complications. *Nature*. 2001;414:813–820.
9. Boyle PJ. Diabetes mellitus and macrovascular disease: mechanisms and mediators. *Am J Med*. 2007 Sep;120(9 Suppl 2): S12–S17.
10. Cavusoglu AC, Bilgili S, Alaluf A, et al. Vascular endothelial growth factor level in the serum of diabetic patients with retinopathy. *Ann Ophthalmol (Skokie)*. 2007;39:205–208.
11. Ryan GJ. New pharmacologic approaches to treating diabetic retinopathy. *Am J Health Syst Pharm*. 2007;64(17 Suppl 12): S15–S21.
12. Zatz R, Dunn BR, Meyer TW, et al. Prevention of diabetic glomerulopathy by pharmacological amelioration of glomerular capillary hypertension. *J Clin Invest*. 1986;77:1925–1930.
13. Gruden G, Zonca S, Hayward A, et al. Mechanical stretch-induced fibronectin and transforming growth factor-beta1 production in human mesangial cells is p38 mitogen-activated protein kinase-dependent. *Diabetes*. 2000;49:655–661.
14. Lassila M, Jandeleit-Dahm K, Seah KK, et al. Imatinib attenuates diabetic nephropathy in apolipoprotein E-knockout mice. *J Am Soc Nephrol*. 2004;15:2125–2138.
15. Izquierdo A, Lopez-Luna P, Ortega A, et al. The parathyroid hormone-related protein system and diabetic nephropathy outcome in streptozotocin-induced diabetes. *Kidney Int*. 2006;69:2171–2177.
16. Wang Y, Zhou J, Minto AW, et al. Altered vitamin D metabolism in type II diabetic mouse glomeruli may provide protection fro diabetic nephropathy. *Kidney Int*. 2006;70:882–891.
17. Zhang Z, Yuan W, Sun L, et al. 1,25 dihydroxy vitamin D3 targeting of NFκB suppresses high glucose-induced MCP-1 expression in mesangial cells. *Kidney Int*. 2007;72:193–201.

18. Zhang Z, Sun L, Wang Y, et al. Renoprotective role of the vitamin D receptor in diabetic nephropathy. *Kidney Int*. 2008;73: 163–167.

19. Earle KS, Walker J, Hill C, et al. Familial clustering of cardiovascular disease in patients with insulin-dependent diabetes and nephropathy. *N Engl J Med*. 1992;325:673–677.

20. Krolewski A, Fogarty D, Warram J. Hypertension and nephropathy in diabetes mellitus: what is inherited and what is acquired? *Diabetes Res Clin Pract*. 1998;39 Suppl:S1–S14.

21. Strojek K, Grzeszczak W, Ritz E. Risk factors for development of diabetic nephropathy: a review. *Nephrol Dial Transplant*. 1997;12(Suppl 2):24–26.

22. Fioretto P, Steffes M, Barbosa J, et al. Is diabetic nephropathy inherited? Studies of glomerular structure in type 1 diabetic sibling pairs. *Diabetes*. 1999;48:865–869.

23. Canani L, Gerchman F, Gross J. Familial clustering of diabetic nephropathy in Brazilian type 2 diabetic patients. *Diabetes*. 1999;48:909–913.

24. Marshall SM. Recent advances in diabetic nephropathy. *Postgrad Med J*. 2004;80:624–633.

25. Krolewski A, Canessa M, Warram J, et al. Predisposition to hypertension and susceptibility to renal disease in insulin-dependent diabetes mellitus. *N Engl J Med*. 1998;318:140–145.

26. Fujita J, Tsuda K, Seno M, et al. Erythrocyte sodium-lithium countertransport activity as a marker of predisposition to hypertension and diabetic nephropathy in NIDDM. *Diabetes Care*. 1994;17:977–982.

27. Lindsay R, Little J, Jaap A, et al. Diabetic nephropathy in associated with an increased familial risk of stroke. *Diabetes Care*. 1999;22:422–425.

28. Freire MB, van Dijk DJ, Erman A, et al. DNA polymorphisms in the ACE gene, serum ACE activity and the risk of nephropathy in insulin-dependent diabetes mellitus. *Nephrol Dial Transplant*. 1998;13:2553–2558.

29. Vleming LJ, van der Pijl JW, Lemkes HH, et al. The DD genotype of the ACE gene polymorphism is associated with progression of diabetic nephropathy to end stage renal failure in IDDM. *Clin Nephrol*. 1999;51:133–140.

30. Miller JA, Scholey JW. The impact of renin-angiotensin system polymorphisms on physiological and pathophysiological processes in humans. *Curr Opin Nephrol Hypertens*. 2004;13:101–106.

31. Mogensen CE. Glomerular filtration rate and renal plasma flow in short-term and long-term juvenile diabetes mellitus. *Scand J Clin Lab Invest*. 1971;28:91–100.

32. Nowack R, Raum E, Blum W, et al. Renal hemodynamics in recent-onset type II diabetes. *Am J Kidney Dis*. 1992;20:342–347.

33. Parving HH, Chaturvedi N, Viberti GC, et al. Does microalbuminuria predict diabetic nephropathy? *Diabetes Care*. 2002;25:406–407.

34. Stephenson JM, Kenny S, Stevens LK, et al. Proteinuria and mortality in diabetes: the WHO multinational study of vascular disease in diabetes. *Diabet Med*. 1995;12:149–155.

35. Sowers JR, Epstein M. Diabetes mellitus and associated hypertension, vascular disease, and nephropathy. *Hypertension*. 1995;26:869–879.

36. Herlitz H, Aurell M, Holm G, et al. Renal degradation of insulin in patients with renal hypertension. *Scand J Urol Nephrol*. 1983;17:109–113.

37. Feneberg R, Sparber M, Veldhuis JD, et al. Altered temporal organization of plasma insulin oscillations in chronic renal failure. *J Clin Endocrinol Metab*. 2002;87:1965–1973.

38. Chimori K, Miyazaki S, Kosaka J, et al. The significance of autonomic neuropathy in the elevation of inactive renin in diabetes mellitus. *Clin Exp Hypertens*. 1987;9:1–18.

39. Oh MS, Carroll HJ, Clemmons JE, et al. A mechanism for hyporeninemic hypoaldosteronism in chronic renal disease. *Metabolism*. 1974;23:1157–1166.

40. Vander AJ. Direct effects of potassium on renin secretion and renal function. *Am J Physiol*. 1970;219:455–459.

41. Sebastian A, Schambelan M, Lindenfeld S, et al. Amelioration of metabolic acidosis with fludrocortisone therapy in hyporeninemic hypoaldosteronism. *N Engl J Med*. 1977;297:576–583.

42. Eurich DT, McAlister FA, Blackburn DF, et al. Benefits and harms of antidiabetic agents in patients with diabetes and heart failure: systematic review. *BMJ*. 2007;335:497.

43. Lincoff AM, Wolski K, Nicholls SJ, Nissen SE. Pioglitazone and risk of cardiovascular events in patients with type 2 diabetes mellitus: a meta-analysis of randomized trials. *J Am Med Assoc*. 2007;298:1180–1188.

44. Singh S, Loke YK, Furberg CD. Long-term risk of cardiovascular events with rosiglitazone: a meta-analysis. *J Am Med Assoc*. 2007;298:1189–1195.

45. DCCT Research Group. Effect of intensive therapy on the development and progression of diabetic nephropathy in the Diabetic Control and Complications Trial. *Kidney Int*. 1995;47:1703–1720.

46. Reichard P, Nilsson BY, Rosenqvist U. The effect of long-term intensified insulin treatment on the development of microvascular complications of diabetes mellitus. *N Eng J Med*. 1993;329:304–309.

47. Tuttle KR, Bruton JL. Effect of insulin therapy on renal hemodynamic response to amino acids and renal hypertrophy in non-insulin-dependent diabetes. *Kidney Int*. 1992;42:167–173.

48. Writing Team for the Diabetes Control and Complications Trial/Epidemiology of Diabetes Interventions and Complications Research Group. Sustained effect of intensive treatment of type 1 diabetes mellitus on development and progression of diabetic nephropathy: the Epidemiology of Diabetes Interventions and Complications (EDIC) study. *J Am Med Assoc*. 2003;290: 2159–2167.

49. UK Prospective Diabetes Study (UKPDS) Group. Intensive blood-glucose control with sulphonylureas or insulin compared with conventional treatment and risk of complications in patients with type 2 diabetes (UKPDS 33). *Lancet*. 1998;352:837–853.

50. Stratton IM, Adler AI, Neil HA, et al. Association of glycaemia with macrovascular and microvascular complications of type 2 diabetes (UKPDS 35): prospective observational study. *Br Med J*. 2000;321:405–412.

51. McCormack J, Greenhalgh T. Seeing what you want to see in randomised controlled trials: versions and perversions of UKPDS data. United Kingdom prospective diabetes study. *BMJ*. 2000;320:1720–1723.

52. Ohkubo Y, Kishikawa H, Araki E, et al. Intensive insulin therapy prevents the progression of diabetic microvascular complications in Japanese patients with non-insulin-dependent diabetes mellitus: a randomized prospective 6-year study. *Diabetes Res Clin Pract*. 1995;28:103–117.

53. Poulsen PL, Ebbehøj E, Hansen KW, et al. Characteristics and prognosis of normoalbuminuric type 1 diabetic patients. *Diabetes Care*. 1999;22(S2):B72–B75.

54. The EUCLID Study Group. Randomised placebo-controlled trial of lisinopril in normotensive patients with insulin-dependent diabetes and normoalbuminuria or microalbuminuria. *Lancet*. 1997;349:1787–1792.

55. Ravid M, Brosh D, Levi Z, et al. Use of enalapril to attenuate decline in renal function in normotensive, normoalbuminuric patients with type 2 diabetes mellitus. A randomized, controlled trial. *Ann Intern Med*. 1998;128:982–988.

56. Adler AI, Stratton IM, Neil HA, et al. Association of systolic blood pressure with macrovascular and microvascular complications of type 2 diabetes (UKPDS 36): prospective observational study. *Br Med J*. 2000;321:412–419.

57. The JNC 7 Report. *J Am Med Assoc*. 2003;289:2560–2572.

58. Hypertension management in adults with diabetes. *Diabetes Care*. 2004;27(S1):S65–S67.

59. Lewis EJ, Hunsicker LG, Bain RP, et al. The effect of angiotensin-converting enzyme inhibition on diabetic nephropathy. *N Engl J Med*. 1993;329:1456–1462.

60. Effects of ramipril on cardiovascular and microvascular outcomes in people with diabetes mellitus: results of the HOPE study and MICRO-HOPE substudy. *Lancet*. 2000;355:253–259.

61. Parving HH, Brenner BM, Cooper ME, et al. The effect of irbesartan on the development of diabetic nephropathy in patients with type 2 diabetes. *N Eng J Med*. 2001;345:870–878.

62. Brenner BM, Cooper ME, de Zeeuw D, et al. RENAAL Study Investigators. Effects of losartan on renal and cardiovascular outcomes in patients with type 2 diabetes and nephropathy. *N Engl J Med*. 2001;345:861–869.

63. Lewis EJ, Hunsicker LG, Clarke WR, et al. Collaborative Study Group. Renoprotective effect of the angiotensin-receptor antagonist irbesartan in patients with nephropathy due to type 2 diabetes. *N Engl J Med*. 2001;345:851–860.

64. UK Prospective Diabetes Study Group. Efficacy of atenolol and captopril in reducing risk of macrovascular and microvascular complications in type 2 diabetes: UKPDS 39. *Br Med J*. 1998;317:713–720.

65. Schrier RW, Estacio RO, Esler A, et al. Effects of aggressive blood pressure control in normotensive type 2 diabetic patients on albuminuria, retinopathy and strokes. *Kidney Int*. 2002;61:1086–1097.

66. Casas JP, Chua W, Loukogeorgakis S, et al. Effect of inhibitors of the renin-angiotensin system and other antihypertensive drugs on renal outcomes: systematic review and meta-analysis. *Lancet*. 2005;366:2026–2033.

67. Green EL, Kren S, Hostetter TH. Role of aldosterone in the remnant kidney model. *JCI*. 1996;98:1063–1068.

68. Sato A, Hayashi K, Naruse M, et al. Effectiveness of aldosterone blockade in patients with diabetic nephropathy. *Hypertension*. 2003;41:64–68.

69. Schjoedt KJ, Anderen S, Rossing P, et al. Aldosterone escape during blockade of the renin–angiotensin–aldosterone system in diabetic nephropathy is associated with enhanced decline in glomerular filtration rate. *Diabetologia*. 2004;47:1936–1939.

70. van den Meiracker AH, Man in 't Veld AJ, Admiraal PJ, et al. Partial escape of angiotensin converting enzyme (ACE) inhibition during prolonged ACE inhibitor treatment: does it exist and does it affect the antihypertensive response? *J Hypertens*. 1992;10:803–812.

71. Hollenberg NK, Osei SY, Lansang MC, et al. Salt intake and non-ACE pathways for intrarenal angiotensin II generation in man. *J Renin Angiotensin Aldosterone Syst*. 2001;2:14–18.

72. Weinberg AJ, Zappe DH, Ashton M, et al. Safety and tolerability of high-dose angiotensin receptor blocker therapy in patients with chronic kidney disease: a pilot study. *Am J Nephrol*. 2004;24:340–345.

73. Mogensen CE, Neldam S, Tikkanen I, et al. Randomised controlled trial of dual blockade of renin-angiotensin system in patients with hypertension, microalbuminuria, and non-insulin dependent diabetes: the candesartan and lisinopril microalbuminuria (CALM) study. *Br Med J*. 2000;321:1440–1444.

74. van den Meiracker AH, Baggen RG, Pauli S, et al. Spironolactone in type 2 diabetic nephropathy: Effects on proteinuria, blood pressure and renal function. *J Hypertens*. 2006;24:2285–2292.

75. Epstein M, Williams GH, Weinberger M, et al. Selective aldosterone blockade with eplerenone reduces albuminuria in patients with type 2 diabetes. *Clin J Am Soc Nephrol*. 2006;1:940–951.

76. Sandhu S, Wiebe N, Fried LF, et al. Statins for improving renal outcomes: a meta-analysis. *J Am Soc Nephrol*. 2006;17:2006–2016.

77. Cholesterol Treatment Trialists (CTT) Collaborators. Efficacy of cholesterol-lowering therapy in 18,686 people with diabetes in 14 randomised trials of statins: a meta-analysis. *Lancet*. 2008;371:117–125.

Chapter 23
Diabetic Neuropathy

Russell L. Chin and Michael Rubin

Introduction

Diabetes mellitus (DM) is estimated to affect approximately 20 million Americans (90% with type 2 and 10% with type 1 DM) and is the most common cause of peripheral neuropathy in the United States. There is evidence to suggest that the incidence of neuropathy increases with the duration and severity of disease, and that strict glycemic control delays its development and progression, particularly in patients with type 1 diabetes.[1–3] The prevalence of neuropathy is estimated to be about 10% at the time of diagnosis, increasing to ≥50% in patients diagnosed for longer than 5 years.[4]

Data on the exact incidence and natural history of neuropathic complications are limited. In the Rochester Diabetic Neuropathy Study, a 1.3% incidence of DM (mostly type 2) was determined in a population of 64,573. Sixty-six percent of patients with type 1 and 59% of patients with type 2 diabetes had some form of neuropathy but only 20% were symptomatic.[5]

Neuropathies in DM are a heterogeneous group of disorders with different mechanisms accounting for the various forms of neuropathy.[6]

Neuropathy is the most common late complication of DM and may lead to a significant burden of disability for the patient including painful foot ulceration, Charcot neuroarthropathy, and symptomatic autonomic dysfunction.[2]

In this chapter, we focus on the clinical characteristics of the most common neuropathies resulting from diabetes, their hypothesized etiopathogenesis, and the available treatment modalities.

Definitions

Neuropathy is a nonspecific term implying an abnormality of nerve. It is often used synonymously and imprecisely with *polyneuropathy* or *peripheral neuropathy*, the latter two being equivalent.

Polyneuropathy or *peripheral neuropathy* identifies a predominantly distal, symmetric abnormality of nerves, that begins in the feet and may gradually ascend. *Mononeuropathy* indicates the presence of an abnormality of a single nerve. *Multiple mononeuropathy* or *mononeuropathy multiplex* describes the presence of an abnormality of more than one nerve. Multiple nerves are involved, usually in a random, asymmetric manner. Note that these terms imply nothing regarding the underlying etiology.

M. Rubin (✉)
Electromyography Laboratory, Weill Cornell Medical College, New York Presbyterian Hospital, New York, NY, USA
e-mail: mprubin@med.cornell.edu

L. Poretsky (ed.), *Principles of Diabetes Mellitus*, DOI 10.1007/978-0-387-09841-8_23,
© Springer Science+Business Media, LLC 2010

Classification

Numerous classifications have been proposed for the various neuropathies which occur in DM, some based on clinical subtype, and others based on pathophysiological mechanisms or both.[6] Recognizing the clinical patterns and the suspected etiopathogenesis allows for more precise prognostication. For example, a distal symmetric sensorimotor polyneuropathy, which is the most common diabetic neuropathy subtype, is indolently progressive and secondary to metabolic derangements, whereas an asymmetric, non-length-dependent neuropathy (e.g., diabetic lumbosacral radiculoplexus neuropathy or DLRPN) is believed to be secondary to a microvasculitic process and has a monophasic course with spontaneous, slow improvement.

For this review, we propose the classification outlined in Table 23.1.

Table 23.1 Classification of diabetic neuropathies

Symmetrical length-dependent neuropathy
1. Diabetic sensorimotor polyneuropathy (DPN)
2. Sensory neuropathies
    Predominantly small fiber +/– impaired glucose tolerance
    Painful distal neuropathy with weight loss, "diabetic cachexia"
    Mixed large and small fiber
3. Diabetic autonomic neuropathy (DAN)

Asymmetrical neuropathies (non-length-dependent)
1. Diabetic radiculoplexus neuropathies or radiculoneuropathy
    Lumbosacral (DLRPN)
    Thoracic (DTRN)
    Cervical (DCRPN)
2. Cranial neuropathy
3. Mononeuropathies

Modified from Dyck et al.[7]

Clinical Characteristics

The most common presenting symptoms of neuropathy are summarized in Table 23.2. A directed line of questioning is essential to thoroughly investigate the patient's problem, which may include more than one diabetes-related process. It is also important to consider other disease processes that could result in similar presentations, but would merit different therapies. (See Table 23.3.)

Table 23.2 Neuropathic symptoms and signs in diabetes mellitus

Sensory
1. Negative symptoms: numbness, deadness, "cotton wool feeling," "thick," "less sensitive," loss of dexterity, painless injuries, ulcers
2. Positive symptoms: burning, prickling, pain, hypersensitivity to light touch, stabbing, electric shock-like, tearing, tight, band-like

Motor
1. Proximal weakness: difficulty rising from a seated position, difficulty climbing stairs, falls secondary to knees "giving out," difficulty raising arms above the shoulders (as in combing or shampooing hair)
2. Distal weakness: difficulty turning keys or opening jars, impaired fine hand coordination, toe scuffing, tripping, foot slapping

Adapted from Windebank and Feldman[8]

Table 23.3 Differential diagnosis of diabetic polyneuropathy

Hereditary neuropathies
    Hereditary motor and sensory neuropathy (e.g., Charcot–Marie Tooth syndrome)
    Hereditary sensory and autonomic neuropathy (e.g., familial dysautonomia)
Acquired neuropathies
    Autoimmune processes (e.g., Sjogren's, vasculitis)
    Infectious (e.g., Lyme, HIV, syphilis, leprosy)
    Demyelinating (e.g., chronic inflammatory demyelinating polyneuropathy)
    Toxic (e.g., medication related)
    Nutritional disorders (e.g., alcohol, B12 deficiency)
    Idiopathic

Modified from Dyck et al.[7]

Diabetic Polyneuropathy (DPN)

More than 80% of patients with clinical diabetic neuropathy have DPN. This neuropathy begins and remains most pronounced in the feet, and a combination of sensory (large and small fiber), motor, and autonomic nerves may be affected. Clinically, the first signs are a reduction or loss of ankle reflexes, accompanied by decreased or absent vibratory sensation in the toes. This may progress to sensory loss involving multiple modalities including pain, temperature, position, and vibration, with positive or negative symptomatology. Weakness and atrophy of the small foot muscles and ankle dorsiflexors, with varying degrees of autonomic dysfunction, may follow. The predominantly distal "stocking and glove" pattern of involvement develops because the distal portions of the longest nerves, being furthest from the nucleus in the dorsal root ganglion or anterior horn cell, are affected first.

The electrodiagnostic findings of DPN (see "Electrodiagnostic Features") include slowed nerve conduction velocities and diminished amplitudes – findings that correlate well with clinical abnormalities.[9] Most patients also have an absent sympathetic skin response and many demonstrate a decreased heart rate response to deep breathing and Valsalva maneuver.[5,10]

The clinical course of DPN is characterized by an insidious onset (usually following several years of hyperglycemia) and a slow course. Although estimated to occur in 54% of type 1 and 45% of type 2, most patients are asymptomatic and painful forms are relatively rare.[6] DPN has been found to be strongly associated with concurrent retinopathy and nephropathy. These points may be useful in differentiating DPN from other diabetic neuropathies.

Sensory Neuropathies

The symptoms of a "small fiber neuropathy" are attributed to involvement of unmyelinated C and thinly myelinated Aδ fibers, resulting in burning pains or thermal allodynia (pain resulting from contact with warm or cold water). Autonomic impairment (such as altered sweating, flushing, and skin discoloration) may also be seen. On examination, pinprick and thermal sensation may be reduced in the feet with normal or minimally abnormal nerve conduction studies. Measurement of epidermal nerve density by skin biopsy is a recognized method for the diagnosis of small fiber neuropathy (see "Other Investigations").[11] Asymptomatic diabetic patients may have a measurable, length-dependent reduction of distal epidermal nerves as an early sign of incipient neuropathy, analogous to the finding of microalbuminuria as an early sign of diabetic nephropathy.[12]

"Pre-diabetes" or impaired glucose tolerance (IGT) is defined to be a fasting glucose level between 110 and 126 mg/dL or a 2-h glucose level between 140 and 199 mg/dL, following a 75-g glucose tolerance test. IGT may be a cause or contribute to the development of small fiber neuropathy.[13]

An acute, painful, small fiber polyneuropathy with cachexia and weight loss (also known as "diabetic cachexia") may be a distinct entity, separate from DPN. It has particular clinical hallmarks (a monophasic course, a lack of association with the duration or severity of diabetes, and an increased incidence in men with type 2 DM) that are more reminiscent of diabetic lumbosacral radiculoplexus neuropathy (DLRPN).[6]

Diabetic Autonomic Neuropathy (DAN)

The prevalence of autonomic impairment is 54% in type 1 and 73% in type 2 DM.[14] The autonomic nerves may be involved in isolation or in combination with other nerve types.

Diabetic autonomic neuropathy (DAN) is associated with increased mortality.[15] Although more commonly associated with long-standing diabetes, it may evolve early in the course of disease. DAN presents mainly in the form of cardiac autonomic neuropathy, but may also affect the gastrointestinal, genitourinary, thermoregulatory, and pupillary systems. The cardiovascular hallmark is reduced heart rate variability with clinical manifestations including light-headedness, orthostatic hypotension, and syncope.[16] Patients with DAN may have complement-fixing autoantibodies to sympathetic and parasympathetic ganglia, but their significance and pathogenic role have yet to be determined. They do not appear to be associated with cardiac dysautonomia.[17]

Presenting symptoms vary depending on the organ system involved (see Table 23.4). Impotence may be an early manifestation of autonomic dysfunction, occurring in 30–60% of male patients. The incidence of gastrointestinal symptoms is reportedly as high as 75% and symptoms of either increased or decreased gastric motility may coexist.[18]

Table 23.4 Autonomic symptoms by organ system

Sudomotor: loss of sweating or excessive sweating in defined areas, gustatory sweating, dry skin
Cardiovascular: postural light-headedness, fainting, micturition syncope, cough syncope, exertional syncope
Pupillary: usually asymptomatic, poor dark adaptation, poor tolerance of bright lights
Sexual: impotence, loss of ejaculation, retrograde ejaculation, inability to reach sexual climax
Urinary: urgency, incontinence, dribbling, hesitancy
Gastrointestinal: nausea, vomiting, early satiety, nocturnal diarrhea

A careful history is crucial. Additionally, bedside testing for dry skin, pupillary reactivity, and heart rate and blood pressure variability in the supine and seated positions are simple screening methods for autonomic dysfunction. Sophisticated quantifiable tests for dysautonomia, including skin sympathetic responses, quantitative sudomotor axon reflex test (QSART), thermoregulatory sweat test, sweat imprints, and pupil edge light cycle testing, are beyond the scope of primary care practices. Management of the more common manifestations of DAN is outlined in Table 23.5.

Table 23.5 Management of DAN-related disorders

1. Impotence:
   Meds: α2-adrenergic receptor blockers (e.g., yohimbine), sildenafil citrate
   Vacuum devices, penile injections or implants
2. Neurogenic bladder:
   Intermittent self-catheterization
3. Gastroparesis:
   Reduce meal size, limit fats, and high calorie foods
   Meds: cisapride, domperidone, erythromycin, metoclopramide
4. Orthostatic hypotension:
   Head elevation at night (prevents Na and water loss and supine hypertension)
   Compression stockings
   Increase salt intake to 10–20 g
   Meds: fludrocortisone, midodrine, phenylpropanolamine, NSAID's (inhibit prostaglandins)

Diabetic Radiculoplexus Neuropathy

This group of asymmetrical, non-length-dependent neuropathies may be divided into three subtypes: lumbosacral radiculoplexus neuropathy (DLRPN), thoracic radiculoneuropathy (DTRN), and cervical radiculoplexus neuropathy (DCRPN).

Diabetic Lumbosacral Radiculoplexus Neuropathy (DLRPN)

DLRPN (also known as diabetic amyotrophy, femoral neuropathy, proximal motor neuropathy, or proximal diabetic neuropathy) is the most common of these asymmetric neuropathies. It consists of a syndrome of subacutely evolving, painful, usually asymmetric, proximal weakness that tends to affect males in their seventh decade. The patient initially complains of deep, aching pains localized to the anterior thigh with occasional involvement of the buttock and lumbar musculature. These are typically worse at night, and the pain is not increased with straight leg raising, mechanical movement, coughing, or sneezing. The pain is followed by weakness and atrophy of the pelvic girdle and thigh musculature, resulting in weakness of hip flexion and knee stabilization, and depressed or absent knee reflexes. It may evolve into a widespread, bilateral paralytic disorder and is associated with weight loss of 4.5 kg or more. The syndrome is monophasic, with spontaneous, slow, and often incomplete recovery.[19] The pain resolves before motor improvement. Although motor predominant, there is unequivocal evidence that autonomic and sensory nerves are also involved, and there may be a coexisting distal polyneuropathy.

The histopathologic findings include ischemic injury and microvasculitis.[20,21] The cerebrospinal fluid protein is usually elevated, supporting an inflammatory process targeting areas of weakness of the blood–nerve barrier.[6] Patients with nondiabetic LRPN have similar clinical and pathologic findings, further supporting an inflammatory etiology rather than one related to hyperglycemia.[21]

There is no proven course-altering treatment for DLRPN. Glycemic control, physiotherapy, and pain control are recommended. Intravenous immunoglobulins have been reported to be beneficial based on anecdotal evidence,[22,23] but are generally reserved for patients with severe, bilateral, progressive deficits.[19] Intravenous methylprednisolone has been recommended as a therapy for patients in the subacute phase, given its role as a first-line agent for other forms of microvasculitis. It may have a role in reducing the pain, but not the disability associated with this condition.[24]

Diabetic Thoracic Radiculoneuropathy (DTRN) and Diabetic Cervical Radiculoplexus Neuropathy (DCRPN)

DTRN (also known as truncal radiculopathy) is characterized by the acute onset of unilateral, aching, or burning pain in a band-like distribution, affecting the lower thoracic or abdominal wall in older men. Patients with both type 1 and type 2 diabetes are susceptible. The pain is worse at night and may be associated with hypersensitivity to touch and profound weight loss.[25] Focal motor weakness, though rare, may occur and result in localized bulging of the abdominal wall resembling a hernia.[26]

Similar to DLRPN, DTRN is not related to the duration or severity of diabetes, not associated with retinopathy and nephropathy (as seen with DPN), and suspected to be secondary to a vasculitic process resulting in ischemic injury.[27] The syndrome also has a relatively acute onset and monophasic course with remission over 6–18 months.

It is important to exclude visceral pathology including myocardial infarction and dissecting abdominal aortic aneurysm. A history of trauma may suggest rib fracture or chest wall muscle strain. Herpes zoster (shingles) in elderly, immunocompromised patients and the rare occurrence of thoracic intervertebral disc herniation should also be excluded.

Electrophysiologic findings include the presence of denervation potentials in the intercostal, anterior abdominal, and paraspinal muscles at the affected level. Coexisting polyneuropathy is also common.[26]

Management of these patients usually involves only supportive care. Steroids or immunosuppressive treatments have not proven effective.

DCRPN has been reported to occur preceding, concurrent with, or following the lumbosacral syndrome.[28]

Cranial Neuropathy

The incidence of cranial neuropathies [particularly the oculomotor (III), abducens (IV), trochlear (VI), and facial (VII) nerves] in patients with DM is not known, but is suspected to be higher than the incidence in the nondiabetic population.

Oculomotor palsy occurs acutely, over several hours, and is marked by pain and ipsilateral headache associated with diplopia and ptosis with sparing of the pupil. The exam is noteworthy for ophthalmoparesis, usually with pupillary sparing, because the pupillomotor fibers travel circumferentially along the surface of the optic nerve and retain their vascular supply in this otherwise diabetic microinfarctive process.[29,30] The pupil may be involved in up to 18% but this should prompt a search for a compressive lesion such as an aneurysm or tumor. Prognosis is generally excellent with recovery within days to a few months.[6,31]

Facial neuropathy (VII), or Bell's palsy, may have an increased association with DM and may have a slower recovery rate when compared with nondiabetic patients.[32]

Entrapment and Compression Neuropathy

Patients with diabetes are at greater risk for external compression or entrapment neuropathy, particularly of the median, ulnar, radial, and peroneal nerves. The reasons for this, however, are unclear.[33,34]

The most commonly associated mononeuropathy is carpal tunnel syndrome (CTS). This has a prevalence in the general population of 3.8% vs. 15–33% in patients with diabetes.

More frequent in women than men, CTS presents initially with sensory changes in a median nerve distribution (particularly digits I–III) and sometimes all five fingers. The patient may develop a "pins and needles" sensation or a deep aching pain in the forearm. This may be followed by weakness and wasting of the thenar muscles. Treatment includes wrist splints, anti-inflammatory medication, and steroid injections, with carpal tunnel surgical release reserved for severe cases. The improvement following surgical release may be less significant than in nondiabetic patients.[35]

Ulnar neuropathy at the elbow is the second most common mononeuropathy associated with DM. Symptoms include pain and paresthesias in the fourth and fifth fingers, often accompanied by pain or tenderness along the medial aspect of the elbow. Weakness and atrophy of ulnar-innervated muscles, particularly the interossei, are common. Nerve conduction studies can confirm the diagnosis. Treatment includes anti-inflammatory medication and avoidance of elbow bending. Surgery is offered for progressive cases.

Peroneal neuropathy is the most common compressive neuropathy of the lower extremity. Involvement at the fibular head results in foot drop and foot eversion (but not inversion) weakness. Numbness over the dorsolateral foot and lower leg may also be seen. Most cases improve spontaneously with conservative management and a foot brace.[36]

Sciatic, lateral femoral cutaneous (meralgia paresthetica), radial, and obturator neuropathies have been reported with diabetes; however, a causal relationship is difficult to prove.

Pathogenesis

Defining a precise cause for diabetic neuropathy has proven difficult. Numerous theories have been offered individually but the overall mechanism may ultimately be multifactorial and complex. A review of these hypotheses is valuable in trying to understand the pathophysiology and different treatment approaches attempted in diabetic neuropathy.

Metabolic Hypothesis: Hyperglycemia is associated with the development of neuropathy. The Diabetes Control and Complications trial demonstrated that intensive control of blood glucose decreases the occurrence of neuropathy by 60% in those without neuropathy, and slows its progression in those already affected.[1] The stricter the glucose control the better but at a cost of more frequent hypoglycemic reactions. Hyperglycemia thus results in neuropathy, but how it does so remains unclear.

A popular hypothesis invokes accumulation of polyols, particularly sorbitol, through the aldose reductase pathway. Aldose reductase converts glucose into sorbitol, accumulation of which lowers intracellular myoinositol (Fig. 23.1). Reduced myoinositol is also associated with impaired sodium–potassium ATPase activity, alteration in protein kinase C (PKC) subunits, and slowed nerve conduction velocities. This hypothesis underlies the rationale for using aldose reductase inhibitors to prevent diabetic neuropathy. However, their success has been mediocre at best. Sorbinil resulted in only small increases in nerve conduction velocities and tolrestat had some clinical benefit but the study involved mild diabetic neuropathy.[37,38] The poor results are not surprising. Study of sural nerve biopsy specimens show no correlation between sorbitol content and neuropathy[39] and dietary myoinositol replacement resulted in no improvement in neuropathy. In fact, PKC subunits in peripheral nerve are distributed and behave in such a manner as to make it uncertain whether their inhibition is to be encouraged or counteracted.[40,41]

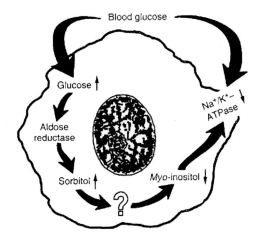

Fig. 23.1 The aldose reductase pathway of glucose metabolism (From Clark and Lee[71]. Reprinted with permission)

Vascular Hypothesis: Nerve ischemia due to small vessel disease is another hypothetical cause for diabetic neuropathy. Work in several areas supports this hypothesis. Blood flow is reduced in diabetic neuropathy and endoneurial hypoxia has been demonstrated.[42,43] Oxygen supplementation prevents, and hyperbaric oxygenation reverses, electrophysiologic and biochemical abnormalities in experimental diabetic neuropathy.[44,45] Pathological study of the sural nerve has shown blood vessel thickening with hyalinization of the vessel walls, reduplication of the basal lamina, and occlusion with platelet aggregates, further supporting a vascular pathogenesis. Focal neuropathy with sudden onset is certainly consistent with this hypothesis but DPN and autonomic neuropathy may also have a vascular basis.

Ischemia per se may directly contribute to the development of neuropathy and explains the benefit of vasodilators in improving nerve conduction velocities. Ischemia also increases oxidative stress and, thus, antioxidants are another avenue of investigation for neuropathy treatment.

Conflicting findings, however, muddy the picture. Sural nerve blood flow was found not to decline with progression of neuropathy, but tended to increase in more severely affected patients.[46] Nerve blood flow was found not to decline in various models of diabetic neuropathy, using a variety of blinded examiners and measurement techniques.[47] Sympathectomy and vasodilation have been associated with worsening of neuropathy rather than improvement.[48] Microvessels in diabetic neuropathy may increase in diameter and demonstrate angiogenesis.[49] Taken together, these findings suggest that clinical trials of vascular endothelial growth factor (VEGF) may be wasteful.

In summary, although diabetic neuropathy is inevitably associated with microvascular abnormalities, the evidence for its exclusive role is questionable.

Mitochondrial Dysfunction: Oxidative stress may target mitochondria and their injury may release cytochrome-c, initiating apoptosis.[50] In support of this mechanism, morphological mitochondrial changes in the form of vacuolization have been reported, but yet may be artifactual.[51]

Immune Hypothesis: Evidence supporting an immune pathogenesis is strongest for diabetic autonomic neuropathy. Autonomic ganglia heavily infiltrated by lymphocytes, plasma cells, and macrophages were found at autopsy in five patients with type 1 diabetes and symptomatic autonomic neuropathy. Striking cervical sympathetic ganglia atrophy was reported in another with severe sensory and autonomic neuropathy.[52]

Autoimmune pathogenesis may be involved in DLRPN as well. Pathologic study revealed polymorphonuclear small vessel vasculitis affecting epineurial vessels with polymorphonuclear transmural infiltration of postcapillary venules in 4 out of 15 patients. IgM deposits were found in affected vessel walls and endoneurium, and activated complement was seen along small vessel endothelium. Perivasculitis was seen in another six and demonstrated findings suggestive of healed vasculitis.[53]

Evidence for an autoimmune basis for the common symmetrical DPN remains sparse.

Altered Protein Synthesis and Axonal Transport: Pathologic findings in human diabetic neuropathy support a distal axonopathy of the dying back variety. Such distal degeneration may result from impaired protein synthesis combined with abnormal axonal transport, both of which have been demonstrated in the experimental diabetic rat model (the streptozocin-treated rat).[54]

Insulin Deficiency and Nerve Growth Factor: Nerve growth factor (NGF) is an endogenous protein necessary for small diameter nerve fiber development and survival. Levels of NGF are decreased in animal models of diabetic neuropathy and NGF was felt to play a role particularly in the development of small fiber painful diabetic neuropathy. Unfortunately, multicenter phase III clinical trials showed no significant benefit of NGF in the treatment of diabetic neuropathy and this avenue of investigation has been halted.

Insulin is itself a potent neuronal growth factor, acting on sensory neuronal and axonal receptors that share signaling cascades with neurotrophin growth factors.[55] Applied near nerve in rats, it reversed sciatic motor velocity slowing, as it did when administered intrathecally, suggesting it has an important role in supporting peripheral nerve.[56] Thus, inadequate insulin dosing may itself play a role in the development of diabetic neuropathy.

Electrodiagnostic Features

Standard nerve conduction studies (NCS) allow the physician to directly measure *large* fiber motor and sensory nerve function. These fibers are involved in position and vibration sensation, deep tendon reflex function, and muscle strength. *Small* diameter fibers, which convey pain and temperature sensation and autonomic function, are not routinely studied. Thus, in diabetes where large fiber nerve function is often impaired, NCS are ideally suited to define the extent and severity of disease.

Motor and sensory nerves are tested individually with NCS but the underlying principle for each is similar. A nerve is stimulated at one or more sites along its course and a recording is made at a second site. If a motor nerve is being studied, the recording electrode is placed over a muscle which the nerve supplies. Sensory nerves, unlike motor nerves, have no end organ from which a recording can easily be made; both the recording and stimulating electrodes are placed over the nerve at some distance apart.

Electromyography (EMG) complements NCS in the study of peripheral nerve function. Indeed, NCS and EMG are often performed in tandem and referred together as "an EMG" – as in "get an EMG." Specifically, EMG is the study of the electrical activity of muscle, performed by means of a needle electrode inserted directly into the muscle. Together with NCS, EMG can distinguish neuropathy from myopathy, localize neuropathic disorders, and quantify and provide prognostic information for nerve and muscle disorders.

Electrophysiologic findings in diabetes are well described. When large diameter nerve fibers are affected in diabetic polyneuropathy, NCS reveal decreased evoked response amplitudes of both motor and sensory nerve fibers with mild conduction velocity slowing. As previously discussed, standard NCS are often normal in purely small fiber neuropathy nature, as these smaller fibers are not measurable by these routine studies. Computers (CASE IV systems) can evaluate small diameter nerve fiber function and, when warranted, patients may be referred to centers where this is available. In most instances, however, this will not be necessary.

As a general rule, electrophysiological deficits, when present, should be symmetrical in the context of a polyneuropathy. If the clinical problem is asymmetrical, the NCS will reflect this as well. For example, NCS in peroneal neuropathy at the fibular head causing unilateral foot drop will show abnormalities limited to the peroneal branch of the sciatic nerve, sparing of the tibial nerve, and slowing of peroneal conduction velocity across the fibular head but not in the distal calf. Similarly, ulnar neuropathy at the elbow or median neuropathy at the wrist (carpal tunnel syndrome) will demonstrate slowing localized to the elbow or wrist, respectively. EMG textbooks should be consulted for details in any specific case.[57]

Other Investigations

In the setting of sensory symptoms and normal electrodiagnostic studies, a skin biopsy can be performed to investigate for a small fiber neuropathy. In this study, a 3-mm diameter circular "punch" biopsy is obtained from the surface skin of the lateral ankle and proximal thigh. The specimens are immunostained with antibodies against markers expressed by peripheral nerve fibers (such as protein gene product 9.5) and the density of epidermal nerve fibers is determined. Qualitative information (such as the orientation of the nerve fibers or the presence of inflammatory cells or congophilic material) may also be useful. Serial biopsies from the same region have been used in research studies to monitor for interval changes or treatment response.[12]

Corneal confocal microscopy is a promising, noninvasive technique that assesses small nerve pathology in vivo.[58]

Treatment

The twin goals of treatment are to (1) halt or slow progression of the neuropathy by targeting the underlying pathophysiological mechanisms (Table 23.6) and (2) manage the clinical symptoms (Table 23.7).

Table 23.6 Management aimed at underlying pathogenic mechanisms

Lifestyle intervention (diet, exercise, weight loss) – Found to result in improved pain and cutaneous innervations in patients with pre-diabetic neuropathy

Glycemic control – Found to reduce clinical and electrophysiologic evidence of neuropathy (particularly in Type 1 DM)

Aldose reductase inhibitors – Found to diminish the reduction in motor nerve conduction velocity. Fidarestat and ranirestat in clinical trials. Epalrestat marketed in Japan. Clinical benefits unclear at this time

Alpha-lipoic acid – Possible effect in reducing somatic and autonomic neuropathies. Dose of 600 mg daily is effective and well tolerated

Gamma-linoleic acid (or evening primrose oil) – An important constituent of membrane phospholipids. Under investigation. One study found benefit at 480 mg daily

Aminoguanidine – Inhibits formation of advanced glycosylation end products. Human trials discontinued secondary to toxicity

Human intravenous immunoglobulin – Anecdotal reports of effectiveness in diabetic neuropathy associated with autoimmunity, e.g., DLRPN

Steroids (methylprednisolone) – May help pain, but not disability in DLRPN

Neurotrophic therapy – Initial positive effects of recombinant human nerve growth factor in sensory neuropathy not borne out in two large multicenter studies

Table 23.7 Treatment options for painful diabetic neuropathy

Agent	Daily dosage	Side effects/remarks
Antidepressants		
1. Tricyclics		
Amitriptyline	25–150 mg	Dry mouth, urinary retention, sedation,
Nortriptyline	25–150 mg	somnolence, postural hypotension
2. SNRIs		
Duloxetine Venlafaxine	60–120 mg	Nausea, dizziness
	150–225 mg	
3. SSRIs		
Citalopram	40 mg	Nausea, vomiting; studied in small series; less
Paroxetine	40 mg	effective than TCAs
Anticonvulsants		
1. Gabapentin	300–3600 mg (divided in 3–4 doses)	NB: renally metabolized; must make adjustment
2. Pregabalin	300–600 mg (divided in 2–3 doses)	Dizziness, somnolence, peripheral edema
4. Carbamazepine	200–600 mg	
5. Oxcarbazepine	1200–1800 mg (600–900 mg bid)	Light-headedness, nausea
6. Topiramate	Titrate from 25 mg up to 400 mg. Typical dose ~100 mg	Diarrhea, weight loss, somnolence
7. Lamotrigine	200–400 mg	Rash, headache; must titrate slowly. Inconsistent benefit
Opioids		
Tramadol (weak opioid)	≤400 mg	Inhibits uptake of monoamines; has low-affinity binding to mu-opioid receptors
Controlled release oxycodone	10–100 mg (average 40 mg/day)	Constipation, cognitive dysfunction
Other agents		
Mexiletine	75–225 mg tid, slow titration	Gastrointestinal distress; Class 1B – antiarrhythmic agent; cardiology clearance required
Topical treatment		
1. Capsaicin cream	Capsaicin 0.075% applied qid	Inhibits substance P uptake at sensory endings

SSRI = selective serotonin reuptake inhibitors
SSNRI = selective serotonin norepinephrine reuptake inhibitors

Management of Underlying Pathogenic Mechanisms

Intensive glycemic control has been shown to slow the progression of DPN in patients with type 1 DM; however, the results in patients with type 2 DM have been variable with intensive therapy resulting in either having partial or no effect. The DCCT showed a 50% reduction in the prevalence rates for clinical or electrophysiologic evidence of neuropathy in patients treated with intensive insulin therapy.[1] Pancreatic transplantation resulting in euglycemia has been associated with a gradual improvement of diabetic polyneuropathy.[59]

Lifestyle modification with changes in diet, exercise, and weight resulted in cutaneous reinnervation (as determined by serial skin biopsies) and improved pain in one study of 32 patients with pre-diabetic neuropathy.[60]

Alpha-lipoic acid has been shown to diminish oxidative stress, and has been studied in intravenous (600 mg/day for 5 weeks) and oral form (600–2400 mg daily). Recently, a dose of 600 mg daily has been determined to be beneficial and without the side effects noted at higher doses.[61]

There is a lack of agreement about the benefits of other treatments that target underlying pathogenic mechanisms. Despite disappointing results to date, there is ongoing interest in the use of aldose reductase inhibitors to prevent excessive sorbitol flux in the nerve. Fidarestat and ranirestat are under investigation,[62] and epalrestat is available in Japan. Ruboxistaurin mesylate has been used as a PKC beta inhibitor in phase II studies with some benefit noted in a subset of patients with less severe DPN.[63] Gamma-linolenic acid may have some benefit at a dose of 480 mg/day.[64]

As discussed, intravenous methylprednisolone may improve pain symptoms, but not disability in DLRPN,[24] and there are only anecdotal reports of benefit with intravenous immunoglobulin.[23]

Management of Neuropathy Symptoms

Current medical management of neuropathic pain includes antidepressants, anticonvulsant medications, opioids, and topical agents. Currently, only duloxetine and pregabalin have FDA approval for management of diabetic neuropathy pain. Careful consideration of comorbidities or risk factors should be given when selecting a therapeutic agent. The treatments are summarized in Table 23.7.[47,65–67]

Tricyclic antidepressants (TCAs) are effective in selected populations, but are less well tolerated and not appropriate for patients with cardiac morbidities. Selective serotonin reuptake inhibitors (SSRIs), such as citalopram and paroxetine, have limited effectiveness, while selective serotonin norepinephrine reuptake inhibitors (SSNRIs), such as duloxetine, have been shown to be helpful.

Gabapentin is at least equally effective as TCAs and is often a first-line treatment given its safer side effect profile. Pregabalin is a more specific alpha-2-gamma ligand with a higher binding affinity and simpler dose titration schedule when compared with gabapentin. There is limited data on the role of carbamazepine for diabetic neuropathy pain and its derivative oxcarbazepine has shown only marginal and inconsistent results. Lamotrigine and topiramate have also produced mixed results, and are not considered first-line therapy.

Opioids have a limited role in diabetic neuropathy pain management. One study found benefit with controlled-release oxycodone versus placebo in a 6-week trial.[68] A role for combination therapy with morphine and gabapentin has also been suggested.[69]

Non-pharmacologic approaches, such as transcutaneous electrical nerve stimulation (TENS) and high-frequency muscle stimulation (HFMS) have been investigated mostly in uncontrolled studies. Frequency-modulated electromagnetic nerve stimulation (FREMS) resulted in pain reduction when compared to placebo stimulation.[70]

Conclusion

The neuropathic complications of diabetes are varied in clinical presentation, presumed pathogenesis, and treatment response. The most frequent complication is a distal, symmetric sensorimotor polyneuropathy, which is usually chronic and progressive. Metabolic derangements are believed to be the cause of this neuropathy, and tight glycemic control has been shown to slow progression, particularly in type 1 DM. The asymmetric neuropathies affect individual nerves (e.g., cranial neuropathies, intercostal or entrapment neuropathies) or groups of nerves in close proximity to each other (e.g., radiculoplexus neuropathies). They typically have a monophasic course with spontaneous improvement and histopathologic findings of ischemic injury and microvasculitis, implicating an immune-mediated etiology.

There is a compelling need for well-designed research into novel and tolerable methods of halting disease progression and treating neuropathic symptoms, which range from numbness to severe pain.

Internet Resources

1. www.aan.com – Homepage of the American Academy of Neurology; features helpful practice advisories for the treatment of most neurological conditions.
2. www.mayohealth.org – Of interest to your patients for general health advice and reviews of neurological conditions.

3. www.ninds.nih.gov/healinfo/nindspub.htm – NINDS site, brief disease description, synopsis and information about NINDS research.
4. www.neuropathy.org – Homepage of the American Neuropathy Association.
5. www.theacpa.org – Homepage of the American Chronic Pain Association.
6. www.neuroland.com – A good page from Baylor College of Medicine for review of neurological diseases; also has a site for patients with links to patient help sources and foundations.
7. www.neuroguide.com – A helpful guide to general neuroscience with numerous links to neurology sites

References

1. Diabetes Control and Complications Trial (DCCT) Research Group. The effect of intensive treatment of diabetes on the development and progression of long-term complications in insulin-dependent diabetes mellitus. *N Engl J Med.* 1993;329: 977–986.
2. Pirart J. Diabetes mellitus and its degenerative complications: a prospective study of 4,400 patients observed between 1947 and 1973. *Diabetes Care.* 1978;1:168–188.
3. Martin CL, Albers J, Herman WH, et al. Neuropathy among the Diabetes Control and Complications Trial Cohort 8 years after trial completion. *Diabetes Care.* 2006;29:340–344.
4. Boulton AJM, Vinik AT, Arezzo JC, et al. Diabetic neuropathies. A statement by the American Diabetes Association. *Diabetes Care.* 2005;28:956–962.
5. Dyck PJ, Karnes JL, O'Brien PC, et al. The Rochester Diabetic Neuropathy Study: reassessment of tests and criteria for diagnosis and staged severity. *Neurology.* 1992;42:1164–1170.
6. Sinnreich M, Taylor BV, Dyck PJB. Diabetic neuropathies. Classification, clinical features, and pathophysiological basis. *Neurologist.* 2005;11:63–79.
7. Melton LJ III, Dyck PJ. Epidemiology. In: Dyck PJ, Thomas PK, et al. (eds). *Diabetic Neuropathy.* 2nd Ed. Philadelphia: WB Saunders; 1999:239–252.
8. Windebank AJ, Feldman EL. Diabetes and the nervous system. In: Aminoff M (ed). *Neurology and General Medicine.* 3rd Ed. Philadelphia: Churchill Livingstone; 2001.
9. Halar EM, Graf RJ, Halter JB, et al. Diabetic neuropathy: a clinical, laboratory, and electrodiagnostic study. *Arch Phys Med Rehabil.* 1982;63:298–303.
10. Niakan E, Harati Y. Sympathetic skin response in diabetic peripheral neuropathy. *Muscle Nerve.* 1988;11:261–264.
11. Lauria G, Lombardi R. Skin biopsy: a new tool for diagnosing peripheral neuropathy. *BMJ.* 2007;334:1159–1162.
12. Umapathi T, Tan WL, Loke SC, et al. Intraepidermal nerve fiber density as a marker of early diabetic neuropathy. *Muscle Nerve.* 2007;35:591–598.
13. Singleton JR, Smith AG, Bromberg MB. Increased prevalence of impaired glucose tolerance in patients with painful sensory neuropathy. *Diabetes Care.* 2001;24:1448–1453.
14. Low PA, Benrud-Larson LM, Sletten DM, et al. Autonomic symptoms and diabetic neuropathy. *Diabetes Care.* 2004;27: 2942–2947.
15. Ewing DJ, Campbell IW, Clarke BF. The natural history of diabetic autonomic neuropathy. *Q J Med.* 1980;49:95–108.
16. Aronson D. Pharmacologic modulation of autonomic tone: implications for the diabetic patient. *Diabetologia.* 1997;40: 476–481.
17. Schnell O, Schwarz A, Becker DM, Standl E. Autoantibodies against autonomic nervous tissues in type 2 diabetes. *Exp Clin Endocrinol Diabetes (Germany).* 2000;108:181–186.
18. Wein TH, Albers JW. Diabetic neuropathies. *Phys Med and Rehab Clinics of North America.* 2001;12(2):307–320.
19. Pascoe MK, Low PA, Windebank AJ, Litchy WJ. Subacute diabetic proximal neuropathy. *Mayo Clin Proc.* 1997;72: 1123–1132.
20. Said G, Goulon-Goeau C, Lacroix C, Moulonguet A. Nerve biopsy findings in different patterns of proximal diabetic neuropathy. *Ann Neurol.* 1994;35:559–569.
21. Dyck PJB, Windebank AJ. Diabetic and nondiabetic lumbosacral radiculoplexus neuropathies: new insights into pathophysiology and treatment. *Muscle Nerve.* 2002;25:477–491.
22. Kawagashira Y, Watanabe H, Oki Y, et al. Intravenous immunoglobulin therapy markedly ameliorates muscle weakness and severe pain in proximal diabetic neuropathy. *J Neurol Neurosurg Psychiatry.* 2007;78:899–901.
23. Schaublin GA, Michet CJ Jr, Dyck PJ, Burns TM. An update on the classification and treatment of vasculitic neuropathy. *Lancet Neurol.* 2005;4:853–865.
24. Dyck JB, O'Brien PC, Bosch EP, et al. Results of a controlled trial of IV methylprednisolone in diabetic lumbosacral radiculoplexus neuropathy (DLRPN): a preliminary indication of efficacy. *J Peripher Nerv Syst.* 2005;10(Suppl 1).
25. Stewart JD. Diabetic truncal neuropathy: topography of the sensory deficit. *Ann Neurol.* 1989;25:233–238.
26. Sun SF, Streib EW. Diabetic thoracoabdominal neuropathy: clinical and electrodiagnostic features. *Ann Neurol.* 1981;9:75.
27. Longstreth GF. Diabetic thoracic polyradiculopathy. *Best Pract Res Clin Gastroenterol.* 2005;19:275–281.

28. Katz JS, Saperstein DS, Wolfe G, et al. Cervicobrachial involvement in diabetic radiculoplexopathy. *Muscle Nerve.* 2001;24:794–798.

29. Goldstein JE, Cogan DG. Diabetic ophthalmoplegia with special reference to the pupil. *Arch Ophthalmol.* 1960;64:592.

30. Jacobson DM. Pupil involvement in patients with diabetes-associated oculomotor nerve palsy. *Arch Ophthalmol.* 1998;116: 723–727.

31. Richards BW, Jones FR, Younge BR. Causes and prognosis in 4,278 cases of paralysis of the oculomotor, trochlear, and abducens cranial nerves. *Am J Ophthalmol.* 1992;113:489.

32. Kanazawa A, Haginomori S, Takamaki A, et al. Prognosis for Bell's palsy: a comparison of diabetic and nondiabetic patients. *Acta Otolaryngol.* 2007;127:888–891.

33. Stamboulis E, Vassilopoulos D, Kalfakis N. Symptomatic focal mononeuropathies in diabetic patients: increased or not? *J Neurol.* 2005;252:448–452.

34. Dahlin LB, Meiri KF, McLean WG, et al. Effects of nerve compression on fast axonal transport in streptozotocin-induced diabetes mellitus. *Diabetologia.* 1986;29:181–185.

35. Ozkul Y, Sabuncu T, Kocabey Y, et al. Outcomes of carpal tunnel release in diabetic and non-diabetic patients. *Acta Neurol Scand.* 2002;106:168–172.

36. Shahani B, Spalding JMK. Diabetes mellitus presenting with bilateral foot-drop. *Lancet.* 1969;2:930–931.

37. Judzewitsch RG, Jaspan JB, Polonsky KS, et al. Aldose reductase inhibition improves nerve conduction velocity in diabetic patients. *N Engl J Med.* 1983;308:119–125.

38. Boulton AJM, Levin SR, Comstock JP. A multicenter trial of the aldose-reductase inhibitor, tolrestat, in patients with symptomatic diabetic neuropathy. *Diabetologia.* 1990;33:433–436.

39. Dyck PJ, Sherman WR, Hallcher LM, et al. Human diabetic endoneurial sorbitol, fructose, and myoinositol related to sural nerve morphometry. *Ann Neurol.* 1980;8:590–596.

40. Yamagishi S, Masuta N, Okamoto K, Yagihashi S. Alterations of protein kinase C activity in the peripheral nerve of STZ-induced diabetic mice overexpressing human aldose reductase (abstract). *Diabetes.* 2001;50:A190.

41. Yamagishi S, Uehara K, Otsuki S, Yagihashi S. Differential influence of increased polyol pathway on protein kinase C expressions between endoneurial and epineurial tissues in diabetic mice. *J Neurochem.* 2003;87:497–507.

42. Newrick PG, Wilson AJ, Jakubowski J, et al. Sural nerve oxygen tension in diabetes. *Br Med J.* 1986;293:1053.

43. Tuck RR, Schmelzer JD, Low PA. Endoneurial blood flow and oxygen tension in the sciatic nerves of rats with experimental diabetic neuropathy. *Brain.* 1984;107:935.

44. Low PA, Tuck RR, Dyck PJ, et al. Prevention of some electrophysiologic and biochemical abnormalities with oxygen supplementation in experimental diabetic neuropathy. *Proc Natl Acad Sci USA.* 1984;81:6894.

45. Low PA, Schmelzer JD, Ward KK, et al. Effect of hyperbaric oxygenation on normal and chronic streptozotocin diabetic peripheral nerves. *Exp Neurol.* 1988;99:201.

46. Theriault M, Dort J, Sutherland G, Zochodne DW. Local human sural nerve blood flow in diabetic and other polyneuropathies. *Brain.* 1997;120:1131–1138.

47. Zochodne DW. Diabetes mellitus and the peripheral nervous system: manifestations and mechanisms. *Muscle Nerve.* 2007;36:144–166.

48. Zochodne DW, Ho LT. The influence of indomethacin and guanethidine on experimental streptozocin diabetic neuropathy. *Can J Neurol Sci.* 1992;19:433–441.

49. Zochodne DW, Nguyen C. Increased peripheral nerve microvessels in early experimental diabetic neuropathy: quantitative studies of nerve and dorsal root ganglia. *J Neurol Sci.* 1999;166:40–46.

50. Halestrap AP. Calcium, mitochondria, and reperfusion injury: a pore way to die. *Biochem Soc Trans.* 2006;34:232–237.

51. Li X-G, Zochodne DW. Microvacuolar neuronopathy is a post-mortem artifact of sensory neurons. *J Neurocytol.* 2003;32: 393–398.

52. Watkins PJ, Gayle C, Alsanjari N, et al. Severe sensory autonomic neuropathy and endocrinopathy in insulin dependent diabetes. *Q J Med.* 1999;88:795–804.

53. Kelkar P, Masood M, Parry GJ. Distinctive pathologic findings in proximal diabetic neuropathy (diabetic amyotrophy). *Neurology.* 2000;55:83–88.

54. Yagihashi S, Kamijo M, Ido Y, et al. Effects of long-term aldose reductase inhibition on development of experimental diabetic neuropathy: ultrastructural and morphometric studies of sural nerve in streptozocin-induced diabetic rats. *Diabetes.* 1990;39:690–697.

55. Xu QG, Li X-Q, Kotecha SA, et al. Insulin as an in vivo growth factor. *Exp Neurol.* 2004;188:43–51.

56. Toth C, Brussee V, Zochodne DW. Remote neurotrophic support of epidermal nerve fibers in experimental diabetes. *Diabetologia.* 2006;49:1081–1088.

57. Kimura J. *Electrodiagnosis in Diseases of Nerve and Muscle: Principles and Practice.* 3rd Ed. New York: Oxford University Press; 2001.

58. Mehra S, Tavakoli M, Kallinikos PA, et al. Corneal confocal microscopy detects early nerve regeneration after pancreas transplantation in patients with type 1 diabetes. *Diabetes Care.* 2007;30:2608–2612.

59. Navarro X, Sutherland DE, Kennedy WR. Long-term effects of pancreatic transplantation on diabetic neuropathy. *Ann Neurol.* 1997;42:727–736.

60. Smith AG, Russell J, Feldman EL, et al. Lifestyle intervention for pre-diabetic neuropathy. *Diabetes Care.* 2006;29:1294–1299.

61. Ziegler D, Ametov A, Barinov A, et al. Oral treatment with α-lipoic acid improves symptomatic diabetic polyneuropathy. *Diabetes Care*. 2006;29:2365–2370.

62. Bril V, Buchanan RA. Long-term effects of ranirestat (AS-3201) on peripheral nerve function in patients with diabetic sensorimotor polyneuropathy. *Diabetes Care*. 2006;29:68–72.

63. Vinik AI, Bril V, Kempler P, et al. Treatment of symptomatic diabetic peripheral neuropathy with the protein kinase C beta-inhibitor ruboxistaurin mesylate during a 1-year, randomized, placebo-controlled, double-blind clinical trial. *Clin Ther*. 2005;27:1164–1180.

64. Keen H, Payan J, Allawi J, et al. Treatment of diabetic neuropathy with gamma-linolenic acid. The gamma-Linolenic Acid Multicenter Trial Group. *Diabetes Care*. 1993;16:8–15.

65. Ziegler D. Treatment of diabetic polyneuropathy. *Ann NY Acad Sci*. 2006;1084:250–266.

66. Vinik A. Clinical review: use of antiepileptic drugs in the treatment of chronic painful diabetic neuropathy. *J Clin Endocrinol Metab*. 2005;90:4936–4945.

67. McKeage K. Treatment options for the management of diabetic painful neuropathy: best current evidence. *Curr Opin Neurol*. 2007;20(5):553–557.

68. Gimbel JS, Richards P, Portenoy RK. Controlled-release oxycodone for pain in diabetic neuropathy: a randomized controlled trial. *Neurology*. 2003;60:927–934.

69. Gilron I, Bailey JM, Tu D, et al. Morphine, gabapentin, or their combination for neuropathic pain. *N Engl J Med*. 2005;352:1324–1334.

70. Bosi E, Conti M, Vermigli C, et al. Effectiveness of frequency-modulated electromagnetic neural stimulation in the treatment of painful diabetic neuropathy. *Diabetologia*. 2005;48:817–823.

71. Clark CM, Lee DA. Prevention and treatment of complications of diabetes mellitus. *N Engl J Med*. 1995;332:1210–1217.

Chapter 24
Peripheral Vascular Disease in Diabetes

Jennifer K. Svahn, Jeffrey S. Kirk, Omar H. Llaguna, and Nancy Habib

Introduction

Diabetes mellitus is a ubiquitous disease which affects millions of Americans (7% of the US population),[1] incurs significant comorbidities, and costs billions annually in health-care dollars. The morbidities associated with diabetes mellitus include a substantial increase in both small vessel (microvascular) and large vessel (macrovascular) diseases. The macrovascular effects of diabetes, causing serious morbidity and mortality, are found in the coronary, cerebral (extra- and intracranial), and peripheral vascular circulation. The focus of this chapter's discussion will be on the lower extremity peripheral vascular complications of diabetes.

The atherosclerotic nature of peripheral vascular disease (PVD) in patients with diabetes is histologically similar to that found in those without diabetes, but tends to be more virulent and aggressive in its behavior and natural history. The early notion of "small vessel disease" unique to diabetes has been disproved. Initially proposed in 1959,[2] it led to the misguided conclusion that patients with diabetes have untreatable micro-occlusive arteriolar disease. This tenet, although subsequently disproved,[3–6] is still espoused by many practitioners today. The very nature of modern vascular surgery and the concept of limb salvage that is so vital to the treatment of the diabetic patients are premised on the knowledge that these patients do not suffer from untreatable occlusive microvascular disease of the lower extremities. Their disease is almost always amenable to infrainguinal and tibial reconstruction for limb salvage, even in the most seemingly dismal circumstances.

There are approximately 21 million individuals with diabetes in the United States. As many as 25% will require medical attention at some point in the course of their disease for diabetes-related foot problems. An astounding 60,000 major amputations are performed annually for these problems. In spite of best efforts, wound failure rates can be as high as 28%, with half of these patients eventually requiring partial amputations of the contralateral limb within 2–5 years.[7]

Pathophysiology of Peripheral Vascular Disease in Diabetes

Exact factors responsible for the development of peripheral vascular disease in diabetes are poorly and incompletely understood (Table 24.1/Fig. 24.1).

The recognition that the vascular endothelium plays a major role in impaired endothelial cell function and the development of diabetic vascular disease is pivotal.[8] The change that does characterize vascular disease in diabetes is most notably a thickening of the capillary basement membrane. This change, however, does not result in capillary narrowing or diminished arteriolar blood flow.[9] Nevertheless, white blood cell migration and response to injury of the diabetic foot may be impeded by thickening of the basement membrane and thus leave the diabetic foot more susceptible to severe infection.[10,11] Patients with diabetes also suffer from an impaired ability to

J.K. Svahn (✉)
Division of Vascular Surgery, Department of Surgery, Beth Israel Medical Center, New York, NY, USA
e-mail: jsvahn@bethisraelny.org

L. Poretsky (ed.), *Principles of Diabetes Mellitus*, DOI 10.1007/978-0-387-09841-8_24,
© Springer Science+Business Media, LLC 2010

Table 24.1 Factors predisposing patient with diabetes to PVD

Thickening of capillary basement membrane
Impaired white blood cell migration
Impaired vasodilatation response to injury
Maldistribution of dermal capillaries
Altered endothelium-derived nitric oxide release
Increased oxygen free radical production
Alteration in function of Na^+–K^+ ATPase

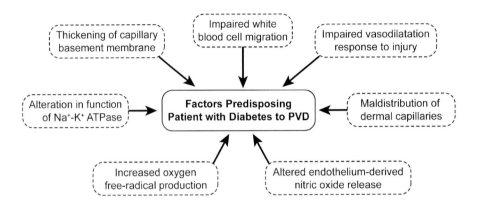

Fig. 24.1

vasodilate in response to injury, with a misdistribution of skin capillaries which results in local skin ischemia, and impaired neurogenic vasodilatory response.[12] This microcirculatory dysfunction occurs in multiple tissue beds long before the onset of atherosclerotic symptoms.[13] All of these changes lead to an increased susceptibility to trauma and subsequently increased risk of infection.

Prolonged and persistent exposure to elevated glucose levels may alter the production, release, and action of endothelium-derived nitric oxide (EDNO) resulting in impaired vasodilation and abnormal relaxation of the vascular smooth muscle.[8] EDNO, previously known as endothelium-derived relaxing factor (EDRF), is a major mediator of endothelium-dependent vasodilation and arterial smooth muscle relaxation,[14,15] two critical protective mechanisms of healthy endothelium.[16] In people with diabetes, impaired synthesis, release, and response to EDNO play a significant role in diabetes-associated atherosclerotic disease.[17] Animal models have shown that eNOS deficiency markedly increases endothelial leukocyte adhesion and accelerates atherosclerotic lesion development.[16] The generation of oxygen-derived free radicals may also be increased in diabetes with a concomitant decrease in free radical scavenger systems which may further impair the activity of EDNO.[18,19] In addition, it has been proposed that endothelium which is chronically exposed to elevated glucose levels produces elevated levels of vasoconstrictive prostanoids. Of note, PVD prevalence increases in individuals with impaired glucose tolerance, with the risk significantly increasing with higher hemoglobin A1c levels.[20,21] For every percentage point above normal, there is a 28% increased risk of PVD, with the severity appearing to be related both to the duration of hyperglycemia and to the glycemic control.[20,22,23] Increase in deleterious free radicals may also exaggerate the effect of hyperglycemia on impaired endothelial relaxation as well as the vasoconstrictive properties of circulating prostanoids. Finally, reduction in the activity of Na^+, K^+ ATPase in the vascular smooth muscle may be yet another factor contributing to the impaired vessel response seen in the diabetic patient.[8]

Additional mechanisms by which hyperglycemia may result in diabetic PVD include the following (Table 24.2): glycation of proteins resulting in dysfunctional or toxic endproducts; interference with the fluid, vascular, and platelet phases of coagulation; hyperglycemia-induced oxidative stress resulting in enhanced peroxidation of arachidonic acid to form biologically active isoprostanes, an important biochemical link between impaired glycemic control and persistent platelet activation; abnormal lipid metabolism, i.e., increased low-density lipoprotein (LDL) cholesterol, elevated triglyceride levels, and decreased levels of high-density

Table 24.2 Mechanisms by which hyperglycemia increases the risk of PVD

Glycation of serum proteins (toxic products)
Alteration in coagulation pathways
Hyperglycemia-induced oxidative stress
Abnormal lipid metabolism
Alteration in insulin/proinsulin levels
Impairment in polymorphonuclear leukocyte
   function/cytokine production

lipoprotein (HDL) cholesterol;[24] abnormal insulin/proinsulin levels; and an impairment in the immune system lymphokine production and polymorphonuclear leukocyte function.[25]

A clear understanding of the exact factors involved in this "glucose toxicity" and the method by which they interact to culminate in the vascular pathophysiology unique to diabetes remain elusive. Ultimately, therapy aimed at reversing these abnormalities could result in minimizing or eliminating the negative effects of hyperglycemia on the vascular system of the diabetic patient.

The Diabetic Foot

Nearly half of all patients with diabetes in the United States will develop some degree of PVD and significant lower extremity ischemia beginning approximately one decade after the onset of their disease. As previously noted, the atherosclerosis in patients with diabetes begins at an early age and is more severe than that in individuals without diabetes. Twenty-five percent of diabetic patients will seek medical attention for a foot lesion. In fact, foot lesions account for the majority of hospitalizations in this group. Patients with diabetes and foot lesions carry a 0.6% risk of major amputation per year, resulting in 60,000 major amputations annually in the country.[26] The likelihood of major amputation is 40 times more likely in the diabetic than nondiabetic population and parallels the risk for vascular disease in general.

Diabetic foot ulcers are the result of a combination of peripheral neurotropic changes, chronic ischemic changes, rigid osseous deformities, infection, and recurring trauma of the lower extremity and foot. Peripheral neuropathy is a significant problem which contributes to and exacerbates the complications of PVD and is discussed in great detail in Chapter 17.

Careful attention to and fastidious care of the diabetic foot is of the utmost importance in an attempt to avoid ulceration, infection, gangrene, and limb loss. Ischemic ulcers are typically located on the digits or heel of the foot and are usually painful. Diabetic neuropathy, however, may dull the sensation of ischemic pain hence the absence of pain does not rule out ischemia. Furthermore, patients may not walk long enough distances for claudication to develop. Neurotropic ulcers are typically found beneath the metatarsal heads on the plantar aspect of the foot and are present often in the setting of a well-perfused foot.[6] Table 24.3 represents a comparison between characteristics of diabetic and ischemic ulcers.

Table 24.3 Comparison of neuropathic versus ischemic ulcers

Diabetic	Ischemic
Metatarsal head	Tips of toes/heel
Painless	Painful
Pulses present (frequently)	Absent pulses

Even extensive infection in the diabetic foot often presents without the classic signs of fever and elevated white blood cell count. A thorough exam and a high degree of suspicion on the part of the physician evaluating the diabetic foot are mandatory to avoid underestimating the extent of infection and the grave consequences of delay in appropriate aggressive therapy.[27] When patients with diabetes mellitus present with foot lesions, early control of the spreading infection and surgical drainage of established infection remain the cornerstone of initial care.[28] Even a seemingly well-perfused diabetic foot with a normal pedal pulse exam may harbor a severe polymicrobial infection and abscess. The most common organisms involved in diabetic foot infections include *Staphylococcus aureus*, *Staphylococcus epidermidis*, *Streptococcus*, peptostreptococci, *Escherichia coli*, *Klebsiella*, *Enterobacter aerogenes*, *Proteus mirabilis*, *Pseudomonas aeruginosa*, and *Bacteroides fragilis*. Pending results of cultures, empiric antibiotic coverage should include a cephalosporin or β-lactam antibiotic (activity against staphylococci and streptococci) and trimethoprim–sulfamethoxazole (activity against MRSA). Alternatively a fluoroquinolone or linezolid is also acceptable. Early complete debridement of infected and devitalized tissue and drainage of abscess cavities in the operating room are required. Immobilization and non-weight bearing on the affected extremity are also necessary. Wound and bone cultures and appropriate antimicrobial therapy in concert with frequent dressing changes, return trips to the operating room for further debridement, and wound care are required to treat the infection, promote tissue healing, and avoid major amputation and limb loss. When indicated, early revascularization should follow initial control of active infection.

Ischemia in the Diabetic Extremity: Assessment and Treatment

Assessment of the degree of peripheral vascular disease present in the diabetic patient is important (Table 24.4). It is not uncommon that the chronically ischemic diabetic foot will require revascularization in order to heal ulcers, control local sepsis, prevent progressive gangrene, and avoid digit, foot, or leg amputation. When physical exam and clinical judgment indicate that ischemia is present in the affected extremity and foot, complete evaluation of the arterial tree is required to plan appropriate intervention and revascularization.

Table 24.4 Assessment of ischemia

History
Physical exam
Noninvasive vascular studies (pulse/volume recordings; ankle–brachial index)
Magnetic resonance angiography
Angiography
Clinical judgment

A thorough history is required when assessing the diabetic patient for evidence of PVD. Patients may describe intermittent claudication as calf pain or heaviness, aching, or fatigue that is reproducible and consistent with ambulation and which is relieved with rest. This pattern of symptoms presents because the gastrocnemius muscle has the highest oxygen consumption of any leg muscle and develops ischemic pain earliest during exercise. More advanced ischemia may be manifested as rest pain when perfusion even in the non-exercising muscle is inadequate. Minimum nutritional requirements of resting skin, muscle, bone, and nerve are not met and lead to rest pain, ulceration, and eventual gangrene. Rest pain in the foot is worse at night with leg elevation in the recumbent position and improved with standing. Patients with severe rest pain often sleep with their leg and foot left dangling over the side of the bed. It is important to keep in mind that neuropathic foot pain may often be confused with ischemic rest pain. Moreover, the insensate diabetic foot may mask the rest pain that is the hallmark typical of severe atherosclerosis in individuals without diabetes.

Physical exam of the diabetic extremity must also be thorough. The examiner should look for signs of trophic changes that are consistent with chronic ischemia. These changes include thin, shiny skin, subcutaneous atrophy, brittle toenails, diminished muscle mass, and poor hair growth. The feet are often pale and cool with sluggish capillary refill, dependent rubor, and weak or absent pedal pulses. In severe ischemia, there is loss of sweating resulting from sympathetic denervation, signs of neuropathy, and signs of tissue loss with ulceration and gangrene. Ulcers are most often located on the tips of toes or on the heel of the foot, with irregular borders and a pale base.[29] Accuracy and success of different examiners in locating the site of arterial obstruction vary considerably with experience. In a study by Baker and String,[30] medical students, resident physicians, and attending surgeons all determined the location of arterial disease based on physical examination. These assessments were then compared to vascular lab and arteriography findings. Residents and students were partially correct 35% of the time and totally correct only 65% of the time, while attending surgeons were accurate 98% of the time. Thus, for most vascular specialists, physical exam is nearly as accurate as the vascular lab and angiography in identifying the level of occlusive disease.

When indicated, noninvasive vascular lab studies and angiography supplement the findings on the physical exam and are important tools in establishing whether or not PVD and ischemia are critical factors in the foot ulcer or infection. The ankle–brachial index (ABI) compares the systolic blood pressure at the ankle with that of the brachial artery (Fig. 24.2). A normal ABI is 1.0–1.1. Progressively diminishing ABIs are found in patients with worsening degrees of PVD – claudication is typically found with ABIs in the range of 0.5–0.9, rest pain is usually experienced with results less than 0.5, and tissue loss is common below 0.3. Pulse volume recordings (PVR) are wave tracings that reflect volume changes in the lower extremity with blood flow. Normally triphasic, the PVR tracing becomes biphasic, monophasic, and eventually flat with progressively more severe vascular disease. When interpreting the results of noninvasive studies in diabetic patients, it is important to keep in mind that medial calcification of tibial vessels may artificially elevate segmental limb pressures and ABI readings as a result of poorly compressible vessels. Absolute ankle pressures of less than 30–40 mmHg are reliable predictors of nonhealing in the diabetic patient. Because digital vessels, unlike tibial vessels, are rarely calcified even in diabetes patient, digital pressure readings may be even more accurate predictors of successful healing.[6] Toe pressures less than 20 mmHg correlate consistently with no healing while toe pressures greater than 40 mmHg predict successful healing.[17]

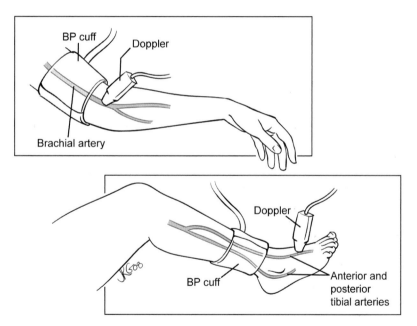

Fig. 24.2 Blood pressure measurements for ankle-brachial index

When the diabetic patient requires revascularization to treat rest pain and/or to heal tissue loss and infection, angiography is indicated. Additionally it is recognized that distal arterial reconstruction and the reversal of hypoxia halt the progression of diabetic nephropathy which is a significant factor in diabetic foot lesions and ulceration. This represents, therefore, another possible indication for angiography.[29] When performing lower extremity angiography, the use of selective digital subtraction angiography with attention to careful pre- and post-angiography hydration to minimize the risk of renal toxicity has proven invaluable. The angiogram must not only demonstrate the more proximal extremity vessels but also define the tibial and pedal vessels to adequately assess the outflow. Only with this complete information can the appropriate intervention to revascularize the diabetic extremity be planned. [28]

Revascularizing the Diabetic Extremity

As noted earlier, lower extremity peripheral vascular disease in the diabetic patient is a result of atherosclerosis which is grossly similar to the atherosclerotic process seen in individuals without diabetes. However, the distribution of vessels involved and the virulence of the atherosclerotic process in diabetic patients are unique. Patients with diabetes classically have atherosclerosis involving the tibial and peroneal arteries with sparing of the relatively normal suprageniculate and foot vessels. Frequently though the diabetic patient also has other risk factors for atherosclerosis (most notably, tobacco smoking) and suffers from atherosclerosis of the more proximal arterial tree in addition to the classic vascular disease below the knee.

When physical exam and clinical judgment indicate that ischemia is present in the affected extremity and foot, complete evaluation of the arterial tree is required to plan appropriate intervention and revascularization (Table 24.5).

Table 24.5 Principles of lower extremity revascularization

Demonstrate necessity for improvement in blood supply
Define vascular anatomy (contrast or magnetic angiography)
Potential vascular anatomy (angioplasty ± stent) as adjunct to surgery
Appropriate choice of conduit (vein, PolyTetraFluoroEthylene)
Careful choice of surgical bypass

While occlusive disease of the proximal large arteries can often be successfully treated nonoperatively with a combination of percutaneous balloon angioplasty and stent placement, smaller vessel disease below the popliteal artery requires surgical bypass to patent distal tibial, peroneal, or foot vessels. Often, a combined cooperative approach between the disciplines affords the patient the best result. Occlusive iliac vessels, for example, can be successfully opened with angioplasty and stent placement by the interventional radiologists thereby providing adequate inflow to the femoral vessels so that the vascular surgeon can perform the lower extremity femoral-to-distal vessel bypass.

Accurate and detailed preoperative information regarding the status of the affected extremity's arterial tree is vital to planning a successful operation. This typically requires contrast angiography or magnetic resonance angiography of the entire inflow and outflow tract, including foot vessels. The classic dictum is that the goal in healing ischemic tissue in the lower extremity or foot is to bring normal pulsatile arterial flow to the level of tissue loss. In the foot, this means attempting to restore palpable pedal pulses. There are certainly cases where tissue healing is achieved without restoring pedal pulses, limiting the operation to more proximal bypasses or simply improving the arterial inflow to the extremity without a distal bypass. These cases, however, are the exception and every attempt should be made to restore palpable distal flow when an acceptable patent outflow vessel exists in a medically suitable patient.

Autogenous greater saphenous vein (left in situ with valvulotomy or reversed ex situ and tunneled) is clearly the conduit of choice in below-the-knee distal bypasses with superior long-term patency and decreased risk of infection as compared to synthetic conduits (PolyTetraFluoroEthylene or PTFE). When the greater saphenous vein is not available for use, autogenous arm vein may also be used as the bypass conduit with good long-term results. However, many surgeons have achieved and described successful operations using a composite graft of autogenous vein and PTFE or PTFE alone.[27]

LoGerfo et al.[28] described the successful decrease in major amputation rates with the application of an increasing rate of dorsalis pedis artery bypass. Bypass to patent dorsalis pedis vessels resulted in a 3-year patency rate of 87% and a limb salvage rate of 92%. Additionally, despite the increased rate of distal bypass surgery, the authors did not experience an increase in mortality in this patient population. Diabetic patients with reconstructable lesions demonstrated on angiography do just as well as nondiabetic individuals in terms of long-term graft patency and limb salvage. Pedal bypass is safe, effective, and durable and should be considered even in "high-risk" patients with critical ischemia before major amputation.[31] That noted, however, there can be a recurrence of diabetic foot ulcers despite patent distal bypasses and adequate blood supply.

Endovascular techniques were originally designed for diagnostic purposes. Today, vascular surgeons are trained to achieve full competence in the endovascular management (i.e., angiography, subintimal dissection, endoluminal stenting) of all vascular disease exclusive of coronary and intracranial pathology.[32] The revascularization paradigm for PVD has shifted strategies from traditional open surgical approaches toward percutaneous endovascular modalities often, but not always, with similar short- and long-term outcomes, and diminished morbidity and mortality.[33] For example, although 30-day mortality is at least two-thirds less with endovascular aortic repair (EVAR) than with open repair,[34] they share the same perioperative mortality risk.[35] The limit of endovascular procedures for PVD is depicted in long-term outcomes. The Bypass versus Angioplasty in Severe Ischemia of the Leg (BASIL) trial was a British multicenter randomized trial that compared an initial strategy of angioplasty versus open surgery in 452 patients with chronic limb ischemia.[36] The primary outcome was time to amputation or death (amputation-free survival). After 6 months, the two treatment strategies did not differ significantly in amputation-free survival.[33] As endovascular therapies continue to develop with improvement in long-term durability and newer technologies to improve long-term outcomes, minimally invasive procedures will continue to replace open surgery.

Summary

"Understanding the pattern of atherosclerotic occlusive disease in patients with diabetes mellitus is the foundation for a successful clinical management plan."[19] Recognizing that the infra-geniculate vessels are involved with atherosclerosis while the pedal vessels, particularly the dorsalis pedis artery, are often spared and are thus amenable to extreme distal revascularization is the cornerstone of successful management. Rejection of the concept of microvascular occlusive disease is stressed. There is no evidence to support the notion of diminished blood flow in the microcirculation as a result of basement membrane thickening – so-called small vessel disease or microangiopathy.[6]

General maintenance and preventive care of the diabetic patient with peripheral vascular disease are mandatory and include the following: control of hyperglycemia and hyperlipidemia and strict avoidance of smoking; a reasonable exercise regimen; close attention to and care of the feet, nails, and skin with avoidance of local trauma; antifungal care when indicated; control of hypertension; and body weight reduction. Additionally, various drugs may be useful adjunctive therapy. Medications which afford the diabetic patient with only PVD varying and inconsistently positive results include hemorrheologic agents (pentoxifylline), antithrombotic therapy, anticoagulants, platelet inhibitors, and thrombolytic drugs.

Together, improved metabolic control, an appreciation of the nature of peripheral vascular disease typical of the diabetic patient and the success of distal bypasses in this population, will lead to decreases in lower extremity amputation and an increase in limb salvage in this patient population. Advances in endovascular techniques have prompted a paradigm shift in the management of PVD toward minimally invasive approaches which have the potential to lessen short- and long-term morbidity and mortality.

Internet Resources

1. www.diabetes.org
2. http://diabetes.niddk.nih.gov
3. http://www.cdc.gov/diabetes

4. http://www.fda.gov/diabetes
5. http://www.who.int/diabetes/en
6. http://www.americanheart.org
7. http://www.mayoclinic.org/peripheral-vascular-disease

References

1. Goldenburg SG, Alex M, Joshi RA, Blementhal HT. Nonatheromatous peripheral vascular disease of the lower extremity in diabetes mellitus. *Diabetes*. 1959;8:261–273.
2. Strandness DE Jr, Priest RE, Gibbons GE. Combine clinical and pathologic study of diabetic and nondiabetic peripheral arterial disease. *Diabetes*. 1964;13:366–372.
3. Conrad MC. Large and small artery occlusion in diabetics and nondiabetics with severe vascular disease. *Circulation*. 1967;36:83–91.
4. Bamer HB, Kaiser GC, William VL. Blood flow in the diabetic leg. *Circulation*. 1971;43:391–394.
5. Ernst CB, Stanley JC, Eds. *Current Therapy in Vascular Surgery*. 3rd Ed. St. Louis, MI: Mosby ; 1995.
6. Cohen RA. Dysfunction of vascular endothelium in diabetes mellitus. *Circulation*. 1993;87:67–76.
7. Parving HH, Viberti GC, Keen H, Christiansen JS, Lassen NA. Hemodynamic factors in genesis of diabetic microangiopathy. *Metabolism*. 1983;32:934–939.
8. Flynn MD, Tooke JE. Aetiology of diabetic ulceration: a role for the microcirculation? *Diabetes Med*. 1992;8: 320–329.
9. Rayman G, Williams SA, Spencer PD, et al. Impaired microvascularhyperemic response to minor skin trauma in type diabetes. *Br Med J*. 1986;292:1295–1298.
10. Parkhouse N, LeQueen PM. Impaired neurogenic vascular response in patients with diabetes and neuropathic foot lesions. *N Engl J Med*. 1998;318:1306–1309.
11. Furchgott RF, Zawadzki JV. The obligatory role of endothelial cells in the relaxation of arterial smooth muscle by acetylcholine. *Nature*. 1980;288:373–376.
12. Palmer RM, Ferrige AG, Moncada S. Nitric oxide release accounts for the biologic activity of endothelium–derived relaxing factor. *Nature*. 1987;327:524–526.
13. Baron AD. The coupling of glucose metabolism and perfusion in the humanskeletal muscle. The potential role of endothelium-derived nitric oxide. *Diabetes*. 1996;45:S105–S109.
14. Wolff SP, Dean RT. Glucose autoxidation and protein modification: the role of oxidative glycosylation in diabetes. *Biochem J*. 1987;245:234–250.
15. Timimi FK, Ting HH, Haley EA, Roddy M, Ganz P, Creager MA. Vitamin C improves endothelium-dependent vasodilation in patients with insulin-dependent diabetes mellitus. *J Am Coll Cardiol*. 1998;31:552–557.
16. Moore WS. *Vascular Surgery: A Comprehensive Review*. 5th ed. Philadelphia, PA: W.B. Saunders co; 1997.
17. Eton D, Weaver F, Eds. *Vascular Disease: A Multi-Specialty Approach to Diagnosis and Management*. Austin, TX: Landes Bioscience; 1998.
18. Akbari CM, LoGerfo FW. Diabetes and peripheral vascular disease. *J Vasc Surg*. 1999;30:373–384.
19. LoGerfo FW, Gibbons GW, Pomposelli FB, et al. Trends in the care of the diabetic foot. *Arch Surg*. 1992;127:617–621.
20. Loscalzo J, Creager MA, Dzau VJ, Eds. *Vascular, Medicine: A Textbook of Vascular Biology and Diseases*. 2nd Edn. Boston: Little, Brown; 1996.
21. Baker WH, String ST, Hayes AC, Turner D. Diagnosis of peripheral occlusive disease: comparison of clinical evaluation and noninvasive laboratory. *Arch Surg*. 1978;113(11):1308–1310.
22. Akbari CM, Gibbons GW, Habershaw GM, et al. The effect of arterial reconstruction on the natural history of diabetic neuropathy. *Arch Surg*. 1997;132:148–152.
23. Gloviczki P, Bower TC, Toomey BJ, et al. Microscope-aided pedal bypass is an effective and low–risk operation to salvage the ischemic foot. *Am J Surg*. 1994;168(2):76–84.
24. Blonde L. State of diabetes care in the United States. *Am J Manag Care*. 2007 Apr;13(Suppl 2):S36–S40.
25. Driver VR, Madsen J, Goodman RA. Reducing amputation rates in patients with diabetes at a military medical center: the limb preservation service model. *Diabetes Care*. 2005 February 1;28(2):248–253.
26. Landmesser U, Hornig B, Drexler H. Endothelial function: a critical determinant in atherosclerosis? *Circulation*. 2004;109(Suppl 1):II27–II33.
27. Regensteiner JG, Wolfel EE, Brass Ep, et al. Chronic changes in skeletal muscle histology and function in peripheral arterial disease. *Circulation* 1993;87:413–421.
28. American Diabetes Association. Peripheral arterial disease in people with diabetes. *Diabetes Care*. 2003;26:3333–3341.
29. Muntner P, Wildman RP, Reynolds K, Desalvo KB, Chen J, Fonseca V. Relationship between HbA1c level and peripheral arterial disease. *Diabetes Care*. 2005;28:1981–1987.

30. Selvin E, Marinopoulos S, Berkenblit G, et al. Meta-analysis: glycosylated hemoglobin and cardiovascular disease in diabetes mellitus. *Ann Intern Med*. 2004;141:421–431.
31. Criqui MH, Denenberg JO, Langer RD, Fronek A. The epidemiology of peripheral arterial disease: importance of identifying the population at risk. *Vasc Med*. 1997;2:221–226.
32. Endovascular training program endorsement essentials. VascularWeb, 2007 [cited Dec 2007]
33. Prinssen M, Verhoeven EL, Buth J, et al. Dutch Randomized Endovascular Aneurysm Management (DREAM) Trial Group. A randomized trial comparing conventional and endovascular repair of abdominal aortic aneurysms. *N Engl J Med*. 2004;351:1607–1618.
34. de Virgilio C, Bui H, Donayre C, et al. Rodney white endovascular vs open abdominal aortic aneurysm repair: a comparison of cardiac morbidity and mortality. *Arch Surg*. 1999;134:947–951.
35. White CJ, Gray WA. Gray endovascular therapies for peripheral arterial disease: an evidence–based review. *Circulation*. 2007;116:2203–2215.
36. Current trials of interventions to prevent radiocontrast-induced nephropathy. *Am J Ther*. 2005 March/April;12(2):127–132.

Chapter 25
The Diabetic Foot

Dennis Shavelson, John S. Steinberg, and Bradley W. Bakotic

Introduction

The importance of the physician's role in examining and assessing the diabetic foot is hard to overstate,[1] yet studies have shown that primary care physicians are rarely performing foot examinations on their diabetic patients during routine visits.[2,3]

Uncontrolled diabetes is the cause of 60% of the 67,000 non-traumatic amputations encountered annually in the United States. The majority of these amputations are preceded by a foot ulcer and are therefore preventable.[4,5]

In 2006, the projected lifetime health-care cost for each patient having undergone a below-knee amputation was $509,275 and the annual cost of these amputations was $600 million. Lost wages and morbidity were estimated at $1 billion, annually.[6]

The United States National Diabetes Advisory Board stated that "the early detection, monitoring and treatment of the risk factors will lead to an 85 percent reduction in lower extremity amputation."[7] Physicians treating diabetic individuals must obtain a foot history and perform a foot examination in the course of office visits. By offering advice and instruction during routine visits, primary care physicians can assist diabetic patients in developing good foot care habits. They must also know when to refer patients to the appropriate specialist for preventive and curative care or to the emergency room for admission and possible urgent surgery. The foot history and exam will enable the physician to classify each patient according to the Relative Risk Factor (RRF) for Lower Extremity Amputation Scale (explained later in the chapter). If the RRF rating is high, a consultation with a podiatrist is in order. It has been found that the preventive care, diagnosis, and treatment of the existing risk factors by a podiatrist are important in determining the health, quality of life, and longevity of diabetic patients' feet and that podiatry is an integral part of the team approach to diabetes.[8]

The Lower Extremity Amputation Prevention Program (LEAPP)[9] consists of five relatively simple activities: annual foot screening, patient education, daily self-inspection of the foot, appropriate footwear selection, and management of simple foot problems (Table 25.1). In addition, it is becoming clear that more aggressive measures are appropriate in order to reduce or remove risk factors for ulcers and amputations. For example, if there is an extremely prominent metatarsal bone that would serve as the site of an eventual neurotrophic ulcer, a foot insert (orthotic) or even a surgical elevation or other mechanical correction should be considered as preventive care before the ulcer or a recurrence develops.[10]

Biomechanics of the Foot

Understanding the inherited biomechanics of feet is important in the evaluation of the diabetic foot. Functional Lower Extremity Biomechanics (FLEB) is the field of knowledge which focuses on the human body from the low

D. Shavelson (✉)
Department of Surgery, Beth Israel Medical Center, New York, NY, USA
e-mail: drsha@lifestylepodiatry.com

L. Poretsky (ed.), *Principles of Diabetes Mellitus*, DOI 10.1007/978-0-387-09841-8_25,
© Springer Science+Business Media, LLC 2010

Table 25.1 Lower Extremity Amputation Prevention (LEAP) Program

1. Annual foot screening
2. Patient education
3. Daily self-inspection of the foot
4. Appropriate footwear selection
5. Management of simple foot problems

back down, when in *closed chain,* e.g., standing [stance] or active [gait] and weightbearing [upon the ground]. Classical medicine studies subjects in *open chain* (on an examining table and not weightbearing).

The etiological forces that must be overcome in managing a patient are the hard unyielding ground, hard unyielding shoeboxes, and the deforming force of the earth's gravity.

Compensating pathological forces from the weightbearing surface into the foot, balancing the posture, and providing functional and safe footwear for the diabetic foot are the biomechanical keys to preventing and treating foot ulcers and gait and balance problems in addition to maintaining quality of life. The use of straps, pads, foot orthotics, therapeutic footwear, and bracing reduces foot ulcers, foot infections, amputations, and hospitalizations in any diabetic population.

Functional Anatomy of the Foot

Biomechanically, the foot is divided into two arched longitudinal segments, the medial dynamic arch, and the lateral dynamic arch. Together, they form the Vault of the Foot (Fig. 25.1).[9]

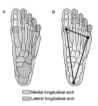

Fig. 25.1 The medial and lateral dynamic arches and the vault of the foot

The Centering Theory of FLEB

If one utilizes architectural engineering to develop a paradigm to diagnose and treat the foot as a supporting and functional entity, then, unlike the architectural arch which has equal pillars, a centered keystone, and symmetrical bases of support, the foot has a short rearfoot pillar, a long forefoot pillar, a keystone that is off-center proximally and has unequal bases of support. In summary, feet lack the centering inherent in architectural arches (Fig. 25.2).

The Use of Centrings in Architecture and the Foot

In architecture, if you want to build an arch, you first build a form in the shape of the arch called a centring. You lay the stones on the centering and set the central keystone and after cementing and drying, you remove the centring and the arch stands forever (Fig. 25.3).

The foot, on the other hand, in order to function as a mobile rigid lever and a functional adaptor to move us about and perform tasks fails as a supporting unit over time and therefore is destined to collapse, deform, degenerate, and perform poorly unless it is supported with a centring underneath (Fig. 25.4).

In summary, in architecture you use a centring to build arches and then remove it while in the foot, you add a centring to support inherited weakness in the arches to prevent collapse and improve performance.

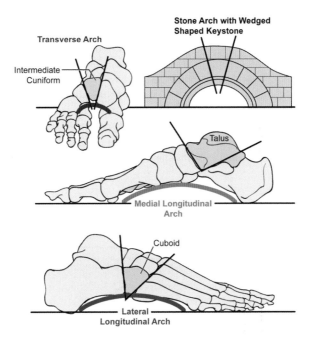

Fig. 25.2 Architectural vs. foot arches

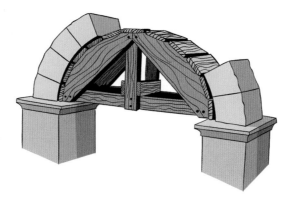

Fig. 25.3 Centring construction of an arch

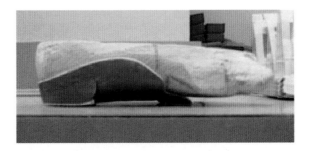

Fig. 25.4 A foot centring orthotic providing arch support

Functional Foot Types® (FFTs)

Some feet have a rigid rearfoot pillar, some a flexible rearfoot pillar, and others fall in between. In addition, some feet have a rigid forefoot pillar, some a flexible forefoot pillar, and others fall in between. Utilizing two rearfoot tests called rearfoot SERM and rearfoot PERM (Serm = Supinatory End Range of Motion and PERM = Pronatory End Range of Motion) and two forefoot tests called forefoot SERM and forefoot PERM, one can classify the feet into four rearfoot types (rigid, stable, flexible, and flat) and four forefoot types (rigid, stable, flexible, and flat) forming 16 possible Functional Foot Types or FFTs.[11] Although there is a matrix of 16 possible FFTs, to date, 9 pure FFTs have been identified. Each Functional Foot Type® has its own characteristic open- and closed-chain presentations, X-ray results, lesion pattern, shoe wear, and foot and postural strengths and weaknesses (Table 25.2).

Table 25.2 The pure Functional Foot Types®

Foot type	Features/callus pattern	Associated problems
Flat RF/flat FF	Flat footed when sitting or standing,	Functional weakness, unable to perform daily tasks
Flexible RF/flexible FF	Flat foot, early bunion callus 2–3 mets, hallux IP jt	Early poor posture, fatigue tired feet, wide feet
Flexible Rf/flat FF	Flat foot, bunions, callus second met, hallux I-P jt	Poor posture, fatigue, second and fifth toe hammertoes
Flexible Rf/rigid Ff	Flat foot, first, fifth callus, hammertoes	
Stable Rf/flexible Ff	Normal arch sitting, flat foot standing	Bunions, heel spurs postural breakdown and problems
Stable FF/stable FF	No callus, normal arch	No problems
Rigid Rf/flexible Ff	High arch sitting, low arch standing callus, second and fifth met, hammertoes	Bunions, thick toenails heel and arch pain, postural pain and problems
Rigid RF/Stable FF	High arch sitting, normal arch standing fifth met callus	Low back pain
Rigid RF/rigid FF	High arch, callus sub 1st met/5th met, 1–5 hammertoes, met-cun exostosis	Low back and shock problems, heel and arch pain

Once a subject's FFT has been determined, foot type-specific care can be rendered. Foot type-specific locations of future deformity, foot and postural breakdown, infections, and ulcerations can be predicted, prevented, and controlled by treating FFTs, resulting in fewer amputations and reduced morbidity in any diabetic population.[12] In addition, a foot type-specific cast and prescription can produce a foot centering orthotic (Fig. 25.5)

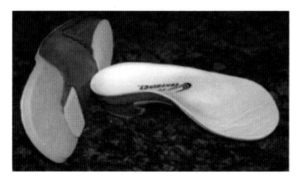

Fig. 25.5 A pair of custom foot centering orthotics

that compensates off-center pathology allowing for improved support and quality of life and preventing ulcers, Charcot feet, and amputations.

The Inclined Posture (TIP)

Since 60% or more of all people have one leg at least 5 mm shorter,[12–14] the balancing of this biomechanical variation is fundamental to treating any unilateral (asymmetrical) foot problem and establishing balanced function, especially in the feet of those suffering from peripheral neuropathy, such as in the diabetic patient.

By testing for asymmetry in ankle dorsiflexion (functional equinus) and subtalar joint inversion (functional varus) between limbs, short limbs can be exposed. This Functional Equinovarus of the Joints of the Ankle or FEJA Test determines if one leg is functionally short.[14] Practitioners can then balance one leg to the other with lifts or physical therapy effectively eliminating a source of biomechanical pathology.

The use of heel lifts or platforms placed on the inside or outside of the short side shoe or incorporated into the short side foot orthotic compensates for TIP if physical therapy fails to stretch soft tissue contractures that may have caused one of the limbs to shorten.

Diabetic Neuropathy

Historically, peripheral arterial disease has been considered the most common complication observed in diabetic lower extremities. However, it is now accepted that the distal symmetric sensory, autonomic, and motor polyneuropathy occurs in up to 60% of patients with long-standing disease.[23] Furthermore, insensitivity coexists with diabetic foot wounds more than 80% of the time.[21] Peripheral nerve dysfunction is significantly associated with both impaired balance and lower extremity impairments.

The Phases of Diabetic Sensory Neuropathy

Diabetic neuropathy may precede other classical signs of diabetes. Its sensory component can be divided into five phases which are often progressive.

Phase I is a tingling sensation in the plantar aspect (bottom) of the foot that may manifest occasionally as a feeling of "bugs crawling" or "bees stinging," and is referred to as fornication.

Phase II has the same symptoms that occur more frequently and are more intense.

Phase III is characterized by a constant burning of the feet that causes disruptions in sleep. This phase usually requires medication for pain control.

Phase IV has increased burning with anesthesia, giving a false sense of improvement from phase III.

Phase V is complete loss of sensation (LOPS).

Corn, Callus, and Poroma Formation

Biomechanical pathology and unhealthy and poorly fitting shoes cause pressure and friction in areas of the foot that are not meant to tolerate such loads. As a result, compensatory protective hyperkeratoses in the form of corns, callus, and porokeratotic (poroma) lesions develop in foot type-specific location. In the diabetic foot, continued pressure causes breakdown of these protective lesions in the form of pressure ulcers and wounds that can become infected. Monitoring and biomechanically controlling compensatory hyperkeratoses and wearing healthy and well-fit shoes are a vital part of preventive diabetic foot care.

The Biomechanics of Charcot Foot

Charcot joint disease or Charcot foot involves a devastating collapse of one of three specific areas of the foot. Since an inherited biomechanical weakness can exist at the midtarsal joint, the tarsometatarsal joint, or the first metatarsal phalangeal joint, it is these areas of the foot that are often affected (as well as the ankle joint). Diabetes is the most commonly underlying disease associated with Charcot foot, end-stage syphilis and leprosy being a distant second and third. Once a Charcot foot develops, morbidity of the foot is permanent and progressive.[13] The patient's lifestyle and his/her ability to walk, work, and wear normal shoes are reduced.

Charcot foot develops in subjects with patent circulation and is composed of a quartet of symptoms:

(1) Patent circulation
(2) Loss of protective sensation (LOPS)
(3) A structurally weak foot type
(4) An active lifestyle, personality, and/or obesity

An individual with intact pain sensation will experience pain and swelling in the area of potential collapse when this area is stressed. Secondary to pain, the patient would likely reduce activity, lose weight, or introduce a biomechanical support, such as a custom foot orthotic, and therefore prevent the potential collapse of the foot. The patient with LOPS in this triad remains pain free and thus does not adjust his or her active lifestyle. Eventually, the weakest link in the biomechanical chain collapses, producing a Charcot foot (Fig. 25.6).

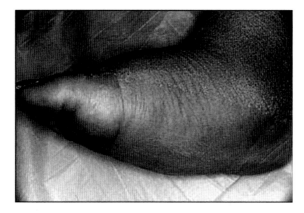

Fig. 25.6 The rocker bottom deformity of a Charcot foot. (Adapted from Sommer,[16] with permission)

There is no successful way to reestablish a normal lifestyle and biomechanics once a Charcot foot occurs. Therefore, it is essential for the physician to detect the impending signs of this quartet and to consider a biomechanical evaluation with a podiatrist for all patients with LOPS before a Charcot foot develops.[12]

The Physician Foot Evaluation

Physicians treating diabetic individuals should obtain a baseline history when it comes to examining the feet of diabetic patients. He or she should then monitor the feet in order to prevent ulcers and amputations and to maintain quality of life. A history of foot and shoe fit problems and quality of life issues should be reviewed. The pedal physical exam should include vascular, neurological, and orthopedic evaluation so that a preventive treatment plan can be developed and monitored. The treatment plan may involve annual examination (if there are no abnormal findings) or more rapid follow-up and consultation with a specialist, such as a podiatrist, if abnormalities are found.

History and Chief Complaint

The patient should be questioned regarding foot and postural problems, including the location and severity of corns, calluses, thick or ingrown toenails, infection and ulceration, as well as ankle, knee, hip, and lower back complaints. Orthopedic deformities, such as bunions and hammertoes, should be noted. Problems with mechanics and posture, such as flat feet or high arches, should be noted, as should a family history of foot and postural problems. Shoe sizing and fit problems must be discussed along with a discussion of lifestyle and activity level. The patient should be asked if he or she is a "slow wound healer," has poor circulation or pedal numbness, burning, tingling, or anesthesia.

The Diabetic Foot Examination

All tests should be performed bilaterally, with asymmetry of complaints, systems, and deformities strongly noted.

Neurological. Touch, cold, and vibratory sense, as well as joint position sense must be tested and the deep tendon reflexes recorded for Achilles and patella. The vibratory sensation should be recorded and, in addition, the time it takes for the sensation of vibration to disappear should be equal in the hands and feet (vibratory dampening). Feet that dampen before the hands should be considered to have reduced proprioception. The Semmes–Weinstein monofilament test (Fig. 25.7)[15] should be taken at least eight sites to determine insensitivity (refer to section on loss of protective sensation).[17]

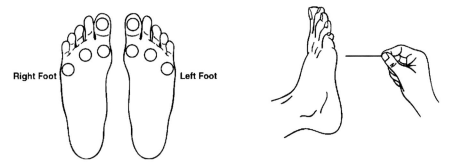

Fig. 25.7 The monofilament sensation test and common test sites. Adapted from LEAPP website www.bphc.hrsa.dhhs.gov/leap/def.htm, with permission

Vascular. Dorsalis pedis and posterior tibial pulses should be recorded. Pedal hair growth, temperature, and skin texture should be examined. Capillary return time/venous filling tests should be performed. The lower extremity should be checked for spider veins, varicosities, and edema. Cuts, abrasions, and wounds should be checked for healing time.

Dermatological. Toenails should be checked for dystrophy, ingrowing, microtrauma, and fungus infection.[18] Skin texture, dryness, and fissures should be appreciated. Skin rashes or even tinea pedis should be noted. Location and severity of corns and callus should be noted. The location and depth of ulcers, wounds, and infections should be determined. Associated skin findings such as yellowish plaques indicative of necrobiosis lipoidica, brown pretibial macules characteristic of diabetic dermopathy, and skin atrophy associated with microvascular compromise should be noted.

Orthopedic. Pedal and digital deformities, such as bunions, hammer toes, and prominent metatarsal heads, should be located and graded. The foot should be examined for intrinsic muscle wasting. The Functional Foot Type® and the existence of the inclined posture should be determined. Shoes should be checked for wear and fit. Gait and postural abnormalities should be noted.

The Diabetic Foot Ulcer Prevention Plan

Risk factors for ulcer development should be determined and utilizing a classification system, a plan of preventive care should be instituted.[19] This type of plan is capable of preventing not only ulceration, but also infection, hospitalization, and amputation.

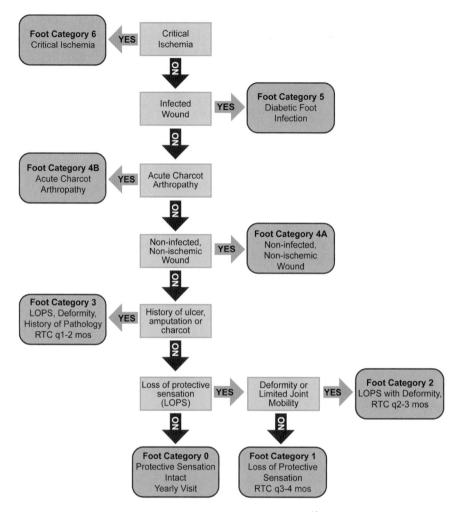

Fig. 25.8 The UT risk classification flowchart (Adapted from Armstrong DG et al.,[18] with permission)

Risk factors include the level of peripheral neuropathy and vascular compromise, the degree of foot deformity and joint mobility, and the existence of current or previous ulceration, infection, or Charcot foot. The University of Texas Risk Classification System (Fig. 25.8) utilizes all of these risk factors to classify diabetic foot ulcer risk. Once the patient is classified, the corresponding level of foot care needed in order to prevent ulceration is instituted. For example, if a patient has a loss of protective sensation and a previous history of ulceration of the foot, he or she would be rated as belonging to the UT foot category 3 and require foot care every 1–2 months. In this manner, an appropriate plan of foot care and monitoring can be established for each patient.

The Team Approach to Diabetic Foot Care

Successful management of the diabetic foot involves the concept of a team approach. The team consists of medical specialists, each focusing on specific risk factors, and commonly includes an endocrinologist, vascular surgeon, neurologist, podiatrist, diabetic nurse educator, and nutritionist.[19]

In successful models, the "captains" of the team include the treating endocrinologist, vascular surgeon, or podiatrist. New patients undergo a diabetic foot history and physical examination and have an initial consultation with the team members. Each specialist provides a baseline report including diagnosis, recommended immediate care, and long term follow-up to the captain who then reports to the patient's primary care physician.

Risk Factors for Amputation

The risk factors for lower extremity amputation are classified into primary and secondary.

The *primary risk factors* include peripheral neuropathy, peripheral vascular disease, structural and functional foot deformities, infection, and ulceration.

The *secondary risk factors* include obesity, impaired vision, improper footwear, lack of a home-based support system, and apparent noncompliance on the patient's part (Table 25.3).

Table 25.3 Risk factors for diabetic foot ulceration and amputation

Primary risk factors
1. Loss of protective sensation (LOPS)
2. Autonomic neuropathy (dryness and fissuring of the skin)
3. Peripheral vascular disease
4. Structural and biomechanical deformities
5. Prior infection
6. Prior ulceration

Secondary risk factors
1. Obesity
2. Impaired vision and retinopathy
3. Nephropathy
4. Poor control of diabetes
5. Poor footwear selection
6. At home noncompliance
7. Lack of adequate home support system

Primary Risk Factors

Peripheral Neuropathy

Peripheral neuropathy is the clinical manifestation of any of a number of potential defects in the physiologic function of the peripheral nervous system. The classic pattern of peripheral neuropathy development is distal to proximal with regard to anatomic location and small to large with regard to the size of the nerves that are involved. In other words, peripheral neuropathy typically begins in the distal lower extremity in a stocking distribution and then progresses proximally. In most cases, the initial nerves that are involved are the smallest and most terminal branches of the peripheral nerves within the epidermis. These myelinated (A-delta) and unmyelinated (c) fibers become diminished in number thereby leading to positive symptoms (pain and paresthesias) and/or negative findings (numbness and coolness). Patients may also experience autonomic deficits (hyperhidrosis, hyperperfusion); however, these rarely are "chief presenting complaints." This early stage of peripheral neuropathy has been designated as "small fiber" peripheral neuropathy. As more proximally located larger nerves become involved the neuropathy becomes "mixed."

Not withstanding the fact that most cases of diabetic peripheral neuropathy begin in the aforementioned distal to proximal pattern, such is not always the case. Patients may also be afflicted by primary large nerve peripheral neuropathy, whether involving single large peripheral nerves or multiple large or medium-sized nerves. The hallmark of large nerve peripheral neuropathy is diminished proprioception, vibratory sensation, and/or conduction velocity.

Loss of Protection Sensation

Insensitivity coexists with diabetic foot wounds more than 80% of the time.[20] The combination of structural foot deformities, biomechanical abnormalities, and poor fitting shoes with a lack of protective sensation in diabetic feet dictates the need for frequent foot examination. Repetitive friction or trauma that would ordinarily cause no more than a painful blister can fester into a lower extremity amputation when LOPS is concomitant.[21]

When a 5.07-mm nylon monofilament (a 10-g force) is pressed against the skin to the point of buckling (Fig. 25.6), patients who cannot feel the filament are at risk for ulceration and require special care. Testing with the monofilament is the most effective screening device and is cost-effective, quick, and easy to perform. Other more time-consuming tests of vibration and thermal sensation are available for identifying patients prone to ulceration.[22] In addition, nylon monofilament testing can potentially register small fiber involvement whereby testing for vibratory sensation is only indicative of large fiber involvement. All patients with diabetes should be tested frequently with this inexpensive, rapidly performed test.

Autonomic Neuropathy

The autonomic component of the diabetic neuropathy produces reduced sweating and fissuring of the skin of the heels and soles and increased sweating in the toe web spaces, making them prone to infection and ulceration. In addition, there is a potential for osseous hyperemia that can be involved in the development of a Charcot foot.

Peripheral Arterial Disease (PAD)

Occlusive arterial disease of the posterior tibial and common peroneal arteries is four times more prevalent in diabetic patients.[23] Reduced pedal pulses, pedal hair loss, claudication, rest and night pain in the arch and calf, cool feet, indurated or shiny skin, dependent rubor, clubbed digits, and thickened toenails, as well as poor healing of cuts and wounds indicate the existence of PAD.[24]

Structural and Biomechanical Deformity

Structural deformities, such as bunions and rigid hammertoes, as well as normal anatomical prominences, such as the fifth metatarsal head and the base of the fifth metatarsal, serve as predictable locations for ulceration in the diabetic patient. It is important to document where these deformities exist for each patient and to instruct the patient to observe these areas carefully for change.

Orthopedic deformities are preceded by underlying biomechanical pathology that reduces weightbearing under one anatomical site thereby producing a compensatory increase in weightbearing in predictable pedal locations. This increased weightbearing creates repetitive injury, callus formation, and ulceration. This is the common mechanism in the creation of plantar metatarsal and great toe ulcers (malum perforans) in the diabetic patient and can be prevented by the use of well-selected and fit shoes and orthotics.

Infection

Diabetic patients tend to have cuts, contusions, and superficial tineal infections that are slow to respond to care. These otherwise minor injuries tend to get infected. Because of concomitant risk factors, multiple aerobic bacteria, yeast, and anaerobic organisms become pathogens in these wounds, making them difficult to control and heal. In addition, because the deep structures in the foot (such as the bone) are actually quite close to the surface, osteomyelitis is more common.[25]

Ulceration

Repetitive microtrauma, repetitive friction, and continuous pressure lead to corn and callus formation which, if left unattended in the insensate foot, leads to sublesional hemorrhage (intracorneal exsanguination) within the keratoses, with eventual ulceration, infection, and amputation.

Ulceration usually occurs in areas of bony prominence that are being irritated by shoe, weightbearing pressure, or excess activity. Without the reflexive repositioning that is necessary to prevent ischemia related to compressive forces over bony prominences, the affected skin is stressed secondary to localized ischemia and is therefore susceptible to ulceration. Thus, ulcerations occur over bony prominences that are irritated by shoe gear or excessive weightbearing pressure.

Secondary Risk Factors

Obesity

Obesity plays an important role in initiating and maintaining type 2 diabetes. It also plays a role in lower extremity amputation since, with obesity, weightbearing increases for all foot structures. The presence of obesity magnifies biomechanical pathology. For this reason, among others, weight reduction must be considered a critical goal in overweight diabetic patients.

Impaired Vision

The demographic characteristics for lower extremity amputation are skewed toward senior citizens with an age greater than 60. This population suffers from age-related vision problems such as cataracts and glaucoma. In addition, these patients may suffer from diabetic retinopathy. Impaired vision prevents patients from self-examination and self-care of the feet. It also impairs the ability of patients to observe their surroundings and plan movements safely.

Improper Footwear

Irritation and pressure from poor sizing and selection of footwear play a critical role in the development of ulcers and infections. Since insensitivity also includes reduced proprioception, patients with diabetes often cannot tell if their shoes are well fit or creating irritation. Therefore, diabetic patients need skilled shoe fitters and ongoing monitoring of their shoes.

Tight shoes, high heels, low toe boxes, and improper fitting (either too small or too large) may press shoes onto bony prominences and contribute to the formation of ulcers. Shoes should be selected and sized with sufficient toe box, width, closing systems, and depth in order to accommodate all existing deformities without being too large. Selecting a larger size, if in doubt, should reduce errors, but it should be noted that as a shoe becomes too large for a patient's foot, balance and gait problems become exposed.

The Congress has tried to address the needs of diabetic patients by initiating The Medicare Therapeutic Shoe Bill in 1996.[26] Under this bill, a physician must certify that a patient has diabetes, is under a treatment plan for diabetes, and has a related foot problem. A professional with shoe prescribing knowledge, such as a podiatrist, may then prescribe a pair of shoes with protective insoles. Medicare will pay for one pair of shoes and three protective insoles or a molded shoe annually.

Shoe Noncompliance at Home

Patients with diabetes and LOPS often do not wear their protective shoes when at home.[27] Since this may be where they spend most of their day, slippers should be dispensed with protective foot inserts (orthotics) and the use of diabetic socks should be considered. If problems with the feet continue, outdoor shoes should be worn at all weightbearing moments, even when at home.

Lack of a Home-Based Support System

The ability to observe and care for a wound and the additional needs of a diabetic patient are enhanced by the support system. Without adequate support from a family member or visiting professional, such as a wound care nurse, wounds that would otherwise heal uneventfully can lead to a lower extremity amputation in a matter of days. The physician must coordinate home support or change the patient's environment in order to prevent such tragedies.

Apparent Noncompliance on the Patient's Part

When working with diabetic feet that are ulcerated or infected, a physician may experience a false sense that the patient is noncompliant. Since the lack of pain sensation can interfere with the patient's compliance, it is the responsibility of the physician to alert all parties involved in the patient's care, including the patient himself or herself, to this problem and to assume adequate monitoring.

Plantar Offloading of the Diabetic Foot

The feet are the foundation of the posture and must accept a lifetime of weightbearing stress. Biomechanics, body weight, and activity level determine the location and timing of areas of potential breakdown. It is necessary to disperse the plantar weightbearing forces away from high stress areas in order to prevent ulceration or to heal an existing wound.

Thermography and computerized pressure scanning can be used to predict sites that will ulcerate on the plantar surface of the diabetic foot. Plantar off-loading of the diabetic foot encompasses the use of pads, inserts (foot orthotics), shoe modifications, pressure-distributing boots, and prophylactic foot surgery to remove or redistribute stress away from areas under extreme pressure.[28]

Principles of Padding

The use of $\frac{1}{4}''$ adhesive felt and other pads to relocate pressure proximally to a problematic area can be a key element of wound care. Given the human gait cycle, pads that are horseshoe or rectangular in shape and placed just proximal to a callus (or ulcer) will reduce pressure under the callused area (or ulceration) without being too bulky. This will prevent the breakdown of a callus (or heal the ulcer). These pads can be adhered directly to the foot or incorporated into the footbed of a shoe. It should be noted that pads placed directly on a pressure area would actually add to the pressure.

Foot Orthotics

Foot orthotics can be *prefabricated* (over-the-counter), *customized prefabricated* (over-the-counter with custom modifications), or *custom* (taken from a cast or scan of the foot). They are made from materials that vary from soft and accommodating to rigid and supportive. Orthotics may be soft, hard, or mixed in nature, depending on their purpose. A rigid device can support and control the arches to prevent collapse. An accommodative device can cushion and give comfort and protection to a weak or diabetic foot that is beyond salvage. A mixed material orthotic, when custom casted, can support the arch while removing pressure from specific overweighted areas.

Since an orthotic can be utilized to improve function and quality of life, as well as to reduce pressure in desired locations, the diabetic foot, especially the insensitive diabetic foot, deserves a custom orthotic shoe bed for safe and maximum performance.

Shoe Modifications

Because of cosmetics, shoe modifications should be a last resort. Today, there is over-the-counter footwear that fills the need for almost all diabetic patients. Depth inlay shoes, therapeutic shoes, Velcro closure shoes, wound healing shoes, walking shoes, and comfort shoes have largely replaced the molded shoe from a cast. Custom modifications, such as rocker bars, lifts, cutouts, and heel and sole wedge, can then be added to overcome specific problems.

Pressure-Distributing Casts and Boots

Non-healing wounds (older than 6 months) can often be healed with total contact casting (TCC). Weekly application of a pressure-distributing cast reduces pressure underneath the wound, yet allows for weightbearing function. This gold standard is slowly being replaced by a new generation of healing boots that reduce pressure under wounds yet, unlike TCC, allow for their removal for inspection, physical therapy, and unencumbered bed rest. While these removable devices are generally better accepted than fixed casting, they do present the added variable of concern over patient compliance.

Prophylactic Foot Surgery

Podiatrists and orthopedic surgeons perform osteotomies, soft tissue balancing procedures, corrective digital procedures, and bony spur excisions on diabetic feet in order to eliminate the occurrence or the recurrence of ulcers and infections. Utilizing the information on foot typing, weightbearing X-rays, thermography, and pressure mat scanning, a surgeon can predict the precise locations that may ulcerate and become infected in the future. In well-selected cases, foot surgeons can prevent a future problem at a time when the vascular system is adequate to allow healing. The same surgical procedures, if performed at a later date, in the face of peripheral vascular disease, may be contraindicated. For example, if a diabetic patient with an insensate foot but adequate circulation has a plantarflexed second metatarsal that is rapidly forming thick callus, a prophylactic dorsiflectory osteotomy of the second metatarsal will prevent a future malum perforans at this site.

Diabetic Neuropathy Testing

Most testing methods that are used in the assessment of peripheral neuropathy have at least one of three important limitations. Foremost is subjectivity that is incorporated into almost all tests involved in the testing of small fiber neuropathy. Secondly, some tests, such as sural nerve biopsies and nerve conduction studies, characterize only large fiber neuropathies and fail to assess the small fiber component. Finally, many available testing methods are performed only at major academic centers.

Epidermal nerves fiber density (EDNF) testing can be used to diagnose peripheral neuropathy. Epidermal nerve fibers are the terminal branches of peripheral nerves which pass into the epidermis as unmyelinated C-fibers or myelinated A-delta fibers. The presence of epidermal nerve fibers has been hypothesized for over a century; however, their existence was not confirmed until the advent of electron microscopy. In persons with small fiber peripheral neuropathy, the number of epidermal nerve fibers is characteristically diminished per area unit. Since the average density of epidermal nerve fibers is consistent for each anatomic location (independent of age or gender), a "normal" range can be determined. [29] An epidermal nerve fiber density below this reference range is consistent with small fiber peripheral neuropathy.

Epidermal nerve fiber density is usually measured within a standard 3-mm cutaneous punch biopsy. By convention samples are obtained from the lower leg and foot, 10 cm proximal to the lateral malleolus and the heel or great toe so that the epidermal nerve fibers within the skin sample may be quantified.

Immunoperoxidase stain PGP 9.5 is employed.[30] This stain uses antibodies that are neuron specific and once applied, it highlights epidermal nerve fibers thereby allowing them to be quantified under light microscopy (Fig. 25.9)

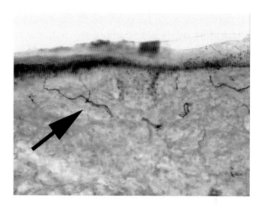

Fig. 25.9 Epidermal nerve fiber test, note epidermal nerve fibers, Dr. Bradley Bakotic

This technique has numerous advantages over others; foremost among them is the fact that it is a wholly objective way to detect peripheral neuropathy. This makes ENFD testing an excellent option for establishing a baseline from which to assess improvement following therapy. Other important advantages are its ease, sensitivity, and specificity. Epidermal nerve fiber density is significantly more sensitive than sural nerve biopsy.[29] Overall, the specificity of ENFD testing is an impressive 97% at the fifth percentile cutoff value, while the specificity is roughly 45%. Maintaining the fifth percentile cutoff value for the ENFD will correctly classify 88% of all tested neuropathy cases.[29] In addition, studies have shown that ENFD can reveal small nerve neuropathy in the precursor of diabetes known as impaired glucose tolerance (IGT) making it a valuable tool in monitoring "borderline" or prediabetic patients.[31] The use of long- and short-acting local anesthetics and cyanocobalamine as common peroneal and posterior tibial nerve "chemical sympathectomies" has been shown to be effective in the treatment of diabetic peripheral neuropathy.[32]

Alternative Treatment

One alternative therapy is based on the evidence of insufficient dietary intake of gamma linoleic acid (GLA) as a possible cause of the diabetic peripheral neuropathy.[30] Normal subjects can convert linoleic acid (LA), which is readily available in our diet, into GLA. However, some diabetic patients have a reduced capacity for this conversion. Evening primrose oil (EPO) seeds, when crushed, are a safe source of GLA. A total of 450 mg, given orally, twice a day, may reverse the signs and symptoms of diabetic neuropathy in 10–14 days in a diabetic individual.[32]

Alpha lipoic acid and L-arginine are two other supplements that may be helpful in some cases. Topical capsaicin cream in low concentration (0.025%) applied sparingly to affected areas may be of some use in subjects that cannot tolerate other treatment.

The use of long- and short-acting local anesthetics and cyanocobalamine as common peroneal and posterior tibial nerve "chemical sympathectomies" has been shown to be effective in the treatment of diabetic peripheral neuropathy.[32] Exercises are generally effective in remobilizing the hammered digits. Toe fists (15X), toe pickups (picking up cotton balls or pencils) (15X), extending the toes over the binding of a book (20X) and toe creeping (crawling with the toes on the ground) (2 min) should be repeated 1–2 times/day.

Surgically, a decompression of the areas where swollen nerves become entrapped is becoming more accepted in relieving late-phase sensory neuropathy.[33]

Cellulitis and Osteomyelitis

Cellulitis and osteomyelitis are still major risk factors for amputation in the diabetic foot. These risks are somewhat reduced due to advances in diagnostic techniques, oral and intravenous antibiotics, and the team approach to care. The bone scan and MRI studies have replaced X-rays as the standard techniques for early diagnosis and monitoring followed by bone biopsy, if necessary. In a vascularized limb, with appropriate antibiotic therapy, cellulitis resolves in a matter of days[31] and 6- to 8-week course of antibiotics will heal osteomyelitic bone. If this protocol fails, the insertion of antibiotic beads can be considered.[32] Since early diagnosis is critical, the physician must react quickly and aggressively when the signs and symptoms of cellulitis and osteomyelitis are apparent.[33]

Non-healing Wound Care

With the evolution of modern antibiotics, diagnostic tools such as MRI, home wound care, and educational programs that allow the physician to make an earlier diagnosis and provide more effective treatment than in the past, most diabetic foot wounds heal uneventfully.[34] However, wounds that have not significantly healed after 3–6 weeks of care can be considered non-healing. They have sparse angiogenesis potential, reduced growth factor release, and are more likely to become infected. These wounds can, however, be converted into acute, healing wounds, with proper management.

After evaluation of the status of the foot and of the wound a clinician can classify a wound according to its depth, size, and healing ability. A multifaceted program of care can then be instituted and monitored.

Clinical attention to many factors involved in healing a wound, rather than focus on a single risk factor, can lead a non-healing wound to improve at a time when it seems to be stagnant. If the status of a particular system or risk is uncertain, then immediate consultation with a specialist (s) is in order.

Evaluation of the Status of the Wound

The wound should be measured and photographed.[35] The wound should be classified according to depth as follows:

1. pre- or post-ulceration, completely epithelialized;
2. superficial and not involving tendon, capsule, or bone;
3. penetrating to tendon or capsule; and
4. penetrating to bone.

The location of the wound is critical and will determine the importance for off-loading. The margins should be examined for redness, heat, swelling. The level of pain should be determined, but since insensitivity of wounds in diabetic patients is the rule, painless wounds should be considered high risk. The epithelial borders of the wound should be assessed. The quality of the base of the wound should be determined. A fresh, granular base is desirable and necrosis and detritus are to be avoided. The presence of bleeding and/or exudate should be recorded. Microbial culture and sensitivity should be obtained and an antibiotic should be started if the wound is showing signs of drainage, infection, or poor healing. It should be noted that even the smallest amount of healing every week will lead to a healed wound but a wound that remains stagnant for more than 2 weeks needs immediate reassessment. Some changes in the treatment regimen or consultation are necessary at this critical time.

Evaluation of the Status of Complications

Wounds should be classified according to the vascular status and the presence of infection:
(1) absence of vascular complications and infection;
(2) presence of infection;
(3) presence of vascular complications; and
(4) presence of both infection and vascular complications.

A vascular and/or infectious disease consultation becomes critical when these complications are present.

Classification of Diabetic Foot Wounds

Once the clinician determines the status of the wound and the foot, it is necessary to utilize this information to classify the wound and establish a treatment protocol. The UT wound classification[36] gives a wound status number (0–3) and a foot status letter (A–D) which gives a final description of the wound. For example, a UT wound classification of C-3 would be a wound penetrating to bone involving an avascular foot. Figure 25.10 shows the University of Texas Wound Classification Flowchart which incorporates both the status of the wound and complications.

Meticulous Debridement

Meticulous debridement is the most important service that a chronic, non-healing wound deserves since wounds that are not aggressively debrided form a callus that masks the clinician's ability to evaluate, treat, and monitor a wound. In a poorly healing wound, the epithelial edges seal and stop growing inward, preventing closure of the wound.

The base of the wound becomes necrotic and infected and growth factors cease to be released (Fig. 25.11). Meticulous debridement utilizes aggressive sterile surgery to remove peripheral callus and make the epithelial edges raw. It eliminates necrotic tissue and detritus as well as free bleeding at the base and periphery of the wound.

Debridement stimulates the release and production of the multiple growth factors that contribute to wound healing.[38] It denudes circumferential epithelial margins so that the skin margins can continue to close instead of "sealing off" at the wound edge. It stimulates angiogenesis and the vascular cascade. Wounds should be measured weekly and debrided using a sterile field and instruments, as they heal. Debridement can be carried out on a weekly basis in the outpatient office or wound healing center setting. In contrast, a deep wound with need for more aggressive tissue dissection and instrumentation should be performed in the operating room.[40,41]

Off-loading of the Non-healing Wound

The use of $1/4''$ adhesive sponge horseshoe-shaped pads just proximal to non-healing wounds reduces plantar pressure on these wounds dramatically. Wound healing shoes and boots with custom insoles to reduce weightbearing pressure are invaluable. If, in spite of these measures, a wound remains resistant to healing, a wheelchair, contact casting, or bed rest must be considered.

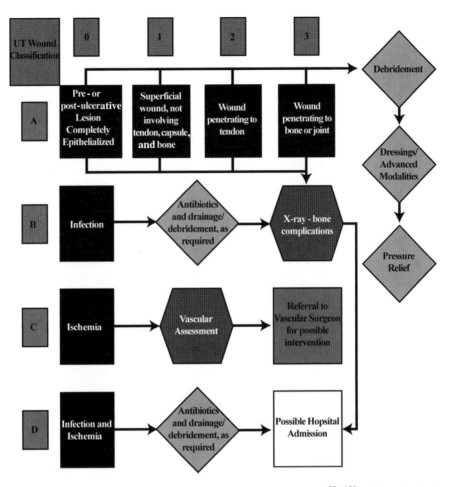

Fig. 25.10   The UT wound classification flowchart. (Adapted from Armstrong DM et al.,[37(p150)] with permission)

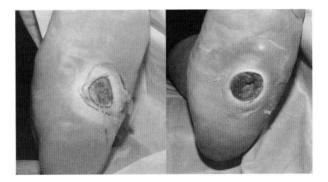

Fig. 25.11   A diabetic ulcer under the cuboid of a Charcot foot, before and after meticulous debridement. (Adapted from Brenner,[1] with permission.)

Advances in Wound Healing

The three most utilized advances in wound care are hyperbaric oxygen treatment,[39] recombinant growth factors,[42] and bioengineered alternative tissues.[43] These modalities are adjunctive to meticulous debridement and off-loading and, although costly, when used in properly selected cases, can reduce the healing time of wounds as well as the overall cost of care.

Hyperbaric oxygen treatment (HBO) uses pressurized 100% oxygen, delivered in a full body chamber. If the PO_2 of the wound surface is low, then HBO may be of benefit. This is of particular benefit in wounds that are complicated by microvascular disease.[44]

Platelet-derived growth factor (PDGF) has been successfully produced in a gel form and, when applied to large and deep noninfected wounds, it can accelerate the healing process.[45] Other growth factors are under investigation and additional products are on the horizon, including vascular endothelial growth factor (VEGF).

Bioengineered alternative tissues (BAT) are a highly specialized group of products that include both living and nonliving applications which can serve as wound healing adjuncts. The most sophisticated products to date include living human keratinocytes and living human dermal fibroblasts derived from neonatal foreskin and propagated in culture.[46,47] These products are easy to apply and, since BAT serves as a substrate for the patient's own skin repair, the end result is a plantar wound covered by plantar tissue.

Vacuum-assisted closure (VAC) is a new dynamic adjunct to the wound healing armamentarium.[48] Also called *negative pressure wound therapy*, this technology is best suited for large, deep wound defects or post-partial foot amputation wounds. Negative pressure wound therapy utilizes an electrically powered suction pump and occlusive dressing system to create a subatmospheric pressure at the wound base. This serves to stimulate angiogenesis, reduce bacterial burden, and efficiently remove exudates from the wound site.

The past decade has brought an enormous number of new topical wound care technologies to this field. Two categories are seeing wider acceptance in wound healing circles. The first is the utilization of slow release topical silver into the wound base for the reduction of bacterial burden and biofilm contaminant that often retard healing or cause clinical wound infection.[49] The second is the use of active honey tested for its antibacterial component topically found only in honey produced from *Leptospermum* (Manuka) rated with a Unique Manuka Factor (UMF) of 10+, even when diluted and in a non-sterile state.[50,51]

Conclusions

Diabetes affects the feet, with regularity as the disease progresses. Complications of the foot are the leading cause for hospital admission in patients with diabetes.

By implementing a foot care program that involves risk classification, biomechanical evaluation, the team approach, and close monitoring, the physician will be able to keep his/her patients active, functional, ulcer and infection free and will reduce the risk of limb loss and maintain a high quality of patient's life.

References

1. Brenner MA, Ed. *Management of the Diabetic Foot (Chapter 6)*. Williams and Wilkins, New York, 1987.
2. Mayfield J. Foot examinations reduce the risk of diabetic amputations. *J Fam Practice*. 1998;49:499–504.
3. American Diabetes Association. Foot care in patients with diabetes mellitus. *Diabetes Care*. 1998;21:54–58.
4. Reiber GE, Raugi GJ. A model for foot care in people with diabetes. *Lancet*. 2005;366:1676–1677, 1719–1724.
5. Boulton AJ, Vileikyte L, Apelqvist J. The global burden of diabetic foot disease. *Lancet*. 2005;366:1719–1724.
6. Einhorn DA. The state of diabetes complications in America. The American Association of Clinical Endocrinologists 16th Annual Meeting and Clinical Congress; May 2007; Seattle, Washington.
7. Ragnarson TG, Apelqvist J. Health and economic consequences of diabetic foot lesions. *Clin Infect Dis*. 2004;39(Suppl 2):S132–S139.
8. Todd WF, Armstrong DG, Liswood PJ. Evaluation and treatment of the infected foot in a community teaching hospital. *J Am Podiatr Med Assoc*. 1996;86:421–426.
9. Lower Extremity Amputation Prevention Project. *Diabetes Care*. 1998;21:23–25.
10. Armstrong DG, Lavery LA, Stern S, et al. Is prophylactic diabetes foot surgery dangerous? *J Foot Ankle Surg*. 1996;35:585–590.
11. Shavelson D. A closer look at neoteric biomechanics. *Podiatry Today*. Sept 2007;9:234–241.
12. Root ML, Orien WP, Weed JH. Normal and abnormal function of the foot. In: *Clinical Biomechanics*, Vol 2, Clinical Biomechanics Corp, Los Angeles, CA, 1977.
13. Inman VT. *The Joints of the Ankle*. Mann RA and Inman VT, Eds. Williams and Wilkins, Baltimore, MD 1976.

14. Shavelson D. The unequal limb syndrome: biomechanical considerations. *J Am Acad Pod Sport Med*. 1983;1:18–23.
15. Caputo GM. The nylon monofilament test for sensation. *New Eng J Med*. 1994;331:854–859.
16. Sommer, TA. Charcot foot, the diagnostic dilemma. Amer Fam Prac 11: 109, 1995.
17. Frykberg R, Ed. *The High Risk Foot in Diabetes*. Churchill Livingstone, New York, 1991.
18. Armstrong DG, Lavery LA, Harkless LB. Who is at risk for diabetic foot ulceration?. *Clin Podiatr Med Surg*. 1998;15:11–19.
19. Frykberg RG. Team approach toward lower extremity amputation prevention in diabetes. *J Am Podiatr Med Assoc*. 1997;87: 5–12.
20. Selby JV, Hang D. Risk factors for lower extremity amputation in persons with diabetes. *Diabetes Care*. 1995;18:509–516.
21. Day MR, Harkless LB. Factors associated with pedal ulceration in patients with diabetes mellitus. *J Am Podiatr Med Assoc*. 1997;87:365–369.
22. Young MJ, Breddy JL, Veves A, et al. The prediction of diabetic neuropathic foot ulceration using vibration perception thresholds. *Diabetes Care*. 1994;17:557–562.
23. McNeely MJ, Boyko EJ, Ahroni JH, et al. The independent contributions of diabetic neuropathy and vasculopathy in foot ulceration. *Diabetes Care*. 1995;18:216–219.
24. Sykes MT, Godsey JB. Vascular evaluation of the problem diabetic foot. *Clin Podiatr Med Surg*. 1998;15:49–83.
25. Apelqvist J. Wound healing in diabetes: outcome and costs. *Clin Podiatr Med Surg*. 1998;15:21–39.
26. The Medicare Therapeutic Shoe Bill. Department of Health and Human Services, Medical Carriers Manual, Section 2134, p2-85.1-2-86. US Gov't Printing Office, Washington, DC, 1994.
27. Armstrong DG, et al. Continuous activity monitoring in persons at high risk for diabetes-related lower extremity amputation. *J Am Podiatr Med Assoc*. 2001;91:451–455.
28. Lavery LA, Vela SA, Lavery DC, et al. Reducing dynamic foot pressures in high-risk diabetic subjects with foot ulcerations. *Diabetes Care*. 1999;19:818–821.
29. McArthur JC, Stocks EA, Hauer P, Cornblath DR, Griffin JW. Epidermal nerve fiber density. Normal reference range and diagnostic efficiency. *Arch Neurol*. 1998;55:1513–1520.
30. Chien HF, Tseng TJ, Lin WM, et al. Quantitative pathology of cutaneous nerve terminal degeneration in the human skin. *Acta Neuropathol*. 2000;102:455–461.
31. Shavelson D Local anesthetics and injectable cortisone. In: T Delauro, Ed. *Clinics in Pod Med & Surg*, Chapter 8, W.B. Saunders, Philadelphia, 1993
32. Jamal GA. The use of gamma linoleic acid in the prevention and treatment of diabetic neuropathy. *Diabetes Medicine*. 1994;11:145–149.
33. Hounsom L, et al. GLA is effective against multiple indices of experimental diabetic neuropathy. *Diabetologia*. 1998;41: 839–843.
34. Mayo Clinic Reports. Alpha Lipoic Acid (ALA) improves symptoms of diabetic neuropathy. *Diabetes Care*. March 2003;26(3): 456–459.
35. Head KA. Peripheral neuropathy: pathogenic mechanisms and alternative therapies. *Altern Med Rev*. Dec 2006;11(4):32–37.
36. Resneck HE, et al. Independent effects of peripheral nerve dysfunction on lower-extremity physical function in old age. *Diabetes Care*. 2000;23:132–138.
37. Armstrong DG, Harkless LB, et al. Validation of a diabetic wound classification system: the importance of depth, infection and ischaemia. *J Am Podiatr Med Assoc*. 1998;79:144–153.
38. Marcinko DE. Antibiotic-impregnated polymethyl methacrylate beads. In: *Infections of the Foot: Diagnosis and Management*. Habershaw GM Ed. Mosby-Year Book Pub, St. Louis, MO, 174–176, 1998.
39. Gibbons GW, Habershaw GM. Diabetic foot infections: anatomy and surgery. *Infect Dis Clin North Am*. 1995;9:131–142.
40. Frykberg RG. Diabetic foot ulcers: current concepts. *J Foot Ankle Surg*. 1998;37:440–446.
41. Sage RA. The management of foot ulcers. In: *Advances in Podiatric Medicine and Surgery*. W Joseph, Ed. Mosby-Year Book Pub, St. Louis, MO 139–153, 1995.
42. Sommer TA. Charcot foot: the diagnostic dilemma. *J Fam Pract*. 2001;11:1591–1599.
43. Poretsky LY, Shavelson DE, et al. The pre-charcot foot. A new clinical entity to prevent Charcot Joint Disease. *Clin Diabetol*. Sept 2006;25(3):24–28.
44. Faglia E, Favales F, Aldeghi A, et al. Adjunctive systemic hyperbaric oxygen therapy in treatment of severe prevalently ischemic diabetic foot ulcer: a randomized study. *Diabetes Care*. 1996;19:1338–1342.
45. Wieman TJ, Smiell JM, Su Y. Efficacy and safety of a topical gel formulation of recombinant human platelet-derived growth factor-BB (becaplermin) in patients with chronic neuropathic diabetic ulcers: a phase III randomized placebo-controlled double-blind study. *Diabetes Care*. 1998;21:822–829.
46. Snyder RJ, Simonson DA. Cadaveric allograft as adjunct therapy for nonhealing wounds. *J Foot Ankle Surg*. 1999;38:93–101.
47. Falanga V. How to use Apligraf to treat venous ulcers. *Skin and Aging*. 1999;2:30–36.
48. Webb LX. New techniques in wound management: vacuum assisted wound closure. *J Am Acad Orthop Surg*. September/October 2002;10(5):303–311.
49. Lansdown ABG. Silver: toxicity in mammals and how its products aid wound repair. *J Wound Care*. 2002;11(5):173–177.
50. Cutting K. Antibacterial honey: in vitro activity against clinical isolates of MRSA, VRE and Pseudomonas aeruginosa. *Wounds*. 2007;19(9):231–236.
51. Molan PC. The evidence supporting the use of honey as a wound dressing. *Int J Low Extrem Wounds*. 2006;5:40–42.

Chapter 26
Male Sexual Dysfunction in Diabetes Mellitus

Barry M. Mason, Albert C. Leung, Michael E. DiSanto, and Arnold Melman

Introduction

Male sexual dysfunction can be classified according to the following categories: erectile dysfunction (ED), orgasmic, ejaculatory dysfunction, priapism, and decreased libido. Of these various disorders, medical therapy for ED is the most advanced. ED, also known as impotence, is defined as the inability to achieve or maintain an erection sufficient for satisfactory sexual function.[1] In recent years, there has been an escalating public awareness of the magnitude of ED, partly attributable to the advent of Viagra[TM], Levitra[TM], and Cialis [TM] and their associated marketing. The impact of ED is significant as its prevalence in men aged 40–70 years old was estimated at 52% by the Massachusetts Male Aging Study. Based on these data and the US population projection for the year 2020 of more than 62 million men 45–84 years old, ED will affect more than 31 million men and millions more over the age of 84.[2,3] The projected worldwide prevalence of ED for the year 2025 will be staggering at 322 million men.[4] Certain patient populations are found to have a significantly higher prevalence of ED; for example, diabetic men have a more than threefold increase in risk of ED compared to their nondiabetic counterparts. Indeed, diabetes mellitus is the single most common cause of ED.[5] More than 50% of diabetic patients are afflicted with some degree of ED, and approximately 50% of the patients evaluated at our Center for Male Sexual Dysfunction are diabetic.

Studies have found ED to be an age-dependent disease process that is accelerated in age-matched diabetic men. The prevalence of ED in diabetic men ranges from 35 to 75%,[3] and correlates positively with patient age, duration of diabetes, and disease severity. Compared to healthy men, the onset of ED occurs 10–15 years earlier on an average in diabetic men, regardless of insulin dependency status.

Etiology

ED is multifactorial in origin, but can be classified as either organic or psychogenic.[6] Organic ED can be secondary to vasculogenic, neurogenic, hormonal, or cavernosal smooth muscle abnormalities. Psychogenic ED is a result of central nervous system inhibition of the erectile mechanism and is most prevalent in younger men. The common causes of the organic component of ED in men with diabetes are autonomic neuropathy and vascular abnormalities. The latter are often associated with diabetes, reflecting disease in major arteries, arterial insufficiency, veno-occlusive dysfunction, and microvascular abnormalities.[7–11] Corporal cavernosal smooth muscle (CCSM) abnormalities, such as enhanced CCSM tone, are also essential factors in diabetes-induced ED. Chronic renal failure and endocrine disorders such as hypogonadism, hyperprolactinemia, hypothyroidism and hyperthyroidism, testicular failure, and estrogen excess may also result in ED. Substances of abuse and certain medications, such as antihypertensives, antidepressants, hormones, diuretics, and cardiac medications, are

A. Melman (✉)

Department of Urology, Montefiore Medical Center/Albert Einstein College of Medicine, Bronx, NY, USA

e-mail: amelman@montefiore.org

L. Poretsky (ed.), *Principles of Diabetes Mellitus*, DOI 10.1007/978-0-387-09841-8_26,
© Springer Science+Business Media, LLC 2010

commonly associated with ED.[6-10] Cummings et al. describe the striking degree of overlap between the risk factors of ED and common comorbidities of diabetes: cardiovascular disease, treated and untreated hypertension, multiple drug therapy, neuropathy, and obesity.[12] Thus the vulnerability of diabetic men to ED is further compounded by their additional need for multiple medications for other diabetes-associated medical conditions. Finally, trauma, irradiation, or pelvic surgery can also result in iatrogenic ED. Table 26.1 summarizes the various processes that contribute to ED.

Table 26.1 Etiology of erectile dysfunction

Systemic diseases	*Penile*
Diabetes mellitus	Peyronie's disease
Atherosclerosis	Epispadias
Arterial hypertension	Priapism
Myocardial infarction	
Scleroderma	*Psychiatric*
Renal failure	Depression
Liver cirrhosis	Widower's syndrome
Idiopathic hemochromatosis	Performance anxiety
Neurogenic	*Nutritional*
Epilepsy	Protein malnutrition
Cerebrovascular accidents	Zinc deficiency
Multiple sclerosis	
Guillain–Barre	*Hematologic*
Alzheimer's disease	Leukemias
Respiratory	
Chronic obstructive pulmonary disease	*Infections*
	Brucellosis
Endocrine	Tuberculosis
Hyperthyroidism	AIDS
Hypothyroidism	Trypanosomiasis
Hypogonadism	

General Penile Erection Physiology

The presentation of diabetic ED can be described in one of three ways: (1) asymptomatic diabetes followed years later by impotence, (2) impotence as a firm sign of diabetes, and (3) temporary impotence resulting from poorly controlled diabetes, which is more likely caused by associated malnutrition and weakness.[13] The onset of organic ED is usually insidious and gradual, initially presenting with the inability to sustain erection, followed by incomplete rigidity and ultimately complete loss of erectile function. In order to appreciate the penile erectile physiology and dysfunction, knowledge of the penile anatomy and hemodynamics of erection is imperative.

The penis originates as separate, paired structures, the crura, which are attached by dense facial fibers to the periosteum of the ischiopubic rami. As the crura course toward the pubic symphysis, they join together and to the corpus spongiosum caudally to form a tripartite structure. The corpora cavernosa are enclosed in a thick fibrous sheath, the tunica albuginea, whose fibers unite medially to form a perforated septum that allows the two bodies to function as a single unit. At the cellular level, the cavernosal tissue contained within the corpora contains a meshwork of interconnected cavernosal spaces known as sinusoidal or lacunar spaces. These are lined by vascular endothelium and separated by trabeculae composed of bundles of CCSM fibers with an extracellular matrix of collagen, elastin, and fibroblasts. Gap junctions, hexamer protein-lined aqueous intercellular channels, connect the CCSM cells and create an efficient syncytial network of those smooth muscle cells.[10-14]

The arterial inflow to the penis is the end terminal of the internal pudendal artery, a branch of the hypogastric or internal iliac artery. Upon emerging from Alcock's canal, the internal pudendal artery gives rise to the common penile artery, which further subdivides into the bulbo-urethral, cavernosal (deep), and dorsal penile end arteries. The cavernosal arteries of the penis give off multiple helicine branches that are tortuous and contracted in the flaccid state and become straight and larger in caliber during erection. While the vascular elements lead to tumescence, it is the intracavernosal pressure that ultimately determines erectile function.

The penis is a complex vascular organ that requires the coordination of vascular, neural, and hormonal factors in order to achieve satisfactory penile erection. Any abnormality that affects the integrity of the penile vasculature may result in ED. Four physiologic mechanisms are necessary to effect penile erections: (1) an intact neuronal innervation, (2) an intact arterial supply, (3) appropriately responsive CCSM with normally functional intercellular communication, and (4) an intact veno-occlusive mechanism. Nonetheless, penile erection and detumescence are principally vascular events coordinated by the relaxation and contraction of CCSM, respectively. In the absence of severe arterial insufficiency, relaxation of the CCSM is sufficient to elicit a sustained erection.[15,16] The CCSM tone is thus a primary determinant of erectile function. In the flaccid state, the cavernosal arteries and cavernosal smooth muscle cells are constricted, permitting venous outflow. In the flaccid state, blood flow via the cavernous arteries into the cavernous spaces is minimal (3–5 mL/min). Sexual stimulation leads to a decrease in peripheral resistance, vasodilation, and a tenfold increased blood flow through the cavernous and helicine arteries. The intracavernous pressure increases without any accompanying increase in systemic pressure. Relaxation of the trabecular smooth muscle causes increased compliance of the cavernosal spaces, leading to penile engorgement and erection. In the fully erect state, compression of the trabecular smooth muscle cells against the fibroelastic tunica albuginea causes closure of the draining emissary veins and accumulation of blood at systemic pressure in the corporal sinusoidal bodies. Detumescence ensues during contraction of the trabecular smooth muscle, with resumption of arterial blood flow at the prestimulation level and reopening of venous outflow channels. The intracavernosal pressure declines leading to the flaccid state. Any interruption or interference in this cascade of vascular events may precipitate ED.[10,17,18]

Pathophysiology of Erectile Dysfunction and Diabetes

Neurological/Biochemical Physiology

The Physiological Problem

The normal state of the penis is flaccidity, i.e, contracted. ED is the inability to achieve sufficient blood flow and relaxation of the CCSM to raise the corporal pressure to mean systemic levels for a prolonged duration. In men with diabetes who have impaired erection, there is the inability to either obtain or maintain a state of penile rigidity sufficient for satisfactory intercourse.

Neurological Changes

The neurotransmitters that mediate penile contraction include noradrenaline and the endothelins. There is a long-standing view that ED in men with diabetes is primarily caused by neurological abnormalities.[7,19,20] Ellenberg attributed the increased incidence of diabetic impotence to autonomic neuropathy.[7,8] Penile erection is under the regulation of the autonomic system. The neurotransmitters that control erection can be grouped into those that mediate contraction (noradrenaline, the endothelins, neuropeptide Y (NPY), prostanoids, angiotensin II, and the RhoA/Rho-kinase system) and those that mediate relaxation (acetylcholine, nitric oxide, vasoactive intestinal polypeptide, calcitonin gene-related peptide, adrenomedullin, adenosine triphosphate (ATP), adenosine, and the prostanoids). Sexual stimuli result in neurological impulses via somatic and autonomic motor tracts to the penis, generating tumescence and erection. Recent studies suggest that the motor control of erection is exerted via both sympathetic and parasympathetic nerve fibers, and that neither a cholinergic nor an adrenergic neurotransmitter system is solely responsible for erectile function. Interestingly, intravenous or intracavernous injection of atropine fails to inhibit penile erection.[21] Moreover, in vitro experiments on human erectile tissue treated with exogenous acetylcholine have demonstrated contraction or relaxation, or no responses at all.

Saenz de Tejado et al. suggest that acetylcholine is probably an inhibitory modulator of adrenergic constrictor nerves and a facilitatory modulator of nonadrenergic noncholinergic relaxation.[22] Studies from Blanco et al. demonstrated an impaired ability of penile cholinergic nerves from impotent diabetic men to synthesize and release acetylcholine. Therefore, they concluded that these patients have dysfunctional penile cholinergic nerves and that this autonomic neuropathy within the corporal tissue worsens with disease duration.[20]

Studies have also suggested a role for adrenergic neurotransmitters in erectile function. High concentrations of norepinephrine have been demonstrated in the blood vessels and CCSM in healthy men. These are significantly decreased in impotent diabetic patients.[23] Animal experiments show that the sympathetic noradrenergic fibers innervating the penis appear to demonstrate neuropathic changes and markedly reduced norepinephrine content in uncontrolled streptozotocin-induced diabetic rats supporting the finding in human studies that noradrenergic sympathetic nerve damage in the penis is a complication of diabetes.[24–27] Our studies also demonstrate that alterations in α-adrenoceptor (phenylephrine) responsiveness are positively correlated with age in diabetic human erectile tissues but not in nondiabetic tissues.[28] However, in an animal model of type 1 diabetes we found that there was no significant alteration in the amount of force produced in response to phenylephrine compared to controls.[29] Nonetheless, it has been observed that the addition of β-adrenergic blockers to isolated corporal tissue strips has no apparent effect on the contractile response to catecholamines, indicating that CCSM relaxation cannot be effectively achieved solely by endogenous catecholamines.[18]

Since neither cholinergic nor adrenergic mechanisms can fully mediate erectile function, the role of nona-drenergic and noncholinergic neurotransmitters (NANC) has been explored. One of the peptides that has been studied as a neurotransmitter in penile physiology is vasoactive intestinal polypeptide (VIP). A potent vasodilator contained in the neurons of the major pelvic ganglion, VIP-immunospecific fibers have been demonstrated in cavernosal tissue.[30] Experiments have demonstrated a dose-dependent relaxation response to VIP,[31] and VIPergic nerves have been found to be depleted in the corpora of diabetic men.[32] Additional data demonstrate a consistent reduction of VIP-like immunoreactivity density in penile disease from streptozotocin-diabetic rats and human diabetic penile tissue when compared with control subjects.[33] Lincoln et al. utilized an immunohistochemical, histochemical, and biochemical investigation of the VIPergic, cholinergic, and adrenergic innervation in penile tissue from impotent patients and provided evidence that all three types may be affected in diabetes.[34]

Endothelial cell-derived modulators, such as endothelin-1 (a potent vasoconstrictor peptide), nitric oxide, and prostanoids, have been identified in the corpus cavernosum.[35,36] Endothelin is one of the most potent vasocon-strictors known. The endothelins (ETs) are a family of 21-amino acid peptides and include ET-1, ET-2, and ET-3,[37] each the product of a separate gene and differing from one another by only a few amino acids.[38] Relative expression of the ET isoforms varies in different tissues with the biological actions of the ETs being determined by their relative binding to ET receptor subtypes.[39] ET-1, the most well characterized and predominant ET in normal plasma,[40] is synthesized by endothelial cells,[37] including corpus cavernosal endothelial cells[36] and CCSM cells.[41] These observations along with the presence of specific binding sites for ET-1 on human CCSM cells, the effect of ET-1 on intracellular calcium levels, and the long-lasting and potent contractile effects of ET-1 on human CCSM strips suggest that ET-1 may serve as a crucial modulator of ED.[42]

Endothelin levels in plasma are elevated in the diabetic state in experimental animal models of both type 1[43] and type 2 diabetes.[44] ET-1 levels are also elevated in diabetic humans. A recent study by Shestakova et al. showed a significant increase in plasma endothelin levels in type 1 diabetic patients. The level of endothelin in the plasma correlated positively with the severity of renal disease.[45] Mokdad et al. reported elevated endothelin levels in type 2 diabetes patients.[46] Data from Francavilla et al. also reveal elevated circulating ET-1 levels in diabetic and nondiabetic men with ED compared with normal men. They also showed elevated ET-1 levels in diabetic impotent patients when compared with nondiabetic impotent individuals, suggesting that diffuse endothelial dysfunction contributes to diabetic ED.[53]

The two main subtypes of ET receptors are referred to as ETA and ETB and are encoded by separate genes.[47,48] Activation of one ETB receptor isoform has been shown to cause a transient vasodilation[49] while activation of either the ETA or the alternative ETB receptor isoform can cause a sustained contraction of SM.[50] Thus, the relative expressions of these endothelin receptors are crucial for defining the SM tone including that of the CCSM. Although both ETA and ETB receptors exist in mammalian CCSM[51] including human;[42] current data support that ET-1-induced CCSM contraction appears to be mediated predominantly by ETA receptors.

Diabetes has been shown to upregulate ETB receptor expression in the STZ-induced type 1 diabetic rat stomach but to have no effect on ETA receptor expression.[52] In contrast, both ETA and ETB receptors are upregulated in type 2 diabetic rats.[44] Mixed results have been reported in the corpus cavernosum with one study demonstrating an upregulation of only the ETA isoform in response to type 1 diabetes[51] and another study finding only an upregulation of the ETB receptor.[54] Our work has revealed an increase in both the ETA and ETB receptors (at both the mRNA and protein levels) but with a more significant upregulation of the ETA receptor isoform in the alloxan-induced model of type 1 diabetes.[29] The same study also showed an increased expression of the ET-1 peptide (via immunohistochemical analysis) in the corpus cavernosum of diabetic rabbits, which correlated with functional changes, including increased sensitivity and maximum force production in response to ET-1 in the CCSM isolated from diabetic compared to normal animals.

Our studies have also suggested that the relevance of ET-1 to corporal smooth muscle physiology may depend on its ability to augment the contractile responses of other vasomodulators present in the human corpora. ET-1 potentiates contractile response of several spasmogens such as norepinephrine, serotonin, and angiotensin II in diverse vasculature and may affect corporal smooth muscle tone via augmentation of underlying $\alpha1$-adrenergic activity.[53] Elevated ET-1 levels may reflect local overproduction of peptide from damaged endothelial cells with plasma spillover secondary to disease processes and cause an increased intracellular calcium level in diabetic cavernosal tissue.[54] Organic ED may thus be fostered through altered regulation of ET-induced vasoconstriction which leads to heightened CCSM tone. As ET-1 levels in serum are easily quantifiable, the potential exists for using ET-1 as a biomarker for ED. These data all suggest that ET-1 is a putative modulator of ED.

Nitric oxide (NO) induces vascular smooth muscle relaxation and is deemed by many to be the putative principal mediator of penile erection. Produced from L-arginine via nitric oxide synthase (NOS), NO is identified in corporal smooth muscle cells, and there is a consensus that endothelium-dependent relaxation in the corpora is achieved by activation of cholinergic receptors on corporal endothelial cells and increased NO production.[35,55,56] NO may be released via other mechanisms; for example, it may be related to mechanical deformation or shear-stress of the endothelial cells subsequent to the increased blood flow produced by helicine arteriole dilatation, or it may be released from nonadrenergic or noncholinergic neurons.[18] NO activates soluble guanylate cyclase which produces cGMP. Several families of phosphodiesterase enzymes are natural feedback inhibitors of that process. Cyclic GMP-specific phosphodiesterase 5 (PDE5) is such an enzyme and is present in the human corpora. Viagra™, Cialis™, and Levitra™ are potent and selective PDE5 inhibitors that revolutionized the field of oral agents in ED treatment. They function by inhibiting the breakdown of cGMP and thereby promoting smooth muscle relaxation. Moreover, advanced glycosylation end products, formed from glucose and amino groups of tissue proteins elevated in diabetic and/or aging patients, may contribute to diabetic ED by binding NO and thereby quenching its supply.[57] The collagen and elastin present in penile smooth muscle and tunica albuginea are suspected to be the target of injury by glycosylated end products formed in diabetic animals.[58,59] Deleterious effect on NO formation and diminished nitrergic innervation of the diabetic rat corpora has also been documented.[60–62] While NO mediates CCSM relaxation and penile erection, studies demonstrate significantly higher NOS activity in diabetic rats when compared with control rats, as well as a marked increase in plasma NO.[63] Despite the elevated NO levels, its action or pathway may be hindered in the diabetic corpora secondary to impaired receptors or transduction mechanism for second messengers, heightened tone of corporal smooth muscle cells, or increased catabolism.[63,64] Miller and associates demonstrate a reduction in the hydrolysis of cAMP and cGMP in diabetic rats and conclude that the increased intracellular cyclic nucleotide levels constitute an adaptive response to counteract the deleterious effects of diabetes.[65] The mechanism leading to the functional blockade of NO in diabetic penile tissues needs further elucidation.

Other investigators have corroborated the original conclusions of Ellenberg and Kolodny et al. that autonomic neuropathy is the primary cause of increased incidence of diabetic impotence.[7,8,22,66,67] ED may not be a late complication of diabetes and ED may be present early during the course of the disease. The diagnosis of ED may also lead to the discovery of otherwise unrecognized diabetes.[68] The correlation of bladder neuropathies or dysfunction in diabetic impotent patients, such as decreased bladder sensation, increased residual urine, and detrusor instability, is crucial in supporting autonomic neuropathy as a cause of diabetic impotence since the bladder and penis both receive autonomic innervation from the hypogastric sympathetic and the pelvic parasympathetic nerves. In our own lab, we have demonstrated detrusor overactivity in the streptozotocin-induced diabetic rat model.[69] Ellenberg and Faerman both reported a high incidence of bladder dysfunction in diabetic impotent patients.[8,70] Neurophysiological, hormonal, and vascular investigations from Bermelmans and associates lead to a conclusion that diabetic urogenital neuropathy along with poor diabetes regulation plays a crucial role in the etiology of diabetic ED while vasculopathy appears to be of secondary importance.[71] Their studies demonstrate significantly lower glycosylated hemoglobin values and plasma glucose levels in potent diabetic men than in impotent ones, suggestive of better diabetic control in the former group. Morphologic abnormalities such as beaded thickenings, vacuolated thickenings, hyperargentophilia, and moniliform thickenings have been shown in the autonomic nerve fibers of diabetic corporal tissue,[70] but our earlier studies showed preserved sympathetic nerves retrieved from the corporal tissue of impotent diabetic men.[72] The host of neurotransmitters implicated in the physiology of penile erection, along with the various neuroeffector systems, also lend support to the notion that diabetic penile neuropathy is the primary origin of diabetic ED. Recently, Schaumburg et al. have shown in both ultrastructural and electrophysiological studies of the STZ-induced diabetic rat that there are morphologic changes of axonal dystrophy only after a prolonged period of hyperglycemia (>8 months).[73] This is in contrast to nerve conduction velocity in the unmyelinated fibers of the cavernous nerve, which is decreased as early as the second month after induction of diabetes. Reduction of intracavernous pressure with cavernous nerve stimulation is observed as early as 1 month after induction of diabetes in those same animals. These findings underscore the fact that gaps remain in our knowledge regarding the exact contribution of diabetic neuropathy to ED at the molecular and cellular levels. Is there a secondary response of the corporal tissue per se or changes in the myocytes when the innervation to the tissue is altered? Current efforts at the Urology Research Laboratory at the Albert Einstein College of Medicine focus on the differential control of smooth muscle cell tone in physiologically distinct tissues such as the bladder and corpora. Our findings in excitable bladder detrusor myocytes and non-excitable corporal smooth muscle indicate that differential organ function is attributable to quantifiable differences in the way that ionic mechanisms participate in the control of myocyte tone. Our data also support the hypothesis that altered neural and/or myocyte function will differentially contribute to diabetic ED and bladder dysfunction and can thus lead to novel therapeutic possibilities by better defining the mechanisms involving diabetic neuropathy or myopathy.

Integrative Corporal Smooth Muscle Physiology

Recent clinical data demonstrate the essential role of the CCSM in modulating penile blood flow during erection with an emerging consensus that the etiologic basis of organic ED lies in the primary changes of CCSM physiology and function.[74] Regardless of the primary defect or abnormality, CCSM relaxation is both necessary and sufficient to elicit an erection in many cases.[74]

The modulation of the CCSM tone is an intricate process necessitating the integration of a host of intracellular events and extracellular signals. Data reveal that the neurotransmitters that participate in erection and detumescence modulate CCSM tone largely via their effects on gap junctions as well as calcium and potassium channels.[74] Figure 26.1 depicts the major mechanisms regulating corporal smooth muscle tone. Broadly, events linked to calcium mobilization and muscle contraction increase the level of intercellular communication while events linked to the activation of cAMP and muscle relaxation decrease the level of intercellular communication.[10]

Potassium channels, ubiquitous in myocytes, appear to exhibit a greater diversity than any other ion channels. At least four distinct subtypes have been identified in the CCSM: calcium-sensitive potassium channel (Maxi-K or K_{Ca}), ATP-dependent potassium channel (K_{ATP}), inwardly rectifying channel (K_{ir}), and voltage-gated potassium channel (K_V). Of these four subtypes, the K_{ATP} and Maxi-K channels are the most thoroughly studied and are physiologically relevant to the control of CCSM tone. The importance of potassium channels to the modulation of CCSM tone is related to the intricate interplay between membrane potential, cellular excitability, and contractility.[75,76] In other words, sustained contractions of CCSM are dependent on continuous transmembrane calcium flux through voltage-dependent calcium channels, and hyperpolarization of CCSM cells via potassium

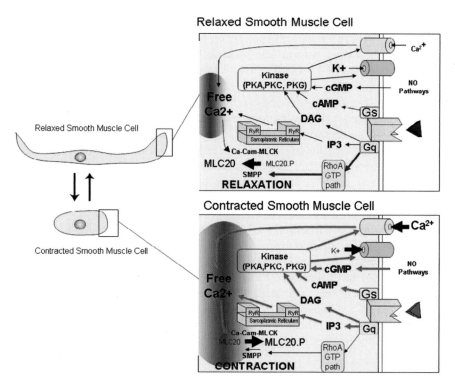

Fig. 26.1 This figure shows cellular enzymatic mechanisms needed to obtain smooth muscle cell relaxation (i.e., erection), as compared to smooth muscle cell contraction (i.e., penile flaccidity). Ca^{2+} = intracellular calcium ion concentration, PKA, PKC, PKG = protein kinases, NO = nitric oxide, MLCK = myosin light chain kinase, MLC = myosin light chain, cAMP = cyclic adenosinemonophosphate, cGMP = cyclic guanosinemonophosphate, DAG = diacylglycerol

channels may represent an important mechanism for modulating corporal muscle tone.[74] Recent studies report that diabetic corporal tissues from patients are less sensitive to relaxation with potassium modulators.

Gap junction proteins play a vital role in the initiation, maintenance, and modulation of CCSM tone.[77–79] The sparse neuronal innervation of CCSM may not explain their synchronized and coordinated relaxation, while the response of the CCSM to locally released or injected neuromodulators is rapid and diffuse. Our studies demonstrate the diffusion of current carrying ions and second messengers (calcium ions and IP3) through gap junctions between coupled CCSM cells in culture.[77] A significant increase in connexin43 mRNA expression in the rat corpora is reported in STZ-induced diabetic rats,[80] and Giraldi et al. reveal a twofold to eightfold variability in connexin43 mRNA in corporal tissue isolated from patients with organic ED,[81] which signifies that the connexin43 mRNA level may be a crucial regulatory point in organic ED. Interestingly, changes in connexin43 mRNA expression are also correlated with physiologically significant alterations in other smooth muscle tissues such as the uterus.[82,83] Gap junction dysfunction may be accountable for the impaired smooth muscle relaxation and contraction coordination in vascular disease due to the presence of collagen fibers between cellular membranes.[84] Thus, there is strong evidence to support a role for intercellular communication in the integration of CCSM tissue responses, and gap junctions play an invaluable role in modulating CCSM tone and consequently penile erection.

Recently it has been shown that CCSM contraction can occur in the absence of changes in $[Ca^{2+}]$ by inhibiting SM myosin phosphatase (SMMP) activity. This process has been termed "calcium sensitization" of SM.[85] One such mechanism of "calcium sensitization" recently identified involves an enzyme known as Rho-kinase (ROK). ROK activity is regulated through a complex molecular pathway. One of the most important regulators of ROK activity is RhoA, a small GTP-binding protein.[86] ROK binds GTP-RhoA at its centrally located Rho-binding domain. This binding of RhoA causes ROK to migrate to the cell membrane where it is maximally active.[87] ROK increases SM myosin phosphorylation (with no change in the intracellular calcium concentration) indirectly by inhibiting the phosphatase (SMMP) responsible for dephosphorylating SMM.[88] Our work has demonstrated a selective upregulation of the ROKβ isoform (compared to ROKα) in the corpus cavernosum of the diabetic rabbits.[29] Increased expression of ROK in an STZ type 1 model of diabetes was later reported by Bivalacqua et al. who also showed that transfection of a dominant negative form of ROK could improve ED.[89]

In contrast to activation by RhoA, Rho-kinase activity is inhibited by cGMP-dependent protein kinase-1 (PKG-1), which has been termed "calcium desensitization" as this reaction does not involve an alteration in the intracellular calcium levels. This decrease in "calcium sensitivity" results either indirectly via PKG-1 phosphorylation and inactivation RhoA (which prevents RhoA from activating ROK)[90,91] or directly via PKG-1 activation of SMMP.[92] The cGMP generated via nitric oxide-induced activation of guanylyl cyclase is considered the main mediator of CCSM relaxation, and preventing its degradation constitutes the mechanism of action of PDE5 inhibitors. The physiological relevance of PKG-1 in SM has been demonstrated by PKG-1 knockout mice. Of particular relevance to this review is that these mice cannot obtain normal erections.[93]

There are two PKG-I isoforms, PKG-Iα (76 kDa) and PKG-Iβ (78 kDa), which arise from the alternative splicing of a single gene[94,95] and differ in their amino-terminal autoinhibitory domains but are similar in their cGMP-binding sites and catalytic domains. Our laboratory has shown that the expression of PKG-1 (most significantly PKG-1α) is reduced in the CC in response to alloxan-induced diabetes in a type 1 diabetic rabbit model.[96] This study showed that the diabetes was associated with significantly decreased PKG-1 activity of CCSM in vitro, correlating with decreased CCSM relaxation. Immunofluorescence microscopy revealed a diabetes-associated decrease in PKG-1 in the CCSM cells. Bivalacqua et al. confirmed the upregulation of PKG-1 in response to diabetes in the STZ-rat and further showed that gene therapy with PKG-1α could restore PKG activity and erectile function in diabetic rats.[97]

Although once thought to merely serve structural roles in cell membranes, lipids are now known to participate in signal transduction pathways. One of the most rapidly emerging bioactive lipids is known as sphingosine-1-phosphate (S1P). This molecule, formed via the reversible phosphorylation of sphingosine and transported in the blood,[98] is emerging as a powerful player in the regulation of a number of important cellular processes including SM contractility and differentiation.[99] By acting on its three main mammalian S1P receptors (S1P1, S1P2, and S1P3), S1P has been shown to regulate a large number of diverse cellular pathways including the endothelin and Rho-kinase (ROK) contractile systems. In general, S1P has been shown to induce vasoconstriction at high doses (> 1 μM) while at lower doses of 10–100 nM, vasodilation has been observed.[100]

Preliminary experiments in our lab have demonstrated the expression of all three S1P receptor isoforms in the rat corpus cavernosum and have shown that S1P, at concentrations greater than 1 μM, cause contraction of rat CCSM. Using high-performance liquid chromatography (HPLC), our laboratory recently found that the serum level of S1P in male Zucker Diabetic Fatty (ZDF) rats (a genetic model of type 2 diabetes) is elevated threefold compared to lean age-matched control rats and correlates with a decrease in erectile function. Di Villa Bianca et al. have reported that human corpus cavernosum also expresses all S1P receptor isoforms and that at low concentrations, S1P activates eNOS and increases acetylcholine relaxation.[101] The relaxation would be presumed to be mediated by the S1P1 receptor, which has been associated with activation of eNOS, rather than the S1P2 and S1P3 receptors, which are more associated with contraction via the RhoA/Rho-kinase pathway.[100] These observations, coupled with the fact that S1P is present at high levels (0.2–4.0 μM) in normal serum, suggest the potential of using S1P serum levels as a biomarker for diabetes-induced ED.

Streptozotocin (STZ)–Induced Diabetic Erectile Dysfunction in a Rat Model

Our recent studies propose that differential organ function is attributable to quantifiable organ-specific differences in the way that ionic mechanisms participate in the control of myocyte tone. We hypothesize that altered neural functions (diabetic peripheral neuropathy), impaired myocyte function (loss or decrease in myocytes), or change in myocyte responsiveness to agonist stimulation (alterations in potassium channels or gap junctions) will differentially contribute to STZ-induced diabetic bladder and erectile dysfunction. These alterations may be related to differences in the severity and duration of diabetes. Isolating the effects of altered myocyte function versus altered neural regulation in our experiments is monumental since a more direct or accurate cause-and-effect relationship can then be elucidated. Development of a more targeted remedy can thus be attempted. Diabetes or hyperglycemia may induce direct effects on myocyte function. It has been demonstrated that alterations in neural and myocyte function are unequivocally related to hyperglycemia and not to a nonspecific effect of STZ.[60,80] The following alterations have been observed in STZ-induced diabetic rats: a significant reduction in penile erectile reflexes, decreased erectile response to cavernous neurostimulation, loss of erectile rigidity similar to the loss of erection in diabetic men, and loss of efferent neurons as evidenced by altered synaptophysin staining.[60,61,102] In addition, preliminary studies in our lab have revealed that there is a diabetes-induced decrease in the number of neurofilaments within the corpora of STZ-induced diabetic rats compared to control rats. This change may be one of the early events in neuronal alteration that leads to ED. Diminished hyperpolarization of the CCSM, possibly secondary to decreased expression of functional potassium channels, may lead to impaired smooth muscle relaxation as hyperpolarization of CCSM cells via potassium channels may be vital in modulating CCSM tone.

Our studies reveal a significant diabetes-related difference in the maximal amplitude of the phenylephrine (PE, equipotent to endogenous norepinephrine on corporal tissue strips)-induced contractile response, and a virtually absent pinacidil-induced relaxation in the corporal tissue strips from STZ-diabetic rats. Moreover, our pharmacological assays that measure the ability of purinergic agonists (ATP and UTP) to induce changes in the intracellular calcium levels have shown a significant reduction in ATP-mediated calcium mobilization in the diabetic corporal tissue and a sevenfold decrease in the sensitivity of the corpora to ATP. This observation may reflect a functional reduction/expression of the P2-receptor, mediator of CCSM relaxation induced by stimulation of the penile purinergic innervation. These changes in purinergic signaling may possibly contribute to diabetic ED.

Through the aforementioned mechanism, STZ-induced alterations in potassium channel activity can manifest as quantifiable changes in their ability to modulate contractility. Based upon research in our lab, we have recently published on sialorphin and its human analogue opiorphin as markers for erectile dysfunction.[103,104] The genes encoding these proteins, Vcsa1 and hSMR3A, respectively, are significantly down-regulated in STZ-induced diabetic rats and humans with ED with or without diabetes. Injection of sialorphin itself directly into diabetic rat corpora was capable of increasing intracavernosal pressures. One possible explanation for this result is that sialorphin's presence is capable of inducing increased activity in the Maxi-K channel, which ultimately leads to relaxation of corporal smooth muscle. A separate study examined the effects of gene transfer of *Slo* (encoding the alpha subunit of Maxi-K) via naked plasma DNA into STZ-induced diabetic rats and how its injection appeared to restore erectile function in these diabetic rats.[105] Analysis in these rats revealed a durable response with increased levels of *Slo* transcript, Maxi-K, for over 4 weeks. This also correlated with increased time of longest erection as well as the intracavernosal pressure to systemic blood pressure ratio. There was also a fourfold increase in sialorphin levels compared to controls. Further work in this area revealed that Cialis[TM], a PDE5 inhibitor, given 2 h prior to erectile measurements, also increases sialorphin expression fourfold. This indicates that PDE5 inhibitors may rapidly induce the expression of sialorphin. With the combination of Cialis[TM] and *Slo*, there is a fivefold increase in sialorphin compared to the individual treatments. These positive results have led to human trials discussed later in this chapter.

Vascular Factors

Vascular abnormalities associated with diabetes mellitus and atherosclerosis constitute a major cause of organic ED. Atherosclerosis is the cause of approximately 40% of ED in men older than age 50, and is characterized by the proliferation of smooth muscle and the deposition of lipid or collagen in the vessel wall. The presence of arteriogenic ED in men older than age 50 is considered by some investigators as an ominous sign for the presence of atherosclerotic disease and microangiopathy in other parts of the body.[106,107] Diabetic retinopathy is often a manifestation of small vessel disease in diabetic patients. Diffuse vascular processes such as atherosclerosis can lead to arteriogenic ED by causing vessel obstruction or arterial insufficiency, commonly of the internal pudendal artery and sometimes of the collaterals, consequently reducing arterial inflow. Thickening of the capillary basement membrane and increased vascular permeability with extravasation of lipoproteins into the vessel walls are considered to be the etiologies of small vessel disease in diabetic patients.[108] Jevtich and associates conclude from their studies that stenosis and obliteration of penile arteries is a primary contributor to diabetic ED.[109] Other studies demonstrate that in patients with leg ischemia, there is significant pudendal arterial stenosis in impotent diabetic and nondiabetic men compared to potent men.[109] Diabetes is also associated with an increased risk of developing hypercholesterolemia and hypercoagulopathy.[110] Hypercholesterolemia may contribute to ED by accelerating atherosclerosis;[107] thus, diabetic patients are subject to compounded risk factors and insults when they develop hypercholesterolemia and atherosclerosis independently. The hypercoagulopathic state, which is induced by increases in coagulation factors such as the von Willebrand factor and tissue plasminogen, is associated with diabetes and can lead to thrombosis and reduced arterial inflow.[111,112] Diabetic impotent patients may also have other vascular risk factors, such as hypertension and cigarette smoking, which can cause atherosclerotic vessel changes.[3,113–115] Corporal veno-occlusive dysfunction associated with atherosclerotic alterations is also implicated in the etiology of ED in diabetic men[116] via structural changes in the fibroelastic components of the corpora.

Diagnostic Modalities

What is the cause of the complaint?
The male sexual response is composed of five phases:

1. Libido
2. Erection
3. Orgasm
4. Ejaculation
5. Refractory period

As the first step in the evaluation process, a complete history and physical examination should be completed. It is imperative that the physician be cognizant of the presenting complaint. Patients may complain of being "impotent" when in reality they may have premature ejaculation, retrograde ejaculation, diminished libido, or a combination of symptoms. The work up and treatments are different for each. In the era of readily available oral agents and the constraints of office time posed by insurance companies and HMOs, it is imperative that the therapy be in harmony with the complaint.

The physical examination should be attentive toward sexual and genital development as well as identifying any vascular, endocrine, or neurologic abnormalities. Approximately 20% of men by history and physical examination alone will be overdiagnosed with organic ED.[117] Any patient who describes overt, rigid, and straight erections (for example, with mistress but not with wife or during masturbation) is likely to have a primary psychological cause of the problem. Referral for conjoint sex therapy is appropriate for such a complaint. A careful neurologic examination is important in a patient whose history is suggestive of peripheral or central neuropathies such as diabetes. The endocrine studies that may be performed for evaluation of impotent men are targeted toward the hypothalamic–pituitary–testicular axis. These assays measure serum testosterone, prolactin, thyroid, and luteinizing hormones. A screening glycosylated hemoglobin A1c or fasting blood sugar should also be obtained to assess for new onset ED as 13% of men with diabetes have ED as their first symptom.

To diagnose the presence of ED, initial tests such as Rigiscan[TM] analysis, visual sexual stimulation, and penile plethysmography (pulse volume recording) can be performed as baseline studies. Rigiscan[TM] analysis monitors nocturnal penile tumescence and rigidity by measuring penile circumference and radial rigidity through loops connected to a microcomputer that is strapped to the patient's thigh. Rigiscan[TM] remains the only objective way of monitoring the presence or absence of erectile ability. Intracavernous pharmacotesting can also serve as a treatment trial to assess the quality of erection. If erection is not achieved, the test should be considered as inconclusive and other diagnostic tests should be sought. Penile plethysmography is a good screening test that measures volume changes with each pulsatile expansion of the penis during flaccidity. Duplex sonography is a minimally invasive initial diagnostic test of vascular impairment.[118,119] The advantages of penile duplex ultrasound include its abilities to visualize penile anatomy, to measure arterial flow velocity or peak systolic velocity, to assess arterial compliance and pharmacologic response, and to evaluate venous efflux.

Although autonomic neuropathy is the primary cause of erectile dysfunction, there is no direct method to assess the autonomic nervous system. Penile biothesiometry simply measures the sensory function or vibration perception threshold of the penis and can be used as an initial screening test. Aging and diabetes accelerate the diminished perception of vibratory sensation.[120] Since first described by Haldeman et al., somatosensory-evoked potential testing has evolved into a promising tool in the evaluation of neurogenically impotent patients.[121,122]

Although no tests can directly measure the autonomic component of erectile function, testing of the autonomic cardiovascular reflexes suggests that abnormal reflexes are associated with aging and organic impotence, indicating the equal importance of autonomic dysfunction in the etiology of erectile failure.[123] Cystometrography and tests of certain vascular functions regulated by the autonomic nervous system, including blood pressure and pulse response to cold, sympathetic skin responses to electrical stimulation, and orthostatic measurements of blood pressure and pulse, have been suggested as ways of identifying autonomic neuropathy in impotent patients.[124]

Therapeutic Options

After the diagnosis of ED is established, a treatment plan should be configured. The applicability of the particular therapeutic option is dependent on the underlying pathology, potential reversibility of the dysfunction, and the wishes of the patient.

No Treatment

Some 25–30% of patients are content to be told of the etiology of their dysfunction, and desire no further treatment.[120]

Medical Therapy

The drug therapies available to induce penile erection are nonspecific and may promote erection in the presence of psychological, hormonal, neurologic, or vascular pathologies. If there is a frank vascular obstruction or vessel stenosis, veno-occlusive dysfunction, corporal fibrosis, severe micro or macro angiopathy, drug treatment will be ineffective, and other noninvasive therapies must be sought.

The introductions of oral sildenafil (Viagra[TM]), tadalafil (Cialis[TM]), and vardenafil (Levitra[TM]) have contributed to increased public awareness of ED. They exert their effect by prolonging the action of cGMP, thereby increasing calcium efflux and consequent corporal smooth muscle relaxation. Impotent patients with a long history of severe poorly controlled diabetes may not optimally benefit from PDE-5 inhibitors because of microangiopathy, altered myocyte function, and impaired neural regulation. Nonetheless Rendell et al. reported improved erections in 57% of diabetic impotent patients receiving sildenafil versus 10% in the placebo group, which is encouraging despite the pathophysiologic alteration diabetes can impose on penile physiology.[125] This study of 268 patients, however, excludes those presenting with more severe diabetic complications such as unstable glucose control and severe autonomic neuropathy. In other words, patients sustaining more severe diabetic complications may not be suited to administration of PDE5 inhibitors, despite the study's conclusion that oral sildenafil is an effective and well-tolerated treatment for men with diabetic ED. Price et al. also reported good efficacy of oral sildenafil in treating diabetic impotence, though only 21 men are included in the study and only 6 have evidence of autonomic neuropathy.[126] Guay has reported that control of diabetes made a difference in response to sildenafil. If the HbA1C was less than 9%, there was a 63% response rate. If the HbA1C was >9%, the response rate dropped to 44%. [127] To reiterate, we believe that oral PDE-5 inhibitors may not be an effective treatment for impotent men suffering from more advanced or severe diabetes-induced pathophysiologic alterations. Nevertheless, the advent of a relatively effective oral agent for ED is encouraging, and since none of its adverse effects exacerbates diabetes, impotent patients with diabetes may be given a trial of an oral PDE5 inhibitor. Common minor side effects include headache, flushing, and blurred vision. The hypotensive effect of PDE-5 inhibitors in patients already receiving nitrates makes them absolutely contraindicated in these patients.

Patients with primary hormonal abnormalities such as severe hypotestosteronemia may benefit from testosterone therapy. Those with hyperprolactinemia induced by prolactin-secreting tumors can utilize oral bromocriptine, radiation, or surgical ablation of the pituitary tumor.

Prostaglandins have been identified in human corporal tissue and are known to modulate autonomic nerve function as well as the effects of vasoactive hormones that contribute to the myogenic tone of vascular smooth muscle.[128] Intraurethral alprostadil, the synthetic formation of prostaglandin E1, administered as a pellet in 500 μg quantities has rapid absorption rates and can induce penile erection in some patients. This "medicated urethral system for erection" or "MUSE" may incur side effects such as urethral pain and bleeding, hypotension, or infection.[129]

Intracorporeal injection of vasoactive agents is a minimally invasive therapy pioneered by Virag in 1983. The pharmacological erection can be induced with an intracavernous injection of 0.20 mL of Trimix (papaverine 30 mg/mL, phentolamine 5 mg, and prostaglandin E1, 25 μg, in 1.2 mL saline) or 10 μg of prostaglandin E1. Papaverine is a nonspecific phosphodiesterase inhibitor that prolongs the action of both intracellular cyclic AMP and cyclic GMP and causes vascular smooth muscle relaxation. This form of therapy works best in patients with good or marginal penile blood supply and properly functioning CCSM and may be used alone or in conjunction with other drugs.

Lastly, the results of the successful transfer of the Maxi-K gene in both the aging and the diabetic rat models that results in normalization of erectile function has led to the first human trial of hMaxi-Kgene transfer in males with ED.[130] In a recently completed phase I trial that enrolled 11 patients, the safety and tolerability of escalating hMaxi-K doses were assessed. No adverse effects were noted. Secondary efficacy objectives were measured primarily by use of the International Index of Erectile Function (IIEF) scale. In two of the patients that were given the two highest doses of 5000 and 7500 μg of the product, clinically significant responses were noted and maintained through the 24-week study period. The successful phase I trial is leading to further work in clinical trials to study the efficacy of this gene therapy.

Vacuum Devices

The external vacuum device offers a relatively safe and nonsurgical alternative for almost all types of ED. When placed over the penis it generates a vacuum, which pulls blood into the corpora creates an erection-like state. A tourniquet or tension band is then placed at the penile base in order to trap blood in the shaft, and the band is left in place for a maximum of 30 min.

Surgical Treatment

Penile prosthesis is an effective surgical alternative for impotent patients with organic or systemic diseases. Either a semi-rigid or inflatable prostheses can be inserted. The primary side effect is infection at the time of surgery, with a reported incidence of about 3%.[131] Studies report that penile prosthesis is effective in diabetic impotent men with low-complication rates.[132,133]

Future Directions in Diabetic Erectile Dysfunction

ED is commonly associated with diabetes, and each disease process by itself incurs debilitating consequences. Diabetes is now the leading cause of new blindness in adults, end-stage renal disease, and lower-extremity amputations not related to injury. It is one of the major contributing factors to cardiac disease and stroke, as well as a host of other comorbidities. The diabetes-related changes observed in ED and bladder function are permanent and require medical therapy to ameliorate the symptoms.[134] Since hyperglycemia is responsible for complications and glucose management remains problematic, development of diagnostic biomarkers and novel therapeutic options continue to be a high priority. There is an impressive reduction in the incidence and progression of microangiopathy and neuropathy with tight glycemic control. Even with rigorous control, however, complications develop. Since the pathophysiology of diabetes is related to the duration and severity of hyperglycemia and its complications,[135] aggressive tight metabolic control from the onset of disease is essential and prevention of diabetes mellitus is key to avoiding ED.

Summary

Recognized since antiquity, diabetes mellitus has become ubiquitous in many developing and newly industrialized countries. Dubbed the silent killer, diabetes causes more deaths per year in the United States than AIDS. Although the effect of diabetes on sexual function in men has been recognized for the last 200 years, the association has been well understood only during the last three decades. The impact of diabetes on male sexual function is emphasized by the fact that more than 50% of patients with diabetes have ED. The most common causes of diabetic ED include autonomic neuropathy and vascular abnormalities often associated with diabetes. Numerous neurotransmitters are implicated in the modulation of penile erection, including vasoactive intestinal polypeptide, endothelin-1, and nitric oxide, strengthening the notion that diabetic neuropathy plays a role in the genesis of diabetic ED. Our current research focuses on the gap junctions and potassium channels at the molecular level. We are working toward deciphering the mechanisms governing penile smooth muscle relaxation and contraction to help guide novel therapeutic options.

Several therapeutic options are offered for ED: medical therapy such as oral PDE-5 inhibitors, intracorporeal pharmacotherapy, vacuum devices, or surgical modalities such as penile prosthesis. The frontier of medical management will undoubtedly include gene therapy as indicated by the positive results in phase I trials of Maxi-K. Despite the advancement and efficacy of such treatments, the biggest hope of patients and physicians alike will be a cure for diabetes and thus the eradication of its associated comorbidities such as ED. As we strive to search for more answers, a cure for diabetes mellitus may be on the horizon.

Acknowledgments We would like to thank Sarah Collins, M.D., Urogynecology Fellow at the Albert Einstein College of Medicine, for making valuable contributions in editing the text.

We also want to thank Kelvin Davies, Ph.D., Associate Professor in the Department of Urology at Albert Einstein College of Medicine, for his diagrammatic representation of smooth muscle physiology.

References

1. NIH Consensus Development. Panel on impotence. NIH Consensus Conference. *J Am Med Assoc.* 1993;270:83.
2. U.S. Census Bureau, 2004, U.S. interim projections by age, sex, race, and hispanic origin, http://www.census.gov/ipc/www/usinterimproj/
3. Feldman HA, Goldstein I, Hatzichristou DG, Krane RJ, McKinlay JB. Impotence and its medical and psychosocial correlates: results of the Massachusetts Male Aging Study. *J Urol.* 1994;151:54–61.
4. AytaçIA, Mckinlay JB, Krane RJ. The likely worldwide increase in erectile dysfunction between 1995 and 2025 and some possible policy consequences. *BJU Int.* 1999;84(1):50–56.
5. Zonszein J. Diagnosis and management of endocrine disorders of erectile dysfunction. *Urol Clin N Am.* 1995;22:789–802.
6. Benet AE, Melman A. The epidemiology of erectile dysfunction. *Urol Clin N Am.* 1995;22:699–709.
7. Ellenberg M. Impotence in diabetes: the neurologic factor. *Ann Intern Med.* 1971;75:213–219.
8. Ellenberg M. Sexual function in diabetic patients. *Ann Intern Med.* 1980;92:331–333.
9. Ryder RE, Close CF, Moriarty KT, Moore KT, Hardisty CA. Impotence in diabetes: aetiology, implications for treatment and preferred vacuum device. *Diabetes Med.* 1992;9:893–898.
10. Melman A, Gingell JC. The epidemiology and pathophysiology of erectile dysfunction. *Urology.* 1999;161:5–11.
11. Buvat J, Lemaire A, Buvat-Herbaut M, et al. Comparative investigations in 26 impotent and 26 nonimpotent diabetic patients. *J Urol.* 1985;133:34–38.

12. Cummings MH, Alexander WD. Erectile dysfunction in patients with diabetes. *Hosp Med*. 1999;60:638–644.

13. Lehman TP, Jacobs JA. Etiology of diabetic impotence. *J Urol*. 1983;129:291–294.

14. Christ GJ, Brink PR, Melman A, Spray DC. The role of gap junctions and ion channels in the modulation of electrical and chemical signals in human corpus cavernosum smooth muscle. *Int J Impot Res*. 1993;5:77.

15. Goldstein I. Impotence (editorial). *J Urol*. 1994;51:1533.

16. Lue TF. Erectile dysfunction associated with cavernous and neurological model (editorial). *Am J Physiol*. 1991;260:H1590.

17. Andersson KE, Wagner G. Physiology of penile erection. *Physiol Rev*. 1995;75:191.

18. Lerner SE, Melman A, Christ CJ. A review of erectile dysfunction new insights and more questions. *J Urol*. 1993;149: 1246–1255.

19. McCulloch DK, Campbell IW, Wu FC, Prescott RJ, Clarke BF. The prevalence of diabetic impotence. *Diabetologia*. 1980;18:279–283.

20. Blanco R, Saenz de Tejada I, Goldstein I, Krane RJ, Wotiz HH, Cohen RA. Dysfunctional penile cholinergic nerves in diabetic impotent men. *J Urol*. 1990;144:278–280.

21. Wagner G, Brindley GS. The effect of atropine, alpha and beta blockers on human penile erection: a controlled pilot study. In: Zorgniotti AW, Rossi G, eds. *Vasculogenic Impotence. Proceedings of the First International Conference on Corpus Cavernosum Revascularization*. Springfield, IL: Charles C Thomas Publishers; 1980:77–81.

22. Saenz de Tejada I, Goldstein I. Diabetic penile neuropathy. *Urol Clin N Am*. 1988;15:17–22.

23. Melman A, Henry DP. The possible role of the catecholamines of the corpora in penile erection. *Urology*. 1979;121: 419–421.

24. Felten DL, Felten SY, Melman A. Noradrenergic innervation of the penis in control and streptozotocin-diabetic rats: evidence of autonomic neuropathy. *Anat Rec*. 1983;206:49–59.

25. Melman A, Henry DP, Felten DL. Catecholamine content of penile corpora in patients with diabetes associated impotence. *Surg Forum*. 1978;29:634–636.

26. Melman A, Henry DP, Felten DL, O'Connor BL. The effect of diabetes mellitus upon the sympathetic nerves of the penile corpora in patients with erectile impotence. *South Med J*. 1980;73:307–309.

27. Melman A, Henry DP, Felten DL, O'Connor BL. Alteration of the nerves of the penile corpora in patients with erectile impotence. *Invest Urol*. 1980;17:474–477.

28. Christ GJ, Maayani S, Valcic M, Melman A. Pharmacological studies of human erectile tissue: characteristics of spontaneous contractions and alterations in alpha-adrenoceptor responsiveness with age and disease in isolated tissues. *Br J Pharmacol*. 1990;101:375–381.

29. Chang S, Hypolite J, Changolkar A, Wein AJ, Chacko S, DiSanto ME. Increased contractility of diabetic rabbit corpora smooth muscle in response to endothelin is mediated via Rho-kinase beta. *Int J Impot Res*. 2003;15:53–62.

30. Gu J, Polak JM, Probert L, Islam KN, et al. Peptidergic innervation of the human male genital tract. *J Urol*. 1983;130:386–391.

31. Adaiken PG, Kottegoda SR, Ratnam SS. Is vasoactive intestinal peptide the principal transmitter involved in human penile erection? *J Urol*. 1986;135:638–640.

32. Gu J, Polak J, Lazarides M, Morgan RJ, et al. Decrease of vasoactive intestinal polypeptide (VIP) in the penises from impotent men. *Lancet*. 1984;2:315–318.

33. Crowe R, Lincoln J, Blacklay FP, Pryor JP, Lumley JS, Burnstock G. Vasoactive intestinal polypeptide-like immunoreactive nerves in diabetic penis. A comparison between streptozocin-treated rats and man. *Diabetes*. 1983;32:1075–1077.

34. Lincoln J, Crowe R, Blacklay PF, Pryor JP, Lumley JS, Burnstock G. Changes in the VIPergic, cholinergic and adrenergic innervation of human penile tissue in diabetic and non-diabetic important males. *J Urol*. 1987;137:1053–1059.

35. Azadzoi K, Kim N, Brown ML, Goldstein I, Cohen RA, Saenz de Tejada I. Endothelium-derived nitric oxide and cyclooxygenase products modulate corpus cavernosum smooth muscle tone. *Urology*. 1992;147:220–225.

36. Saenz de Tejada I, Carson MP, de las Morenas A, Goldstein I, Triash AM. Endothelin: localization, synthesis, activity, and receptor types in human penile corpus cavernosum. *Am J Physiol*. 1991;261:H1078-H1085.

37. Yanagisawa M, Kurihara H, Kimura S, et al. A novel potent vasoconstrictor peptide produced by vascular endothelial cells. [see comments]. *Nature*. 1988;332:411–415.

38. Luscher TF, Barton M. Endothelins and endothelin receptor antagonists: therapeutic considerations for a novel class of cardiovascular drugs. *Circulation*. 2000;102:2434–2440.

39. Firth JD, Ratcliffe PJ. Organ distribution of the three rat endothelin messenger RNAs and the effects of ischemia on renal gene expression. *J Clin Invest*. 1992;90:1023–1031.

40. Usuki S, Kondoh K, Kubo T. Plasma endothelin and LH-RH, LH, FSH, prolactin, progesterone, 17alpha-hydroxyprogesterone, estrone, 17beta-estradiol, delta4-androstenedione, testosterone, active renin, angiotensin-II and ANP levels in blood and LH, estrone and 17beta-estradiol and pregnanediol levels in urine of normal cycling women. *J Cardiovasc Pharm*. 2000;36: S421–S427.

41. Granchi S, Vannelli GB, Vignozzi L, et al. Expression and regulation of endothelin-1 and its receptors in human penile smooth muscle cells. *Mol Hum Reprod*. 2002;8:1053–1064.

42. Christ GJ, Lerner SE, Kim DC, Melman A. Endothelin-1 as a putative modulator of erectile dysfunction: characteristics of contraction of isolated corporal tissue strips. *J Urol*. 1995;153:1998–2003.

43. Makino A, Kamata K. Time-course changes in plasma endothelin-1 and its effects on the mesenteric arterial bed in streptozotocin-induced diabetic rats. *Diabetes Obes Metab*. 2000;2:47–55.

44. Jesmin S, Hattori Y, Maeda S, Zaedi S, Sakuma I, Miyauchi T. The subdepressor dose of benidipine ameliorates diabetic cardiac remodeling accompanied by the normalization of the upregulated endothelin system in rats. *Am J Physiol Heart Circ Physiol*. 2005.

45. Shestakova MV, Jarek-Martynowa IR, Ivanishina NS, et al. Role of endothelial dysfunction in the development of cardiorenal syndrome in patients with type 1 diabetes mellitus. *Diabetes Res Clin Pract*. 2005;68(Suppl1):S65-S72.

46. Migdalis IN, Kalogeropoulou K, Karmaniolas KD, Varvarigos N, Mortzos G, Cordopatis P. Plasma levels of endothelin and early carotid atherosclerosis in diabetic patients. *Res Commun Mol Pathol Pharmacol*. 2000;108:15–25.

47. Nakamuta M, Takayanagi R, Sakai Y, et al. Cloning and sequence analysis of a cDNA encoding human non-selective type of endothelin receptor. *Biochem Bioph Res Co*. 1991;177:34–39.

48. Sakamoto A, Yanagisawa M, Sakurai T, Takuwa Y, Yanagisawa H, Masaki T. Cloning and functional expression of human cDNA for the ETB endothelin receptor. *Biochem Bioph Res Co*. 1991;178:656–663.

49. Matsuda H, Beppu S, Ohmori F, Yamada M, Miyatake K. Involvement of cyclo-oxygenase-generated vasodilating eicosanoid(s) in addition to nitric oxide in endothelin-1-induced endothelium-dependent vasorelaxation in guinea pig aorta. *Heart Vessels*. 1993;8:121–127.

50. Sumner MJ, Cannon TR, Mundin JW, White DG, Watts IS. Endothelin ETA and ETB receptors mediate vascular smooth muscle contraction. *Brit J Pharmacol*. 1992;107:858–860.

51. Bell CR, Sullivan ME, Dashwood MR, Muddle JR, Morgan RJ. The density and distribution of endothelin 1 and endothelin receptor subtypes in normal and diabetic rat corpus cavernosum. *Br J Urol*. 1995;76:203–207.

52. Endo K, Matsumoto T, Kobayashi T, Kasuya Y, Kamata K. Diabetes-related changes in contractile responses of stomach fundus to endothelin-1 in streptozotocin-induced diabetic rats. *J Smooth Muscle Res*. 2005;41:35–47.

53. Francavilla S, Properzi G, Bellini C, Marino G, Ferri C, Santucci A. Endothelin-1 in diabetic and nondiabetic men with erectile dysfunction. *J Urol*. 1997;158:1770–1774.

54. Sullivan ME, Dashwood MR, Thompson CS, Muddle JR, Mikhailidis DP, Morgan RJ. Alterations in endothelin B receptor sites in cavernosal tissue of diabetic rabbits: potential relevance to the pathogenesis of erectile dysfunction. *J Urol*. 1997;158:1966–1972.

55. Kim N, Azadzoi K, Goldstein I, Saenz de Tejada I. A nitric oxide-like factor mediates nonadrenergic-noncholinergic neurogenic relaxation of penile corpus cavernosum smooth muscle. *J Clin Invest*. 1991;88:112–118.

56. Rajfer J, Aronson WJ, Bush PA, Dorey FJ, Ignarro LJ. Nitric oxide as a mediator of relaxation of the corpus cavernosum in response to nonadrenergic, noncholinergic neurotransmission. *N Engl J Med*. 1992;326:90–94.

57. Seftel AD, Vaziri ND, Ni Z, et al. Advanced glycation end products in human penis: elevation in diabetic tissue, site of deposition, and possible effect through iNOS or eNOS. *Urology*. 1997;50:1016–1026.

58. Makita Z, Vlassara H, Cercimi H, Bucola R. Immunochemical detection of advanced glycosylation products in vivo. *J Biol Chem*. 1992;267:5133–5138.

59. Maher E, Bachoo M, Elabbady AA, et al. Vasoactive intestinal peptide and impotence in experimental diabetes mellitus. *Br J Urol*. 1996;77:271–278.

60. Cellek S, Rodrigo J, Lobos E, Fernandez P, Serrano J, Moncada S. Selective nitrergic neurodegeneration of diabetes mellitus – a nitric oxide-dependent phenomenon. *Br J Pharmacol*. 1999;128:1804–1812.

61. el-Sakka AI, Lin CS, Chui RM, Dahiya R, Lue TF. Effects of diabetes on nitric oxide synthase and growth factors genes and protein expression in an animal model. *Int J Impot Res*. 1999;11:123–132.

62. Sullivan M, Thompson CS, Mikhailidis DP, Morgan RJ, Angelini GD, Jeremy JY. Differential alterations of prostacyclin, cyclic AMP and cyclic GMP formation in the corpus cavernosum of the diabetic rabbit. *Br J Urol*. 1998;82:578–584.

63. Elabbady AA, Gagnon C, Hassouna MM, Begin LR, Elhilali MM. Diabetes mellitus increases nitric oxide synthase in penises but not in major pelvic ganglia of rats. *Br J Urol*. 1995;76:196–202.

64. Basar MM, Yildiz M, Soylemezoglu F, et al. Histopathological changes and nitric oxide synthase activity in corpus cavernosum from rats with neurogenic erectile dysfunction. *Br J Urol Int*. 1999;83:101–107.

65. Miller MA, Morgan RJ, Thompson CS, Mikhailidis DP, Jeremy JY. Hydrolysis of cyclic guanosine monophosphate and cyclic adenosine monophosphate by the penis and aorta of the diabetic rat. *Br J Urol*. 1996;78:252–256.

66. Kolodny RC, Kahn CB, Goldstein HH, Barnett DM. Sexual dysfunction in diabetic men. *Diabetes*. 1974;23:306–309.

67. Jensen SB. Sexual dysfunction in insulin-treated diabetes: a six year follow-up study of 101 patients. *Arch Sex Behav*. 1986;15:271.

68. Deutsch S, Sherman L. Previously unrecognized diabetes mellitus in sexually impotent men. *J Am Med Assoc*. 1980;244: 2430–2432.

69. Christ GJ, Hsieh Y, Zhao W, et al. Effects of streptozotocin-induced diabetes on bladder and erectile (dys)function in the same rat in vivo. *BJU Int*. 2006;97:1076–1082.

70. Faerman I, Glocer L, Fox D, Jadzinsky MN, Rapaport M. Impotence and diabetes. Histological studies of the autonomic nervous fibers of the corpora cavernosa in impotent diabetic males. *Diabetes*. 1974;23:971–976.

71. Bermelmans BL, Meuleman EJ, Doesburg WH, Notermans SL, Debruyne FM. Erectile dysfunction in diabetic men: the neurological factor revisited. *J Urol*. 1994;151:884–889.

72. Melman A, Henry DP, Felten DL, O'Connor BL. Effects of diabetes upon penile sympathetic nerves in impotent patients. *South Med J*. 1980;73:307–309.

73. Schaumberg H, Zotova E, Raine C, et al. Experimental autonomic neuropathy. *Ann Neurol*. 2007;62:S65.

74. Christ GJ. The penis as a vascular organ. The importance of corporal smooth muscle tone in the control of erection. *Urol Clin N Am*. 1995;22:727–745.

75. Lee SW, Wang HZ, Christ GJ. Characterization of ATP-sensitive potassium channels in human corporal smooth muscle cells. *Int J Impot Res*. 1999;11:189–199.

76. Lee SW, Wang HZ, Zhao W, Ney P, Brink PR, Christ GJ. Prostaglandin E1 activates the large conductance Kca channel in human corporal smooth muscle. *Int J Impot Res*. 1999;11:179–188.

77. Christ GJ, Moreno AP, Melman A, Spray DC. Gap junction-mediated intercellular diffusion of Ca in cultured human corporeal smooth muscle cells. *Am J Physiol*. 1992;263:C373.

78. Campos de Carvalho AC, Roy C, Moreno AP, et al. Gap junctions formed of connexin 43 are found between smooth muscle cells of human corpus cavernosum. *J Urol*. 1993;149:1568–1575.

79. Christ GJ, Moreno AP, Parker ME, et al. Intercellular communication through gap junctions: potential role in pharmacome-chanical coupling and syncytial tissue contraction in vascular smooth muscle isolated from the human corpus cavernosum. *Life Sci*. 1991;49:PL195.

80. Rehman J, Chenven E, Brink PR, et al. Diminished neurogenic-, but not pharmacologic-induced intracavernous pressure responses in the 3 month Streptozotocin (STZ)-diabetic rat. *Am J Physiol*. 1997;272:H1960–H1971.

81. Giraldi A, Wen Y, Geliebter J, Christ GJ. Differential gap junction mRNA expression in human corpus cavernosum: a significant regulatory event in cell-to-cell communication? *Urology*. 1995;153:508A.

82. Andersen J, Grine E, Eng CL, et al. Expression of connexin-43 in human myometrium and leiomyoma. *Amer J Obst Gyn*. 1993;169:1266–1277.

83. Risek B, Guthrie S, Kumar N, Gilula NB. Modulation of gap junction transcript and protein expression during pregnancy in the rat. *J Cell Biol*. 1990;110:269–282.

84. Persson C, Diederichs W, Lue TF, et al. Correlation of altered penile ultrastructure with clinical arterial evaluation. *J Urol*. 1989;142:1462–1468.

85. Somlyo AP, Wu X, Walker LA, Somlyo AV. Pharmacomechanical coupling: the role of calcium, G-proteins, kinases and phosphatases. *Rev Physiol Biochem Pharmacol*. 1999;134:201–234.

86. Ishizaki T, Maekawa M, Fujisawa K, et al. The small GTP-binding protein Rho binds to and activates a 160 kDa Ser/Thr protein kinase homologous to myotonic dystrophy kinase. *EMBO J*. 1996;15:1885–1893.

87. Leung T, Manser E, Tan L, Lim L. A novel serine/threonine kinase binding the Ras-related RhoA GTPase which translocates the kinase to peripheral membranes. *J Biol Chem*. 1995;270:29051–29054.

88. Kimura K, Ito M, Amano M, et al. Regulation of myosin phosphatase by Rho and Rho-associated kinase (Rho-kinase). [see comments]. *Science*. 1996;273:245–248.

89. Bivalacqua TJ, Champion HC, Usta MF, et al. RhoA/Rho-kinase suppresses endothelial nitric oxide synthase in the penis: a mechanism for diabetes-associated erectile dysfunction. *Proc Natl Acad Sci USA*. 2004;101:9121–9126.

90. Sauzeau V, Le Jeune H, Cario-Toumaniantz C, et al. Cyclic GMP-dependent protein kinase signaling pathway inhibits RhoA-induced Ca^{2+} sensitization of contraction in vascular smooth muscle. *J Biol Chem*. 2000;275:21722–21729.

91. Sawada N, Itoh H, Yamashita J, et al. cGMP-dependent protein kinase phosphorylates and inactivates RhoA. *Biochem Bioph Res Co*. 2001;280:798–805.

92. Surks HK, Mochizuki N, Kasai Y, et al. Regulation of myosin phosphatase by a specific interaction with cGMP- dependent protein kinase Ialpha. *Science*. 1999;286:1583–1587.

93. Hedlund P, Aszodi A, Pfeifer A, et al. Erectile dysfunction in cyclic GMP-dependent kinase I-deficient mice. *Proc Natl Acad Sci USA*. 2000;97:2349–2354.

94. Francis SH, Woodford TA, Wolfe L, Corbin JD. Types I alpha and I beta isozymes of cGMP-dependent protein kinase: alternative mRNA splicing may produce different inhibitory domains. *Sec Mess Phosphoprot*. 1988;12:301–310.

95. Wolfe L, Corbin JD, Francis SH. Characterization of a novel isozyme of cGMP-dependent protein kinase from bovine aorta. *J Biol Chem*. 1989;264:7734–7741.

96. Chang S, Hypolite JA, Velez M, et al. Downregulation of cGMP-dependent protein kinase-1 activity in the corpus cavernosum smooth muscle of diabetic rabbits. *Am J Physiol Regul Integr Comp Physiol*. 2004;287:R950–R960.

97. Bivalacqua TJ, Kendirci M, Champion HC, Hellstrom WJ, Andersson KE, Hedlund P. Dysregulation of cGMP-dependent protein kinase 1 (PKG-1) impairs erectile function in diabetic rats: influence of in vivo gene therapy of PKG1alpha. *BJU Int*. 2007;99(6):1488–1494.

98. Hänel P, Andréani P, Gräler MH. Erythrocytes store and release sphingosine 1-phosphate in blood. *FASEB J*. 2007;21(4):1202–1209.

99. Hait NC, Oskeritzian CA, Paugh SW, Milstien S, Spiegel S. Sphingosine kinases, sphingosine 1-phosphate, apoptosis and diseases. *Biochim Biophys Acta*. 2006;1758(12):2016–2026.

100. Watterson KR, Ratz PH, Spiegel S. The role of sphingosine-1-phosphate in smooth muscle contraction. *Cell Signal*. 2005;17(3):289–298.

101. di Villa Bianca R, Sorrentino R, Sorrentino R, et al. Sphingosine 1-Phosphate Induces Endothelial Nitric-Oxide Synthase Activation through Phosphorylation in Human Corpus Cavernosum. *J Pharmacol Exp Ther* 2006;316:703–708.

102. Vernet D, Cai L, Garban H, et al. Reduction of penile nitric oxidesynthase in diabetic BB/WORdp (type 1) and BBZ/WORdp (type II) rats with erectile dysfunction. *Endocrinol*. 1995;136:5709–5719.

103. Davies KP, Tar M, Rougeot C, Melman A. Sialorphin (the mature peptide product of Vcsa1) relaxes corporal smooth muscle tissue and increases erectile function in the ageing rat. *BJU Int*. 2006.

104. Tong Y, Tar M, Davelman F, Christ G, Melman A, Davies KP. Variable coding sequence protein A1 as a marker for erectile dysfunction. *BJU Int*. 2006;98:396–401.

105. Christ G, Day N, Santizo C, et al. Intracorporal injection of hSlo cDNA restores erectile capacity in STZ-diabetic F-344 rats in vivo. *Am J Physiol Heart Circ Physiol*. Oct 2004;287(4):H1544–H1553.

106. Kaiser FE, Udhoji V, Viosca SP, et al. Cardiovascular stress tests in patients with vascular impotence. *Clin Res*. 1989;37:89A.

107. Virag R, Bouilly P, Frydman D. Is impotence an arterial disorder? *Lancet*. 1984;1:181–184.

108. Jevtich MJ, Edson M, Jarman WD, Herrera HH. Vascular factor in erectile failure among diabetics. *Urology*. 1982;19:163–168.

109. Herman A, Adar R, Rubinstein Z. Vascular lesions associated with impotence in diabetic and nondiabetic arterial occlusive disease. *Diabetes*. 1978;27:975–981.

110. Akoi I, Shimoyama K, Aoki N, et al. Platelet dependent thrombin generation in patients with diabetes mellitus: effects of glycemic control on coagulopathy in diabetes. *J Am Coll Cardiol*. 1996;27:560–566.

111. Jensen T, Bjerre-Knudsen J, Feldt-Rasmussen B, Deckert T. Features of endothelial dysfunction in early diabetic nephropathy. *Lancet*. 1989;1:461–463.

112. Carrier S, Brock G, Kour NW, Lue TR. Pathophysiology of erectile dysfunction. *Urology*. 1993;42:468–481.

113. Rosen MP, Greenfield AJ, Walker TG, et al. Cigarette smoking: an independent risk factor for atherosclerosis in the hypogastric-cavernous arterial bed of men with arteriogenic impotent. *J Urol*. 1991;145:759–763.

114. Hakim LS, Goldstein I. Diabetic sexual dysfunction. *Endocrinol Metab Clin North America*. 1996;25:379–400.

115. Krane RJ, Goldstein I, Saenz de Tejada I. Medical progress: impotence. *N Engl J Med*. 1989;321:1648.

116. Mottonen M, Nieminen K. Relation of atherosclerotic obstruction of the arterial supply of corpus cavernosum to erectile dysfunction. Proceedings of the Sixth Biennial International Symposium on corpus Cavernosum Revascularization and Third Biennial World Meeting on Impotence. Boston: 12, 1988.

117. Davis-Joseph B, Tiefer L, Melman A. Accuracy of the initial history and physical examination to establish the etiology of erectile dysfunction. *Urology*. 1995;45:498–502.

118. Merckx LA, DeBruyne RMG, Goes E, Derde MP, Keuppens F. The value of dynamic color duplex scanning in the diagnosis of venogenic impotence. *J Urol*. 1992;148:318–320.

119. Kropman RF, Schipper J, Oostayen JA, Nijeholt ABL, Meinhardt W. The value of increased end diastolic velocity during penile duplex sonography in relation to pathological venous leakage in erectile dysfunction. *J Urol*. 1992;148:314–317.

120. Melman A, Tiefer L, Pedersen R. Evaluation of first 406 patients in urology department based Center for male sexual dysfunction. *Urology*. 1988;32:6–10.

121. Haberman S, Bradley We, Bhatia NN, Johnson BK. Pudendal evoked responses. *Arch Neurol*. 1982;39:280.

122. Bleustein CB, Eckholdt H, Arezzo JC, Melman A. *J Urol*. 2003;169:2266–2269.

123. Nisen HO, Larsen A, Lindstrom BL, Ruutu ML, Virtanen JM, Alfthan OS. Cardiovascular reflexes in the neurological evaluation of impotence. *Br J Urol*. 1993;71:199–203.

124. Sharlip ID. Evaluation and nonsurgical management of erectile dysfunction. *Urol Clin N Am*. 1988;25:647–659.

125. Rendell MS, Rajfer J, Wicker PA, Smith MD. Sildenafil for treatment of erectile dysfunction in men with diabetes: a randomized controlled trial. Sildenafil Diabetes Study Group. *J Am Med Assoc*. 1999;281:421–426.

126. Price DE, Gingell JC, Gepi-Attee S, Wareham K, Yates P, Boolell M. Sildenafil: study of a novel oral treatment for erectile dysfunction in diabetic men. *Diabetes Med*. 1998;15:821–825.

127. Guay AT. Relation of endothelial cell function to erectile dysfunction: implications for treatment. *Am J Cardiol*. 2005;96(S):52 M-56 M.

128. Melman A. Neural and vascular control of erection. In: Rosen RC, Leiblum SR, eds. *Erectile Disorder: Assessment and Treatment*. New York: The Guilford Press; 1992:55–71.

129. Kim ED, McVary KT. Topical prostaglandin E-1 for the treatment of erectile dysfunction. *Urology*. 1995;153:1828–1830.

130. Melman A, Bar-Chama N, Mccullough A, Davies KP,, Christ G. hMaxi-K gene transfer in males with erectile dysfunction: results of the first human trial. *Hum Gene Ther*. 2006;17:1165–1176.

131. Montague DK, Angermeier KW, Lakin MM. *Int J Impot Res*. 2001;13(6):326–328.

132. Beaser RS, Van der Hoek C, Jacobson AM, Flood TM, Desautels RE. Experience with penile prosthesis in the treatment of impotence in diabetic men. *J Am Med Assoc*. 1982;248:943–948.

133. Scott FB, Fishman IJ, Light JK. An inflatable penile prosthesis for treatment of diabetic impotence. *Ann Intern Med*. 1980;92:340–342.

134. McCulloch DK, Young RJ, Prescott RJ, Campbell IW, Clarke BF. The natural history of impotence in diabetic men. *Diabetologia*. 1984;26:437–440.

135. Klein R, Klein BE, Lee KE, Moss SE, Cruickshank KJ. Prevalence of self-reported erectile dysfunction in people with long-term IDDM. *Diabetes Care*. 1996;19:135–141.

Chapter 27
Gastrointestinal Manifestations of Diabetes

Donald P. Kotler and Stanley Hsu

Introduction

Gastrointestinal (GI) disorders are exceedingly common in diabetics and are reported by as many as 75% of patients.[1] Symptoms may be underappreciated by patients and their physicians, as they are considered minor as compared to retinopathy, nephropathy, and other complications of diabetes. Some patients may be asymptomatic but still have underlying GI dysfunction.

It is important to remember that a diabetic patient may develop the same GI diseases as a nondiabetic patient, e.g., cholecystitis, colon cancer, or inflammatory bowel disease. In some cases, diabetes or its complications may modify the disease presentation or course. This chapter will focus on those gastrointestinal disorders that have been specifically linked to diabetes. Liver diseases related to diabetes are covered elsewhere in this textbook (Chapter 35). Discussion of general gastrointestinal diseases that also might occur in a diabetic patient can be found in a general gastrointestinal textbook.

In order to provide a background for the gastrointestinal problems associated with diabetes, the topics of neurogastroenterology and absorptive physiology will be briefly reviewed, followed by a discussion of disease complications organized by symptom, with a focus on practical methods of assessment and treatment.

The Enteric Nervous System

The enteric nervous system modulates gastrointestinal motility, secretion, visceral perceptions of pain and other sensations, and the absorption of water, electrolytes, and nutrients. The two limbs of the autonomic nervous system, parasympathetic and sympathetic, generally exert opposite effects. For example, parasympathetic stimulation promotes ion and water secretion, while sympathetic stimulation promotes absorption. The parasympathetic system provides excitatory stimuli to non-sphincteric muscles, while the thoracolumbar sympathetic system provides excitatory stimulus to sphincters and inhibitory stimuli to non-sphincteric muscles. Diabetic autonomic neuropathy affects both the vagal input (cholinergic) and the thoracolumbar sympathetic output (adrenergic) of the enteric nervous system. Histopathologic studies in diabetic animals demonstrated axonal neuropathic changes in the sympathetic neurons supplying the gut, the sympathetic ganglia, postganglionic sympathetic nerves, and intramural adrenergic plexuses.[1] Functional alterations in neural and muscular activity also may occur as a long-term consequence of decreased signaling from insulin or insulin-like growth factor 1, as suggested in a murine model.[2]

D.P. Kotler (✉)
Division of Gastroenterology and Liver Disease, Saint Luke's Roosevelt Hospital, Columbia University College of Physician and Surgeons, New York, NY, USA
e-mail: dkotler@chpnet.org

Glycemic control acutely affects many gastrointestinal functions, including gastric emptying, myoelectric activity, and the colonic motor response to feeding. Autonomic nerve damage may affect other neurotransmitters, such as vasoactive intestinal peptide (VIP), which normally promotes proximal intestinal relaxation, and calcitonin G related protein (CGRP), which helps regulate peristalsis. Clinical manifestations of enteric neural dysfunction are related to alterations in lower esophageal sphincter competence, gastric secretion, gastric emptying, small bowel transit, solute and water flux, and colonic motility. The sensory neurons in the enteric nervous system, which are responsible for the perception of pain, also may be affected. This explains why some patients with diabetes do not complain of symptoms despite gastric distention or severe reflux.

Motility of the Gastrointestinal Tract

The esophagus is around 20 cm in length and is composed of skeletal and smooth muscle bordered by the upper esophageal (UES) and lower esophageal (LES) sphincters. The upper esophageal sphincter and the proximal 5% of the esophageal muscle are striated, the middle 40% is mixed, and the distal 60% is composed of smooth muscle. The inner muscularis propria layer is composed of circular muscle, while the outer layer is composed of longitudinal muscle. The myenteric plexus lies between the longitudinal and circular muscles in both the striated and smooth muscle portions of the esophagus. These enteric neurons are the relay neurons between the vagus and the smooth muscle. Meissner's plexus is found between the circular muscle and muscularis mucosa.

The initial event of swallowing is pharyngeal contraction occurring at a time of upper esophageal sphincter relaxation, which pushes the food bolus into the esophagus, at which point peristalsis propels the food bolus into the stomach. The vagus nerve regulates esophageal peristalsis under normal conditions. The neural plexuses of the esophagus control its activity through excitation of circular and longitudinal muscle bundles by muscarinic receptors or inhibition of the circular layer by nitric oxide. When a second swallow occurs during the peristalsis of the first swallow, the contraction induced by the first swallow is inhibited due to the deglutitive effect.

A key feature of the swallowing reflex is early relaxation of the lower esophageal sphincter, which lasts until peristalsis has propelled the food bolus into the stomach, and which is followed by a return to a tonic sphincteric contraction. In addition to primary peristalsis, a secondary peristaltic wave can be initiated by reflux of gastric contents, and can be mimicked by inflating a balloon in the esophageal body. Secondary peristalsis limits the exposure of esophageal mucosa to the acid refluxate.

The stomach's primary role is to store an ingested meal, to grind solid food particles into millimeter-sized bits, and to empty the slurry into the duodenum in a controlled fashion. The gastrointestinal smooth muscle has myoelectric activity that consists of slow waves and recurring cycles of depolarization and repolarization, linked to muscle activity. Slow waves occur at a frequency of three cycles per minute and are thought to originate near the middle corpus along the greater curvature from specialized intramuscular interstitial cells (interstitial cells of Cajal).

A migrating motor complex (MMC) cycles in the stomach approximately every 60–90 min, throughout the day and night in the fasting state, but is inhibited by meals. The complex has three phases: a quiescence phase (phase I) that lasts for 15–30 min, a period of intermittent pressure (phase II) that last 60 min, and an activity phase (phase III) that lasts around 6 min, during which the stomach contracts at the highest frequencies. Gall bladder emptying occurs at the end of phase II and during phase III of the MMC. In healthy adults, gastric emptying of a solid meal occurs with a half-life of 90–120 min, while liquids normally empty with a half-life of 20–30 min. The rate of emptying is influenced by the temperature, osmolality, and caloric density of the ingested liquid. For example, the higher the osmolality or nutrient content of the liquid, the slower the rate of emptying.

The stomach accommodates to a large meal by a process known as receptive relaxation, which is mediated by the vagus nerve. The loss of vagal activity through disease or surgery may increase intragastric pressure and the rate of gastric emptying of liquids. However, since the vagus nerve promotes contractile activity in the antrum, the loss of vagal activity delays the emptying of solids.

The small intestine undergoes regular motor activity, even if removed from all neural and vascular connections. The MMC of the intestine in the fasting state is similar to the stomach, consisting of three phases: quiescent (phase I), discrete clustered contractions (DCC) – small bursts of electrical activity that are uncoordinated and do not propagate (phase II), and prolonged propagated contraction (phase III). In phase III, the frequency of contraction is 11–12 min^{-1} in the duodenum and 8 min^{-1} in the terminal ileum. This activity serves to push luminal debris, including microbes, to the large intestine and is an important innate defense against bacterial overgrowth. Phase III activity is also known as the "intestinal housekeeper". Phase III motility may be impaired in diabetic patients, leading to bacterial overgrowth.

Like smooth muscle throughout the gastrointestinal tract, colonic smooth muscle also shows spontaneous oscillatory electrical activity. This occurs even when all neural input is interrupted. The first type of activity, called myenteric potential oscillations (MPOs), is small in amplitude, with a frequency of 12–20 per minute and originates in the plane of the myenteric plexus. These are responsible for contractions when neurotransmitters are released by the enteric excitatory motor neurons. A second pacemaker is located at the submucosal border of the circular muscle. These are larger amplitude, slower oscillations occurring at 2–4 per minute. The slow waves function predominately to mix the contents with little peristalsis as they can occur up or down the colon.

When stool reaches the rectum, the stretching of the rectal wall leads to a simultaneous activation of the enteric descending inhibitory reflex that causes relaxation of the internal anal sphincter and the extrinsic reflex pathway that leads to the contraction of external anal sphincter. This reflex can be demonstrated by balloon distention of the rectum. Defecation involves a combination of pelvic reflexes coordinated in the medulla and pons. As pressure is exerted at the rectum, the anterior rectal wall flattens, while the puborectalis muscle and the external anal sphincter relax. The levator ani muscles are also activated during the relaxation of the puborectalis muscle, allowing for the expulsion of stool.

Digestion and Absorption of the Gastrointestinal Tract

In the stomach, parietal cells secrete hydrochloric acid. Parietal cells have three stimulating receptors: histamine receptor, muscarinic receptor for acetylcholine release from preganglionic neurons, and cholecystokinin receptor for gastrin released from pylori G cells. Acid secretion occurs in response to sight, smell, or thought of food, and is mediated by the vagus nerve. Vagal stimulation results in the release of histamine from enterochromaffin-like cells, activation of parietal cell, and stimulation of G cell, eliciting a modest release of gastrin. Gastric distention and food also causes G cells to release gastrin. The stomach also secretes other substances including mucus, bicarbonate, intrinsic factor, and pepsinogen. Intrinsic factor is responsible for B12 absorption in the terminal ileum. Pepsinogen I and II are proteolytic proenzymes that are cleaved to form the active product, pepsin, in the presence of acidic pH. Pepsin aids in protein digestion.

The small bowel is approximately 20 ft long and is responsible for the majority of nutrient absorption. Protein digestion is completed in the small intestine by pancreatic proteases including trypsin, chymotrypsin, elastase, and carboxypeptidase. As fat enters the duodenum, secretin and cholecystokinin are released which stimulate pancreatic secretion and gall bladder contraction. Lipase hydrolyzes triglyceride into fatty acids and monoglycerides, which then combine with bile salts to form mixed micelles, which increase fat solubility 100- to 1000-fold. After digestion, mono-and oligosaccharides, amino acids and oligopeptides, fatty acids, and cholesterol are absorbed in the small intestine. Calcium, iron, zinc, folate, and fat-soluble vitamins (A, D, E, and K) also are absorbed in the duodenum and jejunum. Bile salts and vitamin B12 are absorbed in the ileum. Diseases that affect upper intestine, such as celiac disease, may cause impaired absorption of iron or calcium and vitamin D. Ileal resection may cause B12 and bile salt malabsorption.

The intestine also absorbs water, electrolytes, and minerals. In addition to the approximately 2 l of water ingested per day normally, another 9–10 l of fluid enter the intestine from salivary, gastric, pancreatic, biliary, and intestinal secretions. About 90% of this fluid is absorbed in the small intestine. Of the rest about 800–1200 ml of fluid that enters the colon each day, 90% is absorbed during the normal colonic transit time of 24–30 h. Thus, about 80–100 ml of water is excreted each day in feces. If a disease process in the small intestine increases the fluid load, the colon can compensate by absorbing up to 3–4 l in 24 h. Diarrhea occurs when the fluid load exceeds the absorptive capacity of the colon.

Gastrointestinal Symptoms in Diabetic Patients

Many epidemiologic studies have shown that the prevalence of GI symptoms is higher in diabetic patients than in nondiabetic individuals, but that the actual symptoms do not differ. The most prevalent are constipation, diarrhea, epigastric fullness, heartburn, abdominal pain, and fecal incontinence. Many of these symptoms also correlate strongly with psychological distress, though the direction of causality often is not clear.[3] The presence of diabetic neuropathy does not necessarily predict the presence of symptoms.

Dysphagia, Odynophagia, and Chest Pain

About one-third of diabetic patients have symptoms of esophageal disease and may present with dysphagia (difficulty swallowing), odynophagia (painful swallowing), or chest pain. Others may have esophageal dysfunction without symptoms, because of altered sensation. Esophageal symptoms should not be attributed to diabetes until other clinical disorders, including esophageal cancer, have been excluded. Initial workup of dysphagia or odynophagia often includes endoscopic or radiologic examination, especially in the presence of "alarm" symptoms, such as weight loss, hematemesis, odynophagia, or the onset of symptoms after age 50. Because coronary atherosclerosis is common in diabetic patients, the etiology of chest pain should not be attributed to esophageal disease without consideration of cardiac evaluation. In diabetic patients presenting with dysphagia or odynophagia, especially those with poor glycemic control, candida esophagitis and esophageal dysmotility are prominent possibilities.

Candida Esophagitis

Diabetic patients are more prone to candida esophagitis than are the general population. Infection in the oral cavity is promoted by high salivary glucose concentrations that generally correlate with blood glucose levels.[4] In addition, diabetic patients may have defective neutrophil and macrophage functions. This promotes yeast infections since phagocytosis and intracellular killing are important defenses against microbial translocation and systemic invasion. In addition, abnormal esophageal motility, which contributes to stasis, promotes growth of candida. Symptoms of candida esophagitis are odynophagia and/or dysphagia, and if severe lead to decreased caloric intake and to weight loss. The diagnosis of candida esophagitis is readily made by endoscopy, which reveals adherent white plaques lining the esophagus. Biopsy of the esophagus or brushing with cytopathologic analysis confirms the diagnosis; culture is optional. Treatment of candida esophagitis involves administering a systemic antifungal agent such as fluconazole, 100–200 mg po daily for 2–3 weeks. Because the hyphae of candida penetrate the superficial squamous epithelium, topical therapy is not effective.

Esophageal Dysmotility

Up to 50% of diabetic patients have abnormal esophageal motility, including decreased amplitude and number of contractions, slowed esophageal transit, spontaneous contractions, failed peristalsis, and decreased lower esophageal sphincter pressure.[5–7] Patients may present with dysphagia or a feeling of mild chest discomfort with every swallow. The cause of esophageal dysmotility is vagal neuropathy in most cases. The majority of diabetic patients with esophageal motility disorders have coexistent peripheral and autonomic dysfunction. Histologically, the vagus nerve shows signs of damage. However, hyperglycemia itself may also play a role. In healthy subjects, hyperglycemia reversibly decreases lower esophageal sphincter pressure as well as the velocity of peristalsis.[8] Manometric studies can confirm the diagnosis of esophageal dysmotility. Interestingly, although esophageal dysmotility and gastroparesis are both believed to result from impaired vagal function, limited studies have not found an epidemiologic link between the two diseases, suggesting separate pathophysiology of the diseases.[9]

Dyspepsia

Abdominal symptoms such as nausea, vomiting, bloating, postprandial fullness, anorexia, early satiety, heartburn, mild abdominal discomfort are commonly reported by diabetic individuals. Two common and pathophysiologically linked diagnoses are gastroparesis and gastroesophageal reflux disease (GERD).

Gastroparesis

As many as 50% of patients with type 1 diabetes have delayed gastric emptying of solids, or gastroparesis.[10] Gastroparesis is a motility problem caused by a gastric dysrhythmia and, as such, is a form of pseudoobstruction. Gastroparesis is diagnosed more commonly in women than in men. Symptoms are greater after solid meals. Clinical findings in severe cases may include a succussion splash, which is audible through a stethoscope over the gastric area while the trunk is shaken, and which is due to a large gastric residual after an overnight fast, or a meal. In milder cases, objective evidence of slowed gastric emptying may be present with few or nonspecific symptoms.

Because of gastric stasis, diabetic patients are prone to form "bezoars" which are conglomerations of undigested food material.[11] Bezoars can cause epigastric discomfort, and can obstruct the pylorus, further promoting nausea and vomiting. Pylorospasm, i.e., impaired relaxation, and small bowel dysmotility may also contribute to gastric stasis and bezoar formation.[12]

The pathophysiology of gastroparesis is believed to be autonomic dysfunction but the evidence is not fully convincing. No consistent pathologic abnormalities have been reported in diabetic gastroparesis.[32] Some authors have suggested a role for nitric oxide in altered gastric emptying in poorly controlled diabetes, as insulin restores neuronal nitric oxide synthase expression and function in experimental studies, and diabetes is characterized by abnormalities in nitric oxide generation.[13] Prostaglandins have also been implicated in gastric dysmotility, since tachygastria, a gastric dysrhythmia, could be blocked by pretreatment with indomethacin. Elevation of postprandial glucagon levels associated with hyperglycemia also may contribute to the delayed emptying, as this hormone promotes smooth muscle relaxation.

Diabetic gastroparesis should be suspected when a patient presents with compatible clinical symptoms and has no demonstrable disease by endoscopy or barium studies. The diagnosis may be confirmed by the demonstration of a delay in gastric emptying of solids. Measuring the emptying of liquids is of limited use, since this is usually normal, even in diabetic patient with gastroparesis. Gastric scintigraphy, a noninvasive nuclear medicine study, is the "gold standard" test for measuring gastric emptying. The patient ingests a radiolabeled meal of at least 300 kcal and the rate of emptying of the isotope determined over time. The result is reported as the percentage of the meal emptied after 2 or 4 h, or as the time needed to empty 50% of the meal.

Other tests include the measurement of gastric myoelectrical activity, though few centers perform this test. Electrogastrography (EGG) noninvasively measures fasting and postprandial gastric myoelectrical activity via electrodes placed on the skin in the epigastrium. EGG accurately reflects the normal 3 cycles per minute (cpm) electrical rhythm and abnormal gastric dysrythmias termed tachygastria (3.6–9.9 cpm) and bradygastria (1.0–2.4 cpm). Care must be taken to keep the patient still, since artifacts in the EGG signal may be created by patient movement.[14]

For the few most severe, refractory patients who fail all other treatments, direct measurement of antroduodenal motility, done only in major referral centers, has a limited role in assessing diabetic individuals with gastroparesis. Patients with selective abnormality of antral motility may tolerate feeding directly into the small bowel while those with a generalized motility disorder may not tolerate any enteral feeding.[15]

It is prudent to distinguish between acute and chronic gastroparesis. In acute gastroparesis, delay in gastric emptying is often the result of acute hyperglycemia or other metabolic alterations, such as the case with diabetic ketoacidosis. Both delayed gastric emptying and symptoms often improve once glucose control is restored toward normal. In contrast, chronic gastroparesis, which currently appears to be much less common, does not improve markedly with improvement in glucose control.

Several diseases may mimic gastroparesis. The differential diagnosis for gastroparesis includes gastric outlet obstruction caused by peptic ulcer disease, neoplasm, or pyloric stenosis, metabolic derangements, such as ketoacidosis or uremia, and medication toxicities, such as calcium channel blockers and anticholinergic agents.

Cyclic vomiting syndrome is an important differential in the evaluation of recurrent vomiting and possible gastroparesis. In cyclic vomiting syndrome, patients have repeated bouts of vomiting interspersed with periods of normal health. This disease, which is linked to migraine headaches, is more common in children. A subset of children with cyclic vomiting appears to have maternal inheritance and an associated mitochondrial mtDNA variation.[16] Rome III criteria define the disease based on (1) stereotypical acute episodes of vomiting lasting less than a week, (2) three or more discrete episodes of vomiting the year before, (3) absence of nausea and vomiting between episodes. Limited studies have linked cyclic vomiting to other evidence of autonomic dysfunction.[17] Treatment is usually supportive, including antimigraine medicine for headaches. Antidepressants, such as amitriptyline, also may be helpful (Table 27.1).

Table 27.1 Differential diagnosis of gastroparesis

- Mechanical obstruction – bezoar, gastric cancer, pyloric stenosis
- Peptic ulcer disease
- Chronic cholecystitis
- Pancreatitis
- Uremia
- Hypercalcemia – hyperparathyroidism
- Hypokalemia
- Addison's disease
- Hypothyroidism
- Medications – anticholinergics, calcium channel blockers, octreotide
- Cyclic vomiting syndrome

The treatment of gastroparesis depends on its severity. For patients with severe symptoms, liquids are better tolerated than solids. Increasing the nutrient component of the liquid meal can improve nutritional balance. A low fat, low residue diet is also recommended as high residue foods may lead to bezoar formation. A low fat diet (<40 g per day) is recommended, since fats delay gastric emptying. Patients should be encouraged to eat six small meals (snacks) a day rather than one or two large meals to promote a more steady flow of nutrients to the small bowel. Alcohol should be avoided as it can decrease antral contractility. The Gastroparesis Diet created by Dr. Kenneth Koch (Table 27.2) may be a helpful guideline for a diabetic patient with gastroparesis.

Table 27.2 The nausea or vomiting (gastroparesis) diet

Step 1. Rehydration solution (sports drink and bouillon)
  Diet: Small volume of salty liquids to avoid dehydration
  Goal: 1000–1500 ml/day in multiple servings, e.g., 1–2 oz at a time
  Avoid: Citrus and highly sweetened drinks

Step 2. Soup and crackers
  Diet: Soups with noodles or rice and crackers and peanut butter in small amounts in at least six divided meals per day
  Goal: 1500 calories per day; avoid dehydration and maintain weight
  Avoid: Creamy, milk-based liquids

Step 3. Solid food: starches, chicken and fish
  Diet: Starches such as noodles, pastas, potatoes, and rice are easily mixed and emptied by the stomach; chicken breast and fish are usually well tolerated in six divided meals per day; a one-a-day chewable vitamin should be prescribed to be taken with an evening snack; chewable calcium should also be given in the appropriate dose
  Goal: To find common foods that evoke minimal nausea or vomiting
  Avoid: Fatty foods which delay gastric emptying and red meats and fresh vegetables which require maximum trituration

From Koch[18], with permission.

Table 27.3 Medications to stimulate gastric emptying

Drug	Dose	Mechanism	Side effects
Metoclopramide	5–10 mg before meals	D2 antagonist 5-HT4 antagonist (peripheral and central)	Extrapyramidal, anxiety, drowsiness dystonia, hyperprolactinemia
Erythromycin (suspension)	125–250 mg	Motilin agonist	Nausea, diarrhea, cramps, rash
Domperidone[a]	10–20 mg	D2 antagonist (peripheral)	Hyperprolactinemia
Cisapride[a]	5–20 mg AC, hs	5-HT4 agonist (peripheral)	Diarrhea, abdominal discomfort
Tegaserod[a]	6 mg twice daily before meals	5-HT4 receptor agonist	Diarrhea

[a]Not available in United States
D = Dopamine
5-HT4= 5 hydroxytryptamine or serotonin "4" receptor

For symptomatic patients who do not respond to dietary modification alone, prokinetic agents can be used (Table 27.3). The most commonly used agent is metoclopramide (Reglan), starting at 5 mg po qhs, and titrating upward. Metoclopramide is a peripheral cholinergic and anti-dopaminergic agent with central antiemetic activity. It may be slowly increased to QID dosing as needed. Side effects include drowsiness, Parkinson's type movements, and the development of tardive dyskinesia. Sometimes metoclopramide, 5 mg po, at least 30 min before lunch and dinner, is sufficient, especially if the patient is compliant with a low-fat, low-residue diet.[19]

Domperidone (Motilium) is a peripheral dopamine 2 receptor antagonist that increases gastric emptying. The starting dose of domperidone is 10 mg BID. Central nervous system side effects are observed less frequently with domperidone than with metoclopramide, as the drug does not cross the blood–brain barrier to an appreciable extent. Other adverse effects attributed to metoclopramide and domperidone are hyperprolactinemia and galactorrhea. Domperidone is not approved for any indication by the FDA but is available in Canada and elsewhere. Use of this agent may require obtaining a treatment IND from the FDA.

Cisapride (Propulsid) acts as a partial serotonin (5HT$_4$ receptor) agonist. Cisapride enhances gastric emptying but has been withdrawn due to the potential for cardiac dysrythmias. Erythromycin mimics the effects of motilin and stimulates smooth muscle motilin receptors in the antroduodenal area. In most patients, the effect is reduced after 5–7 days due to intolerance or to tachyphylaxis. Tegaserod (Zelnorm) is a 5-HT4 serotonin receptor agonist previously approved for constipation-predominant irritable bowel syndrome. Tegaserod can also increase gastroduodenal motility. However, the drug is currently unavailable because of safety concerns.

The medical treatment of severe gastroparesis (Table 27.4) may involve nasogastric decompression, intravenous fluids, and correction of metabolic derangements (potassium, magnesium, electrolytes, and glucose). Bezoars can be mechanically disrupted at the time of endoscopy. Erythromycin (3 mg/kg body weight intravenously every 8 h) may help gastric emptying acutely. One week of treatment with oral erythromycin, 125–250 mg TID, is worth trying once patients tolerate food. Frequent monitoring of blood glucose is essential during this phase. Surgical intervention should be avoided in gastroparesis. Certain patients may be selected for laparoscopic placement of a jejunal feeding tube, but otherwise should not undergo elective surgery.[20]

Gastroesophageal Reflux Disease and Barrett's Esophagus

Gastroesophageal reflux disease (GERD) is more common in diabetic patients than in nondiabetic individuals, though heartburn is a very common symptom in the general population. Several disorders of esophageal motility have been described in diabetes, and often occur together. These include decreased lower esophageal sphincter (LES) pressure, weak contractions, slowed or absent peristalsis, and prolonged esophageal transit, all of which either promote reflux or decrease esophageal emptying response to reflux, and increase exposure time and esophageal injury.

Table 27.4 Management of diabetic gastroparesis

Gastric decompression if needed
Upper endoscopy to exclude bezoar, outlet obstruction
Diet modification/glucose control
    Liquid supplements if solids not tolerated
    Koch's three step Gastroparesis Diet
    Feeding j-tube (only in carefully selected patients)
    Total parenteral nutrition
Promotility therapy: stimulation of gastric emptying with medication
    Domperidone 10–20 mg po BID, TID, or QID
    Metoclopramide 5–10 mg po qhs or 30 minutes before meals, if tolerated
Antiemetic therapy
    For moderate symptoms:
    Prochlorperazine (Compazine) 5–10 mg po or IV BID PRN or 25 mg rectal suppository q 12 h
        PRN
    Antihistamines
    For hospitalized patients with severe gastroparesis:
    Ondansetron (Zofran) 8–16 mg IV qd
    Halogenated phenothiazines – Haloperidol, 1–2 mg IM or IV bid
Gastric pacing (experimental)

Gastroparesis contributes to acid reflux by increasing gastric residual volume. For this reason, lifestyle modifications that apply to nondiabetic patients with GERD, such as avoiding late night meals, are even more important in the diabetic patient. In some cases, GERD is so severe that ulcerative esophagitis or strictures develop. Due to sensory abnormalities, a diabetic patient may not feel the acid reflux and seek relief with antacid or antisecretory therapy. In addition, failure of secondary peristalsis increases exposure time of the esophageal mucosa to the refluxate, which may be acidic. Such a situation can be diagnosed by assessment of pH in the esophagus over 24 h, using either a tube or tubeless system.

The term "Barrett's esophagus" refers to metaplasia of the esophageal epithelium, from squamous epithelium to gastric or intestinal epithelium. Barrett's esophagus is a precursor lesion for esophageal adenocarcinoma, and many patients with Barrett's esophagus may benefit from endoscopic surveillance regimens. If symptoms of reflux have persisted for more than 5 years in any patient over 40 years of age, endoscopy should be performed to exclude Barrett's esophagus. No data specifically link Barrett's esophagus to diabetes.

The treatment of a diabetic patient with GERD is similar to that of nondiabetic individuals. Current therapy is limited mainly to antisecretory agents because of a lack of agents that increase LES pressure or stimulate effective esophageal peristalsis. Prokinetic agents may be helpful in the presence of gastroparesis. Because effective motility agents are not readily available, lifestyle changes are very important (Table 27.5).

Many patients will respond to lifestyle changes alone. However, others will also need antisecretory therapy. For patients with mild, intermittent reflux, and mild symptoms, the fastest relief occurs with antacids, such as

Table 27.5 Lifestyle changes to improve reflux

– Sit up in a chair whenever eating food and taking pills
– Drink small volumes of liquid throughout the day, between meals
– Eat small frequent meals
– Avoid "trigger" foods such as onions, pepper, garlic, citrus and tomatoes
– Elevate the head of the bed with 3 in. blocks
– Do not eat anything for 3 h before lying supine
– Limit fatty and fried foods
– Drink plenty of water with all pills to avoid pill-induced esophagitis
   especially NSAIDS, iron, digoxin, bisphosphonates
– Avoid carbonated beverages, alcohol, and smoking
– Lose excess weight

calcium carbonate, which can be dissolved in the mouth. Products containing magnesium should be avoided in diabetic patients with renal insufficiency. Histamine type 2 receptor antagonists, such as ranitidine (Zantac), may be helpful but the dose should not exceed 150 mg po daily in patients with renal insufficiency. These agents are appropriate for mild-to-moderate reflux symptoms and can be taken PRN, though there is a lag before symptomatic relief is noted. Tachyphylaxis is common with prolonged therapy.

For more severe or refractory GERD, proton pump inhibitor therapy is indicated. Proton pump inhibitors are most effective when taken around 1 h before the first meal of the day. Consuming a meal is important in promoting binding of the drug to the proton (acid) pump. Proton pump inhibitors must be taken regularly to be maximally effective and do not work well when taken PRN. No proton pump inhibitor has consistently shown significant clinical benefits over another. However, there are some important individual distinctions within this class of drugs. In addition, lansoprazole cannot be given to patients with cirrhosis, omeprazole interacts with coumadin, and pantoprazole can be taken with or without food or antacids, and has been shown to be safe in the elderly.

There are minimally invasive procedures, performed endoscopically, and more invasive surgical procedures that have been or are being developed to treat patients with severe GERD. These techniques have not been proven to be safe and effective in diabetic patients and are not presently recommended in this group of patients.

Abdominal Pain

Diabetic patients are susceptible to the same disorders that cause abdominal pain in nondiabetic individuals. These include mesenteric ischemia, diverticular disease, neoplasms, ovarian cysts and torsion, appendicitis, cholecystitis, diverticulitis, and others. Though all disease entities involving abdominal pain should be considered in a diabetic patient with pain, certain conditions, such as diabetic ketoacidosis, pancreatitis/pancreatic cancer, small intestinal/colonic ischemia, diabetic radiculopathy, biliary colic, and cholecystitis deserve special mention.

Pancreatitis

The incidence of acute pancreatitis is twice as high in diabetic patients compared to nondiabetic individuals. Acute pancreatitis may precipitate ketoacidosis. On the other hand, diabetic patients presenting with ketoacidosis frequently have elevated serum amylase activity and may present with abdominal pain, nausea, and vomiting. Treatment includes aggressive resuscitation with intravenous fluids, nasogastric decompression, avoiding oral intake, and appropriate pain management.

Pancreatic Cancer

There is an association between diabetes and pancreatic cancer though the precise cause and effect relationship is unclear. Two meta-analyses showed that preexisting diabetes led to pancreatic cancer with a pooled relative risk of 1.8–2.1.[21, 22] Insulin was shown in vitro to promote tumor growth.[23] Animal studies have suggested that islet cell proliferation in the pancreas as a result of insulin resistance enhances carcinogenesis.[24] Other studies suggest that pancreatic cancer may precede and promote the development of diabetes. It is not likely to be due to destruction of islet cells, since autopsy description in patients who died of pancreatic cancer showed atrophy of acinar tissue with intact islets and beta cells.[25] Some authors have suggested that pancreatic cancer promotes insulin resistance through the same signals by which it promotes cachexia, i.e., pro-inflammatory cytokines.

Diabetic patients with pancreatic cancer may or may not present with abdominal pain and acute pancreatitis. However, when the diabetic patient presents with significant weight loss, pancreatic cancer should be considered.

Diabetic Ketoacidosis

Hyperglycemia can have a major influence on the motor function and perception of sensations. There is a strong relationship between hyperglycemia and delayed gastric emptying. Hyperglycemia relaxes the fundus and suppresses the frequency and propagation of antral contractions. Disturbances of slow wave activity also occur. Patients with diabetic ketoacidosis may present with nausea, vomiting and abdominal pain, abdominal fullness, and early satiety. Studies also show delayed gastric emptying. Nasogastric drainage may yield a large volume of gastric residual (>1 l). It is important to note that while these findings imply gastroparesis, the abnormality is acute and not chronic, as symptoms and other evidence of delayed emptying usually resolve with effective treatment

Mesenteric Ischemia

The incidence of macrovascular athrerosclerosis in diabetic patients is extremely high. Mesenteric ischemia, which is a medical and surgical emergency, may occur. Small bowel ischemia is life-threatening and needs to be diagnosed quickly. Early diagnosis and intervention can prevent fatal intestinal gangrene. Effective diagnosis is based upon maintaining a high index of suspicion, especially in an older diabetic patient. An important clinical clue is that the pain often is out of proportion to the findings on examination.

Colonic Ischemia

Diabetic patients also are prone to develop colonic ischemia. Dehydration, antihypertensive agents, and diuretics all predispose to low flow states and colonic ischemia. Ischemia usually is self-limited and patients present with painless, bloody diarrhea, though some may have low-grade pain. The symptoms may be transient and patients may not report them to their physicians. In mild cases, ischemic damage is limited to the mucosa, and bleeding occurs with restoration of normal blood flow and complete healing. If the depth of ischemia is greater, the colon may heal with scarring and stricture formation. In the most severe cases, transmural ischemia occurs, and the colon is at risk for gangrene and perforation.

Diabetic Radiculopathy

Uncommonly, chronic abdominal pain may result from diabetic radiculopathy, i.e., peripheral neuropathy affecting the thoracic nerve roots. Electromyographic examination may provide evidence of thoracic or lumbar nerve root impairment. The pain is typically in a girdle distribution and may respond to amitriptyline, 50 mg po qhs. Phenytoin, 100 mg po TID, may also be effective.

Cholelithiasis/Cholecystitis/Cholangitis

Cholelithiasis is more common in diabetic patients than in the general population. The link between cholelithiasis and diabetes is likely multifactorial. While many diabetic patients are obese, other factors also may affect pathogenesis. Ultrasound and scintigraphy showed normal or reduced gallbladder ejection fraction independent of BMI or lipid profile in a group of diabetic subjects.[26] Hyperglycemia also reduces gallbladder emptying. Decreased gallbladder motility and incomplete gallbladder emptying promote stasis and may predispose to gallstone formation. A relative deficiency of cholecystokinin (CCK) receptors has been found in diabetic gallbladder with poor contractility.[27] One study demonstrated improved gall bladder emptying with clonidine, suggesting reduced alpha adrenergic tone.

Cholelithiasis predisposes to the development of acute cholecystitis or cholangitis. Diabetic patients are prone to cholangitis, which may be complicated by sepsis with uncommon organisms such as *Yersinia enterocolitica*. Thus, when the diabetic patient presents with right upper quadrant pain, the possibilities of cholelithiasis, cholecystitis, and cholangitis always should be considered. Surgical morbidity and mortality are increased in diabetic patients, especially when elderly or with vascular disease, due to poor healing. These factors may play a role in the timing of surgery. However, prophylactic cholecystectomy for stable diabetic patients with asymptomatic cholelithiasis is not recommended.

Diarrhea

Diarrhea is a common complaint in diabetic patients, though a higher proportion of patients complain of constipation than diarrhea. It is important to elicit the exact symptom complex during medical history-taking, as individual definitions of diarrhea vary among patients. The most accepted definition includes an alteration in stool consistency with increased water content. However, some patients define diarrhea solely on the basis of stool frequency, and some even confuse diarrhea with incontinence. Most relevant diarrheal conditions are chronic in nature, with the definition of "chronic" typically referring to diarrhea lasting more than 3 weeks. As with abdominal pain and other GI symptoms, diabetic patients may develop the same diarrheal conditions as nondiabetic individuals. In addition, some causes of diarrhea are specifically associated with diabetes.

The evaluation of a patient with diarrhea begins with a detailed review of diet and medication history. Common triggers of osmotic diarrhea are sorbitol, high fructose corn syrup, and antacids that contain magnesium. Drugs such as metformin may cause diarrhea. Although patients often interpret fecal incontinence to be diarrhea, the incontinent stool is usually formed. The presence of anemia, macrocytosis, hypoalbuminemia, or excess stool fat suggests intestinal malabsorption. Quantitation of stool fat is rarely helpful, however. In diabetic patients who present with diarrhea, bacterial overgrowth, celiac sprue, diabetic diarrhea, bile salt diarrhea, and pancreatic insufficiency warrant special consideration.

Bacterial Overgrowth

Diabetic patients with bacterial overgrowth may present with symptoms of periumbilical abdominal discomfort, bloating, gaseous distention, or diarrhea. Chronic bacterial overgrowth may be associated with features of malabsorption such as anemia, osteoporosis, and coagulopathy. For example, bacteria inhabiting the terminal ileum consume Vitamin B_{12}, leading to B_{12} deficiency, which presents as megaloblastic anemia. Bacterial overgrowth results in bile salt deconjugation and fat malabsorption, contributing to diarrhea. Vitamin K malabsorption promotes the development of a coagulopathy manifested as prolonged prothrombin time. In severe, chronic cases, Vitamin D malabsorption may lead to osteomalacia.

The cause of bacterial overgrowth is believed to be dysmotility secondary to autonomic dysfunction. As described above, failure of the intestinal "housekeeper" motility pattern leads to retention of small bowel contents, including microbes, allowing increased time to divide and produce proteases, toxins, and other agents that affect intestinal function. Delayed small bowel transit after a meal also has been described in diabetes mellitus. One study revealed delayed intestinal transit of a liquid meal in 33% of insulin-dependent diabetic patients as evidenced by a delay in the appearance of hydrogen during a breath test.[28]

The gold standard for the diagnosis of bacterial overgrowth is a quantitative culture of jejunal aspirates; a count of more than 10^5 aerobes or $>10^3$ anaerobes/ml is diagnostic, but this test is available in few centers. Alternatively, breath tests can be used measuring the amount of H_2 or $^{14}CO_2$ released after oral ingestion of 50 g of glucose or 1 g of ^{14}C D-xylose, respectively. The sugars, at these doses, normally are absorbed and not metabolized by bacteria, whose fermentation products can be detected in a breath sample. If these tests are not available, a therapeutic trial of antibiotics is appropriate if the clinical suspicion is high. The treatment of bacterial overgrowth includes antibiotics for 10 days to 2 weeks (Table 27.6). The potential for developing antibiotic-associated diarrhea may temper the enthusiasm for therapeutic trials. Newer generations of agents, some of which are nonabsorbable, may find a role in this clinical setting.

Pancreatic Insufficiency

Epidemiologic studies have linked diabetes mellitus to pancreatic exocrine deficiency. Patients with type 1 diabetes may develop pancreatic insufficiency. There is controversy regarding type 2 diabetes. In this situation,

Table 27.6 Treatment of bacterial overgrowth

Metronidazole [Flagyl] 250 mg po TID with meals for 10–14 days (Metronidazole cannot be taken during pregnancy or lactation)
Ciprofloxacin 250 mg BID
Amoxicillin and clavulanate potassium (Augmentin), 875 mg orally twice a day for 14 days
Doxycycline 100 mg po BID for 10–14 days

diabetes precedes the development of pancreatic insufficiency. How the diabetic patient develops pancreatic insufficiency also is unclear. It is possible that autoimmune pancreatitis may play a role in the destruction of both the exocrine and the endocrine portions of the pancreas in some cases.

Patients with long standing chronic pancreatitis may develop diabetes late in the course of their disease. This situation is usually seen in chronic pancreatitis due to alcohol abuse. In these cases patients develop weight loss due to malabsorption and require treatment with pancreatic enzymes as well as insulin. The pancreatic islets are involved in the fibrotic process and are damaged progressively. The loss of islet cells includes all cell types, rather than being limited to beta cells as in the case in type 2 diabetes. In this situation, pancreatic insufficiency precedes the development of diabetes by several years.

If a patient with chronic pancreatitis develops new onset diabetes, carcinoma of the pancreas needs to be carefully excluded. Diabetic patients who drink alcohol have a two to four increased risk of developing adenocarcinoma of the pancreas.[29]

Celiac Disease

Celiac disease is an autoimmune disorder related to gliadin proteins in rye, barley, and wheat and is found more commonly in diabetic patients than in nondiabetic individuals. The prevalence of celiac disease in the general population is 0.4–1% in North America. The prevalence of celiac disease in type I diabetics in tertiary centers ranges from 1 to 7%. Histologically, celiac disease is characterized by small bowel villus atrophy, crypt hyperplasia, and lymphocytic infiltration of the epithelium and lamina propria. Patients with celiac disease often have signs of malabsorption and can present with diarrhea, weight loss, abdominal fullness, mild abdominal pain, and nutritional deficiencies leading to osteopenia, short stature, and edema. Several serological tests are available to aid in diagnosis. Tissue transglutaminase is an enzyme on connective tissue or endomysium that deaminates gliadin to form peptides. IgA antibodies against tissue transglutaminase have a sensitivity and specificity as high as 95%. IgA and IgG antibodies to gliadin yield a sensitivity and specificity between 80 and 90% for most studies. The diagnosis is often confirmed by small bowel biopsy. The mainstay of treatment is consumption of a gluten free diet. Symptoms of abdominal pain and diarrhea typically improve on a gluten free diet. Nonresponse to a gluten free diet usually is due to poor adherence. In others, the development of intestinal lymphoma should be suspected, as this is a well recognized disease complication.

Bile Salt Diarrhea

Bile salt diarrhea or cholerrheic enteropathy is reported to be more common in diabetic than in nondiabetic patients. Bile is normally reabsorbed in the terminal ileum. In diabetic patients, intestinal motility may be fast or slow. Excessively rapid transit may exceed ileal reabsorptive capacity and lead to malabsorption. On the other hand, excessively slow transit may lead to bacterial overgrowth with bile salt deconjugation and malabsorption. In either case, the malabsorbed bile salt stimulates salt and water secretion in the right colon. Unfortunately, there is no standardized, generally available test for detecting bile salt malabsorption in the United States. If bile salt malabsorption is suspected, a therapeutic trial of the intraluminal binding agent, cholestyramine (4–16 g/day), may be undertaken. Antidiarrheal agents, such as loperamide and diphenoxylate, are partially effective for treating the diarrhea, but could promote small bowel bacterial overgrowth.

Diabetic Diarrhea

Diabetic diarrhea is a relatively uncommon gastrointestinal symptom that occurs in poorly controlled diabetic patients with severe autonomic neuropathy.[30] Diabetic diarrhea is watery and painless, generally most severe at night, and is more common in men. The pathogenesis of diabetic diarrhea is believed to be an autonomic neuropathy, specifically of the sympathetic system. Normally, parasympathetic neural activity promotes solute and water secretion, while the sympathetic neural activity promotes solute and water absorption.

The management of diabetic diarrhea is challenging. Treatment should begin with rehydration, correction of electrolyte disturbances, rigorous control of blood glucose, and restoration of positive caloric balance.[31] Antidiarrheal agents, such as loperamide 2–4 mg QID, or codeine 30 mg QID, may be helpful. In one study, clonidine (0.6 mg TID), an alpha 2-adrenoreceptor agonist that stimulates electrolyte and intestinal fluid reabsorption in vitro, was shown to reduce the volume of diarrhea.[32] Significant adverse effects, such as orthostatic hypotension, worsening of gastroparesis, and dry mouth limit the use of this therapy. Topical clonidine may control diarrhea without causing hypotension.[32] Verapamil (40 mg twice daily) also may help diarrhea by increasing colonic transit time, but hypotension can occur with this therapy as well.

For severe, refractory cases, octreotide (a somatostatin analog) has been effective in doses of 50–75 mcg subcutaneously twice a day. Octreotide suppresses the release of GI hormones that promote secretion.[33] Care must be taken when using octreotide since the drug also suppresses exocrine function of the pancreas which can cause maldigestion. In addition, octreotide inhibits gallbladder emptying and may promote gallstone formation.

Constipation

Constipation is a major gastrointestinal complaint among patients with diabetes. The prevalence of constipation is higher in diabetic patients than in the general population. While a few patients have pelvic floor dysfunction which may improve with behavioral or biofeedback, most diabetic individuals with constipation have a diffuse disorder of colonic motility. However, clinical evaluation should be performed to exclude mucosal lesions such as rectocele, rectal prolapse, and pelvic floor dysfunction. Medical disorders such as hypercalcemia, hyperthyroidism, diverticular disease, colonic strictures, and colon neoplasms also need to be excluded as clinically indicated.

Like gastroparesis, the precise pathophysiology of colonic dysmotility in diabetes is not well understood.[34] In one study, the normal postprandial increase in colonic motility was either delayed or absent.[35] These abnormalities were reversed with neostigmine or metoclopramide, suggesting a functional defect in the autonomic nervous system. The content of substance P, but not VIP or somatostatin, was found to be reduced in the rectal mucosa of diabetic patients.[36] Substance P normally stimulates pancreatic secretion, intestinal water and electrolyte secretion, and intestinal motility.

The first step in the treatment of a diabetic patient with constipation, after optimizing blood glucose control, is to increase water intake to 6–8 ounce glasses of water a day, as tolerated. Exercise is very important to stimulate the bowel as well as for the health of the patient. Soluble fiber is encouraged as opposed to insoluble fiber (cabbage, bell peppers) which can predispose to gastric bezoar formation. Some natural forms of soluble fiber are oatmeal, lentil soup, split pea soup, navy bean soup, and black bean soup. One serving of bean soup contains around 15 g of fiber, which is equivalent to at least 2 heads of broccoli. Fiber supplements may be helpful, but may cause excessive flatus, bloating, and cramping.

Pharmacologic therapy should be started with milk of magnesia or other osmotic laxatives. Newer agents that may be tried include a powder form of the nonabsorbable polymer, polyethylene glycol (Miralax), and lubiprostone (Amitiza), an agent that interacts with a chloride channel (Table 27.7).

Incontinence

Fecal incontinence is more frequent in females and in patients with long standing diabetes, especially those with autonomic neuropathy. Incontinence is often mistakenly identified as diarrhea. Diabetic patients with incontinence may have dysfunction in the internal anal sphincter, external anal sphincter, or the rectum.

Table 27.7 The treatment of constipation

1. Diet and lifestyle changes: increase water intake, exercise, functional dietary guidelines (above)
2. Encourage the "p" fruits – pears, papaya, peaches, plums
3. Milk of magnesia may be effective
   a. Contraindicated in the presence of renal dysfunction
4. Polyethylene glycol powder [Miralax]: 1 capful (17 gm) qhs PRN
5. Lubiprostone [Amitiza]
6. Promotility agents: Misoprostil [Cytotec], Tegaserod [Zelnorm]

Sphincter Dysfunction

Diabetic patients with fecal incontinence have been reported to have reduced resting anal sphincter pressure (a function of the internal anal sphincter and sympathetic innervation) but usually normal squeeze pressure (a function of the external sphincter). External anal sphincter function (voluntary) usually is unaffected in diabetes. Although rare in diabetes, external sphincter dysfunction indicates a pudendal neuropathy and may be associated with dysfunction of the urinary bladder. One study ascribed sphincter dysfunction to ischemia. Symptomatic treatment may include codeine, loperamide, and biofeedback aimed at increasing sphincter tone.[37]

Rectal Dysfunction

Incontinent patients with diabetes may demonstrate decreased anorectal sensation and decreased rectal sensation to balloon distention.[38] The decreased awareness of rectal sensation and rectal volume leads to more frequent soiling in diabetic patients. This condition may be improved with biofeedback.

The anorectal examination allows assessment of the resting and squeeze anal sphincter pressure. Lack of sensation in the rectum and perianal skin may indicate the presence of a significant neuropathy. Absence of the cutaneous "wink" reflex indicates sacral root dysfunction. Evaluation of anorectal function should include a rectal ultrasound, especially in women who have had vaginal deliveries, to see if the sphincter is intact. Other patients may benefit from anorectal manometry but electromyography or pudendal nerve conduction tests are used mostly as research tools. Imaging studies during defecation evaluate rectal anatomy and can identify defects in the anal canal, rectoceles, or intussusception and the function of the pelvic floor during the process of defecation.

Summary

Gastrointestinal disorders are common in diabetic patients. Patients often suffer from the same gastrointestinal disorders as nondiabetic individuals. Diseases such as neoplastic, infectious, or inflammatory disorders of the gastrointestinal tract should be excluded before focusing disease related to diabetes. Several disease entities described in this chapter such as esophageal dysmotility, gastroparesis, bacterial overgrowth, and rectal dysfunction are particularly common and pathogenically associated with specifically linked to diabetes. The cause of these disease entities is likely multifactorial but diabetic enteric autonomic neuropathy is believed to be causative. Some gastrointestinal symptoms are the result of hyperglycemia-induced dysmotility and are reversible. Treatment includes making an accurate diagnosis, educating the patient, initiating permanent lifestyle changes and effective pharmacotherapeutic agents.

References

1. Folwaczny C, Riepl R, Tschop M, Landgraf R. Gastrointestinal involvement in patients with diabetes Mellitus: Part I (first of two parts). epidemiology, pathophysiology, clinical findings. *Z Gastroenterol*. 1999;37:803–815.
2. Horvath KV, et al. Reduced stem cell factor links smooth myopathy and loss of interstitial cells of Cajal in murine diabetic gastroparesis. *Gastroenterology*. 2006;130:759–770.

3. Talley SJ, Bytzer P, Hammer J, et al. Psychological distress is linked to gastrointestinal symptoms in diabetes mellitus. *Am J Gastroenterol*. 2001;96(4):1033–1038.
4. Darwazeh AM, MacFarlane TW, McCuish A, et al. Mixed salivary glucose levels and candial carriage in patients with diabetes mellitus. *J Oral Pathol Med*. 1991;20(6):280–283.
5. Loo FD, Dodds WJ, Soergel KH, et al. Multipeaked esophageal peristaltic pressure waves in patients with diabetic neuropathy. *Gastroenterology*. 1985;88:485–491.
6. Faraj J, Melander O, Sundkvist G, et al. Oesophageal dysmotility, delayed gastric emptying and gastrointestinal symptoms in patients with diabetes mellitus. *Diabetes Med*. Nov 2007;24(11):1235–1239.
7. Keshavarzian A, Iber FL, Nasrallah S. Radionuclide esophageal emptying and manometric studies in diabetes mellitus. *Am J Gastroenterol*. 1987;82:625–631.
8. Rayner CK, Samsom M, Jones KL, et al. Relationships of upper gastrointestinal motor and sensory function with glycemic control. *Diabetes Care*. 2001;24(2):371–381.
9. Sargyn M, Uygur-Bayramicli O, Sargyn H, Orbay E, Yavuzer D, Yayla A. Type 2 diabetes mellitus affects eradication rate of Helicobacter pylori. *World J Gastroenterol*. May 2003;9:1126–1128.
10. Horowitz M, Edelbroek M, Fraser R, Maddox A, Wishart J. Disordered gastric motor function in diabetes mellitus: recent insights into prevalence, pathophysiology, clinical relevance, and treatment. *Scand J Gastroenterol*. 1991;26:673–684.
11. Koch KL. Dyspepsia of unknown origin: pathophysiology, diagnosis and treatment. *Dig Dis*. 1997;15:316–329.
12. Mearin F, Camilleri M, Malagelada J-R. Pyloric dysfunction in diabetics with recurrent nausea and vomiting. *Gastroenterology*. 1986;90:1919–1925.
13. Watkins CC, Sawa A, Jaffrey S. Insulin restores neuronal nitric oxide synthase expression and function that is lost in diabetic gastropathy. *J Clin Invest*. 2000;106:373–384.
14. Stern RM, Koch KL, Stewart WR, Vasey MW. Electrogastrography: current issues on validation and methodology. *Psychophysiology*. 1987;24:55–64.
15. Koch KL. Diabetic gastropathy: gastric neuromuscular dysfunction in diabetes mellitus – a review of symptoms, pathophysiology, and treatment. *Dig Dis Sci*. 1999;44(6):1061–1075.
16. Wang Q, Ito M, Adams K, et al. Mitochondrial DNA control region sequence variation in migraine headache and cyclic vomiting syndrome. *Am J Med Genet A*. 2004;131:50–58.
17. Chelimsky TC, Chelimsky GG. Autonomic abnormalities in cyclic vomiting syndrome. *J Pediatr Gastroenterol Nutr*. Mar 2007;44(3):326–330.
18. Koch KL. Therapy of nausea and vomiting. In: MM Wolfe Ed. *Therapy of Digestive Disorders*. Philadelphia: WB Saunders; 2000:731–746.
19. Koch KL. Unexplained nausea and vomiting. *Curr Treatment Opt Gastroenterol*. 2000;3:303–313.
20. Koch KL. Diabetic gastropathy: gastric neuromuscular dysfunction in diabetes mellitus–a review of symptoms, pathophysiology, and treatment. *Dig Dis Sci*. 1999;44(6):1061–1075.
21. Everhart J, Wright D. Diabetes mellitus as a risk factor for pancreatic cancer a meta-analysis. *J Am Med Assoc*. 1995;273:1605–1609.
22. Huxley R, Ansary-Moghaddam A, Berrington de Goonzalez A, et al. Type-II diabetes and pancreatic cancer a meta-analysis of 36 studies. *BR J Cancer*. 2005;92(11):2076–2083.
23. Fisher WE, Boros LG, Schirmer WJ. Insulin promotes pancreatic cancer evidence for endocrine influence on exocrine pancreatic tumors. *J Surg Res*. 1996;63:310–313.
24. Schneider MB, Matsuzaki H, Haorah J, et al. Prevention of pancreatic cancer induction in hamsters by metformin. *Gastroenterology*. 2001;120:1263–1270.
25. Bell ET. Carcinoma of the pancreas. I. A. clinical and pathological study of 609 necropsied cases II. The relation of carcinoma of the pancreas to diabetes. *Am J Pathol*. 1957;33:499.
26. Stone BG, Gavaler JS, Belle SH, et al. Impairment of gallbladder emptying in diabetes mellitus. *Gastroenterology*. 1988;95:170–176.
27. Upp JR, Nealon WH, Singh P, et al. Correlation of cholecystokinin receptors with gallbladder contractility in patients with gallstones. 1987;205:641–648.
28. Keshavarzian A, Iber FL. Intestinal transit in insulin-requiring diabetics. *Am J Gastroenterol*. 1986;81:257–260.
29. Cuzick J, Babiker AG. Pancreatic cancer, alcohol, diabetes mellitus, and gallbladder disease. *Int J Cancer*. 1989;43:415–421.
30. Saslow SB, Camilleri M. Diabetic diarrhea. *Semin Gastrointest Dis*. 1995;6:187.
31. Valdovinos MA, Camilleri M, Zimmerman BR. Chronic diarrhea in diabetes mellitus: mechanisms and an approach to diagnosis and treatment. *Mayo Clin Proc*. 1993;68:691–702.
32. Fedorak RN, Field M, Chang EB. Treatment of diabetic diarrhea with clonidine. *Ann Intern Med*. Feb 1985;102(2):197–199.
33. Von der Ohe MR, Camilleri M, Thomforde GM, et al. Differential regional effects of octreotide on human gastrointestinal motor function. *Gut*. 1995;36:743–748.
34. Camilleri M. Gastrointestinal problems in diabetes. *Endocrin Metab Clin*. 1996;25(2):361–378.
35. Battle WM, Snape WR, Alavi A, et al. Colonic dysfunction in diabetes mellitus. *Gastroenterology*. 1980;79:1217–1221.
36. Lysy J, Karmeli F, Sestieri M, et al. Decreased substance P content in the rectal mucosa of diabetics with diarrhea and constipation. *Metabolism*. 1997;46:730–734.

37. Wald A, Tunuguntla K. Anorectal sensorimotor dysfunction, fecal incontinence and diabetes mellitus. *N Engl J Med.* 1984;310:1282–1287.
38. Schiller LR, Santa Ana CA, Schulen AC, et al. Pathogenesis of fecal incontinence in diabetes mellitus. *N Engl J Med.* 1982;307:1666–1671.

Other Recommended Review Articles

Feldman M, Schiller LR. Disorders of gastrointestinal motility associated with diabetes mellitus. *Ann Intern Med* 1983;98:378–384

Verne GN, Sninsky CA. Diabetes and the gastrointestinal tract. *Gastroenterology Clin.* 1998;27(4):861–874.

Web Sites and Internet Sources for Patient Information

www.amwa-online.com
www.healthology.com
www.IBSvillage.com
www.IBSinformation.com

Chapter 28
Dyslipidemia: Pathogenesis and Management

Om P. Ganda

Introduction

Diabetes is the leading cause of cardiovascular morbidity and mortality around the world. On the basis of a number of epidemiologic studies and clinical trials, diabetes was designated a coronary heart disease (CHD)risk equivalent by the National Cholesterol Education Program's Adult Treatment Panel III (ATPIII).[1] The 10 yr risk of major CHD events in patients with diabetes generally exceeds 20%, which is comparable to that observed in nondiabetic patients with established CHD. This inference has been particularly supported by the data from a population study in Finland[2] and a multinational study, the OASIS[3] from patients with type 2 diabetes who frequently have multiple coexisting risk factors for cardiovascular disease (CVD). In a large meta-analysis of 22 studies, the multivariate-adjusted relative risk for fatal CHD was a highly significant 3.12 in women and 1.99 in men with diabetes, compared to nondiabetic individuals[4] (Fig. 28.1). Moreover, diabetes leads to myocardial infarction (MI) at a much younger age, in both men and women, as shown in a large population database, encompassing more than 379,000 people with, compared to more than 9 million people without diabetes[5] (Fig. 28.2). This was corroborated in another cohort study, which concluded that at age 50 yr, diabetes confers a reduction in life expectancy by 7.5 yr in men, and by 8.2 yr in women.[6] Furthermore, even after an acute MI, patients with diabetes have a worse prognosis, with a 40% increase in 30-day mortality, and a 33% increase in 1-yr mortality, compared to nondiabetic subjects in a multi-trial analysis, involving more than 60,000 patients, of whom more than 10,600 had diabetes.[7]

The increased risk for CHD may precede the clinical diagnosis of diabetes by many years. This was well documented in the long-term study of more than 117,000 women in the Nurses' Health Study, of which close to 6000 developed diabetes during 20 yr of follow-up. There was an approximately 2- to3-fold increased risk for MI or stroke during the "prediabetes" period, compared to women who remained nondiabetic.[8] On the other hand, in MRFIT, an observational analysis of a large number of men ($n = 348,000$, of which 5,163 had diabetes), it was revealed that the presence of diabetes was associated with 3- to 4-fold increased risk for age-adjusted cardiovascular mortality at comparable levels of cholesterol, blood pressure, and cigarette smoking.[9] These observations suggest a rather enhanced susceptibility of diabetic vasculature to the well-established risk factors for CHD.

There is also a gender paradox regarding CVD and total mortality that remains unexplained. During the past three decades, the CVD and total mortality in general population have declined,[10] largely contributed by the reduction in cardiovascular risk factors.[11] However, while a similar trend has been observed in the diabetic men, the CVD and total mortality in women with diabetes has not declined appreciably.[10] Some of the postulated reasons for this paradox might include a delay in diagnosis of atypical symptoms of CHD, a greater prevalence of lipid abnormalities,[12] or suboptimal treatment and control of lipids and other risk factors in women with diabetes, compared to men.[13-15]

O.P. Ganda (✉)
Joslin Diabetes Center, Beth-Israel Deaconess Medical Center, Harvard Medical School, Boston, MA, USA
e-mail: om.ganda@joslin.harvard.edu

L. Poretsky (ed.), *Principles of Diabetes Mellitus*, DOI 10.1007/978-0-387-09841-8_28,
© Springer Science+Business Media, LLC 2010

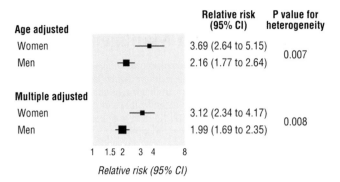

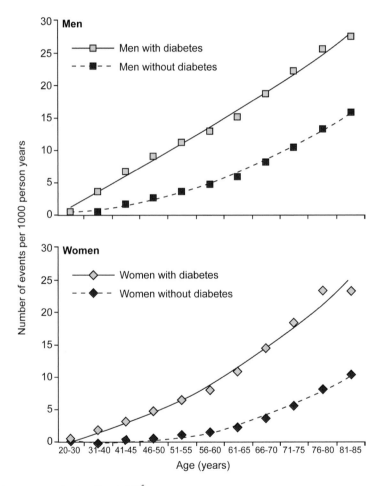

Fig. 28.1 Relative risks for fatal CHD in men and women with and without diabetes in 22 studies[4]

Fig. 28.2 Relation between age and rates of acute MI[5]

Lipoprotein Abnormalities Associated with Diabetes

Diabetes is associated with multiple disturbances in lipoprotein metabolism, triggered by insulin deficiency, insulin resistance, and hyperglycemia. The dyslipidemia of type 2 diabetes is characterized by a number of inter-related atherogenic abnormalities related to insulin resistance and consists of increased levels of triglyceride-rich

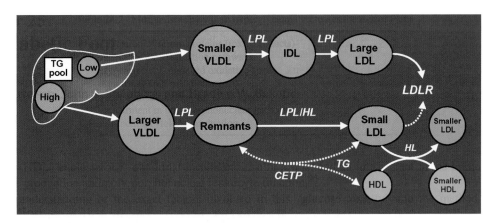

Fig. 28.3 Pathophysiology of dyslipidemia in type 2 diabetes[16]

lipoproteins (very low-density lipoprotein, [VLDL], intermediate-density lipoprotein [IDL], and remnant particles), low levels of high-density lipoprotein-cholesterol (HDL-C), as well as increased levels of small, dense low-density lipoprotein (LDL) particles[16,17] (Fig. 28.3). There is an increase in the lipid-rich, large VLDL (VLDL-1), upregulation of hepatic sterol regulatory element binding protein (SREBP-1), which stimulates de novo lipid synthesis and increased availability of FFA. All of these effects are probably linked with insulin resistance.[17] The activity of lipoprotein lipase (LPL) is suppressed, leading to reduced catabolism of triglyceride-rich particles, while hepatic lipase (HL) activity is increased, facilitating the compositional changes in LDL and HDL particles. In addition, there is enhanced activity of cholesterol ester transfer protein (CETP), which mediates the transfer of triglyceride to LDL and HDL while cholesterol esters from HDL are shunted to the larger triglyceride-rich particles. Thus, hypertriglyceridemia is indirectly linked with changes in the HDL and the LDL composition and associated with increased atherogenesis. This was well documented in a comparative study of young patients (mean age 12–16 yr), where there was a much higher prevalence of obesity, elevated triglycerides, and small, dense LDL with similar LDL- cholesterol levels but elevated apolipoprotein B particle number in patients with type 2, compared to type 1 diabetes[18] (Fig. 28.4). The prevalence of dense LDL also correlated with the level

	Age	BMI	LDL (mg/dl)	TG (mg/dl)	HDL (mg/dl)	ApoB (mg/dl)	Dense LDL (Rf)
Type 1 (n = 7562)	12.6	21.3	100	78	55	76	0.279
Type 2 (n = 345)	16.0*	34.1*	108*	195*	42*	94*	0.256

Prevalence of Elevated Markers

	Elevated Apo B (> 100 mg/dl)	Dense LDL (Rf < 0.237)	LDL-Cholesterol (> 130 mg/dl)
Type 1 (n = 2657)	11	8	12
Type 2 (n = 345)	36	36	23

Fig. 28.4 SEARCH: lipid levels and LDL – composition in type 1 and type 2 diabetes[18]

of glycemic control in that study. The small, dense LDL particles bind to intimal proteoglycans more avidly, are more susceptible to oxidation and glycation, and have impaired binding to LDL receptors.[1,16] All of these factors contribute to enhanced atherosclerosis in patients with diabetes and metabolic syndrome.

Lipoprotein particle size and concentrations were characterized by nuclear magnetic resonance (NMR) in subjects with type 2 diabetes, and nondiabetic individuals with normal or impaired insulin sensitivity characterized by euglycemic, hyperinsulinemic clamp technique.[19] There was a progressive increase in the size of VLDL particles in insulin-sensitive, insulin-resistant, and type 2 diabetes subjects, respectively, as well as a reciprocal decrease in the size of LDL and HDL particles. On the other hand, the cholesterol content in large LDL was increased and that in small LDL was decreased in those with insulin resistance and type 2 diabetes, whereas the calculated LDL-cholesterol was relatively unchanged despite increased LDL particle number (Fig. 28.5).

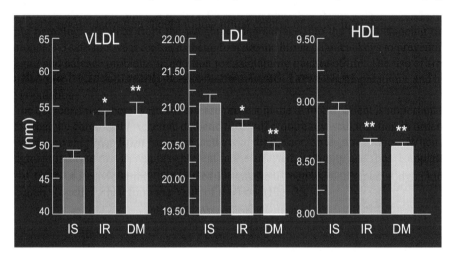

Fig. 28.5 Effect of insulin sensitivity and type 2 diabetes on lipoprotein particle size by nuclear magnetic resonance (*p <0.05; **p< 0.01)[19]

In view of the compositional changes in lipoproteins, the LDL-cholesterol determined in routine assays tends to underestimate the LDL particle number, particularly in patients with hypertriglyceridemia. It has therefore been proposed that direct measurement of apolipoprotein B (apoB) might provide a better estimate of risk than LDL-C in such patients.[20,21,21a] This recommendation was recently endorsed in a joint statement by the American Diabetes Association (ADA) and American College of Cardiology (ACC).[22] The assays for apoB are now better standardized than in the past and becoming more widely available. An alternative proposed by NCEP-ATP III guidelines is the calculation of non-HDL-cholesterol, which estimates the cholesterol content in all atherogenic particles: VLDL, IDL, remnants particles, LDL, and lipoprotein (a) [LP(a)].[1] Non-HDL-C has been shown to be a stronger predictor of CVD risk, compared to LDL-C in several studies.[22–24] However, the proponents of apoB recommend a greater predictive ability of apoB over non-HDL-C, although direct evidence from randomized clinical trials is relatively limited.

Low-Density Lipoprotein-Cholesterol Lowering Trials

Given the heterogeneity of lipoproteins and the complexity of lipoprotein metabolism in patients with diabetes, the evidence-based approach to restore all of the pathophysiologic defects is still not well established. Since the mid 1990s a variety of randomized, controlled trials with HMG-CoA reductase inhibitors (statins) have established the efficacy of these LDL-lowering agents in reducing cardiovascular outcomes.

In an extensive meta-analysis of 14 randomized trials of statin therapy, encompassing 90,056 individuals from various parts of the world, a mean LDL-cholesterol reduction of 1 mmol (~40 mg/dl) over 5 years resulted in a 23% reduction in myocardial infarction (MI) or coronary death (P<0.0001), a 17% reduction in stroke,

Major vascular event and prior diabetes	Events (%)		RR (CI)
	Treatment	Control	
Major coronary event			
Diabetes	776 (8·3%)	979 (10·5%)	0·78 (0·69–0·87)
No diabetes	2561 (7·2%)	3441 (9·6%)	0·77 (0·73–0·81)
Any major coronary event	**3337 (7·4%)**	**4420 (9·8%)**	**0·77 (0·74–0·80)**
Test for heterogeneity within subgroup: χ^2_1=0·1; p=0·8			
Coronary revascularisation			
Diabetes	491 (5·2%)	627 (6·7%)	0·75 (0·64–0·88)
No diabetes	2129 (6·0%)	2807 (7·9%)	0·76 (0·72–0·81)
Any coronary revascularisation	**2620 (5·8%)**	**3434 (7·6%)**	**0·76 (0·73–0·80)**
Test for heterogeneity within subgroup: χ^2_1=0·1; p=0·8			
Stroke			
Diabetes	407 (4·4%)	501 (5·4%)	0·79 (0·67–0·93)
No diabetes	933 (2·7%)	1116 (3·2%)	0·84 (0·76–0·93)
Any stroke	**1340 (3·0%)**	**1617 (3·7%)**	**0·83 (0·77–0·88)**
Test for heterogeneity within subgroup: χ^2_1=0·8; p=0·4			
Major vascular event			
Diabetes	1465 (15·6%)	1782 (19·2%)	0·79 (0·72–0·86)
No diabetes	4889 (13·7%)	6212 (17·4%)	0·79 (0·76–0·82)
Any major vascular event	**6354 (14·1%)**	**7994 (17·8%)**	**0·79 (0·77–0·81)**
Test for heterogeneity within subgroup: χ^2_1=0·0; p=0·9			

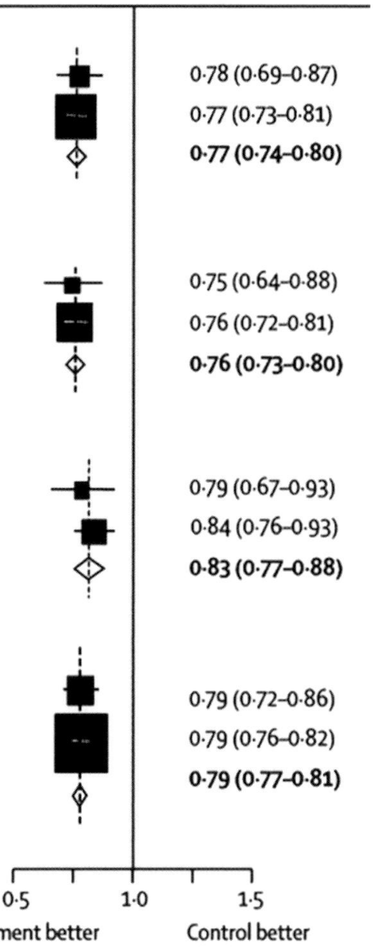

-■- RR (99% CI)
◇ RR (95% CI)

0·5   1·0   1·5
Treatment better   Control better

Fig. 28.6 Major vascular events with or without diabetes: effect per 1 mm/L reduction in LDL-cholesterol[26]

($P<0.001$), and a 12% reduction in all-cause mortality ($P< 0.0001$).[25] Similar improvements in the outcomes were seen in a detailed analyses of patients with diabetes ($n = 18,686$) in that meta-analysis[26] (Fig. 28.6). Moreover, similar significant benefits were seen regardless of age, gender, BMI, smoking status, presence or absence of hypertension, or vascular disease at baseline, and in the 1466 patients with type 1 diabetes. In addition, the total mortality was significantly reduced by 9 and 13%, and total vascular mortality reduced by 13 and 18% respectively, in those with or without diabetes, with no increase in non- cardiovascular mortality (Fig. 28.7).[26]

In another meta-analysis of 12 large, randomized trials, comparing patients with or without diabetes, similar risk reductions of 21–23% in CHD events were found in both populations in primary or secondary prevention.[27] Since the absolute baseline risk in patients with diabetes is greater, the benefit in such patients, with similar decrease in lipid levels, would be correspondingly greater, especially in secondary prevention. For example, in the landmark Heart Protection Study (HPS), among 6000 patients with diabetes, the 5-yr rates of first major vascular event in patients on placebo, ranged from 13% in those with diabetes alone, to 36% in those with diabetes and vascular disease, despite similar lipid levels.[28] Such observations support the concept that the absolute risk of CVD is mainly determined by underlying preexisting disease, rather than lipid levels.

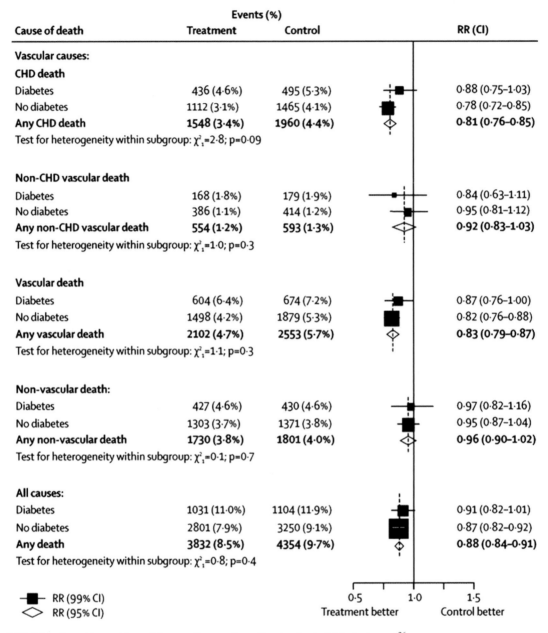

Fig. 28.7 Mortality with or without diabetes: effect per 1 mm/L reduction in LDL-cholesterol[26]

Whether the benefits of statin therapy are greater in patients with metabolic syndrome, in the absence of diabetes, remains controversial in the absence of clinical trials designed to answer this question. This is an important question in view of the lipid defects associated with triglyceride-rich particles and LDL compositional defects associated with insulin resistance as described above. However, subgroup analyses of some of the statin trials suggest that patients with metabolic syndrome may, in fact, have greater benefits, compared to those without metabolic syndrome. The first is the data from 4S trial.[29] In that analysis, those with lipid triad (high LDL, high triglyceride, low HDL) had a CHD event rate of 0.48 (confidence interval [CI], 0.33–0.69) compared to those with isolated high LDL alone (event rate, 0.86; CI, 0.59–1.26). More recently, a reanalysis of the Treat to New Target (TNT) statin trial was carried out according to the presence or absence of metabolic syndrome, as defined by the revised ATPIII criteria.[30] Of the 10,001 patients in this trial, comparing efficacy of Atorvastatin 80 mg vs. 10 mg in patients with clinically stable CHD, 5,584 had metabolic syndrome. Irrespective of treatment assignment, the hazard ratio of CHD events over 5 yr of follow-up in those with metabolic syndrome was 1.35 ($P<0.001$), compared to those without (Fig. 28.8). Furthermore, there was a greater risk reduction in CHD events with Atorvastatin 80 mg vs. 10 mg in patients with metabolic syndrome, in the presence or absence of diabetes, although patients with diabetes and metabolic syndrome were at the highest risk. It is currently debated whether the putative anti-inflammatory effects of statin may account for part of the benefits in patients with metabolic syndrome.[31] However, recent data from the JUPITER (Justification for the Use of statins in Prevention:an Intervention Trial Evaluating Rosuvastatin) trial, a large primary prevention trial are noteworthy. In that trial, where subjects were selected for increased CRP, a proinflammatory marker, at baseline, there was a sustantial 44% reduction in primary outcome, regardless of presence or absence of metabolic syndrome.[31a]

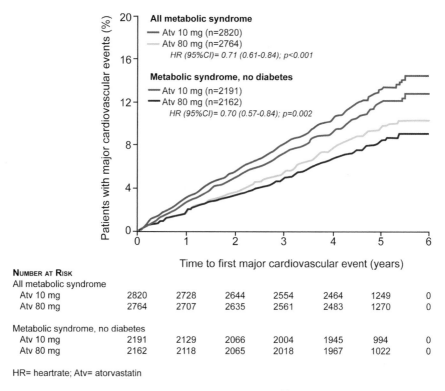

Fig. 28.8 TNT: major cardiovascular events by treatment and metabolic status[30]

Intensive Lipid Lowering with Statins

In view of the markedly increased risk of subsequent cardiovascular events (CHD and stroke) in patients with preexisting CHD, the current updated ATPIII guidelines and AHA guidelines recommend an LDL-cholesterol goal of <70 mg/dl in all patients in this category.[32,33] A meta-analysis included four trials of intensive LDL-lowering therapy in patients with acute coronary syndromes (PROVE-IT and A-to-Z) or stable CAD (TNT and IDEAL), involving 27,548 patients.[34] Of these, 4,379 patients had diabetes. The mean LDL-cholesterol achieved by intensive therapy was 75 mg/dl, compared to 101 mg/dl by standard treatment. This analysis revealed a 16% risk reduction (RR) in coronary death or MI ($P<0.0003$) and an 18% RR in stroke ($P=0.012$) (Fig. 28.9). Similar outcomes were observed in patients with diabetes. However, these analyses were underpowered for effects on cardiovascular or total mortality. Of some concern is the small, but significant increase in hepatic toxicity with

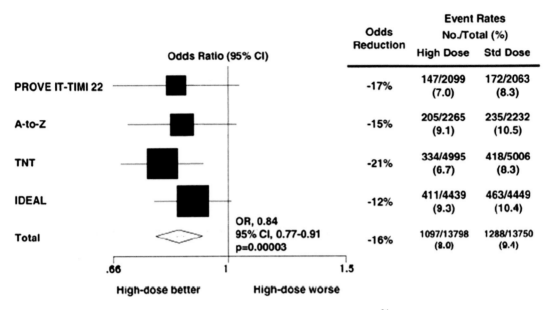

Fig. 28.9 Meta-analysis of intensive statin trials: coronary death or myocardial infarction[34]

more intensive therapy, using 80 mg dosing of both atorvastatin and simvastatin in these trials; however, there was no significant increase in the incidence of myositis or rhabdomyolysis.

In many patients with intolerance to higher dose statins, and consequent difficulty to achieve LDL goal, a combination of lower dose statins with cholesterol absorption inhibitor, ezetimibe, bile acid sequestrants (e.g., cholestyramine, colesevelam), or niacin are very useful strategies.[32,35–37] The efficacy and convenient dosing of ezetimibe in monotherapy and combination therapy with statin is well established. However, some controversy in its use was kindled by the results of a recent 24 month clinical trial, ENHANCE, in 720 patients with familial hypercholesterolemia (baseline LDL-C 319 mg/dl).[37] In that study, the primary outcome of the mean carotid intima-medial thickness (CIMT) increased by 0.0111 vs. 0.0058 mm (P=0.29) on simvastatin 80 mg + ezetimibe, compared to simvastatin 80 mg alone despite a 17% greater reduction in LDL-C and a 19% greater CRP reduction with the combination therapy. On the other hand, in a clinical trial in patients with type 2 diabetes, the intensification of LDL-lowering therapy resulted in a comparable reduction in CIMT, regardless of whether or not ezetimibe was added to a statin to achieve optimal lipid goal.[37a] The relevance of these findings to long-term clinical events is unclear, and the results of an ongoing clinical trial, IMPROVE-IT, with similar drug design in patients with acute coronary syndrome at baseline, are awaited.

Evidence for the Benefits of Triglyceride and HDL Intervention

The triglyceride-rich lipoproteins and low HDL-cholesterol are intimate components of the insulin resistance-mediated pathophysiology. Unlike the evidence from a plethora of trials of CHD risk reduction with statins, the direct evidence from drugs to lower triglycerides or to raise HDL-cholesterol is relatively limited. A meta-analysis of 29 observational studies, encompassing more than 10,000 CHD cases suggested a significant relationship of triglycerides with CHD, even after adjustment for HDL-cholesterol[38] (Fig. 28.10). In many of the statin trials, the residual risk of CHD events after statin treatment was considerably higher in patients with elevated triglycerides and lower HDL-C. In the 4S trial, in post hoc analyses, patients with lipid triad (elevated LDL, elevated triglyceride, and low HDL-cholesterol) had the highest event rates in the placebo arm and the greatest risk reduction with simvastatin.[29] Similarly, the TNT trial sub-analyses[30] strongly suggest increasing CHD risk with number of metabolic syndrome characteristics. Of note, also are similar observations with triglyceride as a

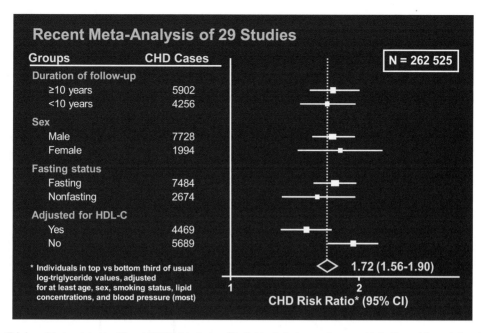

Fig. 28.10 Triglyceride level is significant CVD risk factor. *Individuals in top vs bottom third of usual log-triglyceride values, adjusted for at least age, sex, smoking status, lipid concentrations, and blood pressure (most)[39]

risk factor for CHD events in the sub-analysis of PROVE-IT trial, with a significant 37% lower hazard ratio ($P <$ 0.01) in those with triglycerides <150 vs. >150 mg/dl despite achieving identical LDL-cholesterol, <70 mg/dl.[40] Furthermore, a recent further analysis of TNT trial[41] revealed that in patients achieving an on-treatment LDL-cholesterol of <70 mg/dl, the risk of CHD events differed significantly by HDL-cholesterol quintiles ($P = 0.003$), with a 39% lower hazard ratio in patients in quintile 5 vs. quintile 1 (HDL-cholesterol >55 vs. <38 mg/dl) (Fig. 28.11). Finally, in the INTERHEART study, a large, case–control study of determinants of acute MI in 52

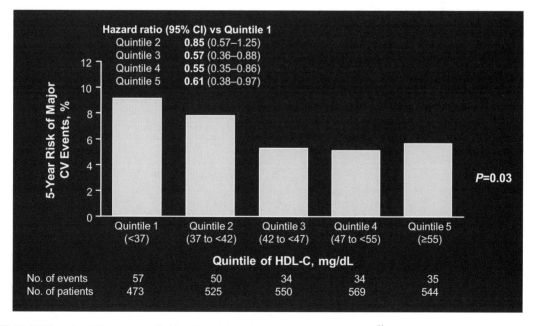

Fig. 28.11 TNT: major CV events stratified by HDL-C in patients with LDL-C <70 mg/dl[41]

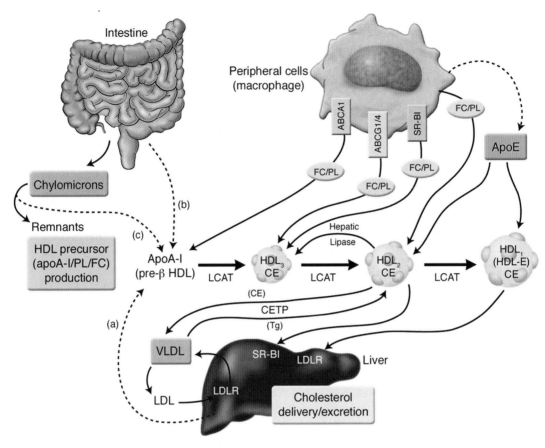

Fig. 28.12 Role of HDL in the redistribution of lipids[43]

countries around the world, apoB/apoA-1 ratio, rather than either of these apolipoprotein alone, was the strongest risk determinant and it outperformed the risk stratifications with total/HDL or LDL/HDL ratios.[42]

HDL is intimately involved in reverse cholesterol transport (Fig. 28.12) and has other crucial effects in the pathogenesis of atherosclerosis[43–45] (Table 28.1). Gene polymorphism for the variations in the antioxidant activity (paroaoxonase-1) may explain some of the association of functional properties of HDL with CVD events.[46] The antioxidant effects of HDL may be impaired in patients with type 2 diabetes,[47] in addition to enhanced activity of cholesterol ester transfer protein (CETP) caused by hypertriglyceridemia and insulin resistance.

Table 28.1 Mechanisms that may mediate the anti-atherogenic effects of HDL

- Reverse cholesterol transport
- Antioxidant effects
- Inhibition of adhesion molecule expression
- Inhibition of platelet activation
- Prostacyclin stabilization
- Promotion of NO production
- Association with increased adiponectin

Table 28.2 summarizes the lipid trials with fibrates in patients with diabetes or metabolic syndrome. In the Helsinki Heart Study, a primary prevention trial, a subgroup of 292 patients achieved a 71% decrease in CHD events with gemfibrozil over 5 yr.[48] In the Bezafibrate Infarction Prevention (BIP) study, the subgroup of 1,470 patients with metabolic syndrome or diabetes had a 29% risk reduction of reinfarction ($P <0.02$).[49] In the St.

Table 28.2   Major cardiovascular trials with fibrates in patients with type 2 diabetes or metabolic syndrome

Trial	Drug	Endpoints	n	CHD	Outcome	P
HHS	Gemfibrozil	Cardiac events/deaths	292	No	68% Reduction	<0.005
BIP	Bezafibrate	Fatal or nonfatal MI	1470	Yes	29% Reduction	0.002
SENDCAP	Bezafibrate	Carotid ultrasound	328	No	No difference*	–
DAIS	Fenofibrate	Coronary stenosis on angiography	418	48% of patients	Reduced lesion progression	0.02
VA-HIT	Gemfibrozil	Fatal/nonfatal MI	769	Yes	32% Reduction	< 0.004
FIELD	Fenofibrate	CHD death or nonfatal MI	9975	No: 7664 Yes: 2131	11% Reduction**	NS**

*60% fewer coronary events ($p=0.01$); ** nonfatal MI reduced by 24% ($p=0.01$) and total CV events reduced by 19% in the primary cohort group ($P=0.004$).
HHS: Helsinki Heart Study; BIP: Bezafibrate Infarction Prevention; SENDCAP: St Mary's Ealing Northwick Park Diabetes Cardiovascular Prevention Study; DAIS: Diabetes Atherosclerosis Intervention Study; VA-HIT: Veterans Administration – HDL Intervention Trial; FIELD: Fenofibrate Intervention and Event Lowering in Diabetes.

Mary's, Ealing, Northwick Park Diabetes Cardiovascular Disease Prevention (SENDCAP) trial, involving 328 patients with type 2 diabetes, intervention with bezafibrate resulted in no significant difference in the primary endpoint of carotid lesions detected by ultrasound, but there were 60% fewer total coronary events over a period of 3 yr ($P < 0.01$).[50] In the Diabetes Atherosclerosis Intervention Study (DAIS), an angiographic regression trial, 418 patients with type 2 diabetes and evidence of CHD on angiography were treated with fenofibrate or placebo over at least 3 yr.[51] The fenofibrate group showed significantly slower progression of disease and a trend toward fewer clinical endpoints (38 vs. 50) in this relatively small trial.

Two major fibrate trials have reported somewhat discrepant results. The Veterans Affairs High-Density Lipoprotein Cholesterol Intervention Trial (VA-HIT) studied 2,531 men with CHD who had LDL-cholesterol <140 mg/dl, HDL-cholesterol lower than 40 mg/dl, and triglyceride <300 mg/dl at baseline. Of these, 769 had evidence of diabetes or metabolic syndrome.[52] Treatment with gemfibrozil for a median duration of 5.1 yr resulted in 24% risk reduction in the combined outcome of CHD death, MI, and stroke despite no change in LDL-cholesterol; HDL-cholesterol in this trial rose by 6% and triglyceride levels decreased by 30%. The diabetes subgroup had a greater reduction in the combined endpoints (32%), compared to the nondiabetic subjects (18%) (Fig. 28.13). Subsequent analyses from the VA-HIT revealed that the outcomes in this trial were not

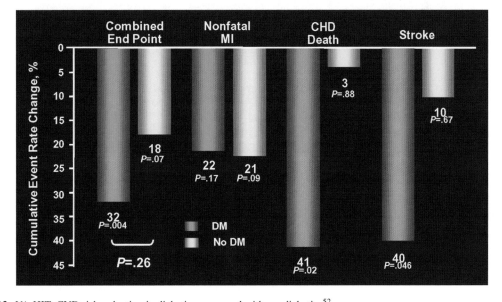

Fig. 28.13   VA-HIT: CVD risk reduction in diabetics compared with nondiabetics[52]

explained by the change in triglycerides and were only partially explained by the rise in HDL-cholesterol.[53] The 5-yr event rates were highly correlated with insulin resistance with or without diabetes, and the event reduction was significantly greater in those with insulin resistance and was independent of the HDL-cholesterol or triglyceride levels before or after treatment.[54] These analyses suggest the possibility that other anti-atherogenic effects of fibrates, mediated by a variety of reported mechanisms (such as changes in LDL composition, peroxisome proliferator-activated receptor α (PPAR-α) agonism, anti-inflammatory effects on vessel walls, and fibrinolysis), may contribute to the event reductions seen in the VA-HIT. Interestingly, evidence from BIP study suggests an insulin sensitizing effect of fibrates.[55]

The largest trial of fibrates, to date, is the FIELD trial with fenofibrate vs. placebo which was conducted in 9,795 patients with type 2 diabetes, of which the majority (7,664) were the primary prevention group. Overall, there was a nonsignificant 11% reduction in primary endpoint of CHD death or nonfatal MI ($P = 0.16$) but a significant 24% reduction in nonfatal MI ($P=0.010$) and a significant 11% reduction in total cardiovascular events ($P = 0.035$).

Of note, 17% of placebo- and 8% of fenofibrate-treated patients were started statins during the trial, thus confounding the statistical analysis (Fig. 28.14).[56] Furthermore, only 38% of the patients had dyslipidemia at baseline, and this subgroup tended to have lower rate of CVD events. Also, the primary prevention majority had a significant 19% reduction in total CVD events ($P = 0.004$). Patients with metabolic syndrome had a higher risk of events but similar event reduction. Of the adverse effects, there was a slight increase in creatinine that resolved after discontinuation after end of the trial. Similarly, homocysteine concentration was higher in the fenofibrate-treated patients by 3.7 mmol/l, but it declined to the same level as in the placebo group after the discontinuation of the drug. Interestingly, there was significantly less progression of retinopathy requiring laser treatment and less progression of albuminuria ($P < 0.003$) despite no differences in mean fasting glucose, HbA1c, or blood pressure.

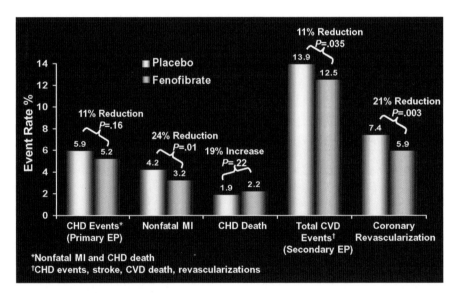

Fig. 28.14 FIELD: primary and secondary endpoints.
*Nonfatal MI and CHD death;
†CHD events, stroke, CVD death, revascularizations[56]

Lipid Management Goals in Diabetes

Diabetes is a CHD risk equivalent, as defined by the ATP III panel of the NCEP recommendations.[1] Based on the evidence from the LDL-lowering clinical trials, most patients with diabetes should have an LDL goal of <100 mg/dl. Following the more recent evidence from the newer statin trials, including the more intensive statin trials summarized above, the ATP III panel updated their current guidelines.[32] It is now recommended that LDL-lowering drug therapy be considered simultaneously with lifestyle changes in high-risk patients if LDL exceeds 100 mg/dl. For patients in very high-risk category such as patients with diabetes and CVD, a therapeutic option is to lower LDL-cholesterol goal to <70 mg/dl, regardless of the baseline LDL-cholesterol. The American Diabetes Association (ADA) has endorsed same recommendations for LDL goal, with an emphasis that statin therapy be used achieve that goal.[57] Moreover, according to the revised ADA guidelines in 2009 (Table 28.3), the intensity of therapy should be sufficient to achieve at least ~30–40% reduction in LDL-cholesterol levels. The evidence for the benefits of lower LDL goals, even for primary prevention in high-risk individuals, continues to mount.[58–60] Individuals with lifelong low LDL, such as those with a loss of function mutation in *PCSK9* gene studied in a 15-yr prospective study, had up to 88% lower risk of CHD events.[58] In a recent trial of intensive lipid therapy in 499 American Indian cohort with type 2 diabetes, the mean LDL of 72 mg/dl, compared to 104 mg/dl, along with optimal blood pressure control, led to a less progression and a greater regression of the carotid IMT.[60] Such observations support the "lower the better" concept engendered from the long-term statin trials.

Table 28.3 ADA Lipid Goals and Recommendations 2009[57]

- Lifestyle modifications
- Primary LDL-C goal <100 mg/dl (A); If CVD:LDL-C <70 mg/dl is an option (E)
- Statin therapy added to lifestyle changes, regardless of baseline LDL, if
  – Overt CVD (A);
  – Without CVD but age >40 yr + one or more other CVD risk factors (A)
- Without overt CVD and age <40 yr
  – Consider statin if LDL-C >100 mg/dl or multiple risk factors, despite lifestyle therapy (E)
- In drug treated patients, a reduction in LDL-C of ~30–40% from baseline, if LDL targets not achieved with maximum tolerated statin therapy (A).
- Triglycerides <150 mg/dl; HDL-C >40 mg/dl (men), >50 mg/dl (women): Desirable (C)
  – Combination therapy to achieve lipid goals may be needed but outcome studies pending (E)

According to ATPIII, when triglyceride levels are elevated (200–499 mg/dl) after achieving LDL goal, non-HDL-cholesterol should be the secondary target of therapy.[1,32] This can be achieved by intensification of LDL – lowering therapy, or by the addition of fibrates or niacin therapy. There is no HDL goal specified in ATPIII, due to the lack of sufficient evidence to specify a goal. It is recommended that if HDL remains low after LDL and non-HDL goals are achieved, or if triglyceride is <200 but HDL is low (isolated low HDL-cholesterol), drugs for the raising HDL can be considered. The ADA recommendations state a desirable triglyceride goal of <150 mg/dl and a HDL-cholesterol goal of >40 mg/dl in men, and >50 mg/dl in women.[57] Of these, achievement of desirable HDL-C with glycemic control along with lifestyle changes remains a major challenge.[22,45]

The ideal lipid marker to identify the CVD risk continues to be controversial. As discussed above, several epidemiolologic studies and clinical trials suggest that LDL-C measurements underestimate the apoB particle number, particularly in patients with hypertriglyceridemia. The Framingham Heart Study and others have recommended Total-C/HDL-C as better determinant of risk,[61] while others have recommended direct non- HDL-C, apoB, LDL-C/HDL-C, TG/HDL-C, or apoB/apoA1.[20–22,42] However, none of these are currently recommended for routine clinical use, although the recent joint consensus statement by the ADA and ACC concludes that apoB might provide a more accurate assessment of risk, after initial treatment to lower LDL-C to goal.[22]

In patients with triglycerides >500 mg/dl or diabetic lipemia (triglyceride above 1000 mg/dl), often associated with underlying genetic disorders, the initial aim is to achieve triglyceride lowering to prevent acute pancreatitis. This requires a combination of very low-fat diet, glycemic control, weight reduction, increased physical activity, and a triglyceride-lowering drug.[62,63] Once triglyceride levels have been lowered to <500 mg/dl, the LDL-C and other lipid targets should be assessed.

Principles of Lipid Management in Diabetes

Treatment of lipid disorders associated with diabetes includes therapeutic lifestyle changes, optimal glycemic control, and pharmacologic agents. The priorities for achieving lipid goals are LDL-cholesterol lowering, non-HDL-cholesterol lowering, followed by triglyceride lowering, and HDL raising, as per recommendations by the ATP III and all diabetes/endocrine organizations. LDL-lowering trials with statins make a persuasive argument for the efficacy and safety of the statin therapy, currently underutilized in this high-risk population. In highly motivated individuals, LDL-cholesterol reductions of ~30%, by dietary approaches, comparable to statins, have been demonstrated.[64] However, in most patients, LDL-cholesterol reductions of >10–15% are not easily achievable by non-pharmacologic approaches. The ATP III therefore recommends simultaneous initiation of statin therapy if LDL-cholesterol is >100 mg/dl.[1,32] The currently available statins provide LDL-cholesterol reductions of up to 50–60%, with rosuvastatin being the most potent[1,32,65] (Table 28.4). However, the simultaneous adherence to dietary measures, including soluble fiber, plant sterols, ruling out secondary causes of dyslipidemia,[62,63,66] and weight management are essential for maintaining lipid goals with lower dosage of drugs. The effectiveness of statins and other lipid-lowering agents in achieving lipid goals in patients with diabetes is comparable to that in the nondiabetic patients.[1,32,57]

Table 28.4 The range of the lipid effects of commonly used drugs

Drug	LDL-cholesterol (%)	HDL-cholesterol (%)	Triglycerides (%)
Statins	–18 to –55	+5 to +15	–7 to –30
Fibrates	+5 to –20	+10 to +20	–20 to –50
Niacin	–5 to –25	+15 to +35	–20 to –50
Bile Acid Sequestrants	–15 to –30	+3 to +5	No change or increa
Ezetimibe	– 15 to –20	+1 to +2	–5 to –10

Approximately 5–15% of patients have significant statin intolerance, generally due to myalgia at higher doses, or other adverse effects,[67,68] but myositis and rhabdomyolysis are extremely rare in the absence of renal disease or other risk factors. Myalgia may be minimized by the use of statins that are not metabolized by CYP 3A4 pathway, such as pravastatin, fluvastatin, and rosuvastatin.[67] According to the data in a recent mechanistic study, some patients may be susceptible to myalgia or myopathy due to overexpression of a mitochondrial gene, Atrogin-1.[69] Other genetic polymorphic loci associated with increased susceptibility to statin- induced myopathy have also been reported.[70] In patients with intolerance to statins or inability to escalate to the optimal dose, other options include bile acid sequestrants, niacin, or a cholesterol absorption inhibitor, ezetimibe.[1,35–37,62] The bile acid sequestrant, cholestyramine, was associated with reduced CHD events in a primary prevention trial in the pre-statin era.[71] The newer sequestrant, Colesevelam, is associated with fewer gastrointestinal side effects and was recently approved by the FDA in patients with type 2 diabetes for its additional, modest glucose-lowering effect as an adjunct to other glucose-lowering drugs.[72] However, sequestrants tend to raise triglycerides and are contraindicated in patients with triglyceride >500 mg/dl. Both sequestrants and ezetimibe enhance LDL-lowering effect in combination with statins, by upregulating the hepatic LDL-receptor activity.[35,73,74]

In patients with LDL-cholesterol of <100 mg/dl at baseline or on treatment, but in the presence of other CVD risk factors, therapeutic options include intensifying the LDL-lowering therapy, adding a drug (fibrate or nicotinic acid) to modify other atherogenic components, and intensifying control of other risk factors, including hypertension and hyperglycemia. Fibrates or niacin would also be indicated in patients with hypertriglyceridemia and/or low HDL-cholesterol, in a patient already at, or close to, LDL goal. In addition to the epidemiologic evidence,[38] recent prospective studies such as the Copenhagen City Heart Study,[75] and the Women's Health Study,[76] reported significant association of non-fasting triglycerides with CHD events, as well as a stronger risk relationship, relative to the fasting triglycerides in the latter. These observations support the atherogenic role of the cholesterol associated with remnant particles, and at the least, the need for a greater reliance on the risk assessment with non-HDL-cholesterol.

Nicotinic acid (niacin) is associated with up to a 20–40% increase in HDL-cholesterol in a dose-dependent manner and is currently considered a drug of choice in patients with low HDL,[1,37,44,45] particularly in combination therapy with other agents. It has a variety of anti-atherogenic effects on all lipoproteins, although its predominant mechanism of action is still not entirely clear in man.[77] It is the only agent moderately effective in lowering Lipoprotein (a) level, a genetic determinant of additional CVD risk.[78,79] The principal concern has been its suboptimal tolerability due to flushing and other side effects, and limited adherence to higher dosage. The niacin-associated flush was reported to be reduced in frequency and severity by gradual titration of dosing, and with the use of an extended-release formulation, Niaspan. Recent multicenter trials have shown no significant effects on glycemic control with up to 3 g of crystalline niacin,[80] or 1–1.5 g of Niaspan.[81] Niacin was shown to reduce the risk of nonfatal MI and stroke by 27% in the Coronary Drug Project (CDP), a secondary prevention trial in the pre-statin era in which 40% of the patients had evidence of abnormal glucose tolerance.[82] In several other studies, niacin was shown to reduce progression of coronary atherosclerotic lesion, in combination with bile acid sequestrants.[32,45,62] Even though a modest increase in blood glucose has been associated with the use of high-dose niacin,[37] similar benefits of niacin on CVD events were seen in the CDP trial, regardless of baseline glycemic status, including those with impaired fasting glucose or diabetes.[83] The non-flush OTC formulations of niacin are ineffective and their use should be discouraged. A combination pill of niacin and DP-1 receptor antagonist, laropiprant (MK-0524) to prevent flushing is currently in clinical trials.

Combination Therapy in Lipid Management

According to the ATP III update[32] and the ADA guidelines,[57] combination therapy with an LDL-lowering drug, preferably a statin, plus fibrates or niacin may be considered in high-risk patients with elevated triglycerides or low HDL-C. However, despite the known pharmacologic effects of fibrates and niacin in ameliorating the underlying defects of diabetic dyslipidemia (increased triglyceride-rich lipoproteins, low HDL-cholesterol, small, dense LDL particles), the clinical trial evidence of the potential benefits of combining these agents with statins in preventing cardiovascular events remains inconclusive, pending the results of ongoing studies.

Trials such as VA-HIT, FIELD, BIP, and DAIS provide some support for the potential benefits of adding fibrates to statins. In short-term studies, statins in combination with fibrates[84,85] or a statin along with niacin[81] have been shown to be more effective in normalizing all lipid abnormalities, including lipid particle distribution, than either agent alone, without significant risk for adverse events, including myositis (Figs. 28.15 and 28.16). However, caution should be exercised in patients with potential drug interactions (e.g., cyclosporine, antifungal agents, protease inhibitors, erythromycin) and in those with renal disease (Table 28.5).[66–68]

A few relatively short-term, small studies with the combination of statin and niacin are noteworthy. In a study of 160 patients with CHD and low HDL-cholesterol, the HDL Atherosclerosis Treatment Study (HATS), combining niacin with simvastatin over 3 years, resulted in an impressive reduction in angiographic progression of lesions and clinical endpoints.[86] A subgroup (16%) of these patients had diabetes. Similarly, in a recent 12-month study, with another 12 months of open-label follow-up, niacin–simvastatin combination therapy, in 167 patients with stable coronary artery disease, resulted in significantly reduced progression of carotid intima-medial thickness, compared to simvastatin alone.[87] However, these studies did not have the power to detect differences in clinical outcomes. Lovastatin in combination with extended-release niacin, in fixed-combination doses of up to 40 mg lovastatin plus 2000 mg extended-release niacin, respectively, was reported to lower LDL-cholesterol and triglyceride by 47 and 41%, respectively, and to increase HDL-cholesterol by 30%.[88] Similar results were reported with the lovastatin–niaspan combination in a 20-week study of patients with type 2 diabetes.[89] Based on similar efficacy and safety results,[90] a combination pill of simvastatin and Niaspan was approved by the FDA. The combination of statins with niacin has also been shown to lead to a significant reduction in small, dense LDL particles, as well as a reduction in LP(a) levels, compared to statins alone or stain in combination with ezetimibe.[91]

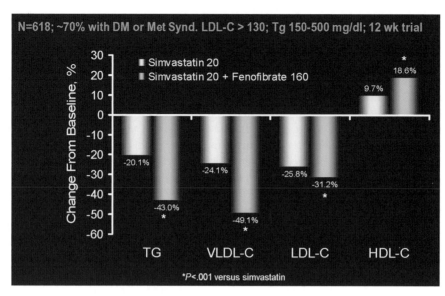

Fig. 28.15 SAFARI: combination therapy in combined hyperlipidemia versus simvastatin. *P<0.001 [84]

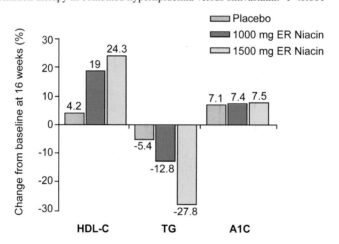

ER niacin= extended-release niacin

Fig. 28.16 ER niacin vs placebo in people with type 2 diabetes: the advent study[81]

Despite the evidence from various studies discussed above, a direct evidence from longer-term clinical trials about the CVD benefits of combination therapy with fibrates and niacin is clearly needed in order to make firm recommendations. In this regard, two major trials are currently ongoing. The ACCORD trial is comparing long-term benefits of simvastatin and fenofibrate, vs. simvastatin in ~6000 patients, of whom 35% had CVD at baseline. AIM-HIGH is comparing simvastatin and niacin, compared to statin alone, in 3300 patients with known cardiovascular disease, and dyslipidemia associated with metabolic syndrome with or without diabetes.

In patients with diabetic lipemia or severe hypertriglyceridemia, a triglyceride-lowering drug is frequently indicated, in addition to several concurrent measures including glycemic control, a very low fat diet, alcohol restriction, physical activity, and weight management. Many such patients are unable to lower triglyceride levels to a safe range (<500 mg/dl) with fibrates alone and require addition of niacin or fish oils, or both. Fish oils are usually required in relatively large doses to provide 3–6 g or more of omega-3 fatty acids – EPA and DHA.[92,93] The mechanism of action is probably multifactorial, including reduced VLDL synthesis via inhibition of DGAT, increased hepatic triglyceride oxidation, and perhaps increased activation of lipoprotein lipase.[92,93]

Table 28.5   Myopathy with statins and fibrates

- Creatine kinase (CK)
  - o Elevation >10× ULN observed in 0.1% of patients at starting doses of statins
  - o Measure at baseline and monitor symptoms
- Rhabdomyolysis (incidence = 1 in 10,000 person-yr). Renal failure may occur if drug continued
- Risk increases with
  Dose escalation, renal disease, hypothyroidism, or in combination with gemfibrozil, cyclosporine, azole antifungals, macrolide antibiotics, nefazodone, verapamil, amiodarone, HIV-protease inhibitors, etc.
- Reversed after discontinuation

Adapted from Graham[67] and Antons[66].

A high potency, ~900 mg, purified omega-3 ethyl ester preparation (Lovaza, formerly known as Omacor) is currently approved for use in patients with triglycerides >500 mg/dl.[93]

An alternative approach to restoring lipid pathophysiology in patients with insulin resistance and type 2 diabetes is the addition of an insulin sensitizer, e.g., a thiazolidinedione (TZD) agent. Both of the available TZDs, rosiglitazone and pioglitazone, raise HDL-cholesterol by up to 10–15% depending upon the baseline HDL levels.[94,95] Pioglitazone has been shown to have more favorable lipid effects including the triglyceride levels and LDL compositional abnormalities associated with insulin resistance.[95] However, the relative value of these agents in overall cardiovascular outcomes is unclear in the absence of additional data.

Novel Lipid Intervention Approaches

With the increased understanding of the genetic and molecular etiology underlying lipid disorders associated with atherosclerosis in humans, a large number of drug targets are being actively pursued.[96] Of these, the novel approaches to augment HDL effects on anti-atherogenesis are under intensive investigation (Table 28.6). CETP inhibitors have been thought to be worth pursuing for a number of years. The CETP inhibition with recently available agents has been shown to increase HDL-cholesterol by 50–100% in dose-ranging studies.[45,97] However, whether the compositional changes in HDL particle brought about by this mechanism (Fig. 28.12) would be pro- or anti-atherogenic remains controversial.[43,97,98] In the genetic studies, the risk of CHD with CETP mutations has been reported to be inconsistent.[98–100] In a population-based prospective study, a common CETP polymorphism was associated with higher HDL-cholesterol but paradoxically with an increased incidence of CHD.[101] A large clinical trial (ILLUMINATE) with torcetrapib, a CETP inhibitor in combination with atorvastatin, was halted due to unexpected increase in adverse CVD outcomes in patients with CHD despite a 72% increase in HDL-C and a 22% decrease in LDL-C compared to atorvastatin alone.[102] A drug- specific, rather than CETP inhibition- specific effect to explain the adverse effects could not be ruled out since torcetrapib resulted in a modest but significant increase in blood pressure and mineralocorticoid activity.[102] To resolve this question, the results from ongoing studies with other CETP antagonists would be of interest.[43,45,103]

An approach to HDL raising with more potent and selective PPAR-α agents or dual PPAR-α–γ agents have been hampered by toxicity issues,[104] while studies with PPAR-δ agents are in preliminary stages. In early studies with a novel PPAR-α–γ agonist, Aleglitazar, a significantly greater efficacy on triglycerides and HDL, alongwith

Table 28.6   Potential HDL therapies

- Cholesterol ester transfer protein (CETP) inhibitors
- Synthetic HDLs
- apoA-1 mimetic peptides
- PPAR-α drugs
- MK-0524A – ER Niacin + DP-1 receptor antagonist

---

a significant decrease in LDL-C was demonstrated, in contrast to currently available PPARγ agents.[104a] The longer-term safety data will be of interest. Finally, the development of apoA-1 based strategies, such as Apo a-1 Milano, based on encouraging short-term trials[105,106] represents an exciting physiologic approach but longer-term studies are awaited.

Summary

Diabetes is associated with an increased incidence of cardiovascular disease. The atherogenic dyslipidemia of type 2 diabetes and insulin-resistance syndrome is characterized by an increase in triglyceride-rich lipoproteins, a decrease in HDL-cholesterol, and compositionally abnormal lipoproteins, including smaller, denser LDL particles. The increase in pro-inflammatory and pro-thrombotic milieu, along with visceral obesity and endothelial dysfunction inherent in cardio-metabolic syndrome, likely contribute to the enhanced atherogenecity in the presence of dyslipidemia. A number of clinical trials with statins have established the benefits of LDL lowering in individuals with increased baseline cardiovascular risk associated with diabetes. This has been best shown in secondary prevention trials thus far. Several epidemiologic studies as well as angiographic regression trials and clinical trials have also documented the benefits of strategies to raise HDL and to lower triglyceride-rich particles. The impact of HDL particle, as a disease modifier, is currently the subject of particularly intense scrutiny. A number of potential newer avenues to increase HDL synthesis and/or inhibit its catabolism are being pursued. Furthermore, it is currently recommended that after achieving LDL-C goal, further attention to other indices of increased risk, such as, non-HDL-cholesterol and apolipoprotein B might provide better assessment of residual risk for events. The potential benefits of combination therapy regimens such as statins plus niacin, or statin plus a fibrate, in producing additional benefits in CVD event reduction, beyond those achieved by statins, are the subject of ongoing clinical trials.

References

1. Executive Summary of the Third Report of the National Cholesterol Education Program (NCEP) Expert panel on detection, evaluation, and treatment of high blood cholesterol in adults (Adult Treatment Panel III). *J Am Med Assoc.* 2001;285(19):2486–2497.
2. Haffner SM, Lehto S, Ronnemaa T, Pyorala K, Laakso M. Mortality from coronary heart disease in subjects with type 2 diabetes and in nondiabetic subjects with and without prior myocardial infarction. *N Engl J Med.* 1998;339(4):229–234.
3. Malmberg K, Yusuf S, Gerstein HC, Brown J, Zhao F, Hunt D, et al. Impact of diabetes on long-term prognosis in patients with unstable angina and non-Q-wave myocardial infarction: results of the OASIS (Organization to Assess Strategies for Ischemic Syndromes) registry. *Circulation.* 2000;102(9):1014–1019.
4. Huxley R, Barzi F, Woodward M. Excess risk of fatal coronary heart disease associated with diabetes in men and women: meta-analysis of 37 prospective cohort studies. *BMJ.* 2006;332(7533):73–78.
5. Booth GL, Kapral MK, Fung K, Tu JV. Relation between age and cardiovascular disease in men and women with diabetes compared with non-diabetic people: a population-based retrospective cohort study. *Lancet.* 2006;368(9529):29–36.
6. Franco OH, Steyerberg EW, Hu FB, Mackenbach J, Nusselder W. Associations of diabetes mellitus with total life expectancy and life expectancy with and without cardiovascular disease. *Arch Intern Med.* 2007;167(11):1145–1151.
7. Donahoe SM, Stewart GC, McCabe CH, Mohanavelu S, Murphy SA, Cannon CP, et al. Diabetes and mortality following acute coronary syndromes. *J Am Med Assoc.* 2007;298(7):765–775.
8. Hu FB, Stampfer MJ, Haffner SM, Solomon CG, Willett WC, Manson JE. Elevated risk of cardiovascular disease prior to clinical diagnosis of type 2 diabetes. *Diabetes Care.* 2002;25(7):1129–1134.
9. Stamler J, Vaccaro O, Neaton JD, Wentworth D. Diabetes, other risk factors, and 12-yr cardiovascular mortality for men screened in the multiple risk factor intervention trial. *Diabetes Care.* 1993;16(2):434–444.
10. Gregg EW, Gu Q, Cheng YJ, Narayan KM, Cowie CC. Mortality trends in men and women with diabetes, 1971 to 2000. *Ann Intern Med.* 2007;147(3):149–155.
11. Ford ES, Ajani UA, Croft JB, Critchley JA, Labarthe DR, Kottke TE, et al. Explaining the decrease in U.S. deaths from coronary disease, 1980–2000. *N Engl J Med.* 2007;356(23):2388–2398.
12. Howard BV, Cowan LD, Go O, Welty TK, Robbins DC, Lee ET. Adverse effects of diabetes on multiple cardiovascular disease risk factors in women. The Strong Heart Study. *Diabetes Care.* 1998;21(8):1258–1265.
13. Wexler DJ, Grant RW, Meigs JB, Nathan DM, Cagliero E. Sex disparities in treatment of cardiac risk factors in patients with type 2 diabetes. *Diabetes Care.* 2005;28(3):514–520.

14. Ferrara A, Mangione CM, Kim C, Marrero DG, Curb D, Stevens M, et al. Sex disparities in control and treatment of modifiable cardiovascular disease risk factors among patients with diabetes: Translating Research Into Action for Diabetes (TRIAD) Study. *Diabetes Care*. 2008;31(1):69–74.

15. Gouni-Berthold I, Berthold HK, Mantzoros CS, Bohm M, Krone W. Sex disparities in the treatment and control of cardiovascular risk factors in type 2 diabetes. *Diabetes Care*. 2008;31(7):1389–1391.

16. Krauss RM. Lipids and lipoproteins in patients with type 2 diabetes. *Diabetes Care*. 2004;27(6):1496–1504.

17. Taskinen MR. Diabetic dyslipidaemia: from basic research to clinical practice. *Diabetologia*. 2003;46(6):733–749.

18. Albers JJ, Marcovina SM, Imperatore G, Snively BM, Stafford J, Fujimoto WY, et al. Prevalence and determinants of elevated apolipoprotein B and dense low-density lipoprotein in youths with type 1 and type 2 diabetes. *J Clin Endocrinol Metab*. 2008;93(3):735–742.

19. Garvey WT, Kwon S, Zheng D, Shaughnessy S, Wallace P, Hutto A, et al. Effects of insulin resistance and type 2 diabetes on lipoprotein subclass particle size and concentration determined by nuclear magnetic resonance. *Diabetes*. 2003;52(2):453–462.

20. Sniderman AD. Non-HDL cholesterol versus apolipoprotein B in diabetic dyslipoproteinemia: alternatives and surrogates versus the real thing. *Diabetes Care*. 2003;26(7):2207–2208.

21. Barter PJ, Ballantyne CM, Carmena R, Castro CM, Chapman MJ, Couture P, et al. Apo B versus cholesterol in estimating cardiovascular risk and in guiding therapy: report of the thirty-person/ten-country panel. *J Intern Med*. 2006;259(3):247–258.

21a. Ganda OP. Refining lipoprotein assessment in diabetes: Apolipoprotein B makes sense. *Endocrine Practice* 2009;15:370–376.

22. Brunzell JD, Davidson M, Furberg CD, Goldberg RB, Howard BV, Stein JH, et al. Lipoprotein management in patients with cardiometabolic risk: consensus statement from the American Diabetes Association and the American College of Cardiology Foundation. *Diabetes Care*. 2008;31(4):811–822.

23. Lu W, Resnick HE, Jablonski KA, Jones KL, Jain AK, Howard WJ, et al. Non-HDL cholesterol as a predictor of cardiovascular disease in type 2 diabetes: the strong heart study. *Diabetes Care*. 2003;26(1):16–23.

24. Liu J, Sempos CT, Donahue RP, Dorn J, Trevisan M, Grundy SM. Non-high-density lipoprotein and very-low-density lipoprotein cholesterol and their risk predictive values in coronary heart disease. *Am J Cardiol*. 2006;98(10):1363–1368.

25. Baigent C, Keech A, Kearney PM, Blackwell L, Buck G, Pollicino C, et al. Efficacy and safety of cholesterol-lowering treatment: prospective meta-analysis of data from 90,056 participants in 14 randomised trials of statins. *Lancet*. 2005;366(9493):1267–1278.

26. Kearney PM, Blackwell L, Collins R, Keech A, Simes J, Peto R, et al. Efficacy of cholesterol-lowering therapy in 18,686 people with diabetes in 14 randomised trials of statins: a meta-analysis. *Lancet*. 2008;371(9607):117–125.

27. Costa J, Borges M, David C, Vaz CA. Efficacy of lipid lowering drug treatment for diabetic and non-diabetic patients: meta-analysis of randomised controlled trials. *BMJ*. 2006;332(7550):1115–1124.

28. Collins R, Armitage J, Parish S, Sleigh P, Peto R. MRC/BHF Heart Protection Study of cholesterol-lowering with simvastatin in 5963 people with diabetes: a randomised placebo-controlled trial. *Lancet*. 2003;361(9374):2005–2016.

29. Ballantyne CM, Olsson AG, Cook TJ, Mercuri MF, Pedersen TR, Kjekshus J. Influence of low high-density lipoprotein cholesterol and elevated triglyceride on coronary heart disease events and response to simvastatin therapy in 4S. *Circulation*. 2001;104(25):3046–3051.

30. Deedwania P, Barter P, Carmena R, Fruchart JC, Grundy SM, Haffner S, et al. Reduction of low-density lipoprotein cholesterol in patients with coronary heart disease and metabolic syndrome: analysis of the Treating to New Targets Study. *Lancet*. 2006;368(9539):919–928.

31. Devaraj S, Chan E, Jialal I. Direct demonstration of an antiinflammatory effect of simvastatin in subjects with the metabolic syndrome. *J Clin Endocrinol Metab*. 2006;91(11):4489–4496.

31a. Ridker PM, Danielson E, Fonseca FA, Genest J, Gotto AM, Jr., Kastelein JJ et al. Rosuvastatin to prevent vascular events in men and women with elevated C-reactive protein. *N Engl J Med* 2008;359(21):2195–2207.

32. Grundy SM, Cleeman JI, Merz CN, Brewer HB Jr., Clark LT, Hunninghake DB, et al. Implications of recent clinical trials for the National Cholesterol Education Program Adult Treatment Panel III guidelines. *Circulation*. 2004;110(2):227–239.

33. Smith SC Jr., Allen J, Blair SN, Bonow RO, Brass LM, Fonarow GC, et al. AHA/ACC guidelines for secondary prevention for patients with coronary and other atherosclerotic vascular disease: 2006 update: endorsed by the National Heart, Lung, and Blood Institute. *Circulation*. 2006;113(19):2363–2372.

34. Cannon CP, Steinberg BA, Murphy SA, Mega JL, Braunwald E. Meta-analysis of cardiovascular outcomes trials comparing intensive versus moderate statin therapy. *J Am Coll Cardiol*. 2006;48(3):438–445.

35. Goldberg AC, Sapre A, Liu J, Capece R, Mitchel YB. Efficacy and safety of ezetimibe coadministered with simvastatin in patients with primary hypercholesterolemia: a randomized, double-blind, placebo-controlled trial. *Mayo Clin Proc*. 2004;79(5):620–629.

36. Hunninghake D, Insull W Jr., Toth P, Davidson D, Donovan JM, Burke SK. Coadministration of colesevelam hydrochloride with atorvastatin lowers LDL cholesterol additively. *Atherosclerosis*. 2001;158(2):407–416.

37. Goldberg RB, Jacobson TA. Effects of niacin on glucose control in patients with dyslipidemia. *Mayo Clin Proc*. 2008;83(4):470–478.

37a. Fleg JL, Mete M, Howard BV, Umans JG, Roman MJ, Ratner RE, et al. Effect of statins alone versus statins plus ezetimibe on carotid atherosclerosis in type 2 diabetes: the SANDS (Stop Atherosclerosis in Native Diabetics Study) trial. *J Am Coll Cardiol* 2008;52(25):2198–2205.

38. Kastelein JJ, Akdim F, Stroes ES, Zwinderman AH, Bots ML, Stalenhoef AF, et al. Simvastatin with or without ezetimibe in familial hypercholesterolemia. *N Engl J Med.* 2008;358(14):1431–1443.

39. Sarwar N, Danesh J, Eiriksdottir G, Sigurdsson G, Wareham N, Bingham S, et al. Triglycerides and the risk of coronary heart disease: 10,158 incident cases among 262,525 participants in 29 Western prospective studies. *Circulation.* 2007;115(4):450–458.

40. Miller M, Cannon CP, Murphy SA, Qin J, Ray KK, Braunwald E. Impact of triglyceride levels beyond low-density lipoprotein cholesterol after acute coronary syndrome in the PROVE IT-TIMI 22 trial. *J Am Coll Cardiol.* 2008;51(7):724–730.

41. Barter P, Gotto AM, LaRosa JC, Maroni J, Szarek M, Grundy SM, et al. HDL cholesterol, very low levels of LDL cholesterol, and cardiovascular events. *N Engl J Med.* 2007;357(13):1301–1310.

42. McQueen MJ, Hawken S, Wang X, Ounpuu S, Sniderman A, Probstfield J, et al. Lipids, lipoproteins, and apolipoproteins as risk markers of myocardial infarction in 52 countries (the INTERHEART study): a case-control study. *Lancet.* 2008;372(9634):224–233.

43. Mahley RW, Huang Y, Weisgraber KH. Putting cholesterol in its place: apoE and reverse cholesterol transport. *J Clin Invest.* 2006;116(5):1226–1229.

44. Barter P. Metabolic abnormalities: high-density lipoproteins. *Endocrinol Metab Clin North Am.* 2004;33(2):393–403.

45. Singh IM, Shishehbor MH, Ansell BJ. High-density lipoprotein as a therapeutic target: a systematic review. *J Am Med Assoc.* 2007;298(7):786–798.

46. Bhattacharyya T, Nicholls SJ, Topol EJ, Zhang R, Yang X, Schmitt D, et al. Relationship of paraoxonase 1 (PON1) gene polymorphisms and functional activity with systemic oxidative stress and cardiovascular risk. *J Am Med Assoc.* 2008;299(11):1265–1276.

47. Mastorikou M, Mackness M, Mackness B. Defective metabolism of oxidized phospholipid by HDL from people with type 2 diabetes. *Diabetes.* 2006;55(11):3099–3103.

48. Koskinen P, Manttari M, Manninen V, Huttunen JK, Heinonen OP, Frick MH. Coronary heart disease incidence in NIDDM patients in the Helsinki Heart Study. *Diabetes Care.* 1992;15(7):820–825.

49. Secondary prevention by raising HDL cholesterol and reducing triglycerides in patients with coronary artery disease: the Bezafibrate Infarction Prevention (BIP) study. *Circulation.* 2000;102(1):21–27.

50. Elkeles RS, Diamond JR, Poulter C, Dhanjil S, Nicolaides AN, Mahmood S, et al. Cardiovascular outcomes in type 2 diabetes. A double-blind placebo-controlled study of bezafibrate: the St. Mary's, Ealing, Northwick Park Diabetes Cardiovascular Disease Prevention (SENDCAP) Study. *Diabetes Care.* 1998;21(4):641–648.

51. Effect of fenofibrate on progression of coronary-artery disease in type 2 diabetes: the Diabetes Atherosclerosis Intervention Study, a randomised study. *Lancet.* 2001;357(9260):905–910.

52. Rubins HB, Robins SJ, Collins D, Nelson DB, Elam MB, Schaefer EJ, et al. Diabetes, plasma insulin, and cardiovascular disease: subgroup analysis from the Department of Veterans Affairs high-density lipoprotein intervention trial (VA-HIT). *Arch Intern Med.* 2002;162(22):2597–2604.

53. Robins SJ, Collins D, Wittes JT, Papademetriou V, Deedwania PC, Schaefer EJ, et al. Relation of gemfibrozil treatment and lipid levels with major coronary events: VA-HIT: a randomized controlled trial. *J Am Med Assoc.* 2001;285(12):1585–1591.

54. Robins SJ, Rubins HB, Faas FH, Schaefer EJ, Elam MB, Anderson JW, et al. Insulin resistance and cardiovascular events with low HDL cholesterol: the Veterans Affairs HDL Intervention Trial (VA-HIT). *Diabetes Care.* 2003;26(5):1513–1517.

55. Tenenbaum A, Fisman EZ, Boyko V, Benderly M, Tanne D, Haim M, et al. Attenuation of progression of insulin resistance in patients with coronary artery disease by bezafibrate. *Arch Intern Med.* 2006;166(7):737–741.

56. Keech A, Simes RJ, Barter P, Best J, Scott R, Taskinen MR, et al. Effects of long-term fenofibrate therapy on cardiovascular events in 9795 people with type 2 diabetes mellitus (the FIELD study): randomised controlled trial. *Lancet.* 2005;366(9500):1849–1861.

57. Executive summary: standards of medical care in diabetes–2009. *Diabetes Care* 2009;32Suppl 1:S6–12.

58. Cohen JC, Boerwinkle E, Mosley TH Jr., Hobbs HH. Sequence variations in PCSK9, low LDL, and protection against coronary heart disease. *N Engl J Med.* 2006;354(12):1264–1272.

59. Crouse JR III, Raichlen JS, Riley WA, Evans GW, Palmer MK, O'Leary DH, et al. Effect of rosuvastatin on progression of carotid intima-media thickness in low-risk individuals with subclinical atherosclerosis: the METEOR Trial. *J Am Med Assoc.* 2007;297(12):1344–1353.

60. Howard BV, Roman MJ, Devereux RB, Fleg JL, Galloway JM, Henderson JA, et al. Effect of lower targets for blood pressure and LDL cholesterol on atherosclerosis in diabetes: the SANDS randomized trial. *J Am Med Assoc.* 2008;299(14):1678–1689.

61. Ingelsson E, Schaefer EJ, Contois JH, McNamara JR, Sullivan L, Keyes MJ, et al. Clinical utility of different lipid measures for prediction of coronary heart disease in men and women. *J Am Med Assoc.* 2007;298(7):776–785.

62. Kreisberg RA, Oberman A. Medical management of hyperlipidemia/dyslipidemia. *J Clin Endocrinol Metab.* 2003;88(6):2445–2461.

63. Brunzell JD. Clinical practice. Hypertriglyceridemia. *N Engl J Med.* 2007;357(10):1009–1017.

64. Jenkins DJ, Kendall CW, Marchie A, Faulkner DA, Wong JM, de Souza R, et al. Effects of a dietary portfolio of cholesterol-lowering foods vs lovastatin on serum lipids and C-reactive protein. *J Am Med Assoc.* 2003;290(4):502–510.

65. Jones PH, Davidson MH, Stein EA, Bays HE, McKenney JM, Miller E, et al. Comparison of the efficacy and safety of rosuvastatin versus atorvastatin, simvastatin, and pravastatin across doses (STELLAR* Trial). *Am J Cardiol.* 2003;92(2):152–160.

66. Antons KA, Williams CD, Baker SK, Phillips PS. Clinical perspectives of statin-induced rhabdomyolysis. *Am J Med.* 2006;119(5):400–409.
67. Graham DJ, Staffa JA, Shatin D, Andrade SE, Schech SD, La Grenade L, et al. Incidence of hospitalized rhabdomyolysis in patients treated with lipid-lowering drugs. *J Am Med Assoc.* 2004;292(21):2585–2590.
68. Jacobson TA. Toward "pain-free" statin prescribing: clinical algorithm for diagnosis and management of myalgia. *Mayo Clin Proc.* 2008;83(6):687–700.
69. Hanai J, Cao P, Tanksale P, Imamura S, Koshimizu E, Zhao J, et al. The muscle-specific ubiquitin ligase atrogin-1/MAFbx mediates statin-induced muscle toxicity. *J Clin Invest.* 2007;117(12):3940–3951.
70. Link E, Parish S, Armitage J, Bowman L, Heath S, Matsuda F, et al. SLCO1B1 variants and statin-induced myopathy – a genomewide study. *N Engl J Med.* 2008;359(8):789–799.
71. The Lipid Research Clinics Coronary Primary Prevention Trial results. II. The relationship of reduction in incidence of coronary heart disease to cholesterol lowering. *J Am Med Assoc.* 1984;251(3):365–374.
72. Davidson MH. The use of colesevelam hydrochloride in the treatment of dyslipidemia: a review. *Expert Opin Pharmacother.* 2007;8(15):2569–2578.
73. Insull W Jr. Clinical utility of bile acid sequestrants in the treatment of dyslipidemia: a scientific review. *South Med J.* 2006;99(3):257–273.
74. Gagne C, Bays HE, Weiss SR, Mata P, Quinto K, Melino M, et al. Efficacy and safety of ezetimibe added to ongoing statin therapy for treatment of patients with primary hypercholesterolemia. *Am J Cardiol.* 2002;90(10):1084–1091.
75. Nordestgaard BG, Benn M, Schnohr P, Tybjaerg-Hansen A. Nonfasting triglycerides and risk of myocardial infarction, ischemic heart disease, and death in men and women. *J Am Med Assoc.* 2007;298(3):299–308.
76. Bansal S, Buring JE, Rifai N, Mora S, Sacks FM, Ridker PM. Fasting compared with nonfasting triglycerides and risk of cardiovascular events in women. *J Am Med Assoc.* 2007;298(3):309–316.
77. Kamanna VS, Kashyap ML. Mechanism of action of niacin. *Am J Cardiol.* 2008;101(8A):20B–26B.
78. Bennet A, Di Angelantonio E, Erqou S, Eiriksdottir G, Sigurdsson G, Woodward M, et al. Lipoprotein(a) levels and risk of future coronary heart disease: large-scale prospective data. *Arch Intern Med.* 2008;168(6):598–608.
79. Danesh J, Collins R, Peto R. Lipoprotein(a) and coronary heart disease. Meta-analysis of prospective studies. *Circulation.* 2000;102(10):1082–1085.
80. Elam MB, Hunninghake DB, Davis KB, Garg R, Johnson C, Egan D, et al. Effect of niacin on lipid and lipoprotein levels and glycemic control in patients with diabetes and peripheral arterial disease: the ADMIT study: a randomized trial. Arterial Disease Multiple Intervention Trial. *J Am Med Assoc.* 2000;284(10):1263–1270.
81. Grundy SM, Vega GL, McGovern ME, Tulloch BR, Kendall DM, Fitz-Patrick D, et al. Efficacy, safety, and tolerability of once-daily niacin for the treatment of dyslipidemia associated with type 2 diabetes: results of the assessment of diabetes control and evaluation of the efficacy of niaspan trial. *Arch Intern Med.* 2002;162(14):1568–1576.
82. Canner PL, Furberg CD, Terrin ML, McGovern ME. Benefits of niacin by glycemic status in patients with healed myocardial infarction (from the Coronary Drug Project). *Am J Cardiol.* 2005;95(2):254–257.
83. Canner PL, Furberg CD, McGovern ME. Benefits of niacin in patients with versus without the metabolic syndrome and healed myocardial infarction (from the Coronary Drug Project). *Am J Cardiol.* 2006;97(4):477–479.
84. Grundy SM, Vega GL, Yuan Z, Battisti WP, Brady WE, Palmisano J. Effectiveness and tolerability of simvastatin plus fenofibrate for combined hyperlipidemia (the SAFARI trial). *Am J Cardiol.* 2005;95(4):462–468.
85. Athyros VG, Papageorgiou AA, Athyrou VV, Demitriadis DS, Kontopoulos AG. Atorvastatin and micronized fenofibrate alone and in combination in type 2 diabetes with combined hyperlipidemia. *Diabetes Care.* 2002;25(7):1198–1202.
86. Brown BG, Zhao XQ, Chait A, Fisher LD, Cheung MC, Morse JS, et al. Simvastatin and niacin, antioxidant vitamins, or the combination for the prevention of coronary disease. *N Engl J Med.* 2001;345(22):1583–1592.
87. Taylor AJ, Sullenberger LE, Lee HJ, Lee JK, Grace KA. Arterial Biology for the Investigation of the Treatment Effects of Reducing Cholesterol (ARBITER) 2: a double-blind, placebo-controlled study of extended-release niacin on atherosclerosis progression in secondary prevention patients treated with statins. *Circulation.* 2004;110(23):3512–3517.
88. Bays HE, Dujovne CA, McGovern ME, White TE, Kashyap ML, Hutcheson AG, et al. Comparison of once-daily, niacin extended-release/lovastatin with standard doses of atorvastatin and simvastatin (the ADvicor Versus Other Cholesterol-Modulating Agents Trial Evaluation [ADVOCATE]). *Am J Cardiol.* 2003;91(6):667–672.
89. Grundy SM, Vega GL, McGovern ME, et al. Comparative effects on lipid and glycemic control of niacin extended-release/lovastatin or fenofibrate in patients with diabetic dyslipidemia. 64th Annual Scientific Sessions, Orlando, FL June 4–8, 2004 # 29–LB
90. Ballantyne CM, Davidson MH, McKenney J, Keller LH, Bajorunas DR, Karas RH. Comparison of the safety and efficacy of a combination tablet of niacin extended release and simvastatin vs simvastatin monotherapy in patients with increased non-HDL cholesterol (from the SEACOAST I study). *Am J Cardiol.* 2008;101(10):1428–1436.
91. McKenney JM, Jones PH, Bays HE, Knopp RH, Kashyap ML, Ruoff GE, et al. Comparative effects on lipid levels of combination therapy with a statin and extended-release niacin or ezetimibe versus a statin alone (the COMPELL study). *Atherosclerosis.* 2007;192(2):432–437.
92. Harris WS, Bulchandani D. Why do omega-3 fatty acids lower serum triglycerides? *Curr Opin Lipidol.* 2006;17(4):387–393.
93. Bays HE, Tighe AP, Sadovsky R, Davidson MH. Prescription omega-3 fatty acids and their lipid effects: physiologic mechanisms of action and clinical implications. *Expert Rev Cardiovasc Ther.* 2008;6(3):391–409.

94. Yki-Jarvinen H. Thiazolidinediones. *N Engl J Med*. 2004;351(11):1106–1118.

95. Goldberg RB, Kendall DM, Deeg MA, Buse JB, Zagar AJ, Pinaire JA, et al. A comparison of lipid and glycemic effects of pioglitazone and rosiglitazone in patients with type 2 diabetes and dyslipidemia. *Diabetes Care*. 2005;28(7):1547–1554.

96. Rader DJ, Daugherty A. Translating molecular discoveries into new therapies for atherosclerosis. *Nature*. 2008;451(7181):904–913.

97. Ansell BJ, Fonarow GC, Fogelman AM. The paradox of dysfunctional high-density lipoprotein. *Curr Opin Lipidol*. 2007;18(4):427–434.

98. Fazio S, Linton MF. Sorting out the complexities of reverse cholesterol transport: CETP polymorphisms, HDL, and coronary disease. *J Clin Endocrinol Metab*. 2006;91(9):3273–3275.

99. Zhong S, Sharp DS, Grove JS, Bruce C, Yano K, Curb JD, et al. Increased coronary heart disease in Japanese-American men with mutation in the cholesteryl ester transfer protein gene despite increased HDL levels. *J Clin Invest*. 1996;97(12):2917–2923.

100. Thompson A, Di Angelantonio E, Sarwar N, Erqou S, Saleheen D, Dullaart RP, et al. Association of cholesteryl ester transfer protein genotypes with CETP mass and activity, lipid levels, and coronary risk. *J Am Med Assoc*. 2008;299(23):2777–2788.

101. Borggreve SE, Hillege HL, Wolffenbuttel BH, de Jong PE, Zuurman MW, van der SG, et al. An increased coronary risk is paradoxically associated with common cholesteryl ester transfer protein gene variations that relate to higher high-density lipoprotein cholesterol: a population-based study. *J Clin Endocrinol Metab*. 2006;91(9):3382–3388.

102. Barter PJ, Caulfield M, Eriksson M, Grundy SM, Kastelein JJ, Komajda M, et al. Effects of torcetrapib in patients at high risk for coronary events. *N Engl J Med*. 2007;357(21):2109–2122.

103. Krishna R, Anderson MS, Bergman AJ, Jin B, Fallon M, Cote J, et al. Effect of the cholesteryl ester transfer protein inhibitor, anacetrapib, on lipoproteins in patients with dyslipidaemia and on 24-h ambulatory blood pressure in healthy individuals: two double-blind, randomised placebo-controlled phase I studies. *Lancet*. 2007;370(9603):1907–1914.

104. Nissen SE, Nicholls SJ, Wolski K, Howey DC, McErlean E, Wang MD, et al. Effects of a potent and selective PPAR-alpha agonist in patients with atherogenic dyslipidemia or hypercholesterolemia: two randomized controlled trials. *J Am Med Assoc*. 2007;297(12):1362–1373.

104a. Henry RR, Lincoff AM, Mudaliar S, Rabbia M, Chognot C, Herz M. Effect of the dual peroxisome proliferator-activated receptor-alpha/gamma agonist aleglitazar on risk of cardiovascular disease in patients with type 2 diabetes (SYNCHRONY): a phase II, randomised, dose-ranging study. *Lancet* 2009;374(9684):126–135.

105. Tardif JC, Gregoire J, L'Allier PL, Ibrahim R, Lesperance J, Heinonen TM, et al. Effects of reconstituted high-density lipoprotein infusions on coronary atherosclerosis: a randomized controlled trial. *J Am Med Assoc*. 2007;297(15):1675–1682.

106. Bloedon LT, Dunbar R, Duffy D, Pinell-Salles P, Norris R, DeGroot BJ, et al. Safety, pharmacokinetics, and pharmacodynamics of oral apoA-I mimetic peptide D-4F in high-risk cardiovascular patients. *J Lipid Res*. 2008;49(6):1344–1352.

Chapter 29
Dermatological Complications of Diabetes Mellitus; Allergy to Insulin and Oral Agents

George I. Varghese, Ellen S. Marmur, and Mathew C. Varghese

Introduction

Long-standing diabetes and/or lack of tight glucose control over time may result in the development of complications affecting many organ systems including the skin. Due to the metabolic nature of the skin, fluctuations in glucose and insulin levels may result in skin changes. In many patients, the first presentation of diabetes may be in the form of skin changes. Therefore, recognition of skin manifestations of diabetes mellitus is an important aspect of the physical examination. Most cutaneous manifestations of diabetes are attributed either to chronic degenerative changes or to metabolic derangement.

Necrobiotic Disorders

Necrobiosis Lipoidica Diabeticorum. Necrobiosis Lipoidica Diabeticorum (NLD, Fig. 29.1) is a chronic and indolent inflammatory skin disease of unknown origin. The incidence of NLD in diabetic patients is 0.3%, but studies of NLD patients show that diabetes was subsequently diagnosed in about two-thirds of patients.[1,2] NLD is three times more common in women than men.[3] NLD, found in both type 1 and type 2 diabetes mellitus, may precede the development of DM in 15% of patients. In 25% of patients both diseases appear simultaneously.[4] NLD usually resolves in 13–19% of patients 6–12 years after onset.[5] The incidence of NLD is independent of glycemic control.

Lesions can appear at any age, but most commonly develop in the third and fourth decades. Lesions may be solitary or multiple. The characteristic lesions of NLD are asymptomatic and are found most commonly bilaterally on the anterior and lateral surfaces of the lower legs. Lesions on other areas of the body are less commonly associated with DM.[6] Early lesions of NLD are small, red elevated nodules with sharply demarcated borders. As the nodule enlarges, it flattens into a plaque with an irregular outline and eventual depression as the dermis becomes atrophic. The lesion changes in color to brownish yellow, with the advancing border remaining red. The lesions coalesce and sometimes cover the pretibial area completely. Telangiectasias are more prominent as the epidermis becomes scaly and atrophic. NLD lesions are often painless due to degeneration of cutaneous nerves in the affected region. However, persistent lesions will develop painful shallow ulcers. Ulcers, which are often preceded by trauma, occur in about 30% of lesions.[7] The differential diagnosis of NLD includes granuloma annulare, sarcoidosis, rheumatoid nodules, and xanthomas in its early stages.

The exact pathogenesis of NLD has not yet been elucidated. However, since NLD is found in both type 1 and type 2 diabetes, genetic factors are an unlikely cause. Diabetic microangiopathy associated with neuropathy has been implicated in playing a role in the necrobiosis of collagen.[3] Histopathology demonstrates zones of degenerated collagen with loss of normal architecture in dermis, granulomatous changes, palisading of histiocytes

M.C. Varghese (✉)

Department of Dermatology, New York Presbyterian Hospital, Weill Medical College of Cornell University, New York, NY, USA

e-mail: mcvargh@med.cornell.edu

L. Poretsky (ed.), *Principles of Diabetes Mellitus*, DOI 10.1007/978-0-387-09841-8_29,
© Springer Science+Business Media, LLC 2010

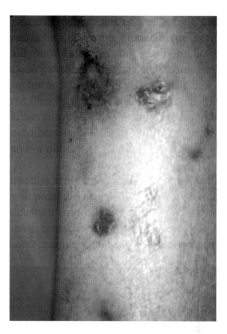

Fig. 29.1 Necrobiosis lipoidica diabeticorum: painful, shallow ulcers, and hyperpigmented, yellowish plaques on the pretibial surface

around the degenerated collagen, obliteration of dermal blood vessels and sclerosis. The etiology of collagen degeneration is currently under investigation. Immunoreactants such as IgM, C3, fibrin, IgG, and IgA have been found in vessels of NLD lesions supporting the theory of an immunologic pathogenesis.[8]

There is no standard of treatment for NLD and effective treatments are still under investigation. Since lesions are independent of glucose levels, glycemic control is ineffective in treatment. Application of topical glucocorticoids under occlusion or by intralesional injections atthe periphery of lesions has been beneficial in active lesions. Ulcerations may be treated with local wound care or excision of the entire lesion. Some authors suggest increased platelet aggregation as a catalyst for vascular changes.[9] Therefore, studies have attempted to show improvement of lesions with the use of aspirin and dipyridamole in which the dosage is a critical factor. The researchers suggest therapeutic doses of aspirin at 3.5 mg/kg every 48–72 h. Clofazimine, nicotinamide, pentoxifylline, and chloroquine have also been reported as a case by case basis in the treatment of NLD.[10] Newer treatment strategies have used immunomodulating agents such as cyclosporine A, infliximab, and tacrolimus, topically or systemically, to decrease the amount of inflammation associated with NLD.[7] These studies help support the hypothesis that T-cell mediated immune processes may be involved in the pathogenesis. More studies are needed to determine efficacy of these treatments.

Generalized Granuloma Annulare. Granuloma Annulare (GA, Fig. 29.2) causes degeneration of collagen in the dermis similarly to NLD, with surrounding areas of inflammation and fibrosis. The etiology of GA is unknown. The correlation between GA and DM remains controversial. Some reports show no relationship between GA and DM[11] while others report an association. Diabetes was found in 21% of patients with generalized granuloma annulare and 10% localized granuloma annulare in a study of 100 patients.[12] Another study reported a relationship between localized granuloma annulare and insulin-dependent diabetes mellitus.[13] Patients develop firm, smooth 1–5 cm shiny dermal papules and plaques, often in an annular or circinate configuration, commonly on the extremities.

Histopathology typically shows a palisade of histiocytes surrounding mucin deposits in the dermis.[14] Treatment for GA is usually unnecessary due to the self-limited nature of the disease. However, intralesional and topical steroids may be beneficial. Other treatments that have been tried include antimalarials, dapsone, cytotoxic drugs, and phototherapy with PUVA.

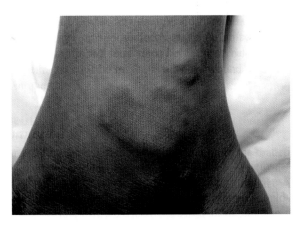

Fig. 29.2 Granuloma annulare (localized): annular erythematous dermal plaque on the extremity

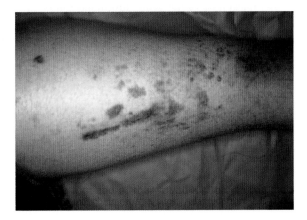

Fig. 29.3 Diabetic dermopathy: asymmetric, atrophic, brown plaques on lower extremities

Diabetic Dermopathy. The most common finding in diabetes is diabetic dermopathy (Fig. 29.3), occurring in 40% of diabetic patients older than 50 years.[15] This condition is not exclusively seen in diabetes; in fact 20% of nondiabetic individuals have demonstrated these lesions. It is twice as common in men as in women. Dermopathy or shin spots commonly occur on the lower legs as well as forearms, thighs, and bony prominences. Shin spots are usually asymmetric, multiple and bilateral, asymptomatic, and well-circumscribed lesions that initially appear as 0.5–1.0 cm oval to round papules that progress to hyperpigmented, atrophic scars. Hemosiderin deposits are in histiocytes adjacent to the vessels causing the discoloration. Additionally, intimal thickening of the dermal arterioles and capillaries and deposition of periodic acid Schiff (PAS) positive material in vessel walls are noted histologically.[103]

Although the etiology is not quite elucidated, microangiopathy and neuropathy have been postulated to play a role in the formation of these lesionsref. However, one recent study measuring blood flow did not show decreased cutaneous blood flow in the area of the lesion, but in fact a paradoxical increase in blood flow to the dermopathic lesions.[16] More studies are needed to validate the hypothesis of ischemic changes to the skin as a result of microangiopathy in diabetic individuals. There is no known correlation between development of lesions, their duration, and severity of diabetes.

Scleredema Diabeticorum. Scleredema diabeticorum found in association with DM is characterized by progressive, painless induration of the skin. Scleredema associated with diabetes has a prevalence of 3% and is more common in obese individuals with vascular complications type 2 diabetes.[17] The posterior, lateral neck, and back are usually involved first with eventual extension to the face, shoulders, anterior neck, arms, and torso. Although the exact pathogenesis has yet to be determined, hypotheses suggest decreased insulin levels as the source of derangement of collagen metabolism. Physical examination shows taut indurated, non-pitting areas of skin with poorly demarcated borders. Histopathology examination reveals marked thickening of collagen bundles that are separated by clear spaces and abundant deposits of mucin in the dermis. There is no effective treatment available for scleredema diabeticorum. Treatment and control of the diabetes have been futile in ameliorating the condition.

Disorders of Increased Skin Thickness. Diabetic thick skin or cheiroarthropathy is present in 30–40% insulin treated diabetic individuals. Prevalence of cheiroarthropathy in diabetes patients who are not on insulin therapy varies from 4 to 70% and is related to retinopathy, nephropathy, and neuropathy. This condition bears no relation to glycemic control, but does increase in incidence with age and duration of diabetes. Patients present with thick, tight, waxy skin, and limited joint mobility (LJM) that may occur before the patient is diagnosed with diabetes.[18,19] This constellation of symptoms is also known as *scleroderma-like syndrome*.[20] The stiffness of the hands in this condition often results in an inability to oppose the two palms. A screening test in which patients are unable to bring their palms completely together due to contractures of proximal and distal interphalangeal joints is called the "prayer sign."[21] Pebbled or rough skin on the interphalangeal joints, called Huntley's papules is another physical sign suggesting thickening of the skin. Ultrasound can be utilized for identification of skin and tendon sheath thickness. The illness can be debilitating due to complications such as frozen shoulder or Dupuytren's contracture. Diagnosis and follow-up is important since these patients are also at an increased risk for retinal and renal disease due to vascular changes. Definitive pathogenesis has not been determined. However, alteration in collagen metabolism via nonenzymatic glycosylation had been suggested. If these hypotheses are correct then tight glucose control may be beneficial in limiting the extent of disease.[22] Research studies for treatment of this condition are rare. One study examined aldose reductase inhibitors in an attempt to reduce the accumulation of sugar alcohols. Researchers found that Sorbinil (400 mg/dl) helped correct the effects of LJM[23] with the 10-year follow-up study[24] showing those patients were free of LJM with minimal side effects. Physical therapy can also play a significant role in those with severe LJM to preserve range of motion.[19]

Infections

It is widely believed that diabetic patients have a greater predisposition for infections. However, this remains controversial. There are no definitive studies that show whether diabetic patients are more susceptible to infection and/or have a more severe course once they are infected.[25] Host-specific factors such as hyperglycemia-related impairment of immune response, vascular insufficiency, sensory peripheral neuropathy, autonomic neuropathy, and increased skin and mucosal colonization of bacteria/yeast have all been hypothesized as potential reasons behind increased diabetic infections.[26] Studies on hyperglycemic patients have shown decreased chemotaxis, phagocytosis, and lysis of organisms in these individuals.[27] Subsequently, a decreased inflammatory and immune response may be the result of thickened capillary walls and compromised vasculature which serves as a physical barrier and impedes diffusion of nutrients and movement of leukocytes to the site of injury.[28] Colonization of staphylococcus, candidiasis, streptococcus, and dermatophytosis are the most frequent infections found in diabetic patients.

Fungal

Candida. Candidal infections are more common in diabetic patients than in normal controls. Candidiasis, often seen in poorly controlled diabetic individuals, may also precede the diagnosis of diabetes. Conversely, good glucose control may improve or prevent candidiasis. These infections may present as thrush in the mouth, chronic paronychia in the nail folds, and intertrigo in the skin folds. One study reported increased glucose levels in the saliva of diabetic patients with oral candidal infections.[29] Candida angular stomatitis is often seen in children with DM. Vulvovaginitis is a common complication of poorly controlled diabetes in women and may be accompanied by vulvar pruritus and inflammatory lesions. Genital candidal infections in men such as balanitis and balanoposthitis are much less common, but may also be the presenting feature of DM. Chronic candidal paronychia usually involves the nail fold and may be associated with inflammation, pain, and loss of the cuticle. Infection between the middle and fourth finger, called erosio interdigitalis blastomycetica is rarer than paronychia.[5] Good glucose control is optimal in the prevention of candidal infections. Topical or systemic anti fungal medications may be required in the management.

Phycomycetes. Phycomycetes infections may develop in diabetic ulcers or in traumatic wounds as a primary infection or a complicating infection. This should be suspected in individuals who do not respond to standard antibacterial or antifungal therapy.[30] Therapy for phycomycetes infections must be aggressive due to the high fatality rate. Treatment must be initiated at the earliest opportunity, and includes debridement of all necrotic tissue, administration of IV amphotericin B as well as correction of acid–base imbalance and control of hyperglycemia.[5]

Mucormycosis (zygomycosis). Zygomycetous are a class of fungi that commonly cause infection in diabetic patients. The most common infection causing organism is from the Rhizopus genera. These organisms thrive in high glucose, acidic conditions due to a ketone reductase enzyme. Patients with diabetic ketoacidosis are more prone to stimulate their growth.[31] Iron overload and deferoxamine also increase the risk of mucormycosis. Serum iron is elevated in diabetic patients due to impaired transferrin binding, increasing their risk of infection.[32]

Rhinocerebral mucormycosis is an example of a rare, mucormycotic infection caused most commonly by *Rhizopus oryzae*. Debilitated patients with diabetic ketoacidosis are predisposed to rhinocerebral form of this infection. The infection presents as an acute sinusitis with fever, nasal stuffiness, purulent nasal discharge, headache, and sinus pain. The infection can spread quickly in the sinuses and once the infection has spread to contiguous structures there is ischemic necrosis of tissue, which is a hallmark sign of invasive disease. The results are palatal eschars, destruction of the turbinates, perinasal swelling, and erythema and cyanosis of the facial skin overlying the involved sinuses. Invasion rapidly progresses to involve the orbit and may lead to periorbital edema, proptosis, and blindness. Facial numbness is frequent and results from infarction of the sensory nerves of the trigeminal nerve. Spread of the infection from the ethmoid sinus to the frontal lobe results in obtundation, while spread from the sphenoid sinuses to the adjacent cavernous sinus can result in cranial nerve palsies, thrombosis of the sinus, and involvement of the carotid artery.[33,34]

Less severe forms of mucormycosis are the cutaneous forms. This is a result of infection of the skin and soft tissues with zygomycetes, which is usually associated with trauma or wounds. Patients with diabetes mellitus are more prone to minor trauma resulting in an increased incidence of infection. Cutaneous mucormycosis usually appears as a single, painful, indurated area of cellulitis that develops into an ecthyma-like lesion. Dissemination or deep tissue involvement are unusual complications of cutaneous mucormycosis.[35]

Treatment for this infection initially involves surgical intervention. Debridement of necrotic tissue should be done as soon as the diagnosis is made. Amphotericin B is used as an adjunctive therapy, but generally other antifungal agents are ineffective against zygomycetes.[36] Control of predisposing factors for infection such as hyperglycemia, metabolic acidosis, and neutropenia is also critical.[35]

Dermatophytosis (Tinea). Although dermatophyte infections occur at a similar prevalence when compared with the general populations,[37] they are more significant when they occur in diabetic patients because the lesions may serve as an accessible route for other, mainly bacterial, infections.[33] When these infections are identified, they should be treated.

Bacterial

Staphylococcus aureus and beta-hemolytic streptococci are usually the most common bacterial pathogens affecting diabetic skin.[102] They may cause impetigo, folliculitis, furuncles, carbuncles, ecthyma, cellulitis, and erysipelas.[37] Bullous lesions leading to diabetic gangrene and necrotizing fasciitis may complicate bacterial infection of the legs.[38] Diabetic patients may also develop gas gangrene that is caused by clostridial organisms. Other organisms that cause gas gangrene include *Escherichia coli*, *Klebsiella*, and *Pseudomonas*.

Necrotizing Fasciitis. Necrotizing fasciitis is an infection of the subcutaneous tissue that results in progressive destruction of fascia and fat, but may spare the skin. There are three types of necrotizing fasciitis that are more common in diabetic patients than others: type I necrotizing fasciitis, nonclostridial anaerobic cellulitis, and synergistic necrotizing cellulitis. These are polymicrobial infections that commonly start in the feet and have rapid extension along the fascia into the leg.[39,40] The early manifestations of necrotizing fasciitis include unexplained pain that increases over time. However, diabetic patients with peripheral neuropathy may have an absence of pain and are at further risk of not detecting tissue necrosis early. Other signs include erythema which may be present diffusely or locally. Within 24–48 h, erythema may darken to a reddish-purple color, frequently with associated blisters and bullae. The bullae are initially filled with clear fluid but rapidly take on a blue or maroon appearance. Once the bullous stage is reached, there is already extensive deep soft tissue destruction and patients usually exhibit fever and systemic toxicity. Necrotizing fasciitis should also be considered in diabetic patients with cellulitis and systemic signs of infection (tachycardia, leukocytosis, hyperglycemia, and acidosis). Treatment involves surgical debridement of necrotic tissue with adjuvant antibiotic therapy.[40]

Malignant Otitis Externa. Diabetic patients may also develop malignant otitis externa due to *Pseudomonas aeruginosa*, which may begin as a cellulitis, but progresses to chondritis, osteomyelitis, and infectious cerebritis.[5] Elderly patients with diabetes are at an overwhelming risk of malignant external otitis. One review showed more than 90% of adults with this disease were found to have some sort of glucose intolerance;[41] however, susceptibility to malignant otitis externa has not been correlated with a level of glucose intolerance.[42] Some studies believe that the infections are due to increased microangiopathy in the ear canal which is more common in the elderly.[42] Another hypothesis states that an increase in pH of cerumen in diabetic patients predisposes them to infection.[43] The classical presentation of malignant external otitis is otalgia and otorrhea with granulation tissue frequently visible in the inferior portion of the external auditory canal at the bone–cartilage junction. Complications such as osteomyelitis and infarction of the cranial nerves can develop when the infection spreads. If untreated, fatal complications of meningitis, brain abscess, and dural sinus thrombophlebitis can potentially occur. First-line treatment of malignant external otitis is antipseudomonal antibiotics.

Erythasma. Corynebacterium minutissimum infection results in erythrasma in diabetic patients. Patients develop erythematous plaques in the upper thigh regions, axilla, submammary creases or torso. Plaques may also be confined to the interdigital spaces of the toes.[44] When the lesions progress they become brown, hyperpigmented plaques with scale. Erythrasma may be elucidated by color of red fluorescence on Wood's lamp and may be treated with topical or systemic antibiotics. The differential diagnosis of erythrasma includes psoriasis, dermatophytosis, candidiasis, and intertrigo.[26]

Miscellaneous

Diabetic Bullae. Diabetic bullae are an uncommon skin condition that is characterized by the appearance of spontaneous blisters that are usually confined to the hands and feet but also occur on the extensor aspect of the forearms and legs. The condition is more common in men than women as well as in patients with a long history of diabetes.[45] The blisters usually appear suddenly and start as tense, non-erythematous lesions that become flaccid as they enlarge over several days. They vary in size, with some being several centimeters. They may take 6 weeks to heal and can recur.[6] Scarring and atrophy may occur in patients with subepidermal blisters.[46] The exact pathogenesis of blister formation is unclear, although one report documented a reduced threshold for suction-induced blistering.[47] Derangements in carbohydrate metabolism are also implicated.[17]

Patients with long-standing history of diabetes may develop bullae as a result of renal failure. Bullae of renal disease or pseudoporphyria resemble porphyria cutanea tarda clinically and histologically and are seen in 1–16% of patients undergoing renal dialysis.[48] These patients most commonly develop blisters on the dorsa of their hands; bullae on other parts of the body are not uncommon. The exact pathogenesis is still unclear, but some proposed etiologic factors include increased serum porphyrin levels,[49] oxidative stress,[50] and photosensitivity.

Acanthosis Nigricans. Acanthosis nigricans is a skin manifestation of insulin resistance in several endocrine disorders, including diabetes mellitus. It is nonspecific for diabetes. In fact, it occurs in a number of benign conditions, in response to medications, and as manifestation of internal disease such as gastric adenocarcinoma.

In diabetic patients, the high levels of insulin are thought to be responsible for the development of acanthosis nigricans.[51] The condition is characterized by hypertrophic, hyperpigmented, black-brown velvety plaques in flexural areas of skin, such as the breast creases, neck-fold, axilla, and groin. Some patients also have involvement of the face, hands, elbows, knees, and abdominal area.[52] The skin changes are usually asymptomatic, but can be painful, malodorous, or macerated. Histopathologically, the lesions are hyperkeratotic, papillomatotic, and acanthotic.[26] It is classified as benign when it occurs in insulin-resistant states.[53] Other benign states include obesity,[54] total lipodystrophy,[55] and polycystic ovarian syndrome.[56] Certain drugs, such as corticosteroids and niacin are also linked to benign acanthosis nigricans as they can cause hyperglycemia and insulin resistance.[57] The pathogenesis of insulin-resistant acanthosis nigricans may be related to the high levels of circulating insulin that cross react and bind with insulin-like growth factor receptors found on keratinocytes and dermal fibroblasts causing proliferation.[58] Although there is no definitive treatment, weight reduction in obesity has shown to decrease insulin resistance and improve the skin lesions.[54] Topical retinoids[59] can be used and those lesions that are malodorous can be treated with antibacterial soaps or topical antibiotics (clindamycin).[53]

Lipoatrophy. The group of uncommon disorders that result in a decrease or total absence of subcutaneous fat is referred to as lipodystrophies or lipoatrophies. These conditions are usually seen in conjunction with insulin-dependent diabetes mellitus and have a higher prevalence in women as compared with men. The lipodystrophies may be congenital or acquired or may result in total or partial loss of subcutaneous fat.

In *total lipoatrophy* of congenital origin, diabetes usually develops in the second decade while the absence of subcutaneous fat is present from birth or develops within the first 2 years of life. If subcutaneous fat is not absent from birth, it usually disappears over several months. These children usually die from cirrhosis of the liver and their condition has been associated with parental consanguinity. *Acquired total lipoatrophy* starts in childhood or early adulthood. Acquired lipoatrophy may manifest itself after bacterial infections, such as pertussis, or after viral infections. Both forms of total lipoatrophy are often referred to as the Lawrence–Seip syndrome and are considered to be variants of the same disorder despite differences in presentation. Due to the syndrome's association with consanguineous marriages and the presence of the condition in siblings, it is presumed to have a recessive mode of inheritance.[60]

The syndrome is characterized by total lipoatrophy, insulin resistance, non-ketotic diabetes, increased consumption of oxygen, acceleration of bone and muscle growth, acanthosis nigricans,[55] hepatomegaly due to fatty infiltration from hypertriglyceridema,[61] and finally hepatic failure. Patients with the congenital form may also have the associated features of hirsutism, genital enlargement, and central nervous system involvement. Additionally, renal disease or cutaneous xanthomas[62] may be seen. The development of insulin-resistant diabetes usually trails the onset of the syndrome by several years.

The cause and pathogenesis of total lipoatrophy have not yet been established. However, hypothalamic dysfunction has been implicated due to its importance in the regulation of glucose and lipid metabolism. Upton and Corbin[63] proposed that the defect in this disorder is related to an abnormality in dopamine beta-hydroxylase activity and successfully treated a patient with pimozide, a cerebral dopaminergic-blocking agent. Subsequently, Oseid et al.[64] reported decreased binding of insulin to its receptor in patients with congenital generalized lipoatrophy.

Partial lipoatrophy develops any time during childhood to early adulthood and is much more common than the total lipoatrophies. The genetic association is uncertain, although some cases appear to be inherited in an autosomal dominant fashion.[62] The disorder may appear after a febrile childhood illness, such as measles or scarlet fever or idiopathically. The face is almost always affected, while neck, arm, and torso involvement may vary. There is no loss of fat from the hips to the lower extremities and an increase in fat around the hips may also be seen in some individuals. There are several uncommon variants of partial lipoatrophy, which may involve only the buttocks, arms, or legs. The adipose loss in lipoatrophy is usually permanent. As with total lipoatrophy, insulin-resistant diabetes may develop several years after partial lipoatrophy has developed. Circulating immune complexes resulting in membranoproliferative glomerulonephritis can be demonstrated in 40–50% of patients.

Localized lipodystrophies are characterized by a loss of subcutaneous fat from small areas of the body and are not a result of insulin resistance or other metabolic abnormalities. Drug-induced lipodystrophy at the site of injection was a frequent complication of insulin therapy. With the advent of purified human insulin this complication is now rare. Other medications, such as glucocorticoids and antibiotics, can also cause localized lipoatrophy.[65]

There are no evidence-based guidelines for treating lipoatrophic syndromes. Reducing insulin-resistant states by decreasing weight, or changing to low-fat diet have been recommended, although there is no diet that will reverse lipoatrophy. Oral diabetic agents such as metformin may reduce hyperglycemia and hypertriglyceridemia.[66] Newer studies have looked at leptin replacement therapy for those that are leptin-deficient. Patients treated with leptin had significant decreases in HbA1C, serum triglyceride concentrations, liver volume, caloric intake, and resting metabolic rate.[67] Further studies are needed to explore the therapeutic role of leptin and its mechanism of action.

Yellow Skin/Xanthoderma. The nature of yellow skin in diabetes is still under debate. Early studies reported carotenemia in over 50% in diabetic patients[68] and related the change in skin color with this finding. However, a more recent study by Hoerer et al.[69] established higher levels of carotene in the blood of nondiabetic controls as compared with diabetics who often had yellow skin, but normal carotene levels. Carotenosis is usually characterized by yellow pigment on the palms, sole, and face. Possible causes of yellow skin include elevated serum carotene and nonenzymatic glycosylation of dermal collagen and other proteins that eventually become yellow.[3] Other endocrine disorders that can be associated with a yellowish complexion are hypothyroidism, hypogonadism, hypopituitarism, as well as bulimia, and anorexia nervosa.[26]

Eruptive Xanthoma. This is an uncommon syndrome in diabetes that is characterized by eruptive xanthomas (Fig. 29.4) that are associated with hyperlipidemia, hyperglycemia, and glycosuria. The lesions are firm, nontender, yellow papules that erupt in crops on the extensor surfaces. The knees elbows, buttocks, and torso are the most common areas for these lesions. Treatment of underlying hyperlipidemia and controlling carbohydrate metabolism will help improve eruptive xanthoma.

Acquired Perforating Dermatosis. Patients with acquired perforating dermatosis (APD, Fig. 29.5) have kidney failure and/or IDDM or NIDDM.[70] Lesions usually occur on the extremities such as the extensor surfaces and the dorsum of the hands, but may also be found on the torso or face. They are usually hyperkeratotic papules and

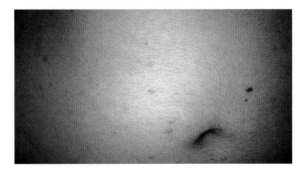

Fig. 29.4 Eruptive xanthoma: firm yellow papules on extensor surfaces

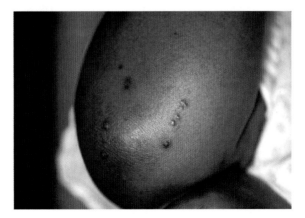

Fig. 29.5 Acquired perforating dermatosis: hyperkeratotic papules on extremities and upper body

less than 1 cm in size that occur after minor trauma. These papules are extremely pruritic and are a feature of APD. Koebner phenomenon can occur and rubbing may cause the papules to coalesce forming a linear pattern. Patients may be treated with keratolytics.

Diabetic Complications

Neuropathy. Diabetic neuropathy is an important condition to diagnose since it may be the presenting manifestation of diabetes in some patients which can be prevented or slowed with tight glucose control. Older patients with insidious onset of disease are especially at risk. Distal symmetric polyneuropathy is the most common diabetic neuropathy, with motor and sensory involvement.[71] Dorsally subluxed digits, distally displaced plantar fat pads, depressed metatarsal heads, hammer toes, and pes cavus (exaggeration of the normal arch) characterize motor neuropathy. Chronic motor neuropathy will gradually affect the intrinsic muscles of the foot creating a lack of opposing force against the larger anterior tibial muscles. This can lead to a subluxation of the proximal interphalangeal-metatarsal joints resulting in a claw toe appearance. This results in increased pressure of the metatarsal heads, which become a target area for ulcer development. Good foot care plays an important role in the care of these patients and may prevent the formation of debilitating, painless, and indolent perforating ulcers (mal perforans).[5] These lesions are circular, punched out ulcers that occur in a callous or other pressure site. Sensory neuropathies result in numbness, tingling, aching, and burning. Restless legs and burning feet may be exacerbated at night. Autonomic nerve damage can lead to decreased sweating in the skin resulting in dry, scaly, and cracked feet, allowing infections to penetrate the skin. There can also be compensatory sweating in other parts of the body that result in erythema, edema, and atrophy in advanced cases.[17]

Immunohistochemical analysis has demonstrated a depletion of neuropeptides in the nerve endings of diabetic patients with neurologic dysfunction.[72] Several serotonin-norepinephrine reuptake inhibitors such as desipramine and amitriptyline have shown some efficacy in treating diabetic neuropathy.[73]

Diabetic Foot. The diabetic foot is the result of a multifactorial pathological process and requires appropriate care. It is now believed that neuropathy plays as much of a contributory role in foot complications as does vascular pathology. The foot complications of diabetic neuropathy often begin with absence of the ankle jerk reflex, loss of normal foot posture, and atrophy of the intrinsic muscles of the foot. As a result, weight is distributed over a much smaller area of plantar skin causing calluses and eventually ulcers.[74] Misalignment of the foot may also lead to ligament tears, minor fractures, loss of bone, and a deformed foot. Subsequently, decreased pain perception and dry skin may result in fissuring, cellulitis, and deep tissue infection that may go unnoticed by the patient.[75] The lifetime risk of a person, either with type 1 or 2 diabetes, developing ulcerations in the diabetic foot is 15% (Fig. 29.6).[76]

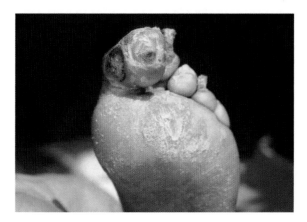

Fig. 29.6 Malalignment of the foot causing calluses, neuropathic ulcers, and dry skin

Ulcers of the foot can become infected. These infections can be divided into superficial and local, soft tissue and spreading (cellulitis), and osteomyelitis.[76] The infection usually begins in the paronychia, around the cracks in the skin, or arising from neuropathic or ischemic ulcers. As the infection progresses, it can be erythematous with swelling and tenderness and even have a purulent discharge. When the infection spreads to soft tissue, it is classified as cellulitis.

Generally, the same signs and symptoms as a local infection are present with potential for serious complications that may occur in necrotizing infections such as cutaneous bullae, soft tissue gas, or purple or black discoloration of the skin. Osteomyelitis is often the result of contiguous spread of a soft tissue foot infection with bony involvement. Again, the clinical features of acute osteomyelitis can appear identical to the clinical features of superficial infections of the foot in the diabetic patient.

In caring for the diabetic patient with peripheral neuropathy of the foot, glucose control is of great importance. Patients should also be educated about the nature of their disease, the recognition of abnormalities and foot care in between regularly scheduled visits to the podiatrist. Skin over pressure points should be kept well hydrated with emollients while ingrown toenails, hallux valgus, and claw toes should be managed surgically.[77] Patients should be instructed not to walk around barefoot and should wear special shoes with adequate support and good weight distribution. Infections of the diabetic foot should be cultured to determine the inciting pathogen(s) and treated appropriately with antibiotics. Recalcitrant ulcers may require debridement, systemic antibiotics, or eventual amputation in the case of extensive bone involvement.

Cutaneous Manifestations of Vascular Abnormalities in DM

The most dramatic and debilitating skin complications of DM are related to compromise of the vascular system. Derangements affect the small and large blood vessels.

Microangiopathy. Some skin changes can be attributed to small vessel damage Small vessels usually demonstrate proliferation of endothelial cells, basement membrane thickening, and the deposition of PAS-positive material resulting in decrease in vessel diameter.[78] Pigmented purpuras, periungual telangiectasias,[79] erysipelas-like erythema, NLD, neuropathy, and dermopathy may result in microangiopathy.[80] Microvascular impairment can be viewed most easily in the nail fold and retina. Examination of the nail folds may reveal telangiectasias. One study showed nail fold capillary dilatation in 49% of diabetic patients free of apparent peripheral vascular disease compared with 10% in healthy controls.[81] The relevance of this clinical sign still requires further investigation. According to some data, the eye is more sensitive and reliable in determining microangiopathy.[82] Retinal venous dilatation, microaneurysms, hemorrhages, exudates, and neovascularization are considered manifestations of retinal microangiopathy.

Pigmented Purpuric Dermatoses. Pigmented purpuric dermatoses (PPD) have been reported in older diabetic patients. Many of these individuals are men with a history of cardiac decompensation; half of these patients have a history of diabetic dermopathy.[83] Whether this condition is a cutaneous marker of microangiopathy is under debate. PPD are caused by erythrocyte extravasation in the superficial vascular plexus. The lesions are usually brown-orange to tan macules or "cayenne pepper" spots in the pretibial area or dorsa of feet.[5]

Gangrene. The foot is the most common location for tissue necrosis and gangrene, due to vascular compromise. Foot gangrene is 50 times more prevalent in diabetic patients compared with nondiabetics over 40 years of age.[5] While the dry form is due to large vessel blockage due to atherosclerosis, wet gangrene is believed to be a late manifestation of microangiopathy. Both may occur in diabetes, but small vessel disease is more common and directly associated with diabetic vascular derangements. Dry gangrene occurs mainly in diabetic patients with concurrent atherosclerosis. Wet gangrene develops when barely satisfactory perfusion in the extremities becomes insufficient as a result of decreased cardiac output or increased oxygen demand by infected tissue.

Diligent foot care is imperative in these patients, since minor abrasions to the skin may lead to infection and gangrene. Tinea pedis should also be treated aggressively as the fissures in the skin may be a nidus for infection.

Erysipelas-Like Erythema. Erysipelas-like erythema is seen most commonly in older individuals with at least a 5-year history of diabetes and is also considered to result from small vessel damage. Well-demarcated red areas without fever, leukocytosis, or elevated sedimentation rate characterize the disease. Some patients have associated bone destruction due to small vessel insufficiency. Lithner reported the development of erythema in diabetic patients after cardiac decompensation or venous thrombosis.[84]

Diabetic Rubeosis. Diabetic rubeosis is a condition seen in patients with a long history of diabetes and is characterized by a reddening of the face and occasionally of the hands and feet. The condition is believed to be related to small vessel disease and decreased vascular tone.[19]

Calciphylaxis. Calciphylaxis is observed in the setting of diabetes, end stage renal disease, and hyperparathyroidism and is associated with angiopathy of small and medium vessels. Vessel calcification from calcium deposits results in progressive cutaneous necrosis. Initially plaques appear red to violaceous with a reticulated pattern. There may be bullae formation and eventually development of a black, bound-down eschar with necrosis of tissues. These lesions may become secondarily infected and are slowly progressive despite medical management. Unfortunately, calciphylaxis has a poor prognosis and high fatality rate.[85]

Macroangiopathy. Large vessel disease is usually seen in diabetes in association with microangiopathy. Conversely, microangiopathy is usually seen alone.[17] Atherosclerosis has been shown to have a higher prevalence and incidence in diabetic patients when compared with the general population.[86] The clinical signs are intermittent claudication, skin atrophy, hair loss, coldness of the toes, nail dystrophy, and pallor upon elevation. When the leg is lowered, venous filling is prolonged, and dependent mottling is observed.[5]

Diabetic Drug Reactions

Oral hypoglycemic agents. Sulfonylureas may cause an allergic drug reaction in 1–5% of patients. The reaction is usually evident within the first two months of therapy. The reaction is often usually in the form of a maculopapular eruption that may be accompanied by generalized erythema or urticarial eruptions. The rash usually disappears on its own while the person continues to maintain the sulfonylurea dose. Rarely, a generalized pruritus may result in a diffuse exfoliative dermatitis, generalized erythema multiforme, Stevens–Johnson syndrome, or toxic epidermal necrolysis that requires immediate discontinuation of the drug.

Insulin. The incidence of allergic reactions caused by insulin may range from 10 to 50% of patients.[86] Some insulin preparations, such as the purified or recombinant types, are much less likely to produce generalized reactions than others. The allergy may be associated with impurities in the insulin, beef versus pork protein, the insulin molecule itself,[87] or zinc.[88]

Most reactions are localized at the site of injection. Localized, immediate reactions start within 15 min – 2 h of injection with pruritic erythema or urticaria and occasional vesiculation.[89] The reaction, which is mediated by IgG antibodies, may be seen soon after starting insulin therapy or many years thereafter.[90] The best treatment option in this event is to change to more purified insulin, which has a lower, but not negligible risk for developing an allergic reaction.[91] Local, delayed reactions are usually most intense 1–2 days after the injection and are characterized by pruritis and burning erythema that is followed by the development of an indurated papule or nodule. Most lesions resolve by a month of continuation of usual insulin administration.[3] Insulin-induced lipoatrophy is most common in children and adolescent girls and may appear at the site of injection within 6–24 months of initial administration. While change of injection site alone does not result in resolution of lipoatrophy, incidence of lipoatrophy is decreased when patients are switched to a pure form of insulin or human recombinant insulin. Some children may also develop painless nodules at sites of repeated injections that contain adipose and fibrous tissue.[90] A recent case study reported allergic reactions to the long-acting insulin analogue detemir. The patient reported a well-circumscribed rash around the injection site, followed by the formation of a small lump that would increase in size with repeated injections.[92]

Systemic allergic reactions to insulin are IgE mediated and may present as generalized urticaria or rarely as angioedema or anaphylaxis in less than 1% of insulin treated patients. Some systemic reactions may be biphasic, developing features of serum-sickness-like reaction.

Lichen Planus

Lichen planus is an uncommon disorder of unknown etiology. It primarily affects the skin, nails, mucous membranes, vulva, and penis. It most commonly presents as an eruption of shiny, flat, violaceous papules with white lacelike patterns on the surface. Most patients experience extreme pruritis with these lesions which can be painful if they ulcerate. There has been an interest in the association between diabetes mellitus and lichen planus. Reports have shown an increased incidence of abnormal glucose tolerance tests in patients with lichen planus[93] as well as an increased incidence of lichen planus in diabetic patients compared with healthy controls.[94] Higher prevalence was also noted in diabetic individuals who smoke and those with a history of oral candidiasis.[3] Oral lichen planus has been associated with diabetes mellitus and hypertension and is known as Grinspan's syndrome. However, anecdotal studies have reported that the oral lichen planus may actually be iatrogenically produced by the drug therapy of diabetes mellitus and hypertension.[95]

Hemochromatosis

Approximately 80% of patients with hemochromatosis eventually develop diabetes.[96] The main symptoms of hemochromatosis are liver disease, hyperpigmentation, joint disease, hypogonadism, and eventually diabetes.[5] The classic skin finding is hyperpigmentation, which is thought to be due to a general increase in epidermal melanization.[97] Other skin findings in hemochromatosis are spider angiomas in 60–80% of patients, palmar erythema, skin atrophy, ichthyosis, and a decrease in body hair.[98]

Vitiligo

Vitiligo is an acquired autoimmune process directed at melanocytes causing depigmentation of the skin. There is usually a symmetrical depigmentation of the skin that often presents on the dorsa of the hands and on the face. The axilla, genitalia, and perianal area also can be involved. Complete depigmentation may occur with progressive involvement. An increased incidence of vitiligo has been reported in polyglandular autoimmune (PGA) syndrome type II. This includes a host of immunoendocrinopathy syndromes which includes type 1 diabetes mellitus. Overall treatment of vitiligo can be difficult and prolonged with limited evidence-based studies for long-term benefits and safety.

Acrochordons (Skin Tags)

Early studies defined an association between skin tags and diabetes mellitus. Skin tags are common benign skin tumors composed of loose fibrous tissue. They are small, soft, pedunculated papules that commonly occur on the neck, eyelids, and axillae. These lesions have a higher prevalence in women and overweight individuals. The etiology of skin tags may be linked to impaired carbohydrate metabolism although there have been conflicting results. Earlier studies have demonstrated that 26% of patients with acrochordons also had overt DM,[99] while other studies have shown that 73% of patients with skin tags also had diabetes mellitus.[100] More recent studies examined the prevalence of diabetes and impaired glucose tolerance in patients with the number of skin tags.[101] They found that patients with increased skin tags had increased fasting plasma glucose and are at a greater risk of developing diabetes mellitus. More studies are needed to further elucidate to establish skin tags as a cutaneous marker in diabetes. Treatment for skin tags are removal of the lesion by cryosurgery, electrodessication or excision.

Summary

The skin manifestations of diabetes mellitus are varied and numerous. Often they can present as the initial manifestation of the disease. Occasionally, these skin conditions may portend progression of the disease. For this reason, it is important to be familiar with the cutaneous aspects of diabetes with respect to both diagnosis and treatment.

Useful internet web sites:

http://dermatlas.med.jhmi.edu/derm/
http://www.dermis.net/dermisroot/en/home/index.htm
http://telemedicine.org/stamford.htm

References

1. Krakowski A, Covo J, Berlin C. Diabetic Scleredema. *Dermatologica*. 1973;146:193–198.
2. Rosenbloom AL, Silverstein JM, Lezotte DC, et al. Limited joint mobility in childhood diabetes mellitus indicates increased risk of microvascular disease. *N Engl J Med*. 1981;305:191–194.
3. Perez MI, Kohn SR. Cutaneous manifestations of diabetes mellitus. *J Am Acad Dermatol*. 1994;30:519–531.
4. Meure M, Szeimies RM. Diabetes mellitus and skin diseases. *Curr Prob*. 1991;20:11–23.
5. Huntley AC. Cutaneous manifestations of diabetes mellitus. *J Am Acad Dermatol*. 1982;7:427–455.
6. Braverman IM. *Skin Signs of Systemic Disease*. Philadelphia: WB Saunders; 1981:654–664.
7. Korber A, Dissemond J. Necrobiosis lipoidica diabeticorum. *CMAJ*. 2007;177:12.
8. Quimby SR, Muller SA, Schroeter AL. The cutaneous immunopathology of necrobiosis lipodica diabeticorum. *Arch Dermatol*. 1988;124:1364–1371.
9. Karkavitsas K, et al. Aspirin in the management of necrobiosis lipodica. *Acta Derm*. 1982;62:183.
10. Freinkel RK. *Diabetes Mellitus in Fitzpatrick's Dermatology in General Medicine*. 5th edition. New York: Mc-Graw Hill; 1999:1969.
11. Dicken CH, Carrington SG, Winkelmann RK. Generalizes granuloma annulare. *Arch Dermatol*. 1969;99:556–563.
12. Dabski K, Winkelmann RK. Generalized granuloma annulare: clinical and laboratory findings in 100 patients. *J Am Acad Dermatol*. 1989;20:39–47.
13. Muhlemann MF, Williams DRR. Localized granuloma annulare is associated with insulin-dependent diabetes. *Br J Dermatol*. 1984;111:325–329.
14. Thyresson HN, Doyle JA, Winkelmann RK. Granuloma annulare: histopathologic and direct immunofluorescence study. *Acta Derm Venereol (Stockh)*. 1980;60:261.
15. Shmer A, Bergman R, Linn S, Kantor Y, Friedman-Birnbaum R. Diabetic dermopathy and internal complications of diabetes mellitus. *Int J Dermatol*. 1998;37:113–115.
16. Wigington G, Ngo B, Rendell M. Skin blood flow in diabetic dermopathy. *Arch Dermatol*. 2004;140:1248–1250.
17. Weissman K. *Skin Disorders in Diabetes Mellitus in Rook/Wilkinson/Ebling's Textbook of Dermatology*. Malden, MA: Blackwell Science, Inc; 1998:2676.
18. Sherry DD, Rothstein RR, Petty RE, et al. Joint contracture preceding insulin-dependent diabetes mellitus. *Arthritis Rheum*. 1982;25:1362–1364.
19. Brik R, Berant M, Vardi P. The scleredema-like syndrome of insulin dependent diabetes mellitus. *Diabetes-Metabolism Reviews*. 1991;7(2):120–128.
20. Yosipovitch G, Loh KC, Hock OB. Medical pearls: scleroderma-like skin changes in patients with diabetes mellitus. *J Am Acad Dermatol*. 2003;48:109–111.
21. Starkman HS, Gleason RE, Rand LI, et al. Limited joint mobility of the hands in patients with diabetes mellitus. *Ann Rheum Dis*. 1986;45:130–135.
22. Lieberman LS, Rosenbloom AC, Riley WJ, et al. Reduced skin thickness with pump administration of insulin. *N engl J Med*. 1980;303:940–941.
23. Eaton P, Sibbitt WL, Harsh A. The effect of an aldose reductase inhibiting agent on limited joint mobility in diabetic patients. *JAMA*. 1985;253:1437–1440.
24. Eaton RP, Sibbitt WL, Shah VO, et al. A commentary on 10 years of aldose reductase inhibition for limited joint mobility in diabetes. *J Diabetes Complications*. 1998;12:34–38.
25. Oakley WG, Pyke DA, Taylor KW. *Diabetes and Its Management*. 3rd ed. Oxford: Blackwell Scientific Publications; 1978:43.

26. Ahmed I, Goldstein B. Diabetes mellitus. *Clin In Dermatol*. 2006;24:237–246.

27. Sabin JA. Bacterial Infections in diabetes mellitus. *Br J Dermatol*. 1974;91:481.

28. Meurer M, Szeimies RM. Diabetes mellitus and skin diseases. *Curr Probl*. 1991;20:11–23.

29. Knight L, Fletcher J. Growth of candida albicans in saliva: stimulation by glucose associated with antibiotics, corticosteroids and diabetes mellitus. *J Infect Dis*. 1971;123:371–377.

30. Tomford JW, Whittlesey D, Ellner JJ, Tomashefski JF. Invasive primary cutaneous phycomycosis in diabetic leg ulcers. *Arch Surg*. 1980;115:770–771.

31. Rashid M, Bari A, Majeed S, et al. Mucormycosis: a devastating fungal infection in diabetics. *J Coll Phys Surg Pak*. 2005;15:43–45.

32. De Locht M, Boelaert JR, Schneider YJ. Iron uptake from ferrioxamine and from ferrirhizoferrin by germinating spores of Rhizopus microsporus. *Biochem Pharmacol*. 1994;47:1843–1850.

33. Lugo_Somolinos A, Sanchez JL. Prevalence of dermatophytosis in patients with diabetes. *J Am Acad Dermatol*. 1991;26: 408–410.

34. Adam RD, Hunter G, DiTomasso J, Comerci G Jr. Mucormycosis: emerging prominence of cutaneous infections. *Clin Infect Dis*. Jul 1994;19(1):67–76.

35. Yohai RA, Bullock JD, Aziz AA, Markert RJ. Survival factors in rhino-orbital-cerebral mucormycosis. *Surv Ophthalmol*. Jul-Aug 1994;39(1):3–22.

36. Spanakis EK, Aperis G, Mylonakis E. New agents for the treatment of fungal infections: clinical efficacy and gaps in coverage. *Clin Infect Dis*. Oct 15 2006;43(8):1060–1068.

37. Alteras I, Saryt E. Prevalence of pathogenic fungi in the toe-webs and toe-nails of diabetic patients. *Mycopathologia*. 1979;67:157–159.

38. Calhoun JH, Mader JT. Infection in the diabetic foot. *Hosp Pract*. 1992;30:81–140.

39. Brook I, Frazier EH. Clinical and microbiological features of necrotizing fasciitis. *J Clin Microbiol*. 1995;33:2382–2387.

40. Wong CH, Chang HC, Pasupathy S, Khin LW, Tan JL, Low CO. Necrotizing fasciitis: clinical presentation, microbiology, and determinants of mortality. *J Bone Joint Surg Am*. Aug 2003;85-A(8):1454–1460.

41. Rubin Grandis J, Branstetter BF 4th, Yu VL. The changing face of malignant (necrotising) external otitis: clinical, radiological, and anatomic correlations. *Lancet Infect Dis*. Jan 2004;4(1):34–39.

42. Rubin J, Yu VL. Malignant external otitis: insights into pathogenesis, clinical manifestations, diagnosis, and therapy. *Am J Med*. Sep 1988;85(3):391–398.

43. Barrow HN, Levenson MJ. Necrotizing malignant" external otitis caused by, *Staphylococcus epidermidis*. *Arch Otolaryngol Head Neck Surg*. 1992;118:94–96.

44. Montes LF, Dobson H, Dodge BG, Knowles WR. Erythrasma and diabetes mellitus. *Arch Dermatol*. 1969;99:674–680.

45. Basarab T, Munn SE, McGrath J, Jones RR. Bullous diabeticorum. A case report and literature review. *Clin Exp Dermatol*. 1995;20:218–220.

46. Bernstein JE, Medenica M, Soltani K, et al. Bullous eruption of diabetes mellitus. *Arch Dermatol*. 1979;115:324–325.

47. Bernstein JE, Levine LE, Medenica MM, et al. Reduced threshold to suction-induced blister formation in insulin-epidermolysis bullosa without immunoreactants. *J Am Acad Dermatol*. 1983;8:790–791.

48. Gilchrest B, Rowe JW, Mihm MC. Bullous dermatosis of hemodialysis. *Ann Intern Med*. 1975;83:480–483.

49. Glynne P, et al. Bullous dermatoses in end-stage renal failure: porphyria or pseudoporphyria? *Amer J Kidney Diseases*. 1999;34:155–160.

50. Vadoud-Sayedi J, et al. Treatment of hemodialysis-associated pseudoporphyria with N-acetycysteine: report of two cases. *Br J Dermatol*. 2000;142:580–581.

51. Rendon MI, Ponciano PD, Sontheimer RD, et al. Acanthosis nigricans: a cutaneous marker of tissue resistance to insulin. *J Am Acad Dermatol*. 1989;21:461–469.

52. Sibbald RG, Schachter RK. The skin and diabetes mellitus. *Int J Dermatol*. 1984;23:567–584.

53. Hermanns-Le T, Scheen A, Pierard GE. Acanthosis nigricans associated with insulin resistance: pathophysiology and management. *Am J Clin Dermatol*. 2004;5:199–203.

54. Veysey E, Ratnavel R. Facial acanthosis nigricans associated with obesity. *Am J Clin Dermatol*. 2005;30:437–439.

55. Simha V, Garg A. Phenotypic heterogeneity in body fat distribution in patients with congenital generalized lipodystrophy caused by mutations in the AGPAT2 or seipin genes. *J Clin Endocrinol Metab*. 2003;88:5433–5437.

56. Apridonidze T, Essah PA, Iuorno MJ, Nestler JE. Prevalence and characteristics of the metabolic syndrome in women with polycystic ovary syndrome. *J Clin Endocrinol Metab*. 2005;90:1929–1935.

57. McKenney JM, Proctor JD, Harris S, Chinchili VM. A comparison of the efficacy and toxic effects of sustained- vs immediate-release niacin in hypercholesterolemic patients. *JAMA*. Mar 2 1994;271(9):672–677.

58. Cruz P Jr, Hud J Jr. Excess insulin binding to insulin-like growth factor receptors: proposed mechanism for acanthosis nigricans. *J Invest Dermatol*. 1992;98:82S.

59. Katz RA. Treatment of acanthosis nigricans with oral isotretinoin. *Arch Dermatol*. 1980;116:110.

60. Pdolsky S. Lipoatrophic diabetes and leprechaunism. In: Podolsky S, Viswanthan M, editors. *The Spectrum of the Diabetic Syndromes*. New York: Raven Press; 1980:335–352.

61. Lawrence RD. Lipodystrophy and hepatomegaly with diabetes, lipemia, and other metabolic disturbances. *Lancet*. 1946;250:724–731.

62. Dunnigan MG. Unusual clinical manifestation of diabetes mellitus. *Practitioner*. 1979;222:321–330.
63. Mabry CC, Hollingsworth DR, Upton CV, Corbin A. Pituitary-hypothalamic dysfunction in generalized lipodystrophy. *Journal of Pediatrics*. 1973;82(4):625–633.
64. Oseid S, Beck-Nielsen H, Pederson O, Sovik O. Decreased binding of insulin to its receptor in patients with congential generalized lipodystrophy. *N Engl J Med*. 1977;296:245–248.
65. Garg A. Lipodystrophies. *Am J Med*. Feb 2000;108(2):143–152.
66. Vantyghem MC, Vigouroux C, Magre J, et al. Late-onset lipoatrophic diabetes. Phenotypic and genotypic familial studies and effect of treatment with metformin and lispro insulin analog. *Diabetes Care*. 1999;22:1374.
67. Oral EA, Simha V, Ruiz E, et al. Leptin-replacement therapy for lipodystrophy. *N Engl J Med*. Feb 21 2002;346(8):570–578.
68. Jelinek JE. The skin in diabetes mellitus: cutaneous manifestations, complications and associations. In: *Year Book of Dermatology, 1970*. Chicago: Year Book Medical Publishers, Inc.; 1970:5–35.
69. Hoerer E, Dreyfuss F, Herzberg M. Carotenemia, skin color and diabetes mellitus. *Acta Diabetol Lat*. 1975;12:202–207.
70. Rapini RP, Herbert AA, Drucker C. Acquired perforating dermatosis: evidence for combined transepidermal elimination of both collagen and elastic fibers. *Arch Dermatol*. 1989;125:1074–1078.
71. Bleich HL, Boro ES. Diabetic polyneuropathy: the importance of insulin deficiency, hyperglycemia and alterations in myoinositol metabolism in its pathogenesis. *N Eng J Med*. 1976;295:1416–1420.
72. Levy DM, Teenghi G, Gu XH. Immunohistochemical measurements of nerves and neuropeptides in diabetic skin: relationship to tests of neurological function. *Diabetologia*. 1992;35:889–897.
73. Max MB, Lynch SA, Muir J, et al. Effects of desipramine, amitriptyline and fluoxetine on pain in diabetic neuropathy. *N Engl J Med*. 1992;326:1250–1256.
74. Ellenberg M. Diabetic foot. *NY State J Med*. 1973;73:2778–2781.
75. Lippman HI, Perotto A, Farrar R. The neuropathic foot of the diabetic. *Bull NY Acad Med*. 1976;52:1159–1178.
76. Jeffcoate WJ, Harding KG. Diabetic foot ulcers. *Lancet*. May 3 2003;361(9368):1545–1551.
77. Editorial. Diabetic foot ulcers. *Lancet*. 1977;1:232–233.
78. Ajam Z, Barton SP, Marks R. Characterization of abnormalities in the cutaneous microvasculature of diabetic subjects. *Br J Dermatol*. 1982;107(Suppl 22):22–23.
79. Huntley AC. Cutaneous manifestations of diabetes mellitus. *Dermatol Clin*. 1989;7:531–546.
80. Grunfeld C. Diabetic foot ulcers: etiology, treatment and prevention. *Adv Intern Med*. 1991;37:103–132.
81. Ditzel J. Functional microangiopathy in diabetes mellitus. *Diabetes*. 1968;17:388–397.
82. Landau J, Davis E. The small blood vessels of the conjunctiva and nailbed in diabetes mellitus. *Lancet*. 1960;2:731–734.
83. Lithner F. Purpura, pigmentation and yellow nails of the lower extremities in diabetes. *Acta Med Scand*. 1976;199:202–208.
84. Lithner J, Hietala SO. Skeletal lesions of the feet in diabetics and their relationship to cutaneous erythema with or without necrosis of the feet. *Acta Med Scand*. 1976;200:155–161.
85. Fitzpatrick TB, et al. *Color Atlas and Synopsis of Clinical Dermatology*. New York: McGraw-Hill; 2001:417–418.
86. Jegasothy BV. Allergic reactions to insulin. *Int J Dermatol*. 1980;19:139–147.
87. Galloway JA, Davidson JK. Clinical use of insulin. In: Rifkin H, Raskin P, editors. *Diabetes Mellitus*. Bowie: RJ Brady Co. vol 5; 1981:117–127.
88. Feinglos MN, Jegasothy BV. "Insulin" allergy due to zinc. *Lancet*. 1979;1:122–124.
89. Galloway JA, Bressler R. Insulin treatment in diabetes. *Med Clin North Am*. 1978;62:663–680.
90. Grammer LC, Metzger BE, Patterson R. Cutaneous allergy to human (recombinant DNA) insulin. *JAMA*. 1984;251: 1459–1460.
91. Edidin DV. Cutaneous manifestations of diabetes mellitus in children. *Pediator Dermatol*. 1985;2:161–179.
92. Ghosh S, McCann V, Bartle L, Collier A, Malik I. Allergy to insulin detemir. *Diabetic Medicine*. 2007;24:1305–1307.
93. Halevy S, Feuerman EJ. Abnormal glucose tolerance associated with lichen planus. *Acta Derm Venereol*. 1979;59:167–170.
94. Albrecht M, Banoczy J, Dinya E, et al. Occurrence of oral leukoplakia and lichen planus in diabetes mellitus. *J Oral Pathol*. 1992;21:364–366.
95. Lamey PJ, Gibson J, Barclay SC, Miller S. Grinspan's syndrome: a drug-induced phenomenon? *Oral Surg Oral Med Oral Pathol*. Aug 1990;70(2):184–185.
96. Muller SA. Dermatologic disorders associated with diabetes mellitus. *Mayo clin Proc*. 1966;41:689–703.
97. Pinkus H, Mehregan AH. *A Guide to Dermatohistopathology*. New York: Appleton-Century-Crofts; 1976:417.
98. Chevrant-Breton J, Simon M, Bourel M, Ferrand B. Cutaneous manifestations of idiopathic hemochromatosis. *Arch Dermatol*. 1977;113:161–165.
99. Kahana M, Grossman E, Feinstein A, et al. Skin tags: a cutaneous marker for diabetes mellitus. *Acta Derm Venereol*. 1986;67:175–177.
100. Demir S, Demir Y. Acrochordon and impaired carbohydrate metabolism. *Acta Diabetol*. Jun 2002;39(2):57–59.
101. Rasi A, Soltani-Arabshahi R, Shahbazi N. Skin tag as a cutaneous marker for impaired carbohydrate metabolism: a case-control study. *Int J Dermatol*. 2007;46:1155–1159.
102. Celestin R, Brown J, Kihiczak G, Schwartz RA. Erysipelas; a common potentially dangerous infection. *Acta Dermatoven APA*. 2007;16(3):123–127.
103. Morgan AJ, Schwartz RA. Diabetic dermopathy: a subtle sign with grave implications. *J Am Acad Dermatol*. [Epub ahead of print] 2007.

Part VII
Related Disorders

Chapter 30
Obesity – Genetics, Pathogenesis, Therapy

William C. Hsu, Kalliopi M. Arampatzi, and Christos S. Mantzoros

Introduction

The prevalence of obesity is increasing at alarming rates across all sociodemographic groups in industrialized and developing nations alike. Obesity poses a tremendous clinical challenge, as it contributes to significant morbidity and mortality and carries a staggering economic cost. In this chapter, we examine the current understanding of the epidemiology, etiology, pathophysiology, and treatment of obesity.

Definition and Measurement of Obesity

Obesity is formally defined as an excess of fat mass resulting from the chronic accumulation and storage of excess energy. Although accurate methods of determining the quantity of body fat (including underwater densitometry, dual-energy x-ray absorptiometry, total body water estimate, total body potassium measurement, and bioelectrical impedance) have been developed, for practical purposes obesity is classified according to the body mass index (BMI), a ratio of weight in kilograms over height in meters squared. Overweight is defined as a BMI of 25–29.9 kg/m^2 and class I obesity as a BMI of 30–34.9 kg/m^2, class II obesity as a BMI of 35–39.9 kg/m^2; and class III obesity as a BMI of >40 kg/m^2. For children and adolescents, overweight is defined as a body mass index for age at or above the 95th percentile of a specified reference population.

A quarter of the American adults are obese[1] and approximately 60% of US adults are either overweight or obese. Minority populations and those with low incomes or low education are especially susceptible. However, in the past decade, an increase was observed in all ages, genders, races, and educational levels with the highest magnitude of rise in those who are in their twenties, those with some college education, and those of Hispanic ethnicity.[2] More importantly, almost a quarter of the children and adolescents between ages 6 through 17 years are overweight and many have already developed obesity-related complications, such as type 2 diabetes.

Increasing prevalence of obesity has been a worldwide phenomenon, and it is estimated that obesity and its complications, including diabetes, will be the epidemic of the twenty first century.[3]

Consequences of Obesity

Obesity now exceeds smoking and poverty as the leading health risk in the United States and is linked to the development of many chronic diseases (Table 30.1). In general, higher BMIs are associated with higher risk of developing obesity-related comorbidities, as well as with a direct role in shortening life expectancy, especially among subjects who develop obesity early in life.[4] For example, a woman with a BMI of 25 has a 5-fold relative

W.C. Hsu (✉)
Joslin Diabetes Center, Harvard Medical School, Boston, MA, USA
e-mail: cmantzor@bidmc.harvard.edu

L. Poretsky (ed.), *Principles of Diabetes Mellitus*, DOI 10.1007/978-0-387-09841-8_30,
© Springer Science+Business Media, LLC 2010

Table 30.1 Medical morbidities associated with obesity

Cardiovascular	*Pulmonary*
Congestive heart failure	Hypoventilation syndrome
Coronary heart disease	Sleep apnea
Dyslipidemia	
Hypertension	*Endocrine*
Proinflammatory state	Diabetes – type 2
	Gestational diabetes
Gynecological/Obstetrical	Hirsutism
Breast cancer	
Endometrial cancer	*Renal*
Complications of pregnancy	Renal cell cancer
Menstrual irregularities	
Polycystic ovary syndrome	*Gastrointestinal*
	Colon cancer
Cerebrovascular	Gallstones
Stroke	Gall bladder cancer
Musculoskeletal	*Urologic*
Osteoarthritis	Prostate cancer
Gout	Stress incontinence
Dermatologic	
Abdominal striae	
Acanthosis nigricans	

risk of developing type 2 diabetes than a woman with a BMI of less than 22; a 28-fold higher risk, if the BMI is increased to 30; and a 93-fold higher risk with a BMI of 35 or greater.[5] All-cause mortality rises from a BMI nadir of just below 25 kg/m^2 and escalates at a BMI above 30 kg/m^2, accounting for approximately 280,000–325,000 deaths annually in the United States.[6]

Obesity is a highly stigmatized disease. Negative attitudes toward the obese are common and are evident in employment, marriage, and educational opportunities.[7] Furthermore, obese patients often experience discrimination from their health care providers, and are less likely to receive preventive care, including screening for cervical and breast cancer.

Given the emphasis on being slim in our society, nearly 40% of Americans attempt to lose weight at any given time, a phenomenon translated into a 30 billion dollar diet industry. Furthermore, the direct medical cost for treating obesity-related diseases was estimated to be 51.6 billion in 1995. Combined with the economic value of productivity lost due to obesity-related morbidity and mortality, the total economic burden of obesity amounts to a staggering 100 billion dollars per year.[8]

Etiolology of Obesity

Obesity results from complex interactions between genetic factors and environmental influences. Adoption studies suggest that the BMIs of the adoptees have stronger correlations with the BMIs of the biologic parents, than with that of the adoptive parents. Furthermore, twin studies have shown that identical twins, even when reared apart, have BMIs that are more tightly correlated than fraternal twins. Overall, the genetic contribution to BMI has been estimated to be between 50 and 90%.[9] In addition to long recognized genetic syndromes (Table 30.2), such as Prader–Willi, Cohen, and Bardet–Biedl, several monogenic defects due to genetic mutations in the locus of leptin, leptin receptor,[10] proopiomelanocortin (POMC) or other enzymes, and neuropeptides have recently been recognized as important causes of obesity (Table 30.3).[11] However, they explain only a distinct minority of common obesity. For example, mutations of the melanocortin-4 (MC4) receptor,[12] which, despite the fact that available data are limited, are considered to be one of the most prevalent mutations responsible for monogenic

Table 30.2 Genetic syndromes

1. Albright Hereditary Osterodystrophy (short stature, round facies, brachydactyly, ectopic soft tissue ossification, resistance to several hormones including PTH)
2. Alström (diabetes mellitus, insulin resistance, neurosensory deficits, subset with dilated cardiomyopathy, hepatic dysfunction, hypothyroidism, male hypogonadism, short stature, mild to moderate developmental delay)
3. Bardet–Biedl (mental retardation, dysmorphic extremities, retinal dystrophy or pigmentary retinopathy, hypogonadism or hypogenitalism [male], renal abnormalities)
4. Borjeson-Forssman-Lehmann (mental retardation, epilepsy, hypogonadism, gynecomastia)
5. Carpenter (mental retardation, male hypogonadism, acrocephaly, polydactyly, syndactyly)
6. Cohen (mental retardation, microcephaly, characteristic facial features, progressive retinochoroidal dystrophy)
7. Fragile X (mental retardation, macroorchidism, large ears, macrocephaly, prominent jaw, high-pitched speech)
8. Prader–Willi (diminished fetal activity, hypotonia, mental retardation, short stature, central hypogonadism)
9. Ulnar-Mammary (developmental abnormalities in limbs, teeth, hair, apocrine glands, and genitalia)
10. WAGR (Wilm's tumor, anorexia, ambiguous genitalia, mental retardation)

Table 30.3 Monogenic disorders

  i. Leptin deficiency
 ii. POMC deficiency
iii. Prohormone convertase 1 mutation
 iv. Human MC4R deficiency
  v. Mutation in the Neurotrophin receptor TrkB

obesity known to date, are found in approximately 4–5% of obese children and/or adults with a BMI above 40 kg/m^2.

Given the relative rarity of the above as causes of obesity, it has recently been suggested that in the majority of obese subjects the genetic contribution is due to the effect of multiple genes acting in concert, i.e., that obesity is a "polygenic" disease state. For example, loci on the *FTO* (fat mass and obesity) gene on chromosome 16 have recently been directly associated with body mass index, obesity, and consequently type 2 diabetes.[13,14] It is expected that, in this respect, more genes will be discovered in the future.

Moreover, the rapidly rising prevalence of obesity in the last decades strongly suggests that environmental factors also play an important role since our genetic makeup has not been altered significantly during this short period. In this regard, recently published data linking obesity with social networks, underline the effect of the interactions between environmental and social factors on food intake and energy expenditure and, as a result, obesity.[15] Given the availability of dense caloric food served in ever-larger portions, it is surprising that the correlation between dietary intake and obesity has not been firmly established. In contrast, physical inactivity strongly predicts weight gain in both cross-sectional and longitudinal studies.[16] Other environmental factors, such as smoking cessation and drugs, may also contribute to obesity in susceptible individuals. Smoking cessation is associated with an average weight gain of 3–5 kg due to an increase in appetite and a decline in metabolic rate.[17] Medications, such as tricyclic antidepressants, phenothiazines, and certain selective serotonin receptor inhibitors (SSRI) such as paroxetine, are commonly associated with weight gain. Among neuroleptic drugs, "atypical" antipyschotic agents appear to cause greater weight gain than conventional agents[18] (Table 30.4). However, two atypical antipsychotic agents, aripiprazol and ziprasidone, are considered weight neutral, do not increase risk for diabetes, and/or do not worsen lipid profile.[19]

Table 30.4 Common drugs that increase weight

Antipsychotic
Atypical neuroleptics (clozapine, olanzapine, risperidone, quetiapine)
Conventional neuroleptics
    a. Phenothiazines (e.g., chlorpromazine , thioridazine)
    b. Butyrophenones (e.g., haloperidol)

Antidepressant
MAO inhibitors[a] (e.g., phenelzine)
Lithium
Trazadone
Tricyclics (e.g., amitryptyline, immipramine, desipramine)
SSRIs[a] (e.g., paroxetine)
a-2 antagonist (e.g., mitrazapine)

Antiepileptic
Carbamazepine
Valproic Acid
Gabapentin

Antidiabetic
Insulin
Sulfonylurea
Thiazolidinediones

Steroids
Corticosteroids
Megesterol acetate

Others
Hormonal contraceptives
Progestational agents
Antihistamines
β-blockers (e.g., propranolol), α-blockers (e.g., terazosin)

[a]MAO inhibitors = Monoamine Oxidase Inhibitors, SSRIs = Selective
Serotonin Reuptake Inhibitors

Mechanisms Underlying Weight Regulation

Our understanding of the system integrating genetic and environmental factors to regulate energy homeostasis has been greatly advanced by the discovery of leptin, the 167-amino acid product of *ob* gene, discovered in 1994 by positional cloning using the leptin-deficient *ob/ob* mouse model of obesity.[20] Leptin, an anorexigenic hormone mainly produced by adipocytes, is a member of the cytokine family. Leptin circulates in both free and bound form. Serum leptin levels increase exponentially with an increase in fat mass and decrease in response to food deprivation and low fat mass.[21] Leptin acts by crossing the blood-brain barrier to bind to specific receptors in the hypothalamus that in turn modulate the expression of orexigenic and anorexigenic neuropeptides responsible for regulating appetite and energy expenditure. For example, the binding of hypothalamic leptin receptors downregulates the anabolic pathways by inhibiting the expression of orexigenic neuropeptides, including neuropeptides Y (NPY) and agouti-related protein (AgRP), and upregulates the catabolic pathways by stimulating the expression of anorexigenic neuropeptides such as melanocyte stimulating hormone (α-MSH), corticotropin-releasing hormone (CRH), and cocaine-and amphetamine-regulated transcript (CART) in the hypothalamus [22] (Table 30.5) (Fig. 30.1). In contrast, inhibition of the leptin system, in response to energy deprivation, results in stimulation of appetite, activation of the pituitary-adrenal axis to mobilize energy stores and suppression of both the pituitary-hypothalamic-thyroidal and gonadal axis as well as thermogenesis.[23] The net outcome is a coordinated effort to restore energy balance and return the body to its initial weight. Activation of the leptin system also affects energy expenditure through the stimulation of the sympathetic autonomic nervous system in mice and has recently been linked with the activation of uncoupling protein (UCP-1) in the mitochondria of brown

Table 30.5 Hypothalamic neuropeptides regulating appetite

Anorexigenic	Orexigenic
α-MSH (alpha-melanocyte stimulating hormone)[a]	AGRP (agouti-related protein)[a]
CART (cocaine amphetamine-regulated transcript)[a]	Galanin
CNTF (ciliary neurotrophic factor)	Ghrelin[a]
CRH (corticotrophin-releasing hormone)[a]	MCH (melanin-concentrating hormone)
GLP-1 (glucagon-like peptide-1)[a]	Noradrenaline
Serotonin	NPY (neuropeptide-Y)[a]
TRH (thyrotropin releasing hormone)[a]	Orexin

[a]Indicates neuropeptides modulated by leptin action

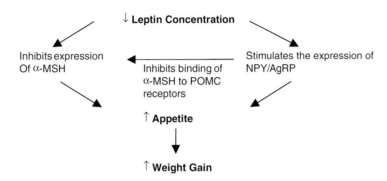

Fig. 30.1 Decreased leptin concentration activates the orexigenic pathway (NPY/AgRP) in the arcuate nucleus and concurrently inhibits the anorexigenic pathway (α-MSH and POMC neurons), together resulting in an increase in food intake

adipose tissue in mice and of muscle and fat (UCP-2, UCP-3) in humans.[24] In the animal models, UCP uncouples the cellular oxidation of fuels from the generation of ATP, thereby releasing food energy in the form of heat, a process also known as thermogenesis. The sympathetic nervous system appears to activate thermogenesis by stimulating the beta-adrenergic receptors. Specifically, treatment of multiple animal species with selective agonist of the beta-3 adrenergic receptors caused an increase in energy expenditure. Whether the resulting alterations in thermogenesis are effective for weight loss in human remains the focus of intense investigation.

To a certain extent interacting with the leptin system, monoamine neurotransmitters have long been recognized to modulate food intake.[25] The serotonin pathway has traditionally been the target of several antiobesity drugs that increase serotoninergic signaling and suppress food intake. The stimulation of serotonin (HT) receptors, particularly the 5-HT$_{2c}$ receptors, decreases food intake, and the knock out of this receptor in rodents results in modest obesity. Stimulation of the noradrenergic receptors in the paraventricular nuclei or other hypothalamic areas contributes to hyperphagia and has been the target of current amphetamine-based anorexic agents. Similarly, the stimulation of dopaminergic (Dop) receptors in the dorsomedial and arcuate nuclei of the hypothalamus decreases food intake whereas mesolimbic dopaminergic pathways may be involved in the pleasurable aspects of feeding. Moreover, pharmacologic depletion and genetic disruption of the dopaminergic pathways results in profound feeding deficits.

In addition, several hormones secreted by the gastrointestinal tract such as glucagon-like peptide-1 (GLP-1) and Ghrelin as well as pancreatic hormones such as amylin and pancreatic polypeptide may also play very important roles in energy homeostasis, by providing input from the gastrointestinal tract and the pancreas to CNS centers regulating energy homeostasis. These molecules and/or their analogues are now being tested in clinical trials in humans.

Despite clear evidence linking obesity and its complications, such as hypertension and type 2 diabetes, the mechanism by which obesity is related to insulin resistance remains largely elusive. Adipocyte secreted factors, such as leptin and tumor necrosis factor-α, have traditionally been considered to be the mediators of metabolic comorbidities associated with obesity whereas recent data indicate that reduced production of adiponectin,[21,26]

Table 30.6 Conditions associated with obesity

Endocrine
Polycystic ovary syndrome (women)
Hypogonadism
Hypothyroidism/hyperthyroidism
Cushing's syndrome
Insulinoma
Growth hormone deficiency

Hypothalamic
Injuries
Infections
Tumors
Infiltrative disease

a recently discovered adipocyte secreted hormone, may also be potential link between obesity and the development of insulin resistance and diabetes.

Evaluation of Obese Patients

Despite the fact that physicians have unique opportunities to play a major role in the prevention and treatment of obesity, concerns about drug safety, the lack of a permanently effective treatment and poor reimbursement have contributed to reluctance of physicians to treat obesity.

BMI is most frequently utilized for the clinical evaluation of obese patients, but it overestimates adiposity in individuals with very short stature or very muscular built and underestimates it in the elderly due to loss of lean body mass. It has also been proposed that abdominal obesity, independent of body weight, maybe a stronger predictor for the development of coronary heart disease. In certain populations, such as Asian Americans, waist circumference may correlate better with morbidity or mortality than the currently established cutoff points for BMI. While a waist circumference of >94 cm in men or >80 cm in women confers increased health risks, when the waist circumference reaches 102 cm in men and 88 cm in women, intervention is definitely justified.[27]

In addition to quantifying the degree of obesity, patient's motivation, expectations, and adherence pattern should also be carefully assessed. Obtaining a dietary, smoking, and activity history, screening for psychiatric disorders, eating disorders, and depression are integral parts of the evaluation. Identifying physical features suggestive of secondary causes of obesity (Table 30.6), and detecting and quantifying obesity-related comorbidities including diabetes, hyperlipidemia, or hypertension are important components of a comprehensive assessment. Finally, since the use of drug therapy for weight loss is contraindicated in pregnancy, a pregnancy test should be considered and contraception recommended for every woman of child-bearing age considering pharmacological therapy.

Establishing Weight Goals

Despite initial success, almost all weight loss is regained within 3–5 years of completing treatment in more than 90% of treated patients. This common occurrence underlies much of the frustration and fatalism of both patients and clinicians towards obesity treatment, especially when the goal for weight loss has been to achieve ideal body weight. Yet, a weight reduction as little as 5–10% body weight significantly improves blood pressure, lipids, body fat distribution, insulin resistance, and glycemic control and may be easier to maintain;[28] therefore, it represents a better goal from the medical point of view. Finally, modest weight loss prevents the development of osteoarthritis and hypertension in normotensive obese subjects and improves the quality of life. Since obesity is a chronic condition, the goal for treatment is not only to reduce weight but also to maintain the reduced weight with the ultimate aim of improving overall health. Given that many obese individuals lose weight for cosmetic reasons, convincing them to set a realistic weight goal and to continue treatment indefinitely is very challenging but also imperative.

Current Treatment Options

Obesity is a chronic disease and requires lifelong treatment. Lifestyle modification should be encouraged in all patients who are overweight or obese and specific recommendations[29] have been developed to aid clinicians in the appropriate use of pharmacotherapy or bariatric surgery.

In general, lifestyle modification (diet and exercise) is recommended for all individuals with a BMI >25 kg/m^2. Patients with BMI >30 kg/m^2 or >27 kg/m^2 with comorbidities (e.g., diabetes, dyslipidemia, hypertension, cardiovascular disease, sleep apnea) are eligible for pharmacotherapy. For severely obese patients with BMI of >40 kg/m^2 or BMI > 35 kg/m^2 with serious comorbidities and acceptable operative risks who failed previous weight loss attempts, bariatric surgery is indicated.

Dietary Therapy

All randomized, controlled studies have documented the efficacy of caloric restriction in weight loss but it remains to be conclusively shown whether food composition has an impact on weight loss as long as calories are fixed. In general, a deficit of 500 kcal/day will result in a weight loss of 1/2 to 1 lb per week. Although for subjects with a BMI greater than 35, a higher caloric deficit of 500–1000 kcal/day may be required, a low calorie diet (LCD), defined as consumption of 1000–1500 kcal/day, generally results in a mean of 8–10% weight reduction during a period of 6–12 months. A very low caloric diet (VLCD), i.e., 400–800 kcal/day, produces rapid and significant weight loss during the initial phase but is contraindicated in patients with cardiovascular, hepatic, renal disease, and those with eating disorders. It does not achieve a greater weight loss than LCD at 1 year, is associated with high attrition rate and higher cost, and may be associated with nutritional deficiency, electrolyte imbalance, gout, gallstones, and cardiac complications including sudden death.[30]

Exercise Therapy

Exercise, when combined with dietary therapy, results in more weight loss than with either therapy alone but most obese patients find it difficult to start a regular exercise program until they have lost first some weight from dieting. In addition to the maintenance of weight loss and the prevention of further weight gain, increasing physical activity results in reduction of abdominal fat, increase in cardiorespiratory fitness, and improvement in insulin resistance. Before initiating exercise in obese patients, musculoskeletal and cardiovascular risks must be carefully considered and the intensity and duration should be increased gradually up to the goal of 30 min of moderate-intensity physical activity (i.e., walking at 3–4 mph) every day, a recommendation endorsed by the Surgeon General, National Institutes of Health and American Heart Association.

Behavior Therapy

Techniques and methodologies designed to improve weight management involve accountability and support through group sessions, keeping food diaries and exercise logs to document caloric intake and energy expenditure, stress management to prevent adverse behaviors that lead to weight gain, and stimulus control, and cognitive restructuring that deals with constructing an appropriate self-image and setting realistic weight goal. Behavior strategies, designed to reinforce dietary and exercise treatment, generally produce about a 10% reduction in weight within 1 year. The fear of weight gain may also be an important barrier to smoke cessation, especially among women and teenage smokers, but the emphasis should be placed on the overwhelming health benefits of quitting smoking over the risks associated with the weight gained during cessation.[31]

Drug Therapy

At current development, the role of pharmacotherapy remains supportive to lifestyle modification.[32] If 6-months of lifestyle modification fails to produce adequate weight loss, pharmacotherapy should be considered in patients with a BMI >30 or a BMI between 27 and 29.9 kg/m^2 with coexisting comorbidities such as hypertension, hyperlipidemia, coronary heart disease, type 2 diabetes, and sleep apnea. Currently, the FDA has approved two medications in U.S., orlistat and sibutramine, for long-term obesity treatment, but the safety and added efficacy of combination drug therapy, although theoretically plausible, has not yet been tested in large randomized trials.

Orlistat

Orlistat (Xenical) is a pentanoic acid ester that inhibits reversibly pancreatic and gastric lipase. Therefore, about 30% of ingested dietary fat is excreted instead of hydrolyzed to fatty acids and glycerol before they are absorbed. The current recommended dose is 120 mg three times a day with meals and can be omitted if a meal is skipped. In the first meta-analysis of 22 randomized trials that used orlistat in addition to dietary interventions and reported 1 year data,[33] the orlistat treated group had an average placebo subtracted weight loss of 2.9 kg. By the end of the second year, orlistat treatment results in a smaller weight regain than the placebo group and in a 1-year trial greater weight maintenance after dieting. Other studies have shown beneficial effects on low-density lipoprotein cholesterol, insulin levels, and abdominal circumference as well as significant improvement in glycemic control in diabetes.

Orlistat is minimally absorbed and generally well tolerated but is contraindicated in chronic malabsorption, cholestasis, and hypersensitivity reaction to its components. Flatulence and steatorrhea are the most common adverse effects and absorption of fat-soluble vitamins may be slightly reduced. Thus, vitamin supplementation is recommended at least 2 h before or after taking orlistat to avoid malabsorption. The amount of initial weight loss predicts the long-term response. Thus, patients who fail to lose at least 4 lbs after 4–8 weeks of treatment can be considered treatment failures and the medication can be stopped at that time.

Sibutramine

Sibutramine reduces food intake by selectively inhibiting postsynaptic norepinephrine and serotonin reuptake and to a lesser degree dopaminergic reuptake, whereas earlier drugs such as fenfluramine and dexfenfluramine increased serotonin release. This agent is available in 5, 10, and 15 mg tablets, with a usual initial starting dose of 10 mg and titration up accordingly. In a large randomized multicenter trial lasting 24 weeks, sibutramine was shown to produce weight loss in a dose dependent fashion, ranging from 6.1 up to 9.4% reduction of initial weight.[34] Use of sibutramine for 2 years showed that 43% of the sibutramine-hypocaloric diet group maintained 80% or more of their original weight loss compared in contrast to 16% in the hypocaloric group alone.[35] Sibutramine is also helpful in decreasing and maintaining long-term weight loss achieved by VLCD (220–800 kcal/day).

The use of sibutramine is contraindicated in patients with arrhythmias, coronary artery disease, stroke, congestive heart failure, and poorly controlled hypertension, as well as in patients taking monoamine oxidase inhibitors or selective serotonin reuptake inhibitors. Sibutramine has been associated with a small increase of diastolic blood pressure compared with the placebo group and a small increase in the pulse rate. Common side effects of sibutramine are dry mouth, headache, anorexia, constipation, and insomnia and are mostly related to sympathomimetic properties of the drug. Similar to orlistat the initial weight loss can predict the long-term response. Thus, patients who fail to lose at least 4 lbs after 4–8 weeks of treatment can be considered treatment failures and the medication can be stopped at that time.

Table 30.7 Drugs that have weight loss effect

Serotoninergic	*Pancreatic lipase inhibitor*
Dexfenfluramine	Orlistat[a]
Fenfluramine	
Fluoxetine	*Hormone*
	Thyroxine
Sympathomimetic	
Benzphetamine [a,b]	*Antidiabetic*
Bupropion	*Metformin*
Diethylpropion[a,b]	
Ephedrine	
Mazindol[a,b]	
Phendimetrazine [a,b]	
Phenopropanolamine	
Phentermine[a,b]	
Sibutramine[a]	

[a]Indicates drugs approved by the FDA for weight loss
[b]Indicates drug enforcement agency (DEA) scheduled drugs

Rimonabant

Rimonabant acts as a selective antagonist of the CB1 cannabinoid receptor. According to recent studies this agent demonstrates beneficial effects on waist circumference and metabolic parameters, including HDL and triglyceride levels, with no or minimal effects on LDL or blood pressure. Its most common adverse effects include nausea, dizziness, and depression. Although this medication has been approved in Europe, approval has not been granted in the USA.

Other Agents

Anorexants (phentermine, diethylpropion) currently scheduled as controlled substances, stimulate the adrenergic system by either inhibiting postsynaptic reuptake of norepinephrine or by directly stimulating the presynaptic release of noreprinephrine. These agents are indicated only for short-term use (up to 3 months) and are limited by development of tolerance, whereas weight regain is common after discontinuation of their use.

Fenfluramine and dexfenfluramine cause valvular heart disease and pulmonary hypertension resulting in their withdrawal from the market. Phenylpropanolamine, an over-the-counter product for nasal congestion resulting in appetite suppression, was recently linked to the development of hemorrhagic stroke and is being withdrawn from the market. Ephedrine and caffeine induce weight loss by stimulating thermogenesis. Psychotropic medications acting as 5-HT$_{1b}$, 5-HT$_{2c}$, and Dop-2 receptor agonists or as selective serotonin reuptake inhibitors, such as fluoxetine, have weight reducing effects but their action may not be sustainable in the long term. Thyroxine stimulates thermogenesis and reduces body fat but should not be used as an antiobesity agent since it also leads to significant side effects, including the loss of lean body mass, the development of cardiac arrhythmias, and osteoporosis. Metformin, an insulin sensitizer, induces anorexia and some weight loss in humans but, due to its rather limited weight reducing effect and potential side effects, its use as antiobesity agent in the nondiabetic population is not advocated. See Table 30.7 for a list of drugs with weight loss effect.

Diet and currently available pharmacotherapies result in significant improvements in insulin resistance and cardiovascular risk factors. Long-term data on other obesity comorbidities and/or mortality are needed.

Surgical Therapy

Individuals with a BMI exceeding 40 or between 35 and 40 with comorbidities are potential candidates for bariatric surgery after careful evaluation by a multidisciplinary team including internist, surgeon, nutritionist, and psychiatrist.

There are two major categories of weight loss surgery: gastric restriction and intestinal malabsorption techniques. Restrictive operations create a small neogastric pouch and a gastric outlet and reduce body weight by decreasing food intake. Malabsortive procedures aim at rearranging the small intestine in order to decrease the functional length or efficiency of the intestinal mucosa for nutrient absorption. Although the malabsortive approach produces more rapid and profound weight loss than restrictive methods, it is currently less commonly performed since it also poses risks of metabolic complications, such as vitamin deficiencies and protein–energy malnutrition.[36]

Gastric restriction or gastroplasty involves stapling or banding the stomach to decrease the storage capacity of the stomach by constructing a small proximal reservoir with outlet restriction (Fig. 30.1). Gastric bypass involves the partitioning of the stomach by stapling, with an outlet formed by a loop of small intestine proceeding from the proximal stomach, bypassing the distal stomach, duodenum, and proximal portion of jejunum (Roux-en-Y) (Fig. 30.1). Biliopancreatic Diversion (BPD) is a malabsortive procedure in which a distal gastrectomy and Roux-en-Y configuration is created with a short common limb. It is effective in inducing weight loss particularly in "super obese" patients (BMI >50 kg/m^2), but it is also associated with significant complications.[37,38] Also, sleeve gastrectomy, although new, is a procedure currently used as a bridge for surgery in patients with super extreme obesity (BMI >50 kg/m^2).

Long-term weight loss with gastric bypass procedure is considered generally superior. With rapid advances in minimally invasive surgery, laparoscopic gastric bypass may become the procedure of choice in selected patients. Currently, the immediate operative mortality rate has been estimated to be approximately 1%, and early postoperative complications, such as wound infections, deep thrombophlebitis, and pulmonary complications can be as high as 10%.[39] After discharge from the hospital, most patients are maintained on liquid diet initially, and are gradually advanced to a full diet. In addition to behavioral modification, exercise, and dietary counseling, medical follow-up should be regularly scheduled postoperatively, to monitor for the development of nutrient deficiencies (B12, folate, iron), depression, gastritis, anastomotic ulcer, and cholelithiasis.

Bariatric surgery can achieve an average of excess weight reduction of 50% as far as 10 years after surgery. Maximum weight loss is reached approximately 2 years after the operation with significant amount of patients experiencing resolution of the type 2 diabetes, hypertension, hypertriglyceridemia, and obesity hypoventilation syndrome. However, 20–25% of the patients experience weight loss failures mostly due to dietary indiscretion and insufficient follow-up (Fig. 30.2)

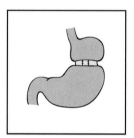 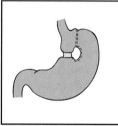 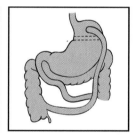

Fig. 30.2 Common procedures of bariatric surgery. *Left* – gastric banding. *Middle* – vertical banded gastroplasty. *Right* – Gastric bypass (Roux-en-Y)

Recently published studies provide valuable information on the long-term effect of weight loss on mortality. One prospective, controlled, interventional study suggests that bariatric surgery (including gastric bypass, vertical banded gastroplasty, and banding) for severe obesity results in long-term weight loss and is associated with decreased overall mortality.[40] According to another recently published retrospective cohort study total mortality after gastric bypass surgery is significantly reduced during a mean follow-up of 7.1 years (overall 40%, 37.6 vs. 57.1 deaths per 10,000 person-years). Reduced mortality is mainly due to decreased death rates from coronary artery disease (56%, 2.6 vs. 5.9 per 10,000 person-years), diabetes (92%, 0.4 vs. 3.4 per 10,000 person-years), and cancer (60%, 5.5 vs. 13.3 per 10,000 person-years), although the rate of death from causes other than disease (such as accidents or suicide) was higher in the surgery group than in the control group (58%, 11.1 vs. 6.4 per 10,000 person-years).[41] Study limitations discussed in these papers in combination with the complex nature of obesity and the multitude of weight loss methods currently available emphasize the need for more intensive research, data accumulation and analyses, as well as further long-term follow-up studies.

Finally, the overwhelming majority of studies have found that bariatric surgery improves quality of life. In general, improvements in psychosocial markers correspond to the magnitude of weight loss, but it has been suggested that the socioeconomic impact of morbid obesity persists long after a reduction in weight and improvement in quality of life.[42]

Future Directions

New advances in understanding the mechanisms regulating body weight have intensified research efforts and are expected to lead to the development of new treatment options for obesity in the near future.

Leptin and Leptin Analogs

Although leptin administration has been effective in the limited subjects with absolute leptin deficiency resulting in morbid obesity, common obesity is believed to be associated with high leptin levels and leptin resistance.[43] The apparent resistance may be related to a defect in leptin transport through the brain–blood barrier, binding defect to its receptors, over-expression of hypothalamic inhibitors of leptin action or defective signaling pathways downstream of leptin receptor.

Thus, the majority of human obesity is a leptin resistant state. Therefore, efforts to overcome leptin resistance focus on designing leptin agonists that have higher potency, longer serum half-life and ability to cross the blood–brain barrier easier.

Hypothalamic Neuropeptides

The successful weight loss effects in animal models targeting anorexigenic pathways downstream of the leptin receptor by using melanocortin receptor agonists, such as α-MSH or novel MC3R and MC4R agonists, have generated much interest for their potential use in humans. Alternatively, inhibitors of centrally acting orexigenic molecules, such as AGRP, melanin-concentrating hormone, orexin, opioid receptors, and ghrelin are being studied for their potential pharmacological value.

Peripheral Satiety Signals

Molecules such as cholecystokinin, bombesin, amylin, PYY, and glucagon-like peptide-1 that are secreted by the gastrointestinal tract convey satiety signals to the brain. Their analogues may also have suppressive effects on appetite and may be effective against obesity but development of most of these agents is still in the preclinical phase. Medications like long acting GLP-1 analogues (e.g., exanetide, liraglutide) amylin analogues (e.g., pramlintide) decrease body weight when used for the treatment of diabetes. In contrast, inhibitors of dipeptidyl peptidase IV (DPP IV), the enzyme that breaks down GLP-1, cause normal, but no higher than normal circulating GLP-1 levels, and thus do not alter body weight, despite their beneficial effect on diabetes.

Fat Absorption and Metabolism

Blocking molecules in fat digestion or absorption, such as fatty acid transporters in the intestine, or using energy-free substitutes, such as olestra, may reduce contribution of dietary fat to weight gain. Another strategy currently being exploited by pharmaceutical companies is to design drugs that inactivate key molecules in fat metabolism.

Thermogenesis

To increase energy expenditure through heat loss, specific beta-3 adrenergic receptor agonists have been tested in multiple animal species and are currently being evaluated for use in humans, whereas the development of drugs that enhance the expression of uncoupling proteins involved in dissipation of energy to heat is still in very early phases.

The Look AHEAD Study

Despite all the above recent developments, uncertainty still exists with respect to the optimal efficacy and cost-effectiveness of currently available treatments and/or combinations thereof.

A national multicenter clinical trial, the "Look AHEAD" study, currently examines the long-term effects of an intensive lifestyle intervention program designed to achieve and maintain weight loss by decreasing caloric intake and increasing physical activity, along with use of approved medications as appropriate, in overweight volunteers with type 2 diabetes. Although primary outcomes of the study include cardiovascular morbidity and mortality, important information on other complications of diabetes and obesity is also collected. Results of this large, multicenter trial are expected to provide important insights into the efficacy and cost-effectiveness of currently available treatment options for obesity among patients with diabetes.

Summary

Obesity, a chronic disease, has reached epidemic proportions, is associated with overwhelming morbidity, mortality, and health care costs. Human and animal studies reveal that energy homeostasis is tightly regulated by highly redundant and complex systems of neuropeptides and neuropathways modulating appetite and energy expenditure. The unmasking of latent genetic predisposition for energy conservation brought on by environmental factors that promote inactivity and high calorie diet is largely responsible for the explosive rise in obesity in recent years. Current treatment options, though limited, are effective in reducing health risks associated with obesity A comprehensive clinical evaluation and setting realistic goals of weight loss are the cornerstones of treatment of obese patients since even a modest weight reduction of 5–10% provides significant health benefits and is reasonably attainable and sustainable. Dietary changes, exercise, behavior modification, pharmacotherapy, and surgical therapy are useful tools to achieve this goal, but require lifelong efforts to maintain the reduced body weight. As we are entering a new era in understanding the mechanisms of weight regulation, new discoveries hold promise for the development of novel therapeutic agents that will eventually provide tangible benefits to those who are struggling to control excessive body weight.

References

1. Flegal KM, Carroll MD, Kuczmarski RJ, Johnson CL. Overweight and obesity in the United States: prevalence and trends. *Int J Obes Relat Metab Disord*. 1998;22:39–47.
2. Mokdad AH, Serdula MK, Dietz WH, Bowman BA, Marks JS, Koplan JP. The Spread of the obesity epidemic in the United States. 1991–1998. *J Am Med Assoc*. 1999;282:1519–1522.
3. Ogden CL, Yanovski SZ, Carrol MD, Flegal KM. The epidemiology of obesity. *Gastroenterology*. May 2007;132(6):2087–2102.
4. Fontaine KR, Redden DT, Wang C, et al. Years of life lost due to obesity. *J Am Med Assoc*. 2003;289:187–193.
5. Colditz GA, Willett WC, Rotnitzky A, Manson JE. Weight gain as a risk factor for clinical diabetes mellitus in women. *Ann Intern Med*. 1995;122:481–486.
6. Allison DB, Fontaine KR, Manson JE, Stevens J, VanItallie TB. Annual deaths attributable to obesity in the United States. *J Am Med Assoc*. 1999;282:1530–1538.
7. Gortmaker SL, Must A, Perrin JM, Sobol AM, Dietz WH. Social and economic consequences of overweight in adolescence and young adulthood. *N Engl J Med*. 1993;329:1008–1012.
8. Wolf AM, Colditz GA. Current estimates of the economic cost of obesity in the United States. *Obes Res*. 1998;6:97–106.

9. Maes HH, Neale MC, Eaves LJ. Genetic and environmental factors in relative body weight and human adiposity. *Behav Genet.* 1997;27(4):325–351.

10. Faraoqi IS, Wangensteen T, Collins S, et al. Clinical and molecular genetic spectrum of congenital deficiency of the leptin receptor. *N Engl J Med.* 2007;356:237–247.

11. Farooqi S, O'Rahily S. Genetics of obesity in humans. *Endocr Rev.* 2006;27(7):710–718.

12. Farooqi IS, Keogh JM, Yeo GS, Lank EJ, Chetam T, O'Rahilly S. Clinical spectrum of obesity and mutations in the melanocortin 4 receptor gene. *N Engl J Med.* 2003;348:1085–1095.

13. Hampton T. Common gene variant linked to obesity. *J Am Med Assoc.* May 16, 2007;297(19):2063–2064.

14. Frayling TM, et al. A common variant in the FTO gene is associated with body mass index and predisposes to childhood and adult obesity. *Science.* May 11, 2007;316(5826):889–894.

15. Christakis NA, Fowler JH. Spread of obesity in a large social network over 32 years. *N Engl J Med.* Jul 26, 2007;357(4):370–379.

16. Williamson DF, Madans J, Anda RF, Kleinman JC, Kahn HS, Byers T. Recreational physical activity and ten-year weight change in a US national cohort. *Int J Obes Relat Metab Disord.* 1993;17:279–286.

17. Williamson DF, Madans J, Anda RF, Kleinman JC, Giovino GA, Byers T. Smoking cessation and severity of weight gain in a national cohort. *N Engl J Med.* 1991;324:739–745.

18. Allison DB, Mentore JL, Moonseong H, et al. Antipsychotic-induced weight gain: a comprehensive research synthesis. *Am J Psychiatry.* 1999;156:1686–1696.

19. Newcomer JW. Metabolic considerations in the use of antipsychotic medications: a review of recent evidence. *J Clin Psychiatry.* 2007;68(Suppl 1):20–27, Review.

20. Zhang Y, Proenca R, Maffei M, Barone M, Leopold L, Friedman JM. Positional cloning of the mouse obese gene and its human homologue. *Nature.* 1994;372:425–432.

21. Gale SM, Castracane VD, Mantzoros CS. Energy homeostasis, obesity and eating disorders: recent advances in endocrinology. *J Nutr.* Feb 2004;134(2):295–298, Review.

22. Ahima RS, Saper CB, Flier JS, Elmquist JK. Leptin regulation of neuroendocrine systems. *Front Neuroendocrinol.* 2000;21:263–307.

23. Mantzoros CS. The role of leptin in human obesity and disease: a review of current evidence. *Ann Intern Med.* 1999;130:671–680.

24. Lowell BB, Speigelman BM. Towards a molecular understanding of adaptive thermogenesis. *Nature.* 2000;404:652–660.

25. Schwartz MW, Woods SC, Porte D Jr, Seeley RJ, Baskin DG. Central nervous system control of food intake. *Nature.* 2000;404:661–670.

26. Brennan AM, Mantzoros CS. Leptin and adiponectin: their role in diabetes. *Curr Diab Rep.* Feb 2007;7(1):1–2.

27. National Institutes of Health. Clinical guidelines on the identification, evaluation, and treatment of overweight and obesity in adults: the evidence report. *Obes Res.* 1998;6:51S-209S.

28. Knowler WC, Barrett-Connor E, Fowler SE, et al. Reduction in the incidence of type 2 diabetes with lifestyle intervention or metformin. *N Engl J Med.* 2002;346:393–403.

29. Bray GA, Ryan DH. Medical approaches to treatment of the obese patient. In: CS Mantzoros, Ed. *Obesity and Diabetes.* Totowa: Humana Press, Inc.; 2006:457–469.

30. Gilden Tsai A, Wadden TA. The evolution of very-low-calorie diets: an update and meta-analysis. *Obesity (Silver Spring).* Aug 2006;14(8):1283–1293, Review.

31. Thompson WG, Cook DA, Clark MM, et al. Treatment of obesity. *Mayo Clin Proc.* 2007;82:93–101.

32. Li Z, Maglione M, Tu W, et al. Meta-analysis: pharmacologic treatment of obesity. *Ann Intern Med.* 2005;142:532–546.

33. Sjostrom L, Rissanen A, Andersen T, Boldrin M, Golay A, Koppeschaar HPF, et al. Randomized placebo-controlled trial of orlistat for weight loss and prevention of weight regain in obese patients. The European Multicentre Orlistat Study Group. *Lancet.* 1998;352:167–172.

34. Hollander P, Elbein S, Hirsch I, Kelley D, McGill J, Taylor T, et al. Role of orlistat in the treatment of obese patients with type 2 diabetes: a randomized double-blind study. *Diabetes Care.* 1998;21:1288–1294.

35. James WPT, Astrup A, Finer N, et al. Effect of sibutramine on weight maintenance after weight loss: a randomized trial. *Lancet.* 2000;356:2119–2125.

36. Blackburn GL, Mun EC. Weight loss surgery and major cardiovascular risk factors. *Nat Clin Pract Cardiovasc Med.* 2005;2:585–591.

37. Gagner M, Matteotti R. Laparoscopic biliopancreatic diversion with duodenal switch. *Surg Clin North Am.* 2005;85:141–149.

38. Kelly J, Tarnoff M, Shikora S, et al. Expert panel on weight loss surgery. Best practice recommendations for surgical care in weight loss surgery. *Obes Res.* Feb 2005;13(2):227–233.

39. NIH Consensus Development Conference. Gastrointestinal surgery for severe obesity. *Nutrition.* 1996;12:397–402.

40. Sjöström L, Narbo K, Sjöström D, et al. Effects of bariatric surgerz on Mortalitz in Swedish obese subjects. *N Engl J Med.* Aug 2007;357(8):741–752.

41. Adams T, Gress E, Smith S, et al. Long-term mortality after gastric bypass surgery. *N Engl J Med.* Aug 2007;357:8.

42. Sarwer DB, Fabricatore AN. Psychosocial and behavioral aspects of bariatric surgery. *Obes Res.* 2005;13:639–648.

43. Brennan AM, Mantzoros CS. Drug insight: the role of leptin in human physiology and pathophysiology-emerging clinical applications. *Nat Clin Pract Endocrino Metab.* Jun 2006;2(6):318–327.

Helpful Internet Sources for Additional Information on Obesity

- NIH clinical guidelines on obesity (http://www.nhlbi.nih.gov/guidelines/obesity/ob_home.htm)
- Prevalence of overweight and obesity among adults: United States, 1999. National Center for Health Statistics web site. (www.cdc.gov/nchs/products/pubs/pubd/hestats/obese/obse99.htm).
- web site: Look Ahead – Action for Health in Diabetes
- https://www.lookaheadtrial.org/public/home.cfm?CFID=48926&CFTOKEN=33c88afd544566b7-5D487FFC-1143-5817-64C4F62EC7CADCD6

Chapter 31
Hypertension

Samy I. McFarlane, Ho Won Lee, Sara Choudhry, and Nathaniel Winer

Introduction

Hypertension is a major risk factor for cardiovascular disease (CVD). It substantially increases the risk for coronary heart disease (CHD), stroke, and nephropathy. There is a positive association between hypertension and insulin resistance and the evidence of a causal link is growing. When hypertension coexists with diabetes, as it commonly does, the risk of stroke or CVD is doubled and the risk for developing end-stage renal disease increases to 5–6 times, compared to hypertensive patients without diabetes. In this chapter we discuss the interaction of hypertension, insulin resistance, and other CVD risk factors in the context of the metabolic syndrome, emphasizing the unique aspects of hypertension in patients with diabetes. Therapy for hypertension is discussed in the light of the major prospective trials available to date, such as the HOPE, RENAAL, IDNT, and IRMA.

Hypertension and CVD in Patients with Diabetes

CVD is the major cause of mortality in patients with diabetes. Risk factors for CVD that cluster with diabetes (Table 31.1) include hypertension, central obesity, dyslipidemia, microalbuminuria, and coagulation abnormalities.[1]

Among these risk factors, hypertension is approximately twice as frequent in patients with diabetes compared to those without the disease and accounts for up to 75% of CVD risk. Conversely, patients with hypertension are more likely to have diabetes than are normotensive persons.[2] In a prospective study of 12,550 adults, the development of type 2 diabetes was nearly 2.5 times as frequent in patients with hypertension as in their normotensive counterparts after adjustment for age, sex, race, education, adiposity, family history of diabetes, physical activity, and other health-related behavior.[3]

The association of hypertension, insulin resistance, and the resultant hyperinsulinemia was shown in several studies. In untreated essential hypertensive patients, fasting and postprandial insulin levels were higher than in normotensive controls, regardless of body mass index (BMI), and plasma insulin correlated directly with blood pressure (BP), suggesting that essential hypertension is an insulin-resistant state.[4] Another study of 24 adults documented that those with hypertension, whether treated or untreated, were insulin resistant, hyperglycemic, and hyperinsulinemic compared to a well-matched control group.[5] Insulin resistance and hyperinsulinemia also exist in rats with genetic hypertension such as Dahl hypertensive and spontaneously hypertensive rat (SHR) strains.[6,7] In contrast, the absence of an association between insulin resistance and essential hypertension in secondary hypertension[8] suggests a common genetic predisposition for essential hypertension and insulin resistance, a concept that is also supported by the finding of altered glucose metabolism in normotensive offspring

S.I. McFarlane (✉)
Division of Endocrinology, Diabetes and Hypertension, State University of New York, Downstate Medical Center and Kings County Hospital Center, Brooklyn, NY, USA
e-mail: smcfarlane@downstate.edu

L. Poretsky (ed.), *Principles of Diabetes Mellitus*, DOI 10.1007/978-0-387-09841-8_31,
© Springer Science+Business Media, LLC 2010

Table 31.1 CVD risk factors associated with diabetes

1. Hypertension
2. Obesity
3. Hyperinsulinemia/insulin resistance
4. Endothelial dysfunction
5. Microalbuminuria
6. Low HDL cholesterol levels
7. High triglyceride levels
8. Small, dense LDL cholesterol particles
9. Increased apo-lipoprotein B levels
10. Increased fibrinogen levels
11. Increased plasma activator inhibitor-1 levels
12. Increased C-reactive protein and other inflammatory markers
13. Absent nocturnal dipping of blood pressure and pulse
14. Salt sensitivity
15. Left ventricular hypertrophy
16. Premature coronary artery disease

of hypertensive patients.[9,10] Therefore, hypertension in patients with diabetes must be viewed in the context of the metabolic syndrome. This has important implications in understanding the principles of management of these patients as discussed later. Detailed discussion of the metabolic syndrome (Syndrome X) is presented in Chapter 43.

Unique Aspects of Hypertension in Patients with Diabetes

Hypertension in patients with diabetes has unique features, such as increased salt sensitivity, volume expansion, isolated systolic BP elevation, loss of nocturnal dipping of BP and pulse, increased propensity to proteinuria, and orthostatic hypotension.[2] Most of these features are considered risk factors for CVD (Table 31.1) and are relevant to the selection of appropriate antihypertensive medications, for example, low-dose diuretics to reduce volume expansion, and angiotensin-converting enzyme inhibitors (ACEs) or angiotensin receptor blockers (ARBs) to minimize proteinuria.

Salt Sensitivity and Volume Expansion

Alterations in sodium balance and extracellular fluid volume have varying effects on BP in both normotensive and hypertensive subjects. The rise of BP in response to dietary salt intake is greatest in hypertensive African-American and elderly patients who have diabetes, obesity, renal insufficiency, and low plasma renin activity. Similarly, salt sensitivity in normotensive subjects is also associated with a greater age-related increase in BP. Thus, in the management of hypertension in patients with diabetes, age is especially important among the factors affecting salt sensitivity, since the prevalence of both diabetes and salt sensitivity increases in the elderly.

Isolated Systolic Hypertension

The earlier onset and accelerated progression of atherosclerosis in patients with diabetes leads to the loss of elasticity and the "cushioning" effect in larger arteries, causing an increase in systolic BP. The more rapid runoff of blood during the systolic ejection phase of the cardiac cycle results in a lower diastolic BP, producing a widened pulse pressure and isolated systolic hypertension, which is more common and occurs at a relatively younger age in patients with diabetes.[2]

Loss of Nocturnal Decline of BP

In normotensive individuals, BP shows a reproducible circadian pattern during 24-h ambulatory monitoring. BP is highest during daytime hours and typically falls by 10–15% during sleep, a pattern termed nocturnal "dipping." A nocturnal decline in BP <10% compared to daytime BP values (non-dipping)[11] has been observed in patients with diabetes. The loss of nocturnal dipping increases risk for stroke and myocardial infarction and is consistent with data showing the superiority of ambulatory BP compared to office BP in predicting target organ involvement, such as left ventricular hypertrophy.[11] Since about 30% of myocardial infarctions and 50% of strokes occur between 6:00 AM and noon it is mandatory to design dosing strategies which use antihypertensive medications that provide consistent, sustained 24 h BP control.[12]

Microalbuminuria

There is considerable evidence that hypertension in type 1 diabetes is a consequence, rather than a cause, of renal disease and that nephropathy precedes the rise in BP.[2] Persistent hypertension in patients with type 1 diabetes is often a manifestation of diabetic nephropathy as indicated by concomitant elevation of urinary albumin. Both hypertension and nephropathy appear to exacerbate each other. In type 2 diabetes, microalbuminuria is correlated with insulin resistance,[13] salt sensitivity, loss of nocturnal dipping, and left ventricular hypertrophy.[14] Elevated systolic BP is a significant determining factor in the progression of microalbuminuria. Indeed, there is increasing evidence that microalbuminuria is an integral component of the metabolic syndrome associated with hypertension.[14] Therefore, in hypertensive patients with diabetes, antihypertensive medications should have the dual effect of reducing proteinuria and lowering blood pressure as seen with the use of ACE inhibitors and ARBs. Agents which block the renin–angiotensin–aldosterone system (RAAS) have evolved as increasingly important tools in reducing the progression of nephropathy in such patients.

Orthostatic Hypotension

Pooling of blood in dependent veins during rising from a recumbent position normally leads to decrease in stroke volume and systolic BP with reflexogenic sympathetic response and resultant increases in systemic vascular resistance and heart rate. In patients with diabetes and autonomic dysfunction, excessive venous pooling can cause immediate or delayed orthostatic hypotension that might cause reduction in cerebral blood flow leading to intermittent lightheadedness, fatigue, unsteady gait, and syncope.[15] Orthostatic hypotension in patients with diabetes and concomitant hypertension has several diagnostic and therapeutic implications. For example, discontinuation of diuretic therapy and volume repletion might be necessary. Also α-adrenergic receptor blockers may be less desirable as second-line agents. In the subset of patients with "hyperadrenergic" orthostatic hypertension, manifested by excessive sweating and palpitation, the use of low-dose clonidine may blunt excess sympathetic response.[16] Finally, for patients with diabetes who are at risk for orthostatic hypertension, doses of all antihypertensive agents must be titrated more carefully.

Management of Hypertension in Patients with Diabetes

The Seventh Report of the Joint National Committee on Prevention, Detection, Evaluation, and Treatment of High Blood Pressure (JNC VII)[17] characterizes hypertension and concomitant diabetes as a high-risk condition and a compelling indication for specific pharmacologic therapy. The Report notes that the combined prevalence of diabetes and impaired fasting glucose in subjects over age 20 is 14.4% and that diabetes is the leading cause of blindness, end-stage renal disease, and nontraumatic amputations. Type 2 diabetes, per se, increases the likelihood of premature death from CVD or stroke by 70–80%, but with concurrent hypertension, CVD, stroke, progression of renal disease, and retinopathy are greatly accelerated. Randomized controlled trials that have included large diabetic populations (UKPDS[18], HOT[19], SHEP[20], Syst EUR[21], HOPE[22], MICRO-HOPE[22], LIFE[23], and ALLHAT[24]) have shown improved CVD outcomes if BP was controlled to 130/80 mmHg or lower. In view of studies of chronic kidney disease in patients with diabetes, defined by albuminuria (albumin >300 μg/day or >200 μg/g creatinine in a random urine) or renal insufficiency (estimated GFR <60 mL/min, corresponding to serum creatinine >1.5 mg/dL in men and 1.3 mg/dL in women) showing that the rate of decline of renal function varies continuously with BP, down to a level of 125–130/75–80 mmHg, JNC 7 recommended a BP target <130/80 mmHg in patients with diabetes, consistent with guidelines advocated by the American Diabetes Association (ADA),[25] the National Kidney Foundation (NKF),[26] and the Canadian Hypertension Society.

The question of which class of antihypertensive agents should constitute first-line therapy is largely academic since most patients with diabetes and hypertension will require at least two agents to achieve target BP levels. Indeed, in our study of 1372 patients with hypertension and diabetes, an average of 3.1 medications was required to achieve a target BP ≤130/85 mmHg,[27] consistent with results from other major studies such as UKPDS, MDRD, HOT, and ABCD[28] mentioned above, where more than two medications were often required for optimal control of BP. Diuretics, ACE inhibitors, ARBs, beta blockers (BBs), and calcium channel blockers (CCBs) have been shown to be beneficial in treating hypertension in patients with diabetes. For patients at high-CVD risk, such as those with diabetes presenting with BP>20/10 mmHg above target, JNC 7 recommends that antihypertensive therapy should be initiated with two agents, one of which would typically be a diuretic. Low-dose combinations were found to produce BP reductions that were additive, but as doses of the components were increased, BP reduction was less than additive, even though overall BP was reduced.

The following treatment algorithm (Fig. 31.1) reflects the new treatment goal of BP <130/80 mmHg as well as the latest recommendations regarding drug therapy.[29][30]

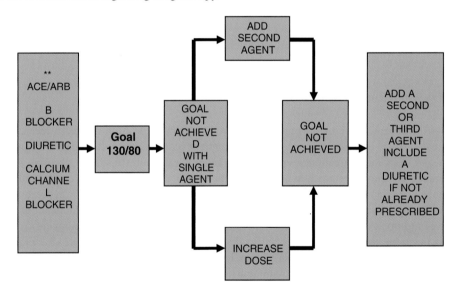

Fig. 31.1 Management of hypertension in patients with diabetes. In patients with >1 g proteinuria and renal insufficiency the treatment goal is BP <125/75 mmHg. **ARBs = angiotensin receptor blockers

Dietary and Lifestyle Modifications

Lifestyle and dietary modifications are an integral part of the management of hypertension in patients with diabetes. Attempts to modify other CVD risk factors such as smoking, inactivity, and elevated LDL cholesterol should be made.[25] Dietary and lifestyle modifications recommended for patients with hypertension are listed in Table 31.2.

Table 31.2 Dietary and lifestyle modifications recommended for management of hypertension

1. Weight loss
2. Exercise (aerobic physical activity) 30–45 min at least three times a week
3. Reduced sodium intake to 100 mmol (2.4 g) per day
4. Smoking cessation
5. Adequate intake of dietary potassium, calcium, and magnesium.
6. Reduced alcohol intake to < 1 oz of ethanol (24 oz of beer) per day.
7. Diet rich in fruits and vegetables but low in fat[a]

[a]Based on the results of the dietary approaches to stop hypertension (DASH) study,[31,32] the reduction of sodium intake to levels below the current recommendation of 100 mmol per day and the DASH diet both lower BP substantially, with greater effects in combination than each of these approaches used alone.[32]

Dietary management and exercise in patients with diabetes are discussed in detail in Chapters 41 and 42, respectively. It is important to integrate the above lifestyle and dietary modifications for hypertension in the overall nutritional and lifestyle management of these patients.

Pharmacological Therapy for Hypertension in Patients with Diabetes

Angiotensin-Converting Enzyme Inhibitor

ACE inhibitors were first introduced in the early 1980s as antihypertensive agents. Subsequently, their ability to attenuate albuminuria and renal disease progression led to their use as renoprotective agents in diabetic nephropathy.[33] More recently, randomized controlled trials have shown that ACE inhibitors provide cardiovascular and microvascular benefits and may also improve insulin resistance. These cardiovascular benefits were greater than those attributable to the decrease in blood pressure alone, and were particularly demonstrated in people with diabetes.[22] However, the beneficial effect of ACE-inhibition in preventing diabetes was not confirmed in the DREAM trial in which treatment of 5269 patients with impaired plasma fasting glucose or glucose intolerance over 3 years with the ACE inhibitors, ramipril, failed to reduce the incidence of new-onset diabetes, compared to the insulin-sensitizing agent, rosiglitazone.[34] In patients with type 1 diabetes and proteinuria, ACE inhibitor treatment was associated with a 50% reduction in the risk of the combined end points of death, dialysis, and transplantation.[33] Furthermore, ACE inhibitors provide considerable benefits in diabetic patients with heart failure. In the Studies of Left Ventricular Dysfunction (SOLVD) trial, ACE inhibitors reduced left ventricular mass and left ventricular dilation and significantly reduced mortality and hospitalization for heart failure.[35] ACE inhibitors have also been reported to slow the progression of diabetic retinopathy.[36]

With these clearly proven benefits, ACE inhibitors form the cornerstone of therapy for patients with hypertension and diabetes, particularly for those with proteinuria as well as for those with heart failure.

Treatment with ACE inhibitors is associated with cough in a substantial minority of patients (up to 15%), probably secondary to accumulation of bradykinin or substance P in the upper airways (Fig. 31.2). Angioedema is a rare, unpredictable, and potentially life-threatening adverse effect, particularly if the upper airway is involved, and requires immediate discontinuation and supportive care, including airway protection. ACE inhibitors reduce aldosterone secretion (Fig. 31.2) and may cause hyperkalemia, especially at the initiation of therapy. Patients with diabetes and mild renal insufficiency and those on potassium-sparing diuretics are at greater risk. Aldosterone antagonists, such as spironolactone and eplerenone, should be used with caution. Concomitant use of thiazide or loop diuretics and limitation of dietary potassium intake should allow the use of ACE inhibitors without inducing hyperkalemia. In patients with normal renal function, ACE inhibitors have little effect on glomerular filtration rate (GFR), but with reduced renal function, these agents may precipitate uremia. In patients with diabetes, a decrease in GFR of up to 25% from reduced efferent arteriolar tone and decreased intraglomerular pressure may be used as an indicator of the adequacy of ACE inhibition. ACE inhibitors are relatively contraindicated in patients with known bilateral renal artery stenosis and unilateral stenosis with a solitary kidney because of the risk of renal failure.

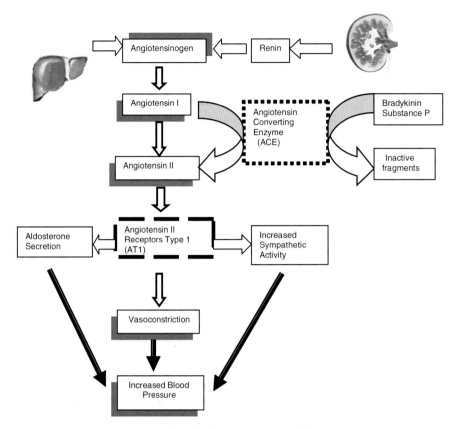

Fig. 31.2 Renin–angiotensin–aldosterone system (RAAS). Site of action for ACE inhibitors and of angiotensin receptor blockers (ARBs)

Angiotensin II Receptor Blockers

There are at least four types of angiotensin II receptors: AT1, AT2, AT3, and AT4. Of these, the AT1 receptors mediate most of the effects of angiotensin II, including vasoconstriction, cardiomyocyte and vascular smooth muscle hypertrophy, aldosterone release, increased sympathetic outflow, and stimulation of sodium reabsorption. ARBs selectively inhibit the binding of angiotensin II to the AT1 receptors; therefore, they are also called AT1 receptor blockers. Unlike ACE inhibitors, ARBs have no effects on bradykinin (Fig. 31.2) and are therefore well tolerated with a lower incidence of side effects such as cough. Angioedema may occur rarely (probably an idiosyncratic reaction), but much less commonly than with ACE inhibitors. Although there are no specific recommendations, ARBs should not be used in patients with a history of ACE inhibitor-related angioedema, since angioedema is a potentially life-threatening condition. In addition, because of inhibition of aldosterone release by ARBs, hyperkalemia is a concern especially in those with renal insufficiency and, as with ACE inhibitors, progressive azotemia and renal failure might occur in those with bilateral renal artery stenosis or those with renal artery stenosis in a solitary kidney.

Recently, the first orally active renin inhibitor, aliskerin, became available. This agent blocks the renin–angiotensin system by inhibiting the rate-limiting step in angiotensin II (Ang II) biosynthesis. Unlike ACE inhibitors or ARBs which block either Ang II production or action and increase plasma renin activity, renin inhibitors suppress the generation of renin, but lead to elevation of the renin precursors, preprorenin and prorenin. Initially prorenin was thought to be biologically inactive, but the recent discovery of a renin receptor which can be activated by both renin and prorenin suggests that there may be separate pathways by which renin and prorenin can stimulate formation of Ang II.[37] Whether increased levels of prorenin may have a deleterious cardiovascular effect in individuals with diabetes is unknown. Initial clinical studies indicate that aliskerin has a longer duration of action than ACE inhibitors or ARBs and has antihypertensive efficacy equal to that of ACE inhibitors and ARBs either as monotherapy or in combination with diuretics.[38,40] Outcome data from clinical trials in high-risk hypertensive patients, especially in those with diabetes, are pending.

JNC 7 recommended the use of ARBs as one of several alternative first-line therapies for patients with hypertension who cannot tolerate or do not respond to the recommended first-line medications. In addition, ARBs were also recommended as an initial therapy for those who could not tolerate ACE inhibitors (usually because of cough) and in whom ACE inhibitors are recommended as first-line drugs, such as patients with diabetes and proteinuria, heart failure, systolic dysfunction, post myocardial infarction, and those with mild renal insufficiency. However, data from randomized controlled trials in patients with type 2 diabetes suggest that ARBs may be considered equal to ACE inhibitors for renal protection.[41] Indeed, the reduction of endpoints in type 2 diabetes mellitus with the angiotensin losartan[42] (RENAAL), irbesartan in Diabetic Nephropathy Trial[43] (IDNT), and irbesartan in patients with type 2 Diabetes and Microalbuminuria Study Group[44] (IRMA trials) demonstrated that angiotensin II receptor blocker combined with conventional antihypertensive treatment as needed confers significant renal protection in patients with type 2 diabetes and nephropathy. In the RENAAL trial, the risk of the primary end point (a composite of doubling of serum creatinine, end-stage renal disease, or death from any cause) was reduced by 16% with losartan. In the same study, the risk of doubling of serum creatinine was reduced by 25% and the risk of end-stage renal disease was reduced by 28% over a follow-up period of 3.4 years. The study also documented reduction in the initial hospitalization for heart failure. These benefits were above and beyond those attributable to BP reduction alone.

Beta Blockers

BBs may be useful antihypertensive agents in the treatment of hypertension in patients with diabetes[2] when used as part of a multidrug regimen, but their value as monotherapy is less clear, according to JNC 7. In the UKPDS study, atenolol reduced microvascular complications of diabetes by 37%, strokes by 44%, and death related to diabetes by 32%. In that study, the efficacy of the BB and atenolol was equivalent to that of the ACE inhibitor, captopril, in reducing the micro- and macrovascular complications of diabetes, most probably secondary to their ability to modulate the RAAS system. In a nonrandomized study, hypertensive patients receiving BBs had a 28% higher risk of diabetes than untreated subjects. In contrast, patients with hypertension who received thiazide diuretics, ACE inhibitors, or CCBs were not found to be at increased risk for subsequent development of diabetes compared to patients receiving no medication.[3] However, increased risk for the development of diabetes with BB therapy was not found in other randomized studies.[45] Despite the possible adverse metabolic effects of BBs and their potential to mask symptoms of hypoglycemia, they have shown significant long-term favorable effects on CVD in hypertensive patients with diabetes and therefore, should be used in patients with diabetes, particularly those with coronary artery disease.

Calcium Channel Blockers

To achieve a target BP $\leq$130/80 mmHg, clinical trials suggest that at least 65% of patients require two or more antihypertensive agents. Additional therapies in people with diabetes (besides ACE inhibitors and diuretics) may include long-acting CCBs. A non-dihydropyridine CCB, such as verapamil or diltiazem, may have more beneficial effects on proteinuria than a dihydropyridine CCB, such as nifedipine. However, with the use of ACEs (or ARBs) with a diuretic as first-line treatment, the addition of a long-acting dihydropyridine such as amlodipine, nifedipine, or felodipine reduces both proteinuria and CVD event rates. If the targeted BP is still not achieved, a low-dose BB or an alpha/beta blocker can be added. It is important to note that both the ABCD[28] and AASK[46] trials demonstrated the superiority of ACEs over CCBs in prevention of CVD events; however, in the ABCD trial, the difference was likely the result of the beneficial effects of the ACE inhibitors rather than a negative effect of the CCB. The use of CCBs is particularly helpful in achieving the target BP, especially in patients with isolated systolic BP not responding to the addition of low-dose diuretic therapy.

Diuretics

Low-dose diuretics are effective antihypertensive agents in patients with diabetes as these patients often have expanded plasma volume. They may be used as monotherapy but are more often combined with ACE inhibitors, ARBs, BBs, or CCBs. Combination tablets may have advantages of cost, convenience, and patient adherence. In the ALLHAT diabetic subgroup, regimens containing the diuretic, chlothalidone, were as effective as ACE inhibitor- or CCB-based regimens in reducing fatal CHD and MI.[47] In contrast, the Second Australian National Blood Pressure trial reported a better prognosis in patients randomly assigned to an ACE-based treatment compared to a diuretic-based therapy.[48] The differences in outcomes may have reflected the ethnicity of the populations studied. Of concern in ALLHAT was the higher incidence of new-onset diabetes in the diuretic group, which over time could have substantial health consequences. Conversely, a report of 12,500 hypertensive adults did not find any influence of thiazide diuretics on the development of diabetes.[49] Hypokalemia has been observed with the use of large doses of hydrochlorothiazide (e.g., 50–200 mg) but is less likely in daily doses less than 25 mg.

Diuretics are also effective in the treatment of isolated systolic hypertension, which is common and occurs at a younger age in people with diabetes as discussed above. The systolic hypertension in the elderly program (SHEP) showed that small doses of chlorothalidone are not only safe but also effective, as evidenced by the reduced rate of major CVD events, fatal and nonfatal strokes, and all cause mortality in patients with diabetes.[2050] In addition, diuretics are often a necessary component of combination antihypertensive therapy in people with diabetes who often require three or more medications to achieve target BP.

Fixed-Dose Combination

The use of a fixed-dose combination therapy has the potential of enhancing compliance, reducing side effects, and cost of medications. Several diuretic-based combinations are available. These include those with beta blocker, ACE inhibitor, and ARB. These agents are being used increasingly. Our above-mentioned report indicates that 23% of patients with diabetes and hypertension are on a fixed-dose combination. Long-term benefits from these fixed-dose combinations remain to be seen. However, a combination of particular interest is that of a dihydropyridine CCB (amlodipine) and an ACE inhibitor (benazapril). Less pedal edema was reported with this combination than with CCB alone. This observation supports the notion that combination therapy might reduce side effects. In the above case, CCBs, being mainly arteriolar vasodilators, may induce pedal edema, but the addition of an ACE inhibitor with a balanced arterial and venous dilation reduces edema formation. This combination also showed enhanced rate of response compared to either placebo or each component given separately.

Summary

Rigorous treatment of hypertension, a common comorbid condition in patients with diabetes, is very important to reduce both microvascular and microvascular complications in this population. Combination therapy is often required to achieve and maintain blood pressure at the target level. The currently recommended target BP for patients with diabetes is 130/80 mmHg.

Based on the current evidence from randomized controlled trials, ACE inhibitors or ARBs are recommended as initial therapeutic agents with the addition of other agents as necessary to achieve and maintain target blood pressure.

References

1. McFarlane SI, Banerji M, Sowers JR. Insulin resistance and cardiovascular disease. *J Clin Endocrinol Metab.* 2001;86:713–718.
2. Sowers JR, Epstein M, Frohlich ED. Diabetes, hypertension, and cardiovascular disease: an update. *Hypertension.* 2001;37:1053–1059.

3. Gress TW, Nieto FJ, Shahar E, Wofford MR, Brancati FL. Hypertension and antihypertensive therapy as risk factors for type 2 diabetes mellitus. Atherosclerosis Risk in Communities Study. *N Engl J Med.* 2000;342:905–912.
4. Ferrannini E, Buzzigoli G, Bonadonna R, et al. Insulin resistance in essential hypertension. *N Engl J Med.* 1987;317:350–357.
5. Shen DC, Shieh SM, Fuh MM, Wu DA, Chen YD, Reaven GM. Resistance to insulin-stimulated-glucose uptake in patients with hypertension. *J Clin Endocrinol Metab.* 1988;66:580–583.
6. Kotchen TA, Zhang HY, Covelli M, Blehschmidt N. Insulin resistance and blood pressure in Dahl rats and in one-kidney, one-clip hypertensive rats. *Am J Physiol.* 1991;261:E692–E697.
7. Reaven GM, Chang H. Relationship between blood pressure, plasma insulin and triglyceride concentration, and insulin action in spontaneous hypertensive and Wistar-Kyoto rats. *Am J Hypertens.* 1991;4:34–38.
8. Sechi LA, Melis A, Tedde R. Insulin hypersecretion: a distinctive feature between essential and secondary hypertension. *Metabolism.* 1992;41:1261–1266.
9. Beatty OL, Harper R, Sheridan B, Atkinson AB, Bell PM. Insulin resistance in offspring of hypertensive parents. *BMJ.* 1993;307:92–96.
10. Grunfeld B, Balzareti M, Romo M, Gimenez M, Gutman R. Hyperinsulinemia in normotensive offspring of hypertensive parents. *Hypertension.* 1994;23:I12–I15.
11. Verdecchia P, Porcellati C, Schillaci G, et al. Ambulatory blood pressure. An independent predictor of prognosis in essential hypertension. *Hypertension.* 1994;24:793–801.
12. White WB. A chronotherapeutic approach to the management of hypertension. *Am J Hypertens.* 1996;9:29S–33S.
13. Bianchi S, Bigazzi R, Quinones Galvan A, et al. Insulin resistance in microalbuminuric hypertension. Sites and mechanisms. *Hypertension.* 1995;26:789–795.
14. Mitchell TH, Nolan B, Henry M, Cronin C, Baker H, Greely G. Microalbuminuria in patients with non-insulin-dependent diabetes mellitus relates to nocturnal systolic blood pressure. *Am J Med.* 1997;102:531–535.
15. Streeten DH, Auchincloss JH Jr., Anderson GH Jr., Richardson RL, Thomas FD, Miller JW. Orthostatic hypertension. Pathogenetic studies. *Hypertension.* 1985;7:196–203.
16. Streeten DH. Pathogenesis of hyperadrenergic orthostatic hypotension. Evidence of disordered venous innervation exclusively in the lower limbs. *J Clin Invest.* 1990;86:1582–1588.
17. Chobanian AV, Bakris GL, Black HR, et al. The seventh report of the Joint National Committee on prevention, detection, evaluation, and treatment of high blood pressure: the JNC 7 report. *JAMA.* 2003;289:2560–2572.
18. Adler AI, Stratton IM, Neil HA, et al. Association of systolic blood pressure with macrovascular and microvascular complications of type 2 diabetes (UKPDS 36): prospective observational study. *BMJ.* 2000;321:412–419.
19. Hansson L, Zanchetti A, Carruthers SG, et al. Effects of intensive blood-pressure lowering and low-dose aspirin in patients with hypertension: principal results of the hypertension optimal treatment (HOT) randomised trial. HOT Study Group. *Lancet.* 1998;351:1755–1762.
20. Prevention of stroke by antihypertensive drug treatment in older persons with isolated systolic hypertension. Final results of the Systolic Hypertension in the Elderly Program (SHEP). SHEP Cooperative Research Group. *JAMA.* 1991;265:3255–3264.
21. Staessen JA, Fagard R, Thijs L, et al. Randomised double-blind comparison of placebo and active treatment for older patients with isolated systolic hypertension. The Systolic Hypertension in Europe (Syst-Eur) Trial Investigators. *Lancet.* 1997;350: 757–764.
22. Effects of ramipril on cardiovascular and microvascular outcomes in people with diabetes mellitus: results of the HOPE study and MICRO-HOPE substudy. Heart outcomes prevention evaluation study investigators. *Lancet.* 2000;355:253–259.
23. Lindholm LH, Ibsen H, Dahlof B, et al. Cardiovascular morbidity and mortality in patients with diabetes in the losartan intervention for endpoint reduction in hypertension study (LIFE): a randomised trial against atenolol. *Lancet.* 2002;359:1004–1010.
24. Major outcomes in high-risk hypertensive patients randomized to angiotensin-converting enzyme inhibitor or calcium channel blocker vs diuretic: The Antihypertensive and Lipid-Lowering Treatment to Prevent Heart Attack Trial (ALLHAT). *JAMA.* 2002;288:2981–2997.
25. Standards of medical care for patients with diabetes mellitus. *Diabetes Care.* 2003;26(Suppl 1):S33–S50.
26. Bakris GL, Williams M, Dworkin L, et al. Preserving renal function in adults with hypertension and diabetes: a consensus approach. National Kidney Foundation Hypertension and Diabetes Executive Committees Working Group. *Am J Kidney Dis.* 2000;36:646–661.
27. McFarlane SI, Jacober SJ, Winer N, et al. Control of cardiovascular risk factors in patients with diabetes and hypertension at urban academic medical centers. *Diabetes Care.* 2002;25:718–723.
28. Estacio RO, Jeffers BW, Hiatt WR, Biggerstaff SL, Gifford N, Schrier RW. The effect of nisoldipine as compared with enalapril on cardiovascular outcomes in patients with non-insulin-dependent diabetes and hypertension. *N Engl J Med.* 1998;338: 645–652.
29. Sowers JR, Williams M, Epstein M, Bakris G. Hypertension in patients with diabetes. Strategies for drug therapy to reduce complications. *Postgrad Med.* 2000;107:47–54.
30. Bakris G, Sowers J, Epstein M, Williams M. Hypertension in patients with diabetes. Why is aggressive treatment essential? *Postgrad Med.* 2000;107(53–6)61–64.
31. Conlin PR, Chow D, Miller ER 3rd, et al. The effect of dietary patterns on blood pressure control in hypertensive patients: results from the Dietary Approaches to Stop Hypertension (DASH) trial. *Am J Hypertens.* 2000;13: 949–955.

32. Sacks FM, Svetkey LP, Vollmer WM, et al. Effects on blood pressure of reduced dietary sodium and the dietary approaches to stop hypertension (DASH) diet. DASH-Sodium Collaborative Research Group. *N Engl J Med*. 2001;344:3–10.

33. Lewis EJ, Hunsicker LG, Bain RP, Rohde RD. The effect of angiotensin-converting-enzyme inhibition on diabetic nephropathy. The Collaborative Study Group. *N Engl J Med*. 1993;329:1456–1462.

34. Bosch J, Yusuf S, Gerstein HC, et al. Effect of ramipril on the incidence of diabetes. *N Engl J Med*. 2006;355:1551–1562.

35. Shindler DM, Kostis JB, Yusuf S, et al. Diabetes mellitus, a predictor of morbidity and mortality in the Studies of Left Ventricular Dysfunction (SOLVD) Trials and Registry. *Am J Cardiol*. 1996;77:1017–1020.

36. Randomised placebo-controlled trial of lisinopril in normotensive patients with insulin-dependent diabetes and normoalbuminuria or microalbuminuria. The EUCLID Study Group. *Lancet*. 1997;349:1787–1792.

37. Nguyen G, Delarue F, Burckle C, Bouzhir L, Giller T, Sraer JD. Pivotal role of the renin/prorenin receptor in angiotensin II production and cellular responses to renin. *J Clin Invest*. 2002;109:1417–1427.

38. Oh BH, Mitchell J, Herron JR, Chung J, Khan M, Keefe DL. Aliskiren, an oral renin inhibitor, provides dose-dependent efficacy and sustained 24-hour blood pressure control in patients with hypertension. *J Am Coll Cardiol*. 2007;49:1157–1163.

39. Birkenhager WH, Staessen JA. Dual inhibition of the renin system by aliskiren and valsartan. *Lancet*. 2007;370:195–196.

40. Villamil A, Chrysant SG, Calhoun D, et al. Renin inhibition with aliskiren provides additive antihypertensive efficacy when used in combination with hydrochlorothiazide. *J Hypertens*. 2007;25:217–226.

41. Kaplan NM. Management of hypertension in patients with type 2 diabetes mellitus: guidelines based on current evidence. *Ann Intern Med*. 2001;135:1079–1083.

42. Brenner BM, Cooper ME, de Zeeuw D, et al. Effects of losartan on renal and cardiovascular outcomes in patients with type 2 diabetes and nephropathy. *N Engl J Med*. 2001;345:861–869.

43. Lewis EJ, Hunsicker LG, Clarke WR, et al. Renoprotective effect of the angiotensin-receptor antagonist irbesartan in patients with nephropathy due to type 2 diabetes. *N Engl J Med*. 2001;345:851–860.

44. Parving HH, Lehnert H, Brochner-Mortensen J, Gomis R, Andersen S, Arner P. The effect of irbesartan on the development of diabetic nephropathy in patients with type 2 diabetes. *N Engl J Med*. 2001;345:870–878.

45. Grimm RH Jr., Flack JM, Grandits GA, et al. Long-term effects on plasma lipids of diet and drugs to treat hypertension. Treatment of Mild Hypertension Study (TOMHS) Research Group. *JAMA*. 1996;275:1549–1556.

46. Norris K, Bourgoigne J, Gassman J, et al. Cardiovascular outcomes in the African American Study of kidney disease and hypertension (AASK) Trial. *Am J Kidney Dis*. 2006;48:739–751.

47. Whelton PK, Barzilay J, Cushman WC, et al. Clinical outcomes in antihypertensive treatment of type 2 diabetes, impaired fasting glucose concentration, and normoglycemia: antihypertensive and lipid-lowering treatment to prevent heart attack trial (ALLHAT). *Arch Intern Med*. 2005;165:1401–1409.

48. Wing LM, Reid CM, Ryan P, et al. Second Australian National Blood Pressure Study (ANBP2). Australian Comparative Outcome Trial of ACE inhibitor- and diuretic-based treatment of hypertension in the elderly. Management Committee on behalf of the High Blood Pressure Research Council of Australia. *Clin Exp Hypertens*. 1997;19:779–791.

49. Barzilay JI, Davis BR, Cutler JA, et al. Fasting glucose levels and incident diabetes mellitus in older nondiabetic adults randomized to receive 3 different classes of antihypertensive treatment: a report from the Antihypertensive and Lipid-Lowering Treatment to Prevent Heart Attack Trial (ALLHAT). *Arch Intern Med*. 2006;166:2191–2201.

50. Hall WD. The systolic hypertension in the elderly program: implications for the management of older hypertensive patients. *Am J Geriatr Cardiol*. 1992;1:15–23.

Chapter 32
Coronary Artery Disease and Cardiomyopathy

Richard B. Devereux

Introduction

Cardiovascular disease (CVD) is the leading cause of death in patients with type 2 diabetes. Epidemiological studies have shown that diabetes mellitus is a potent independent risk factor for cardiovascular disease.[1,2] It has been recognized for several decades that diabetic patients have a 2- to 3-fold higher risk for CVD than their nondiabetic counterparts. CVD accounts for up to 80% of deaths in patients with diabetes, approximately 75% of which are due to ischemic heart disease. More than 25% of diabetic patients have evidence of CVD at diagnosis. Therefore, the American Heart Association has stated that "diabetes is a cardiovascular disease."[3]

Although the cardiovascular disease burden is obvious, the causal pathways are incompletely understood. Two major effects of diabetes on the heart are accelerated coronary artery disease and specific diabetic cardiomyopathy. This chapter reviews the clinical implications of these manifestations of diabetic heart disease and the impact of treatment on cardiovascular mortality and morbidity based on clinical trials.

Coronary Artery Disease

The Burden of Coronary Artery Disease in Diabetic Patients. Accelerated coronary artery disease (CAD), accounts for 75–80% of deaths and hospitalizations in diabetic individuals and a heavy burden of disability and expense.[4] A large body of epidemiological data documents that diabetes is an independent risk factor for CAD in men and especially in women, who seem to lose most of their inherent protection against CAD.[1,2,5] Diabetic patients with no history of CAD have, on average, long-term rates of myocardial infarction and cardiovascular death comparable to those of nondiabetic patients with prior myocardial infarction.[6] To make matters worse, when patients with diabetes develop clinical CAD, their survival is worse than that of nondiabetic CAD patients.[7] Although cardiovascular mortality is declining in the general US population due to reduction in cardiovascular risk factors and improved treatment of heart disease, the decline is smaller in diabetic men (–13% vs. –36%), and, worse yet, cardiovascular mortality has actually increased in diabetic women (–23% vs. + 27%).[8] While overall heart disease mortality decreased by 52% from 1970 to 2002, the death rate associated with diabetes rose by 45%.[9]

Myocardial Infarction: Patients with diabetes are at increased risk of myocardial infarction (MI) compared with the general population. In fact, the incidence of MI among patients with diabetes who did not have CAD was similar to patients without diabetes who had preexisting CAD.[6] Diabetes is associated with a 1.2- to 2.0-fold increase in mortality risk after acute MI after adjusting for known confounding variables (Fig. 32.1).

The 1-year mortality after an MI is also significantly higher in diabetic than in nondiabetic individuals (24% vs. 14% in men and 33% vs. 11% in women). In addition, the pre-hospitalization mortality rate from acute CHD

R.B. Devereux (✉)
Laboratory of Echocardiography, New York Presbyterian Hospital, Weill Medical College of Cornell University, New York , USA
e-mail: rbdevere@med.cornell.edu

L. Poretsky (ed.), *Principles of Diabetes Mellitus*, DOI 10.1007/978-0-387-09841-8_32,
© Springer Science+Business Media, LLC 2010

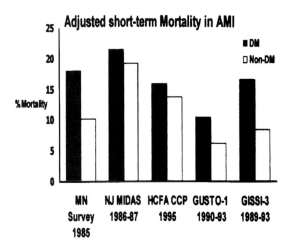

Fig. 32.1 Diabetes and acute myocardial infarction (AMI) outcomes. Diabetes is associated with a 1.2- to 2.0-fold increase in mortality after AMI (Adapted from McGuire DK et al.[10], with permission)

is higher in diabetic than in nondiabetic subjects. Diabetic patients with MI are more likely to die before reaching the hospital (sudden deaths) than nondiabetic patients with MI.[11] The explanation for this high risk is not entirely clear, but may in part be due to a specific coexisting diabetic heart muscle disease which, independent of CAD, impairs myocardial relaxation and contractility. This diabetic cardiomyopathy is discussed later in this chapter.

Silent Ischemia. Myocardial ischemia due to coronary atherosclerosis commonly occurs without symptoms in diabetic patients. As a result, multivessel atherosclerosis often is present before ischemic symptoms occur and treatment is instituted. Diabetic patients have higher prevalences of asymptomatic ischemia on both exercise stress test and 48 h ambulatory ECG monitoring in most,[12,13] but not all[14] studies. The increased rate of silent ischemic episodes is likely due to autonomic neuropathy associated with DM, characterized by loss of sympathetic and parasympathetic innervation to the heart. Therefore, impaired pain perception makes angina a poor discriminating symptom in many diabetic patients with ischemic heart disease. In a series of asymptomatic patients with type 2 diabetes studies by myocardial perfusion imaging, coronary calcium scoring, and multislice computed tomographic coronary arteriography, 20–25% had evidence of significant coronary artery disease detected by each modality, with minor evidence of coronary artery disease in even larger, additional proportions of patients.[15] In the DIAD-2 study of 358 diabetic patients who underwent adenosine-stress myocardial perfusion imaging at baseline and after 3 years of follow-up, the number with abnormal perfusion scans decreased from 71 to 43, associated with significant increases in the use of statins, aspirin, and ACE inhibitors, suggesting that asymptomatic ischemia in diabetic patients can be reversed by aggressive medical management.[16]

Pathophysiology/Risk Factors

The increased cardiovascular event rate in diabetes is partially due to independent contributions of the other major cardiovascular risk factors.[1,2,17] Most patients with type 2 DM have the insulin resistance syndrome, also known as the metabolic syndrome, characterized by clustering of metabolic risk factors including hypertension, hyperinsulinemia, glucose intolerance, and dyslipidemia.[18–21]

Diabetes is also associated with coagulopathy and endothelial dysfunction, predisposing to thrombosis and vasospasm on top of atherogenesis promoted by the coexisting risk factor of hyperglycemia. The relations among diabetes, other established risk factors, and the risk of cardiovascular events are, however, complex. In older analyses in populations with modest prevalences of diabetes, it appeared to have a multiplying effect on cardiovascular risk in the presence of other cardiovascular risk factors. However, more recent studies in large populations of diabetic individuals have demonstrated a strong gradient of rates of subsequent cardiovascular

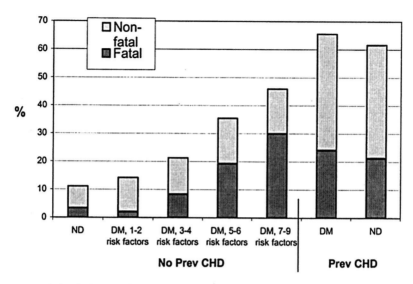

Fig. 32.2 The 10-year cumulative incidence of CHD by numbers of risk factors (men and women combined). Baseline risk factors include sex, LDL cholesterol >100 mg/dl, albuminuria (>300 mg/g creatinine), hypertension, HDL <40 mg/dl, triglycerides >150 mg/dl, current smoking, fourth quartile of fibrinogen (>352 mg/dl), and diabetes duration >20 years. DM, diabetes; ND, no diabetes; Prev, previous[22]

events, from low levels in the presence of one or no other risk factors to levels approaching those seen in non-diabetic adults with overt coronary heart disease in the presence of three or more concomitant risk factors[22,23] (Fig. 32.2).

Dyslipidemia. The Multiple Risk Factor Intervention Trial (MRFIT) showed a curvilinear relationship between total cholesterol and coronary heart disease mortality in diabetic men that was parallel but with about 4-fold greater risk than that in men without diabetes (Fig. 32.3).

Type 2 diabetic patients have an atherogenic dyslipidemia characterized by three lipoprotein abnormalities: elevated levels of very-low density lipoprotein (VLDL) triglycerides; small, dense low-density lipoprotein (LDL) cholesterol particles; and decreased level of high-density lipoprotein (HDL) cholesterol. Evidence suggests that

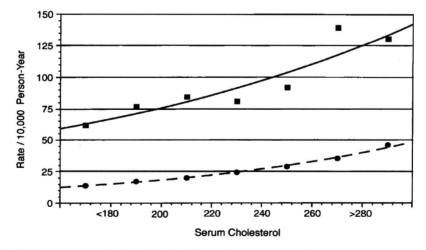

Fig. 32.3 Relationship between serum cholesterol and cardiovascular mortality in diabetic subjects in a 12-year follow-up study from the Multiple Risk Factor Intervention Trial (MRFIT). (Adapted from Goldberg[24] with permission)

all elements of diabetic dyslipidemia are atherogenic independent of the commonly elevated serum LDL choles-terol level. Because of frequent changes of glycemic control of diabetic patients and their effects on lipoprotein levels, the American Diabetes Association has recommended that fasting levels of LDL, HDL, total cholesterol, and triglycerides be measured annually in adult patients.

Intervention Trials: No clinical trials have been designed to test specifically whether lipid-lowering treatment reduces CHD events in diabetic patients. Data from subanalyses of clinical trials with lipid-lowering treatment provide some insight into the benefit of treating hyperlipidemia in diabetes. The Helskinski Heart Study found a nonsignificant trend toward lower CHD incidence in diabetic subjects (3.4% vs. 10.5%, p = NS) treated with gemfibrozil as compared to placebo[25] especially in the subset with high triglycerides and low HDL cholesterol. In addition to the known risks of elevated LDL cholesterol in diabetic as well as nondiabetic patients, diabetes is associated with small, denser LDL cholesterol particles that are especially atherogenic. In subgroup analyses of Scandinavian Simvastatin Survival Study (4S)[26] and the Cholesterol and Recurrent Events (CARE) trial,[27] aggressive LDL lowering therapy reduced recurrent CVD events by 22–25 % in patients with type 2 diabetes. A recent meta-analysis examined the effect of statin treatment on cardiovascular outcomes in 18,686 diabetic participants and 71,370 without diabetes in 14 randomized trials of statin therapy.[28] During a mean follow-up of 4.3 years, there were 3247 major vascular events in people with diabetes. There was a 9% proportional reduction in all-cause mortality per mmol/L reduction in LDL cholesterol in participants with diabetes (p = 0.02), which was similar to the 13% reduction in those without diabetes (p < 0.0001). This finding reflected a significant 13% reduction in vascular mortality (p = 0.008) in participants with diabetes. There were significant 21% proportional reductions in major vascular events per mmol/L reduction in LDL cholesterol in people with or without diabetes (both p < 0.0001). In diabetic participants there were reductions in myocardial infarction or coronary death by 22%, coronary revascularization by 25%, and stroke by 21% (all p < 0.0003). After 5 years, 42 (95% CI 30–55) fewer people with diabetes had major vascular events per 1000 allocated statin therapy.

Based on the most recent National Cholesterol Education Program (Adult Treatment Panel III) guidelines, diabetes is regarded as equivalent to established CHD due to the high risk of new CHD within 10 years. Thus, the primary goal of lipid management in diabetes is to reduce LDL cholesterol to ≤100 mg/dl.[19] This goal should be achieved by addition of drug therapy after maximal dietary therapy. Statins are first-line drug therapy for LDL cholesterol reduction. Triglyceride levels >200 mg/dl should be treated with fibrate therapy. Whether to combine a statin and a fibrate in the treatment of combined hyperlipidemia needs to be carefully considered, given the documented, although infrequent, occurrence of rhabdomyolysis with this combination. Although nicotinic acid can effectively reduce triglyceride and raise HDL levels, its potential to worsen hyperglycemia raises a concern about its use, although the mildly increased glucose levels did not reduce the reduction of MI by nicotinic acid in the Coronary Drug Project.[29]

Hypertension. Hypertension is a well-established major risk factor for CVD. The prevalence of hyperten-sion in diabetic patients is at least 2-fold increased compared to the nondiabetic population. In addition to the increased risk for coronary events, hypertension also increases the risk of stroke, nephropathy, and retinopathy in diabetes. MRFIT demonstrated that the rate of CVD mortality was increased by nearly 3-fold at each level of systolic blood pressure in diabetic as compared to nondiabetic hypertensive men[24] (Fig. 32.4).

Thus, not only is hypertension more prevalent in the diabetic population, it also has a greater impact on the risks of CAD. Clinical trials in hypertensive patients with type 2 diabetes have shown that blood pressure control using several classes of medication is an extremely effective and important preventive therapy.

Of interest, several large, recent, and randomized hypertension treatment trials have shown greater rates of new-onset diabetes in patients treated by regimens based on beta blockers or diuretics than in patients receiving regimens based on renin-angiotensin-aldosterone system inhibitors or calcium channel blockers[30–32] (LIFE, ALLHAT, ASCOT). In one large series of treated hypertensive patients, moderate self-reported physical activity (>30 min twice a week) was associated with a 34% lower rate of new-onset diabetes, independent of the type of treatment and other risk factors for diabetes.[33]

Intervention Trials. Clinical trial data all support the need to treat hypertension in patients with type 2 dia-betes. The Hypertension Optimal Treatment[34] trial evaluated the effect of aggressive lowering of diastolic blood pressure using a calcium channel blocking agent, felodipine. A 51% reduction in cardiovascular events was seen in diabetic patients when diastolic pressure was treated to a mean of 82.6 mmHg as compared to those treated

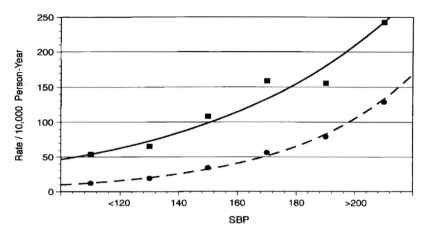

Fig. 32.4 Relationship between systolic blood pressure and cardiovascular mortality in diabetic subjects in a 12-year follow-up study from the Multiple Risk Factor Intervention Trial (MRFIT). (Adapted from Goldberg[24] with permission)

to a diastolic pressure of 90 mmHg. In the Systolic Hypertension in the Elderly Trial,[35] antihypertensive treatment with chlorthalidone produced a 34% reduction in CVD events in the diabetic population. A study of tight blood pressure control within the UKPDS[36] showed that a difference of 10/5 mmHg was associated with a 24% reduction in combined microvascular and macrovascular end points. The Appropriate Blood Pressure Control in Diabetes Trial (ABCD)[37] and the Fosinopril Versus Amlopidipine Cardiovascular Events Randomized Trial (FACET)[38] found that the incidence of CVD events was lower by 8% ($p = 0.01$) and 7% ($p = 0.03$) respectively, in those randomized to an angiotensin-converting enzyme (ACE) inhibitor than in those treated with dihydropyridine calcium channel blockers. In fact, the ABCD trial was terminated 1 year earlier than scheduled on the basis of recommendations from the independent Data and Safety Monitoring Committee. The committee became concerned with the marked disparity between the two treatment arms in the number of major coronary events that appeared after several years of treatment. The Heart Outcomes Prevention Evaluation (HOPE) and the MICRO-HOPE substudy[39] demonstrated that ACE inhibitors lowered the risk of cardiovascular death by 37% and total mortality by 24% in patients with diabetes. After adjusting for the changes in blood pressure, the risk of cardiovascular and total mortality was still reduced by 25% ($p = 0.0004$). Similarly, in the LIFE study, treatment based on the angiotensin-receptor blocker losartan was associated with a 25% reduction in overall cardiovascular morbidity and mortality and a 40% reduction in CV death compared to treatment based on the beta-blocker atenolol.[40] Smaller, albeit still beneficial, reductions by 9–14% in a spectrum of micro- and macrovascular events was seen with a fixed ACE inhibitor-diuretic combination in the ADVANCE study.[41]

The HOPE study also demonstrated that ACE inhibitors reduced the risk of overt nephropathy (by 24%) as well as microalbuminuria ($p = 0.02$). Albuminuria is not only a marker of nephropathy, but its presence also reflects a higher CVD risk.[42] Another finding, confirmed in subsequent studies using treatment regimens using ACE inhibitors or angiotensin-receptor blockers,[30–32] is that there was a reduction by one-third in the new-onset diabetes in those not diabetic at baseline over the 4.5 years of the study. Although ACE inhibitors may worsen renal function in patients with bilateral renal artery stenosis and may cause hyperkalemia, they can be used safely with careful titration and measurement of electrolytes and creatinine. Given the powerful protective effect on a range of important cardiovascular outcomes and renal function, ACE inhibitors are emerging as first-line antihypertensive treatment in the diabetic population. Recent reports have demonstrated that angiotensin II receptor antagonists also have strong renoprotective effects in patients with type 2 diabetes.[43,44] However, future studies are needed to determine whether they have similar cardiovascular protective effects.

Independent of the agent used, aggressive blood pressure control should be a high priority. Current guidelines in the US and Europe recommend a target blood pressure of less than 130/85 mmHg, where possible, in subjects with diabetes. However, the continued high rates of CV events in individuals with diabetes despite current approaches to treatment has stimulated investigation of whether treatment to lower goals for both blood pressure and LDL cholesterol would be of clinical benefit. While the large ACCORD study has not yet reported its findings with regard to CV outcomes, the SANDS study has documented that treatment over 3 years to more aggressive goals of LDL cholesterol ≤70 mg/dl and systolic blood pressure ≤115 mmHg resulted in regression vs. progression of carotid intimal medial thickness and greater regression of LV hypertrophy than treatment to goals espoused in current guidelines[45] (Table 32.1).

Hyperglycemia. Chronic hyperglycemia can directly impair vascular endothelial function, which is thought to be one of the underlying mechanisms of increased microvascular and macrovascular events in diabetes. Accumulation of advanced glycation end products (AGEs), formed by the glycation of proteins and lipoproteins, in the vessel wall leads to increased vessel stiffness, lipoprotein binding, macrophage recruitment, reduced nitric oxide production, and proliferation of vascular smooth muscle cells.[46] All of these contribute to abnormal vasomotion and increased atherogenesis which can lead to arterial thrombosis. Data from clinical trials show that the degree of hyperglycemia in diabetic patients correlates with the risk and severity of microvascular complications, and improving hyperglycemia reduces this risk incrementally. However, the relationship between glycemic control and macrovascular complications is less close. Early observational studies that have addressed the relationship of hyperglycemia and the risk of CVD in the diabetic population yielded conflicting results,[47–51] as summarized in Table 32.2.

Early data from the Diabetes Control and Complications Trial (DCCT)[52] found a trend toward reduction in cardiovascular events in the intensive treatment group as compared to conventional treatment group (0.5 event per 100 patient-years vs. 0.8 event, 95% CI, –10 to 68%). However, the study was conducted among relatively young patients with type 1 diabetes and was not powered to test the hypothesis. The study did find a significant reduction in the microvascular complications in the intensively treated group (76% risk reduction in the development of retinopathy, 39% reduction in microalbuminuria and 60% reduction in clinical neuropathy). The UKPDS, initiated in the 1970s, reported the effects of intensive treatment of hyperglycemia using sulfonylurea agents, insulin, or metformin in newly diagnosed type 2 diabetic patients over a 10-year period.[53] Despite the fact that the hemoglobin A1c was lower in the intensively treated group (7.0% vs. 7.9%, approaching the American Diabetes Association goal of <7%), the reductions in myocardial infarction (14.7 events per 1000 patient-years vs. 17.4 events; $p = 0.052$) and stroke (5.6 events per 1000 patient-years vs. 5.0 events ; $p = 0.52$) did not attain significance compared with the conventional treatment group. The development of microvascular disease was however, significantly reduced (25%, $p < 0.01$). This study was powered to demonstrate whether improved glycemic control would reduce cardiovascular events, but demonstrated only a modest reduction in myocardial infarction and none for stroke.

More recent randomized studies with greater power have yielded divergent results with regard to the effect of intensive long-term glycemic control on cardiovascular events. In the ACCORD study,[54] 10,251 patients with type 2 diabetes (mean age, 62.2 years) with a median glycated hemoglobin level of 8.1% were randomly assigned to receive intensive therapy (targeting a glycated hemoglobin level below 6.0%) or standard therapy (targeting a level from 7.0 to 7.9%). The primary outcome was a composite of nonfatal myocardial infarction, nonfatal stroke, or death from cardiovascular causes. At 1 year, stable median glycated hemoglobin levels of 6.4 and 7.5% were achieved in the intensive-therapy group and the standard-therapy group, respectively. During follow-up, the primary outcome occurred in 352 patients in the intensive-therapy group, as compared with 371 in the standard-therapy group (hazard ratio, 0.90; 95% confidence interval [CI], 0.78 to 1.04; $p = 0.16$). At the same time, 257 patients in the intensive-therapy group died, as compared with 203 in the standard-therapy group (hazard ratio, 1.22; 95% CI, 1.01 to 1.46; $p = 0.04$). Hypoglycemia requiring assistance and weight gain of more than 10 kg were more frequent in the intensive-therapy group ($p < 0.001$). Thus, in this population, the use of intensive therapy to target normal glycated hemoglobin levels for 3.5 years increased mortality and did not significantly reduce major cardiovascular events. Contrasting results were obtained in the ADVANCE study[55] of 11,140 patients with type 2 diabetes randomized to either standard glucose control or intensive glucose control (to achieve a glycated hemoglobin value of 6.5% or less). After a median of 5 years of follow-up, the mean glycated hemoglobin level was lower in the intensive-control group (6.5%) than in the standard-control group (7.3%). Intensive control reduced the incidence of combined major macrovascular and microvascular events (18.1%, vs. 20.0% with standard control; hazard ratio, 0.90; 95% confidence interval [CI], 0.82 to 0.98;

Table 32.1 Baseline and follow-up carotid and cardiac measures

| | Mean (95% confidence interval) | | | |
	Aggressive	Standard	Difference	p Value
Carotid (N = 499)				
Intimal medial thickness, mm				
Baseline	0.808 (0.78 to 0.83)	0.797 (0.78 to 0.82)		
18 mo	0.802 (0.78 to 0.82)	0.804 (0.78 to 0.83)		
36 mo	0.796 (0.77 to 0.82)	0.837 (0.81 to 0.86)		
Mean change, 18 mo	−0.006 (−0.02 to 0.008)	0.007 (−0.01 to 0.02)		
Mean change, 36 mo	−0.012 (−0.03 to 0.003)[a]	0.038 (0.02 to 0.06)[a,b]	0.05	<0.001[c]
Arterial cross-sectional area, mm^2				
Baseline	17.36 (16.7 to 18.0)	17.33 (16.8 to 17.9)		
18 mo	17.22 (16.6 to 17.8)	17.53 (17.0 to 18.1)		
36 mo	17.53 (17.0 to 18.1)	18.39 (17.8 to 19.0)		
Mean change, 18 mo	−0.13 (−0.42 to 0.15)	0.20 (−0.13 to 0.53)		
Mean change, 36 mo	−0.02 (−0.33 to 0.30)[a]	1.05 (0.73 to 1.38)[a,b]	1.07	<0.001[d]
Plaque score (0–8)				
Baseline	1.85 (1.64 to 2.05)	1.84 (1.64 to 2.03)		
18 mo	2.02 (1.82 to 2.23)	2.02 (1.82 to 2.22)		
36 mo	2.38 (2.17 to 2.59)	2.34 (2.13 to 2.55)		
Mean change, 18 mo	0.18 (0.07 to 0.29)	0.18 (0.05 to 0.32)		
Mean change, 36 mo	0.54 (0.39 to 0.68)[b]	0.50 (0.36 to 0.65)[b]	0.03	0.75
Plaque, %				
Baseline	74.6 (69 to 80)	76.5 (71 to 82)		
18 mo	81.0 (76 to 86)	81.4 (77 to 86)		
36 mo	86.5 (82 to 91)	84.2 (80 to 89)		
Point change, 18 mo	6.3 (1 to 13.5)	4.9 (−2 to 12)		
Point change, 36 mo	11.9 (5 to 19)[b]	7.7 (1 to 15)[e]		
Cardiac (N = 453)				
Left ventricular mass, g				
Baseline	156.7 (152 to 162)	156.1 (151 to 161)		
18 mo	143.2 (139 to 148)	148.3 (143 to 154)		
36 mo	149.3 (145 to 154)	152.5 (147 to 157)		
Mean change, 18 mo	−14.0 (−17 to −11)	−7.1 (−10.6 to −3.6)		
Mean change, 36 mo	−8.0 (−10.9 to −5.1)[b]	−3.3 (−6.2 to −0.35)[e]	4.8	0.02
Left ventricular mass index, g/m$^{2.7}$				
Baseline	41.2 (40 to 42)	40.5 (40 to 42)		
18 mo	37.6 (37 to 39)	38.8 (38 to 40)		
36 mo	38.9 (37.8 to 40.1)	39.4 (38.2 to 40.6)		
Mean change, 18 mo	−3.7 (−4.4 to −2.9)	−1.7 (−2.7 to −0.8)		
Mean change, 36 mo	−2.4 (−3.2 to −1.6)[b]	−1.2 (−1.9 to −0.4)[b]	1.3	0.03
Ejection fraction, %				
Baseline	60.5 (60 to 61)	59.8 (59 to 61)		
18 mo	60 (59 to 60.4)	58.7 (58 to 60)		
36 mo	59.7 (59 to 60.3)	59.1 (58 to 60)		
Mean change, 18 mo	−0.9 (−1.5 to −0.2)	−1.2 (−2 to −0.5)		
Mean change, 36 mo	−0.7 (−1.4 to 0)	−0.74 (−1.5 to 0)	0.03	0.95

[a]The changes at 36 mo in intimal medial thickness and in arterial cross-sectional area remained significantly different between the 2 groups under the Bonferroni-adjusted significance level 0.007 (=0.05/7).
[b]Significant within-group change (p value <0.01).
[c] p values from the worst-rank analyses for intimal medial thickness were 0.691 at 18 mo and <0.0001 at 36 mo.
[d]p values from the worst-rank analyses for arterial cross-sectional area were 0.194 at 18 mo and <0.0001 at 36 mo.
[e]Significant within-group change (p value <0.05).
From Howard et al.[45] by permission.

Table 32.2 Hyperglycemia and the risk of CVD

Study	No. of diabetic subjects (N)	Results
WHO Multinational Study[47]	3,583	Neither the degree of hyperglycemia or the duration of diabetes was related to the onset of CVD
Framingham Study[48]	239	No relationship between hyperglycemia and CVD incidence
The Whitehall Study[49]	178	Similar risk for CAD in newly diagnosed and previously diagnosed diabetic subjects, suggesting that neither duration nor severity had a major impact on the development of CAD
Finnish Elderly Study[50]	229	The degree of hyperglycemia was independently correlated with CVD occurrence
The Winsconsin Epidemiological Study of Diabetic Retinopathy[51]	10,135	A 1% decrease in hemoglobin A1c predicted 10% fall in CVD events but 50% reduction in retinopathy occurrence of progression, without adjustment for other CVD risk factors

$p = 0.01$), as well as that of major microvascular events (9.4% vs. 10.9%; hazard ratio, 0.86; 95% CI, 0.77 to 0.97; $p = 0.01$), primarily because of a reduction in the incidence of nephropathy (4.1% vs. 5.2%; hazard ratio, 0.79; 95% CI, 0.66 to 0.93; $p = 0.006$), with no significant effect on retinopathy ($p = 0.50$) or on major macrovascular events, death from cardiovascular causes, or death from any cause (hazard ratios with intensive control, 0.88 to 0.93, $p = 0.12$ to 0.32). In the PROACTIVE study,[56] patients randomized to receive pioglitazone on top of their existing glucose-lowering and cardiovascular medications, had an 18% lower incidence of a composite endpoint of all-cause mortality, nonfatal myocardial infarction, nonfatal stroke or acute coronary syndromes in the more aggressively treated patient group. A recent meta-analysis[57] of 29 randomized studies of tight glucose control versus usual care in 8,432 adult intensive care unit patients found no impact of tighter glucose control on mortality or need for dialysis, but did identify a 24% reduction in the risk of septicemia and a 5-fold increase in the risk of hypoglycemia requiring treatment. Aggressive treatment of hyperglycemia in diabetes has been shown to be extremely beneficial in prevention of microvascular disease. However, whether reducing HgA1c to <7% will reduce the excess risk of cardiovascular disease in diabetic patients over and above the benefit of aggressively treating all risk factors remains uncertain.

Procoagulant State. Multiple abnormalities in platelet function, coagulation, fibrinolysis, and blood viscosity have been described in diabetic patients. Abnormal platelet adhesion and aggregation, increased fibrinogen, factor VII, and increased plasminogen activator inhibitor-1 levels are well recognized.[58] These alterations in the coagulation system are particularly seen in those with the metabolic syndrome or Syndrome X. For these reasons, the American Diabetes Association has recommended that aspirin treatment be considered in diabetic patients with two or more risk factors in addition to those with established cardiovascular disease.

Cigarette Smoking, Obesity, and Physical Activity. Cigarette smoking is a leading risk factor for CVD. In MRFIT[2], cigarette smoking was a powerful determinant of CVD mortality in men with diabetes and had an additive effect when superimposed on either risk factor. Among over 11,000 participants in the Swedish National Diabetes Register, current smoking and higher body mass index both strongly predicted the occurrence of nearly 1,500 incident CV events (both p <0.002), independent of effects of other risk factors.[59] Weight reduction and regular physical activity have beneficial effects on glycemic control, hypertension, dyslipidemia, and insulin resistance.

Management of Coronary Artery Disease in Diabetic Patients. Available data, reviewed above, indicates that optimal control of arterial pressure and lipid levels are of substantial benefit, for prevention of coronary artery disease events in diabetic patients. Use of aspirin and nephroprotection by ACE inhibitors also appear to reduce CAD risk. After CAD has become manifested by myocardial infarction, optimal glucose control with insulin therapy in diabetic patients was shown to produce a significant 30% reduction in mortality at 12 months as compared to usual glycemic control.[60] Beta blockers are also effective in mortality reduction after myocardial infarction in diabetic patients. Pooled trial results show a 37% reduction in CVD mortality in diabetic patients compared with 13% found in all treated groups.[61] Thus, the management of diabetic patients with acute myocardial infarction should include optimum glycemic control with insulin, immediate coronary reperfusion, aspirin, and early beta blockade.

Coronary Revascularization. Coronary artery bypass graft surgery (CABG) and percutaneous coronary angioplasty (PTCA) are both effective revascularization strategies in patients with diabetes. Diabetes is not associated with increased perioperative mortality during bypass graft surgery, although the frequency of wound infection and the length of hospital stay are increased. Although the initial rate of success of PTCA is similar in diabetic and nondiabetic individuals, there is an increased rate of restenosis during the next 6 months. The mechanism of restenosis is thought to be due to exaggerated neointimal hyperplasia rather than increased vessel remodeling.[62] Whether the use of more technologically advanced procedures, such as stenting, will lead to improved outcomes in diabetes remains to be answered by future clinical trials.

Several trials have examined the outcome of PTCA compared to CABG in diabetic patients with multivessel CAD. The Bypass Angioplasty Revascularization Investigation (BARI)[63] demonstrated that 5-year survival was only 65.5% in diabetic patients randomly assigned to PTCA compared to 80.6% survival in the CABG group. For patients without diabetes, the 5-year mortality rates were virtually identical. After 10 years of follow-up in the BARI study,[64] in the subgroup of patients with no treated diabetes, survival rates were nearly identical by randomization (PTCA 77.0% vs. CABG 77.3%, $p = 0.59$). In the subgroup with treated diabetes, the CABG assigned group continued to have higher survival than the PTCA assigned group (PTCA 45.5% vs. CABG 57.8%, $p = 0.025$). One limitation of the study, however, was the lack of the use of stents in the angioplasty group, since stenting may improve outcomes in patients with diabetes; the question of whether use of stents has improved the relative benefit of angioplasty versus bypass surgery for diabetic patients is being addressed in the ongoing randomized BARI-2 study.[65] One explanation for the higher mortality associated with PTCA is that diabetes is usually associated with more diffuse coronary disease and the vessels are of small caliber. It is also likely that angioplasty leaves a higher proportion of myocardium ischemic than does bypass grafting. The issue of whether the findings of the BARI trial are consistent with other revascularization trials has been raised. The Emory Angioplasty Versus Surgery Trial (EAST)[66] found no difference in mortality in diabetic patients treated with PTCA compared with coronary bypass surgery. However, diabetic patients fared no worse than nondiabetic patients in general, which suggest that the diabetic patients in this study represent an unusually low risk group. Also, EAST involved fewer diabetic patients than did BARI and had limited statistical power to detect a treatment difference.

In a recent meta-analysis of 13 randomized clinical trials and 16 registries including over 12,500 diabetic patients comparing treatment with the two major types of drug-eluting stents,[67] there were similar, moderate rates of subsequent target vessel revascularization (5.8–8.6%) or major adverse cardiac events (10.1–15.4%) with both types of drug-eluting stents. However, this analysis was limited by lack of comparative data for outcomes with coronary bypass surgery. The conclusion which can be drawn from the above studies is that the form of revascularization for the treatment of multivessel coronary disease in diabetes can be individually tailored to patients, taking into account the clinical and angiographic suitability for each procedure. Those patients with more severe disease should undergo surgery and those with milder form of disease can be treated with angioplasty plus stenting.

Cardiomyopathy

One reason for the poor prognosis in patients with diabetes after myocardial infarction is the increased susceptibility to develop heart failure. Diabetic men have more than twice the frequency of heart failure than nondiabetic cohorts, while diabetic women have a 5-fold increased risk of developing heart failure.[68] This excessive risk of heart failure persists despite correcting for age, hypertension, obesity, hypercholesterolemia, other conventional risk factors, and recognized coronary artery disease at baseline. However, it remained unclear whether the excess incidence of heart failure in diabetic individuals was due to their high rate of myocardial infarction.

Recently de Simone et al.[69] documented in a large population-based sample that diabetes was associated with a 1.5-fold higher incidence of heart failure after accounting for incident myocardial infarction as a competing risk, in addition to control for a wide array of established risk factors. It has been proposed that a specific diabetic cardiomyopathy exists, independent of coronary artery disease or other coexisting confounding factors, characterized by alteration of left ventricular (LV) structure and function. There are now considerable experimental, pathological, and epidemiological data to support the existence of "diabetic cardiomyopathy." The existence of a subclinical or early form of diabetic cardiomyopathy is suggested by documentation of abnormal LV structure and function, detected by echocardiography, in newly diagnosed type 2 diabetes.[70] The process of alteration of the myocardium may occur before the degree of abnormality of glucose metabolism reaches the criteria level for the diagnosis of diabetes. Features of this diabetic cardiomyopathy are discussed below.

Left Ventricular Hypertrophy. The association of LV hypertrophy and risk of cardiovascular morbidity and mortality is well established.[71] In one landmark study, LV hypertrophy was associated with a greater relative risk for all-cause mortality than the number of stenotic coronary arteries or the LV ejection fraction.[72] In animal models,[73] rats with streptozotocin induced diabetes demonstrate increased LV mass. The combination of hypertension and diabetes mellitus is synergistic in rats, leading to higher mortality, as it does in humans. This finding is confirmed in pathologic studies which showed that human diabetic hearts have higher LV mass, unrelated to the extent of coronary artery disease and hypertension.[74] Other abnormalities noted in human diabetic hearts include microvascular constriction, interstitial fibrosis, and edema.

In epidemiological studies, diabetes has been shown to be independently associated with higher prevalences of LV hypertrophy in both the Framingham population and the Strong Heart Study.[75,76] In the latter study, the combination of hypertension and diabetes, which frequently coexist, was associated with a higher prevalence of LV hypertrophy (38%) than found in individuals with either diabetes or hypertension (19–24%) or with neither (11%).[77] In 1,950 hypertensive patients in the population-based HyperGEN study,[78] the 386 (20%) with diabetes had a higher prevalence of LV hypertrophy (38 vs. 26%, $p = 0.03$) and lower LV midwall shortening ($p < 0.001$). Recently, evaluation of a population-based sample of adolescents and young adults has shown that diabetes is associated with an increased prevalence of LV hypertrophy even at young ages.[79] In a population of 1,810 diabetic adults, CV mortality was significantly higher (OR $= 2.36$, 95% CI 1.18–4.69) in DM participants with as opposed to those without echocardiographic LV hypertrophy, after adjusting for age, gender, body mass index, hypertension, smoking, and plasma creatinine.[80] Furthermore, electrocardiographic repolarization abnormalities that are influenced by LV hypertrophy as well as underlying coronary artery disease have been shown to predict CV and all-cause mortality.[81] In addition to increasing LV mass, diabetes also impacts cardiac remodeling, with an associated increase in relative wall thickness, a measure of concentricity of the left ventricle.[76]

The association between diabetes and left ventricular hypertrophy may be bidirectional. Recent analyses in a large population of patients with moderately severe hypertension have shown that individuals with diabetes and baseline left ventricular hypertrophy had less reduction of left ventricular hypertrophy – whether measured by electrocardiography[82] or echocardiography[83] – than their nondiabetic counterparts despite even greater reduction of blood pressure in the former group. Conversely, it has recently been shown in this same population that regression of electrocardiographic left ventricular hypertrophy was associated with a 26% lower incidence of new diabetes, after adjustment for multiple risk factors for diabetes.[84]

Left Ventricular Function. Diabetes is associated with systolic and diastolic dysfunction, independent of coronary artery disease or hypertension. Hemodynamic, biochemical, and histological studies in alloxan induced diabetic dogs demonstrated a lower stroke volume despite normal LV end-diastolic pressure. Chamber stiffness was increased in diabetic dogs compared to control dogs.[85] Isolated papillary muscle studies in diabetic rats indicate prolongation of contraction, prolonged relaxation, and a reduced rate of shortening.[73] A wide range of abnormal biochemical changes have been described in the hearts of diabetic rats including alterations in ATPase, impaired calcium ion transport and alterations in carbohydrate, lipid, and adenine nucleotide metabolism.

In clinical studies, Jain et al. found increased chamber stiffness in diabetic as compared to nondiabetic subjects. In addition, epidemiological studies have found that adults with diabetes have lower fractional shortening (by a mean of 0.7%) and midwall fractional shortening (an index of myocardial contractility) by a mean of 0.9%.[86] Hildebrandt et al.[87] showed in a large series of hypertensive patients with ECG LV hypertrophy that participants who also had diabetes had lower LV systolic chamber and myocardial function, as well as lower mean stroke volume than their nondiabetic counterparts. Of note, LV mass was similar in diabetic and nondiabetic patients, indicating that the observed functional abnormalities are independent of the degree of hypertrophy. Impaired LV systolic function is the strongest predictor of morbid cardiac events in coronary artery disease.[88] Diabetes is also associated with diastolic dysfunction, which appears to predate the onset of systolic dysfunction. The severity of diabetes-associated abnormal LV relaxation is similar to the well known impaired relaxation associated with hypertension.[89] The combination of both diabetes and hypertension induces more severe abnormal LV relaxation than does either condition alone. In addition, abnormal relaxation in subjects with diabetes is associated with worse glycemic control and positively associated with duration of diabetes. Evidence of impaired LV relaxation is associated with higher cardiovascular and all-cause mortality in diabetes.[90] Evidence of diabetic cardiomyopathy is seen early in the course of the disease, often at the onset of diabetes.[70]

Potential Mechanisms. The etiology of diabetic cardiomyopathy characterized by increased LV mass, concentric remodeling, systolic dysfunction, and impaired LV relaxation is not entirely clear. One hemodynamic mechanism that has been identified in several studies is increase in arterial stiffness, which may augment central arterial pressure and thus the load placed on the LV and also on the coronary and cerebral arterial trees.[87] It has been proposed that additional pathogenic mechanisms may involve impact of metabolic alterations due to hyperglycemia. Interstitial accumulation of advanced-glycated end products (AGES), collagen deposition, and fibrosis in the myocardium have been reported in human diabetic hearts.[74] Animal studies have found p-aminosalicyclic acid-positive material among the muscle fibers and cholesterol and triglyceride deposition in the myocardium.[73] These tissue alterations can increase end-diastolic myocardial stiffness as well as LV mass, and impair systolic function.

The pathogenic mechanism underlying these changes in myocardial tissue composition is unclear. We have reported that albuminuria, a strong predictor of cardiovascular mortality and morbidity, is independently associated with increased LV mass and systolic and diastolic dysfunction among diabetic patients.[91] Albuminuria has been proposed to represent a marker of a generalized vascular dysfunction[92] and has been associated with renal alterations, proliferative retinopathy, and cardiovascular disease in diabetic and nondiabetic populations. Albuminuria reflects a renal and systemic transvascular albumin leakage that is perhaps due to low vessel wall content of heparin sulfate which has been shown not only in the glomerular basement membrane but also in the atherosclerotic aorta and coronary arteries.[93] This generalized increase of vascular permeability can also cause leakiness of collagen, cholesterol, and advanced glycated end products that have been reported in the myocardium of human hearts .[85] Furthermore, this change in permeability causing insudation of lipoproteins into the intima of large vessels can lead to atherosclerosis of the epicardial coronary arteries as well as small arterioles of the heart. Small vessel disease can lead to subendocardial ischemia causing systolic and diastolic myocardial dysfunction. The microvascular changes in the heart are the same as those throughout the rest of the body such as interstitial fibrosis, perivascular thickening and fibrosis, and micro-aneurysm formation.

Conclusions

The high rates of morbidity and mortality associated with diabetes are, most notably due to cardiovascular disease. The risk of developing new coronary heart disease is high in diabetes, in part because of its frequent association with other risk factors for coronary artery disease. In addition, diabetes is associated with higher morbidity and mortality after myocardial infarction. Diabetes is also often associated with a distinct cardiomyopathy which may partially mediate the high mortality associated with coronary heart disease and congestive heart failure. Management goals for the diabetic patient should focus on optimal glucose control and intense modification of coronary disease risk factors, especially optimal control of arterial pressure and lipids. In addition, evaluation to detect subclinical or early clinical evidence of atherosclerosis and diabetic cardiomyopathy may be warranted to target especially intensive intervention most accurately.

References

1. Garcia MJ, McNamara M, Gordon T, Kannel WB: 16 year follow-up study. Morbidity and mortality in diabetics in the Framingham population. *Diabetes*. 1974;23:105–111.
2. Kannel WB, McGee DL. Diabetes and cardiovascular disease; The Framingham Study. *J Am Med Assoc*. 1979;241:2035–2038.
3. Grundy SM, Benjamin IJ, Burke GL, et al. Diabetes and cardiovascular disease: a statement for healthcare professionals from the American Heart Association. *Circulation*. 1999;100:1134–1146.
4. Laakso M, Lehto S. Epidemiology of macrovascular disease in diabetes. *Diabetes Rev*. 1997;5:294–315.
5. Brezinka V, Padmos I. Coronary heart disease risk factors in women. *Eur Heart J*. 1994;15:1571–1584.
6. Haffner SM, Lehto S, Ronnemaa T, et al. Mortality from coronary heart disease in subjects with type 2 diabetes and in nondiabetic subjects with and without prior myocardial infarction. *N Engl J Med*. 1998;339:229–234.
7. Donahoe SM, Stewart GC, McCabe CH, et al. Diabetes and mortality following acute coronary syndromes. *J Am Med Assoc*. 2007;298:765–775.
8. Gu K, Cowie CC, Harris MI. Diabetes and decline in heart disease mortality in US adults. *J Am Med Assoc*. 1999;281: 1291–1297.
9. Jemal A, Ward E, Hao Y, et al. Trends in the leading causes of death in the United States, 1970–2002. *J Am Med Assoc*. 2005;294:1255–1259.
10. McGuire DK et al. Diabetes and ischemic heart disease. *Am Heart J*. 1999;138:S366–S375.
11. Miettinen H, Lehto S, Salomaa V, et al. Impact of diabetes on mortality after the first myocardial infarction. *Diabetes Care*. 1998;21:69–75.
12. Naka M, Hiramatsu K, Aizawa T, et al. Silent myocardial ischemia in non-insulin dependent diabetes mellitus as judged by treadmill exercise testing and coronary angiography. *Am Heart J*. 1992;123:46–52.
13. Langer A, Freeman M, Josse R, et al. Detection of silent myocardial ischemia in diabetes mellitus. *Am J Cardiol*. 1991;67: 1073–1078.
14. Caracciolo EZ, Chaitman BR, Forman SR, et al. Diabetics with coronary disease have a prevalence of asymptomatic ischemia during exercise treadmill testing and ambulatory ischemia monitoring similar to that of non-diabetic patients. *Circulation*. 1996;93:2097–2105.
15. Scholte AJ, Schuijf JD, Kharagjitsingh AV, et al. Different manifestations of coronary artery disease by stress SPECT myocardial perfusion imaging, coronary calcium scoring, and multislice CT coronary angiography in asymptomatic patients with type 2 diabetes mellitus. *J Nucl Cardiol*. 2008;15:503–509.
16. Wackers FJ, Chyun DA, Young LH, et al. Detection of Ischmeia in Asymptomatic Diabetics (DIAD) Investigators. Resolution of asymptomatic myocardial ischemia in patients with type 2 diabetes in the Detection of Ischemia in Asymptomatic Diabetics (DIAD) study. *Diabetes Care*. 2007;30:2892–2898.
17. Stamler J, Vaccaro O, Neaton JD, et al. Diabetes, other risk factors and 12-year cardiovascular mortality in men screened in the Multiple Risk Factor Intervention Trial (MRFIT). *Diabetes Care*. 1993;16:434–444.
18. WHO. Definition of metabolic syndrome in definition, diagnosis and classification of diabetes and its complications. Report of a WHO consultation. Part 1: Diagnosis and classification of diabetes mellitus. WHO/NCD/NCS/99.2. 1999. Geneva, World Health Organization - Department of Noncommunicable Disease Surveillance.
19. Third Report of the National Cholesterol Education Program (NCEP) Expert Panel on Detection, Evaluation, and Treatment of High Blood Cholesterol in Adults (Adult Treatment Panel III) final report. *Circulation*. 2002;106:3143–3421.
20. Balkau B, Charles MA, Drivsholm T, et al. Frequency of the WHO metabolic syndrome in European cohorts, and an alternative definition of an insulin resistance syndrome. *Diabetes Metab*. 2002;28:364–376.
21. Einhorn D, Reaven GM, Cobin RH, et al. American College of Endocrinology position statement on the insulin resistance syndrome. *Endocr Pract*. 2003;9:237–252; Alberti G. Introduction to the metabolic syndrome. Eur Heart J Suppl 2005;7:3–5.
22. Howard BV, Best LG, Galloway JM, et al. Coronary heart disease risk equivalence in diabetes depends on concomitant risk factors. *Diabetes Care*. 2006;29:391–397.
23. Folsom AR, Chambless LE, Duncan BB, et al. The Atherosclerosis Risk in Communities Study Investigators: Prediction of coronary heart disease in middle-aged adults with diabetes. *Diabetes Care*. 2003;26:2777–2784.
24. Goldberg RB. Cardiovascular disease in diabetic patients. *Med Clin North Am*. 2000;84(1):81–93.
25. Koskinen P, Manttari M, Manninen V, et al. Coronary heart disease incidence in NIDDM patients in the Helsinki Heart Study. *Diabetes Care*. 1992;15:820–825.
26. Pyprala K, Pedersen TR, Kjekshus J, et al. Cholesterol lowering with simvastatin improves prognosis of diabetic patients with coronary heart disease. A subgroup analysis of the Scandinavian Simvastatin Survival Study (4S). *Diabetes Care*. 1997;20: 614–620.
27. Goldberg RB, Mellies MJ, Sacks FM, et al. For the CARE Investigators. Cardiovascular events and their reduction with pravastatin in diabetic and glucose intolerant myocardial infarction survivors with average cholesterol levels: subgroup analyses in the Cholesterol and Recurrent Events (CARE) trial. *Circulation*. 1998;98:2513–2519.
28. Kearney PM, Blackwell L, Collins R, et al. Efficacy of cholesterol lowering therapy in 18,686 people with diabetes in 14 randomised trials of statins: a meta-analysisCholesterol Treatment Trialists' (CTT) Collaborators. *Lancet*. 2008;371: 117–125.

29. Canner PL, Furberg CD, Terrin ML, et al. Benefits of niacin by glycemic status in patients with healed myocardial infarction (from the Coronary Drug Project). *Am J Cardiol.* 2005;95:254–257.

30. Dahlöf B, Devereux RB, Kjeldsen SE, et al. For the LIFE study group. Cardiovascular morbidity and mortality in the Losartan Intervention for Endpoint reduction in hypertension study (LIFE): a randomised trial against atenolol. *Lancet.* 2002;359: 995–1003.

31. Barzilay JI, Davis BR, Cutler JA, et al. Fasting glucose levels and incident diabetes mellitus in older nondiabetic adults randomized to receive 3 different classes of antihypertensive treatment: A report from the Antihypertensive and Lipid-Lowering Treatment to Prevent Heart Attack Trial (ALLHAT). *Arch Intern Med.* 2006;166:2191–2201.

32. Dahlöf B, Sever PS, Pulter NR, et al. Prevention of cardiovascular events with an antihypertensive regimen of amlodipine adding perindopril as required versus atenolol adding bendroflumethiazide as required, in the Anglo-Scandinavian Cardiac Outcomes Trial-Blood Pressure Lowering Arm (ASCOT-BPLA): a multicentre randomized controlled trial. *Lancet.* 2005;366: 895–906.

33. Fossum E, Gleim GW, Kjeldsen SE, et al. The effect of baseline physical activity on cardiovascular outcomes and new-onset diabetes in patients treated for hypertension and left ventricular hypertrophy: the LIFE study. *J Intern Med.* 2007;262:439–448.

34. Hansson L, Zanchetti A, Carruthers SG, et al. Effects of intensive blood-pressure lowering and low-dose aspirin in patients with hypertension: principal results of the Hypertension Optimal Treatment (HOT) randomized trial. Hot Study Group. *Lancet.* 1998;351:1755–1762.

35. Curb JD, Pressel SL, Cutler JA, et al. For the Systolic Hypertension in the Elderly Program Cooperative Research Group. Effect of diuretic-based antihypertensive treatment on cardiovascular disease risk in older diabetic patients with isolated systolic hypertension. *J Am Med Assoc.* 1996;276:1886–1892.

36. UK Prospective Diabetes Study Group. Tight blood pressure control and risk of macrovascular and microvascular complications in type 2 diabetes. UKPDS 38. *Br Med J.* 1998;317:703–713.

37. Estacio RO, Jeffers BW, Hiatt WR, et al. The effect of nisoldipine as compared with enalapril on cardiovascular outcomes in patients with non-insulin dependent diabetes and hypertension. *N Engl J Med.* 1998;338:645–652.

38. Tatti P, Pahor M, Byrington RB, et al. Outcome results of the Fosinopril versus Amlodipine Cardiovascular Events Randomized Trial (FACET) in patients with hypertension and NIDDM. *Diabetes Care.* 1998;21:597–603.

39. Heart Outcomes Prevention Evaluation Study Investigators: Effects of ramipril on cardiovascular and microvascular outcomes in people with diabetes mellitus: results of the HOPE study and MICRO-HOPE substudy. *Lancet.* 2000;355:253–259.

40. Lindholm LH, Ibsen H, Dahlöf B, et al. for the LIFE study group: Cardiovascular morbidity and mortality in hypertensive patients with diabetes: The LIFE Study. *Lancet.* 2002;359:1004–1010.

41. Patel A, ADVANCE Collaborative Group, MacMahon S, Chalmers J, et al. Effects of a fixed combination of perindopril and indapamide on macrovascular and microvascular outcomes in patients with type 2 diabetes mellitus (the ADVANCE trial): a randomised controlled trial. *Lancet.* 2007;370:829–840.

42. Mogensen CE. Microalbuminuria predicts clinical proteinuria and early mortality in maturity-onset diabetes. *N Engl J Med.* 1994;310:356–360.

43. Brenner BM, Cooper ME, de Zeeuw D, et al. Effects of losartan on renal and cardiovascular outcomes in maturity-onset diabetes. *N Engl J Med.* 2001;345:861–869.

44. Parving H-H, Lehnert H, Brochner-Mortensen J, et al. The effect of irbesartan on the development of diabetic nephropathy in patients with type 2 Diabetes. *N Engl J Med.* 2001;345:870–878.

45. Howard BV, Roman MJ, Devereux RB, et al. Effect of lower targets for blood pressure and LDL cholesterol on atherosclerosis in diabetes: the SANDS randomized trial. *J Am Med Assoc.* 2008;299:1678–1689.

46. Brownlee M. Glycation and diabetic complications. *Diabetes.* 1994;43:836–841.

47. West KM, Ahuja MM, Bennet PH, et al. The role of circulating glucose and triglyceride concentrations and their interactions with other "risk factors" as determinants of arterial disease in nine diabetic population samples from the WHO Multinational Study. *Diabetes Care.* 1983;6:361–369.

48. Wilson PW, Cupples LA, Kannel WB. Is hyperglycemia associated with cardiovascular disease? The Framingham Study. *Am Heart J.* 1991;121(2 Pt 1):586–590.

49. Jarrett RJ, Shipley MJ. Type 2 (non-insulin dependent) diabetes mellitus and cardiovascular disease. Putative associations via common antecedents. Further evidence from the Whitehall Study. *Diabetologia.* 1988;31:737–740.

50. Kuusisto J, Mykkänen L, Pyorala K, et al. NIDDM and its metabolic control predict coronary heart disease in elderly subjects. *Diabetes.* 1994;43:960–967.

51. Klein R. Kelly West Lecture 1994. Hyperglycemia and microvascular and macrovascular disease in diabetes. *Diabetes Care.* 1995;18:258–268.

52. Diabetes Control and Complications Trial Research Group (DVVT): The effect of intensive treatment of diabetes on the development and progression of long-term complications in insulin-dependent diabetes mellitus. *N Engl J Med.* 1993;329: 977–986.

53. UK Prospective Diabetes Study (UKPDS) Group: Intensive blood-glucose control with sulfonylureas or insulin compared with conventional treatment and risk of complications in patients with type 2 diabetes (UKPDS33). *Lancet.* 1998;352: 837–852.

54. Action to Control Cardiovascular Risk in Diabetes Study Group, Gerstein HC, Miller ME, Byington RP, et al. Effects of intensive glucose lowering in type 2 diabetes. *N Engl J Med.* 2008;358:2545–2559.

55. ADVANCE Collaborative Group, Patel A, MacMahon S, Chalmers J, et al. Intensive blood glucose control and vascular outcomes in patients with type 2 diabetes. *N Engl J Med.* 2008;358:2560–2572.
56. Wilcox R, Kupfer S, Erdmann E; PROactive Study investigators. Effects of pioglitazone on major adverse cardiovascular events in high-risk patients with type 2 diabetes: results from PROspective pioglitAzone Clinical Trial In macro Vascular Events (PROactive 10). *Am Heart J.* 2008;155:712–717.
57. Soylemez Wiener R, Wiener DC, Larson RJ. Benefits and risks of tight glucose control in critically ill adults: a meta-analysis. *J Am Med Assoc.* 2008;300:933–944.
58. Colwell JA. Aspirin therapy in diabetes. *Diabetes Care.* 1997;20:1767–1771.
59. Cederholm J, Eeg-Olofsson K, Eliasson B, et al. On behalf of the Swedish National Diabetes Register. Risk prediction of cardiovascular disease in type 2 diabetes: A risk equation from the Swedish National Diabetes Register (NDR). *Diabetes Care.* 2008 Jun 30. [Epub ahead of print].
60. Malmberg K, Ryden L, Efendic S, et al. Randomized trial of insulin-glucose infusion followed by subcutaneous insulin treatment in diabetic patients with acute myocardial infarction (DIGAMI Study): effects on mortality at 1 year. *J Am Coll Cardiol.* 1995;26:57–65.
61. Kendall MJ, Lynch KP, Hjalmarson A, et al. Beta-blockers and sudden cardiac death. *Ann Intern Med.* 1995;123:358–367.
62. Komowski R, Mintz GS, Kent KM, et al. Increased restenosis in diabetes mellitus after coronary interventions is due to exaggerated intimal hyperplasia. *Circulation.* 1997;95:1366–1369.
63. The Bypass Angioplasty Revascularization Investigation (BARI) Investigators: Comparison of coronary bypass surgery with angioplasty in patients with multivessel disease. *N Engl J Med.* 1996;335:217–225.
64. BARI Investigators. The final 10-year follow-up results from the BARI randomized trial. *J Am Coll Cardiol.* 2007;49: 1600–1606.
65. King SB, Lembo NJ, Weintraub WS, et al. For the Emory Angioplasty Versus Surgery Trial (EAST). A randomized trial comparing coronary angioplasty with coronary bypass surgery. *N Engl J Med.* 1994;331:1044–1050.
66. Brooks MM, Grye RL, Genuth S, et al. Hypotheses, design and methods for the Fypass Angioplasty Revascularization Investigation 2 Diabetes (BARI 2D) Trial. *Am J Cardiol.* 2006;12(Suppl 1):9–19.
67. Mahmud E, Bromberg-Marin G, Palakodeti V, et al. Clinical efficacy of drug-eluting stents in diabetic patients: a meta-analysis. *J Am Coll Cardiol.* 2007;49:1600–1606.
68. Abbott RD, Donahue RP, Kannel WB, et al. The impact of diabetes on survival following myocardial infarction in men vs. women. The Framingham Study. *J Am Med Assoc.* 1988;260:3456–3460.
69. de Simone G, Devereux RB, Chinali M, et al. Diabetes and incident congestive heart failure: The Strong Heart Study. *Circulation.* 2007;116(Suppl II):II-835.
70. Liu JE, Robbins DC, Sosenko J, et al. Abnormal left ventricular structure and function are associated with recent conversion from normal glucose tolerance to diabetes mellitus – the Strong Heart Study. *Diabetes.* 2001;50(suppl 2):s147.
71. Levy D, Garrison RJ, Savage DD, et al. Prognostic implications of echocardiographically determined left ventricular mass in the Framingham Heart Study. *N Engl J Med.* 1990;322:1561–1566.
72. Liao Y, Cooper RS, McGee DL, et al. The relative effects of left ventricular hypertrophy, coronary artery disease, and ventricular dysfunction on survival among black adults. *J Am Med Assoc.* 1995;273:1592–1597.
73. Fein FS, Sonnenblick EH. Diabetic cardiomyopathy. *Cardiovascular Drugs Ther.* 1994;8:65–73.
74. Van Hoeven KH, Factor SM. A comparison of the pathological spectrum of hypertensive, diabetic and hypertensive-diabetic heart disease. *Circulation.* 1990;82:848–855.
75. Galderisi M, Anderson KM, Wilson PW, et al. Echocardiographic evidence for the existence of a distinct diabetic cardiomyopathy (The Framingham Heart Study). *Am J Cardiol.* 1991;68:85–89.
76. Devereux RB, Roman MJ, Paranicas M, et al. Impact of diabetes on cardiac structure and function: The Strong Heart Study. *Circulation.* 2000;101:2271–2276.
77. Bella JN, Devereux RB, Roman MJ, et al. Separate and joint cardiovascular effects of hypertension and diabetes: The Strong Heart Study. *Am J Cardiol.* 2001;87:1260–1265.
78. Palmieri V, Bella JN, Arnett DK, et al. Impact of Type II Diabetes on Left Ventricular Geometry and Function: The Hypertension Genetic Epidemiology Network (HyperGEN) Study. *Circulation.* 2001;103:102–107.
79. De Marco M, de Simone G, Russell M, et al. Metabolic and cardiovascular characteristics of diabetes in adolescents and young adults: the Strong Heart Study. *Circulation.* 2008;118 (Suppl 2):s1116.
80. Liu JE, Palmieri V, Roman MJ, et al. Cardiovascular disease and prognosis in adults with glucose disorders: The Strong Heart Study. *J Am Coll Cardiol.* 2000;35:263A.
81. Okin PM, Devereux RB, Lee ET, et al. Electrocardiographic repolarization complexity and abnormality predict all-cause and cardiovascular mortality in diabetes: The Strong Heart Study. *Diabetes.* 2004;53:434–440.
82. Okin PM, Gerdts E, Snapinn SM, et al. The impact of diabetes on regression of electrocardiographic left ventricular hypertrophy and the prediction of outcome during antihypertensive therapy: The LIFE Study. *Circulation.* 2006;113: 1588–1596.
83. Gerdts E, Okin PM, Omvik P, et al. Impact of concomitant diabetes on changes in left ventricular structure and systolic function during long-term antihypertensive treatment in hypertensive patients with left ventricular hypertrophy (the LIFE study). *Nutr Metab Cardiovasc Dis.* 2009;19:306–312.

84. Okin PM, Harris KE, Jern S, et al. In-treatment resolution or absence of electrocardiographic left ventricular hypertrophy is associated with decreased incidence of new-onset diabetes mellitus in hypertensive patients: The LIFE Study. *Hypertension.* 2007;50:984–990.
85. Regan TJ, Wu CF, Yeh CK, et al. Myocardial composition and function in diabetes: the effect of chronic insulin use. *Circ Res.* 1981;49:1268–1277.
86. Jain A, Avendano G, Dharamsey S, et al. Left ventricular diastolic function in hypertension and role of plasma glucose and insulin. Comparison with diabetic heart. *Circulation.* 1996;93:1396–1402.
87. Hildebrandt P, Wachtell K, Dahlöf B, et al. Impairment of cardiac function in hypertensive patients with type 2 diabetes. A LIFE study. *Diabet Med.* 2005;22:1005–1011.
88. Mock MB, Ringqvist I, Fischer LD, and Participants in the Coronary Artery Surgery Study (CASS) Registry. Survival of medically treated patients in the Coronary Artery Study (CASS) registry. *Circulation.* 1982;66:562–571.
89. Liu JE, Palmieri V, Roman MJ, et al. The impact of glycemia and diabetes on left ventricular filling pattern: The Strong Heart Study. *J Am Coll Cardiol.* 2001;37:1943–1949.
90. Bella JN, Palmieri V, Liu JE, et al. Mitral E/A ratio as a predictor of mortality in middle-aged and elderly adults: The Strong Heart Study. *Circulation.* 2002;105:1928–1933.
91. Liu JE, Robbins DC, Palmieri V, et al. Association of albuminuria with systolic and diastolic left ventricular dysfunction in type 2 diabetes: The Strong Heart Study. *J Am Coll Cardiol.* 2003;41:2022–2028.
92. Deckert T, Feldt-Rasmussen B, Borch-Johnsen K, et al. Albuminuria reflects widespread vascular damage – The Steno Hypothesis. *Diabetologia.* 1989;32:219–226.
93. Yla-Herrtuala S, Sumuvuori H, Karkola K, et al. Glycosoaminoglycans in normal and atherosclerotic human coronary arteries. *Lab Invest.* 1986;61:231–236.

Chapter 33
Polycystic Ovary Syndrome

Susan B. Zweig, Marsha C. Tolentino, Marina Strizhevsky, and Leonid Poretsky

Definition, Clinical Manifestations, and Prevalence

Polycystic ovary syndrome (PCOS) is a common disorder affecting (depending on the population studied and the definition of the syndrome) between 5 and 20% of reproductive age women.[1] If the middle of this range is considered as a realistic prevalence, then PCOS may be the most prevalent endocrine disorder in women. In spite of the widespread presence of PCOS, its precise definition still eludes both investigators and practitioners. Most consensus definitions describe PCOS as a disorder characterized by *chronic anovulation* and the presence of some degree of *hyperandrogenism,* with the exclusion of specific disorders that may lead to similar phenotypes, particularly, 21-hydroxylase deficiency and other forms of congenital adrenal hyperplasia. The definition proposed in 1990 by the National Institutes of Health Conference on PCOS requires a minimum of two criteria: menstrual abnormalities due to oligo- or anovulation, and hyperandrogenism of ovarian origin. Other disorders, such as 21-hydroxylase deficiency, androgen secreting tumors, hypothyroidism, Cushing's syndrome, and hyperprolactinemia, must be excluded.[2] In 2003 in Rotterdam a revised consensus on the diagnosis of PCOS was proposed. The new criteria require two out of the three following features once exclusion of other causes of hyperandrogenism has been made: oligo- or amenorrhea, hyperandrogenism (clinical or biochemical), and polycystic ovary morphology on ultrasound.[3,4]

Clinical manifestations vary widely among women with this disorder. Chronic anovulation may present as infertility or some form of menstrual irregularity, such as amenorrhea, oligomenorrhea, or dysfunctional uterine bleeding. Signs of hyperandrogenism include hirsutism, seborrhea, acne, and alopecia. Evidence of virilization, including clitoromegaly, may be present in severe cases. Obesity and acanthosis nigricans are clinical features that are commonly seen in PCOS women and are associated with insulin resistance.

Epidemiological data and prospective controlled studies have reported an increased prevalence of insulin resistance, impaired glucose tolerance, and undiagnosed type 2 diabetes mellitus in these women.[5] Increased risk for dyslipidemia, cardiovascular disease, and endometrial carcinoma has also been observed in this population.[6,7] In this chapter, we will discuss the role of insulin resistance in the pathogenesis of PCOS, the risk of diabetes mellitus in this population and the role of insulin-sensitizing agents, oral contraceptive pills and antiandrogens in treating patients with polycystic ovary syndrome.

Stein–Leventhal Syndrome

Although reports of disorders resembling PCOS date prior to the seventeenth century, the first clear description belongs to Chereau, who in 1844 described "sclerocystic degeneration of the ovaries."[8] The modern era of PCOS began with a report by two gynecologists, Irving F. Stein and Michael L. Leventhal, who in 1935 described a

L. Poretsky (✉)

Division of Endocrinology, Beth Israel Medical Center, Albert Einstein College of Medicine, New York, USA

e-mail: lporetsk@chpnet.org

L. Poretsky (ed.), *Principles of Diabetes Mellitus*, DOI 10.1007/978-0-387-09841-8_33,
© Springer Science+Business Media, LLC 2010

syndrome of amenorrhea, hirsutism, and enlarged polycystic ovaries in anovulatory women. After observing the restoration of menstruation following ovarian biopsies in patients with this syndrome, Stein and Leventhal performed one-half to three-fourths wedge resection of each ovary in seven women. During the operation the ovarian cortex containing the cysts was removed. All of the patients who underwent wedge resection in Stein and Leventhal's series experienced the return of their menses and two became pregnant.

Stein and Leventhal established both the term "polycystic ovary syndrome" and the theory attributing the origin of this disorder to endocrine abnormalities.[9] In 1949, Culiner and Shippel coined the term "hyperthecosis ovarii" for polycystic ovaries comprised of nests of theca cells. Wedge resection performed in patients with this condition did not result in amelioration of hyperandrogenism. These women were masculinized, and often had diabetes and hypertension. The hyperthecosis ovarii was characterized by familial clustering. The polycystic ovaries in these patients were found to have not only hyperplasia of the theca cells but also atretic follicles.[10]

Hormonal studies in PCOS women were performed only after the clinical manifestations and anatomical abnormalities of this disorder were well reported. In one of the first studies that measured hormone levels in PCOS patients, McArthur et al., in 1958, reported increased urinary levels of luteinizing hormone (LH).[11] Reports of elevated circulating androgen levels followed.[12]

During the last two decades PCOS has been identified as a metabolic disorder in which underlying insulin resistance and consequent hyperinsulinemia contribute to hyperandrogenism.

Genetics in PCOS

It has been proposed that the development of PCOS is dependent on the combination of both genetic and environmental factors. Familial aggregation of PCOS phenotypes has been reported in as early as the1960s.[13] Multiple studies have evaluated the association of various genes and PCOS. Some of these studies support the association while others do not. The genes that have been evaluated can be divided into those involved in adrenal or ovarian steroidogenesis; gonadotropin action and regulation; insulin action and secretion; chronic inflammation; and energy homeostasis.[14] The genes which are potential candidates for the pathogenesis of PCOS are CYP 11a, CYP 17, sex hormone-binding globulin (SHBG), insulin (with variable tandem repeats [VNTR] polymorphism), peroxisome proliferator-activated receptor-gamma (PPAR-γ), and plasminogen activator inhibitor-1 (PAI-1). In summary, studies evaluating the genetic association of PCOS, have presented conflicting results. Further research is required to have a more conclusive proof of the relationship between genetic inheritance and PCOS (Table 33.1).

Table 33.1 Genes implicated in polycystic ovary syndrome and linked to insulin signaling pathway or insulin resistance

Mechanisms	Genes
Insulin action and secretion	Insulin (VNTR polymorphism)
	Insulin receptor
	Insulin receptor substrate (IRS-1 or IRS-2)
Energy homeostasis	Leptin gene and receptor
	Adiponectin
	PPAR-γ (Pro12Ala polymorphism)

Main Hormonal Abnormalities

The two main endocrine theories of PCOS attribute its pathogenesis to the primary role of either central (hypothalamic, pituitary) or ovarian hormonal abnormalities.[15]

The central theory proposes that the initial pathogenic event is an abnormally increased pulsatile secretion of gonadotropin releasing hormone (GnRH) from the hypothalamus that causes a tonically increased secretion of LH instead of the normal pulsatile pattern with a surge during ovulation.[16] It has been proposed that LH levels may rise further because of hyperandrogenism: after androstenedione is converted in the peripheral fat to estrone by aromatase, estrone enhances LH secretion by increasing LH-producing gonadotroph sensitivity to GnRH.[17] In response to increased LH, ovarian thecal cells undergo hypertrophy and their androgen secretion is further increased, thus establishing a vicious cycle. On the contrary, follicle stimulating hormone (FSH) secretion is normal or decreased due to negative feedback from increased estrogen levels produced through aromatization of androgens. Thus, the LH:FSH ratio is often increased.

The ovarian theory attributes primary pathogenic role in the development of PCOS to the ovary, where the production of androgens is increased.[15] According to this theory, dysregulation of the enzyme cytochrome P450c17-alpha, which comprises 17-hydroxylase and 17/20 lyase activities, results in increased amount of androgens. Increased levels of androstenedione and estrone could also be secondary to reduced levels of the enzyme 17-ketosteroid reductase, which converts androstenedione to testosterone and estrone to estradiol.[18]

When ovarian theca cells from women with PCOS were propagated in vitro, it was shown that the activity of 17 α-hydroxylase/C17,20 lyase and 3β-hydroxysteroid dehydrogenase levels were elevated. This results in increased production of testosterone precursors, and, ultimately, causes increased testosterone production. Thus, thecal cells from PCOS patients, when cultured in vitro, possess intrinsic ability to produce increased amounts of testosterone.[19]

In summary, main hormonal abnormalities in PCOS include elevated androgen and estrogen levels and commonly, although not always, an elevated LH:FSH ratio. Hyperinsulinemia, commonly observed in patients with PCOS, contributes to the development of these hormonal abnormalities.[20]

Insulin Resistance in PCOS

In 1921, Archard and Thiers described "the diabetes of bearded women," the first reference to an association between abnormal carbohydrate metabolism and hyperandrogenism.[21] Since then, several syndromes of extreme insulin resistance have been described in patients with distinctive phenotypes which include acanthosis nigricans, hyperandrogenism, polycystic ovaries, or ovarian hyperthecosis and, sometimes, diabetes mellitus. These syndromes (described in detail in Chapter 17) are rare and include leprechaunism, type A and B syndromes of insulin resistance, lipoatrophic diabetes and, Rabson–Mendenhall syndrome. Severe insulin resistance observed in these rare syndromes can be due to a mutation of the insulin receptor gene or other genetic defects in insulin action. In the type B syndrome of insulin resistance, anti-insulin receptor autoantibodies have been identified as a cause of severe insulin resistance.[22–24]

Euglycemic hyperinsulinemic glucose/insulin clamp studies are used to quantify insulin resistance. After a priming dose of insulin, euglycemia is maintained by a constant dose of insulin infusion and simultaneous glucose infusion, the rate of which is adjusted to achieve normal circulating glucose levels. When stable glucose levels are achieved, the rate of peripheral glucose utilization, measured in grams glucose/m^2 of body surface area, is equal to the rate of glucose infusion. Insulin clamp studies in PCOS subjects have demonstrated significant reduction in insulin-mediated glucose disposal similar to that seen in type 2 diabetes mellitus, thus proving that many patients with PCOS are insulin resistant.[25]

Insulin sensitivity is affected by several independent parameters, including obesity, muscle mass, and the site of body fat deposition (central versus peripheral obesity).[25] When insulin clamp studies are performed in PCOS women who are matched to non-PCOS controls for body mass index and body composition, insulin resistance is demonstrated in PCOS women independent of these parameters. Thus, lean PCOS women are more insulin resistant than lean controls. However, body fat does have a synergistically negative effect on insulin sensitivity in PCOS, so that lean PCOS women are usually less insulin resistant than the obese PCOS subjects. Central obesity is the characteristic form of obesity in PCOS and it magnifies insulin resistance and hyperinsulinemia in PCOS patients.[26] The etiology of insulin resistance in polycystic ovary syndrome is unknown, although abnormalities of insulin receptor signaling have been reported in some patients.[27]

Two theories of the pathogenesis of insulin resistance, one involving free fatty acids (FFAs) and another involving tumor necrosis factor-α (TNF-α) have been proposed. First, increased FFA flux into the liver decreases hepatic insulin extraction, increases gluconeogenesis, produces hyperinsulinemia, and reduces glucose uptake by the skeletal muscle.[28–30] Second, TNF-α, produced by adipose tissue, leads to insulin resistance by stimulating phosphorylation of serine residues of the insulin receptor substrate-1 (IRS-1), which leads to the inhibition of insulin receptor cascade.[31,32] Elevated circulating levels of FFA and TNF-α have been reported in PCOS patients.[33–35]

It has been hypothesized that elevated serum insulin levels in patients with PCOS result in excessive ovarian androgen production, as well as ovarian growth and cyst formation. Several in vitro studies have demonstrated the presence of insulin receptors in the ovary[36–38] and the stimulation of androgen production in ovarian cells by insulin.[39] Continuous stimulation of the ovary by hyperinsulinemia in synergism with LH over a prolonged period of time may produce morphological changes in the ovary, such as ovarian growth and cyst formation.[40] The effects of insulin on the ovary can be mediated by the binding of insulin to its own receptor or to the type 1 IGF receptor in what is known as the "specificity spillover" phenomenon. The latter could be an important mechanism in cases of extreme insulin resistance with severe hyperinsulinemia.[41,42]

Role of Insulin in Ovarian Function

Despite Joslin's early observations of abnormal ovarian function in women with type 1 diabetes mellitus,[43] insulin was not thought to play a significant role in ovarian function until the late 1970s, when patients with extreme forms of insulin resistance were described.[22,23] Manifestations of ovarian hypofunction (primary amenorrhea, late menarche, anovulation, and premature ovarian failure) in untreated type 1 diabetes mellitus can be understood if it is accepted that insulin is necessary for the ovary to reach its full steroidogenic and ovulatory potential. Thus, patients with insulin deficiency commonly exhibit hypothalamic-pituitary and ovulatory defects, but not hyperandrogenism.[20,44] On the other end of the clinical spectrum, women with syndromes of severe insulin resistance and consequent hyperinsulinemia exhibit anovulation associated with hyperandrogenism, as discussed above.

If insulin is capable of stimulating ovarian androgen production in insulin resistant patients, one has to postulate that ovarian sensitivity to insulin in these patients is preserved, even in the presence of severe insulin resistance in the classical target organs, such as liver, muscle, and fat.[42] To explain this paradox, we will briefly review cellular mechanisms of insulin action in the ovary and the relationships between insulin, insulin-like growth factors (IGFs), and their receptors.

The term "insulin-related ovarian regulatory system" has been proposed to describe a complex system of ovarian regulation by insulin and IGFs.[15] The components of this system include insulin, insulin receptors, insulin-like growth factor I (IGF-I), insulin-like growth factor II (IGF-II), type 1 IGF receptors, type 2 IGF receptors, IGF binding proteins (IGFBPs) 1-6, and IGFBP proteases. The relationships among the various components of this system are illustrated in Fig. 33.1 and are discussed in detail in Poretsky et al.[15]

Insulin receptors are widely distributed in the ovaries. These ovarian insulin receptors are structurally and functionally similar to insulin receptors found in other organs (see Chapter 5). Regulation of insulin receptor expression, however, may be somewhat different in the ovaries compared to other target tissues. While in classical target tissues insulin receptors are down-regulated by hyperinsulinemia, there is evidence that circulating factors other than insulin may regulate insulin receptor expression in the ovaries of premenopausal women.[45,46] These factors may include sex steroids, gonadotropins, IGFs, and IGFBPs. The phenomenon of differential regulation of ovarian insulin receptors, with their preservation on cell membrane in spite of hyperinsulinemia, may provide one explanation for the ovarian responsiveness to insulin in premenopausal women with insulin resistance in peripheral target organs.[46]

The ovarian insulin receptors have heterotetrameric $\alpha_2\beta_2$ structure, possess tyrosine kinase activity, and may stimulate the generation of inositolglycans. After insulin binds to the α-subunits of the insulin receptor, the β-subunits are activated via phosphorylation of the tyrosine residues and acquire tyrosine kinase activity, e.g., the ability to promote phosphorylation of other intracellular proteins. The intracellular proteins phosphorylated

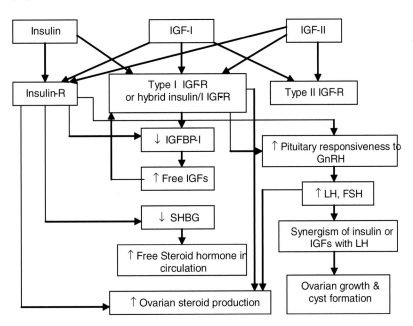

Fig. 33.1 The relationships among the various components of the insulin-related ovarian regulatory system. Insulin, IGF-I, and IGF-II, acting through insulin receptors or type I IGF receptors, increase pituitary responsiveness to GnRH; stimulate gonadotropin secretion directly; stimulate ovarian steroidogenesis; inhibit IGFBP-1 and SHBG production; and act synergistically with gonadotropins to promote ovarian growth and cyst formation. (Adapted, with permission, from L. Poretsky et al.[15] ©The Endocrine Society)

under the influence of the insulin receptor tyrosine kinase are the insulin receptor substrates (IRS) (see Chapter 5).

The insulin receptor activation and IRS phosphorylation result in the activation of phosphatidylinositol-3 kinase (PI-3-kinase). This activation is necessary for transmembrane glucose transport. Mitogen-activated protein kinase (MAPK), responsible for DNA synthesis and gene expression, is also activated by insulin; MAPK activation does not require activation of PI-3-kinase.

Tyrosine kinase activation is the earliest postbinding event and is necessary for many of the effects of insulin. Although it is believed to be the main signaling mechanism of the insulin receptor, an alternative-signaling pathway involving the generation of inositolglycan second messengers has been described[47,48] (see Fig. 33.2). This alternative pathway has been found to mediate several of the effects of insulin, including, possibly, ovarian steroid production. Thus, activation of MAP-kinase and inositolglycan signaling cascades follows pathways that are distinct from those involved in glucose transport. This phenomenon of postreceptor divergence of insulin signaling pathways helps explain how some of the effects of insulin may be normally preserved, or even over-expressed, in the presence of hyperinsulinemia observed in insulin resistant states. In fact, it has been demonstrated that some of the ovarian effects of insulin are PI-3-kinase independent.[49]

Finally, the ovaries may remain sensitive to the actions of insulin in the presence of insulin resistance because, as mentioned above, insulin, when present in high concentration, can activate type 1 IGF receptors. This pathway of insulin action may be operative in patients with syndromes of extreme insulin resistance whose insulin receptors are rendered inactive by a mutation or by anti-insulin receptor antibodies. There is evidence that type 1 IGF receptors may be up-regulated in the presence of hyperinsulinemia both in animal models and in women with PCOS.[50-52]

Recent studies suggested yet another pathway which explains preserved insulin sensitivity in the ovary by invoking insulin-induced activation of PPAR-γ gene. This activation was shown to have direct and indirect effects in the ovary (Table 33.2). Activation of PPAR-γ by PPAR-γ agonists, thiazolidinediones (TZD) (rosiglitazone or pioglitazone), has been shown to produce direct effects in the ovary, which can be both insulin-independent and

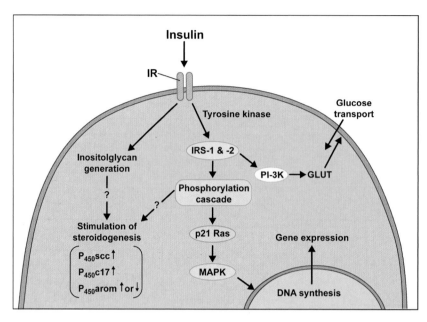

Fig. 33.2 Insulin receptor, its signaling pathways for glucose transport, and hypothetical mechanisms of stimulation or inhibition of steroidogenesis. The main pathways for the propagation of the insulin signal include the following events: after insulin binds to the insulin receptor α-subunits, the β-subunit tyrosine kinase is activated; IRS-1 and -2 are phosphorylated; PI-3 kinase is activated; GLUT glucose transporters are translocated to the cell membrane, and glucose uptake is stimulated. An alternative-signaling system may involve generation of inositolglycans at the cell membrane after insulin binding to its receptor. This inositolglycan signaling system may mediate insulin modulation of steroidogenic enzymes. (Adapted, with permission, from L. Poretsky et al.[15] ©The Endocrine Society)

Table 33.2   Effects of TZDs related to ovarian function (adapted with permission from Seto-Young et al.[53])

1. Direct Can be observed in vitro, may be present in vivo	2. Indirect Observed in vivo; are due to systemic insulin-sensitizing action and reduction of hyperinsulinemia
A. Insulin-independent	
↑ Progesterone production	↓ Testosterone production
↓ Testosterone production	↓ Estradiol production
↓ Estradiol production	↑ IGFBP-1 production
↑ IGFBP-1 production in the absence of insulin	↑ SHBG ↓free T
B. Insulin sensitizing (enhanced insulin effect)	
↓ IGFBP-1 production	
↑ Estradiol production (in vivo, in a setting of high-dose insulin infusion)	

insulin sensitizing.[53] Another study demonstrated an interaction between PPAR-γ and insulin signaling pathways with steroidogenic acute regulatory (StAR) protein, thus, suggesting that PPAR-γ may represent a novel human ovarian regulatory system.[54]

In summary, the paradox of preserved ovarian sensitivity to insulin in insulin resistant states can be explained by differential regulation of insulin receptors in the ovaries of premenopausal women; by activation of signaling pathways distinct from those involved in glucose transport (inositolglycan and MAP-kinase pathways, rather than tyrosine kinase and PI-3 kinase pathways); by the activation of type 1 IGF receptors which may be up-regulated in the presence of hyperinsulinemia; and by activation of PPAR-γ gene leading to improvement in insulin sensitivity

Table 33.3 Possible mechanisms of preserved ovarian sensitivity to insulin in insulin resistant states

1. Differential regulation of ovarian insulin receptors in premenopausal women
2. Activation of alternative insulin signaling pathways (MAP-kinase and inositolglycan), rather than PI-3 kinase pathway of glucose transport
3. Activation of type 1 IGF receptors which may be up-regulated by hyperinsulinemia
4. Activation of PPAR-γ

either by direct or indirect effects in the ovary (Table 33.3). In conclusion, in PCOS patients, ovarian sensitivity to insulin appears to be preserved and the insulin signaling pathways do not exhibit hypersensitivity.[55]

Insulin Effects Related to Ovarian Function

Potential mechanisms underlying the gonadotropic activity of insulin include direct effects on steroidogenic enzymes, synergism with FSH and LH, enhancement of pituitary responsiveness to GnRH, and effects on SHBG and on the IGF/IGFBP systems (see Table 33.4). Investigations focused on these mechanisms have provided insights not only into normal ovarian physiology, but also into the pathogenesis of ovarian dysfunction in a wide spectrum of clinical entities, such as obesity, diabetes mellitus, PCOS, and syndromes of extreme insulin resistance.

Table 33.4 Insulin effects related to ovarian function

Effect	Organ
Directly stimulates steroidogenesis	Ovary
Acts synergistically with LH and FSH to stimulate steroidogenesis	Ovary
Stimulates 17 α-hydroxylase	Ovary
Stimulates or inhibits aromatase	Ovary, adipose tissue
Up-regulates LH receptors	Ovary
Promotes ovarian growth and cyst formation synergistically with LH/hCG	Ovary
Down-regulates insulin receptors	Ovary
Up-regulates type I IGF receptors or hybrid insulin/type I IGF receptors	Ovary
Inhibits IGFBP-I production	Ovary, liver
Potentiates the effect of GnRH on LH and FSH	Pituitary
Inhibits SHBG production	Liver
Up-regulates PPAR-γ	Ovary
Activates StAR protein	Ovary

Adapted, with permission, from L. Poretsky et al.[15] ©The Endocrine Society

Effects on steroidogenesis. In vitro, insulin acts on the granulosa and thecal cells to increase production of androgens, estrogens, and progesterone. This action is likely mediated by the interaction of insulin with its receptors. Several in vitro studies, however, have demonstrated that supraphysiologic concentrations of insulin are needed to achieve this steroidogenic effect on the ovary, suggesting that, under some circumstances, insulin action may be mediated via the type 1 IGF receptor.[20,42]

Studies that attempted to determine whether insulin stimulates or inhibits aromatase or 17-α-hydroxylase have resulted in contradictory conclusions. For example, Nestler et al. reported that 17-α-hydroxylase activity appears to be stimulated by insulin,[56] but Sahin et al. in a later study found no relation between insulin levels and 17-hydroxyprogesterone (17-OHP) after treatment with GnRH agonist.[57] One study showed that, after gonadotropin infusion, hyperinsulinemic women with PCOS had an increased estradiol/ androstenedione ratio compared with women with PCOS and normal insulin levels,[58] thus suggesting insulin's stimulatory effect on aromatase. However, in other studies increased circulating levels of androstenedione were found during insulin infusions, suggesting that insulin inhibits aromatase.[59,60]

Ovarian androgen production in response to insulin has also been extensively studied in vivo both directly, in the course of insulin infusions, and indirectly, after a reduction of insulin levels by insulin sensitizers or other agents, such as diazoxide. While insulin infusion studies did not produce consistent evidence of increased androgen production, reduction of insulin levels has consistently resulted in decreased androgen levels.[15]

Synergism with LH and FSH on the stimulation of steroidogenesis. At the ovarian level, insulin has been demonstrated to potentiate the steroidogenic response to gonadotropins.[20,52] This effect is possibly caused by an increase in the number of LH receptors that occurs under the influence of hyperinsulinemia.[20,61]

Enhancement of pituitary responsiveness to GnRH. Another area of uncertainty is whether insulin enhances the sensitivity of gonadotropes to GnRH in the pituitary. Several investigators have demonstrated increased responsiveness of gonadotropes to GnRH in the presence of insulin in cultured pituitary cells.[62,63] Nestler and Jakubowicz showed decreased circulating levels of LH in patients treated with insulin sensitizers.[64] But in another study, gonadotropin responsiveness to GnRH did not change after insulin infusion.[65] Similarly, in rats with experimentally produced hyperinsulinemia, response of gonadotropins to GnRH does not appear to be altered.[50]

The effect on SHBG. Insulin has been shown to suppress hepatic production of sex hormone-binding globulin (SHBG).[66–69] Lower levels of SHBG result in increased serum levels of unbound steroid hormones, such as free testosterone. In PCOS and other hyperinsulinemic insulin resistant states, insulin may increase circulating levels of free testosterone by inhibiting SHBG production. When insulin sensitizers are used, SHBG levels rise, thereby decreasing free steroid hormone levels.[64]

The effect on IGFBP-1. Insulin has been found to regulate insulin-like growth factor-binding protein-1 (IGFBP-1) levels. In both liver and ovarian granulosa cells, insulin inhibits IGFBP-1 production.[41,70,71] Lower circulating and intraovarian IGFBP-1 concentrations result in higher circulating and intraovarian levels of free IGFs that may contribute to increased ovarian and adrenal steroid secretion.[15,72]

Type 1 IGF receptor. Insulin increases ovarian IGF-I binding in rats, suggesting an increase in the expression of ovarian type 1 IGF receptors or hybrid insulin/type 1 IGF receptors.[37] In these studies, ovarian type 1 IGF receptors are up-regulated even though insulin receptors are either down-regulated or preserved. Studies in women with PCOS appear to confirm this phenomenon.[51,73]

PPAR-γ. Insulin increases expression of PPAR-γ in vitro in human ovarian cells. Activation of PPAR-γ enhances steroidogenesis via activation of StAR protein (Fig. 33.3).[54]

StAR protein. In addition to being activated through PPAR-γ, StAR protein can be also activated by insulin directly via insulin signaling pathway (Fig. 33.3).[54]

Ovarian growth and cyst formation. It has been shown that insulin enhances theca-interstitial cell proliferation in both human and rat ovaries.[74–78] In a report of a patient with the type B syndrome of insulin resistance, infusion of insulin resulted in a significant increase of ovarian volume with sonogram demonstrating that the ovaries doubled in size.[79] Experimental hyperinsulinemia in synergism with hCG produces significant increase in ovarian size and development of polycystic ovaries in rats (Fig. 33.4).

In summary, in a number of in vitro animal and human ovarian cell systems and in vivo experiments in animals and in women a variety of insulin effects related to ovarian function have been demonstrated. These effects can account for many features of PCOS in hyperinsulinemic insulin resistant women.[15] Insulin effects related to ovarian function are summarized in Table 33.4.

Risk of Diabetes Mellitus; Prevention of Diabetes

A major risk factor for the development of type 2 diabetes mellitus in PCOS is insulin resistance. However, a defect in pancreatic β-cell function resulting in deficient insulin secretion has also been reported in PCOS patients.[80]

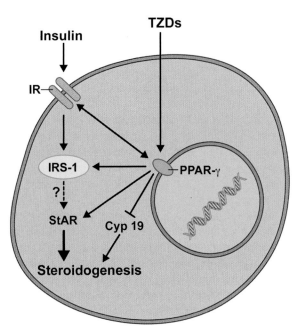

Fig. 33.3 Proposed interactions among PPAR-γ, insulin receptor (IR), IRS-1, and StAR protein in human ovarian cells. Both insulin (by activating primarily insulin receptor) and TZDs (by activating primarily PPAR-γ) lead to stimulation of StAR protein expression. In addition TZDs activate insulin receptor expression while insulin activates expression of PPAR-γ, thus, further enhancing StAR protein expression and stimulating steroidogenesis. Both insulin and TZDs activate a downstream component of insulin signaling pathway, IRS-1. This effect of TZDs may be mediated with or without activation of the insulin receptor (adapted with permission from Seto-Young et al.[54])

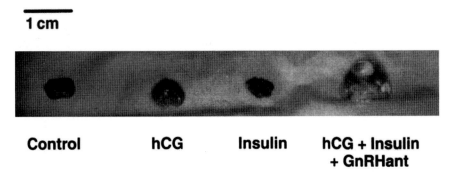

Fig. 33.4 The effects of 23 days of daily injections of normal saline (control), hCG, insulin, or insulin plus hCG and GnRHant on gross ovarian morphology in rats. Female Sprague-Dawley rats were randomized into the following treatment groups: vehicle; high-fat diet (to control for the effects of weight gain); insulin; hCG; GnRH antagonist (to control for possible central effects of insulin vs. direct effects on the ovary); GnRHant and hCG; insulin and GnRHant; insulin and hCG; insulin, hCG, and GnRHant. Ovarian morphology in the group treated with insulin and hCG (not shown) did not differ from that seen in the group treated with insulin, hCG, and GnRHant (shown above). [Reproduced with permission from L. Poretsky et al.[40] ©W.B. Saunders Co.]

    The prevalence and predictors of risk for type 2 diabetes mellitus have been studied in PCOS women. In prospective studies of glucose tolerance in women with hyperandrogenism and chronic anovulation, the prevalence of undiagnosed diabetes mellitus was 7.5% and that of impaired glucose tolerance (IGT) was 31.1%. Further analysis of the non-obese subgroup demonstrated that the risk for diabetes decreased to 1.5% and for IGT to 10.3%. However, these rates were still significantly increased compared to a population-based study of age-matched women in the United States in whom the prevalence rate of undiagnosed diabetes mellitus was 1.0% and that of IGT was 7.8%.[81]

A study of women with previous history of gestational diabetes revealed a greater prevalence of polycystic ovaries (PCO) compared to controls (39.4% versus 16.7%), higher serum levels of adrenal androgens, and significantly impaired glucose tolerance. Oral glucose tolerance testing in these women uncovered a decreased early phase insulin response while euglycemic clamp studies demonstrated impaired insulin sensitivity. The investigators theorized that a dual component of insulin resistance plus impaired pancreatic insulin secretion could explain the vulnerability of PCOS patients to diabetes.[82]

PCOS, and not PCO (in which the polycystic ovarian morphology is not associated with hyperandrogenism or anovulation), has been found to be a substantially more significant risk factor for diabetes mellitus than race or ethnicity.[81] Factoring in obesity, age, family history of diabetes, and waist/hip ratios, the prevalence of glucose intolerance increases. This suggests that the pathogenesis of diabetes mellitus in PCOS is a result of underlying genetic defects, resulting in insulin resistance and pancreatic β-cell dysfunction, and an interplay of various environmental factors.

Primary prevention of type 2 diabetes mellitus was the focus of the Diabetes Prevention Program (DPP). The DPP, a National Institutes of Health-sponsored clinical study, targeted preventive measures at specific individuals or groups at high risk for the future development of type 2 diabetes (see Chapter 50). The study interventions included intensive lifestyle modification or pharmacological intervention versus placebo. The primary outcome was the development of diabetes mellitus in these high-risk groups. The results of this study showed that both lifestyle modification and treatment with metformin prevented or delayed the onset of type 2 diabetes in individuals with impaired glucose tolerance (IGT).[83,84] Thus, specific interventions may be implemented at an early enough time period to prevent the development of diabetes mellitus and its accompanying complications in high-risk individuals. PCOS, with its dual defect of insulin resistance and β-cell dysfunction, is a significant risk factor for diabetes mellitus. When effective protocols for prevention of diabetes mellitus are established, PCOS patients may become one target group for such measures.

Role of Insulin Sensitizers

There are numerous treatment modalities for signs and symptoms of PCOS. However, traditional approaches, although often successful, do not address insulin resistance.

Hyperandrogenism and its consequences, such as hirsutism and acne, have many treatment modalities. Hirsutism can be treated with depilatories, shaving, waxing, electrolysis, or laser therapy. Oral contraceptives and anti-androgen medications, such as spironolactone[85] or cyproterone acetate,[86] may be used to reduce androgen levels and manifestations of hyperandrogenism.

Oral contraceptive pills may also be used to treat menstrual irregularities. This treatment leads to a reduction in LH and an increase in SHBG. The increased SHBG binds the excess androgens, thereby decreasing the amount of free circulating androgens.[87] Progestins may be used to regulate the menstrual cycle, however they do not affect the hair growth or metabolic abnormalities.

Weight loss, when successful, is a very effective measure which addresses insulin-related abnormalities of PCOS by decreasing insulin resistance and circulating insulin levels. One report studied 18 obese women who were hyperandrogenic and insulin resistant. A weight reduction diet resulted in a decrease in plasma androstenedione and testosterone levels.[88] Pasquali et al. found decreased concentrations of LH, fasting insulin, and testosterone levels after weight loss in 20 obese women with hyperandrogenism and oligo-ovulation.[89] In another study, 67 obese anovulatory women were treated with weight reduction. Sixty of these women ovulated and 18 became pregnant.[90]

When weight loss is not achieved, insulin resistance can be reduced with the help of insulin sensitizers, such as biguanides or thiazolidinediones. The goal of these approaches is to decrease the amount of circulating insulin, thereby decreasing insulin's stimulatory effect on androgen production and gonadotropin secretion. Circulating levels of SHBG and IGFBP-1 are increased, leading to clinical improvement via mechanisms described above.[91]

Metformin decreases hepatic gluconeogenesis and increases fat and muscle sensitivity to insulin. There are many reports showing meformin's efficacy in PCOS, however, most of the studies have been short-term only.

One long-term study followed women with PCOS treated with metformin (500 mg tid) for 6–26 months. These women not only had a reduction in insulin and androgen levels, independent of any change in weight, but also a sustained increase in menstrual regularity.[92]

Nestler and coworkers showed that when insulin secretion is decreased by metformin administration either alone or in combination with clomiphene in obese women with PCOS, the ovulatory response is increased.[93] In an analysis of 14 studies of metformin treatment of PCOS, 57% of women had ovulatory improvement with metformin.[94] The improvement in ovulation may have been only due to weight loss. However, *lean* women with PCOS, who had increased P450c17-alpha activity and whose circulating insulin levels were reduced while on metformin, experienced a decline in P450c17-alpha activity and improvement in hyperandrogenism.[56] In another study, women with PCOS who were given metformin demonstrated decreased circulating levels of LH, free testosterone, and a decreased LH/FSH ratio, as well as a reduced body mass index (BMI).[95]

In one study of women with PCOS given metformin, improved endometrial function and intrauterine environment were found. This observation suggests that metformin can be used to improve implantation and pregnancy maintenance in women with PCOS.[96] Treatment of infertility using either metformin or clomiphene citrate in anovulatory PCOS women has been successful. In the study by Legro et al. clomiphene was shown to be superior to metformin in achieving live births.[97] Later in a smaller study by Palomba et al., both agents have been found to be equally effective.[98]

A thiazolidinedione (TZD) troglitazone, an insulin-sensitizing agent, was the first in its class to improve insulin action in patients with PCOS.[99] Studies with troglitazone in patients with PCOS showed improvements in ovulation, insulin resistance, hyperandrogenemia, and hirsutism.[100] However, troglitazone was taken off the market because of hepatotoxicity. Since other members of TZD family (rosiglitazone and pioglitazone) became available, multiple studies evaluating their efficacy in PCOS patients have been published. Studies of overweight and non-obese females treated with rosiglitazone showed an improvement in ovulation, glucose tolerance, insulin sensitivity, hirsutism,[100] and a decrease in hyperinsulinemia and androgen levels, as well as a small increase in BMI.[101,102] Pioglitazone in PCOS patients showed similar effects (increased insulin sensitivity, ovulation rate, and SHBG levels and decreased insulin secretion and free androgen index) but BMI remained unchanged.[103,104] While assessing the effects of TZDs in such studies, it is important to remember that TZDs exhibit both systemic insulin-sensitizing action and direct insulin-independent effects in the ovary (Table 33.2).[53]

Some of the medications were evaluated in a head-to-head comparison to determine the best therapy of PCOS. When metformin was compared with spironolactone, both medications increased frequency of menstrual cycles and decreased testosterone, DHEA-S, and hirsutism score. Spironolactone produced more significant changes, but metformin improved glucose tolerance and insulin sensitivity.[105] In another study, metformin was compared with rosiglitazone in obese and lean women with PCOS.[106] Women taking these agents exhibited decrease in insulin resistance and increase in insulin sensitivity but only rosiglitazone group showed significant reduction in androgen levels as well as small but significant increase in BMI (metformin had significant decrease in BMI). Pioglitazone was compared with metformin in yet another study.[107] Both medications were equally effective in improving insulin sensitivity and hyperandrogenism (hirsutism and androgen levels) despite an increase in BMI in pioglitazone group.

Single medication therapy (monotherapy) sometimes is not sufficient to ameliorate the symptoms of PCOS. Various studies have explored the effects of combination therapies. One study involved combination therapy of metformin and oral contraceptive pills (OCPs). When a combination of metformin and OCP (ethinyl estradiol-cyproterone acetate) was compared to OCP alone, the group using combination therapy had more dramatic reduction in androstenedione and increase in SHBG.[108,109] This group, unlike OCP group, also had significant decrease in BMI, waist-to-hip ratio, and fasting insulin level; however, these differences between the groups did not reach statistical significance. There was significant increase in total cholesterol in OCP group, while the rest of the lipid panel remained unchanged in both groups. Elter et al. suggested that insulin sensitivity (glucose-to-insulin ratio) improved in combination therapy group but these results were not supported by the study of Cibula et al. which used more definitive test (euglycaemic hyperinsulinaemic clamp). Another combination therapy that has been studied involved rosiglitazone with OCP. In the study by Lemay et al. overweight women with PCOS and insulin resistance were divided into two groups to receive either rosiglitazone or ethinyl estradiol/cyproterone acetate for the first 6 months and then a combination therapy for an additional 6 months.[110] Women receiving combination therapy had greater reduction in androgens and increase in SHBG and HDL than either agent alone. Improved insulin sensitivity and increased triglycerides were found in only one of the two combination groups. In summary, combination therapies of oral contraceptives and insulin sensitizers have small but beneficial effect on androgen levels.

Patients and physicians should be aware that at this time there is no medical therapy which is approved by the Food and Drug Administration for the treatment of PCOS. Women with PCOS who think that they are infertile and therefore do not use contraception may become pregnant while on these medications. Thus, it is important to discuss contraception before prescribing any of these medications.

Conclusions

PCOS is a compilation of multiple endocrine and metabolic abnormalities. The main features of PCOS include chronic anovulation, hyperandrogenemia, and polycystic ovaries. Many patients have insulin resistance and hyperinsulinemia of unknown etiology, although often related to obesity. Besides the hirsutism, acne, and infertility, these women are at an increased risk for diabetes.

New therapeutic strategies addressing insulin resistance in PCOS are developing. As research elucidates specific ovarian effects of insulin and specific pathways of insulin signaling in the ovary, new targets will be identified for emerging therapies.

References

1. Knochenhauer ES, Key TJ, Kahsar-Miller M, Waggoner W, Boots LR, Azziz R. Prevalence of the polycystic ovarian syndrome in unselected black and white women of the Southeastern United States: a prospective study. *J Clin Endocrinol Metab.* 1998;83:3078–3082.
2. Zawadzki JK, Dunaif A. Diagnostic criteria for polycystic ovary syndrome: towards a rational approach. In: Dunaif A ed. *Polycystic Ovary Syndrome.* Boston: Blackwell Scientific; 1995:337–384.
3. Rotterdam ESHRE/ASRM – Sponsored PCOS Concensus Workshop Group, "Revised 2003 consensus on diagnostic criteria and long-term health risks related to polycystic ovary disease," Fertil Steril, vol 81, 19–25, 2004
4. Rotterdam ESHRE/ASRM – Sponsored PCOS Concensus Workshop Group, "Revised 2003 consensus on diagnostic criteria and long-term health risks related to polycystic ovary disease," Human reproduction, vol 19, 41–47, 2004
5. Dunaif A. Hyperandrogenic anovulation (PCOS): a unique disorder of insulin action associated with an increased risk of non-insulin-dependent diabetes mellitus. *Am J Med.* 1995;98([Suppl]):33S–39S.
6. Legro RS. Polycystic ovary syndrome and cardiovascular disease: premature association? *Endocr Rev.* 2003;24:302–312.
7. Hardiman P, Pillay OS, Atiomo W. Polycystic ovary syndrome and endometrial carcinoma. *Lancet.* 2003;361:1810–1812.
8. Chereau A. *Mémoires pour servir a l'étude des maladies des ovaries.* Paris: Fortin, Masson and Cie; 1844.
9. Stein IF, Leventhal ML. Amenorrhea associated with bilateral polycystic ovaries. *Am J Obstet Gynecol.* 1935;29:181–186.
10. Culiner A, Shippel S. Virilism and thecal cell hyperplasia of the ovary syndrome. *J Obstet Gynaecol Br Comm.* 1949;56: 439–445.
11. McArthur JW, Ingersoll FW, Worcester J. The urinary excretion of interstitial-cell and follicle-stimulating hormone activity by women with diseases of the reproductive system. *J Clin Endocrinol Metab.* 1958;18:1202–1215.
12. De Vane GW, Czekala NM, Judd HL, Yen SS. Circulating gonadotropins, estrogens, and androgens in polycystic ovarian disease. *Am J Obstet Gynecol.* 1975;121:496–500.
13. Cooper H, Spellacy W, Prem K, Cohen W. Hereditary factors in the Stein-Leventhal syndrome. *Am J Obstet Gynecol.* 1968;100:371–387.
14. Unluturk U, Harmanci A, Kocaefe C, Yildiz B. The genetic basis of the polycystic ovary syndrome: a literature review including discussion of PPAR-g. *PPAR Res.* 2007:49109.
15. Poretsky L, Cataldo N, Rosenwaks Z, Giudice L. The insulin-related ovarian regulatory system in health and disease. *Endocr Rev.* 1999;20:535–582.
16. Zumoff B, Freeman R, Coupey S, Saenger P, Markowitz M, Kream J. A chronobiologic abnormality in luteinizing hormone secretion in teenage girls with the polycystic-ovary syndrome. *N Engl J Med.* 1983;309:1206–1209.
17. McLachlan RI, Healy DL, Burger HG. The ovary. In: Felig P, Baxter JD, Broadus AE, Frohman LA, eds. *Endocrinology and Metabolism.* 2nd ed. New York: McGraw-Hill Book Company; 1987:951–983.
18. Pang S, Softness B, Sweeney WJ, New MI. Hirsutism, polycystic ovarian disease, and ovarian 17-ketosteroid reductase deficiency. *N Engl J Med.* 1987;316:1295–1301.

19. Nelson VL, Qin K-N, Rosenfeld RL, et al. The biochemical basis for increased testosterone production in theca cells propagated from patients with polycystic ovary syndrome. *J Clin Endocrinol Metab*. 2001;86:5925–5933.

20. Poretsky L, Kalin M. The gonadotropic function of insulin. *Endocr Rev*. 1987;8:132–141.

21. Archard C, Thiers J. Le virilisme pilaire et son association a l'insuffisance glycolytique (diabete des femmes a barbe. *Bull Acad Nat Med*. 1921;86:51.

22. Kahn CR, Flier JS, Bar RS, et al. The syndromes of insulin resistance and acanthosis nigricans: insulin-receptor disorders in man. *N Engl J Med*. 1976;294:739–745.

23. Flier JS, Kahn CR, Roth J, Bar RS. Antibodies that impair insulin receptor binding in an unusual diabetic syndrome with severe insulin resistance. *Science*. 1975;190:63–65.

24. Taylor SI, Moller DE. Mutations of the insulin receptor gene. In: Moller DE ed. *Insulin Resistance*. New York: John Wiley & Sons; 1993:83–121.

25. Dunaif A. Insulin resistance and the polycystic ovary syndrome: mechanism and implications for pathogenesis. *Endocr Rev*. 1997;18:774–800.

26. Salehi M, Bravo-Vera R, Sheikh A, Gouller A, Poretsky L. Pathogenesis of polycystic ovary syndrome: what is the role of obesity? *Metabolism*. 2004;53:358–376.

27. Dunaif A, Book CB, Schenker E, Tang Z. Excessive insulin receptor serine phosphorylation in cultured fibroblasts and in skeletal muscle: a potential mechanism for insulin resistance in the polycystic ovary syndrome. *J Clin Invest*. 1995;96:801–810.

28. Svedberg J, Bjorntorp P, Smith U, et al. Free-fatty acid inhibition of insulin binding, degradation, and action in isolated rat hepatocytes. *Diabetes*. 1990;39:570–574.

29. Boden G. Role of fatty acids in the pathogenesis of insulin resistance and NIIDM. *Diabetes*. 1997;46:3–10.

30. Kelley DE. Skeletal muscle triglycerides: an aspect of regional adiposity and insulin resistance. *Ann N Y Acad Sci*. 2002;967:135–145.

31. Hotamisligil GS, Peraldi P, Budavari A. IRS-1-mediated inhibition of insulin receptor tyrosine kinase activity in TNF-alpha and obesity-induced insulin resistance. *Science*. 1996;271:665–668.

32. Hrebicek A, Rypka M, Chmela Z, et al. Tumor necrosis factor alpha in various tissues and of insulin-resistant obese Koletsky rats: relations to insulin receptor characteristics. *Physiol Res*. 1999;48:83–86.

33. Holte J, Bergh T, Berne C, et al. Serum lipoprotein lipid profile in women with the polycystic ovary syndrome: relation to anthropometric, endocrine and metabolic variables. *Clin Endocrinol*. 1994;41:463–471.

34. Ek I, Arner P, Ryden M, et al. A unique defect in the regulation of visceral fat cell lipolysis in the polycystic ovary syndrome as an early link to insulin resistance. *Diabetes*. 2002;51:484–492.

35. Escobar-Morreale HF, Calvo RM, Sancho J, et al. TNF-alpha hyperandrogenism: A clinical, biochemical, and molecular genetic study. *J Clin Endocrinol Metab*. 2001;86:3761–3767.

36. Poretsky L, Smith D, Seibel M, Pazianos A, Moses AC, Flier JS. Specific insulin binding sites in the human ovary. *J Clin Endocrinol Metab*. 1984;59:809–811.

37. Poretsky L, Grigorescu F, Seibel M, Moses AC, Flier JS. Distribution and characterization of the insulin and IGF-I receptors in the normal human ovary. *J Clin Endocrinol Metab*. 1985;61:728–734.

38. El-Roeiy A, Chen X, Roberts VJ, et al. Expression of the genes encoding the insulin-like growth factors (IGF-I and II), the IGF and insulin receptors, and IGF-binding proteins 1-6 and the localization of their gene products in normal and polycystic ovary syndrome ovaries. *J Clin Endocrinol Metab*. 1994;78:1488–1496.

39. Barbieri RL, Makris A, Ryan KJ. Effects of insulin on steroidogenesis in cultured porcine ovarian theca. *Fertil Steril*. 1983;40:237–241.

40. Poretsky L, Clemons J, Bogovich K. Hyperinsulinemia and human chorionic gonadotropin synergistically promote the growth of ovarian follicular cysts in rats. *Metabolism*. 1992;41:903–910.

41. Poretsky L, Chandrasekher YA, Bai C, Liu HC, Rosenwaks Z, Giudice L. Insulin receptor mediates inhibitory effect of insulin, but not of insulin-like growth factor (IGF)-1, on binding protein 1 (IGFBP-1) production in human granulosa cells. *J Clin Endocrinol Metab*. 1996;81:493–496.

42. Poretsky L. On the paradox of insulin-induced hyperandrogenism in insulin-resistant states. *Endocr Rev*. 1991;12:3–13.

43. Joslin EP, Root HF, White P. The growth, development and prognosis of diabetic children. *J Am Med Assoc*. 1925;85:420–422.

44. Zumoff B, Miller L, Poretsky L, et al. Subnormal follicular-phase serum progesterone levels and elevated follicular-phase serum estradiol levels in young women with insulin-dependent diabetes. *Steroids*. 1990;55:560–564.

45. Poretsky L, Bhargava G, Kalin MF, Wolf SA. Regulation of insulin receptors in the human ovary: in vitro studies. *J Clin Endocrinol Metab*. 1988;67:774–778.

46. Poretsky L, Bhargava G, Saketos M, Dunaif A. Regulation of human ovarian insulin receptors in vivo. *Metabolism*. 1990;39:161–166.

47. Saltiel AR. Second messengers of insulin action. *Diabetes Care*. 1990;13:244–256.

48. Nestler JE, Jakubowicz DJ, De Vargas AF, Brik C, Quintero N, Medina F. Insulin stimulates testosterone biosynthesis by human thecal cells from women with polycystic ovarian syndrome by activating its own receptor and using inositolglycan mediators as the signal transduction system. *J Clin Endocrinol Metab*. 1998;83:2001–2005.

49. Poretsky L, Seto-Young D, Shrestha A, et al. Phosphatidyl-inositol-3 kinase-independent insulin action pathway(s) in the human ovary. *J Clin Endocrinol Metab*. 2001;86:3115–3119.

50. Poretsky L, Glover B, Laumas V, Kalin M, Dunaif A. The effects of experimental hyperinsulinemia on steroid secretion, ovarian [^{125}I] insulin binding, and ovarian [^{125}I] insulin-like growth factor I binding in the rat. *Endocrinology*. 1988;122: 581–585.

51. Samoto T, Maruo T, Matsuo H, Katayama K, Barnea ER, Mochizuki M. Altered expression of insulin and insulin-like growth factor-I receptors in follicular and stromal compartments of polycystic ovarian ovaries. *Endocr J*. 1993;40:413–424.

52. Willis D, Mason H, Gilling-Smith C, Franks S. Modulation by insulin of follicle-stimulating hormone and luteinizing hormone actions in human granulosa cells of normal and polycystic ovaries. *J Clin Endocrinol Metab*. 1996;81:302–309.

53. Seto-Young D, Paliou M, Schlosser J, et al. Thiazolidinedione action in the human ovary: insulin-independent and insulin-sensitizing effects on steroidogenesis and insulin-like growth factor binding protein-1 production. *J Clin Endocrinol Metab*. 2005;90:6099–6105.

54. Seto-Young D, Avtanski D, Strizhevsky M, et al. Interactions among peroxisome proliferators activated receptor-g, insulin signaling pathways, and steroidogenic acute regulatory protein in human ovarian cells. *J Clin Endocrinol Metab*. 2007;92:2232–2239.

55. Poretsky L. Commentary: polycystic ovary syndrome-increased or preserved ovarian sensitivity to insulin? *J Clin Endocrinol Metab*. 2006;91:2859–2860.

56. Nestler JE, Jakubowicz DJ. Decreases in ovarian cytochrome P450c17 alpha activity and serum free testosterone after reduction of insulin secretion in polycystic ovary syndrome. *N Engl J Med*. 1996;335:617–623.

57. Sahin Y, Ayata D, Kelestimur F. Lack of relationship between 17-hydroxyprogesterone response to buserelin testing and hyperinsulinemia in polycystic ovary syndrome. *Eur J Endocrinol*. 1997;136:410–415.

58. Fulghesu AM, Villa P, Pavone V, et al. The impact of insulin secretion on the ovarian response to exogenous gonadotropins in polycystic ovarian syndrome. *J Clin Endocrinol Metab*. 1997;82:644–648.

59. Stuart CA, Nagamani M. Acute augmentation of plasma androstenedione and dehydroepiandrosterone by euglycemic insulin infusion: evidence for a direct effect of insulin on ovarian steroidogenesis. In: Dunaif A, Givens JR, Haseltine FP, Merriam GR eds. *Polycystic Ovary Syndrome*. Boston: Blackwell Scientific Publications; 1992:279–288.

60. Stuart CA, Prince MJ, Peters EJ, Meyer WJ. Hyperinsulinemia and hyperandrogenemia: in vivo androgen response to insulin infusion. *Obstet Gynecol*. 1987;69:921–925.

61. Poretsky L, Piper B. Insulin resistance, hypersecretion of LH, and a dual-defect hypothesis for the pathogenesis of polycystic ovary syndrome. *Obstet Gynecol*. 1994;84:613–621.

62. Adashi EY, Hsueh AJW, Yen SSC. Insulin enhancement of luteinizing hormone and follicle-stimulating hormone release by cultured pituitary cells. *Endocrinology*. 1981;108:1441–1449.

63. Soldani R, Cagnacci A, Yen SS. Insulin, insulin-like growth factor I (IGF I) and IGF-II enhance basal and gonadotropin-releasing hormone-stimulated luteinizing hormone release from rat anterior pituitary cells in vitro. *Eur J Endocrinol*. 1994;131:641–645.

64. Nestler JE, Jakubowicz DJ. Lean women with polycystic ovary syndrome respond to insulin reduction with decreases in ovarian P450c17 alpha activity and serum androgens. *J Clin Endocrinol Metab*. 1997;82:4075–4079.

65. Dunaif A, Graf M. Insulin administration alters gonadal steroid metabolism independent of changes in gonadotropin secretion in insulin-resistant women with polycystic ovary syndrome. *J Clin Invest*. 1989;83:23–29.

66. Plymate SR, Matej LA, Jones RE, Friedl KE. Inhibition of sex hormone-binding globulin production in the human hepatoma (HepG2) cell line by insulin and prolactin. *J Clin Endocrinol Metab*. 1988;67:460–464.

67. Peiris AN, Stagner JL, Plymate SR, Vogel RL, Heck M, Samols E. Relationship of insulin secretory pulses to sex hormone-binding globulin production in normal men. *J Clin Endocrinol Metab*. 1993;76:279–282.

68. Fendri S, Arlot S, Marcelli JM, Dubreuil A, Lalau JD. Relationship between insulin sensitivity and circulating sex hormone-binding globulin levels in hyperandrogenic obese women. *Int J Obes Relat Metab Disord*. 1994;18:755–759.

69. Nestler JE, Powers LP, Matt DW, et al. A direct effect of hyperinsulinemia on serum sex hormone-binding globulin levels in obese women with the polycystic ovary syndrome. *J Clin Endocrinol Metab*. 1991;72:83–89.

70. Pao CI, Farmer PK, Begovic S, et al. Regulation of insulin-like growth factor-I (IGF I) and IGF-binding protein I gene transcription by hormones and provision of amino acids in rat hepatocytes. *Mol Endocrinol*. 1993;7:1561–1568.

71. Lee PD, Giudice LC, Conover CA, Powell DR. Insulin-like growth factor binding protein-1: recent findings and new directions. *Proc Soc Exp Biol Med*. 1997;216:319–357.

72. Giudice LC. Insulin-like growth factors and ovarian follicular development. *Endocr Rev*. 1992;13:641–669.

73. Nagami M, Stuart CA. Specific binding sites for insulin-like growth factor I in the ovarian stroma of women with polycystic ovarian disease and stromal hyperthecosis. *Am J Obstet Gynecol*. 1990;163:1992–1997.

74. Duleba AJ, Spaczynski RZ, Olive DL, Behrman HR. Effects of insulin and insulin-like growth factors on proliferation of rat ovarian theca-interstitial cells. *Biol Reprod*. 1997;56:891–897.

75. Duleba AJ, Spaczynski RZ, Olive DL. Insulin and insulin-like growth factor I stimulate the proliferation of human ovarian theca-interstitial cells. *Fertil Steril*. 1998;69:335–340.

76. Watson H, Willis D, Mason H, Modgil G, Wright C, Franks S. The effects of ovarian steroids, epidermal growth factor (EGF), insulin (I), and insulin-like growth factor-1 (IGF-I), on ovarian stromal cell growth. Program of the 79th Annual Meeting of the Endocrine Society, Minneapolis, MN, (Abstract 389), 1997.

77. Bogovich K, Clemons J, Poretsky L. Insulin has a biphasic effects on the ability of human chorionic gonadotropin to induce ovarian cysts in the rat. *Metabolism*. 1999;48:995–1002.

78. Damario M, Bogovich K, Liu HC, Rosenwaks Z, Poretsky L. Synergistic effects of IGF-I and human chorionic gonadotropin in the rat ovary. *Metabolism.* 2000;49:314–320.

79. De ClueT J, Shah SC, Marchese M, Malone JI. Insulin resistance and hyperinsulinemia induce hyperandrogenism in a young type B insulin-resistant female. *J Clin Endocrinol Metab.* 1991;72:1308–1311.

80. Dunaif A, Finegood DT. Beta-cell dysfunction independent of obesity and glucose intolerance in the polycystic ovary syndrome. *J Clin Endocrinol Metab.* 1996;81:942–947.

81. Legro R, Kunselman A, Dodson W, Dunaif A. Prevalence and predictors of risk for type 2 diabetes mellitus and impaired glucose tolerance in polycystic ovary syndrome: a prospective, controlled study in 254 affected women. *J Clin Endocrinol Metab.* 1999;84:165–169.

82. Koivunen RM, et al. Metabolic and steroidogenic alterations related to increased frequency of polycystic ovaries in women with a history of gestational diabetes. *J Clin Endocrinol Metab.* 2001;86:2591–2599.

83. The Diabetes Prevention Program Research Group. The Diabetes Prevention Program: baseline characteristics of the randomized cohort. *Diabetes Care.* 2000;23(11):1619–1629.

84. Fujimoto W. Background and recruitment data for the U.S. Diabetes Prevention Program. *Diabetes Care.* 2000;23:B11–B13.

85. Board JA, Rosenberg SM, Smeltzer JS. Spironolactone and estrogen-progestin therapy for hirsuitism. *South Med J.* 1987;80:483–486.

86. Falsetti L, Gamera A, Tisi G. Efficacy of the combination ethinyl oestradiol and cyproterone acetate on endocrine, clinical and ultrasonographic profile in polycystic ovarian syndrome. *Hum Reprod.* 2001;16:36–42.

87. Dewis P, Petsos P, Newman M, Anderson DC. The treatment of hirsuitism with a combination of desogestrel and ethinyl oestradiol. *Clin Endocrinol.* 1985;22:29–36.

88. Bates GW, Whitworth NS. Effect of body weight reduction on plasma androgens in obese infertile women. *Fertil Steril.* 1982;38:406–409.

89. Pasquali R, Antenucci D, Casimirri F, Venturoli S, Paradisi R, Fabbri R, et al. Clinical and hormonal characteristics of obese and amenorrheic women before and after weight loss. *J Clin Endocrinol Metab.* 1989;68:173–179.

90. Clark AM, Thornley B, Tomlinson L, Galletley C, Norman RJ. Weight loss in obese infertile women results in improvement in reproductive outcome for all forms of fertility treatment. *Hum Reprod.* 1998;13:1502–1505.

91. Crave JC, Fimbel S, Lejeune H, Cugnardey N, DeChaud H, Pugeat M. Effects of diet and metformin administration on sex hormone-binding globuliln, androgens, and insulin in hirsute and obese women. *J Clin Endocrinol Metab.* 1995;80:2057–2062.

92. Moghetti P, Castello R, Negri C, et al. Metformin effects on clinical features, endocrine and metabolic profiles, and insulin sensitivity in polycystic ovary syndrome: a randomized, double-blind, placebo-controlled 6-month trial, followed by open, long-term clinical evaluation. *J Clin Endocrinol Metab.* 2000;85:139–146.

93. Nestler JE, Jakubowicz DJ, Evans WS, Pasquali R. Effects of metformin on spontaneous and clomiphene-induced ovulation in the polycystic ovary syndrome. *N Engl J Med.* 1998;338:1876–1880.

94. Bloomgarden ZT, Futterwiet W, Poretsky L. The use of insulin-sensitizing agents in patients with polycystic ovary syndrome. *Endocr Pract.* 2001;7:279–286.

95. Velazquez E, Acosta A, Mendoza SG. Menstrual cyclicity after metformin therapy in polycystic ovary syndrome. *Obstet Gynecol.* 1997;90:392–395.

96. Jakubowicz DJ, Seppala M, Jakubowicz S, et al. Insulin reduction with metformin increases luteal phase serum glycodelin and insulin-like growth factor-binding protein 1 concentrations and enhances uterine vascularity and blood flow in the polycystic ovary syndrome. *J Clin Endocrinol Metab.* 2001;86:1126–1133.

97. Legro R, Barnhart H, Schlaff W, et al. Clomiphene, metformin, or both for infertility in the polycystic ovary syndrome. *N Engl J Med.* 2007;356:551–566.

98. Palomba S, Orio F, Falbo A, Russo T, Tolino A, Zullo F. Clomiphene citrate versus metformin as first-line approach for the treatment of infertile patients with polycystic ovary syndrome. *J Clin Endocrinol Metab.* 2007;92:3498–3503.

99. Dunaif A, Scott D, Finegood D, Quintana B, Whitcomb R. The insulin-sensitizing agent troglitazone improves metabolic and reproductive abnormalities in the polycystic ovary syndrome. *J Clin Endocrinol Metab.* 1996;81:3299–3306.

100. Azziz R, Ehrmann D, Legro RS, et al. Troglitazone improves ovulation and hirsutism in the polycystic ovary syndrome: a multicenter, double blind, placebo-controlled trial. *J Clin Endocrinol Metab.* 2001;86:1626–1632.

101. Dereli D, Dereli T, Bayraktar F, Ozgen A, Yilmaz C. Endocrine and metabolic effects of rosiglitazone in non-obese women with polycystic ovary disease. *Endocr J.* 2005;52:299–308.

102. Rautio K, Tapanainen JS, Ruokonen A, Morin-Papunen LC. Endocrine and metabolic effects of rosiglitazone in overweight women with PCOS: a randomized placebo-controlled study. *Hum Reprod.* 2006;21:1400–1407.

103. Brettenthaler N, De Geyter C, Huber P, Keller U. Effect of insulin sensitizer pioglitazone on insulin resistance, hyperandrogenism, and ovulatory dysfunction in women with polycystic ovary syndrome. *J Clin Endocrinol Metab.* 2004;89:3835–3840.

104. Garmes H, Tambascia M, Zantut-Wittmann D. Endocrine-metabolic effects of the treatment with pioglitazone in obese patients with polycystic ovary syndrome. *Gynecol Endocrinol.* 2005;21:317–323.

105. Ashraf Ganie M, Khurana M, Eunice M, Gulati M, Dwivedi S, Ammini A. Comparison of the efficacy of spironolactone with metformin in the management of polycystic ovary syndrome: an open-labeled study. *J Clin Endocrinol Metab.* 2004;89:2756–2762.

106. Yilmaz M, et al. The effect of rosiglitazone and metformin on insulin resistance and serum androgen levels in obese and lean patients with PCOS. *J Endocrinal Invest.* 2005;29:1003–1009.

107. Ortega-Gonzalez C, Luna S, Hernandez L, et al. Responses of serum androgen and insulin resistance to metformin and pioglitazone in obese, insulin-resistant women with polycystic ovary syndrome. *J Clin Endocrinol Metab.* 2005;90: 1360–1365.

108. Elter K, Imir G, Durmusoglu F. Clinical, endocrine and metabolic effects of metformin added to ethinyl estradio-cyproterone acetate in non-obese women with polycystic ovary syndrome: a randomized controlled study. *Hum Reprod.* 2002;17: 1729–1737.

109. Cibula D, Fanta M, Vrbikova J, et al. The effect of combination therapy with metformin and combined oral contraceptives (COC) versus COC alone on insulin sensitivity, hyperandrogenaemia, SHBG and lipids in PCOS patients. *Hum Reprod.* 2005;20:180–184.

110. Lemay A, Dodin S, Turcot L, Dechene F, Forest J-C. Rosiglitazone and ethinyl estradiol/cyproterone acetate as single and combined treatment of overweight women with polycystic ovary syndrome and insulin resistance. *Hum Reprod.* 2006;21: 121–128.

Chapter 34
Insulin Resistance and the Metabolic Syndrome

Mary Ann Banerji and Rochelle L. Chaiken

Introduction

This chapter focuses on insulin resistance and its role in diabetes, obesity, and cardiovascular (CV) disease. There is significant evidence that both CV disease and diabetes have common metabolic antecedents.[1,2] The metabolic syndrome and its relation to insulin resistance, cardiovascular disease, and diabetes will be critically reviewed with a focus on current clinical controversies.

Insulin Action and Insulin Secretion

To maintain normal glucose homeostasis, there must be adequate insulin secretion synchronized with target tissue insulin responsiveness. Following the ingestion of a meal, insulin, secreted from the pancreas, permits the circulating blood glucose to be transported to muscle and adipose cells for metabolism or storage and also suppresses the release of glucose from the liver.[3]

Insulin acts to increase glucose uptake for storage and metabolism in muscle and adipose cells via the tissue-specific glucose transporter glut-4 and in liver via glut-2. Insulin also decreases lipolysis and promotes lipogenesis. In liver, insulin decreases gluconeogenesis and glycolysis and promotes glycogen synthesis. Insulin also regulates amino acid uptake and protein synthesis, has important actions on the vasculature and endothelial cells and, among its least understood functions, acts on the brain to integrate fuel and energy homeostasis.

Insulin activates its receptor by binding to its two alpha subunits[4,5] (Figure 34.1). This auto-phosphorylates and activates *tyrosine kinases* intrinsic to the beta subunits, to promote phosphorylation of other tyrosines on downstream molecules known as insulin receptor substrates (IRS) and Shc. The IRS family of molecules consists of tissue-specific subtypes, for example, IRS-1 in muscle and IRS-2 in liver. IRS and Shc in turn activate phosphatidylinositol-3 kinase (PI-3-kinase) and mitogen-activated protein kinase (MAP kinase). The PI-3-kinase path is involved with metabolic activity and glucose transport via Glut-4 transporters in muscle and the MAP kinase pathway regulates mitogenesis and growth. Other metabolic activities controlled by the PI-3-kinase pathway include glycogen synthesis, lipolysis, fatty acid, and protein syntheses. Defects in this pathway are likely to reflect a combination of genetic and acquired defects.[6,7] One example of a defect in the pathways involves phosphorylation of serine or threonine residues of the IRS-1 complex instead of tyrosine which results in decreased downstream insulin receptor activity.

M.A. Banerji (✉)
VP Medical Affairs, Pfizer Inc., SUNY Downstate Medical Center, New York, State University of New York, Brooklyn, NY, USA
e-mail: mbanerji@downstate.edu

L. Poretsky (ed.), *Principles of Diabetes Mellitus*, DOI 10.1007/978-0-387-09841-8_34,
© Springer Science+Business Media, LLC 2010

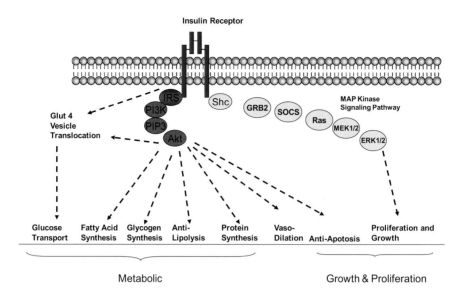

Fig. 34.1 Conceptual pathways of insulin receptor signaling show a simplified scheme for key insulin receptor pathways for metabolic actions and growth and proliferative action. *Dashed lines* represent intermediates which are not shown. (modified from ref [4,5])

Physiological Effects of Insulin Resistance

Resistance to insulin's effects may occur in different tissues.[8] In muscle, decreased insulin-mediated glucose uptake causes elevated blood glucose. Usually, a compensatory increase in insulin secretion develops which results in hyperinsulinemia sufficient to maintain normal glucose homeostasis. Without this, hyperglycemia and diabetes ensue. This compensatory increase in insulin or hyperinsulinemia while perfectly appropriate for maintaining the blood glucose level, may result in the enhancement of other actions of insulin.[9,10]

In the liver, a decreased insulin effect results in a lower suppression of hepatic glucose output and may lead to increased blood glucose. In adipose tissue, increased lipolysis and free fatty acids occur. Increased blood glucose and free fatty acid in turn promote further beta-cell dysfunction, decreased insulin secretion, and action. This negative amplification is also known as glucose toxicity and lipotoxicity.[11] In the brain, insulin resistance may be involved in altered feeding and energy regulation. In endothelial cells, insulin action via the PI-3-kinase pathway promotes the release of nitric oxide from endothelial cells. Nitric oxide, a *vasodilator*, increases blood flow and aids in peripheral glucose uptake. In contrast, insulin, working through the MAP kinase pathway, also promotes the release of endothelin-1 which is a potent *vasoconstrictor.* Normally, the vasodilator and vasoconstrictor aspects of insulin are in balance. However, in insulin resistance, hyperinsulinemia sufficient to maintain normal blood glucose through the PI-3-kinase and glut-4 pathway overactivates the MAP kinase pathway resulting in vasoconstriction. Activation of MAP kinase also promotes proliferation of vascular smooth muscle cells, an early vascular abnormality.[12,13]

Measuring Insulin Action in Humans

Although insulin regulates many physiological functions, our understanding of defects in insulin action in humans centers around muscle glucose uptake which has become a defining feature. Dynamic measures of insulin action include the euglycemic insulin clamp,[14,15] the insulin suppression test with steady-state plasma glucose determination,[16] the frequently sampled intravenous glucose tolerance test,[17–22] and the insulin tolerance test. Estimates of insulin sensitivity can also be obtained during an oral glucose tolerance test and include the Avignon, Matzuda, Gutt, and Stumvoll indices and the $IS_{0,120}$.[23–26] Static measures use fasting plasma insulin

Table 34.1 Measurements of insulin sensitivity

	Direct steady-state measurements
Hyperinsulinemic euglycemic clamp	Glucose infusion rate at steady state $= M$
	Possible variations include use of specific tracers for endogenous glucose output or lipid metabolism and adjustments for actual insulin concentrations achieved
Insulin sensitivity test	Steady-state plasma glucose concentration during constant infusions of insulin and glucose with suppressed endogenous insulin secretion
	Direct non-steady-state measurements
Insulin tolerance test	Measures a disappearance rate (k) of glucose following an intravenous bolus of insulin
Minimal model analysis of FSIVGTT[a]	The minimal model identifies model parameters that determine a best fit to glucose disappearance during the modified FSIVGTT. S_I: fractional glucose disappearance per insulin concentration unit; S_G: ability of glucose itself to facilitate its own disposal and inhibit hepatic glucose production in the absence of an incremental insulin effect (i.e., when insulin is at basal levels)
	Indices derived from fasting conditions
G/I ratio	Ratio of fasting plasma glucose (mg/dl) and insulin (μU/ml)
HOMA	HOMA-IR $= ([I_{0\,\mu U/ml}] \times [G_{0\,mmol/l}])/22.5$
QUICKI	QUICKI $= 1/[\log(I_{0\,\mu U/ml}) + \log(G_{0\,mg/dl})]$
	Indicies derived from oral glucose tolerance test
Matsuda index	$10{,}000/[(G_{0\,(mg/dl)} \times I_{0\,(mU/l)}) \times (G_{mean} \times I_{mean})]$
Gutt index	$75{,}000 + (G_0{-}G_{120})_{(mg/dl)} \times 0.19 \times BW/120 \times G_{mean(0,120)\,(mmol/l)} \times \log(I_{mean(0,120)})$ $_{(mU/l)}$
Stumvoll index	$0.157{-}4.576 \times 10^{-5} \times I_{120\,(pmol/l)} - 0.000299 \times I_{0\,(pmol/l)} - 0.00519 \times G_{90\,(mmol/l)}$

[a]FSIVGTT $=$ frequently sampled intravenous glucose tolerance test
BW $=$ body weight in kilograms
$G_0 =$ fasting plasma glucose
$G_{120} =$ plasma glucose at 120 min after 75 g oral glucose ingestion
$G_{90} =$ plasma glucose at 120 min after 75 g oral glucose ingestion
$I =$ plasma insulin; $I_0 =$ fasting plasma insulin

alone or, together with glucose values, result in indices such as the insulin/glucose ratio, HOMA-IR, and the QUICKI. All correlate to varying degrees with clamp-derived insulin sensitivity[27–34] (Table 34.1).

The euglycemic insulin clamp, considered the gold standard, involves infusing a constant amount of insulin and a variable amount of glucose over time so that the plasma glucose concentration remains constant.[14,15] By quantitating the amount of glucose required, the effect of insulin on whole-body glucose uptake is determined and reported as milligrams of glucose per kg body weight (or lean body mass) per minute. The higher the number of mg/kg/min of glucose infused, the greater the sensitivity at any particular insulin infusion. Adjustments may be made for plasma insulin concentration. Usually data from the last 30 min are used to calculate glucose disposal after a steady-state plasma glucose has been achieved. In its simplest form, the euglycemic insulin clamp method measures whole-body glucose uptake largely in *muscle*. In general, a glucose uptake above 5 mg/kg/min during a 1 mU/kg/min insulin infusion, which achieves a circulating insulin concentration of approximately 100 μU/ml, is usually considered normal insulin sensitivity, although this should be determined in individual populations. The choice of insulin dose infused during the clamp depends upon the hypothesis being tested. Liver glucose output is suppressed at low insulin concentrations while glucose uptake in muscle occurs at higher insulin concentrations. By combining this method with tracer techniques (labeled glucose or glycerol), the effect of insulin on the liver (suppression of hepatic glucose production, gluconeogenesis) and adipose tissue (lipolysis) can also be determined.[35,36] The procedure is reproducible, time consuming, and requires a degree of experience. A variation on the euglycemic insulin clamp, popularized by Reaven, involves the infusion of a fixed dose of insulin and glucose and the resultant steady state plasma glucose is the measure of insulin sensitivity with suppressed insulin secretion.[16]

The frequently sampled intravenous glucose tolerance test (FSIVGTT) relies on a rise of endogenous insulin in response to a bolus infusion of intravenous glucose (0.3 g/kg of 50% dextrose) delivered over 1 min with plasma samples obtained at 0, 2, 3, 4, 5, 6, 8, 10, 12, 14, 16, 22, 25, 30, 40, 50, 60, 70, 80, 90, 100, 120, 140,

160, 180 min.[17–22] The minimal model mathematical analysis of the kinetics of the resulting plasma glucose and insulin concentrations determines the fractional glucose disappearance rates per unit of insulin, termed S_I. Another parameter describes the effect of glucose on its own disposal at basal insulin concentrations, termed S_G. Parameters from the standard FSIVGTT correlate moderately well with clamp-derived insulin sensitivity.[8] One limitation is its reliance on release of endogenous insulin which may not be robust in patients with diabetes. Thus, a modification of the technique evolved which uses a bolus of insulin (30 mU/kg) 20 min after the test begins. This improves the *overall* correlation of the FSIVGTT parameters with the clamp technique ($r=0.62$, $p<0.0001$). Subgroups with impaired glucose tolerance or diabetes may not correlate as well ($r=0.48$, $p=0.016$ and $r=0.41$, $p=0.03$, respectively).[18,20,22]

Measures based on the oral glucose tolerance test, the Avignon, Matsuda, Stromvoll, and Gutt indexes,[23–26] are simpler to perform but may be affected by different and variable rates of gastric emptying and incretin effects. Measures which rely on a fasting glucose and/or insulin are simplest and lend themselves to large population studies.

Correlations of fasting plasma insulin with clamp-derived insulin sensitivity show coefficients of 0.56, $p=0.01$.[33] The HOMA-IR or homeostatic model assessment is calculated using the following formula: fasting plasma glucose mmol/l $\times$ fasting plasma insulin μU/ml/22.5. The number 22.5 is a factor derived from the product of a normal glucose of 4.0 mmol/l and a normal insulin 5.0 μU/ml. Thus the value of 1.0 would be found in a "normal" individual and higher numbers indicate insulin resistance. HOMA-IR correlates well with clamp-derived insulin sensitivity, $r=0.88$, $p<0.0010$.[30] The HOMA-IR is less accurate in diabetes and, because fasting insulin and glucose reflect liver metabolism, this test assumes that hepatic and peripheral insulin resistance are comparable. The log of HOMA-IR provides more consistent results (correlation with clamp data produces in healthy controls $r=-46$, $p=0.056$ and in obese subjects $r=-0.79$, $p<0.0001$). Another variation is the QUICKI or the Quantitative Insulin Sensitivity Check Index $=1/(\log$ insulin (μU/ml) $+ \log$ glucose (mg/dl)).[31] It demonstrates a good correlation with clamp-derived data but appears to be less robust in non-obese subjects (overall $r=0.78$, $p<0.00001$; normal, $r=0.49$, $p=0.01$; obese, $r=0.8$, $p<0.008$; diabetics, $r=0.7$, $p<0.0001$). Modifications of QUICKI include free fatty acid or glycerol determinations and improve the relationship with the euglycemic clamp-derived insulin sensitivity: QUICKI FFA $= 1/(\log$ fasting insulin [μl/ml] $+ \log$ fasting glucose [mg/dl] $+ \log$ fasting FFA [mmol/l]).[32,34] Limitations may include decreased ability to measure *change* in insulin sensitivity and reduced accuracy in uncontrolled diabetes. Thus, there are numerous ways to determine insulin sensitivity, each with its own advantages and limitations. The key is choosing one that is both feasible and best addresses the hypothesis being tested.

Insulin Resistance, Type 2 Diabetes, and Metabolic Abnormalities: Physiological Studies

Following the discovery of the radioimmunoassay technique by Berson and Yalow,[37,38] insulin resistance was identified as important in type 2 diabetes. It is present in the majority of type 2 patients with type 2 diabetes, their first-degree relatives, individuals with impaired glucose tolerance and obesity.[39–44] For years debates raged about whether insulin resistance or insulin secretion was more important in the pathogenesis of diabetes.[39] Most arguments supported insulin resistance since most patients and their relatives were insulin-resistant and nondiabetic individuals without diabetic relatives were not. Fewer arguments supported defective insulin secretion, although it was known that when matched for obesity, patients with type 2 diabetes had lower insulin responses than nondiabetic obese individuals. An important concept was the hyperbolic nature of the relationship between insulin resistance and insulin secretion in maintaining normal glucose tolerance: beta cell function varied reciprocally with the degree of insulin resistance as a constant, called a "disposition index" or DI. Thus mis-matches of beta cell function relative to insulin requirements were predicted to result in hyperglycemia and the development of diabetes.[45]

Longitudinal studies tracking the progression from normal to impaired to diabetic glucose tolerance provided clearer answers.[46–49] Among insulin-resistant Pima Indians, who were followed for 5 years, individuals who remained with normal glucose tolerance developed a slight worsening of insulin resistance and a complementary increase in insulin secretion. In contrast, in those individuals who developed diabetes, there was a slight worsening of insulin resistance but a very dramatic decrease in insulin secretion. Thus, even in the presence of insulin resistance, the key and essential physiological abnormality leading to hyperglycemia was a relative or absolute *decrease in insulin secretion* relative to insulin requirements.

Studies in a different ethnic group further illustrate this concept of insulin deficiency in diabetes. Among African-Americans, type 2 diabetes is heterogeneous: there are insulin-resistant *and* insulin-sensitive variants.[50] Nearly 30% of African-Americans with a BMI < 28.5 kg/m^2 exhibit the *unusual insulin-sensitive variant*.[51] Individuals with the insulin-sensitive variant had fasting plasma insulin levels markedly lower than that in those with the insulin-resistant variant. Postprandial insulin levels were also lower in the insulin-sensitive subgroup suggesting that insulin deficiency was a significant defect in this group. Insulin responses in the typical insulin-resistant variant were lower than that in controls leading to the conclusion that this group had at least two defects, insulin resistance and insulin deficiency, similar to the Pima Indians.

Several important metabolic features distinguish the *variants*. The insulin-resistant variant is associated with metabolic abnormalities including high plasma triglyceride and low plasma HDL cholesterol levels[52] while the insulin-sensitive variant exhibits normal plasma triglycerides, HDL cholesterol, and free fatty acid levels. Body composition also distinguishes the variants. There is a greater amount of visceral adipose tissue volume in the insulin-resistant variant compared with the BMI and age-matched insulin-sensitive variant.[53] Increased visceral adipose tissue is inversely associated with insulin-mediated glucose disposal while total subcutaneous adipose tissue is not (Figure 34.2). Increased visceral adipose tissue volume is also associated with increased plasma triglyceride levels, intramyocellular fat, and liver fat[54–56]. These and other data show that the insulin-resistant form of type 2 diabetes is characterized by increased cardiovascular risk factors with fat in abnormal locations.

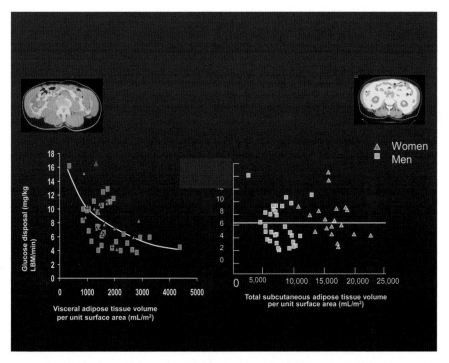

Fig. 34.2 *Left Panel* shows the inverse nonlinear relationship of insulin action to visceral adipose tissue ($r = -0.58$, Pp < 0.0001; men $r = -0.60$ (*squares*) and women $r = -0.59$ (*triangles*); the slope and intercept were not different in men and women). *Right panel* shows there is no significant relationship between insulin-mediated glucose disposal and total subcutaneous adipose tissue volume. *Insets* shown above the *left* and *right panel*, respectively, are a cross section of an abdominal CT image highlighted to show a small compared to a large visceral adipose tissue area.[62]

Insulin resistance and increased myocellular fat are also associated with abnormalities in muscle mitochondria number, size, and function.[57,58] Myocellular ATP production is decreased somewhat in the fasting state and abolished during insulin stimulation in individuals with type 2 diabetes, in their relatives, in obesity and nutrient overload.[59] Both increased FFA and glucose may decrease mitochondrial fitness and expression of genes for oxidative phosphorylation, including PGC-1α.[60,61] It is difficult to determine whether the fundamental cellular decrease in energy production is a result or a cause of obesity or insulin resistance.

There are population differences in the prevalence of insulin resistance in type 2 diabetes. For example, among Japanese, the insulin-sensitive form has a high frequency (~60%) with decreased non-traditional cardiovascular risk factors.[63] In contrast, South Asian Indians have a high prevalence of insulin resistant diabetes.[64] In the US NHANES data, 85% are insulin resistant and only 15% are insulin sensitive.[65]

Insulin resistance has been associated with multiple metabolic abnormalities (Table 34.2), several of which are traditional CV risk factors (high LDL cholesterol, hypertension, obesity, and diabetes), while the rest are known as nontraditional CV risk factors. Because of the link between insulin resistance and these CV risk factors,[66,67] it has been attractive to consider that insulin resistance is the underlying pathophysiological cause of increased CV disease in diabetes and obesity. These metabolic abnormalities include increased inflammatory markers such as increased hsCRP (highly sensitive C-reactive protein), interleukin-6, increased plasminogen activator inhibitor-1 (PAI-1) and increased fibrinogen (predisposing to thrombosis), increased uric acid and endothelial dysfunction with increased microalbuminuria and homocysteine levels.[63–77] The association between insulin resistance and hypertension appears to be population specific as it is not present in all ethnic groups[78–80] and because among individuals with essential hypertension, only 50% are insulin resistant. Many of these metabolic changes found in insulin resistance are also observed with obesity and will be discussed below. It is difficult to know which is of primary importance, obesity or insulin resistance.

Table 34.2 Insulin resistance syndrome and its components

Obesity[a]
Central obesity
Increased liver fat
Increase muscle fat
Glucose intolerance and type 2 diabetes[a]
Altered lipids
High triglyceride concentrations
Low HDL cholesterol concentrations
Dense LDL cholesterol[a] particles
Hypertension[a] – variable expression
Increased inflammation – CRP and others
Increased coagulation
Increased PAI-1
Increased fibrinogen
Increased vascular disease
Microalbuminuria
Endothelial dysfunction

[a]Traditional cardiovascular risk factors

Insulin Resistance and Obesity

In the 1940s and 1950s, Jean Vague of France described two types of obesity, both occurring in men and women: android or central obesity and gynoid or peripheral obesity.[81] The android form was associated with increased rates of diabetes, hypertension, and coronary artery disease while the gynoid form was not.

Obesity is excess of body fat and is most simply defined by a body mass index (BMI) or weight in kilograms divided by the height in meter squared [(weight (kg)/height (m)^2]. By convention, an individual with a BMI of less than 25 kg/m^2 is lean, with a BMI of 25–29.9 kg/m^2 is overweight, and with a BMI greater than 30 kg/m^2 is obese. Because of racial differences in body composition in South Asian Indians, an individual with a BMI

< 23 is defined as normal, 23–25 is defined as overweight, and > 25 is defined as obese. The BMI is an imperfect measure and for a greater understanding of obesity and its relationship to metabolism, it is important to describe body composition. Total body fat can be estimated by body volume (using an underwater or an air displacement method), density, and weight or by using dual photon absorptiometry (DXA). Visceral and subcutaneous fat and muscle are measured using computed tomography or magnetic resonance imaging and in vivo measurement of metabolic activity of muscle can be obtained by NMR spectroscopy.

Obesity is related to insulin resistance.[82,83,87] In studies of obese persons (BMI 30–34.9), McLaughlin[84] showed that insulin-resistant individuals compared to insulin sensitive, had significantly higher systolic and diastolic blood pressures and serum triglyceride levels and low HDL cholesterol levels as well as a higher prevalence of impaired glucose tolerance (48% vs 2%). However, not all obese individuals are insulin resistant[84,85] as highlighted in Ruderman's concept of the metabolically "obese" normal-weight individual.[86] The European Group for the Study of Insulin Resistance (EGIR) examined the relationship of insulin resistance measured by the euglycemic insulin clamp and hyperinsulinemia in healthy European individuals without hypertension over a wide range of body mass indices.[85] Similarly, EGIR reported that only 25% of nondiabetic obese persons (BMI> 25 kg /m^2; mean of 29 kg /m^2) were insulin resistant based on the euglycemic insulin clamp measurements. This unexpected result suggests that 75% of obese (or non-lean) individuals are insulin sensitive. After correcting for age, sex, and BMI, the waist circumference and waist–hip ratio were no longer associated with insulin resistance. This is not surprising as the waist is highly correlated with BMI and reflects both the visceral and the subcutaneous adipose tissue compartments.

Whether visceral or the subcutaneous adipose tissue is most important relative to insulin resistance has been the subject of considerable debate. In a comprehensive review of studies in adults, correlating subcutaneous and visceral adipose tissue measurements made by CT or MRI to insulin resistance measured using either the euglycemic clamp or the steady-state plasma glucose by insulin sensitivity index, Reaven found that the majority (11 of 18 studies) showed that visceral adipose tissue was most highly correlated with insulin resistance in men and women, blacks, whites, and South Asians (with correlation coefficient ranging from –0.33 to –0.60). However five studies reported that subcutaneous adipose tissue had higher correlation coefficients and two had equivalent correlations between the two fat depots. In favor of subcutaneous adipose tissue is an observation that most circulating free fatty acids derive from this depot and have adverse metabolic effects on both insulin secretion and action and promote inflammation. Although, most of these cross-sectional studies suggest the importance of visceral adipose tissue, several well-constructed intervention studies and one longitudinal one provide the most convincing evidence that excess visceral fat has adverse effects.

An initial report from Goodpaster et al. noted that the subcutaneous but not visceral adipose tissue was most significantly correlated with insulin resistance (r= –0.61 vs –0.52).[88] Subsequently, these authors reported that, after diet-induced weight loss, it was the decrease in visceral (not subcutaneous) adipose tissue which correlated most significantly with the improvement in insulin sensitivity.[89] Thus, the visceral adipose tissue depot was clearly critical in determining insulin resistance. Lemieux followed a group of women for 7 years and reported on changes in body composition and insulin resistance.[90] Comparisons of two subgroups with similar increases in visceral fat despite large differences in subcutaneous fat showed that there was no difference in metabolic parameters including glucose levels and insulin secretion. Moreover, individuals with the largest increase in visceral adipose tissue had significant deterioration in glucose tolerance and increase in insulin levels. A different approach – surgically removing subcutaneous adipose tissue - leads to the same conclusion. Klein studied the effects of subcutaneous adipose tissue liposuction on cardiovascular and metabolic risk factors and insulin action in obese diabetic and nondiabetic patients, before and 10 weeks after the procedure.[91] The nondiabetic subjects had 10.5 kg of fat or 28% of the abdominal subcutaneous fat removed and the patients with type 2 diabetes had 9.1 kg of fat removed (44% of this depot); baseline BMIs were 39.9 and 35.1 kg/m^2, respectively. Visceral adipose tissue volume did not change. Klein reported that despite a substantial weight loss there was no improvement in metabolic parameters including lipids, glucose, insulin, adiponectin, insulin resistance measured by the euglycemic insulin clamp method or other measures of inflammation including hsCRP, interleukin-6, and tumor necrosis factor alpha (TNF-α). A follow-up study, performed to evaluate long-term metabolic and CV benefit possibly overlooked in the earlier data, showed nearly identical results.[92] Improved glycemic and metabolic control seen during the treatment of type 2 diabetes with thiazolidiendiones is frequently associated with increases in subcutaneous fat and decreases in liver, visceral and blood fat suggesting specific roles of different fat depots.[95] Finally, a 10 year longitudinal study in Japanese Americans showed that visceral fat measured using the gold standard CT scanning was independently associated with the development of insulin resistance whereas total fat or subcutaneous fat was not.[93] The importance of a longitudinal study in well characterized subjects cannot be over emphasized.

Since human studies cannot always provide definitive information, a study in an animal model serves to clarify the role of *subcutaneous* adipose tissue. In female Syrian hamsters, surgical removal of greater than 50% of the subcutaneous adipose tissue, followed by a high-fat diet, resulted in a marked increase in serum triglycerides and visceral fat as well as a worsening of glucose tolerance and increase in serum insulin levels.[94] This demonstrates both the beneficial role of subcutaneous adipose tissue as a metabolic sink for excess calories and the adverse effects of storing calories in the viscera and in blood.[95]

Visceral adipose tissue has several unique metabolic properties. It demonstrates a high turnover, is more susceptible to catecholamine-induced lipolysis than subcutaneous adipose tissue,[96,97] and is under different sex hormone regulation. 1-Beta hydroxysteroid dehydrogenase type 1 activity may also differ. This enzyme converts inactive cortisone to cortisol and thus may cause local tissue changes in hormonal milieu.[98] Increased visceral adipose tissue is frequently associated with increased plasma triglyceride level, liver fat, and intramyocellular lipid.[55–101] These data suggest that ectopic fat (or fat in the "wrong places") may trigger inflammation with subsequent deleterious effects.

Adipose tissue is metabolically active and contributes to many factors which play a role in the adverse outcomes of obesity including insulin resistance, diabetes, and CV disease. These factors include increased resistin, increased visfatin, decreased adiponectin, increased inflammation, oxidative stress and increased reactive oxygen species[102–113] as well as free fatty acids, plasminogen activator-1 (PAI-1), fibrinogen, and uric acid. While weight loss decreases many of these biomarkers and suggests their importance, the finding that the adipose tissue-derived pro-inflammatory cytokines such as tumor necrosis factor α (TNF-α) can directly trigger inflammation points to a mechanism.[102] Several intracellular mediators of these inflammatory stimuli involve IKKβ/ NF-κB and the JNK pathways. Stimuli that activate the IKKβ/ NF-κB and JNK pathways include free fatty acid, glucose, reactive oxygen species, interleukin-6, ceramides, TNF-α, and advanced glycosylated end products (AGEs), as well as viral or bacterial elements. Activation of the pathways results in increased transcription of inflammatory moieties and the perpetuation of inflammation. Increased inflammation is associated with serine/threonine phosphorylation of IRS-1 and contributes to insulin resistance. Activation of macrophage can set in motion an inflammatory cascade of events leading to the vascular atheroma development and CV disease. In this context, two studies serve as proof of concept. Dandonna showed that treatment with insulin immediately after a myocardial infarction decreased inflammation (hsCRP and interleukin-6) and improved cardiac outcomes.[114] Goldfine treated obese nondiabetic individuals with salsalate, an anti-inflammatory agent, and reported a decrease in inflammation as well as a decrease in C-peptide and glucose suggesting that decreasing inflammation improves insulin resistance.[115] These data show some of the interrelationships of obesity, inflammation, insulin resistance, and CV disease.

Insulin Resistance, Obesity: Metabolic Heterogeneity

Insulin resistance and obesity are associated and are frequently assessed using the surrogate, hyperinsulinemia, especially in population studies. The European Group for the Study of Insulin Resistance (EGIR),[85] which reported on insulin resistance measured by the euglycemic insulin clamp and hyperinsulinemia in healthy European individuals as mentioned earlier, defined insulin resistance as the bottom 10% of the insulin lean group and hyperinsulinemia as the top 10% of fasting plasma insulin. Obesity was defined as a BMI > 25 kg/m^2. Insulin resistance was found in only 26% of obese subjects (mean BMI 29 kg/m^2), far fewer than anticipated. Hyperinsulinemia was observed in 41% of the obese subjects and *both* hyperinsulinemia and insulin resistance were present only among 14% of the obese subjects compared to 1.6% of the lean. The frequency of insulin resistance was low in obese individuals and was exceeded by hyperinsulinemia. Thus, hyperinsulinemia may result not only from obesity and insulin resistance but also through other possibly central nervous system signals as well. Hyperinsulinemia, therefore, is not a precise surrogate for insulin resistance and the obese phenotype is heterogeneous in terms of insulin resistance and its metabolic abnormalities.

The heterogeneity of the obese phenotype is further demonstrated in the NHANES data of 5440 participants without known CV disease. Metabolic parameters assessed included fasting plasma glucose and insulin, insulin resistance measured by HOMA-IR, inflammation measured by hsCRP, lipids and blood pressure. Several interesting observations emerged. In the age-standardized group with *normal* body weight (BMI< 25 kg/m^2), 30%, were metabolically *unhealthy* with two or more abnormalities while in the groups which were *overweight* (BMI 25–29.9 kg/m^2) or *obese* (BMI $\geq$ 30 kg/m^2), 48.8, and 29%, respectively, were *metabolically normal* with 0–1 abnormalities. Racial sub-analyses were similar. Correlates of 0–1 metabolic abnormalities were younger age, black race/ethnicity, higher physical activity levels, and smaller waist circumference (Figures 34.3 and 34.4,[116]). A separate report confirms that obese individuals with high percent body fat can have favorable metabolic profiles characterized by normal insulin sensitivity, lack of high blood pressure, normal lipids, and adiponectin levels.[117] These subjects had less liver, visceral and muscle fat, as well as less intima–media thickness, a surrogate for CV disease. Finally, an intervention study of diet-induced weight loss suggested that the two phenotypes might respond differently: the metabolically

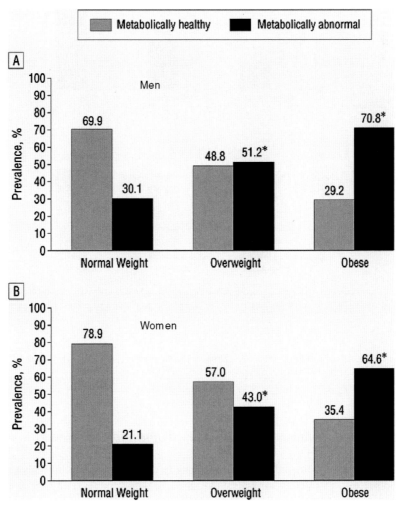

Fig. 34.3 Age-standardized prevalence of cardiometabolic abnormalities by body size and sex (A, men; B, women). *p <.001 for proportion metabolically abnormal vs normal weight. (modified from ref[116])

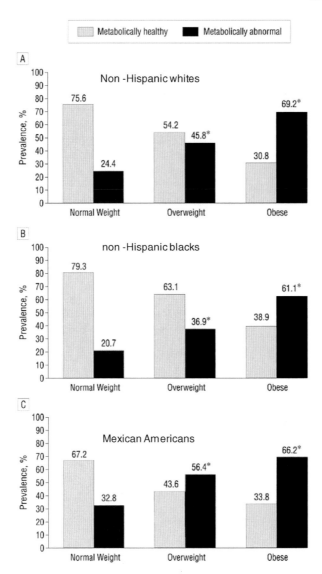

Fig. 34.4 Age- and sex-standardized prevalence of cardiometabolic abnormalities by body size and race/ethnicity. A, non-Hispanic whites; B, non-Hispanic blacks; and C, Mexican Americans. *p <.001 for proportion metabolically abnormal vs normal weight. (modified from ref[116])

adverse group *improved* insulin sensitivity by 26% while in contrast, the metabolically normal group's sensitivity deteriorated by 11%.[118] Whether similarly divergent responses accompany exercise is not known.

Insulin Resistance and Cardiovascular Disease – Population Studies

A prodigious number of population studies have tested the hypothesis that insulin resistance is a risk factor for cardiovascular disease in an attempt to understand the 2- to 4-fold increase in CV disease mortality with diabetes.[119–121] Most used fasting plasma insulin or HOMA-IR to measure insulin resistance.

Small studies, using the euglycemic insulin clamp, showed a positive relationship between insulin resistance and CV disease. In a report of 208 persons followed for 6 years, those in the highest compared to the lowest tertile had increased CV disease.[122] A report on the 6-year follow-up of 73 persons noted that CHD, hypertension, and microalbuminuria were increased in those with insulin resistance.[123]

Reports using the HOMA-IR showed variable results. The San Antonio Heart study which followed 2569 individuals for 7.5 years with 187 CV events. They reported an odds ratio (OR) of CV disease for the lowest versus the highest tertile of insulin resistance of 1.94 (95% CI 1.05–3.59) after adjustments for multiple confounders including sex, age, ethnicity, smoking alcohol use, physical activity, waist, blood pressure, HDL and LDL cholesterol, and triglycerides.[124] The VA HT study[125], The Study of Elderly Men[127] and the DECODE[126], the latter of which followed more than 10,000 individuals for 8.8 years also showed a positive association between insulin resistance and CVD.[126,127] In contrast, the Strong Heart Study and the Framingham Offspring Study did not show a relationship of insulin resistance and CVD[128,129]

The relationship of insulin to CV disease is not as strong as it was initially hypothesized. In 1998, Ruige's review showed an overall hazard ratio (HR) for insulin and CV disease of 1.18 (95% CI 1.08–1.29) for each 50 pmol/l of fasting plasma insulin and highlighted ethnic/racial heterogeneity.[130] In whites the association of insulin and CV disease showed a HR of 1.4 (95% CI 1.23–1.65) compared to non-whites (Nauruans and Pima Indians) of 1.04 (95% CI 0.93–1.16). Whites were older, with clinical outcomes of death or myocardial infarction instead of ECG changes. Several specific studies are worthy of review. The ARIC study of 13,446 men and women with 305 events followed over 6 years showed no relationship of fasting plasma insulin to CV disease.[131] Further follow-up revealed a relationship of fasting insulin to incident stroke with a HR of 1.54 (95% CI 1.01–1.3) for each 50 pmol/l of fasting insulin.[132] In contrast, the Helsinki Policeman study of 970 men followed up to 22 years did *not* show a relationship of hyperinsulinemia to stroke after adjustment for age and other CV disease risk factors [HR 1.54 (95% CI 0.9–2.64)] while blood pressure, upper body obesity, and smoking were significantly predictive [HR 1.36 (95% CI 1.18–3.06), 1.59 (95% CI 1.26–2.00), 1.88 (95% CI 1.16–3.04), respectively]. This study highlights an interesting aspect of long-term follow-up. After adjustment for age and other CV disease risk factors, hyperinsulinemia (defined as the highest quintile of insulin area under the curve during an OGTT) was associated with a HR for major incident coronary heart disease at 5, 10, and 15 years [HR 2.36 (95% CI 1.00–5.57), 2.29 (95% CI 1.31–4.02), 1.76 (95% CI 1.09–2.82), respectively] but not at 22 years [HR 1.32 (95% CI 0.89–1.97)]. This attenuation of effect suggests a changing relationship of insulin to CV risk over time. The concept of a changing temporal relationship of a risk factor to a disease as the pathogenesis evolves may explain the varied findings in different studies.[133,134] The Caerphilly study of 1056 subjects over 12 years with 127 events showed no relationship of fasting plasma insulin to CV disease.[135] Among elderly men born between 1913 and 1923, the risk of coronary heart disease increased 2.4-fold in those in the highest compared to the lowest quintile of fasting plasma insulin after 13-year follow-up.[136] The DECODE Study mentioned above,[126] also reported that the risk of *death* was predicted by the highest compared to the lowest tertile of fasting insulin [HR 2.66 (95% CI 1.45–4.9) for women and 1.54 (95% CI 1.16–2.03) for men].The HOMA-IR results were significantly similar [HR 2.35 (95% CI 1.16–2.03) for women and 1.58 (95% CI 1.2–2.09) for men].

A recent meta-analysis of 19 studies in Western populations with 3600 events showed an overall modest predictive effect of insulin on incident coronary heart disease. For fasting insulin, the RR was 1.2 (95% CI 0.98–1.28) and for non-fasting insulin the RR was 1.35 (95% CI 1.14–1.6). Figure 34.5 shows the effect of insulin for all the studies.[137]

Metabolic Syndrome: Risk for Type 2 Diabetes and Predictor of CV Disease

Although previously described, in 1988 Gerald Reaven's Banting Lecture popularized the "metabolic syndrome," linking insulin resistance as central to, if not the primary cause of a cluster of abnormalities including glucose intolerance, hypertension, and a distinct lipid profile of high triglyceride and low HDL cholesterol levels.[8,136–145] The "syndrome" was a plausible explanation linking diabetes and cardiovascular disease. Diabetes, like obesity, is associated with a 2- to 4-fold increase in CV mortality and since most people with diabetes are obese and insulin resistant, clarifying the contribution of the components of each to cardiovascular disease is challenging.

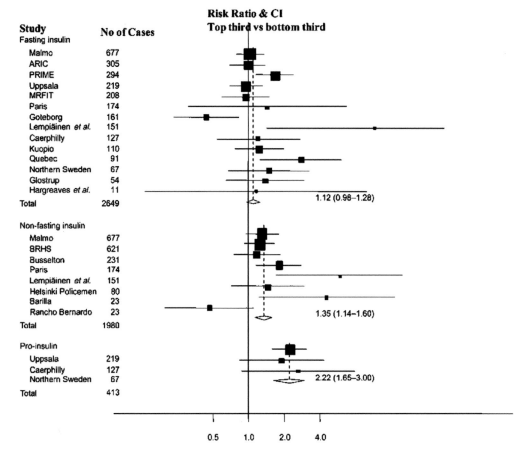

Fig. 34.5 Prospective studies of concentrations of circulating insulin markers and coronary heart disease (CHD) (nonfatal MI or coronary death) in Western populations in 19 prospective studies involving a total of about 3600 incident CHD cases. It shows the risk ratio (RR) for CHD and confidence intervals (CI) for the top third vs the bottom third for fasting insulin (1.12 [95%C 0.98–1.28] for raised fasting insulin) and for non-fasting insulin (1.35 [95% CI 1.14–1.60] for raised non-fasting insulin).[137] The *left inset* shows RR of various study characteristics. Specifically, *top* and *bottom insets* show RR of CHD: 1.12 [95% CI 0.98–1.28] for raised fasting insulin, 1.35 (1.14–1.60) for raised non-fasting insulin, respectively

Reaven presented the metabolic syndrome as a testable hypothesis and ever since, the challenge has been met with an avalanche of articles.

Metabolic Syndrome – WHO, ATP III, and IDF Criteria

The central feature of the Reaven's metabolic syndrome was insulin resistance measured by an insulin clamp. Since the insulin clamp was unwieldy, simpler measures were developed to assess if insulin resistance and metabolic syndrome were predictive of diabetes and increased CV. Various professional organizations devised clinically measurable but arbitrary sets of criteria as surrogates which were initially based on diabetes or insulin resistance. In chronological order these were the following: the World Health Organization (WHO, 1999), European Group for the Study of Insulin Resistance (EGIR, 1999), the National Cholesterol Education Panel (NCEP) of the American Heart Association (AHA), Adult Treatment Panel (ATP III) criteria (2001), the American Association of Clinical Endocrinologists (AACE) (2003), the revised AHA criteria (2005), and the International Diabetes Federation (IDF, 2005) (Tables 34.3 and 34.4).[146–151]

Table 34.3 Different definitions of the metabolic syndrome (modified from ref[150])

Clinical measure	WHO (1998)	EGIR	ATP III (2001)	AACE (2003)	IDF (2005)	AHA 2005
Insulin resistance	IGT, IFG, T2DM, or lowered insulin sensitivity[a] plus any two of the following	Plasma insulin >75th percentile plus any two of the following	None, but any of the following five features	IGT or IFG plus any of the following based on clinical judgment	None	Any three of the following five features
Body weight	Men: waist-to-hip ratio >0.90; women: waist-to-hip ratio >0.85 and/or BMI > 30 kg/m²	WC ≥ 94 cm in men or ≥ 80 cm in women	WC ≥ 102 cm in men or ≥ 88 cm in women	BMI ≥ 25 kgm²	Increased WC (population specific)[b] plus any two of the following	WC ≥ 102 cm men WC ≥ 88 cm women
Lipid	TG ≥ 150 mg/dl and/or HDL-C < 35 mg/dl in men or < 39 mg/dl in women	TG ≥ 150 mg/dl and/or HDL-C < 39 mg/dl in men or women	TG ≥ 150 mg/dl HDL-C < 40 mg/dl in men or < 50 mg/dl in women	TG ≥ 150 mg/dl and HDL-C < 40 mg/dl in men or < 50 mg/dl in women	TG ≥ 150 mg/dl or on TG Rx HDL-C < 40 mg/dl in men or < 50 mg/dl in women or ion HDL-C Rx	TG ≥ 150 mg/dl HDL-C < 40 mg/dl in men or < 50 mg/dl in women or treatment[c]
Blood pressure	≥ 140/90 mmHg	≥ 140/90 mmHg or on hypertension Rx	≥130/85 mmHg	≥130/85 mmHg	≥130 mmHg systolic of ≥ 85 mmHg diastolic or on hypertension Rx	BPs ≥ 130 or BPd ≥ 85 mmHg or treatment
Glucose	IGT, IFG, or T2DM[d]	IGT or IFG (but not diabetes)	> 110 mg/dl (includes diabetes)[d]	IGT or IFG (but not diabetes)	≥ 100 mg/dl (includes diabetes)	> 100 mg/dl
Other	Microalbuminuria			Other features of insulin resistance[e]		

[a]Insulin sensitivity measured under hyperinsulinemic euglycemic conditions, glucose uptake below lowest quartile for background population studied.

[b]See Table 344.

[c]HDL-C =HDL cholesterol, TG = triglyceride. Fibrates and nicotinic acid are the most commonly used drugs for elevated TG and reduced HDL-C. Patients taking one of these drugs are presumed to have high TG and low HDL.

[d]IGT = impaired glucose tolerance, IFG = impaired fasting glucose;T2DM = type 2 diabetes mellitus

The 2001 definition identified fasting plasma glucose of 110 mg/dl (6.1 mmol/l) as elevated. This was modified in 2004 to be 100 mg/dl (5.6 mmol/l), in accordance with the American Diabetes Association's updated definition of IFG

[e]Includes family history of type 2 diabetes mellitus, polycystic ovary syndrome, sedentary lifestyle, advancing age, and ethnic groups susceptible to type 2 diabetes mellitus

WC = waist circumference. To measure, locate top of right iliac crest. Place a measuring tape in a horizontal plane around abdomen at level of iliac crest. Before reading tape measure, ensure that tape is snug but does not compress the skin and is parallel to floor. Measurement is made at the end of a normal expiration.

Some US adults of non-Asian origin (e.g., white, black, Hispanic) with marginally increased waist circumference [e.g., 94–101 cm (37–39 in.) in men and 80–87 cm (31–34 in.) in women] may have strong genetic contribution to insulin resistance and should benefit from changes in lifestyle habits, similar to men with categorical increases in waist circumference. Lower waist circumference cutpoint [e.g., 90 cm (35 in.) in men and 80 cm (31 in.) in women] appears to be appropriate for Asian Americans.

Table 34.4 Population-specific waist circumference

Country/ethnic group	Waist circumference (WC)
Europids In the USA, the ATP III values (102 cm male; 88 cm female) – likely to continue in use for clinical purposes	Male ≥ 94 cm; female ≥ 80 cm
South Asians Based on a Chinese, Malay, and Asian-Indian population	Male ≥ 90 cm; female ≥ 80 cm
Chinese	Male ≥ 90 cm; female ≥ 80 cm
Japanese	Male ≥ 90 cm; female ≥ 80 cm
Ethnic South and Central Americans	Use South Asian recommendations until more specific data are available
Sub-Saharan Africans	Use European data until more specific data are available
Eastern Mediterranean and Middle East (Arab) populations	Use European data until more specific data are available

While the WHO and the EGIR were centered on diabetes, glucose intolerance, or insulin resistance, plus several other factors, the NCEP–ATP III version was developed by cardiologists with the express goal of targeting individuals at high risk for CV disease prevention. In NCEP–ATP III, three out of five equally weighted criteria defined the metabolic syndrome. Neither diabetes nor insulin resistance were necessary for the diagnosis of metabolic syndrome. In the IDF version, the central criterion was a high waist circumference (adjusted for differences in ethnic groups) plus two of four other elements. On the surface, these appear similar but the WHO, EGIR, AACE, and IDF are anchored hierarchically in diabetes/glucose intolerance/ insulin resistance or central obesity while in NCEP–ATP III all criteria are equal. Although conceptually NCEP–ATP III proposal appears simple, a large number of combinations of three out of five criteria raise the question of whether all combinations equally predict CV disease.[152]

Prevalence and Stability Over Time of the Metabolic Syndrome

The prevalence of metabolic syndrome varies by definition, population, and gender; reports suggest that its stability differs among populations. Its prevalence based on the NCEP–ATP III criteria was ~24% in the US NHANES population of 1988–1994 and rose to ~34% in 1999–2002 survey (Figure 34.6)[153,154]

The San Antonio Heart study followed two cohorts over 10 and 7 years and reported an increased prevalence of the metabolic syndrome by the NCEP–ATP III criteria.[155] Among nondiabetic individuals, percent rate increases were from 15.5 to 25.8% and 23.3 to 30.4% in men and 10.8 to 22.6% and 23.3 to 30.4 in women in the first and second cohorts. In diabetics these rates were significantly higher, ranging from 79 to 85% in the second cohort in men and 66 to 87% in both cohorts of women. In contrast, in Mexico, the rate in men was 38.9% without change over 7 years while in women there was no change over 3 years and a slight decrease (65–59%) over the final 4-year study interval.[156] A Finnish cross-sectional study done 10 years apart (1992 and 2002) shows the increasing prevalence of NCEP–ATP III metabolic syndrome (1992 and 2002); men had a higher prevalence of metabolic syndrome compared to women at baseline but only women had a significant increase in incidence over time (32–38% for women and 48.8–52.6% for men).[157] Among adolescents, the diagnosis of the metabolic syndrome is reported to fluctuate.[158]

Several important issues should be examined. (1) Is the metabolic syndrome useful in identifying individuals at high risk for diabetes and/or and increased CV disease in nondiabetic and diabetic populations? (2) Is insulin resistance the basis for the metabolic syndrome?

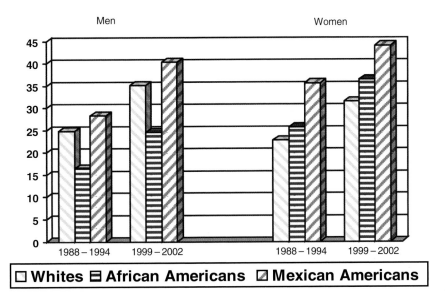

Fig. 34.6   Increase in metabolic syndrome over time in whites, African-Americans, and Mexican Americans

Does the Metabolic Syndrome Predict Diabetes in Nondiabetes Populations?

The metabolic syndrome strongly predicts diabetes. This may not be surprising because one component is an elevated blood glucose which alone has a similar predictive value.[159,160] Indeed, metabolic syndrome accounts for up to half of the new cases of diabetes in the Framingham offspring study among those who did not have diabetes at baseline and were followed for 8 years.[161] While the metabolic syndrome strongly predicts diabetes (HR ~4–6), fasting plasma glucose is far more predictive (HR ~18). The reader is referred to a recent review for more details.[162]

Does the Metabolic Syndrome Predict CV Disease in Nondiabetic Populations?

Early studies[143] enthusiastically reported robust associations of insulin resistance and CV disease but subsequent more rigorous examinations adjusting for components of the metabolic syndrome found it less informative.

   Ford summarized 17 prospective studies from 1998 to 2002, and after adjusting for confounders, the metabolic syndrome by WHO and NCEP–ATP III criteria modestly and similarly predicted CV disease (RR for WHO was 1.93 (95% CI 1.39–2.07) and NCEP was 1.65 (95% CI 1.38–1.00) and all-cause mortality (RR for WHO was 1.37 (95% CI 1.09–1.74) and for NCEP was 1.27 (95% CI 0.09–1.78)). In contrast, metabolic syndrome was a much more robust predictor of diabetes (RR 2.60–2.99).[163] Among elderly Finns, followed for 13.5 years, Wang reported on the relationship of all the different definitions of metabolic syndrome and their ability to predict diabetes or CV mortality and disease.[164] WHO and IDF criteria predicted CHD and CV disease mortality significantly in men [(HR 1.97 (95% CI 1.27–3.05) and 1.70 (95% CI 1.19–2.43) and 1.58 (95% CI 1.02–2.44) and 1.34 (0.94–1.93)], respectively. None predicted all-cause mortality. The individual components themselves significantly predicted disease by a similar magnitude as the metabolic syndrome: impaired glucose tolerance [HR 1.55 (95% CI 1.17–2.0)] in WHO, IDF, and ATP III metabolic syndrome; low HDL cholesterol (<1 mmol/l) [HR 1.50 (95% CI 1.12–2.01)] and microalbuminuria (albumin creatinine ratio greater than 3.39 mg/mmol) [HR 1.86 (95% CI 1.40–2.47)] in metabolic syndrome by WHO. In another publication of the same population followed for 14 years,[165] metabolic syndrome predicted stroke with hazard ratios varying from 1.52 to 1.72 depending on the criteria used. This analysis also demonstrated that the individual components had nearly the same predictive value as the metabolic syndrome in predicting for outcomes and for CV disease risk.

The Malmo study followed over 5,000 Swedes for 11 years and showed a HR for a composite endpoint of MI and stroke of 1.11 (95% CI 0.86–1.44), 1.59 (1.25–2.03), and 1.35 (1.05–1.74), respectively, for the IDF, ATP III, and EGIR metabolic syndrome after adjusting for confounders.[166] Only the NCEP–ATP III criteria were predictive for men but not for women. Individual components had significant hazard ratios of a similar order of magnitude: 2.97, 2.01, 1.81, and 1.75 for blood pressure, HDL cholesterol, obesity, and current smoking. NCEP–ATP III was most predictive of CV disease; however, other studies showed IDF to be equivalent to NCEP–ATP III[167] and the DECODE study showed that WHO was better.[168]

Unlike the other studies, DECODE was a collaborative *mortality* analysis of 11 European studies of over 10,000 individuals, followed for 7–16 years.[168] The prevalence rates of metabolic syndrome for men and women in the WHO were 27% and 19% NCEP, 25.9%, 23.4%; NCEP revised, 32.2% and 28.5%; IDF, 35.9% and 34.1%, respectively. In men the likelihood of CV mortality was 2.09 (95% CI 1.59–2.76), 1.74 (95% CI 1.31–2.3), 1.72 (95% CI 1.31–2.26), and 1.5 (95% CI 1.15–1.99) for WHO, NCEP, NCEP revised, and IDF metabolic syndrome, respectively; the corresponding values in women were weaker: 1.60 (95% CI 1.01–2.51), 1.39 (95% CI 0.89–2.18), 1.09 (95% CI 0.7–1.69), 1.53 (95% CI 0.99–2.39), respectively. Individual components were predictive of CV mortality in men and women with similar orders of magnitude (e.g., for blood pressure, HR was 2.3 for men, for triglyceride HR was 1.68).

Sattar reported on two studies in the elderly in Britain.[169] One was the PROSPER study which randomized 4,812 nondiabetic individuals, age 70–82 years, to placebo or 40 mg pravastatin and followed them for 3.2 years; there were 774 incident cases of CV events and 287 of diabetes. The NCEP–ATP III criteria of metabolic syndrome did not predict CV events [HR 1.07 (95% CI 0.86–1.32)] nor did BMI > 30 g/m^2, triglyceride levels > 1.69 mmol/l, fasting glucose > 6.1 mmol/l, or blood pressure > 130/80 (adjusted for confounders including treatment allocation). Positive predictors included age, male sex, prior CV disease, and low HDL cholesterol. A second study of 2,737 men, age 60–79, reported in the same paper, showed similar negative findings. In contrast, both studies showed that metabolic syndrome was a robust predictor of diabetes [HR 4.41 (95% CI 3.33–5.84) and 7.47 (95% CI 4.90–11.46), respectively]; however, the FPG was a nearly 4-fold better predictor [HR 18.0 (95% CI 13.9–24.5)]. Fasting plasma glucose and waist as dichotomized variables did not predict CV disease. Overall, metabolic syndrome was of no benefit in CV disease risk stratification for the elderly.

Similarly, Gami's meta-analysis of 37 studies representing 172,572 middle age individuals without CV disease reported only a modest effect of metabolic syndrome in predicting CV risk with a HR of 1.49 (95% CI 1.37–1.61).[170] Gami concluded that metabolic syndrome did not enhance risk prediction beyond that of the Framingham algorithm.

The prospective Framingham Heart Offspring Study[161] followed 3323 individuals for 8 years and showed a more positive relationship of metabolic syndrome and CV disease. Of the 2649 with neither diabetes nor CV at baseline, there was a higher prevalence rate of NCEP–ATP III in men than women (26.8% vs 16.1%). Men had an age-adjusted HR of 2.88 (95% CI 1.96–4.16) for CV disease and 2.59 (95% CI 1.62–3.98) for CHD disease which was higher than that for women [HR 2.2 (95% CI 1.31–3.88) and 1.54 (95% CI 0.68–3.5)]. The population-attributable risk was 34 and 29% in men and 16 and 8% in women for CV disease and CHD, respectively, thus accounting for nearly a third of new CV disease cases in 8 years.

Does the Metabolic Syndrome Predict CV Disease in Diabetic Populations?

The evidence is mixed and suggests that metabolic syndrome does not uniquely predict incident CV disease or mortality over and above its components.

Three studies show a positive predictive value of the metabolic syndrome.[171–173] Bonora[171] studied over 900 individuals with diabetes and found that > 90% had the metabolic syndrome by the WHO criteria. Baseline CV disease was more common in patients with the metabolic syndrome than without (32.9% vs 17.8%); among a group without CV disease at baseline, metabolic syndrome was an independent predictor of incident CV disease with an OR of almost 5-fold over 4.5 years and 2-fold for prevalent CV disease. Guzder[172] reported that in new onset type 2 diabetes, metabolic syndrome by ATP III criteria was present in 82% and predicted 2- and

4-fold increases in incident and prevalent CV disease. Tong[173] reported on 4350 Chinese individuals followed for 7.1 years and found that metabolic syndrome by ATP III criteria (but not IDF criteria) predicted a 2.5-fold increase in CHD. This study also noted that micro- and macroalbuminuria, hypertension, and HDL cholesterol were all significant predictors of CV disease. The frequency of metabolic syndrome by NCEP–ATP III or IDF was 65%.

In contrast, three studies show that the metabolic syndrome has no clear predictive value for CV disease.[174–176] Studies by Sone[174] from Japan and Bruno[175] from Italy showed similar results in approximately 1550 patient each followed for 8.9 and 11 years, respectively. Sone's study in type 2 diabetes without baseline CV disease reported 51% with metabolic syndrome by WHO criteria and 45% with metabolic syndrome by ATP III criteria.[174] ATP III was not predictive of CV disease in men or women. WHO was predictive only in women. In men, other factors such as triglycerides or HDL cholesterol were better or equivalent. Bruno's study reported 75% with metabolic syndrome (WHO) but with no difference in mortality in patients with and without the metabolic syndrome (~50% in each group) over 11 years.[175] As with Sone's study, metabolic syndrome with one or more components compared to zero components conferred an ~2-fold increase in CV disease but the individual components were equally predictive. Finally, in 2007, Cull reported on the 10.3-year follow-up of 4,542 new onset type 2 diabetes patients in the UKPDS study.[176] Metabolic syndrome was determined in four ways resulting in different prevalence rates: by ATP III 61%, by WHO 38%, by IDF 54%, and by EGIR 24%. The HR for CV disease was 1.3, 1.45, 1.23, and 1.0, respectively. Metabolic syndrome did not predict microvascular disease. The positive predictive value for CV disease was poor and ranged from 18 to 20%. Furthermore, in 47% of individuals *without metabolic syndrome,* there was a 10-year estimated CV disease risk of > 20% and in 37% of those *with metabolic syndrome* there was a 10-year estimated CV disease risk of < 20%.

Despite positive reports, overall, the metabolic syndrome is a rather poor predictor of CV disease in type 2 diabetes.

Why Does Not the Metabolic Syndrome Predict CV Disease in Type 2 Diabetes?

There are several potential explanations for the lack of predictive power of the MS for CV disease in patients with diabetes.[176] The metabolic syndrome uses dichotomized variables while in fact these variables have a continuous relationship with CV disease (e.g., triglyceride and HDL). Not all the elements of the metabolic syndrome are equivalent in determining CV risk even though in the NCEP–ATP III criteria all are given equal weight. In fact, fasting plasma glucose of greater than 6.1 mmol/l is very strongly associated with CV disease risk.[177,178] Diabetes is a greater risk factor for mortality and CV disease than metabolic syndrome (HR 5 and 3.6 vs 3.5 and 2.7, respectively),[179] and the excess CV mortality in patients with known CV disease associated with metabolic syndrome is due mostly to diabetes; this excess disappears after controlling for diabetes.[180,181]

Does the Combination of Metabolic Syndrome and Insulin Resistance Predict CV Disease?

Although the elements do cluster, the metabolic syndrome does not improve the ability to identify a high CV risk cohort. In the current context, it is not clear whether this is because insulin resistance is not an antecedent CV risk factor or because metabolic syndrome does not capture insulin resistance. Another very real issue is that each component may have several causes besides insulin resistance. It is not clear if insulin resistance serves as an etiology for traditional or nontraditional CV disease risk factors.

Studies using the euglycemic insulin clamp (or FSIVGTT) showed that insulin resistance was present in only 33% of subjects with the metabolic syndrome[182,183] and its sensitivity varied from 20 to 66%. Thus, metabolic syndrome may have a low sensitivity for identifying insulin resistance.

Several population studies bear on this question. The 11-year follow-up report of the Framingham Heart Offspring Study analyzed the impact of insulin resistance (measured using HOMA-IR) on CV disease and diabetes in a subset of people with and without the metabolic syndrome.[184] Using ATP III criteria, approximately one quarter had metabolic syndrome (27.8%) and over half of these were insulin resistant, while in those without metabolic syndrome, 12.8% were insulin resistant. The study found that compared to those with neither the metabolic syndrome nor insulin resistance, metabolic syndrome alone or insulin resistance alone did not predict CV disease [HR 1.2 (95% CI 0.7–1.9)] and 1.3 (95% CI 0.9–1.19)] but both together doubled the risk [HR 2.3 (95% CI 1.7–3.1)] with a population-attributable risk for both men and women of 18% compared to neither metabolic syndrome nor insulin resistance (Figure 34.7). Thus, insulin resistance adds to the CV disease risk beyond just metabolic syndrome and confirms earlier reports that insulin resistance and metabolic syndrome are not identical but describe different subsets of population risk. In contrast, insulin resistance, metabolic syndrome, or both are increasingly predictive for diabetes.

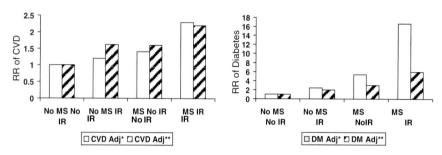

Fig. 34.7 Relative risk of incident CVD (*left panel*) or diabetes (*right panel*) and 8-year follow-up based on the presence of ATP III metabolic syndrome (MetS) or insulin resistance (IR) in the Framingham Heart Offspring Study. On both panels, *open bars* reflect data adjusted for age and sex. *Hatched bars* are adjusted for CV risks factors (*left panel*): age, sex, LDL cholesterol, and smoking and for diabetes risk factors (*right panel*): age, sex, family history of diabetes, BMI, and 2-h glucose during oral glucose tolerance testing. (modified from ref[184])

To conclude, although the metabolic syndrome may add to the prediction of CV risk, overall its magnitude is not as great as was once thought. Nevertheless, the metabolic syndrome is likely to be not more than the sum of its parts after adjusting for standard CV risk factors.

Summary: Insulin

Resistance and the Metabolic Syndrome: The Debate Continues

From its popular inception in 1988, the metabolic syndrome, aka the insulin resistance syndrome, was presented as a testable hypothesis. Initially, insulin resistance was hypothesized to be the physiological basis for the observed clustering of metabolic variables including diabetes, lipid abnormalities, blood pressure, increased cardiovascular disease, and central obesity. It captured the imagination of thousands of scientific investigators and the lay public as the incidence of obesity and diabetes increased to epidemic proportions. Although a great deal of scientifically exciting and valid knowledge has been generated to understand how the variables are related, there is still no unifying consensus that links them.

In 2001, this scientific hypothesis was used as the basis to create a simple clinical screening tool to prevent cardiovascular disease. The presence of three of five variables defined the ATP III metabolic syndrome which was given the stamp of approval by the American Heart Association. It was a novel approach to the old problem of cardiovascular risk and set off a worldwide frenzy of investigations resulting in hundreds of papers, reviews and chapters. It was formally legitimized by an International Classification of Diseases (ICD-9) code. Many competing definitions of the "metabolic syndrome" developed. In 2005, the American Diabetes Association and the European Association for the Study of Diabetes concluded that the metabolic syndrome was an emperor with no clothes. A calculating look revealed that it did not provide sufficient predictive power for CV disease beyond conventional risk factors or the individual components of the metabolic syndrome. Although metabolic syndrome was strongly predictive of diabetes, the fasting plasma glucose was markedly better. The darling of two decades had lost favor.

In 2008, the Endocrine Society published a Clinical Practice Guideline for the Primary Prevention of CV disease or coronary heart disease.[185] Expert opinion recommended that the metabolic syndrome could be used to identify an early likelihood of developing CV disease. Since the variables of the metabolic syndrome are CV risk factors and do cluster, the presence of any one should raise awareness to determine 10 years' absolute risk for cardiovascular disease using the Framingham, PROCAM, or SCORE algorithms. Treatment should be initiated based on this with a focus on apoB-containing lipoproteins [LDL and VLDL cholesterol (triglyceride)], hypertension, increased blood glucose, enlarged waist, a prothrombotic, and a pro-inflammatory state. The guideline further advises that patients with metabolic risk initiate preventive measures with priority given to lifestyle modifications. The metabolic syndrome has risen again.

In the final analysis, what is needed is a way to identify individuals at high risk for cardiovascular disease who might benefit from prevention of the first CV event (primary prevention). Currently, the absolute prevalence rates of CV events are low, at $\sim$2–3% and in a recent trial of primary prevention of CV disease, only 1 individual benefited out of 100 treated with a statin.[186] Given these data, most "healthy" individuals choose not to adhere to long-term preventive strategies, whether lifestyle or pharmacologic. It is obvious that the metabolic syndrome is not a robust marker and neither are the usual risk factors such as LDL cholesterol.

In order to identify individuals who are at risk before they have an event, future novel approaches might involve genomic analyses of CV risk. Another potential approach is to develop the concept of the vascular system phenotype or condition of the vascular using structural measures. This would enrich the target population for primary prevention of CV disease. With the advent of new technology such as ultrasound or CT, can we develop a better correlation between the structure of the vasculature and the risk for CV events? This would also identify a population enriched for risk of CV disease and an effective target for primary prevention. It is likely that these novel approaches would increase compliance, adherence, and cost-effectiveness of CV disease prevention.

References

1. Reaven G. The metabolic syndrome or the insulin resisvntance syndrome? Different names, different concepts, and different goals. *Endocrinol Metab Clin North Am*. 2004;33:283–303.
2. DeFronzo RA. Banting Lecture: from the triumvirate to the ominous Octet June 2008, American Diabetes Association. http://www.diabetesconnect.org/storetemplate/webcast_list.aspx?ses=902
3. Bergman RN, Finegood DT, Kahn SE. The evolution of beta-cell dysfunction and insulin resistance in type 2 diabetes. *Eur J Clin Invest*. 2002;32(Suppl 3):35–45.
4. Taguchi A, White MF. Insulin-like signaling, nutrient homeostasis and life span. *Ann Rev Physiol*. 2008;70:191–212.
5. Taniguchi CM, Emalnuelli B, Kahn CR. Critical nodes in signaling pathways: insights into insulin action. *Nat Rev Mol Cell Biol*. 2006;7:85–96.
6. Chen Y, et al. Variations in DNA elucidate molecular networks that cause disease. *Nature*. 2008;452:429–435.
7. Muoio DM, Newgard CB. Molecular and metabolic mechanisms of insulin resistance and beta-cell failure in type 2 diabetes. *Nat Rev Mol Cell Biol*. 2008;9:193–205.
8. Reaven G. Banting lecture. Role of insulin resistance in human disease. *Diabetes*. 1988;37:15.
9. Lebovitz HE. Insulin resistance – a common link between type 2 diabetes and cardiovascular disease. *Diabetes Obes Metab*. 2006;8:237–249. Review.
10. Cusi K, Maezono K, Osman A, et al. Insulin resistance differentially affects the PI 3-kinase- and MAP kinase-mediated signaling in human muscle. *J Clin Invest*. 2000;105:311–320.
11. Schwartz EA, Reaven PD. Molecular and signaling mechanisms of atherosclerosis in insulin resistance. *Endocrinol Metab Clin North Am*. 2006;35:525–549.
12. Fröjdő S, Vidal H, Pirola L. Alterations of insulin signaling in type 2 diabetes: a review of the current evidence from humans. *Biochem Biophy Acta*. 2009;1792(2):83–92. Review.
13. Leroith D, Accili D. Mechanisms of disease: using genetically altered mice to study concepts of type 2 diabetes. *Nat Clin Pract Endocrinol Metab*. 2008;4:164–172.

14. DeFronzo RA, Tobin JD, Andres R. Glucose clamp technique: a method for quantifying insulin secretion and resistance. *Am J Physiol Endocrinol Metab Gastrointest Physiol*. 1979;237:E214–E223.

15. Sherwin RS, Kramer KJ, Tobin JD, et al. A model of the kinetics of insulin in man. *J Clin Invest*. 1974;53:1481–1492.

16. Shen SW, Reaven GM, Farquhar JW. Comparison of impedance to insulin-mediated glucose uptake in normal subjects and in subjects with latent diabetes. *J Clin Invest*. 1970;49:2151–2160.

17. Bergman RN, Phillips LS, Cobelli C. Physiologic evaluation of factors controlling glucose tolerance in man: measurement of insulin sensitivity and beta cell glucose sensitivity from the response of intravenous glucose. *J Clin Invest*. 1981;68:1456–1467.

18. Bergman RN, Prager R, Volund A, Olefsky JM. Equivalence of the insulin sensitivity index in man derived by the minimal model method and the euglycemic glucose clamp. *J Clin Invest*. 1987;79:790–800.

19. Bergman RN, Ider YZ, Bowden CR, Cobelli C. Quantitative estimation of insulin sensitivity. *Am J Physiol*. 1979;236:E667–E677.

20. Yang YJ, Youn JH, Bergman RN. Modified protocols improve insulin sensitivity estimation using the minimal model. *Am J Physiol Endocrinol Metab*. 1987;253:E595–E602.

21. Beard JC, Bergman RN, Ward WK, Porte D Jr. The insulin sensitivity index in nondiabetic man. Correlation between clamp-derived and IVGTT-derived values. *Diabetes*. 1986;35:362–369.

22. Finegood DT, Hramiak IM, Dupre J. A modified protocol for estimation of insulin sensitivity with the minimal model of glucose kinetics in patients with insulin-dependent diabetes. *J Clin Endocrinol Metab*. 1990;70:1538–1549.

23. Stumvoll M, Mitrakou A, Pimenta W, et al. Use of the oral glucose tolerance test to assess insulin release and insulin sensitivity. *Diabetes Care*. 2000;23:295–330.

24. Matsuda M, DeFronzo RA. Insulin sensitivity indices obtained from oral glucose tolerance testing: comparison with the euglycemic insulin clamp. *Diabetes Care*. 1999;22:1462–1470.

25. Gutt M, Davis CL, Spitzer SB, et al. Validation of the insulin sensitivity index [ISI(0,120)]: comparison with other measures. *Diabetes Res Clin Pract*. 2000;47:177–184.

26. Avignon A, Boegner C, Mariano-Goulart D, Colette C, Monnier L. Assessment of insulin sensitivity from plasma insulin and glucose in the fasting or post oral glucose-load state. *Int J Obes Relat Metab Disord*. 1999;23:512–517.

27. Laakso M. How good a marker is insulin level for insulin resistance? *Am J Epidemiol*. 1993;137:959–965.

28. Yeni-Komshian H, Carantoni M, Abbasi F, Reaven GM. Relationship between several surrogate estimates of insulin resistance and quantification of insulin-mediated glucose disposal in 490 healthy, nondiabetic volunteers. *Diabetes Care*. 2000;23:71–175.

29. Hanson RL, Pratley RE, Bogardus C, et al. Evaluation of simple indices of insulin sensitivity and insulin secretion for use in epidemiologic studies. *Am J Epidemiol*. 2000;151:190–198.

30. Matthews DR, Hosker JP, Rudenski AS, Naylor BA, Treacher DF, Turner RC. Homeostasis model assessment: insulin resistance and beta-cell function from fasting plasma glucose and insulin concentrations in man. *Diabetologia*. 1985;28:412–419.

31. Katz A, Nambi SS, Mather K, et al. Quantitative insulin sensitivity check index: a simple, accurate method for assessing insulin sensitivity in humans. *J Clin Endocrinol Metab*. 2000;85:2402–2410.

32. Rabasa-Lhoret R, Bastard JP, Jan V, et al. Modified quantitative insulin sensitivity check index is better correlated to hyper-insulinemic glucose clamp than other fasting-based index of insulin sensitivity in different insulin-resistant states. *J Clin Endocrinol Metab*. 2003;88:4917–4923.

33. Burén J, Lindmark S, Renström F, Eriksson JW. In vitro reversal of hyperglycemia normalizes insulin action in fat cells from type 2 diabetes patients: is cellular insulin resistance caused by glucotoxicity in vivo? *Metabolism*. 2003;52:239–245.

34. Perseghin G, Caumo A, Caloni M, Testolin G, Luzi L. Incorporation of the fasting plasma FFA concentration into QUICKI improves its association with insulin sensitivity in nonobese individuals. *JCEM*. 2001;86:4776–4781.

35. Radziuk J. Insulin sensitivity and its measurement: structural commonalities among the methods. *J Clin Endocrinol Metab*. 2000;85:4426–4433.

36. Finegood DT, Bergman RN, Vranic M. Estimation of endogenous glucose production during hyperinsulinemic-euglycemic glucose clamps. Comparison of labeled and unlabeled exogenous glucose infusates. *Diabetes*. 1987;36:914–924.

37. Hales CN, Randle PJ. Immunoassay of insulin with insulin-antibody precipitate. *Biochem J*. 1963;88:137–146.

38. Kahn CR, Roth J. Berson, Yalow, and the JCI: the agony and the ecstasy. *J Clin Invest*. 2004;114:1051–1054.

39. Ferrannini E. Insulin resistance versus insulin deficiency in non-insulin-dependent diabetes mellitus: problems and prospects. *Endocr Rev*. 1998;19:477–490.

40. Ginsberg H, Kimmerling G, Olefsky JM, Reaven GM. Demonstration of insulin resistance in untreated adult onset diabetic subjects with fasting hyperglycemia. *J Clin Invest*. 1975;55:454–461.

41. Gautier JF, Wilson C, Weyer C, et al. Low acute insulin secretory responses in adult offspring of people with early onset type 2 diabetes. *Diabetes*. 2001;50:1828–1833.

42. Warram JH, Martin BC, Krolewski AS, Soeldner JS, Kahn CR. Slow glucose removal rate and hyperinsulinemia precede the development of type II diabetes in the offspring of diabetic parents. *Ann Intern Med*. 1990;113:909–914.

43. Lillioja S, Mott DM, Spraul M, et al. Insulin resistance and insulin secretory dysfunction as precursors of non-insulin-dependent diabetes mellitus. *N Engl J Med*. 1993;329:1988–1992.

44. DeFronzo RA. Lilly lecture 1987. The triumvirate: beta-cell, muscle, liver. A collusion responsible for NIDDM. *Diabetes*. 1988;37:667–687.

45. Kahn SE, Prigeon RL, McCulloch DK, Boyko EJ, Bergman RN, Schwartz MW, Neifing JL, Ward WK, Beard JC, Palmer JP, et al. Quantification of the relationship between insulin sensitivity and beta-cell function in human subjects. Evidence for a hyperbolic function. *Diabetes*. 1993;42:1663–1672.

46. Cnop M, Vidal J, Hull RL, et al. Progressive loss of beta-cell function leads to worsening glucose tolerance in first-degree relatives of subjects with type 2 diabetes. *Diabetes Care*. 2007;30:677–682.

47. Weyer C, Bogardus C, Mott DM, Pratley RE. The natural history of insulin secretory dysfunction and insulin resistance in the pathogenesis of type 2 diabetes mellitus. *J Clin Invest*. 1999;104:787–794.

48. Weyer C, Tataranni PA, Bogardus C, Pratley RE. Insulin resistance and insulin secretory dysfunction are independent predictors of worsening of glucose tolerance during each stage of type 2 diabetes development. *Diabetes Care*. 2001;24:89–94.

49. Ferrannini E, Natali A, Bell P, Cavallo-Perin P, Lalic N, Mingrone G. Insulin resistance and hypersecretion in obesity. European Group for the Study of Insulin Resistance (EGIR). *J Clin Invest*. 1997;100:1166–1173.

50. Banerji MA, Lebovitz HE. Insulin-sensitive and insulin-resistant variants in NIDDM. *Diabetes*. 1989;38:784–792.

51. Chaiken RL, Banerji MA, Pasmantier RM, Huey H, Hirsch S, Lebovitz HE. Patterns of glucose and lipid abnormalities in Black NIDDM subjects. *Diabetes Care*. 1991;14:1036–1042.

52. Banerji MA, Lebovitz HE. Coronary heart disease risk factor profiles in Black patients with non-insulin dependent diabetes mellitus. *Am J Med*. 1991;91:51–58.

53. Banerji MA, Chaiken RL, Gorden D, Kral JG, Lebovitz HE. Does intra- abdominal adipose tissue in Black men determine whether NIDDM is insulin resistant or insulin-sensitive. *Diabetes*. 1995;44:141–146.

54. Petersen KF, Dufour S, Savage DB, et al. The role of skeletal muscle insulin resistance in the pathogenesis of the metabolic syndrome. *Proc Natl Acad Sci USA*. 2007;104:12587–12594.

55. Banerji MA, Buckley C, Chaiken RL, Gordon D, Lebovitz HE, Kral JG. The relationship of liver fat, triglycerides and visceral adipose tissue in insulin-resistant and insulin-sensitive black men with NIDDM. *Int J Obesity*. 1995;19:846–850.

56. Hwang JH, Stein DT, Barzilai N, et al. Increased intrahepatic triglyceride is associated with peripheral insulin resistance: in vivo MR imaging and spectroscopy studies. *Am J Physiol Endocrinol Metab*. 2007;293:E1663–E1669.

57. Morino K, Petersen KF, Shulman GI. Molecular mechanisms of insulin resistance in humans and their potential links with mitochondrial dysfunction. *Diabetes*. 2006;55(Suppl 2):S9–S15. Review.

58. Ritov VB, Menshikova EV, He J, Ferrell RE, Goodpaster BH, Kelley DE. Deficiency of subsarcolemmal mitochondria in obesity and type 2 diabetes. *Diabetes*. 2005;54:8–14.

59. Lowell BB, Shulman GI. Mitochondrial dysfunction and type 2 diabetes. *Science*. 2005;307:384–387.

60. Patti ME, Butte AJ, Crunkhorn S, et al. Coordinated reduction of genes of oxidative metabolism in humans with insulin resistance and diabetes: potential role of PGC1 and NRF1. *Proc Natl Acad Sci USA*. 2003;100:8466–8471.

61. Szendoeli J, Roden M. Mitochondrial fitness and insulin sensitivity in humans. Review. *Diabetelologia*. 2008;51:2155–2167.

62. Banerji MA, Lebowitz J, Chaiken RL, Gordon D, Kral JG, Lebovitz HE. Relationship of visceral adipose tissue and glucose disposal is independent of sex in black NIDDM subjects. *Am J Physiol*. 1997;273:E425–432.

63. Taniguchi A, Fukushima M, Sakai M, et al. The role of the body mass index and triglyceride levels in identifying insulin-sensitive and insulin-resistant variants in Japanese non-insulin-dependent diabetic patients. *Metabolism*. 2000;49:1001–1005.

64. Banerji MA, Faridi N, Atluri R, Chaiken RL, Lebovitz HE. The relationship of body composition, insulin resistance and leptin in Asian Indian men. *J Clin Endocrinol Metab*. 1999;84:137–144.

65. Haffner SM, Mykkänen L, Festa A, Burke JP, Stern MP. Insulin-resistant prediabetic subjects have more atherogenic risk factors than insulin-sensitive prediabetic subjects: implications for preventing coronary heart disease during the prediabetic state. *Circulation*. 2000;101:975–980.

66. Pischon T, Boeing H, Hoffmann K, et al. General and abdominal adiposity and risk of death in Europe. *N Engl J Med*. 2008;359:2105–2120.

67. Flegal KM, Graubard BI, Williamson DF, Gail MH. Excess deaths associated with underweight, overweight and obesity. *J Am Med Assoc*. 2005;293:1861–1867.

68. Weyer C, Yudkin JS, Stehouwer CD, Schalkwijk CG, Pratley RE, Tataranni PA. Humoral markers of inflammation and endothelial dysfunction in relation to adiposity and in vivo insulin action in Pima Indians. *Atherosclerosis*. 2002;161:233–242.

69. Stefan N, Vozarova B, Funahashi T, et al. Plasma adiponectin concentration is associated with skeletal muscle insulin receptor tyrosine phosphorylation, and low plasma concentration precedes a decrease in whole-body insulin sensitivity in humans. *Diabetes*. 2002;51:1884–1888.

70. Vozarova B, Weyer C, Hanson K, Tataranni PA, Bogardus C, Pratley RE. Circulating interleukin-6 in relation to adiposity, insulin action, and insulin secretion. *Obes Res*. 2001;9:414–417.

71. Shoelson SE, Lee J, Goldfine AB. Inflammation and insulin resistance. *J Clin Invest*. 2006;116:1793–1801. Review.

72. Salmenniemi U, Ruotsalainen E, Pihlajamäki J, et al. Multiple abnormalities in glucose and energy metabolism and coordinated changes in levels of adiponectin, cytokines, and adhesion molecules in subjects with metabolic syndrome. *Circulation*. 2004;110:3842–3848.

73. Schenk S, Saberi M, Olefsky JM. Insulin sensitivity: modulation by nutrients and inflammation. *J Clin Invest*. 2008;118:2992–3002. Review.

74. Steinberg HO, Chaker H, Leaming R, Johnson A, Brechtel G, Baron AD. Obesity/insulin resistance is associated with endothelial dysfunction: implications for the syndrome of insulin resistance. *J Clin Invest*. 1996;97:2601–2610.

75. Kim JA, Montagnani M, Koh KK, Quon MJ. Reciprocal relationships between insulin resistance and endothelial dysfunction: molecular and pathophysiological mechanisms. *Circulation*. 2006;113:1888–1904.

76. Qasim A, Mehta NN, Tadesse MG, et al. Adipokines, insulin resistance, and coronary artery. *J Am Coll Cardiol*. 2008;52: 231–236.

77. Kelley DE, He J, Menshikova EV, Ritov VB. Dysfunction of mitochondria in human skeletal muscle in type 2 diabetes. *Diabetes*. 2002;51:2944–2950.

78. Reaven GM. Insulin resistance/compensatory hyperinsulinemia, essential hypertension, and cardiovascular disease. *J Clin Endocrinol Metab*. 2003;88:2399–2403.

79. Saad MF, Lillioja S, Nyomba BL, et al. Racial differences in the relation between blood pressure and insulin resistance. *N Engl J Med*. 1991;324:733–739.

80. Ferrannini E, Natali A, Capaldo B, Lehtovirta M, Jacob S, Yki-Järvinen H; for the European Group for the Study of Insulin Resistance (EGIR). Insulin resistance, hyperinsulinemia, and blood pressure. Role of age and obesity. *Hypertension*. 1992;30:1144–1149.

81. Vague J. The degree of masculine differentiation of obesities: a factor determining predisposition to diabetes, atherosclerosis, gout, and uric calculous disease. *Am J Clin Nutr*. 1956;4:20–34.

82. McLaughlin T, Allison G, Abbasi F, Lamendola C, Reaven G. Prevalence of insulin resistance and associated cardiovascular disease risk factors among normal weight, overweight, and obese individuals. *Metabolism*. 2004;53:495–499.

83. Bogardus C, Lillioja S, Mott DM, Hollenbeck C, Reaven G. Relationship between degree of obesity and in vivo insulin action in man. *Am J Physiol*. 1985;248(3 Pt 1):E286–E291.

84. McLaughlin T, Abbasi F, Lamendola C, Reaven G. Heterogeneity in the prevalence of risk factors for cardiovascular disease and type 2 diabetes mellitus in obese individuals: effect of differences in insulin sensitivity. *Arch Int Med*. 2007;167:642–648.

85. Ferrannini E, Natali A, Bell P, Cavallo-Perin P, Lalic N, Mingrone G. Insulin resistance and hypersecretion in obesity. European Group for the Study of Insulin Resistance, EGIR. *J Clin Invest*. 1997;100:1166–1173.

86. Ruderman N, Chisholm D, Pi-Sunyer X, Schneider S. The metabolically obese, normal-weight individual revisited. *Diabetes*. 1998;47:699–713. Review.

87. Reaven GM. Insulin resistance: the link between obesity and cardiovascular disease. *Endocrinol Metab Clin North Am*. 2008;37:581–601.

88. Goodpaster BH, Thaete FL, Simoneau J-A, Kelley DE. Subcutaneous abdominal fat and thigh muscle composition predict insulin sensitivity independently of visceral fat. *Diabetes*. 1997;46:1579–1585.

89. Effects of weight loss on regional fat distribution and insulin sensitivity in obesity. *Diabetes*. 1999;48:839–847.

90. Lemieux S, Després J-P, Moorjani S, et al. Are gender differences in cardiovascular disease risk factors explained by the level of visceral adipose tissue? *Diabetologia*. 1994;37:757–764.

91. Klein S, Fontana L, Young VL, et al. Absence of an effect of liposuction on insulin action and risk factors for coronary heart disease. *N Engl J Med*. 2004;350:2549–2557.

92. Mohammed BS, Cohen S, Reeds D, Young VL, Klein S. Long-term effects of liposuction on metabolic risk factors for coronary heart disease. *Obesity (Silver Spring)*. 2008;16:2648–51. Epub 2008 Sep 25.

93. Ford ES, Giles WH, Dietz WH. Prevalence of the metabolic syndrome among US adults: findings from the third National Health and Nutrition Examination Survey. *JAMA*. 2002;287:356–359.

94. Weber RV, Buckley C, Fried SK, Kral JG. Subcutaneous lipectomy causes a metabolic syndrome in hamsters. *Am J Physiol Regul Integr Comp Physiol*. 2000;279:R936–R943.

95. Banerji M, Tiewala M, Catanzaro J, Lebovitz HE. Decreased plasma free fatty acids improve insulin sensitivity in African-American patients with type 2 diabetes treated with rosiglitazone. *Presented in the 86th Annual Meeting of the Endocrine Society in New Orleans*. 2004, Poster P1-330.

96. Lundgren M, Burén J, Lindgren P, Myrnäs T, Ruge T, Eriksson JW. Sex- and depot-specific lipolysis regulation in human adipocytes: interplay between adrenergic stimulation and glucocorticoids. *Horm Metab Res*. 2008;40:854–860.

97. Wajchenberg BL, Giannella-Neto D, da Silva ME, Santos RF. Depot-specific hormonal characteristics of subcutaneous and visceral adipose tissue and their relation to the metabolic syndrome. *Horm Metab Res*. 2002;34:616–621.

98. Tomlinson JW, Finney J, Gay C, Hughes BA, Hughes SV, Stewart PM. Impaired glucose tolerance and insulin resistance are associated with increased adipose 11β-hydroxysteroid dehydrogenase type 1 expression and elevated hepatic 5α-reductase activity. *Diabetes*. 2008;57:2652–2660.

99. Lettner A, Roden M. Ectopic fat and insulin resistance. *Curr Diab Rep*. 2008;8:185–191. Review.

100. Forouhi NG, Jenkinson G, Thomas EL, et al. Relation of triglyceride stores in skeletal muscle cells to central obesity and insulin sensitivity in European and South Asian men. *Diabetologia*. 1999;42:932–935.

101. Pan DA, Lillioja S, Kriketos AD, et al. Skeletal muscle triglyceride levels are inversely related to insulin action. *Diabetes*. 1997;46:983–988.

102. Hotamisligil GS, Shargill NS, Speigelman BM. Adipose expression of tumor necrosis factor – alpha: direct role in obesity-linked insulin resistance. *Science*. 1993;259:87–91.

103. Arkan MC, Hevener AL, Greten FR, et al. IKK-β links inflammation to obesity-induced insulin resistance. *Nat Med*. 2005;11:191–198.

104. Hirosumi J, Tuncman G, Chang L, et al. A central role for JNK in obesity and insulin resistance. *Nature*. 2002;420:333–336.

105. Ozcan U, Cao Q, Yilmaz E, et al. Endoplasmic reticulum stress links obesity, insulin action, and type 2 diabetes. *Science*. 2004;306:457–461.

106. Shimomura I, Funahashi T, Takahashi M, et al. Enhanced expression of PAI-1 in visceral fat: possible contributor to vascular disease in obesity. *Nat Med*. 1996;2:800–803.

107. Itani SI, Ruderman NB, Schmieder F,, Boden G. Lipid-induced insulin resistance in human muscle is associated with changes in diacylglycerol, protein kinase C, and IkappaB-alpha. *Diabetes*. 2002;51:2005–2011.

108. Tripathy D, Mohanty P, Dhindsa S, et al. Elevation of free fatty acids induces inflammation and impairs vascular reactivity in healthy subjects. *Diabetes*. 2003;52:2882–2887.

109. Summers SA. Ceramides in insulin resistance and lipotoxicity. *Prog Lipid Res*. 2006;45:42–72.

110. Pickup JC, Mattock MB, Chusney GD, Burt D. NIDDM as a disease of the innate immune system: association of acute-phase reactants and interleukin-6 with metabolic syndrome X. *Diabetologia*. 1997;40:1286–1292.

111. Yamauchi T, Kamon J, Waki H, et al. The fat-derived hormone adiponectin reverses insulin resistance associated with both lipoatrophy and obesity. *Nat Med*. 2001;7:941–946.

112. Trujillo ME, Scherer PE. Adipose tissue-derived factors: impact on health and disease. *Endocr Rev*. 2006;27:762–778.

113. Wellen KE, Hotamisligil GS. Inflammation, stress, and diabetes. *J Clin Invest*. 2005;115:1111–1119.

114. Chaudhuri A, Janicke D, Wilson MF, et al. Anti-inflammatory and profibrinolytic effect of insulin in acute ST-segment-elevation myocardial infarction. *Circulation*. 2004;109:849–854.

115. Fleischman A, Shoelson SE, Bernier R, Goldfine AB. Salsalate improves glycemia ad inflammatory parameters in obese young adults. *Diabetes Care*. 2008;3:289–294.

116. Wildman RP, Munter P, Reynolds K, et al. The obese without cardiometabolic risk factors clustering and the normal weight with cardiovascular risk factor clustering: prevalence and correlates of 2 phenotypes among the US population (NHANES 1999–2004). *Arch Int Med*. 2008;168:1617–1724.

117. Stefan N, Kantartzis K, Maachan J, et al. Identification and charcterization of metabolically benign obesity in humans. *Arch Int Med*. 2008;168:1609–1616.

118. Karelis AD, Messier V, Brochu M, Rabasa-Lhoret R. Metabolically healthy but obese women: effect of an energy-restricted diet. *Diabeteologia*. 2008;51:1752–1754.

119. Kannel WB, McGee DL. Diabetes and cardiovascular disease. The Framingham Study. *JAMA*. 1979;241:2035–2038.

120. Hu FB, Stampfer MJ, Solomon CG, et al. The impact of diabetes mellitus on mortality from all causes and coronary heart disease in women: 20 years of follow-up. *Arch Intern Med*. 2001;23(161):1717–1723.

121. Huxley R, Barzi F, Woodward M. Excess risk of fatal coronary heart disease associated with diabetes in men and women: meta-analysis of 37 prospective cohort studies. *BMJ*. 2006;322:73–78. Review.

122. Facchini FS, Hua N, Abbasi F, Reaven GM. Insulin resistance as a predictor of age-related diseases. *JCEM*. 2001;86:3574–3578.

123. Nosadini R, Manzato E, Solini A, et al. Peripheral, rather than hepatic, insulin resistance and atherogenic lipoprotein phenotype predict cardiovascular complications in NIDDM. *Eur J Clin Invest*. 1994;24:258–266.

124. Hanley AJ, Williams K, Stern MP, Haffner SM. Homeostasis model assessment of insulin resistance in relation to the incidence of cardiovascular disease: the San Antonio Heart Study. *Diabetes Care*. 2002;25:1177–1184.

125. Robins SJ, Rubins HB, Faas FH, et al.; Veterans Affairs HDL Intervention Trial (VA-HIT). Insulin resistance and cardiovascular events with low HDL cholesterol: the Veterans Affairs HDL Intervention Trial (VA-HIT). *Diabetes Care*. 2003;26:1513–1517.

126. The DECODE Insulin Study Group. Plasma insulin and cardiovascular mortality in non diabetic European men and women: a metanalysis of data from eleven prospective studies. *Diabeteologia*. 2004;47:1245–1256.

127. Kuusisto J, Lempiäinen P, Mykkänen L, Laakso M. Insulin resistance syndrome predicts coronary heart disease events in elderly type 2 diabetic men. *Diabetes Care*. 2001;24:1629–1633.

128. Resnick HE, Jones K, Ruotolo G, et al. String Heart Study, Insulin resistance, the metabolic syndrome and risk of incident cardiobvascular disease in non-diabeteic American Indians: The Strong Heart Study. *Diabetes Care*. 2003;26:861–867.

129. Rutter MK, Meigs JB, Sullivan LM, D'Agostino RB Sr, Wilson PW. Insulin resistance, the metabolic syndrome, and incident cardiovascular events in the Framingham Offspring Study. *Diabetes*. 2005;54:3252–3257.

130. Ruige JB, Assendelft WJ, Dekker JM, Kostense PJ, Heine RJ, Bouter LM. Insulin and risk of cardiovascular disease: a meta-analysis. *Circulation*. 1998;97:996–1001.

131. Folsom AR, Szklo M, Stevens J, Liao F, Smith R, Eckfeldt JH. A prospective study of coronary heart disease in relation to fasting insulin, glucose and diabetes. The Atherosclerosis Risk in Communities (ARIC) Study. *Diabetes Care*. 1997;20:935–942.

132. Folsom AR, Rasmussen ML, Chambless LE, et al. Prospective associations of fasting insulin, body fat distributin, and diabetes with risk of ischemic stroke: The Atherosclerosis Risk in Communities (ARIC) Study. *Diabetes Care*. 1999;22:1077–1083.

133. Pyörälä M, Miettinen H, Laakso M, Pyörälä K. Hyperinsulinemia predicts coronary heart disease risk in healthy middle-aged men: the 22-year follow-up results of the Helsinki Policemen Study. *Circulation*. 1998;98:398–404.

134. Pyörälä M, Miettinen H, Laakso M, Pyörälä K. Hyperinsulinemia and the risk of stroke in healthy middle-aged men: the 22-year follow-up results of the Helsinki Policemen Study. *Stroke*. 1998;29:1860–1866.

135. Yarnell JW, Patterson CC, Bainton D, Sweetnam PM. Is metabolic syndrome a discrete entity in the general population? Evidence from the Caerphilly and Speedwell population studies. *Heart*. 1998;79:248–252.

136. Welin L, Bresäter LE, Eriksson H, Hansson PO, Welin C, Rosengren A. Insulin resistance and other risk factors for coronary heart disease in elderly men. The Study of Men Born in 1913 and 1923. *Eur J Cardiovasc Prev Rehabil*. 2003;10:283–288.

137. Sarwar N, Sattar N, Gudnason V, Danesh J. Circulating concentrations of insulin markers and coronary heart disease: a quantitative review of 19 Western prospective studies. *Eur Heart J*. 2007;28:2491–2497. Review.

138. Chen W, Srinivasan SR, Li S, Xu J, Berenson GS. Metabolic syndrome variables at low levels in childhood are beneficially associated with adulthood cardiovascular risk: the Bogalusa Heart Study. *Diabetes Care*. 2005;28:126–131.

139. Modan M, Halkin H, Almog S, et al. Hyperinsulinemia. A link between hypertension obesity and glucose intolerance. *J Clin Invest*. 1985;75:809–817.

140. Reaven GM, Lerner RL, Stern M, et al. Role of insulin in hypertriglyceridemia. *J Clin Invest*. 1974;57:551–560.

141. Jeppesen J, Hollenbeck CB, Zhou M.-Y, et al. Relation between insulin resistance, hyperinsulinemia, postheparin plasma lipoprotein lipase activity, and postprandial lipemia. *Arterioscler Thromb Vasc Biol*. 1995;15:320–324.

142. Tobey TA, Greenfield M, Kraemer F, Reaven GM. Relationship between insulin resistance, insulin secretion, very low density lipoprotein kinetics and plasma triglyceride levels in normotriglyceridemic man. *Metabolism*. 1981;30:165–171.

143. Zavaroni I, Bonora E, Pagliara M, Dall'Aglio E, Luchetti L, Buonanno G, et al. Risk factors for coronary artery disease in healthy persons with hyperinsulinemia and normal glucose tolerance. *N Engl J Med*. 1989;320:702–706.

144. Eckel RH, Grundy SM, Zimmet PZ. The metabolic syndrome. *Lancet*. 2005;365:1415–1428.

145. Reaven GM. The individual components of the metabolic syndrome: is there a raison d'etre? *J Am Coll Nutr*. 2007;26: 191–195.

146. WHO Consultation *Definition, Diagnosis and Classification of Diabetes Mellitus and Its Complications. Part 1: Diagnosis and Classification of Diabetes Mellitus*. Geneva: World Health Organization; 1999.

147. Balkau B, Charles MA. Comment on the provisional report from the WHO consultation. European Group for the Study of Insulin Resistance (EGIR). *Diab Med*. 1999;16:442–443.

148. Executive Summary of the Third Report of The National Cholesterol Education Program (NCEP) Expert panel on detection, evaluation, and treatment of high blood cholesterol in adults (Adult Treatment Panel III). *J Am Med Assoc*. 2001;285: 2486–2497.

149. Einhorn D, Reaven GM, Cobin RH, et al. American College of Endocrinology position statement on the insulin resistance syndrome. *Endocr Pract*. 2003;9:237–252.

150. Grundy SM, Cleeman JI, Daniels SR, et al. Diagnosis and management of the metabolic syndrome: an American Heart Association/National Heart, Lung, and Blood Institute Scientific Statement. *Circulation*. 2005;112:2735–2752.

151. Alberti KG, Zimmet P, Shaw J. Metabolic syndrome—a new world-wide definition: a consensus statement from the International Diabetes Federation. *Diab Med*. 2006;23:469–480. Also International Diabetes Federation. The IDF consensus worldwide definition of the metabolic syndrome. Available at: http://www.idf.org/wedata/docs/Meta_def-final.pdf. Accessed December 6, 2008.

152. Kahn R, Buse J, Ferrannini E, Stern M. The metabolic syndrome: a time for critical reappraisal-joint statement from the Americal Diabetes Association and the European Association for the Study of Diabetes. *Diabetes Care*. 2005;28:2289–2304.

153. Ford ES. Prevalence of the metabolic syndrome defined by the International Diabetes Federation among adults in the U.S. *Diabetes Care*. 2005;28:2745.

154. Ford ES, Giles WH, Mokdad AH. Increasing prevalence of the metabolic syndrome among U.S. adults. *Diabetes Care*. 2004;27:2444–2449.

155. Lorenzo C, Williams K, Hunt KJ, Haffner SM. Trend in the prevalence of the metabolic syndrome and its impact on cardiovascular disease incidence: the San Antonio Heart Study. *Diabetes Care*. 2006;29:625–630.

156. Lorenzo C, Williams K, Gonzalez-Villalpando C, Haffner SM. The prevalence of the metabolic syndrome did not increase in Mexico City between 1990–1992 and 1997–1999 despite more central obesity. *Diabetes Care*. 2005;28:2480–2485.

157. Hu G, Lindström J, Jousilahti P, et al. The increasing prevalence of metabolic syndrome among Finnish men and women over a decade. *J Clin Endocrinol Metab*. 2008;93:832–836.

158. Goodman E, Daniels SR, Meigs JB, Dolan LM. Instability in the diagnosis of metabolic syndrome in adolescents. *Circulation*. 2007;115:2316–2322.

159. Wilson PW, Meigs JB, Sullivan L, Fox CS, Nathan DM, D'Agostino RB Sr. Prediction of incident diabetes mellitus in middle-aged adults: the Framingham Offspring Study. *Arch Intern Med*. 2007;28(167):1068–1074.

160. Lorenzo C, Williams K, Hunt KJ, Haffner SM. The National Cholesterol Education Program-Adult Treatment Panel III, International Diabetes Federation, and World Health Organization definitions of the metabolic syndrome as predictors of incident cardiovascular disease and diabetes. *Diabetes Care*. 2007;30:8–13.

161. Wilson PW, D'Agostino RB, Parise H, Sullivan L, Meigs JB. Metabolic syndrome as a precursor of CV disease and type 2 diabetes mellitus. *Circulation*. 2005;112:3066–3072.

162. Ford ES, Li C, Sattar N. Metabolic syndrome and incident diabetes: current state of the evidence. *Diabetes Care*. 2008;31:1898.

163. Ford ES. Risks for all-cause mortality, cardiovascular disease, and diabetes associated with the metabolic syndrome: a summary of the evidence. *Diabetes Care*. 2005;28:1769–1778.

164. Wang J, Ruotsalainen S, Moilanen L, Lepistö P, Laakso M, Kuusisto J. The metabolic syndrome predicts cardiovascular mortality: a 13-year follow-up study in elderly non-diabetic Finns. *Eur Heart J*. 2007;28:857–864.
165. Wang J, Ruotsalainen S, Moilanen L, Lepistö P, Laakso M, Kuusisto J. The metabolic syndrome predicts incident stroke: a 14-year follow-up study in elderly people in Finland. *Stroke*. 2008;39:1078–1083.
166. Nilsson PM, Engström G, Hedblad B. The metabolic syndrome and incidence of cardiovascular disease in non-diabetic subjects – a population-based study comparing three different definitions. *Diab Med*. 2007;24:464–472.
167. Katzmarzyk PT, Janssen I, Ross R, Church TS, Blair SN. The importance of waist circumference in the definition of metabolic syndrome: prospective analyses of mortality in men. *Diabetes Care*. 2006;29:404–409.
168. Qiao Q; DECODE Study Group. Comparison of different definitions of the metabolic syndrome in relation to cardiovascular mortality in European men and women. *Diabetologia*. 2006;49:2837–2846.
169. Sattar N, McConnachie A, Shaper AG, et al. Can metabolic syndrome usefully predict cardiovascular disease and diabetes? Outcome data from two prospective studies. *Lancet*. 2008;371:1927–1935.
170. Gami AS, Witt BJ, Howard DE, et al. Metabolic syndrome and risk of incident cardiovascular events and death: a systematic review and meta-analysis of longitudinal studies. *J Am Coll Cardiol*. 2007;49:403–414.
171. Bonora E, Targher G, Formentini G, et al. The metabolic syndrome is an independent predictor of cardiovascular disease in type 2 diabetic subjects. Prospective data from the Verona Diabetes Complications Study. *Diab Med*. 2004;21:52–58.
172. Guzder RN, Gatling W, Mullee MA, Byrne CD. Impact of metabolic syndrome criteria on cardiovascular disease risk in people with newly diagnosed type 2 diabetes. *Diabetologia*. 2006;49:49–55.
173. Tong PC, Kong AP, So WY, et al. The usefulness of the International Diabetes Federation and the National Cholesterol Education Program's Adult Treatment Panel III definitions of the metabolic syndrome in predicting coronary heart disease in subjects with type 2 diabetes. *Diabetes Care*. 2007;30:1206–1211.
174. Sone H, Mizuno S, Fujii H, et al.; Japan Diabetes Complications Study. Is the diagnosis of metabolic syndrome useful for predicting cardiovascular disease in asian diabetic patients? Analysis from the Japan Diabetes Complications Study. *Diabetes Care*. 2005;28:1463–1471.
175. Bruno G, Merletti F, Biggeri A, et al.; Casale Monferrato Study. Metabolic syndrome as a predictor of all-cause and cardiovascular mortality in type 2 diabetes: the Casale Monferrato Study. *Diabetes Care*. 2004;27:2689–2694.
176. Cull CA, Jensen CC, Retnakaran R, Holman RR. Impact of the metabolic syndrome on macrovascular and microvascular outcomes in type 2 diabetes mellitus: United Kingdom Prospective Diabetes Study 78. *Circulation*. 2007;116:2119–2126.
177. Hunt KJ, Resendez RG, Williams K, Haffner SM, Stern MP. NCEP versus WHO metabolic syndrome in relation to all cause and CV mortality in the San Antonio Heart Study. *Circulation*. 2004;110:1251–1257.
178. Wilson PW, D'Agostino RB, Parise H, Sullivan L, Meigs JB. Metabolic syndrome as a precursor of CV disease and type 2 diabetes mellitus. *Circulation*. 2005;112:3066–3072.
179. Malik S, Wong ND, Franklin SS, et al. Impact of the metabolic syndrome on mortality from CHD, CVD and all causes in United States adults. *Circulation*. 2004;110:1245–1250.
180. Stern MP, William K, Hunt KJ. Impact of diabetes/metabolic syndrome in patients with established CVD. *Atherosclerosis Suppl*. 2005;6:3–6.
181. Stern MP, Williams K, Gonzalez-Villalpando C, Hunt KJ, Haffner SM. Does the metabolic syndrome improve identification of individuals at risk of type 2 diabetes and/or cardiovascular disease? *Diabetes Care*. 2004;27:2676–2681.
182. Cheal KL, Abbasi F, Lamendola C, McLaughlin T, Reaven GM, Ford ES. Relationship to insulin resistance of the adult treatment panel III diagnostic criteria for identification of the metabolic syndrome. *Diabetes*. 2004;53:1195.
183. Liao Y, Kwon S, Shaughnessy S, et al. Critical evaluation of adult treatment panel III criteria in identifying insulin resistance with dyslipidemia. *Diabetes Care*. 2004;27:978–983.
184. Meigs JB, Rutter MK, Sullivan LM, Fox CS, D'Agostino RB Sr, Wilson PW. Impact of insulin resistance on risk of type 2 diabetes and cardiovascular disease in people with metabolic syndrome. *Diabetes Care*. 2007;30:1219–1225.
185. Rosenzweig JL, Ferrannini E, Grundy SM, et al. Primary prevention of cardiovascular disease and type 2 diabetes in patients at metabolic risk: an endocrine society clinical practice guideline. *J Clin Endocrinol Metab*. 2008;93:3671–3689.
186. Ridker PM, Danielson E, Fonseca FA, et al.; JUPITER Study Group. Rosuvastatin to prevent vascular events in men and women with elevated C-reactive protein. *N Engl J Med*. 2008;359:2195–2207.
187. Hayashi T, Boyko EJ, McNeely MJ, Leonetti DL, Kahn SE, Fujimoto WY. Visceral adiposity, not abdominal subcutaneous fat area, is associated with an increase in future insulin resistance in Japanese Americans. *Diabetes*. 2008;57:1269–1275. Epub 2008 Feb 25.

Chapter 35
Diabetes and Liver Disease

Douglas F. Meyer and Henry C. Bodenheimer, Jr.

Introduction

The prevalence of type 2 diabetes, in the United States, has increased in association with the increase in the mean weight of Americans indicative of the epidemic of obesity in this country. Complications of type 2 diabetes can be expected to rise in the near future. These complications include vascular, renal, ophthalmologic, and importantly liver disease. Hepatic complications include nonalcoholic fatty liver disease (NAFLD), cirrhosis, hepatocellular carcinoma (HCC), acute liver failure, and post-liver transplantation diabetes. There is, additionally, a relationship between type 2 diabetes and chronic hepatitis C infection with type 2 diabetes being considered an extrahepatic manifestation of chronic hepatitis C infection. The association of diabetes and liver disease is being increasingly recognized. The morbidity and mortality of acute and chronic liver disease in patients with diabetes, particularly type 2 diabetes, will continue to rise in Americans in the immediate and near future.

Nonalcoholic Fatty Liver Disease

Epidemiology and Natural History of NAFLD

NAFLD is the most prevalent chronic liver disease in the United States and will be increasingly prevalent due to the pandemics of obesity and diabetes in the Unites States.[1] Furthermore, NAFLD is the most prevalent chronic liver disease seen in patients with diabetes, particularly type 2 diabetes. NAFLD is a spectrum of disease ranging from bland hepatic steatosis to nonalcoholic steatohepatitis (NASH) and steatofibrosis to cirrhosis. The diagnosis of NAFLD requires histological confirmation, which includes steatosis, ballooning degeneration, and lobular inflammation with the exclusion of other chronic liver diseases, in particular alcohol-related liver disease.[2] Patients with NAFLD may or may not have elevated hepatic aminotransferase activities.[3,4] In late-stage disease, the histological features of steatosis and necroinflammation may be replaced by fibrosis and present as cryptogenic cirrhosis.[5]

NAFLD is the hepatic manifestation of the metabolic syndrome, which includes central obesity, type 2 diabetes, hypertension, and hyperlipidemia.[6] The pathogenesis of metabolic syndrome, in particular NAFLD and type 2 diabetes, is theorized to be secondary to insulin resistance.[7] NAFLD can present in non-obese nondiabetic patients, particularly males and Asians, and is similarly theorized to be the result of insulin resistance.[8] Hypertension and hyperlipidemia including hypertriglyceridemia have also been shown to be independent risk factors for NAFLD.[9,10]

The prevalence of NAFLD in the United States is approximately 30% and prevalence of NASH is approximately 5%.[3] The prevalence rate varies along racial lines and is higher in type 2 diabetes and obese patients.[3,11]

H.C. Bodenheimer, Jr. (✉)
Department of Medicine, Beth Israel Medical Center and Albert Einstein College of Medicine, New York, NY, USA
e-mail: hbodenheimer@chpnet.org

L. Poretsky (ed.), *Principles of Diabetes Mellitus*, DOI 10.1007/978-0-387-09841-8_35,
© Springer Science+Business Media, LLC 2010

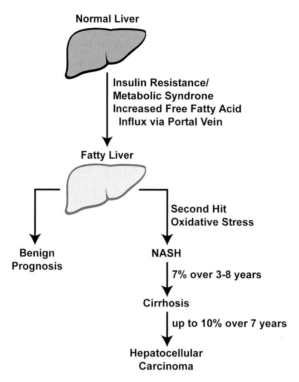

Fig. 35.1 Natural history of non-alcoholic fatty liver disease

African-Americans have a lower prevalence of NAFLD compared to Caucasians and Hispanics. The prevalence by gender appears equal but occurs earlier in white males than females.[12] The prevalence of NAFLD has been reported to be greater than 60% in patients with type 2 diabetes and approximately 90% in obese patients.[13,14] The prevalence of NASH is greater than 35% in obese patients.[14]

The natural history of NAFLD is not well defined (see Fig. 35.1). The clinical course of NAFLD can be predicted by the findings seen in the liver biopsy. Bland steatosis has a relatively benign course.[2,15] Follow-up of patients with hepatic steatosis alone has revealed that 3% will eventually develop cirrhosis over time.[2,15] The life expectancy in patients with benign steatosis is similar to the general population.[15] NASH, in contrast, has a progressive course, where a sizable subset of patients will develop fibrosis and cirrhosis.[2,16] NASH affects approximately 3–5% of the US adult population and up to 25% of people with obesity.[17,18] Over a 3- to 8.3-year period, 7% of subjects followed developed cirrhosis.[16,19,20] The rate of progression to cirrhosis varies among patients with NASH.[21] One study of the natural history of NAFLD found type 2 diabetes and high body mass index (BMI) to be predictive of an increased rate of disease progression.[22] There is increased mortality rate seen in patients with NASH in contrast to benign hepatic steatosis. Patients with NASH, who develop cirrhosis, have 30–40% liver-related mortality over a 10-year follow-up period similar to patients with chronic hepatitis C-related cirrhosis and there is an even higher mortality rate in obese patients.[5,23]

Patients with NASH-related cirrhosis can develop complications of cirrhosis including hepatocellular carcinoma (HCC).[24] Patients who present with cryptogenic cirrhosis, which is a possible presentation of end-stage NAFLD, can also develop HCC.[5] The vast majority of patients with cryptogenic cirrhosis have features of metabolic syndrome, in particular obesity and type 2 diabetes, leading to the belief that these patients in effect have end-stage NAFLD.[5,25] Studies following patients with NASH-related cirrhosis reveal that up to 10% developed HCC over 7–7.6 years.[23,24] Survival is relatively poor when HCC develops in patients with obesity and type 2 diabetes.[26] As a result, screening for HCC in NASH-related or cryptogenic cirrhosis should be considered particularly since the incidence of HCC in these patients will increase as the prevalence of obesity and type 2 diabetes in the United States continues to rise.

Risk Factors for NAFLD

Type 2 diabetes is an independent risk factor for the development of NAFLD.[13] The prevalence of type 2 diabetes is 30–50% in patients with NAFLD.[2,13,16,27] The prevalence differed depending on the diagnostic criteria of diabetes used in the study. One study, performed in newly diagnosed type 2 diabetics, found that 62% met ultrasound criteria for NAFLD.[13] Another study reported that the risk of NAFLD in patients with type 2 diabetes is four times that of nondiabetic non-obese patients.[28] Type 2 diabetes is a recognized risk factor for increased fibrosis in patients with NAFLD.[22,29] Furthermore, type 2 diabetes is an independent risk factor for increased liver-related and overall mortality in a case–cohort study of patients with NAFLD.[29] The higher mortality rate in patients with type 2 diabetes and cirrhosis is due to liver-related not vascular-related complications. The standardized mortality ratio for liver-related death in type 2 diabetics with cirrhosis was even higher than mortality due to cardiovascular complications.[30]

The prevalence of NAFLD in the obese ranges from 25 to 93% and in the morbidly obese patients it is greater than 80%.[2,13,16,18,31] In a large prospective study of liver biopsies performed during bariatric surgery, steatosis was seen in over 85%, fibrosis in approximately 75%, NASH in approximately 25%, and cryptogenic cirrhosis in 2%.[31] The prevalence of NAFLD in the morbidly obese is also associated with type 2 diabetes.[32] Hyperglycemia and obesity are independent predictors of elevated serum aminotransferase activity.[33] In addition, more advanced liver disease was seen in those patients with morbid obesity with type 2 diabetes as compared to those with normal serum glucose levels.[34] The presence of obesity and type 2 diabetes in patients with metabolic syndrome has an additive effect on the prevalence and severity of chronic liver disease.[35] Central obesity is an independent risk factor for NAFLD. Lean individuals with a low or normal BMI and central obesity are at higher risk for developing NAFLD than people with high BMI and no central obesity.[36]

Pathogenesis of NAFLD

The most commonly accepted hypothesis of the pathogenesis of NASH is the two-hit hypothesis.[37] The first hit is insulin resistance, which leads to the accumulation of fat in the liver.[7] Hepatic steatosis is considered to have a benign natural history.[5,234] A subset of patients with NAFLD will develop NASH.[38] In these patients, there is a second hit possibly in the form of endotoxin or another insult to the hepatic steatosis triggering oxidative stress, which generates reactive oxygen species resulting in lipid peroxidation and cytokine release ultimately leading to inflammation and hepatic fibrosis (see Fig. 35.2).[39,40]

While obesity is strongly associated with NAFLD, in animal models it is insulin resistance that is the first hit in the development of NAFLD.[7] However, in humans, increased fat mass plays an essential role in the pathogenesis of NAFLD since weight loss has been shown to improve NAFLD.[41–43] Body fat is an active endocrine organ secreting cytokines, in particular tumor necrosis factor-alpha (TNF-α) and IL-6.[44] There is also secretion of adipokines leptin, resistin, and adiponectin.[45,46] Increased secretion of angiotensinogen and free fatty acids also probably plays a role in the development of NAFLD.[47,48] Obesity and hepatic steatosis are associated with an inflammatory state and the generation of pro-inflammatory cytokines.

TNF-α is increased in obese patients.[49] This cytokine along with IL-6 is believed to result in insulin resistance by producing the upregulation of suppressor of cytokine signaling proteins (SOCS) 1 and 3.[49–51] These proteins interfere with insulin's ability to activate its signaling pathway by binding to JAK tyrosine kinase, thus decreasing the ability of JAK protein to phosphorylate. Normally, insulin binds to its receptor, which is phosphorylated thus producing the activation of insulin receptor substrates. These substrates form complexes, which result in the transport of glucose into the muscle cell and hepatocyte. TNF-α interferes with the phosphorylation of the insulin receptor substrates.[50] The increase in TNF-α level with subsequent insulin resistance precedes the development of NAFLD. Antibodies to TNF-α have been shown to improve insulin resistance and eliminate hepatic steatosis.[7]

Leptin is an adipokine secreted by adipocytes. Insulin resistance and hepatic steatosis naturally occur in the ob/ob mice model.[52] These mice are genetically deficient in leptin. In humans, particularly those that are

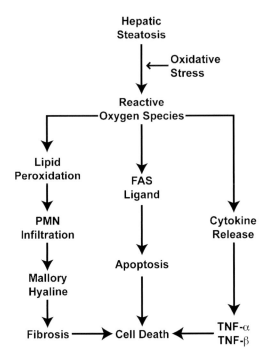

Fig. 35.2 Development of non-alcoholic steatohepatitis

obese, there is an increase in leptin levels suggesting that leptin resistance not deficiency leads to insulin resistance and hepatic steatosis.[53] Leptin may also induce insulin resistance by the upregulation of pro-inflammatory cytokines.[54] Adiponectin is another important adipokine secreted by adipocytes; however, its level is actually decreased in NAFLD despite increased fat mass seen in the disease.[55] Adiponectin increases fatty acid oxidation and suppresses gluconeogenesis in the liver.[56] In addition, adiponectin downregulates TNF-α and is anti-fibrotic by reducing hepatic stellate cell activation and proliferation.[57] There is an association between decreased adiponectin levels, insulin resistance, and NAFLD.

Metabolic consequences of visceral and peripheral fat differ.[58] Central obesity is associated with NAFLD.[6,59] Central obesity along with increased lipolysis of the visceral tissue results in increased delivery of free fatty acids to the liver leading to hepatic steatosis, the first hit in the development of NAFLD.[60] It is central obesity consisting of upper body fat and subcutaneous tissue that supplies the fat deposited in the liver. The contribution of hepatic fat deposition from the splanchnic bed, dietary fat, or de novo lipogenesis is relatively minor.[61] Central obesity, therefore, not total fat is the risk factor for hepatic steatosis and elevated hepatic aminotransferases levels. NAFLD is now considered part of the metabolic syndrome, which includes hyperglycemia, hypertension, central obesity, hypertriglyceridemia, and low HDL level.[6] The number of component diseases comprising the metabolic syndrome present in a patient is predictive of NAFLD and its severity.[31]

Insulin resistance decreases the uptake of glucose into muscle and increases lipolysis of visceral fat, resulting in increased delivery of free fatty acids to the liver.[60] Hepatic steatosis, besides being the result of increased delivery of free fatty acids to the liver, is also contributed to by increased hepatic lipogenesis and decreased export of lipids from the liver despite increased beta oxidation of fats in the liver (see Fig. 35.3).[62] There is net accumulation of fat in the liver. The primary site of insulin resistance appears to be at the muscle with hepatic steatosis being a secondary result.[63]

Hepatic steatosis once developed in a patient can take two different clinical paths. In the first path, hepatic steatosis may have a benign course where pro-inflammatory forces are balanced by cyto-protective processes.[64] In the second path, a subset of patients develop NASH.[38] In these patients, a second hit in the form of endotoxin, reactive oxygen species, and environmental agents results in the production of pro-inflammatory cytokines,

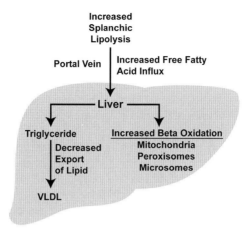

Fig. 35.3 Development of hepatic steatosis

oxidative stress, lipid peroxidation, and even fibrosis formation that is no longer balanced by cyto-protective processes.[39,40]

The second hit in the development of NASH is oxidative stress due to endotoxin, cytokines, and environmental toxins.[7,39,40] Studies have shown increased bacterial overgrowth in the small intestines of patients with NAFLD.[65] Bacterial overgrowth may increase endogenous production of alcohol and activate pro-inflammatory cytokines via endotoxin.[66] The intestinal flora contributes to this process and treatment with probiotics may help reduce the production of pro-inflammatory cytokines, particularly TNF-α.[66,67]

Increased lipid peroxidation is present in patients with NASH.[59,68] In these patients, there is increased delivery of free fatty acids to the liver, which is a source of oxidative stress.[6,59] Free fatty acids bind PPAR-α receptors and result in the upregulation of beta oxidation of free fatty acids.[69] Reactive oxygen species are produced during beta oxidation of free fatty acids, which subsequently can cause lipid peroxidation. In patients with NASH there is increased beta oxidation of free fatty acids in the mitochrondria with upregulation of microsomal enzymes CYP2E1 and CYP4A producing reactive oxygen species.[70]

In NASH, there is mitochondrial injury as a result of oxidative stress.[59] Identified structural abnormalities include megamitochondria, paracrystalline inclusion bodies, and change in mitochondrial location within the hepatocyte cytosol.[71] Mitochondrial function is decreased due to reduced activity of the respiratory chain enzymes and increased uncoupling protein 2 resulting in decreased ATP production.[72] These changes result in the production of reactive oxygen species further promoting lipid peroxidation.

The by-products of lipid peroxidation attract neutrophils and activate hepatic stellate cells via transforming growth factor-beta leading to hepatic fibrosis.[73] In addition, there is increased secretion of TNF-α in NASH further impairing mitochondrial function.[73,74] Free fatty acids, besides increasing free fatty acid oxidation and lipid peroxidation, can directly activate the NF-κB pathway via IKK-β. This activation results in increased production of TNF-α, further promoting insulin resistance leading to a higher prevalence of type 2 diabetes in NAFLD-associated cirrhosis.[75]

There is increasing evidence that hepatocyte apoptosis via increased caspase expression and FAS death receptor activation may play a role in the progression of hepatic steatosis to NASH.[76] Increasing apoptosis is seen in NASH with positive correlation between apoptosis and stage of steatofibrosis via hepatic stellate cell activation.

The role of iron overload in the production of reactive oxygen species and lipid peroxidation in NAFLD is controversial. Iron is pro-oxidant and can damage mitochondria.[77] Iron may be a substrate for oxidative stress in NAFLD leading to disease progression.[78,79] Some studies support the role of iron overload in NASH but most do not.[78,79] There is an association between insulin resistance and hepatic iron deposition.[80] Reduction of iron via phlebotomy has been shown to improve the histology of NAFLD and improve insulin resistance in some patients with diabetes.[81]

There is a decreased amount of endogenous antioxidants including glutathione in patients with NAFLD.[82] The expression of three genes involved in the production of endogenous antioxidants glutathione, superoxide dismutase, and catalase is decreased in patients with NAFLD-associated cirrhosis.[83] In animal models of NAFLD there is a defect in the methionine metabolism pathway, which normally replenishes glutathione stores.[84] The rate-limiting step controlling the conversion of methionine to *S*-adenosylmethionine (SAMe) is affected.[85] Betaine which serves as a methyl donor for the synthesis of methionine from homocysteine was shown to be beneficial in the treatment of NAFLD.[86] Clinical trials in humans evaluating whether treatment with betaine and SAMe are efficacious in NAFLD are ongoing.

Familial clustering of the disorders comprising the metabolic syndrome is apparent. The prevalence of NAFLD varies among different ethnic groups suggesting that genetics plays a role in NAFLD.[87] The isolation of a single gene responsible for insulin resistance has been difficult and probably does not exist. At least 23 genes have been found to be associated with NAFLD.[88] Insulin resistance and metabolic syndrome appear to have polygenic transmission and there is likely an interaction between genetic and environmental factors.

Clinical Presentation and Diagnosis of NAFLD

The most common clinical presentation of NAFLD is the asymptomatic patient with abnormal aminotransferase levels and/or a fatty-appearing liver on abdominal imaging study.[89] A subset of patients with NAFLD even when associated with cirrhosis have normal aminotransferase levels.[90] The most common symptoms are fatigue or right upper quadrant abdominal discomfort. The patient with advanced liver disease may present with hepatic decompensation with fluid overload, variceal bleeding, or hepatic encephalopathy. On physical examination, there may be hepatomegaly, splenomegaly, or stigmata of chronic liver disease.[91]

History, physical examination, and laboratory testing are important tools in making the diagnosis of NAFLD. Other etiologies of chronic liver disease must be excluded, in particular, excessive alcohol consumption of over 10 g daily in women and over 20 g daily in men.[91] Increased serum aminotransferase activities are helpful in making the diagnosis of NAFLD; however, these levels can be normal even in patients with advanced liver disease.[90] The presence of thrombocytopenia, hypoalbuminemia, prolonged INR, and/or elevated bilirubinemia may indicate the presence of cirrhosis. The AST/ALT ratio, in cases of advanced fibrosis, can become greater than 1.[27] Blood tests can also identify risk factors for NAFLD such as dyslipidemia, hyperglycemia, and insulin resistance, which help support the diagnosis.

Abdominal imaging studies are useful, but cannot definitively make the diagnosis of NAFLD, and pathology is needed to define the presence of NASH.[92] Abdominal ultrasound is a noninvasive procedure without radiation, which can assess hepatic steatosis by revealing a bright echo pattern within the liver. Abdominal ultrasound is insensitive in making the diagnosis of mild hepatic steatosis. Abdominal ultrasound can also reveal hepatomegaly or evidence of advanced liver disease including a cirrhotic-appearing liver and splenomegaly.

Abdominal CT scan is also useful in supporting the diagnosis of hepatic steatosis.[93] As the amount of steatosis in the liver increases, there is a decreased density of the liver. Similar to abdominal ultrasound, hepatosplenomegaly can be visualized. Abdominal MRI imaging can provide more accurate assessment of hepatic steatosis based on the shift in signaling of T1 images.[94] However, all of the abdominal imaging modalities cannot differentiate between benign hepatic steatosis and NASH.[92] The abdominal imaging studies cannot determine the degree of fibrosis in the liver. In the future, newer technology such as transient elastography may be able to measure the stiffness of the liver in order to noninvasively assess hepatic fibrosis.[95]

The most accurate means of diagnosing NAFLD is a liver biopsy.[91] Liver biopsy can reveal Mallory hyaline, hepatocellular ballooning degeneration, and lobular inflammation, defining the presence of steatohepatitis.[2] Sometimes liver biopsy can diagnose an unexpected etiology of liver disease. In addition, a liver biopsy of adequate size provides staging of hepatic fibrosis.[96] While liver biopsy is the current gold standard for the diagnosis of NAFLD, sampling error limits sensitivity and specificity.[97] Liver biopsy is an invasive procedure with inherent risks to the patient.[98] Furthermore, experts differ in the histological criteria necessary for the diagnosis of NASH and there is significant interobserver variation among pathologists in making this diagnosis.[99]

Serum adipokine levels may differentiate between bland hepatic steatosis and NASH.[100] Three serum adipokines leptin, adiponectin, and resistin were measured in a study of 10 patients with bland hepatic steatosis and 10 patients with NASH. Patients with NASH had significantly higher serum levels of leptin and resistin and lower levels of adiponectin. The cutoff levels for leptin of 40 ng/ml and resistin of 1.1 ng/ml had a sensitivity of 100%, specificity of 90%, and negative predictive value of 100% in differentiating NASH patients from patients with simple steatosis. These interesting data may render the biopsy obsolete in differentiating NASH from benign hepatic steatosis. In addition, since there is no approved medical intervention for the treatment of NASH, both patients and physicians have been reluctant to perform liver biopsies. Since current noninvasive abdominal imaging cannot differentiate between the relatively benign hepatic steatosis and the potentially progressive NASH, the liver biopsy continues to provide clinical utility in directing management and assessing severity of disease. Liver biopsy is recommended in patients with metabolic syndrome and persistently elevated aminotransferase levels despite treatment of hyperlipidemia, type 2 diabetes, and obesity.[91]

There are predictive risk factors for increased fibrosis in patients with nonalcoholic fatty liver disease, which include elevated BMI, age greater than 50, AST/ALT ratio greater than 2, elevated triglycerides, and diabetes.[27,101] Serum markers for assessment of fibrosis in the liver have been evaluated in chronic hepatitis C patients but have not yet been validated in patients with NAFLD.[102] In the future, the combination of abdominal imaging and serum markers may prove to be of great clinical benefit in the management of patients with NAFLD.

Treatment of NAFLD

Treatment of NAFLD often has consisted of weight reduction and exercise.[42,103] Lifestyle modifications, including dieting and exercise, improve hepatic aminotransferase levels.[103] Weight reduction of 10% or more results in improved histological findings in patients with NASH.[41] Rapid weight loss or starvation, in contrast, has been associated with worsening liver histology possibly related to massive release of free fatty acids from central fat into the splanchnic bloodstream and the liver.[104] Gradual weight loss is recommended, but in order to be sustained, dieting should be combined with exercise and behavior modifications.

The majority of studies evaluating medical therapy in the treatment of NAFLD have been open-label uncontrolled pilot studies carried out over a short period of time.[105–110] As a result, no specific medical therapy has been approved for the treatment of NASH. Orlistat, an enteric lipase inhibitor, improved hepatic aminotransferase levels and liver histology in a small study.[105] Both sibutramine, a selective serotonin uptake inhibitor, and orlistat resulted in significant weight loss, improvement in hepatic aminotransferase activities, and abdominal imaging findings of hepatic steatosis.[111] The durability of weight loss obtained with these antiobesity medications is uncertain.

Since NASH is theorized to be the result of insulin resistance and oxidative stress, clinical studies have evaluated treatment aimed at improving insulin sensitivity or decreasing oxidative stress.[106–110,112–118] Small open-label studies evaluated whether peroxisome proliferator-activated receptor-gamma (PPAR-γ) ligands, which have been shown to improve insulin sensitivity in diabetics, are effective in the treatment in NASH.[106–108] The first PPAR-γ ligand to be studied in patients with NASH was troglitazone, which did show improvement in the biochemical liver test results; however, the medication was withdrawn due to severe hepatotoxicity.[106] Subsequent open-label studies have shown improvement in aminotransferase levels and liver histology with rosiglitazone and pioglitazone, respectively.[107,108] The improvements in aminotransferase levels reverted to baseline after discontinuing the medications. Diet and pioglitazone in a small placebo-controlled study resulted in improvement in metabolic and histological features of NASH.[112] Pioglitazone and vitamin E were found to be of greater benefit than vitamin E alone in the treatment of NASH.[113] PPAR-γ ligand usage has been associated with weight gain and peripheral edema. Rosiglitazone usage may be associated with increased cardiotoxicity.[119] Metformin, a biguanide used in the treatment of diabetes, has not been shown to have significant benefit in the treatment of NASH.[109,110,114,115] In contrast to PPAR-γ ligands, metformin use is not associated with weight gain.

Studies evaluating antioxidants vitamins E and C have not consistently shown efficacy in the treatment of NASH, although randomized trials are ongoing.[116–118] One study comparing ursodiol to combination of vitamins E and C in the treatment of NASH did not show a significant benefit of ursodiol over the combination of vitamins E and C.[118] Betaine did show improvement in histology of NASH patients but only in a small, open-labeled pilot study.[86] Multicenter randomized double-blind studies evaluating medical therapy of NASH are needed before a standard of care is adopted.

Significant sustained weight loss is obtained in the morbidly obese via bariatric surgery.[120] Bariatric surgery, however, is an invasive procedure associated with significant perioperative morbidity and mortality. There is lower morbidity and mortality with gastric banding compared to gastric bypass procedures; however, there may be less resultant weight loss. There has been postsurgical improvement with both bypass and banding procedures in features of the metabolic syndrome including hepatic steatosis, steatohepatitis, and fibrosis.[120,121]

Hepatocellular Carcinoma

Hepatocellular carcinoma (HCC) is the fifth leading cause of cancer worldwide and accounts for more than 500,000 deaths annually.[122] The incidence of HCC in the United States is increasing. Chronic hepatitis B and C infections, alcohol-related liver disease, and hereditary hemochromatosis are recognized as etiologies of liver disease predisposing to HCC, usually in the setting of cirrhosis.[122,123] NAFLD has recently been recognized as a predisposing risk factor for the development of HCC, also probably mediated via cirrhosis.[124] There is an increased risk of HCC as high as two to three times in patients with type 2 diabetes as compared to nondiabetics after accounting for age, gender, ethnicity, and etiology of chronic liver disease.[125,126] Higher BMI in type 2 diabetes further increases the risk of HCC.[127] Type 2 diabetes synergistically increases the risk of developing HCC with etiologies of chronic liver disease other than NAFLD.[126,128] Type 2 diabetes, in the context of chronic liver disease, should be considered a risk factor for the development of HCC.

The temporal relationship between type 2 diabetes and the development of HCC was shown in a large prospective VA cohort study.[127] The incidence of HCC was twice as high in patients with type 2 diabetes as compared to nondiabetics. The mechanism by which type 2 diabetes may promote the development of HCC is believed to be due to hyperinsulinemia via activation of growth factors. Insulin binds both insulin-like growth factor-1 (IGF-1) and its own receptor.[129] Insulin binding activates mitogen-activated kinases leading to the phosphorylation of insulin receptor substrate-1 (IRS-1), a key player in cellular proliferation.[130] In the setting of cirrhosis, overexpression of IRS-1 may prevent transforming growth factor-β (TGF-β)-mediated apoptosis.[131] Furthermore, insulin resistance via lipid peroxidation generates reactive oxygen species, which results in tumor suppressor gene mutations and upregulates pro-inflammatory cytokines particularly TNF-α leading to anti-apoptosis actions.[132,133]

Hepatic resection as treatment of HCC in patients with type 2 diabetes compared to those without diabetes is associated with increased risk of complications mostly due to hepatic decompensation.[134,135] There are decreased survival rates, which may be due to complications of type 2 diabetes since there was no difference in the tumor recurrence rates between patients with type 2 diabetes compared to those without diabetes.[135,136] Decreased survival due to hepatic decompensation is also seen in previously compensated patients with cirrhosis with type 2 diabetes undergoing transarterial chemoembolization (TACE) and percutaneous ethanol injections (PEI) in the treatment of HCC.[137]

Liver Transplantation

Type 2 Diabetes and Liver Transplantation

In liver transplant recipients, type 2 diabetes can develop pre- or post-liver transplantation. Type 2 diabetes is highly prevalent in patients with chronic liver disease, particularly chronic hepatitis C infection.[138,139] The prevalence of type 2 diabetes in patients with cirrhosis ranges from 1 to 25%.[140–142] The prevalence is even higher if type 2 diabetes is defined by formal glucose tolerance testing.[143]

The effect of type 2 diabetes on survival outcomes post-liver transplantation has been evaluated in patients with pre- and post-liver transplantation diabetes. Earlier studies of patients with pre-transplantation type 2 diabetes showed no difference in patient survival post-transplantation; however, infectious complications and renal dysfunction were increased in pre-transplant diabetics.[144,145] A subsequent large case–control study did reveal decreased patient and graft survival in pre-transplant type 2 diabetics, particularly with alcohol-related liver disease.[146] Survival was further decreased in patients with type 2 diabetes requiring insulin. One case–control study revealed the difference in survival between pre-transplantation type 2 diabetics and nondiabetics began at 5 years post-transplant while analysis of the UNOS database shows patients with pre-transplant type 2 diabetes have lower patient and graft survival starting at year 1 post-liver transplantation.[140,147] These patients have more acute rejection episodes and post-transplantation cardiovascular complications.[147] These data do not include the patients with type 2 diabetes with cirrhosis who have severe vascular complications who were deemed not to be transplant candidates.[148] Diabetics who undergo liver transplantation do not have macrovascular disease. Overall the results of liver transplantation, in patients with type 2 diabetes, appear to be acceptable but stringent testing for macrovascular and even microvascular disease pre-transplantation is mandatory.

Post-liver transplantation, the development of type 2 diabetes is common ranging from 4 to 31% of liver transplant recipients.[144,149–152] Risk factors for the development of post-transplantation type 2 diabetes include pre-transplant type 2 diabetes, alcoholic and hepatitis C cirrhosis, male gender, body mass index, alcohol usage, and type of immunosuppressive agent.[144,151–154] Post-transplantation type 2 diabetes is also increased in patients who have multiple episodes of steroid-resistant rejection.[145] Patients with cirrhosis who require insulin for their type 2 diabetes pre-transplantation almost always require insulin for their type 2 diabetes post-transplantation.[144,155] Patients with type 2 diabetes on oral hypoglycemic agents pre-transplantation may require insulin post-transplantation.[156] However, in de novo post-liver transplantation type 2 diabetes, the prevalence of insulin usage decreases from 26% at year 1 to 1% at year 3.[144]

Chronic hepatitis C infection is an independent risk factor for the development of de novo type 2 diabetes post-liver transplantation similar to development of type 2 diabetes in hepatitis C patients pre-liver transplantation.[151,157] The prevalence of type 2 diabetes post-liver transplantation is higher in patients transplanted for chronic hepatitis C infection than for other etiologies of end-stage liver disease.[151] Furthermore, the hepatitis C patients who develop post-liver transplantation type 2 diabetes have a higher mortality rate than hepatitis C patients who do not develop type 2 diabetes, possibly related to more rapid liver disease progression.[158]

Tacrolimus has been associated with higher rates of development of type 2 diabetes post-liver transplantation than those observed in patients receiving cyclosporine.[149,151,155,159] Tacrolimus may inhibit the synthesis and secretion of insulin.[160] Resolution of tacrolimus-associated type 2 diabetes by changing to cyclosporine has been reported.[161] Corticosteroids are diabetogenic due to increased insulin resistance in a dose-dependent fashion.[148] Chronic hepatitis C patients who receive prednisone boluses post-liver transplantation are at increased risk for developing type 2 diabetes.[141] Other immunosuppressive agents such as azathioprine, mycophenolate mofetil, and sirolimus do not promote the development of diabetes.[148]

The development of de novo type 2 diabetes post-liver transplantation can lead to cardiac, retinal, neurological, and infectious complications.[149] The data regarding patient survival after the development of de novo type 2 diabetes post-liver transplantation revealed that patient survival at 1, 2, and 5 years does not appear to be affected by the development of de novo type 2 diabetes.[149]

Treatment of type 2 diabetes developed de novo post-liver transplantation is similar to treatment in non-transplantation type 2 diabetes.[148] Reduction of body weight and exercise are recommended in overweight liver transplantation patients to decrease risk of insulin resistance. Blood glucose levels should be rigorously monitored and controlled.[162] Caution must be used with thiazolidinediones since these medications result in weight gain and rosiglitazone has been associated with increased risk of cardiac events.[119] Metformin should be used with caution in liver transplantation recipients with renal insufficiency due to lactic acidosis. However, there is no concern about drug interactions with oral hypoglycemic agents and immunosuppressive agents. [148] Education about type 2 diabetes is important particularly in the patients who develop de novo type 2 diabetes post-liver transplantation. Another method to treat post-transplantation type 2 diabetes is steroid withdrawal or steroid-free immunosuppression.[163] Mycophenolate mofetil and sirolimus may be used to spare the usage of the calcineurin inhibitors in post-liver transplantation patients with type 2 diabetes.

NAFLD and Liver Transplantation

Recurrent NAFLD occurs post-liver transplantation. Charlton and coworkers reported on 16 patients transplanted for NASH where 60% developed hepatic steatosis post-transplantation in the allograft.[164] One-third of those with hepatic steatosis developed NASH and 12.5% developed cirrhosis. Recurrent NAFLD has been seen early post-liver transplantation. Kim and coworkers reported on eight patients transplanted for NAFLD-associated cirrhosis where 75% developed hepatic steatosis between 3 weeks and 2 years post-transplantation.[165] Half of these patients developed NASH. De novo NAFLD may occur following liver transplantation.[166] Risk factors for development of de novo NAFLD in post-liver transplantation patients are common including type 2 diabetes, hypertension, hyperlipidemia, and obesity. Immunosuppressive agents particularly the calcineurin inhibitors and corticosteroids predispose post-liver transplantation patients to the metabolic syndrome.[167] The long-term prognosis of these patients with recurrent or de novo NAFLD post-liver transplantation is not yet established and requires long-term follow-up studies.

Approximately 7–10% of the liver transplants performed annually in the United States are for cryptogenic cirrhosis according to UNOS database. The vast majority of the patients with cryptogenic cirrhosis have the metabolic syndrome characterized by obesity and type 2 diabetes.[25,168] Since these characteristics are similar to patients with NASH, cryptogenic cirrhosis is believed to represent the end stage of NAFLD. Approximately 40% of patients who are transplanted for cryptogenic cirrhosis develop hepatic steatosis in the allograft, which is a greater rate than those transplanted for other etiologies of liver disease, supporting the concept that these patients had advanced NAFLD pre-liver transplantation.[167,169] The rate of development of hepatic steatosis increases over time post-liver transplantation. In one study, approximately 100% of patients transplanted for cryptogenic cirrhosis with metabolic syndrome developed hepatic steatosis.[169]

Acute Liver Failure

Persons with type 2 diabetes experience a higher rate of acute liver failure at 2.31 cases per 10,000 person-years as compared to the overall rate of 1.44 cases per 10,000 person-years in the U.S. general population.[170] Patients with type 2 diabetes have an excess of 130 cases of acute liver failure over 10–15 years of follow-up. Another study, which was a retrospective cohort study, revealed the rate of acute liver failure to be 1 per 10,000 person-years in diabetics.[171] The mechanism for an increased rate of acute liver failure in type 2 diabetes may be due to increased susceptibility of fatty liver to further hepatotoxic insult.

Chronic Hepatitis C Infection

Prevalence of Diabetes in Chronic Hepatitis C Infection

Hepatitis C virus (HCV) has infected approximately 2% of the US adult population.[172] HCV not only replicates inside the hepatocyte but may replicate also in other cell types. Through its effect on the host immune system or by direct viral cytotoxicity, HCV infection may result in extrahepatic manifestations of disease such as type II mixed cryoglobulinemia, lymphoproliferative disorders, and membranoproliferative glomerulonephritis.[173,174] Type 2 diabetes is theorized to be another extrahepatic manifestation of chronic hepatitis C infection because retrospective and prospective studies show the prevalence of diabetes in chronic hepatitis C patients to be two to five times that of the general population.[175,176] The third NHANES data revealed the prevalence of type 2 diabetes in patients with chronic HCV infection to be increased 3-fold as compared to those without HCV infection.[175] A prospective case–cohort study of 5-year duration found that HCV patients at high risk for the development of type 2 diabetes were 11-fold more likely to develop type 2 diabetes than high-risk individuals without chronic HCV infection.[177] Overall, patients with chronic HCV infection were two times more likely to develop type 2 diabetes than matched controls. Furthermore, the prevalence of type 2 diabetes is higher in chronic HCV patients as compared to patients with hepatitis B infection and alcohol-related liver disease.[138,176] Harrison and coworkers, in a retrospective study of patients with chronic HCV infection, found the prevalence of insulin resistance to be 69%.[178] Lecube and coworkers found nondiabetic chronic HCV patients significantly more likely to be insulin resistant as compared to matched controls without chronic HCV infection.[179]

Pathogenesis of Diabetes and Insulin Resistance in Chronic Hepatitis C

The pathogenesis of the increased association between chronic HCV infection and type 2 diabetes may be related to insulin resistance developing in the setting of cirrhosis.[180] The prevalence of type 2 diabetes in HCV patients with cirrhosis is higher than that in patients with cirrhosis not infected with HCV.[138,181] There is decreased hepatic uptake of glucose and clearance of insulin by the cirrhotic liver leading to insulin resistance and the metabolic syndrome. Whether cirrhosis is an independent predictor of type 2 diabetes remains controversial.

Petit and coworkers noted that insulin resistance in HCV patients occurred prior to the development of cirrhosis.[182] Hui and coworkers also showed that insulin resistance is independent of fibrosis.[183] Insulin resistance may be due to a diabetogenic effect of HCV itself. Insulin resistance occurs in a mouse model at an early stage of HCV infection via hepatitis C core protein binding to the hepatocyte suppressing the insulin signaling proteasome activator 28-gamma-dependent pathway inducing insulin resistance.[184,185] Insulin resistance developed prior to hepatic steatosis or fibrosis in the liver in the mouse model.[186] In addition, TNF-α promoter is activated by the binding of hepatitis C core protein.[185] As mentioned previously, TNF-α interferes with the insulin signaling pathway via upregulation of SOCS proteins 1 and 3 and decreased expression of IRS proteins 1 and 2 in hepatitis C genotype 1 patients.[187] The administration of antibody to TNF-α restores insulin sensitivity in experimental models.[184] In the presence of hepatitis C core protein, there is increased oxidative stress in the hepatocyte due to mitochondrial dysfunction resulting in increased oxidation of mitochondrial glutathione, reduced electron transport function, and increased reactive oxygen species.[188]

Insulin resistance in HCV patients can occur in the absence of advanced fibrosis and cirrhosis.[182,183] Leptin levels are increased in patients with chronic hepatitis C infection as compared to healthy controls.[189] Leptin may induce insulin resistance via upregulation of pro-inflammatory cytokines. Adiponectin levels are decreased in chronic HCV infection similar to patients with obesity and type 2 diabetes.[190] Adiponectin downregulates pro-inflammatory cytokines TNF-α.

Studies of liver tissue of patients with chronic HCV infection demonstrate defects in the insulin signaling pathway at the level of IRS-1 protein.[191] Insulin resistance improved in HCV patients who were successfully treated with interferon therapy.[192] After sustained viral response to hepatitis C therapy, there is 3-fold increased expression of IRS-1 and IRS-2 proteins with resultant improved insulin sensitivity.

Not every patient with chronic HCV develops type 2 diabetes. Clinical predictors of type 2 diabetes in chronic HCV patients include older age, male gender, obesity, African-American ethnicity, severe fibrosis, and family history of type 2 diabetes.[181,182] Transgenic mice developed only type 2 diabetes if there was associated weight gain.[184] The risk of developing type 2 diabetes is increased greater than 10-fold in chronic HCV patients with risk factors for type 2 diabetes as compared to those chronic HCV patients without risk factors.[177] Host factors and the virus act synergistically in the development of type 2 diabetes.

Hepatic Steatosis and Chronic Hepatitis C Infection

Hepatic steatosis resulting from both viral and host factors occurs in approximately 50% of chronic HCV-infected patients, which is greater than that expected in the general population.[193] Clinical predictors for hepatic steatosis in hepatitis C patients include high body mass index, older age, central adiposity, insulin resistance, and diabetes.[194] The mechanism of hepatic steatosis in hepatitis C patients is not clearly understood, but the mouse model shows that the overexpression of hepatitis C core protein interferes with the assembly and secretion of triglyceride-rich VLDL in hepatocytes.[195] Decreased expression of PPAR-α pathway in hepatitis C genotype 1 patients promotes the development of hepatic steatosis.[196] PPAR-α regulates fatty acid delivery into the mitochondria and beta oxidation of fatty acids.

Hepatitis C genotype 3 virus is associated with greater prevalence and severity of hepatic steatosis as compared to hepatitis C non-genotype 3 virus.[197] In genotype 3-infected patients, the extent of hepatic steatosis correlates with viral load and not with metabolic factors. Genotype 3 core protein upregulates the fatty acid synthase promoter to a greater degree than does the non-genotype 3 core protein, resulting in greater de novo synthesis of hepatic lipid.[198] In addition, the activity of the microsomal triglyceride transfer protein in the livers of genotype 3 patients is significantly reduced as compared to non-genotype 3 patients.[199] Hepatic steatosis in genotype 3 patients resolves after sustained loss of the virus in response to interferon therapy.[200] Hepatic steatosis recurs post-liver transplantation in the allograft if not successfully eradicated prior to transplantation.

HCV patients with hyperglycemia have a higher prevalence of hepatic steatosis and faster rate of liver disease progression.[201] A large meta-analysis showed hepatic steatosis to be an independent risk factor for the prevalence and severity of hepatic fibrosis.[194] An association between worsening steatosis and progression of fibrosis over a 2-year period was found in a study with paired liver biopsies from treatment naïve chronic HCV patients.[202] This association was even greater in genotype 3 patients with hepatic steatosis.[203] Insulin resistance without hepatic steatosis is also an independent predictor of fibrosis. [183,204]

HCV patients with insulin resistance, obesity, and hepatic steatosis have a decreased response rate to interferon-based therapy.[205,206] Hepatic steatosis is an independent risk factor for poor response to interferon therapy even after adjusting for viral load, genotype, and fibrosis.[207] Harrison and coworkers, in a retrospective study evaluating the response rates to standard or pegylated interferon and ribavirin in HCV patients with greater than 33% hepatic steatosis and/or NASH, showed a response rate of 28% compared to 44% in those without NAFLD.[205] The difference was greater in those with genotypes 2 and 3 with sustained viral response of 42% versus 78%. A recent prospective study by Westin and coworkers found the sustained viral response to be 46% versus 65% in HCV patients with hepatic steatosis versus those without hepatic steatosis.[208] However, there was no significant difference in the genotype 3 patients with sustained viral response of 88% versus 100% in patients with hepatic steatosis versus those without. Insulin resistance may be the reason for the decreased response rate to interferon therapy in chronic HCV-infected patients. The sustained viral response in one study was 60% in patients without insulin resistance and 20% in those with a HOMA-IR score greater than 4.[206]

The potential mechanism for this decreased response rate to interferon-based HCV therapy may be that obesity, and insulin resistance lead to upregulation of pro-inflammatory cytokines, TNF-α, and IL-6 resulting in oxidative stress.[209] There is, in turn, decreased interferon-α signaling due to decreased phosphorylation of the JAK-STAT pathway similar to the mechanism in which pro-inflammatory cytokines interfere with the insulin signaling pathway.[210] There is increased expression of SOCS-1 and SOCS-3 by TNF-α further inhibiting interferon-α activation of the JAK-STAT pathway and the transcription of interferon-stimulated genes.[187] NAFLD, is independently associated with increased fibrosis formation leading to a further decrease in response to interferon therapy. Obesity may lead to decreased bioavailability of subcutaneously administered interferon due to decreased lymphatic uptake or by under-dosing of patients by body weight.[211,212]

Modification of metabolic factors in chronic HCV patients may improve outcomes to interferon-based therapy. A 3-month weight loss program was shown to improve serum ALT and fasting insulin levels and to reduce both hepatic steatosis and fibrosis.[213] Fifteen HCV genotype 1 infected patients compared to 17 control patients were placed on a low-calorie diet for 3 months with a goal of 10% reduction of weight prior to initiating HCV therapy.[214] The end of treatment response rates were 60% in the treatment group versus 17% in the control group. Insulin resistance was significantly improved in the diet group.

There are studies in progress assessing whether medications that improve insulin sensitivity will also improve response rates to HCV therapy in genotype 1 patients with insulin resistance. A prospective trial assessing whether the addition of pioglitazone prior to and along with pegylated interferon and ribavirin improves response rate is being conducted. Studies are ongoing in Europe evaluating whether the addition of metformin improves the efficacy of pegylated interferon and ribavirin in hepatitis C patients with insulin resistance.

The HCV virus may use the low-density lipoprotein (LDL) receptor as a means to enter the hepatocyte.[215] Use of lipid-lowering agents may downregulate the number of LDL receptors on the hepatocyte surface, inhibiting entry of the virus into the cell. Ikeda and coworkers showed that statin compounds except for pravastatin exhibit anti-hepatitis C activity in vitro.[216] Another study however found that atorvastatin 20 mg daily for 12 weeks was not associated with significant decrease in hepatitis C viral levels from baseline.[217] Studies are needed to assess whether the adjunct use of statin agents with pegylated interferon and ribavirin results in improved efficacy of antiviral therapy. Alternatively, high serum LDL levels may inhibit cell entry of HCV and improve treatment outcome.[218]

Type 1 Diabetes and Liver Disease

Type 2 diabetes, via insulin resistance and the metabolic syndrome, is associated with NAFLD and its associated complications. In addition, type 2 diabetes but not type 1 diabetes is associated with chronic HCV infection. However, there are case reports of type 1 diabetes developing as a result of interferon-based therapy for chronic hepatitis C infection.[219] In contrast type 1 diabetes is more associated with hereditary and autoimmune liver disease. Late-onset type 1 diabetes has been shown to have higher prevalence of homozygotes for the gene mutation most responsible for hereditary hemochromatosis than controls.[220] In addition the homozygotes had elevated transferrin saturations and serum ferritin levels. There are autoantibodies associated with type 1 diabetes such as anti-SOX13 and anti-GAD65. The frequency of Anti-SOX13 is 18% in type 1 diabetes, 18% in primary biliary cirrhosis (PBC), and 13% in autoimmune hepatitis; however, the autoantibody is not significantly associated with rheumatoid arthritis or systemic lupus erythematosus.[221] There is a case report of a patient with PBC, which was complicated by insulin-dependent diabetes as confirmed by positive anti-GAD65.[222] There are case reports revealing patients with autoimmune hepatitis with other autoimmune diseases and syndromes including type 1 diabetes confirmed by autoantibodies.[223]

The prevalence of elevated serum hepatic aminotransferase levels is not only higher in type 2 diabetes but also higher in type 1 diabetes than in the general population. In one study the prevalence of elevated serum hepatic aminotransferase levels was 9.5% in type 1 diabetes and 12.1% in type 2 diabetes.[224] No risk factor for type 1 diabetes was identified in multivariable analysis, but elevated serum hepatic aminotransferase levels were more common in men with microalbuminuria and dyslipidemia. There are case reports of abnormal serum liver tests in type 1 diabetes associated with the finding of hepatic glycogenosis in the absence of significant NAFLD on liver biopsy usually in the setting of poorly controlled diabetes. Hepatic glycogenosis usually resolves with control of the diabetes.[225]

Conclusions

The prevalence of NAFLD in the United States will continue to rise in the near future in conjunction with the pandemics of obesity and type 2 diabetes. There will be a predictable increase in the total number of patients with NAFLD with a subset who will develop the more serious NASH and cirrhosis. NAFLD, in the future, will surpass chronic hepatitis C infection as the leading indication for liver transplantation and contribute to a further increase in the incidence of HCC in this country. NAFLD, as the hepatic manifestation of the metabolic syndrome, is preventable and treatable. Education and public awareness about NAFLD needs to be promoted. Better therapeutic modalities targeting insulin resistance will have to be proven to be effective in the treatment of NASH in large multicenter trials before therapeutic algorithms are adopted.

Internet Sites

http//www.aasld.org
http//www.gastro.org
http//www.easl.ch

References

1. Mokdad AH, Bowman BA, Ford ES, et al. The continuing epidemics of obesity and diabetes in the United States. *J Am Med Assoc*. 2001;286:1195–1200.
2. Matteoni CA, Younossi ZM, Gramlich T, et al. Nonalcoholic fatty liver disease: a spectrum of clinical and pathological severity. *Gastroenterology*. 1999;116:1413–1419.
3. Browning JD, Szczepaniak LS, Dobbins R, et al. Prevalence of hepatic steatosis in an urban population in the United States: impact of ethnicity. *Hepatology*. 2004;40:1387–1395.
4. Ekstedt M, Franzen LE, Mathiesen UL, et al. Long-term follow-up of patients with NAFLD and elevated liver enzymes. *Hepatology*. 2006 Oct;44(4):865–873.
5. Ratziu V, Bonyhay L, DiMartino V, et al. Survival, liver failure and hepatocellular carcinoma in obesity-related cryptogenic cirrhosis. *Hepatology*. 2002;35:1485–1493.
6. Marchesini G, Brizi M, Bainchi G, et al. Nonalcoholic fatty liver disease: a feature of the metabolic syndrome. *Diabetes*. 2001;50:1844–1850.
7. Li Z, Clark J, Diehl AM. The liver in obesity and type 2 diabetes mellitus. *Clin Liver Dis*. 2002 Nov;6(4):867–877.
8. Vikram NK, Pandey RM, Misra A, et al. Non-obese (body mass index < 25 kg/m^2) Asian Indians with normal waist circumference have high cardiovascular risk. *Nutrition*. 2003;19:503–509.
9. Ikai E, Ishizaki M, Suzuki Y, et al. Association between hepatic steatosis, insulin resistance and hyperinsulinaemia as related to hypertension in alcohol consumers and obese people. *J Hum Hypertens*. 1995 Feb;9(2):101–105.
10. Assy N, Kaita K, Mymin D, et al. Fatty infiltration of liver in hyperlipidemic patients. *Dig Dis Sci*. 2000 Oct;45(10):1929–1934.
11. Weston SR, Leyden W, Murphy R, et al. Racial and ethnic distribution of nonalcoholic fatty liver in persons with newly diagnosed chronic liver disease. *Hepatology*. 2005;41:372–379.
12. Ruhl CE, Everhart JE. Determinants of the association of overweight with elevated serum alanine aminotransferase activity in the United States. *Gastroenterology*. 2003;124:71–79.
13. Jimba S, Nakagami S, Takahashi M, et al. Prevalence of nonalcoholic fatty liver disease and its association with impaired glucose metabolism in Japanese Adults. *Diabet Med*. 2005;22:1141–1145.
14. Machado M, Marques-Vidal P, Cortez-Pinto H, et al. Hepatic histology in obese patients undergoing bariatric surgery. *J Hepatol*. 2006;45:600–606.
15. Teli MR, James OF, Burt AD, et al. The natural history of nonalcoholic fatty liver disease. A follow-up study. *Hepatology*. 1995;22:1714–1719.
16. Powell EE, Cooksley WG, Hanson R, et al. The natural history of nonalcoholic steatohepatitis: a follow-up study of forty-two patients for up to 21 years. *Hepatology*. 1990;11:74–80.
17. Wanless IR, Lentz JS. Fatty liver hepatitis (steatohepatitis) and obesity: an autopsy study with analysis of risk factors. *Hepatology*. 1990;12:1106–1110.
18. Dixon JB, Bhathal PS, O'Brien PE. Nonalcoholic fatty liver disease: predictors of nonalcoholic steatohepatitis and liver fibrosis in the severely obese. *Gastroenterology*. 2001;121(1):91–100.
19. Evans CD, Oien KA, MacSween RN, et al. Nonalcoholic steatohepatitis: a common cause of progressive chronic liver injury? *J Clin Pathol*. 2002;55:689–692.
20. Adams LA, Keach JC, Batts K, et al. Time course of fibrosis progression in patients with nonalcoholic fatty liver disease. *Hepatology*. 2003;38:206–7.
21. Harrison SA, Torgerson S, Hayashi PH, et al. The natural history of nonalcoholic fatty liver disease: a clinical histopathological study. *Am J Gastroenterol*. 2003;98:1915–1917.
22. Adams LA, Sanderson S, Lindor KD, et al. The histological course of nonalcoholic fatty liver disease: a longitudinal study of 103 patients with sequential liver biopsies. *J Hepatol*. 2005 Jan;42(1):132–138.
23. Hui JM, Kench JG, Chitturi S, et al. Long-term outcomes of cirrhosis in nonalcoholic steatohepatitis compared with hepatitis C. *Hepatology*. 2003;35:1485–1493.
24. Adams LA, Lymp JF, St. Sauver J, et al. The natural history of nonalcoholic fatty liver disease: a population-based cohort study. *Gastroenterology*. 2005;129:113–121.
25. Caldwell SH, Oelsner DH, Lezzoni JC, et al. Cryptogenic cirrhosis: clinical characterization and risk factors for underlying disease. *Hepatology*. 1999;29:664–669.
26. Bugianesi E. Non alcoholic steatohepatitis (NASH) and cancer. *Clin Liver Dis*. 2007;11:136–150.

27. Angulo P, Keach JC, Batts KP, et al. Independent predictors of liver fibrosis in patients with nonalcoholic steatohepatitis. *Hepatology*. 1999;30:1356–1362.

28. Roesch-Dietlen F, Dorantes-Cuellar A, Carrillo-Toledo MG, et al. Frequency of NAFLD in a group of patients with metabolic syndrome in Veracruz, Mexico. *Rev Gastroenterol Mex*. 2006 Oct-Dec;71(4):446–452.

29. Younossi ZM, Gramlich T, Matteoni CA, et al. Nonalcoholic fatty liver disease and type 2 diabetes. *Clin Gastroenterol Hepatol*. 2004;2:262–265.

30. de Marco R, Locatelli F, Zoppini G, et al. Cause-specific mortality in type 2 diabetes. The Verona Diabetes Study. *Diabetes Care*. 1999 May;22(5):756–761.

31. Marceau P, Biron S, Hould FS, et al. Liver pathology and the metabolic syndrome X in severe obesity. *J Clin Endocrinol Metab*. 1999 May;84(5):1513–1517.

32. Silverman JF, Pories WJ, Caro J. Liver pathology in diabetes mellitus and morbid obesity. Clinical, pathological, and biochemical considerations. *Pathol Annu*. 1989;24(Pt 1):275–302.

33. Marchesini G, Avagnina S, Barantani G, et al. Aminotransferase and gamma-glutamyltranspeptidase levels in obesity are associated with insulin resistance and the metabolic syndrome. *J Endocrinol Invest*. 2005 Apr;28(4):333–339.

34. Papadia FS, Marinari GM, Camerini G, et al. Liver damage in severely obese patients: a clinical-biochemical-morphologic study on 1,000 liver biopsies. *Obes Surg*. 2004 Aug;14(7):952–958.

35. Marchesini G, Bugianesi E, Forlani G, et al. Non-alcoholic steatohepatitis in patients cared in metabolic units. *Diabetes Res Clin Pract*. 2004 Feb;63(2):143–151.

36. Marchesini G, Marzocchi R. Metabolic syndrome and NASH. *Clin Liver Dis*. 2007 Feb;11(1):105–117.

37. Day CP, James UF. Steatohepatitis: a tale of two "hits"? *Gastroenterology*. 1998 Apr;114(4):842–845.

38. Chitturi S, Farrell G. Etiopathogenesis of nonalcoholic steatohepatitis. *Semin Liver Dis*. 2001;21(1):27–41.

39. Yang SQ, Lin HZ, Lane MD, et al. Obesity increases sensitivity to endotoxin liver injury: implications for the pathogenesis of steatohepatitis. *Proc Natl Acad Sci USA*. 1997 Mar 18;94(6):2557–2562.

40. Dong W, Simeonova PP, Galluci R, et al. Cytokine expression in hepatocytes: role of oxidant stress. *J Interferon Cytokine Res*. 1998 Aug;18(8):629–638.

41. Palmer MA, Schaffner F. Effect of weight reduction on hepatic abnormalities in overweight patients. *Gastroenterology*. 1990;99:1408–1413.

42. Ueno T, Sugawara H, Sujaku K. Therapeutic effects of restricted diet and exercise in obese patients with fatty liver. *J Hepatol*. 1997;27:103–107.

43. Dixon JB, Bhathal PS, Hughs NR, et al. Nonalcoholic fatty liver disease: improvement in liver histological analysis with weight loss. *Hepatology*. 2004;39:1647–1654.

44. Rajala MW, Scherer PE. The adipocyte at the crossroads of energy, homeostasis, inflammation and atherosclerosis. *Endocrinology*. 2003;144:3765–3773.

45. Uygun A, Kadayifci A, Yesilova Z, et al. Serum leptin levels in patients with nonalcoholic steatohepatitis. *Am J Gastroenterol*. 2000;95:3584–3589.

46. Pajvani UB, Scherer PE. Adiponectin: systemic contributor to insulin sensitivity. *Curr Diab Rep*. 2003;3:207–213.

47. Aihand G, Teboul M, Massiera F. Angiotensinogen, adipocyte differentiation and fatty mass enlargement. *Curr Opin Clin Nutr Metab Care*. 2002;5:385–389.

48. Boden G, Cheung P, Stein TP, et al. FFA cause hepatic insulin resistance by inhibiting insulin suppression of glycogenolysis. *Am J Physiol Endocrinol Metab*. 2002;283:E12–E19.

49. Katsuki A, Sumida Y, Murashima S, et al. Serum levels of tumor necrosis factor-α are increased in obese patients with non-insulin dependent diabetes mellitus. *J Clin Endocrinol Metab*. 1998;83:859–862.

50. Ueki K, Kondo T, Tseng YH, et al. Central role of suppressors of cytokine signaling proteins in hepatic steatosis, insulin resistance and the metabolic syndrome of the mouse. *Proc Natl Acad Sci USA*. 2004;101:10422–10427.

51. Hotamisligil GS, Peraldi A, Budavari A, et al. IRS-1 mediated kinase activity in TNF-α and obesity induced insulin resistance. *Science*. 1996;272:665–668.

52. Friedman JM, Leibel R, Siegel DS, et al. Molecular mapping of the mouse ob mutation. *Genomics*. 1991 Dec;11(4):1054–1062.

53. Cohen P, Zhao C, Cai X, et al. Selective deletion of leptin receptor in neurons leads to obesity. *J Clin Invest*. 2001 Oct;108(8):1113–1121.

54. Kern PA, Saghizadeh M, Ong JM, et al. The expression of tumor necrosis factor in human adipose tissue. Regulation by obesity, weight loss, and relationship to lipoprotein lipase. *J Clin Invest*. 1995 May;95(5):2111–2119.

55. Spranger J, Kruke A, Mohlig M, et al. Adiponectin and protection against type 2 diabetes mellitus. *Lancet*. 2003;361:226–228.

56. Yamauchi T, Kamon J, Minokoshi Y, et al. Adiponectin stimulates glucose utilization and fatty-acid oxidation by activating AMP-activated protein kinase. *Nat Med*. 2002;8:1288–1295.

57. Ding X, Saxena NK, Lin S, et al. The roles of leptin and adiponectin: a novel paradigm in adipocytokine regulation of liver fibrosis and stellate cell biology. *Am J Pathol*. 2005 Jun;166(6):1655–1669.

58. Arner P. Not all fat is alike. *Lancet*. 1998;351:1301–1302.

59. Sanyal AJ, Campbell-Sargent C, Mirashahi F, et al. Nonalcoholic steatohepatitis: association of insulin resistance and mitochondrial abnormalities. *Gastroenterology*. 2001 Apr;120(5):1183–1192.

60. Nielsen S, Guo Z, Johnson CM, et al. Splanchnic lipolysis in human obesity. *J Clin Invest*. 2004;113:1582–1588.

61. Donnelly Kl, Smith CI, Schwarzenberg SJ, et al. Sources of fatty acids stored in the liver and secreted via lipoproteins in patients with nonalcoholic fatty liver disease. *J Clin Invest*. 2005;115:1343–1350.

62. Diraison F, Moulin P, Beylot M. Contribution of hepatic de novo lipogenesis and reesterification of plasma non esterified fatty acids to plasma triglyceride synthesis during non-alcoholic fatty liver disease. *Diabetes Metab*. 2003 Nov;29(5):478–485.

63. Bugianesi E, Gastadelli A, Vanni E, et al. Insulin resistance in non-diabetic patients with non-alcoholic fatty liver disease: sites and mechanisms. *Diabetologia*. 2005 Apr;48(4):634–642.

64. Washington K, Wright K, Shyr Y, et al. Hepatic stellate cell activation in nonalcoholic steatohepatitis and fatty liver. *Hum Pathol*. 2000 Jul;31(7):822–828.

65. Wigg AJ, Roberts-Thompson IC, McCarthy PJ, et al. The role of small intestinal bacterial overgrowth, intestinal permeability, endotoxaemia, and tumour necrosis factor alpha in the pathogenesis of non-alcoholic steatohepatitis. *Gut*. 2001 Feb;48(2):206–211.

66. Solga SF, Diehl AM. Non-alcoholic fatty liver disease: lumen-liver interactions and possible role for probiotics. *J Hepatol*. 2003 May;38(5):681–687.

67. Li Z, Yang S, Lin H, et al. Probiotics and antibodies to TNF inhibit inflammatory activity and improve nonalcoholic fatty liver disease. *Hepatology*. 2003 Feb;37(2):343–350.

68. Koruk M, Taysi S, Savas MC. Oxidative stress and enzymatic antioxidant status in patients with nonalcoholic steatohepatitis. *Ann Clin Lab Sci*. 2004 Winter;34(1):57–62.

69. Mavrelis PG, Ammon HV, Gleysteen JJ, et al. Hepatic free fatty acids in alcoholic liver disease and morbid obesity. *Hepatology*. 1983 Mar-Apr;3(2):226–231.

70. Chalasani N, Gorski C, Asghar MS, et al. Hepatic cytochrome P450 2E1 activity in nondiabetic patients with nonalcoholic steatohepatitis. *Hepatology*. 2003 Mar;37(3):544–550.

71. Caldwell SH, Swerdlow RH, Khan EM, et al. Mitochondrial abnormalities in non-alcoholic steatohepatitis. *J Hepatol*. 1999 Sep;31(3):430–434.

72. Perez-Carreras M, Del Hoyo P, Martin MA, et al. Defective hepatic mitochondrial respiratory chain in patients with nonalcoholic steatohepatitis. *Hepatology*. 2003 Oct;38(4):999–1007.

73. Poli G. Pathogenesis of liver fibrosis: role of oxidative stress. *Mol Aspects Med*. 2000 Jun;21(3):49–98.

74. Crespo J, Cayon A, Fernandez-Gil P, et al. Gene expression of tumor necrosis factor alpha and TNF-receptors, p55 and p75, in nonalcoholic steatohepatitis patients. *Hepatology*. 2001 Dec;34(6):1158–1163.

75. Feldstein AE, Werneburg NW, Canbay A, et al. Free fatty acids promote hepatic lipotoxicity by stimulating TNF-alpha expression via a lysosomal pathway. *Hepatology*. 2004 Jul;40(1):185–194.

76. Feldstein AE, Gores GJ. Apoptosis in alcoholic and nonalcoholic steatohepatitis. *Front Biosci*. 2005 Sep;1(10):3093–3099.

77. LeMasters JJ. Rusty notions of cell injury. *J Hepatol*. 2004 Apr;40(4):696–698.

78. George DK, Goldwurm S, MacDonald G, et al. Increased hepatic iron concentration in nonalcoholic steatohepatitis is associated with increased fibrosis. *Gastroenterology*. 1998 Feb;114(2):311–318.

79. Bonkovsky HL, Jawaid Q, Tortorelli K, et al. Non-alcoholic steatohepatitis and iron: increased prevalence of mutations of the HFE gene in non-alcoholic steatohepatitis. *J Hepatol*. 1999 Sep;31(3):421–429.

80. MacDonald GA, Powell LW. More clues to the relationship between hepatic iron and steatosis: an association with insulin resistance? *Gastroenterology*. 1999 Nov;117(5):1241–1244.

81. Riquelme A, Soza A, Nazal L, et al. Histological resolution of steatohepatitis after iron depletion. *Dig Dis Sci*. 2004 Jun;49(6):1012–1015.

82. Vendemiale G, Grattagliano I, Caraceni P, et al. Mitochondrial oxidative injury and energy metabolism alteration in rat fatty liver: effect of the nutritional status. *Hepatology*. 2001 Apr;33(4):808–815.

83. Edmison J, McCullough AJ. Pathogenesis of non-alcoholic steatohepatitis: human data. *Clin Liver Dis*. 2007 Feb;11(1): 75–104.

84. McClain CT, Hill DB, Song Z, et al. S-Adenosylmethionine, cytokines, and alcoholic liver disease. *Alcohol*. 2002 Jul;27(3):185–192.

85. Mato JM, Alvarez L, Ortiz P, et al. S-adenosylmethionine synthesis: molecular mechanisms and clinical implications. *Pharmacol Ther*. 1997;73(3):265–280.

86. Abdelmalek MF, Angulo F, Jorgensen SA, et al. Betaine, a promising new agent for patients with nonalcoholic steatohepatitis: results of a pilot study. *Am J Gastroenterol*. 2001 Sep;96(9):2711–2717.

87. Falck-Ytter Y, Younossi ZM, Marchesini G, et al. Clinical features and natural history of nonalcoholic steatosis syndrome. *Semin Liver Dis*. 2001;21:17–26.

88. Younossi ZM, Baranova A, Ziegler K, et al. A genomic and proteomic study of the spectrum of nonalcoholic fatty liver disease. *Hepatology*. 2005 Sep;42(3):665–674.

89. Skelly MM, James PD, Ryder SD. Findings on liver biopsy to investigate abnormal liver function tests in the absence of diagnostic serology. *J Hepatol*. 2001;35(2):195–199.

90. Mofrad P, Contos MJ, Haque M, et al. Clinical and histologic spectrum of nonalcoholic fatty liver disease associated with normal ALT values. *Hepatology*. 2003;37:1286–1292.

91. Nugent C, Younossi ZM. Evaluation and management of obesity-related nonalcoholic fatty liver disease. *Nat Clin Pract Gastroenterol Hepatol*. 2007;4:432–441.

92. Saadeh S, Younossi ZM, Remer EM, et al. The utility of radiological imaging in non-alcoholic fatty liver disease. *Gastroenterology*. 2002;123:745–750.

93. Limanond P, Raman SS, Ghobrial RM, et al. Macrovesicular hepatic steatosis in living related donors: correlation between CT and histological findings. *Radiology*. 2004;230:276–280.

94. Fishbein M, Castro F, Cheruku S, et al. Hepatic MRI for fat quantitation: its relationship to fat morphology, diagnosis and ultrasound. *J Clin Gastroenterol*. 2005;39:619–625.

95. Foucher J, Chanteloup E, Vergniol J, et al. Diagnosis of cirrhosis by transient elastography (FibroScan): a prospective study. *Gut*. 2006;55:403–408.

96. Schiano TD, Azeem S, Bodian CA, et al. Importance of specimen size in accurate needle liver biopsy evaluation of patients with chronic hepatitis C. *Clin Gastroenterol Hepatol*. 2005 Sep;3(9):930–935.

97. Ratzui V, Charlotte F, Heurtier A, et al. Sampling variability of liver biopsy in nonalcoholic fatty liver disease. *Gastroenterology*. 2005;128:1898–1906.

98. Piccinino F, Sagnelli E, Pasquale G, et al. Complications following percutaneous liver biopsy. A multicentre retrospective study on 68,276 biopsies. *J Hepatol*. 1986;2:165–173.

99. Kleiner DE, Brunt EM, Van Natta M, et al. Nonalcoholic Steatohepatitis Clinical Research Network. Design and validation of a histological scoring system for nonalcoholic fatty liver disease. *Hepatology*. 2005;41:1313–1321.

100. Gawrieh S, Rosado B, Lindor M, et al. Adipokine levels are predictive of histology in patients with nonalcoholic fatty liver disease. *Hepatology*. 2004;40(S4):237A.

101. Ratziu V, Giral P, Charlotte F, et al. Liver fibrosis in overweight patients. *Gastroenterology*. 2000 Jun;118(6):1117–1123.

102. Ratziu V, Massard J, Charlotte F, et al. Diagnostic value of biochemical markers (FibroTest-FibroSURE) for the prediction of liver fibrosis in patients with non-alcoholic fatty liver disease. *BMC Gastroenterol*. 2006 Feb;14(6):6.

103. Andersen T, Gluud C, Franzmann NB, et al. Hepatic effects of dietary weight loss in morbidly obese subjects. *J Hepatol*. 1991 Mar;12(2):224–229.

104. Friis R, Vazin ND, Akbarpour F, et al. Effect of rapid weight loss with supplemented fasting on liver tests. *J Clin Gastroenterol*. 1987 Apr;9(2):204–207.

105. Harrison SA, Fincke C, Helinski D, et al. A pilot study of orlistat treatment in obese, non-alcoholic steatohepatitis patients. *Aliment Pharmacol Ther*. 2004 Sep 15;20(6):623–628.

106. Caldwell SH, Hespenheide EE, Redick JA, et al. A pilot study of a thiazolidinedione, troglitazone, in nonalcoholic steatohepatitis. *Am J Gastroenterol*. 2001 Feb;96(2):519–525.

107. Neuschwander-Tetri BA, Brunt EM, Wehmeier KR, et al. Improved nonalcoholic steatohepatitis after 48 weeks of treatment with the PPAR-gamma ligand rosiglitazone. *Hepatology*. 2003 Oct;38(4):1008–1017.

108. Promrat K, Lutchman G, UwaifoG I, et al. A pilot study of pioglitazone treatment for nonalcoholic steatohepatitis. *Hepatology*. 2004 Jan;39(1):188–196.

109. Marchesini G, Brizi M, Bianchi G, et al. Metformin in non-alcoholic steatohepatitis. *Lancet*. 2001 Sep 15;358(9285):893–894.

110. Nair S, Diehl AM, Wiseman M, et al. Metformin in the treatment of non-alcoholic steatohepatitis: a pilot open label trial. *Aliment Pharmacol Ther*. 2004 Jul 1;20(1):23–28.

111. Sabuncu T, Nazligul Y, Karaoglanoglu M, et al. The effects of sibutramine and orlistat on the ultrasonographic findings, insulin resistance and liver enzyme levels in obese patients with non-alcoholic steatohepatitis. *Rom J Gastroenterol*. 2003 Sep;12(3):189–192.

112. Belfort R, Harrison SA, Brown K, et al. A placebo-controlled trial of pioglitazone in subjects with nonalcoholic steatohepatitis. *N Engl J Med*. 2006 Nov 30;355(22):2297–2307.

113. Sanyal AJ, Mofrad PS, Contos MJ, et al. A pilot study of vitamin E versus vitamin E and pioglitazone for the treatment of nonalcoholic steatohepatitis. *Clin Gastroenterol Hepatol*. 2004 Dec;2(12):1107–1115.

114. Uygun A, Kadayifci A, Yesilova Z, et al. Metformin in the treatment of patients with non-alcoholic steatohepatitis. *Aliment Pharmacol Ther*. 2004 Mar 1;19(5):537–544.

115. Duseja A, Murlidharan R, Bhansali A, et al. Assessment of insulin resistance and effect of metformin in nonalcoholic steatohepatitis – a preliminary report. *Indian J Gastroenterol*. 2004 Jan-Feb;23(1):12–15.

116. Harrison SA, Torgerson S, Hayashi P, et al. Vitamin E and vitamin C treatment improves fibrosis in patients with nonalcoholic steatohepatitis. *Am J Gastroenterol*. 2003 Nov;98(11):2485–2490.

117. Hasegawa T, Yoneda M, Nakamura K, et al. Plasma transforming growth factor-beta1 level and efficacy of alpha-tocopherol in patients with non-alcoholic steatohepatitis: a pilot study. *Aliment Pharmacol Ther*. 2001 Oct;15(10):1667–1672.

118. Ersoz G, Gunsar F, Karazu Z, et al. Management of fatty liver disease with vitamin E and C compared to ursodeoxycholic acid treatment. *Turk J Gastroenterol*. 2005 Sep;16(3):124–128.

119. Nissen SE, Wolski K. Effect of rosiglitazone on the risk of myocardial infarction and death from cardiovascular causes. *N Engl J Med*. 2007 Jun 14;356(24):2457–2471.

120. Dixon JB. Surgical treatment for obesity and its impact on non-alcoholic steatohepatitis. *Clin Liver Dis*. 2007 Feb;11(1): 141–154.

121. Silverman EM, Skinner JS, Fisher ES. Regression of hepatic steatosis in morbidly obese persons after gastric bypass. *Am J Clin Pathol*. 1995 Jul;104(1):23–31.

122. El-Serag HB, Mason AC. Rising incidence of hepatocellular carcinoma in the United States. *N Engl J Med*. 1999;340:745–750.

123. Bosch FX, Ribes J, Diaz M, et al. Primary liver cancer worldwide incidence and trends. *Gastroenterology*. 2004;127:5–16.

124. Bugianesi E, Leone N, Vanni E, et al. Expanding the natural history of nonalcoholic steatohepatitis from cryptogenic cirrhosis to hepatocellular carcinoma. *Gastroenterology*. 2002;32:689–692.

125. El-Serag HB, Tran T, Everhart JE. Diabetes increases the risk of chronic liver disease and hepatocellular carcinoma. *Gastroenterology*. 2004 Feb;126(2):460–468.

126. Davila JA, Morgan RO, Shaib Y, et al. Diabetes increases the risk of hepatocellular carcinoma in the United States: a population based case control study. *Gut*. 2005 Apr;54(4):533–539.

127. Coughlin SS, Calle EE, Teras LR, et al. Diabetes mellitus as a predictor of cancer mortality in a large cohort of US adults. *Am J Epidemiol*. 2004 Jun 15;159(12):1160–1167.

128. El-Serag HB, Richardson PA, Everhart JE, et al. The role of diabetes in hepatocellular carcinoma: a case-control study among United States Veterans. *Am J Gastroenterol*. 2001 Aug;96(8):2462–2467.

129. Moore MA, Park CB, Tsuda H. Implications of the hyperinsulinemia-diabetes-cancer link for preventive efforts. *Eur J cancer Prev*. 1998;7:89–107.

130. Kim SO, Park JG, Lee YI. Increased expression of the insulin-like growth factor 1 (IGF-1) receptor gene in hepatocellular carcinoma cell lines: implications of IGF-1 receptor gene activation by hepatitis B virus X gene products. *Cancer Res*. 1996;56:3831–3836.

131. Tanaka S, Wands JR. Insulin receptor substrate -1 overexpression in human hepatocellular carcinoma cells prevents transforming growth factor beta 1-induced apoptosis. *Cancer Res*. 1996 Aug 1;56(15):3391–3394.

132. Hu W, Feng Z, Eveleigh J, et al. The major lipid peroxidation product, trans-4-hydroxy-2-nonenal, preferentially forms DNA adducts at codon 249 of human p53 gene, a unique mutational hotspot in hepatocellular carcinoma. *Carcinogenesis*. 2002;23:1781–1789.

133. Pikarsky E, Porat RM, Stein I, et al. NF-kappa B functions as a tumor promoter in inflammation-associated cancer. *Nature*. 2004;431:461–466.

134. Ikeda Y, Shimada Y, Hasegawa H, et al. Prognosis of hepatocellular carcinoma with diabetes mellitus after hepatic resection. *Hepatology*. 1998 Jun;27(6):1567–1571.

135. Huo TI, Lui WY, Huang YH, et al. Diabetes mellitus is a risk factor for hepatic decompensation in patients with hepatocellular carcinoma undergoing resection: a longitudinal study. *Am J Gastroenterol*. 2003 Oct;98(10):2293–2298.

136. Toyoda H, Kumada T, Nakano S, et al. Impact of diabetes mellitus on the prognosis of patients with hepatocellular carcinoma. *Cancer*. 2001 Mar 1;91(5):957–963.

137. Huo TI, Wu JC, Lui WY, et al. Differential mechanism and prognostic impact of diabetes mellitus on patients with hepatocellular carcinoma undergoing surgical and nonsurgical treatment. *Am J Gastroenterol*. 2004 Aug;99(8):1479–1487.

138. Mason AL, Lau JY, Hoang N, et al. Association of diabetes mellitus and chronic hepatitis C infection. *Hepatology*. 1999;29(2):328–333.

139. Lecube A, Hernandez C, Genesca J, et al. Glucose abnormalities in patients with hepatitis C virus infection: Epidemiology and pathogenesis. *Diabetes Care*. 2006 May;29(5):1140–1149.

140. Yoo HY, Thulvath PJ. The effect of insulin-dependent diabetes mellitus on outcome of liver transplantation. *Transplantation*. 2002;74:1007–1012.

141. Baid S, Cosimi AB, Farrell ML, et al. Posttransplant diabetes mellitus in liver transplant recipients: risk factors, temporal relationship with hepatitis C virus allograft hepatitis, and impact on mortality. *Transplantation*. 2001;72(6):1066–1072.

142. Zein NN, Abdulkarim AS, Weisner RH, et al. Prevalence of diabetes mellitus in patients with end-stage liver cirrhosis due to hepatitis C, alcohol, or cholestatic disease. *J Hepatol*. 2000;32(2):209–217.

143. Petrides AS, DeFronzo RA. Glucose metabolism in cirrhosis: a review with some perspectives for the future. *Diabetes Metab Rev*. 1989 Dec;5(8):691–709.

144. Navasa M, Bustamante J, Marroni C, et al. Diabetes mellitus after liver transplantation: prevalence and predictive factors. *J Hepatol*. 1996;25:64–71.

145. Trail KC, Strata RJ, Larsen JL, et al. Results of liver transplantation in diabetic recipients. *Surgery*. 1993;114:650–658.

146. Shields PL, Tang H, Neuberger JM, et al. Poor outcome in patients with diabetes mellitus undergoing liver transplantation. *Transplantation*. 1999;68:530–535.

147. John PR, Thulvath PJ. Outcome of liver transplantation in patients with diabetes mellitus: a case-control study. *Hepatology*. 2001;34:889–895.

148. Reuben A. Long-term management of the liver transplant patient: diabetes, hyperlipidemia, and obesity. *Liver Transpl*. 2001 Nov;7(11 Suppl 1):S13–S21.

149. John PR, Thulvath PJ. Outcomes of patients with new-onset diabetes mellitus after liver transplantation compared with those without diabetes mellitus. *Liver Transpl*. 2002;8:708–713.

150. Krentz AJ, Dmitrewski J, Mayer D, et al. Postoperative glucose metabolism in liver transplant recipients: a two-year prospective randomized study of cyclosporine versus FK 506. *Transplantation*. 1994;57(11):1666–1669.

151. AlDosary AA, Ramji AS, Elliot TG, et al. Post-liver transplantation diabetes mellitus: an association with hepatitis C. *Liver Transpl*. 2002;8(4):356–361.

152. Saab S, Shpaner A, Zhao Y, et al. Prevalence and risk factors for diabetes mellitus in moderate term survivors of liver transplantation. *Am J Transplant*. 2006;6(8):1890–1895.

153. Knobler H, Stagnaro-Green A, Wallenstein S, et al. Higher incidence of diabetes in liver transplant recipients with hepatitis C. *J Clin Gastroenterol*. 1998;26:30–33.

154. Scantlebury V, Shapiro R, Fung J, et al. New onset diabetes in FK506 vs cyclosporine-treated kidney transplant recipients. *Transplant Proc*. 1991;23:3169–3170.

155. Stegall MD, Everson G, Schroter G, et al. Metabolic complications after liver transplantation, diabetes, hypercholesterolemia, hypertension, and obesity. *Transplantation*. 1995;60(9):1057–1060.

156. Wahlstrom HE, Cooper J, Gores G, et al. Survival after liver transplantation in diabetics. *Transplant Proc*. 1991;23:1565–1566.

157. Soule JL, Olyaei AJ, Boslaugh TA, et al. Hepatitis C infection increases the risk of new onset diabetes after transplantation in liver allograft recipients. *Am J Surg*. 2005 May;189(5):552–557.

158. Foxton MR, Quaglia A, Muiesan P, et al. The impact of diabetes mellitus on fibrosis progression in patients transplanted for hepatitis C. *Am J Transplant*. 2006;6(8):1922–1929.

159. Ericzon B, Groth C, Bismuth H, et al. Glucose metabolism in liver transplant recipients treated with FK506 or cyclosporine in the European multicentre study. *Transpl Int*. 1994;7(Suppl 1):S11–S14.

160. Rilo HL, Zeng Y, Alejandro R, et al. Effect of FK 506 on function of human islets of Langerhans. *Transplant Proc*. 1991 Dec;23(6):3164–3165.

161. Kanzler S, Lohse AW, Schirmacher P, et al. Complete reversal of FK 506 induced diabetes in a liver transplant recipient by change of immunosuppression to cyclosporine A. *Z Gastroenterol*. 1996 Feb;34(2):128–131.

162. Davidson J, Wilkinson A, Dantal J, et al. New-onset diabetes after transplantation: 2003 international consensus guidelines. *Transplantation*. 2003;75(10 Suppl):S3–s24.

163. Stegall MD, Everson GT, Schroter G, et al. Prednisone withdrawal late after adult liver transplantation reduces diabetes, hypertension, and hypercholesterolemia without causing graft loss. *Hepatology*. 1997 Jan;25(1):173–177.

164. Charlton MC, Kasparova P, Weston S, et al. Frequency of nonalcoholic steatohepatitis as a cause of advanced liver disease. *Liver Transpl*. 2001;7(7):608–614.

165. Kim WR, Poterucha JJ, Porayko MK, et al. Recurrence of nonalcoholic steatohepatitis following liver transplantation. *Transplantation*. 1996;62:1802–1805.

166. Liu LU, Schiano TD. Long-term care of the liver transplant recipient. *Clin Liver Dis*. 2007 May;11(2):397–416.

167. Burke A, Lucey MR. Non-alcoholic fatty liver disease, non-alcoholic steatohepatitis and orthotopic liver transplantation. *Am J Transplant*. 2004 May;4(5):686–693.

168. Poonawala A, Nair SP, Thuluvath PJ, et al. Prevalence of obesity and diabetes in patients with cryptogenic cirrhosis: a case control study. *Hepatology*. 2000;32:689–693.

169. Cantos MJ, Cales W, Sterling RK, et al. Development of nonalcoholic fatty liver disease after orthotopic liver transplantation for cryptogenic cirrhosis. *Liver Transpl*. 2001;7:363–373.

170. El-Serag HB, Everhart JE. Diabetes increases the risk of acute liver failure. *Gastroenterology*. 2002;122:1822–1828.

171. Chan KA, Truman A, Gurwitz JH, et al. A cohort study of the incidence of serious acute injury in diabetic patients treated with hypoglycemic agents. *Arch Intern Med*. 2003;163:728–734.

172. Alter MJ, Kruszon-Moran D, Nainan OV, et al. The prevalence of hepatitis C virus infection in the United States, 1988 through 1994. *N Engl J Med*. 1999 Aug 19;341(8):556–562.

173. Ferri C, Monti M, LaCivita L, et al. Infection of peripheral blood mononuclear cells by hepatitis C virus in mixed cryoglobulinemia. *Blood*. 1993 Dec 15;82(12):3701–3704.

174. Blackard JT, Kemmer N, Sherman KE. Extrahepatic replication of HCV: insights into clinical manifestations and biological consequences. *Hepatology*. 2006 Jul;44(1):15–22.

175. Mehta SH, Brancati FL, Sulkowski MS, et al. Prevalence of type 2 diabetes mellitus among persons with hepatitis C virus infection in the United States. *Ann Intern Med*. 2000;133:592–599.

176. Knobler H, Schihmanter R, Ziforni A, et al. Increased risk of type 2 diabetes in noncirrhotic patients with chronic hepatitis C virus infection. *Mayo Clin Proc*. 2000 Apr;75(4):355–359.

177. Mehta SH, Brancati FL, Strathdee SA, et al. Hepatitis C virus infection and incident type 2 diabetes. *Hepatology*. 2003;38: 50–56.

178. Harrison SA. Correlation between insulin resistance and hepatitis C viral load. *Hepatology*. 2006 May;43(5):1168.

179. Lecube A, Hernandez C, Genesca J, et al. Proinflammatory cytokines, insulin resistance, and insulin secretion in chronic hepatitis C patients: A case-control study. *Diabetes Care*. 2006 May;29(5):1096–1101.

180. Lecube A, Hernandez C, Genesca J, et al. High prevalence of glucose abnormalities in patients with hepatitis C virus infection: a multivariate analysis considering the liver injury. *Diabetes Care*. 2004 May;27(5):1171–1175.

181. Thuluvath PJ, John PR. Association between hepatitis C, diabetes mellitus, and race. A case-control study. *Am J Gastroenterol*. 2003 Feb;98(2):438–441.

182. Petit JM, Bour JB, Galland-Jos C, et al. Risk factors for diabetes mellitus and early insulin resistance in chronic hepatitis C. *J Hepatol*. 2001 Aug;35(2):279–283.

183. Hui JM, Sud A, Farrell GC, et al. Insulin resistance is associated with chronic hepatitis C virus infection and fibrosis progression. *Gastroenterology*. 2003 Dec;125(6):1695–1704.

184. Shintani Y, Fujie H, Miyoshi H, et al. Hepatitis C virus infection and diabetes: direct involvement of the virus in the development of insulin resistance. *Gastroenterology*. 2004 Mar;126(3):840–848.

185. Miyamoto H, Moriishi K, Moriya K, et al. Involvement of the PA28gamma-dependent pathway in insulin resistance induced by hepatitis C virus core protein. *J Virol*. 2007 Feb;81(4):1727–1735.

186. Moriya K, Yotsuyangi H, Shintani Y, et al. Hepatitis C virus core protein induces hepatic steatosis in transgenic mice. *J Gen Virol.* 1997 Jul;78(Pt 7):1527–1531.

187. Walsh MJ, Jonsson JR, Richardson MM, et al. Non-response to antiviral therapy is associated with obesity and increased hepatic expression of suppressor of cytokine signaling 3 (SOCS-3) in patients with chronic hepatitis C, viral genotype 1. *Gut.* 2006 Apr;55(4):529–535.

188. Castera L, Chouteau P, Hezode C, et al. Hepatitis C virus-induced hepatocellular steatosis. *Am J Gastroenterol.* 2005 Mar;100(3):711–715.

189. Widjaja A, Wedemeyer H, Tillman HL, et al. Hepatitis C and the leptin system: bound leptin levels are elevated in patients with hepatitis C and decrease during antiviral therapy. *Scand J Gastroenterol.* 2001 Apr;36(4):426–431.

190. Tsochatzis E, Papatheodoridis GV, Archimandritis AJ. The evolving role of leptin and adiponectin in chronic liver diseases. *Am J Gastroenterol.* 2006 Nov;101(11):2629–2640.

191. Aytug S, Reich D, Sapiro LE, et al. Impaired IRS-1/PI3-kinase signaling in patients with HCV: a mechanism for increased prevalence of type 2 diabetes. *Hepatology.* 2003 Dec;38(6):1384–1392.

192. Kawaguchi T, Ide T, Taniguchi E, et al. Clearance of HCV improves insulin resistance, beta-cell function, and hepatic expression of insulin receptor substrate 1 and 2. *Am J Gastroenterol.* 2007 Mar;102(3):570–576.

193. Asselah T, Rubbia-Brandt L, Marcellin P, et al. Steatosis in chronic hepatitis C: why does it really matter? *Gut.* 2006 Jan;55(1):123–130.

194. Leandro G, Mangia A, Hui J, et al. Relationship between steatosis, inflammation, and fibrosis in chronic hepatitis C: a meta-analysis of individual patient data. *Gastroenterology.* 2006 May;130(6):1636–1642.

195. Perlemuter G, Sabile A, Letteron P, et al. Hepatitis C virus core protein inhibits microsomal triglyceride transfer protein activity and very low density lipoprotein secretion: a model of viral-related steatosis. *FASEB.* 2002 Feb;16(2):185–194.

196. Dharancy S, Malapel M, Perlemuter G, et al. Impaired expression of the peroxisome proliferator-activated receptor alpha during hepatitis C virus infection. *Gastroenterology.* 2005 Feb;128(2):334–342.

197. Adinolfi L, Gambardella M, Andreana A, et al. Steatosis accelerates the progression of liver damage of chronic hepatitis C patients and correlates with specific HCV genotype and visceral obesity. *Hepatology.* 2001 Jun;33(6):1358–1364.

198. Jackel-Cram C, Babiuk L, Liu Q, et al. Up-regulation of fatty acid synthase promoter by hepatitis C virus core protein: genotype-3a core has a stronger effect than genotype-1b core. *J Hepatology.* 2007 Jun;46(6):999–1008.

199. Mirandola S, Realdon S, Iqbal J, et al. Liver microsomal triglyceride transfer protein is involved in hepatitis C liver steatosis. *Gastroenterology.* 2006 May;130(6):1661–1669.

200. Kumar D, Farrell GC, Fung C, et al. Hepatitis C virus genotype 3 is cytopathic to hepatocytes: Reversal of hepatic steatosis after sustained therapeutic response. *Hepatology.* 2002 Nov;36(5):1266–1272.

201. Ratziu V, Munteanu M, Charlotte F, et al. Fibrogenic impact of high serum glucose in chronic hepatitis C. *J Hepatol.* 2003 Dec;39(6):1049–1055.

202. Castera L, Hezode C, Roudot-Thoraval F, et al. Worsening of steatosis is an independent factor of fibrosis progression in untreated patients with chronic hepatitis C and paired liver biopsies. *Gut.* 2003 Feb;52(2):288–292.

203. Westin J, Nordlinder H, Lagging M, et al. Steatosis accelerates fibrosis development over time in hepatitis C virus genotype 3 infected patients. *J Hepatol.* 2002 Dec;37(6):837–842.

204. D'Souza R, Sabin C, Foster GR. Insulin resistance plays a significant role in liver fibrosis in chronic hepatitis C and in the response to antiviral therapy. *Am J Gastroenterol.* 2005 Jul;100(7):1509–1515.

205. Harrison SA, Brunt EM, Qazi RA, et al. Effect of significant histologic steatosis or steatohepatitis on response to antiviral therapy in patients with chronic hepatitis C. *Clin Gastroenterol Hepatol.* 2005 Jun;3(6):604–609.

206. Romero-Gomez M, Del Mar Viloria M, Andrade R, et al. Insulin resistance impairs sustained response rate to peginterferon plus ribavirin in chronic hepatitis C patients. *Gastroenterology.* 2005 Mar;128(3):636–641.

207. Poynard T, Ratziu V, McHutchison J, et al. Effect of treatment with peginterferon or interferon alfa-2b and ribavirin on steatosis in patients infected with hepatitis C. *Hepatology.* 2003 Jul;38(1):75–85.

208. Westin J, Lagging M, Dhillon AP, et al. Impact of hepatic steatosis on viral kinetics and treatment outcome during antiviral treatment of chronic HCV infection. *J Viral Hepat.* 2007 Jan;14(1):29–35.

209. Choi J, Ou JH. Mechanisms of liver injury. III. Oxidative stress in the pathogenesis of hepatitis C virus. *Am J Physiol Gastrointest Liver Physiol.* 2006 May;290(5):G847–G851.

210. DiBona D, Cippitelli M, Fionda C, et al. Oxidative stress inhibits IFN-alpha-induced antiviral gene expression by blocking the JAK-STAT pathway. *J Hepatol.* 2006 Aug;45(2):271–279.

211. Charlton MR, Pockros PJ, Harrison SA. Impact of obesity on treatment of chronic hepatitis C. *Hepatology.* 2006 Jun;43(6):1177–1186.

212. Fried M, Jensen D, Rodriguez-Torres M, et al. Improved sustained virological response (SVR) rates with higher, fixed doses pf peginterferon alfa-2A (40KD) plus ribavirin in patients with difficult to cure characteristics. *Hepatology.* 2006;44:314A.

213. Hickman IJ, Clouston AD, Macdonald GA, et al. Effect of weight reduction on liver histology and biochemistry in patients with chronic hepatitis C. *Gut.* 2002 Jul;51(1):89–94.

214. Tarantino G, Conca P, Ariello M, et al. Does a lower insulin resistance affect antiviral therapy response in patients suffering from HCV related chronic hepatitis? *Gut.* 2006 Apr;55(4):585.

215. Monazahian M, Bohme I, Bonk S, et al. Low density lipoprotein receptor as a candidate receptor for hepatitis C virus. *J Med Virol.* 1999 Mar;57(3):223–229.

216. Ikeda M, Abe K, Yamada M, et al. Different anti-HCV profiles of statins and their potential for combination therapy with interferon. *Hepatology*. 2006 Jul;44(1):117–125.

217. O'Leary JG, Chan JL, McMahon CM, et al. Atorvastatin does not exhibit antiviral activity against HCV at conventional doses: a pilot clinical trial. *Hepatology*. 2007 Apr;45(4):895–898.

218. Gopal K, Johnson T, Gopal S, et al. Correlation between Beta-lipoprotein levels and outcome of hepatitis C treatment. *Hepatology*. 2006;44:335–340.

219. Eibl N, Gschwantler M, Ferenci P, et al. Development of insulin-dependent diabetes mellitus in a patient with chronic hepatitis C during therapy with interferon-alpha. *Eur J Gastroenterol*. 2001 Mar;13(3):295–298.

220. Ellervik C, Mandrup-Poulsen T, Nordestgaard BG, et al. Prevalence of hereditary haemochromatosis in late-onset type 1 diabetes mellitus: a retrospective study. *Lancet*. 2001 Oct 27;358(9291):1405–1409.

221. Fida S, Myers MA, Whittingham S, et al. Autoantibodies to the transcriptional factor SOX13 in primary biliary cirrhosis compared with other diseases. *J Autoimmun*. 2002 Dec;19(4):251–257.

222. Nakasone H, Kinjo K, Yamashiro M, et al. A patient with primary biliary cirrhosis complicated with slowly progressive insulin-dependent diabetes mellitus. *Intern Med*. 2003 Jun;42(6):496–499.

223. Oki K, Yamane K, Koide J, et al. A case of polyglandular autoimmune syndrome type III complicated with autoimmune hepatitis. *Endocr J*. 2006 Oct;53(5):705–709.

224. West J, Brousil J, Gazis A, et al. Elevated serum alanine transaminase in patients with type 1 or type 2 diabetes mellitus. *QJM*. 2006 Dec;99(12):871–876.

225. Sayuk GS, Elwing JE, Lisker-Melman M. Hepatic glycogenosis: an underrecognized source of abnormal liver function tests? *Dig Dis Sci*. 2007 Apr;52(4):936–938.

Chapter 36
The Increased Risk of Cancer in Obesity and Type 2 Diabetes: Potential Mechanisms

Emily Jane Gallagher, Ruslan Novosyadlyy, Shoshana Yakar, and Derek LeRoith

Introduction

Theories on a connection between diabetes, obesity, and cancer have existed for over a century. In 1910, despite their elusive etiologies, Maynard hypothesized that a correlation between diabetes and cancer could exist, as both conditions were increasing in prevalence and had similar age distributions.[1] Kessler's review of the medical literature in 1971 proposed an association between diabetes and cancer of the pancreas and endometrium, with possible links to breast, prostate, thyroid, and some hematological cancers.[2] Evidence from animal studies by Morechi, in 1909 and subsequent studies by Rous in 1914 and Tannenbaum in the 1940s, suggested that restriction of caloric intake inhibited carcinogenesis.[3] More recent epidemiological studies have convincingly demonstrated a greater risk of developing cancer at multiple sites in obese individuals.[4] Subjects with type 2 diabetes also appear to be at increased risk of various cancers, while data on type 1 diabetes is conflicting.[5,13] Indeed the cancer risk associated with type 2 diabetes appears to be independent of body mass index (BMI), suggesting that other factors may be involved, above and beyond the effects of obesity.[5,7,8,14] Accordingly, the global epidemic of obesity and type 2 diabetes causes yet another concern: the incidence of certain cancers may also increase. Therefore, it behooves investigators to determine the relationships between obesity, type 2 diabetes, and cancer in order to impede the potential escalation in cancer prevalence.

In this chapter we will present the epidemiological data that propose the relationship between type 2 diabetes, obesity, and cancer risk, followed by a brief review of some insights from human and animal studies that were undertaken primarily to demonstrate these relationships and to determine the mechanisms involved.

Epidemiological Studies

Diabetes and Cancer

Accumulating evidence from case control and observational studies advocates an association between type 2 diabetes and cancer at multiple sites (Table 36.1). The American Cancer Society Cancer Prevention Study (CPS) II reported that, irrespective of BMI, adults with diabetes had a mortality risk from breast, colon, pancreatic, and liver cancers in excess of those without diabetes.[5] Comparable studies from Korea and Europe concluded that there is an increased incidence and mortality from non-Hodgkin's lymphoma and esophageal cancer in men and bladder, lung, and cervical cancers in women, in addition to breast, colon, pancreatic, and liver cancers, in those with diabetes.[14,15] Although obesity in the Korean population was much less prevalent than that in usual Western

D. LeRoith (✉)
Division of Endocrinology, Diabetes & Bone Disease, Department of Medicine, Mount Sinai School of Medicine, New York, NY, USA
e-mail: derek.leroith@mssm.edu

Table 36.1 Cancer mortality by site associated with diabetes and obesity

	RR with DM	References	RR with obesity	References
Increased risk with both diabetes and obesity				
Breast	1.2	5,18,32	1.12–2.12	4,18
Endometrial	1.33–2.0	5,11,34	2.0–4.0	4
Pancreatic	1.5	5,21	1.12–1.49	4,69
Colon	1.2–1.5	5,54,55	1.4	54
Renal cell	1.12	5	1.6–4.75	4

	RR with obesity	References		
Increased risk with obesity				
Esophageal and gastric adenocarcinoma	1.2–2.78	4,66		
Ovarian	1.16–1.5	4,39		
Prostate	1.05–1.22	46		
Cervical adenocarcinoma	1.2–3.2	4		
Hematological (myeloma, B cell lymphoma)	2.4 (myeloma)	4,4		
Uncertain association				
Biliary				
Lung				

populations, the cancer risk was again independent of BMI.[7] Further studies from Europe have had inconsistent findings, with some studies showing no association between cancer and diabetes.[8,16]

The discrepancy in data from the epidemiological studies is thought to be related to different study designs and methodology employed. Many studies report cancer mortality, whereas others report cancer incidence. This creates conflicting results as many cancers are treatable, so patients may be cured or may die with, rather than from, the tumor. Most of the studies rely on self-reporting of diabetes and other demographic factors from the participants. A number of studies neglect to distinguish between type 1 and type 2 diabetes and report diabetes cases in the initial population but not later diagnoses of diabetes over the follow-up period. Several studies overlook other risk factors for certain cancers, such as hepatitis prevalence in populations with liver cancer. Some studies assess overall cancer risk, but not site-specific cancers, and more fail to account for the temporal relationship between the onset of diabetes and cancer. In an attempt to clarify some of these issues a number of meta-analyses have been published on the topic. From these meta-analyses, it was concluded that there is sufficient evidence to infer a positive association between diabetes and risk of breast, colorectal, pancreatic, and bladder cancers, but an inverse association with that of prostate cancer.[11,17–22]

Obesity and Cancer

The epidemic of obesity is occurring not only in the United States, but worldwide.[23] At present, 32% of US adults are classified as obese, with a body mass index (BMI) ≥ 30 kg/m^2, and twice as many (66%) are overweight (BMI ≥ 25 kg/m^2).[24] Globally, the prevalence of obesity is on the rise.[23] In certain ethnic groups BMI does not necessarily reflect the level of visceral adiposity, an important factor in the pathophysiology of insulin resistance and its complications.[25]

Studies on the contribution of obesity to cancer have shown it to be associated with a significant increase in the risk of cancer incidence and mortality at various sites (Table 36.1).[4,26–28] Current statistics from the American Cancer Society (ACS) estimate that there are almost 1.5 million new cancer cases a year and over 500,000 cancer deaths per year.[29] For the population, it has been estimated that 14% of cancer deaths in men and 20% in women are attributable to obesity.[4] Furthermore, combined, overweight and obesity are allegedly accountable for 90,000 (6%) of deaths from cancer annually in the United States.[4] Regarding new cancer cases, Canadian and European studies have estimated that 5–8% are contributed to by obesity and overweight, while the NHANES (National Health and Nutrition Examination Survey) reported that obesity alone contributed to 3.2% of new cases in 2002.[27,28,30] Along with adiposity, high calorie and protein consumption and low physical activity are also associated with the increased cancer risk.[31]

Specific Cancer Sites

Breast Cancer

Obesity and diabetes are consistently and independently associated with an increased risk of breast cancer in postmenopausal women.[4,7,32] For diabetes, American, European, and Asian population studies estimate this excess risk of breast cancer incidence and mortality to be approximately 20%.[7,18,32] Most data refute a link between diabetes and premenopausal breast cancer, while the strongest link has been reported between diabetes and estrogen receptor-positive (ER) breast cancer.[32] As there are multiple well-recognized risk factors involved in breast cancer development, including family history, parity, menopausal status, and hormone use, calculations were adjusted for these potential confounders. The excess risk associated with diabetes is not negated following correction for these factors.[32] The CPS II analysis reported a rise in breast cancer mortality correlating with an increase in BMI above 25 kg/m^2, culminating in those with a BMI over 40 kg/m^2 having twice the risk of normal-weight individuals.[4] Accrual of data from US, European, and Asian studies deduced that approximately 30–50% of breast cancer deaths are attributable to overweight and obesity.[33]

Genitourinary Malignancies

Endometrial, ovarian, and cervical cancers in women, prostate cancer in men, as well as renal cell and bladder cancer in both have been related to diabetes and obesity.

Approximately 40% of endometrial cancer in affluent societies is ascribed to overweight or obesity, considered due to an overall increase in exposure to endogenous estrogens related to obesity.[4] Although there are discordant reports on diabetes and its links to endometrial cancer, there is evidence of a cumulative risk in individuals with diabetes, obesity, and low physical activity: a 2-fold increased risk is seen in those with diabetes alone, a 6-fold increase in those with diabetes and obesity, and a 10-fold increase in those with diabetes, obesity, and low physical activity, compared with nondiabetic, lean, physically active individuals.[34] Type 1 diabetes may also convey an increased risk of endometrial cancer, although data are limited.[10]

Obesity conveys a 36% greater risk of ovarian cancer according to some studies, although there is debate surrounding the extent of this risk, if any.[4,35–39] It appears that obese individuals are more likely to have localized tumors; however in those with advanced disease, obesity is associated with reduced time to recurrence and overall survival.[38] There is a paucity of data on diabetes and ovarian cancer, with most studies showing paltry associations; however, a study of type 1 diabetes did report a significant link.[6,40–42]

While obesity appears to increase the probability of developing cervical cancer, there is minimal evidence of an elevated risk with type 2 or type 1 diabetes.[4,6,7,10] Notably, obesity has been associated with adenocarcinoma of the cervix, which is on the rise in the United States.[43,44]

Conflicting results have been published on prostate cancer and its association with obesity and diabetes. Data from studies in the United States and Europe propose that 4% of prostate cancer cases could be attributable to obesity.[4,30] Although it seems that obesity is associated with a negligible or reduced risk of low-grade cancer, it conveys an increased risk of high-grade disease, potentially related to the androgen sensitivity of the tumor.[30,45,46] There is evidence that obesity carries a greater risk of disease recurrence and mortality after treatment of prostate cancer.[47] Much of the conflicting data regarding prostate cancer are due to differences in study methodology. Some studies report cancer mortality rates, but others report incidence rates. Some studies detect prostate cancer by screening for elevated prostate-specific antigen (PSA), while others include only individuals with clinically evident disease.[46] For diabetes, most studies report an inverse relationship with prostate cancer incidence and mortality.[17,20,45,48] Although African-American men are at greater risk of both diabetes and prostate cancer, studies have failed to demonstrate an association or in fact have shown an inverse relationship between the two diseases.[49,50]

Links between obesity, diabetes, and renal cell cancer have been described.[4-6,30,51-53] The correlation with obesity is strongest with the addition of poor diet and low physical activity. Although the mechanism is uncertain, the link is more consistent in women than men, leading to the hypothesis that it may be related to estrogenic effects. There are limited data suggesting that diabetes carries an increased risk of bladder cancer.[19]

Gastrointestinal Malignancies

Multiple epidemiological studies have consistently reported positive associations between colorectal cancer and both diabetes and obesity in men and women.[22,54,55] Even after adjusting for confounders such as BMI, family history, physical activity, smoking, alcohol, red meat consumption, exogenous hormone and aspirin use, this excess risk persists.[55] Waist circumference appears to be a stronger predictor of colorectal cancer than BMI.[56] The association is greater in men than in women. This may be related to estrogen, which is believed to be protective against colorectal cancer.[57,58] A lifestyle with a diet rich in fats, red meat, low in fiber, fruits, and vegetables, with a sedentary lifestyle is also associated with a higher risk of colon and rectal cancers.[59-61] Furthermore, it is linked with a higher risk of cancer recurrence and mortality in patients with advanced colon cancer.[62]

Adenocarcinoma of the esophagus and, to a lesser extent, the stomach is on the rise in the United States.[63] Obesity has been linked with an increased risk of gastric cardia and esophageal cancers in Western and Asian populations.[4,26,64,65] The mechanism behind this is thought, in part, to be mechanical due to gastroesophageal reflux disease (GERD) causing Barrett's esophagus.[64,66] The association between diabetes and gastric or esophageal cancer is not as strong as that with obesity, but may vary with ethnic background.[5-7,67,68]

The relationship between pancreatic cancer and diabetes is a matter of interest. As although widely associated with pancreatic cancer, whether diabetes is a consequence of this neoplasm or induces its development is the subject of speculation.[5-7,69-73] Reports of a very high risk in some studies may in actuality be an overestimation, in view of the reverse causality between diabetes and pancreatic cancer. One percent of those with newly diagnosed diabetes of ≥ 50 years will develop pancreatic cancer within 3 years.[21,74] There is evidence that pancreatic tumor cells express insulin receptors and their growth is promoted by insulin. However, there is also a hypothesis that these tumor cells have endocrine effects that actually cause hyperglycemia.[69] As regards obesity, central adiposity more so than BMI is a risk factor for pancreatic cancer.[75] Cigarette smoking which is one of the main risk factors associated with pancreatic cancer tends to be inversely related to BMI, but is associated with central adiposity.[76,77]

Hepatocellular carcinoma (HCC) has been consistently linked with both obesity and diabetes.[4,5,7,67,78] There is some difficulty in interpreting rates of HCC as many studies do not account for the prevalence of hepatitis B (HBV) and hepatitis C (HCV) or the prevalence of cirrhosis in the study population. It has been suggested that type 2 diabetes may not be a significant risk factor in populations with a high prevalence of hepatitis. A large Chinese study found that type 2 diabetes had a more important influence on the development of HCC in the absence of HCV than in those infected with HCV.[79]

Biliary tract carcinoma, although rare in the United States, has a poor prognosis. While the incidence of extrahepatic cholangiocarcinoma is stable, intrahepatic cholangiocarcinoma is increasing in incidence. Among other factors, such as HCV and alcoholic liver disease, obesity and diabetes may be contributing to this escalating incidence of intrahepatic cholangiocarcinoma.[80,81] Studies of gallbladder and extrahepatic cholangiocarcinoma have reported an increased risk with obesity, but not diabetes.[4,5,30,82]

Hematological Cancers

Non-Hodgkin's lymphoma, multiple myeloma, and certain leukemias have been associated with obesity.[4,83-85] Obesity appears specifically to be connected with large B cell lymphoma and myeloma in men.[84-86] In children with acute lymphoblastic leukemia, obesity has been reported to be related to decreased disease-free survival.[87] Diabetes is in some studies linked with an increased incidence and a poorer prognosis in non-Hodgkin's lymphoma, but not all studies concur with this finding.[67,88]

Lung Cancer

Many studies report an inverse correlation between BMI and lung cancer.[4] However, in women, a waist circumference >99 cm, irrespective of smoking status, is associated with an increased risk of lung cancer, with an augmented risk for current smokers.[89] No particular connection has been identified in the majority of studies examining diabetes and lung cancer risk.[5,53,67,90] This may be due to the strong correlation between lung cancer and smoking overshadowing other weaker correlations.[76,91] It is worth noting that epidemiological studies from Japan and Korea, with very high rates of non-smoking in females (>80 and >90%, respectively), demonstrated an increased risk of lung cancer in women with diabetes.[7,92]

Summary of Epidemiological Data

As summarized in Table 36.1, it appears that both type 2 diabetes and obesity are linked to an increased risk of breast, endometrial, colon, pancreatic, hepatic, and renal cell cancers. There is evidence that obesity contributes to an augmented risk of esophageal and gastric adenocarcinomas, along with certain hematological cancers, ovarian cancer, and cervical adenocarcinoma, but there is no substantial link with diabetes. Data are contradictory for either obesity or diabetes having an association with prostate, biliary, and lung cancers. From limited studies of type 1 diabetes, there are suggestions that it may carry an excess risk of cervical, gastric, and endometrial cancers. Further studies are necessary to demystify remaining issues. Confounding factors, such as smoking, with lung and pancreatic cancers, hepatitis with HCC, and hormone therapy with breast and ovarian cancers should be identified and excluded from studies, where possible. Uncertainty still exists as to whether pancreatic cancer predisposes to diabetes or occurs as a consequence. Also, more consistent endpoints of either cancer incidence or mortality are required, in order to clearly establish whether diabetes and obesity convey greater cancer risk. Given the high and rising prevalence of both diabetes and obesity in the population, along with their well-known participation in the development of cardiovascular disease, these disorders may emerge as principal players in cancer development.

Mechanisms of Cancer Development

The factors contributing to cancer development in obesity and type 2 diabetes, as they are currently understood, are outlined in Fig. 36.1. Growth hormone (GH), insulin, insulin-like growth factor (IGF), along with other hormones, adipokines, and cytokines have been implicated in tumorigenesis.

Excess adipose tissue causes increased production of free fatty acid (FFA), the peptide leptin, and cytokines, such as tumor necrosis factor α (TNFα) and interleukin-6 (IL-6), with decreased production of the peptide adiponectin. These metabolic alterations from obesity, along with decreased physical activity and elevated triglycerides, lead to hyperinsulinemia and insulin resistance, which are closely related to type 2 diabetes. Obesity and hyperinsulinemia are associated with alterations in the levels of GH and IGF-I. GH stimulates tissue growth through the actions of IGF-I, the synthesis of which is dependent on the action of GH on GH receptors (GHR). Insulin increases the quantity of hepatic GHR and so hyperinsulinemia leads to the production of larger amounts of IGF-I that through signaling pathways leads to cell growth and proliferation.[93–95] Obesity, hyperinsulinemia, and elevated IGF-I also result in reduced hepatic synthesis of sex hormone-binding globulin (SHBG), therefore allowing greater bioavailability of estrogen. In addition, estrogen synthesis is increased by higher levels of aromatase in adipose tissue of obese individuals.[31]

In this section, we will explain how each of these factors is incorporated into the mechanism of cancer development in obesity and diabetes.

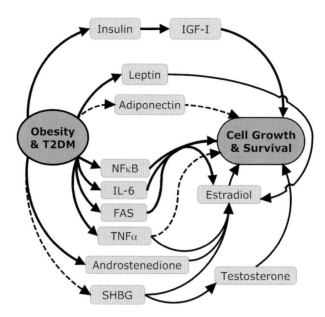

Fig. 36.1 The components involved in obesity, diabetes, and cancer. *Solid lines* indicate a positive influence on the subsequent entity; *dotted lines* indicate an inhibitory effect on the subsequent factor

Insulin-Like Growth Factors

IGF-I and IGF-II exist in the circulation in free form and also bound to insulin-like growth factor-binding proteins (IGFBPs).[96] There are in total six IGFBPs, sequentially IGFBP-1 to IGFBP-6, that bind IGF-I and IGF-II but not insulin. IGFBP-3 is the predominant binding protein in the serum and binds approximately 75% of IGF-I and also binds IGF-II in a ternary complex with acid-labile subunit (ALS). Both IGFBP-3 and IGFBP-5 have effects on cell proliferation, migration, and sensitivity to apoptosis.[97]

While IGFBPs control IGF-I and IGF-II activities by protecting them from degradation, thereby increasing their half-lives and controlling their availability for receptor binding, there is evidence that the interactions between IGFs and IGFBPs are more complex. It seems that IGFBP-3 may protect against downregulation of the IGF-I receptor (IGF-IR) that occurs in response to IGF-I, thereby enhancing the cellular response to IGF-I.[95,97,98] Certain IGFBPs have been shown to have mitogenic effects and cellular interactions independent of IGFs, but as yet these mechanisms remain unclear.[97]

Epidemiological studies measuring IGF-I and IGFBP levels in individuals, to assess their association with cancer, have given contradictory results. IGF-I has been shown to have a positive association with lung, colorectal, premenopausal breast, and advanced-stage prostate cancers.[99–101] The opposite has been reported in other studies.[102] Data on IGFBP levels are conflicting, with variable levels of IGFBP-2 and IGFBP-3 reported in relation to colorectal and postmenopausal breast cancer (IGFBP-2) and with prostate, pre- and postmenopausal breast cancers (IGFBP-3).[101–108]

In rat models, colonic abnormalities are increased by insulin injections, but decreased by caloric restriction.[109,110] In humans, epidemiological studies have suggested an increased risk of cancer related mortality in individuals taking exogenous insulin and insulin secretagogues.[111] Clinical trials using inhaled recombinant insulin demonstrated an increased association with lung cancer. Other epidemiological and tumor cell line studies have suggested that certain insulin analogues may have increased mitogenic effects, possibly related to prolonged binding to the IR or cross-rectivity with the IGF-IR.[112,113] Rodents with high levels of IGF-I exhibit an increased incidence of mammary tumors and epidermal hyperplasia in skin.[114,115] Low circulating levels of IGF-I in mice, caused by energy-restricted diets, led to a significant decrease in cancer incidence.[116,117] Similarly, IGF-I-deficient rodents show a decreased rate of growth of primary and metastatic tumors.[118–123] These effects were reversed by treatment with recombinant hIGF-I.[116,118,124] The production of angiogenic factors in cecal tumors was dependent on circulating concentrations of IGF-1.[118]

IGF Signaling

IGF-I binds with high affinity to the IGF-IR (a transmembrane tyrosine kinase growth factor receptor) and with low affinity to the insulin receptor (IR). Although the IGF-IR and IR are highly homologous, insulin binding to the IR results primarily in a metabolic response, while IGF-I binding to the IGF-IR results in cellular growth responses.[125] IGF-II binds to the IGF-IIR leading to endocytosis and is thought to function as a clearance receptor for IGF-II.

Variations of IR and IGF receptors also exist, with altered affinity for insulin and IGFs. Hybrid receptors resulting from the dimerization of the IR and IGF-IR "hemireceptors" retain their affinity for IGF-I, but exhibit a low affinity for insulin. Therefore, if present in sufficient quantities, these hybrid receptors will lead to a decreased cellular response to insulin but not IGF-I. During gene transcription the *IR* gene is subject to alternative splicing that results in different IR isoforms, IR-A and IR-B. IR-A has a higher affinity for IGF-II and initiates proliferative signaling pathways, whereas IR-B binding predominantly leads to metabolic signaling.[126]

Upon binding of IGFs to the IGF-IR, autophosphorylation and activation of the receptor tyrosine kinase occur, resulting in the recruitment of insulin receptor substrates (IRS) and adaptor proteins, which then incorporate and coordinate the activity of downstream intermediates. These events finally lead to the activation of two principal signaling cascades: the mitogen-activated protein kinase pathway (MAPK) that plays a pivotal role in cell growth and proliferation and the phosphatidylinositol triphosphate kinase (PI3K) pathway, which is mainly involved in mediating metabolic and anti-apoptotic effects. One of the intermediates activated by the PI3K pathway is protein kinase B (Akt), which has many substrates including apoptosis-regulating transcription factors. Activated (phosphorylated) Akt moves to the cell nucleus where it phosphorylates these pro-apoptotic transcription factors, resulting in their removal from the nucleus into the cytoplasm and inhibition of their activity. The activity of PI3K is counteracted by PTEN (phosphatase and tensin homologue deleted on chromosome 10) which, after p53, is the most frequently mutated tumor suppressor gene.[95,127–130] IRS-1 appears to be an intermediate in the signaling pathways of cytokines and integrins. Similarly in some cell types, IGF-II can directly phosphorylate kinases involved in cytokine signaling. Therefore, crosstalk between different signaling systems can occur.[130–132]

Genetic Abnormalities in the Insulin/IGF Pathway

The insulin gene (INS) is located on the short arm of chromosome 11 (Ch 11p15.5) in humans.[133] At the 5′ flanking region of *INS* is a polymorphic region composed of a variable number of tandem repeats (VNTR) of 14 base pairs. This VNTR locus is located next to the transcription start site and is believed to have a direct effect on insulin regulation.[134] In addition to the VNTR, single nucleotide polymorphisms (SNPs) have been identified throughout the *INS* gene, including the VNTR locus.[135–137] The SNP on *INS* is a marker for the 3′ untranslated region (UTR) of *INS* RNA. The 3′-UTR of *INS* suppresses translation, stabilizes mRNA, and acts with the 5′UTR to increase glucose-induced proinsulin biosynthesis. Therefore, polymorphisms in this region may have a functional effect on the expression of *INS*. Two studies of individuals with certain SNPs in this region showed a 2-fold increased risk of prostate cancer.[138,139] The IGF1 gene is expressed on Ch 12q22– 24.1.[137] There is a CA repeat (10–23) near the IGF-I transcription site, believed to regulate IGF-I levels.[140] Polymorphisms in the number of these CA repeats have been associated with an increased risk of colorectal carcinoma, with inconsistent results in prostate and breast cancers.[141–145] Other SNPs in the IGF1 gene have been correlated with an increased risk of prostate and breast cancers.[144,146,147]

The IGF2 gene is also located on Ch 11p15.5, in relatively close linkage to *INS*.[137] The IGF2 gene is an imprinted gene, expressed only from the paternally inherited chromosome.[137] Loss of imprinting (LOI) of IGF2, and the resultant biallelic expression, has been shown in studies of Beckwith Weidman syndrome, a congenital overgrowth syndrome and was first identified in association with Wilm's tumor. LOI is now known to occur in many tumors and is considerably more frequent in lymphocytes of colorectal cancer compared to normal bowel.[148,149]

A SNP in the *IRS1* gene has been reported with metabolic abnormalities including type 2 diabetes insulin resistance has also been investigated as a polymorphism associated with prostate cancer.[140,150–153] Studies investigating the association of abnormalities in IGFBP genes and cancer have, as with their serum levels, been variable.[142,147,154,155] A UK study of Caucasians included 1529 lung cancer cases and 2707 controls and identified 64 SNPs that influenced susceptibility to lung cancer, from which 11 mapped to genes of the GH/IGF axis.[156]

Cellular Glucose and Protein Availability

In order to drive cell growth and proliferation, the cell needs to have the ability to increase protein synthesis.[129] This is regulated in the cell by a pathway associated with the protein kinase mTOR (mammalian target of rapamycin) that increases ribosomal protein synthesis. This is positively affected by glucose and amino acids and equally, in the absence of glucose protein synthesis, is inhibited by inactivating mTOR activity. Involved in the mTOR pathway are the tumor suppressor genes TSC1 that encodes the protein hamartin and TSC2 that encodes the protein tuberin. Tuberous sclerosis, a syndrome characterized by a pleiotropic array of hamartomas that are rarely malignant, but give rise to neurological disease, skin lesions, cardiac dysfunction, kidney and lung failure, has been mapped to mutations of these two tumor suppressor genes.[129] The hamartin and tuberin proteins form a complex (TSC1–TSC2) that potently inhibits mTOR and therefore prevents protein synthesis. The absence of glucose in the cell leads to increased levels of cellular AMP kinase (AMPK), which upregulates the activity of TSC1–TSC2 complex and subsequently inhibits mTOR-mediated protein synthesis.[129] Low glucose levels increase p53-mediated cell autophagy through inhibition of mTOR.[129] The IGF-1 signaling pathway also influences mTOR activity. Akt releases the inhibition of TSC1–TSC2 complex on mTOR and promotes growth.[129,157]

p53

p53 is a tumor suppressor protein that activates the expression of genes leading to cell cycle arrest, DNA repair, and cellular apoptosis.[129] Mutations or deletions of the p53 gene prevent the expression of these growth inhibitors, so cells progress into mitosis.[158] Cellular stress signals that cause DNA damage often leads to cell cycle arrest and cellular apoptosis, mediated by p53.[159,160]

Integration of IGF-I/mTOR/p53 Pathways in Cancer

Elements of the insulin signaling pathway have been recognized for many years to be involved in tumorigenesis.[161] In more primitive organisms such as the nematode *Caenorhabditis elegans*, prolongation of life is associated with mutations that allow the organism to withstand stress, similar to rapidly growing cells in tumors. p53 activation, for example, accelerates aging, whereas p53 mutations are common in many cancers and also regulate metabolism. In the presence of abundant nutrients, mTOR is activated and mTOR inhibitor rapamycin is being used to treat cancers.[162,163]

IGF-I has been shown to have anti-apoptotic effects and influences p53 activity.[164] Inhibition of apoptosis by IGF-I appears to coincide with a reduction in p53 expression and upregulation of p53 inhibitors.[165] Therefore, IGF-I may interfere with the pro-apoptotic tumor suppressor activities of p53, either through direct effects on p53 or indirectly through regulation of its inhibitors.[130,165] Mutations in p53 result in upregulation of the IGF-IR, which has been seen in breast and colon cancer cells.[128,166] Studies in mice demonstrated that mutations leading to inhibition of IGF-IR activity resulted in a marked increase in apoptotic cell lines and inhibition of tumor growth.[130] In patients with acute myeloid leukemia (AML), IGF-IR expression correlated negatively with the apoptotic index in bone marrow samples.[167]

Peutz–Jeghers syndrome, which is associated with multiple gastrointestinal polyps and epithelial cancers, including breast cancer, is the result of germ-line mutations of the gene for a serine/threonine kinase (STK11). The STK11 gene functions as a tumor suppressor gene and regulates the apoptotic pathways of p53.[168,169] As well as being implicated in PJS, mutations of STK11 are linked with the development of metastatic laryngeal and pharyngeal cancers, lung adenocarcinoma, pancreatic cancer, and malignant melanomas.[170–172] In the absence of glucose, STK11-associated AMPK activity is increased and leads to inhibition of mTOR.[157] Metformin has been found to inhibit hepatic gluconeogenesis by activation of AMPK, through a STK11-dependent mechanism in the liver.[173] Studies of diabetic populations have suggested that those individuals treated with metformin have a lower risk of cancer-specific mortality compared to those on alternative diabetic medications.[174,175] In breast cancer cells it also seems that metformin upregulates AMPK activity and inhibits mTOR activation and downstream events.[176]

Progressive tumor growth and metastasis requires new blood vessel formation and the ability of cells to migrate. The IGF system may also be involved in angiogenesis. IGF-I appears to have a direct effect on vascular endothelial cells, binding to the subendothelial extracellular matrix, where it may play a role in cell survival and stability. IGF-II expression is induced by hypoxia and leads to activation of transcription factors such as epidermal growth factor, which promotes neovascularization in tumors and is one target of new cancer therapies.[177] Integrins are transmembrane glycoprotein receptors that mediate cell-matrix or cell–cell adhesion and transduce signals that regulate gene expression and cell growth. IGF-I activation causes integrins to relocate to the edge of migrating cells.[178] IGF-I also induces extension of lamellipodia in neuroblastoma cell lines, another factor associated with metastases. In specific cancers, it has been shown that IGF-I disrupts the cell adhesion E-cadherin/catenin complex and its association with the cytoskeleton. E-cadherin and catenin form cellular adhesion junctions, mutations are associated with dysfunctional cell adhesion, tumor invasion, and metastases.[179]

Summary of Insulin Signaling Pathway and Cancer

Therefore, cell growth and survival is regulated by GH and IGF-I, under the influence of many other factors associated with cell stress from DNA damage and nutrient availability. Abnormalities in this system are associated with cancer syndromes such as tuberous sclerosis and Peutz–Jeghers syndrome. We also appreciate that genetic abnormalities can increase the risk of both tumor formation and other related disorders, such as diabetes. Dysregulation of a number of elements in this intricate arrangement of cellular signals can therefore lead to upregulation of cell survival and proliferation intermediates, resulting in tumor formation.

Adipokines

Leptin

Leptin and adiponectin are peptides produced by adipocytes and released into the circulation. The absence of leptin leads to extreme obesity, as demonstrated in the *ob/ob* mice and humans with congenital leptin deficiency.[180,181] Most obese individuals will, however, have elevated leptin levels with resistance to its appetite-suppressing effects.[182] Insulin exerts positive feedback on the expression of the leptin *ob* gene to suppress appetite. IGF-I, in contrast, is a negative feedback regulator. Leptin is linked to marked insulin resistance and is increased with Western dietary patterns as well as in conditions causing chronic systemic inflammation.[183–185]

The leptin receptor is part of the cytokine receptor family. There are variants of the leptin receptor that result in activation of cellular cascades involved in cellular growth and proliferation through IGF-I and cytokine pathways. Leptin has been shown to stimulate cellular proliferation in esophageal, breast, prostate, colon, and bone marrow cancer cell lines.[186] It is also pro-angiogenic in vivo and in vitro. In prostate cancer cell lines, specifically androgen-independent prostate cancer cells, leptin stimulates proliferation, but it does not in androgen-dependent cells even though both cell types express functional leptin receptors.[187] Caloric restriction results in decreased tumor growth and decreased leptin levels in rat models of colon cancer.[186,188–191] Leptin also stimulates estrogen biosynthesis by induction of aromatase activity which may explain its connection with breast cancer.[192]

Adiponectin

Adiponectin levels, in contrast to leptin, are reduced in states of insulin resistance such as obesity. Adiponectin is an anti-inflammatory adipokine, produced by adipocytes that act through its two receptors Adipo R1 and Adipo R2. It is decreased in obese patients and increased in lean persons, has anti-inflammatory properties (reducing production of pro-inflammatory and increasing anti-inflammatory cytokines) and insulin-sensitizing action.[193,194] Stimulation of glucose utilization and fatty acid oxidation by adiponectin occurs through activation of AMPK.[195] Adiponectin therefore indirectly suppresses mTOR.

Adiponectin has anticancer potential via its anti-inflammatory effects. An inverse relationship exists between breast cancer and adiponectin levels in both premenopausal and postmenopausal women. The inhibitory effect of adiponectin was also seen in gastric cancer cell lines in culture.[196,197] Local injection of adiponectin markedly inhibited the growth of these cells. Similarly, the continuous intraperitoneal infusion of adiponectin effectively suppressed the development of peritoneal metastasis in these cancer cell lines.[198] It is also a negative regulator of angiogenesis.[199] Rodent models have suggested that adipokines may not be essential for the growth of the cancers, but exert their effects through hyperglycemia, hyperinsulinemia, elevated IGF-I levels, or pro-inflammatory cytokines.[200]

Fatty Acid Synthase

Fatty acid synthase (FAS) is an anabolic enzyme required for the conversion of dietary carbohydrate to fatty acids. The gene expression of FAS in adipose tissue is related to visceral fat accumulation, hyperinsulinemia, insulin resistance, IL-6, leptin, and retinol-binding protein 4 (RBP4), suggesting an important role of lipogenic pathways in the relationship between excess energy intake and the development of obesity and type 2 diabetes.[201] While a high-carbohydrate/low-fat diet upregulates FAS, exercise and energy restriction cause downregulation (through AMPK) and a missense mutation of the FAS gene is protective against obesity.[202] Breast, prostate, and a number of other cancers have been shown to express high levels of FAS, which is associated with a poor prognosis.[203] In colorectal carcinoma FAS overexpression is associated with microsatellite instability (MSI). MSI refers to the altered lengths of short nucleotide repeat sequences in tumor DNA, which occur to a high degree in approximately 15% of colorectal tumors.[202] Overexpression of FAS in breast and ovarian cancers is associated with more aggressive tumors. In breast cancer cell lines, inhibiting FAS was found to downregulate HER2 oncogene expression.[204] Oleate, a monounsaturated free fatty acid, promotes the proliferation of breast cancer cells by PI3K activation.[205] Both cerulenin (an antibiotic) and orlistat (a lipase inhibitor drug) inhibit FAS and inhibit growth of breast and prostate cell lines.[204,206] One possible requirement of cancer cells is fatty acids for membrane phospholipids synthesis, to maintain aggressive behavior. Thus increased dietary intake of saturated fats commonly seen in overweight individuals may cultivate the tumors through this pathway.[204]

Cytokines

Hyperinsulinemia and visceral adiposity are associated with the increased production of inflammatory cytokines, such as interleukin-6 (IL-6) and tumor necrosis factor α (TNFα), by adipocytes and macrophages within adipose tissue. Inflammation has been linked to the growth and spread number of cancers including breast and colon.

IL-6

Interleukins are members of a group of cytokines, typically produced by leucocytes, with a wide range of biological functions, including the regulation of inflammatory and immune responses. Human adipocytes secrete significant amounts of IL-6 correlating with BMI.[187] The activities of IL-6 relate to insulin resistance, angiogenesis, and tumor cell biology. Along with insulin, leptin, and TNF-α, IL-6 can stimulate estrogen biosynthesis by the induction of aromatase activity.[192] In one study of breast cancer patients, IL-6 values were found to be higher in breast cancer patients in association with insulin resistance compared to other groups. Estradiol, IL-6 levels, and insulin resistance in the ER-positive group were significantly higher than those of the ER-negative group.[207] In prostate cancer, serum IL-6 levels are remarkably elevated in patients with clinically evident hormone-resistant prostate cancer as compared with those with hormone-dependent cancer.[187] Consistent with this clinical result, IL-6 is secreted by androgen-independent prostate cancer cells but not by androgen-dependent cells. Therefore, IL-6 appears to be elevated as a cause and effect of prostate cancer.[187] IL-6 levels are correlated with obesity; therefore, genetic susceptibility to obesity may be related to genetic susceptibility to multiple myeloma through inheritance of elevated IL-6 levels. One possible candidate locus is the gene encoding IL-6. A SNP in the IL-6 promoter gene has been associated with a 2-fold increase in plasma cell neoplasms. IL-6 is necessary for the differentiation of immature plasmablasts into mature antibody-producing plasma cells in the bone marrow. Myeloma cells in culture do not survive without IL-6 and an IL-6 antibody inhibits myeloma cell proliferation in vitro and in vivo. High levels of IL-6 have been linked to higher stage and poorer prognosis of both multiple myeloma and plasmacytoma. In addition, IL-6 induces polyclonal B cell activation, which can lead to hypergammaglobulinemia.[208]

TNFα

TNFα is a pro-inflammatory cytokine released from macrophages and monocytes in response to inflammatory stimuli and leads to apoptotic or necrotic cell death. Increased expression of TNFα is seen in acute sepsis and chronic inflammatory states such as cancer, HIV and AIDS, rheumatoid arthritis, ankylosing spondylitis, as well as obesity and diabetes.[209] The pro-apoptotic effects of TNFα are mediated through IκB kinase (IKK) and MAPK pathways, leading to inhibition of mTOR and protein synthesis; however under certain circumstances TNFα may also lead to anti-apoptotic signaling through NFκB and increased Akt promoting protein synthesis.[210] In obesity, TNFα has been positively correlated with waist circumference and insulin resistance; it is overexpressed by adipocytes and infiltrating macrophages.[211] Rodents with a genetic lack of TNFα function are protected against obesity-related reductions in insulin signaling, which is the result of TNFα inhibition of insulin receptor tyrosine kinase signaling and IRS-1 and IRS-2 phosphorylation.[212,213] TNFα also stimulates estrogen biosynthesis by way of aromatase induction and angiogenesis.[192]

Other Inflammatory Markers

NFκB is a transcription factor that functions both in cytokine signaling and in cell survival. Its expression is induced by a multitude of different extracellular stimuli, including bacteria, virus, interleukins, growth factors, chemotherapeutic agents, and various stress stimuli. Similarly, activated NFκB promotes the expression of numerous target genes, such as those involved in cellular proliferation, anti-apoptosis, cell migration, and

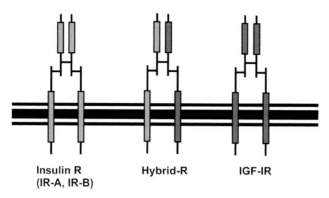

Fig. 36.2 Insulin and IGF-I receptors. Both the insulin receptor (IR) and the IGF-I receptors (IGF-IR) are transmembrane tyrosine kinase receptors that are expressed on the cell surface as preformed oligomers. Traditionally, it has been believed that IR mediates metabolic functions and IGF-IR mediates mitogenic functions. In addition, hybrids may form between IR and IGF-IRs when both are expressed in the same cell. Furthermore, the IR is expressed as two subtypes IR-A and IR-B; two slicing variants with exon 11 included or excluded in the finally expressed protein. IR-A binds insulin and IGF-II and mediates mitogenic actions and IR-B binds insulin primarily and mediates traditional metabolic functions

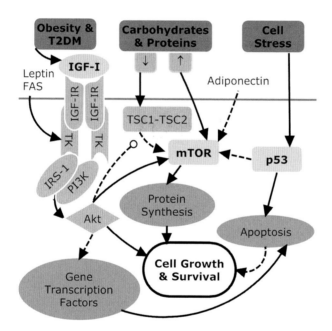

Fig. 36.3 The integration of diabetes, obesity, nutrition, and cell stress in cell survival pathways. *Solid lines* indicate a positive effect and *dotted lines* an inhibitory effect on the next element. Tumors have been seen to upregulate levels of IGF-IR, which results in increased signaling through the TK (tyrosine kinase) pathway with the end result of suppression of pro-apoptotic gene transcription factors. Increased nutritional availability allows for protein synthesis via mTOR, a pathway that is also stimulated by Akt. p53 is a tumor suppressor gene that leads to cell cycle arrest and apoptosis. It also inhibits mTOR. Mutations in p53 are common in tumors and lead to loss of its pro-apoptotic effects and loss of its inhibitory effect on mTOR

angiogenesis. NFκB is strongly associated with abdominal obesity, insulin resistance, and adiponectin levels.[214] It mediates the anti-apoptotic effects of IGF-1 in colon cancer cells and delivers positive feedback to insulin. It is overexpressed in the majority of breast cancers.[215] In ER-negative breast cancer cells, an NFκB antagonist blocked epidermal growth factor-induced NFκB activation and caused apoptotic death. They also showed that the NFκB antagonist inhibited the growth and caused extensive regression of ER-mouse mammary epithelial tumors.[216] Similarly, reduction of NFκB activity correlated with decreased breast tumor cell proliferation.[216]

A strong association between inflammation and obesity has been previously observed. In individuals with a BMI >30 kg/m^2, high levels of hs-CRP were reported in 35% of men and 60% of women.[217] Increased CRP has been associated with increased risk of colorectal cancer and ovarian cancer.[218,219]

Hormones

Obese postmenopausal women have higher circulating levels of estrogens, which are accepted as part of the mechanism by which obesity is associated with breast and endometrial cancers.[220] Adipose tissue is the main source of estrogen in men and postmenopausal women. It expresses several sex steroid-metabolizing enzymes, including aromatase, and is therefore involved in the formation of estrogens from androgenic precursors.[31] Estrogen levels in obese postmenopausal women are 50–100 times higher than those of normal-weight individuals. It is believed that estrogen-sensitive tissues are therefore exposed to more estrogen and undergo more rapid growth. Obese premenopausal women do not have higher levels of plasma estrogens, presumably because their extraglandular production is small relative to the amount of estrogens arising from the premenopausal ovaries. Androstenedione is produced in greater quantity in women with abdominal obesity; consequently more substrate is available for aromatization to yield estrone, which is then converted to estradiol. In addition, in obesity the biologically available fraction of circulating estradiol is elevated due to reduced synthesis of sex hormone-binding globulin (SHBG), likely secondary to the suppressive effect of insulin on its hepatic production.[221] Dietary restriction can rapidly restore the serum SHBG levels to normal. Estrogen bioactivity is tightly regulated, with 30–50% of the plasma estradiol being strongly bound to the SHBG and therefore biologically inactive. As certain cancers are hormone dependent, this may affect cancer growth. Breast and other cancers that are ER positive respond to estradiol with significant cross talk between ER, insulin, and IGF-IR in an additive and even synergistic manner.[221] The Endogenous Hormone and Breast Cancer Collaborative Group reported a protective effect of SHBG in postmenopausal women and an increased risk in those with higher non-SHBG-bound estradiol concentration.[222] Similar findings have been reported with endometrial cancer.[220] In colon cancer, it has been reported that estrogen is inversely related to cancer risk, particularly in colonic tumors with MSI. One study shows that estrogen exposure protects against MSI and a lack of estrogen in older women may increase the risk.[223]

Reduced SHBG also allows for increased free testosterone levels. In prostate cancer, high levels of testosterone and low normal SHBG have been associated with an increased risk of prostate cancer.[224] In obese men, however, who may have lower circulating testosterone, there is evidence suggesting that they develop more aggressive tumors which are androgen independent.[47]

Conclusion

Our understanding of cancer development is rapidly evolving. While the incidence rates of many cancers are falling, it is concerning that those tumors related to obesity and type 2 diabetes are increasing in prevalence. Through recognizing this association, our insights into mechanisms of cancer development and possible novel therapeutic targets have progressed. But while the obesity epidemic continues to infiltrate our modern society, bringing with it as much risk as that associated with cigarette smoking, it is in our interest to prevent the cause of disease in preference to treating the consequences.

Online Resources

1. National Cancer Institute Factsheet: http://www.cancer.gov/cancertopics/factsheet/Risk/obesity
2. American Cancer Society Cancer Statistics http://www.cancer.org/docroot/stt/stt_0.asp
3. Endocrinology online text http://www.endotext.org

References

1. Maynard GD. A statistical study in cancer death-rates. *Biometrika*. 1910;7:276–304.
2. Kessler II. Cancer and diabetes mellitus a review of the literature. *J Chronic Dis*. 1971;23:579–600.
3. Sell C. Caloric restriction and insulin-like growth factors in aging and cancer. *Horm Metab Res*. 2003;35:705–711.
4. Calle EE, Rodriguez C, Walker-Thurmond K, Thun MJ. Overweight, obesity, and mortality from cancer in a prospectively studied cohort of U.S. adults. *N Engl J Med*. 2003;348:1625–1638.
5. Coughlin SS, Calle EE, Teras LR, Petrelli J, Thun MJ. Diabetes mellitus as a predictor of cancer mortality in a large cohort of US adults. *Am J Epidemiol*. 2004;159:1160–1167.
6. Inoue M, Iwasaki M, Otani T, Sasazuki S, Noda M, Tsugane S. Diabetes mellitus and the risk of cancer: results from a large-scale population-based cohort study in Japan. *Arch Intern Med*. 2006;166:1871–1877.
7. Jee SH, Ohrr H, Sull JW, Yun JE, Ji M, Samet JM. Fasting serum glucose level and cancer risk in Korean men and women. *JAMA*. 2005;293:194–202.
8. Stattin P, Bjor O, Ferrari P, et al. Prospective study of hyperglycemia and cancer risk. *Diabetes Care*. 2007;30:561–567.
9. Saydah SH, Loria CM, Eberhardt MS, Brancati FL. Abnormal glucose tolerance and the risk of cancer death in the United States. *Am J Epidemiol*. 2003;157:1092–1100.
10. Zendehdel K, Nyren O, Ostenson C-G, Adami H-O, Ekbom A, Ye W. Cancer incidence in patients with type 1 diabetes mellitus: a population-based cohort study in Sweden. *J Natl Cancer Inst*. 2003;95:1797–1800.
11. Friberg E, Orsini N, Mantzoros CS, Wolk A. Diabetes mellitus and risk of endometrial cancer: a meta-analysis. *Diabetologia*. 2007;50:1365–1374.
12. Wolf I, Sadetzki S, Catane R, Karasik A, Kaufman B. Diabetes mellitus and breast cancer. *Lancet Oncol*. 2005;6: 103–111.
13. Hjalgrim H, Frisch M, Ekbom A, Kyvik KO, Melbye M, Green A. Cancer and diabetes – a follow-up study of two population-based cohorts of diabetic patients. *J Intern Med*. 1997;241:471–475.
14. Rapp K, Schroeder J, Klenk J, et al. Obesity and incidence of cancer: a large cohort study of over 145,000 adults in Austria. *Br J Cancer*. 2005;93:1062–1067.
15. Verlato G, Zoppini G, Bonora E, Muggeo M. Mortality from site-specific malignancies in type 2 diabetic patients from Verona. *Diabetes Care*. 2003;26:1047–1051.
16. Kath R, Schiel R, Müller UA, Höffken K. Malignancies in patients with insulin-treated diabetes mellitus. *J Cancer Res Clin Oncol*. 2000;126:412–417.
17. Kasper JS, Giovannucci E. A meta-analysis of diabetes mellitus and the risk of prostate cancer. *Cancer Epidemiol Biomarkers Prev*. 2006;15:2056–2062.
18. Larsson SC, Mantzoros CS, Wolk A. Diabetes mellitus and risk of breast cancer: a meta-analysis. *Int J Cancer*. 2007;121: 856–862.
19. Larsson SC, Orsini N, Brismar K, Wolk A. Diabetes mellitus and risk of bladder cancer: a meta-analysis. *Diabetologia*. 2006;49:2819–2823.
20. Bonovas S, Filioussi K, Tsantes A. Diabetes mellitus and risk of prostate cancer: a meta-analysis. *Diabetologia*. 2004;47:1071–1078.
21. Huxley R, Ansary-Moghaddam A, Berrington de Gonzalez A, Barzi F, Woodward M. Type-II diabetes and pancreatic cancer: a meta-analysis of 36 studies. *Br J Cancer*. 2005;92:2076–2083.
22. Larsson SC, Orsini N, Wolk A. Diabetes mellitus and risk of colorectal cancer: a meta-analysis. *J Natl Cancer Inst*. 2005;97:1679–1687.
23. Zimmet PZ, Alberti KGMM. Introduction: globalization and the non-communicable disease epidemic. *Obesity*. 2006;14:1–3.
24. Ogden CL, Carroll MD, Curtin LR, McDowell MA, Tabak CJ, Flegal KM. Prevalence of overweight and obesity in the united states, 1999–2004. *JAMA*. 2006;295:1549–1555.
25. Lear SA, Humphries KH, Kohli S, Chockalingam A, Frohlich JJ, Birmingham CL. Visceral adipose tissue accumulation differs according to ethnic background: results of the multicultural community health assessment trial (M-CHAT). *Am J Clinl Nutr*. 2007;86:353–359.
26. Kubo A, Corley DA. Body mass index and adenocarcinomas of the esophagus or gastric cardia: a systematic review and meta-analysis. *Cancer Epidemiol Biomarkers Prev*. 2006;15:872–878.
27. Pan SY, Johnson KC, Ugnat A-M, Wen SW, Mao Y. Association of obesity and cancer risk in Canada. *Am J Epidemiol*. 2004;159:259–268.
28. Polednak AP. Trends in incidence rates for obesity-associated cancers in the US. *Cancer Detect Prev*. 2003;27:415–421.
29. Jemal A, Siegel R, Ward E, Murray T, Xu J, Thun MJ. Cancer statistics, 2007. *CA Cancer J Clin*. 2007;57:43–66.
30. Bergstrom A, Pisani P, Tenet V, Wolk A, Adami HO. Overweight as an avoidable cause of cancer in Europe. *Int J Cancer*. 2001;91:421–430.
31. Calle EE, Kaaks R. Overweight, obesity and cancer: epidemiological evidence and proposed mechanisms. *Nat Rev Cancer*. 2004;4:579–591.
32. Michels KB, Solomon CG, Hu FB, et al. Type 2 diabetes and subsequent incidence of breast cancer in the Nurses' Health Study. *Diabetes Care*. 2003;26:1752–1758.

33. Petrelli JM, Calle EE, Rodriguez C, Thun MJ. Body mass index, height, and postmenopausal breast cancer mortality in a prospective cohort of US women. *Cancer Causes Control*. 2002;13:325–332.

34. Friberg E, Mantzoros CS, Wolk A. Diabetes and risk of endometrial cancer: a population-based prospective cohort study. *Cancer Epidemiol Biomarkers Prev*. 2007;16:276–280.

35. Engeland A, Tretli S, Bjorge T. Height, body mass index, and ovarian cancer: a follow-up of 1.1 million Norwegian women. *J Natl Cancer Inst*. 2003;95:1244–1248.

36. Rodriguez C, Calle EE, Fakhrabadi-Shokoohi D, Jacobs EJ, Thun MJ. Body mass index, height, and the risk of ovarian cancer mortality in a prospective cohort of postmenopausal women. *Cancer Epidemiol Biomarkers Prev*. 2002;11: 822–828.

37. Anderson JP, Ross JA, Folsom AR. Anthropometric variables, physical activity, and incidence of ovarian cancer: the Iowa Women's Health Study. *Cancer*. 2004;100:1515–1521.

38. Pavelka JC, Brown RS, Karlan BY, et al. Effect of obesity on survival in epithelial ovarian cancer. *Cancer*. 2006;107: 1520–1524.

39. Olsen CM, Green AC, Whiteman DC, Sadeghi S, Kolahdooz F, Webb PM. Obesity and the risk of epithelial ovarian cancer: a systematic review and meta-analysis. *Euro J Cancer*. 2007;43:690–709.

40. Adler AI, Weiss NS, Kamb ML, Lyon JL. Is diabetes mellitus a risk factor for ovarian cancer? A case-control study in Utah and Washington (United States). *Cancer Causes Control*. 1996;7:475–478.

41. Weiderpass E, Ye W, Vainio H, Kaaks R, Adami H-O. Diabetes mellitus and ovarian cancer (Sweden). *Cancer Causes Control*. 2002;13:759–764.

42. Swerdlow AJ, Laing SP, Qiao Z, et al. Cancer incidence and mortality in patients with insulin-treated diabetes: a UK cohort study. *Br J Cancer*. 2005;92:2070–2075.

43. Lacey J, Frisch M, Brinton L, et al. Associations between smoking and adenocarcinomas and squamous cell carcinomas of the uterine cervix (United States). *Cancer Causes Control*. 2001;12:153–161.

44. Smith HO, Tiffany MF, Qualls CR, Key CR. The rising incidence of adenocarcinoma relative to squamous cell carcinoma of the uterine cervix in the United States – A 24-year population-based study. *Gynecol Oncol*. 2000;78:97–105.

45. Gong Z, Neuhouser ML, Goodman PJ, et al. Obesity, diabetes, and risk of prostate cancer: results from the prostate cancer prevention trial. *Cancer Epidemiol Biomarkers Prev*. 2006;15:1977–1983.

46. Freedland SJ, Platz EA. Obesity and prostate cancer: making sense out of apparently conflicting data. *Epidemiol Rev*. 2007;29:88–97.

47. Palma D, Pickles T, Tyldesley S. Obesity as a predictor of biochemical recurrence and survival after radiation therapy for prostate cancer. *BJU Int*. 2007;100:315–319.

48. Calton B, Chang S, Wright M, et al. History of diabetes mellitus and subsequent prostate cancer risk in the NIH-AARP Diet and Health Study. *Cancer Causes Control*. 2007;18:493–503.

49. Beebe-Dimmer JL, Dunn RL, Sarma AV, Montie JE, Cooney KA. Features of the metabolic syndrome and prostate cancer in African-American men. *Cancer*. 2007;109:875–881.

50. Coker AL, Sanderson M, Zheng W, Fadden MK. Diabetes mellitus and prostate cancer risk among older men: population-based case-control study. *Br J Cancer*. 2004;90:2171–2175.

51. Lindblad P, Chow WH, Chan J, et al. The role of diabetes mellitus in the aetiology of renal cell cancer. *Diabetologia*. 1999;42:107–112.

52. Chow W-H, Gridley G, Fraumeni JF, Jarvholm B. Obesity, hypertension, and the risk of kidney cancer in Men. *N Engl J Med*. 2000;343:1305–1311.

53. Wideroff L, Gridley G, Mellemkjaer L, et al. Cancer incidence in a population-based cohort of patients hospitalized with diabetes mellitus in Denmark. *J Natl Cancer Inst*. 1997;89:1360–1365.

54. Sturmer T, Buring JE, Lee IM, Gaziano JM, Glynn RJ. Metabolic abnormalities and risk for colorectal cancer in the Physicians' Health Study. *Cancer Epidemiol Biomarkers Prev*. 2006;15:2391–2397.

55. Hu FB, Manson JE, Liu S, et al. Prospective study of adult onset diabetes mellitus (type 2) and risk of colorectal cancer in women. *J Natl Cancer Inst*. 1999;91:542–547.

56. Larsson SC, Wolk A. Obesity and colon and rectal cancer risk: a meta-analysis of prospective studies. *Am J Clinl Nutr*. 2007;86:556–565.

57. Chlebowski RT, Wactawski-Wende J, Ritenbaugh C, et al. Estrogen plus progestin and colorectal cancer in postmenopausal women. *N Engl J Med*. 2004;350:991–1004.

58. Kanaya AM, Herrington D, Vittinghoff E, et al. Glycemic effects of postmenopausal hormone therapy: the heart and estrogen/progestin replacement study: a randomized, double-blind, placebo-controlled trial. *Ann Intern Med*. 2003;138:1–9.

59. Friedenreich CM, Orenstein MR. Physical activity and cancer prevention: etiologic evidence and biological mechanisms. *J Nutr*. 2002;132:3456S–64S.

60. Bingham SA, Norat T, Moskal A, et al. Is the association with fiber from foods in colorectal cancer confounded by folate intake? *Cancer Epidemiol Biomarkers Prev*. 2005;14:1552–1556.

61. Norat T, Bingham S, Ferrari P, et al. Meat, fish, and colorectal cancer risk: the European prospective investigation into cancer and nutrition. *J Natl Cancer Inst*. 2005;97:906–916.

62. Meyerhardt JA, Niedzwiecki D, Hollis D, et al. Association of dietary patterns with cancer recurrence and survival in patients with stage III colon cancer. *JAMA*. 2007;298:754–764.

63. Devesa SS, Blot WJ, Fraumeni JF Jr. Changing patterns in the incidence of esophageal and gastric carcinoma in the United States. *Cancer*. 1998;83:2049–2053.

64. Mayne ST, Navarro SA. Diet, obesity and reflux in the etiology of adenocarcinomas of the esophagus and gastric cardia in humans. *J Nutr*. 2002;132:3467S–3470.

65. Ji BT, Chow WH, Yang G, et al. Body mass index and the risk of cancers of the gastric cardia and distal stomach in Shanghai, China. *Cancer Epidemiol Biomarkers Prev*. 1997;6:481–485.

66. Hampel H, Abraham NS, El-Serag HB. Meta-analysis: obesity and the risk for gastroesophageal reflux disease and its complications. *Ann Intern Med*. 2005;143:199–211.

67. Rousseau MC, Parent ME, Pollak MN, Siemiatycki J. Diabetes mellitus and cancer risk in a population-based case-control study among men from Montreal, Canada. *Int J Cancer*. 2006;118:2105–2109.

68. Rubenstein JH, Davis J, Marrero JA, Inadomi JM. Relationship between diabetes mellitus and adenocarcinoma of the oesophagus and gastric cardia. *Aliment Pharmacol Ther*. 2005;22:267–271.

69. Wang F, Herrington M, Larsson J, Permert J. The relationship between diabetes and pancreatic cancer. *Mol Cancer*. 2003;2:4.

70. Noy A, Bilezikian JP. Clinical review 63: diabetes and pancreatic cancer: clues to the early diagnosis of pancreatic malignancy. *J Clin Endocrinol Metab*. 1994;79:1223–1231.

71. Gapstur SM, Gann PH, Lowe W, Liu K, Colangelo L, Dyer A. Abnormal glucose metabolism and pancreatic cancer mortality. *JAMA*. 2000;283:2552–2558.

72. Everhart J, Wright D. Diabetes mellitus as a risk factor for pancreatic cancer. A meta-analysis. *JAMA*. 1995;273:1605–1609.

73. Calle EE, Murphy TK, Rodriguez C, Thun MJ, Heath CW Jr. Diabetes mellitus and pancreatic cancer mortality in a prospective cohort of United States adults. *Cancer Causes Control*. 1998;9:403–410.

74. Chari ST, Leibson CL, Rabe KG, Ransom J, de Andrade M, Petersen GM. Probability of pancreatic cancer following diabetes: a population-based study. *Gastroenterology*. 2005;129:504–511.

75. Patel AV, Rodriguez C, Bernstein L, Chao A, Thun MJ, Calle EE. Obesity, recreational physical activity, and risk of pancreatic cancer in a large U.S. cohort. *Cancer Epidemiol Biomarkers Prev*. 2005;14:459–466.

76. Canoy D, Wareham N, Luben R, et al. Cigarette smoking and fat distribution in 21,828 British men and women: a population-based study. *Obesity Res*. 2005;13:1466–1475.

77. Coughlin SS, Calle EE, Patel AV, Thun MJ. Predictors of pancreatic cancer mortality among a large cohort of United States adults. *Cancer Causes Control*. 2000;11:915–923.

78. Adami HO, Chow WH, Nyren O, et al. Excess risk of primary liver cancer in patients with diabetes mellitus. *J Natl Cancer Inst*. 1996;88:1472–1477.

79. Lai MS, Hsieh MS, Chiu YH, Chen TH. Type 2 diabetes and hepatocellular carcinoma: A cohort study in high prevalence area of hepatitis virus infection. *Hepatology*. 2006;43:1295–1302.

80. Welzel TM, Graubard BI, El-Serag HB, et al. Risk factors for intrahepatic and extrahepatic cholangiocarcinoma in the United States: a population-based case-control study. *Clin Gastroenterol Hepatol*. 2007;5:1221–1228.

81. Shaib YH, El-Serag HB, Davila JA, Morgan R, McGlynn KA. Risk factors of intrahepatic cholangiocarcinoma in the United States: a case-control study. *Gastroenterology*. 2005;128:620–626.

82. Ahrens W, Timmer A, Vyberg M, et al. Risk factors for extrahepatic biliary tract carcinoma in men: medical conditions and lifestyle: results from a European multicentre case-control study. *Eur J Gastroenterol Hepatol*. 2007;19:623–630.

83. Larsson SC, Wolk A. Body mass index and risk of multiple myeloma: a meta-analysis. *Int J Cancer*. 2007;121:2512–2516.

84. Larsson SC, Wolk A. Obesity and risk of non-Hodgkin's lymphoma: a meta-analysis. *Int J Cancer*. 2007;121:1564–1570.

85. Lim U, Morton LM, Subar AF, et al. Alcohol, smoking, and body size in relation to incident Hodgkin's and non-Hodgkin's lymphoma risk. *Am J Epidemiol*. 2007;166:697–708.

86. Birmann BM, Giovannucci E, Rosner B, Anderson KC, Colditz GA. Body mass index, physical activity, and risk of multiple myeloma. *Cancer Epidemiol Biomarkers Prev*. 2007;16:1474–1478.

87. Butturini AM, Dorey FJ, Lange BJ, et al. Obesity and outcome in pediatric acute lymphoblastic leukemia. *J Clin Oncol*. 2007;25:2063–2069.

88. Chiu BCH, Gapstur SM, Greenland P, Wang R, Dyer A. Body mass index, abnormal glucose metabolism, and mortality from hematopoietic cancer. *Cancer Epidemiol Biomarkers Prev*. 2006;15:2348–2354.

89. Olson JE, Yang P, Schmitz K, Vierkant RA, Cerhan JR, Sellers TA. Differential association of body mass index and fat distribution with three major histologic types of lung cancer: evidence from a cohort of older women. *Am J Epidemiol*. 2002;156:606–615.

90. Hall GC, Roberts CM, Boulis M, Mo J, MacRae KD. Diabetes and the risk of lung cancer. *Diabetes Care*. 2005;28:590–594.

91. Kanashiki M, Sairenchi T, Saito Y, Ishikawa H, Satoh H, Sekizawa K. Body mass index and lung cancer: a case-control study of subjects participating in a mass-screening program. *Chest*. 2005;128:1490–1496.

92. Kuriki K, Hirose K, Tajima K. Diabetes and cancer risk for all and specific sites among Japanese men and women. *Eur J Cancer Prev*. 2007;16:83–89.

93. Renehan AG, Frystyk J, Flyvbjerg A. Obesity and cancer risk: the role of the insulin-IGF axis. *Trends Endocrinol Metab*. 2006;17:328–336.

94. Frystyk J, Skjaerbaek C, Vestbo E, Fisker S, Orskov H. Circulating levels of free insulin-like growth factors in obese subjects: the impact of type 2 diabetes. *Diabetes Metab Res Rev*. 1999;15:314–322.

95. LeRoith D, Roberts CT. The insulin-like growth factor system and cancer. *Cancer Lett*. 2003;195:127–137.

96. Baxter RC. Insulin-like growth factor (IGF)-binding proteins: interactions with IGFs and intrinsic bioactivities. *Am J Physiol Endocrinol Metab*. 2000;278:E967–E976.

97. Firth SM, Baxter RC. Cellular actions of the insulin-like growth factor binding proteins. *Endocr Rev*. 2002;23:824–854.

98. Chen JC, Shao ZM, Sheikh MS, et al. Insulin-like growth factor-binding protein enhancement of insulin-like growth factor-I (IGF-I)-mediated DNA synthesis and IGF-I binding in a human breast carcinoma cell line. *J Cell Physiol*. 1994;158: 69–78.

99. Morris JK, George LM, Wu T, Wald NJ. Insulin-like growth factors and cancer: no role in screening. Evidence from the BUPA study and meta-analysis of prospective epidemiological studies. *Br J Cancer*. 2006;95:112–117.

100. Renehan AG, Zwahlen M, Minder C, O'Dwyer ST, Shalet SM, Egger M. Insulin-like growth factor (IGF)-I, IGF binding protein-3, and cancer risk: systematic review and meta-regression analysis. *Lancet*. 2004;363:1346–1353.

101. Chen C, Lewis SK, Voigt L, Fitzpatrick A, Plymate SR, Weiss NS. Prostate carcinoma incidence in relation to prediagnostic circulating levels of insulin-like growth factor I, insulin-like growth factor binding protein 3, and insulin. *Cancer*. 2005;103:76–84.

102. Janssen JAMJL, Wildhagen MF, Ito K, et al. Circulating free insulin-like growth factor (IGF)-I, total IGF-I, and IGF binding protein-3 levels do not predict the future risk to develop prostate cancer: results of a case-control study involving 201 patients within a population-based screening with a 4-year interval. *J Clin Endocrinol Metab*. 2004;89:4391–4396.

103. Kaaks R, Toniolo P, Akhmedkhanov A, et al. Serum C-peptide, insulin-like growth factor (IGF)-I, IGF-binding proteins, and colorectal cancer risk in women. *J Natl Cancer Inst*. 2000;92:1592–1600.

104. Jenab M, Riboli E, Cleveland RJ, et al. Serum C-peptide, IGFBP-1 and IGFBP-2 and risk of colon and rectal cancers in the European prospective investigation into cancer and nutrition. *Int J Cancer*. 2007;121:368–376.

105. Baglietto L, English DR, Hopper JL, Morris HA, Tilley WD, Giles GG. Circulating insulin-like growth factor-I and binding protein-3 and the risk of breast cancer. *Cancer Epidemiol Biomarkers Prev*. 2007;16:763–768.

106. Severi G, Morris HA, MacInnis RJ, et al. Circulating insulin-like growth factor-I and binding protein-3 and risk of prostate cancer. *Cancer Epidemiol Biomarkers Prev*. 2006;15:1137–1141.

107. Allen NE, Key TJ, Appleby PN, et al. Serum insulin-like growth factor (IGF)-I and IGF-binding protein-3 concentrations and prostate cancer risk: results from the European prospective investigation into cancer and nutrition. *Cancer Epidemiol Biomarkers Prev*. 2007;16:1121–1127.

108. Krajcik RA, Borofsky ND, Massardo S, Orentreich N. Insulin-like growth factor I (IGF-I), IGF-binding proteins, and breast cancer. *Cancer Epidemiol Biomarkers Prev*. 2002;11:1566–1573.

109. Tran TT, Gupta N, Goh T, et al. Direct measure of insulin sensitivity with the hyperinsulinemic-euglycemic clamp and surrogate measures of insulin sensitivity with the oral glucose tolerance test: correlations with aberrant crypt foci promotion in rats. *Cancer Epidemiol Biomarkers Prev*. 2003;12:47–56.

110. Koohestani N, Chia MC, Pham NA, et al. Aberrant crypt focus promotion and glucose intolerance: correlation in the rat across diets differing in fat, n-3 fatty acids and energy. *Carcinogenesis*. 1998;19:1679–1684.

111. Bowker SL, Majumdar SR, Veugelers P, Johnson JA. Increased cancer-related mortality for patients with type 2 diabetes who use sulfonylureas or insulin. *Diabetes Care*. 2006;29(2):254–258.

112. Smith U, Gale EA. Does diabetes therapy influence the risk of cancer? Diabetologia. 2009;52(9):1699–1708.

113. Novosyadlyy R, Vijayakumar A, Lann D, Fierz Y, Kurshnan N, LeRoith D. Physical and functional interaction between polyoma virus T antigen and insulin and IGF-I receptors is required for oncogene activation and tumor initiation. *Oncogene*. 2009;doi:10.1038/onc.2009.209.

114. Bol DK, Kiguchi K, Gimenez-Conti I, Rupp T, DiGiovanni J. Overexpression of insulin-like growth factor-1 induces hyperplasia, dermal abnormalities, and spontaneous tumor formation in transgenic mice. *Oncogene*. 1997;14: 1725–1734.

115. Pollak M, Blouin MJ, Zhang JC, Kopchick JJ. Reduced mammary gland carcinogenesis in transgenic mice expressing a growth hormone antagonist. *Br J Cancer*. 2001;85:428–430.

116. Dunn SE, Kari FW, French J, et al. Dietary restriction reduces insulin-like growth factor I levels, which modulates apoptosis, cell proliferation, and tumor progression in p53-deficient mice. *Cancer Res*. 1997;57:4667–4672.

117. Thissen JP, Ketelslegers JM, Underwood LE. Nutritional regulation of the insulin-like growth factors. *Endocr Rev*. 1994;15:80–101.

118. Wu Y, Yakar S, Zhao L, Hennighausen L, LeRoith D. Circulating insulin-like growth factor-I levels regulate colon cancer growth and metastasis. *Cancer Res*. 2002;62:1030–1035.

119. Yang X-F, Beamer WG, Huynh H, Pollak M. Reduced growth of human breast cancer xenografts in hosts homozygous for the lit mutation. *Cancer Res*. 1996;56:1509–1511.

120. Deitel K, Dantzer D, Ferguson P, et al. Reduced growth of human sarcoma xenografts in hosts homozygous for the lit mutation. *J Surg Oncol*. 2002;81:75–79.

121. Wu Y, Cui K, Miyoshi K, et al. Reduced circulating insulin-like growth factor i levels delay the onset of chemically and genetically induced mammary tumors. *Cancer Res*. 2003;63:4384–4388.

122. Ramsey MM, Ingram RL, Cashion AB, et al. Growth hormone-deficient dwarf animals are resistant to dimethylbenzanthracene (DMBA)-induced mammary carcinogenesis. *Endocrinology*. 2002;143:4139–4142.

123. Swanson SM, Unterman TG. The growth hormone-deficient Spontaneous Dwarf rat is resistant to chemically induced mammary carcinogenesis. *Carcinogenesis*. 2002;23:977–982.

124. Dunn SE, Hardman RA, Kari FW, Barrett JC. Insulin-like growth factor 1 (IGF-1) alters drug sensitivity of HBL100 human breast cancer cells by inhibition of apoptosis induced by diverse anticancer drugs. *Cancer Res.* 1997;57: 2687–2693.

125. Yakar S, Pennisi P, Kim CH, et al. Studies involving the GH-IGF axis: lessons from IGF-I and IGF-I receptor gene targeting mouse models. *J Endocrinol Invest.* 2005;28:19–22.

126. LeRoith D, Werner H, Beitner-Johnson D, Roberts CT Jr. Molecular and cellular aspects of the insulin-like growth factor I receptor. *Endocr Rev.* 1995;16:143–163.

127. Le Roith D, Bondy C, Yakar S, Liu J-L, Butler A. The somatomedin hypothesis: 2001. *Endocr Rev.* 2001;22:53–74.

128. Yakar S, LeRoith D, Brodt P. The role of the growth hormone/insulin-like growth factor axis in tumor growth and progression: lessons from animal models. *Cytokine Growth Factor Rev.* 2005;16:407–420.

129. Levine AJ, Feng Z, Mak TW, You H, Jin S. Coordination and communication between the p53 and IGF-1-AKT-TOR signal transduction pathways. *Genes Dev.* 2006;20:267–275.

130. Kooijman R. Regulation of apoptosis by insulin-like growth factor (IGF)-I. *Cytokine Growth Factor Rev.* 2006;17:305–323.

131. White MF. The IRS-signalling system: A network of docking proteins that mediate insulin action. *Mol Cell Biochem.* 1998;182:3–11.

132. Kisseleva T, Bhattacharya S, Braunstein J, Schindler CW. Signaling through the JAK/STAT pathway, recent advances and future challenges. *Gene.* 2002;285:1–24.

133. Owerbach D, Bell GI, Rutter WJ, Shows TB. The insulin gene is located on chromosome 11 in humans. *Nature.* 1980;286: 82–84.

134. Kennedy GC, German MS, Rutter WJ. The minisatellite in the diabetes susceptibility locus IDDM2 regulates insulin transcription. *Nat Genet.* 1995;9:293–298.

135. Lucassen AM, Julier C, Beressi J-P, et al. Susceptibility to insulin dependent diabetes mellitus maps to a 4.1 kb segment of DNA spanning the insulin gene and associated VNTR. *Nat Genet.* 1993;4:305–310.

136. Bennett ST, Todd JA. Human type 1 diabetes and the insulin gene: principles of mapping polygenes. *Annu Rev Genet.* 1996;30:343–370.

137. Rodriguez S, Gaunt T, Day I. Molecular genetics of human growth hormone, insulin-like growth factors and their pathways in common disease. *Hum Genet.* 2007;122:1–21.

138. Ho GY, Melman A, Liu SM, et al. Polymorphism of the insulin gene is associated with increased prostate cancer risk. *Br J Cancer.* 2003;88:263–269.

139. Claeys GB, Sarma AV, Dunn RL, et al. INSPstI polymorphism and prostate cancer in African-American men. *Prostate.* 2005;65:83–87.

140. Neuhausen SL, Slattery ML, Garner CP, Ding YC, Hoffman M, Brothman AR. Prostate cancer risk and IRS1, IRS2, IGF1, and INS polymorphisms: strong association of IRS1 G972R variant and cancer risk. *The Prostate.* 2005;64: 168–174.

141. Morimoto LM, Newcomb PA, White E, Bigler J, Potter JD. Insulin-like growth factor polymorphisms and colorectal cancer risk. *Cancer Epidemiol Biomarkers Prev.* 2005;14:1204–1211.

142. Chen C, Freeman R, Voigt LF, Fitzpatrick A, Plymate SR, Weiss NS. Prostate cancer risk in relation to selected genetic polymorphisms in insulin-like growth factor-I, insulin-like growth factor binding protein-3, and insulin-like growth factor-I receptor. *Cancer Epidemiol Biomarkers Prev.* 2006;15:2461–2466.

143. Tsuchiya N, Wang L, Suzuki H, et al. Impact of IGF-I and CYP19 gene polymorphisms on the survival of patients with metastatic prostate cancer. *J Clin Oncol.* 2006;24:1982–1989.

144. Cheng I, Stram DO, Penney KL, et al. Common genetic variation in IGF1 and prostate cancer risk in the multiethnic cohort. *J Natl Cancer Inst.* 2006;98:123–134.

145. Wagner K, Hemminki K, Försti A. The GH1/IGF-1 axis polymorphisms and their impact on breast cancer development. *Breast Cancer Res Treatment.* 2007;104:233–248.

146. Johansson M, McKay JD, Stattin P, et al. Comprehensive evaluation of genetic variation in the IGF1 gene and risk of prostate cancer. *Int J Cancer.* 2007;120:539–542.

147. Al-Zahrani A, Sandhu MS, Luben RN, et al. IGF1 and IGFBP3 tagging polymorphisms are associated with circulating levels of IGF1, IGFBP3 and risk of breast cancer. *Hum Mol Genet.* 2006;15:1–10.

148. Murrell A, Heeson S, Cooper WN, et al. An association between variants in the IGF2 gene and Beckwith-Wiedemann syndrome: interaction between genotype and epigenotype. *Hum Mol Genet.* 2004;13:247–255.

149. Cui H, Cruz-Correa M, Giardiello FM, et al. Loss of IGF2 imprinting: a potential marker of colorectal cancer risk. *Science.* 2003;299:1753–1755.

150. Sigal RJ, Doria A, Warram JH, Krolewski AS. Codon 972 polymorphism in the insulin receptor substrate-1 gene, obesity, and risk of noninsulin-dependent diabetes mellitus. *J Clin Endocrinol Metab.* 1996;81:1657–1659.

151. Marini MA, Frontoni S, Mineo D, et al. The Arg972 variant in insulin receptor substrate-1 is associated with an atherogenic profile in offspring of type 2 diabetic patients. *J Clin Endocrinol Metab.* 2003;88:3368–3371.

152. Perticone F, Sciacqua A, Scozzafava A, et al. Impaired endothelial function in never-treated hypertensive subjects carrying the Arg972 polymorphism in the insulin receptor substrate-1 gene. *J Clin Endocrinol Metab.* 2004;89:3606–3609.

153. Hribal ML, Federici M, Porzio O, et al. The Gly->Arg972 amino acid polymorphism in insulin receptor substrate-1 affects glucose metabolism in skeletal muscle cells. *J Clin Endocrinol Metab.* 2000;85:2004–2013.

154. Canzian F, McKay JD, Cleveland RJ, et al. Polymorphisms of genes coding for insulin-like growth factor 1 and its major binding proteins, circulating levels of IGF-I and IGFBP-3 and breast cancer risk: results from the EPIC study. *Br J Cancer*. 2006;94:299–307.

155. Deal C, Ma J, Wilkin F, et al. Novel promoter polymorphism in insulin-like growth factor-binding protein-3: correlation with serum levels and interaction with known regulators. *J Clin Endocrinol Metab*. 2001;86:1274–1280.

156. Rudd MF, Webb EL, Matakidou A, et al. Variants in the GH-IGF axis confer susceptibility to lung cancer. *Genome Res*. 2006;16:693–701.

157. Reiling JH, Sabatini DM. Stress and mTORture signaling. *Oncogene*. 2006;25:6373–6383.

158. Vogelstein B, Kinzler KW. p53 function and dysfunction. *Cell*. 1992;70:523–526.

159. Oliner JD, Kinzler KW, Meltzer PS, George DL, Vogelstein B. Amplification of a gene encoding a p53-associated protein in human sarcomas. *Nature*. 1992;358:80–83.

160. Shieh S-Y, Ikeda M, Taya Y, Prives C. DNA damage-induced phosphorylation of p53 alleviates inhibition by MDM2. *Cell*. 1997;91:325–334.

161. Sugimoto Y, Whitman M, Cantley LC, Erikson RL. Evidence that the Rous sarcoma virus transforming gene product phosphorylates phosphatidylinositol and diacylglycerol. *Proc Natl Acad Sci USA*. 1984;81:2117–2121.

162. Ogg S, Paradis S, Gottlieb S, et al. The Fork head transcription factor DAF-16 transduces insulin-like metabolic and longevity signals in *C. elegans*. *Nature*. 1997;389:994–999.

163. Greer EL, Dowlatshahi D, Banko MR, et al. An AMPK-FOXO pathway mediates longevity induced by a novel method of dietary restriction in *C. elegans*. *Curr Biol*. 2007;17:1646–1656.

164. Shen W-H, Zhou J-H, Broussard SR, Freund GG, Dantzer R, Kelley KW. Proinflammatory cytokines block growth of breast cancer cells by impairing signals from a growth factor receptor. *Cancer Res*. 2002;62:4746–4756.

165. Heron-Milhavet L, LeRoith D. Insulin-like growth factor I induces MDM2-dependent degradation of p53 via the p38 MAPK pathway in response to DNA damage. *J Biol Chem*. 2002;277:15600–15606.

166. Tanno S, Tanno S, Mitsuuchi Y, Altomare DA, Xiao G-H, Testa JR. AKT activation up-regulates insulin-like growth factor I receptor expression and promotes invasiveness of human pancreatic cancer cells. *Cancer Res*. 2001;61: 589–593.

167. Qi H, Xiao L, Lingyun W, et al. Expression of type 1 insulin-like growth factor receptor in marrow nucleated cells in malignant hematological disorders: correlation with apoptosis. *Ann Hematol*. 2006;85:95–101.

168. Giardiello FM, Brensinger JD, TersmetteS AC, et al. Very high risk of cancer in familial Peutz-Jeghers syndrome. *Gastroenterology*. 2000;119:1447–1453.

169. Karuman P, Gozani O, Odze RD, et al. The Peutz-Jegher gene product LKB1 is a mediator of p53-dependent cell death. *Mol Cell*. 2001;7:1307–1319.

170. Su GH, Hruban RH, Bansal RK, et al. Germline and somatic mutations of the STK11/LKB1 Peutz-Jeghers gene in pancreatic and biliary cancers. *Am J Pathol*. 1999;154:1835–1840.

171. Rowan A, Bataille V, MacKie R, et al. Somatic mutations in the Peutz-Jegners (LKB1//STKII) gene in sporadic malignant melanomas. *J Invest Dermatol*. 1999;112:509–511.

172. Guervos MA, Marcos CA, Hermsen M, Nuno AS, Suarez C, Llorente JL. Deletions of N33, STK11 and TP53 are involved in the development of lymph node metastasis in larynx and pharynx carcinomas. *Cell Oncol*. 2007;29:327–334.

173. Shaw RJ, Lamia KA, Vasquez D, et al. The kinase LKB1 mediates glucose homeostasis in liver and therapeutic effects of metformin. *Science*. 2005;310:1642–1646.

174. Evans JMM, Donnelly LA, Emslie-Smith AM, Alessi DR, Morris AD. Metformin and reduced risk of cancer in diabetic patients. *BMJ*. 2005;330:1304–1305.

175. Bowker SL, Majumdar SR, Veugelers P, Johnson JA. Increased cancer-related mortality for patients with type 2 diabetes who use sulfonylureas or insulin. *Diabetes Care*. 2006;29:254–258.

176. Zakikhani M, Dowling R, Fantus IG, Sonenberg N, Pollak M. Metformin is an AMP kinase-dependent growth inhibitor for breast cancer cells. *Cancer Res*. 2006;66:10269–10273.

177. Fukuda R, Hirota K, Fan F, Jung YD, Ellis LM, Semenza GL. Insulin-like growth factor 1 induces hypoxia-inducible factor 1-mediated vascular endothelial growth factor expression, which is dependent on MAP kinase and phosphatidylinositol 3-kinase signaling in colon cancer cells. *J Biol Chem*. 2002;277:38205–38211.

178. Canonici A, Steelant W, Rigot V, et al. Insulin-like growth factor-I receptor, E-cadherin and alphav integrin form a dynamic complex under the control of alpha-catenin. *Int J Cancer*. 2008;1:572-582.

179. Becker K-F, Atkinson MJ, Reich U, et al. E-cadherin gene mutations provide clues to diffuse type gastric carcinomas. *Cancer Res*. 1994;54:3845–3852.

180. Zhang Y, Proenca R, Maffei M, Barone M, Leopold L, Friedman JM. Positional cloning of the mouse obese gene and its human homologue. *Nature*. 1994;372:425–432.

181. Farooqi IS, Jebb SA, Langmack G, et al. Effects of recombinant leptin therapy in a child with congenital leptin deficiency. *N Engl J Med*. 1999;341:879–884.

182. Maffei M, Fei H, Lee GH, et al. Increased expression in adipocytes of ob RNA in mice with lesions of the hypothalamus and with mutations at the db locus. *Proc Natl Acad Sci USA*. 1995;92:6957–6960.

183. Fung TT, Rimm EB, Spiegelman D, et al. Association between dietary patterns and plasma biomarkers of obesity and cardiovascular disease risk. *Am J Clinl Nutr*. 2001;73:61–67.

184. Sandhu MS, Dunger DB, Giovannucci EL. Insulin, insulin-like growth factor-I (IGF-I), IGF binding proteins, their biologic interactions, and colorectal cancer. *J Natl Cancer Inst*. 2002;94:972–980.

185. Hutley L, Prins JB. Fat as an endocrine organ: relationship to the metabolic syndrome. *Am J Med Sci*. 2005;330:280–289.

186. Konopleva M, Mikhail A, Estrov Z, et al. Expression and function of leptin receptor isoforms in myeloid leukemia and myelodysplastic syndromes: proliferative and anti-apoptotic activities. *Blood*. 1999;93:1668–1676.

187. Onuma M, Bub JD, Rummel TL, Iwamoto Y. Prostate cancer cell-adipocyte interaction: leptin mediates androgen-independent prostate cancer cell proliferation through c-Jun NH2-terminal kinase. *J Biol Chem*. 2003;278:42660–42667.

188. Somasundar P, Riggs D, Jackson L, Vona-Davis L, McFadden DW. Leptin stimulates esophageal adenocarcinoma growth by nonapoptotic mechanisms. *Am J Surg*. 2003;186:575–578.

189. Hu X, Juneja SC, Maihle NJ, Cleary MP. Leptin – a growth factor in normal and malignant breast cells and for normal mammary gland development. *J Natl Cancer Inst*. 2002;94:1704–1711.

190. Okumura M, Yamamoto M, Sakuma H, et al. Leptin and high glucose stimulate cell proliferation in MCF-7 human breast cancer cells: reciprocal involvement of PKC-[alpha] and PPAR expression. *Biochim Biophys Acta*. 2002;1592:107–116.

191. Hardwick JCH, Van Den Brink GR, Offerhaus GJ, Van Deventer SJH, Peppelenbosch MP. Leptin is a growth factor for colonic epithelial cells. *Gastroenterology*. 2001;121:79–90.

192. Rose DP, Komninou D, Stephenson GD. Obesity, adipocytokines, and insulin resistance in breast cancer. *Obes Rev*. 2004;5:153–165.

193. Kim C-H, Pennisi P, Zhao H, et al. MKR mice are resistant to the metabolic actions of both insulin and adiponectin: discordance between insulin resistance and adiponectin responsiveness. *Am J Physiol Endocrinol Metab*. 2006;291:E298–E305.

194. Tsatsanis C, Zacharioudaki V, Androulidaki A, et al. Peripheral factors in the metabolic syndrome: the pivotal role of adiponectin. *Ann N Y Acad Sci*. 2006;1083:185–195.

195. Yamauchi T, Kamon J, Minokoshi Y, et al. Adiponectin stimulates glucose utilization and fatty-acid oxidation by activating AMP-activated protein kinase. *Nature Med*. 2002;8:1288–1295.

196. Kelesidis I, Kelesidis T, Mantzoros CS. Adiponectin and cancer: a systematic review. *Br J Cancer*. 2006;94:1221–1225.

197. Marshall S. Role of insulin, adipocyte hormones, and nutrient-sensing pathways in regulating fuel metabolism and energy homeostasis: a nutritional perspective of diabetes, obesity, and cancer. *Sci STKE*. 2006;2006:re7.

198. Ishikawa M, Kitayama J, Yamauchi T, et al. Adiponectin inhibits the growth and peritoneal metastasis of gastric cancer through its specific membrane receptors AdipoR1 and AdipoR2. *Cancer Sci*. 2007;98:1120–1127.

199. Brakenhielm E, Veitonmaki N, Cao R, et al. Adiponectin-induced antiangiogenesis and antitumor activity involve caspase-mediated endothelial cell apoptosis. *Proc Natl Acad Sci U.S.A.* 2004;101:2476–2481.

200. Hursting SD, Nunez NP, Varticovski L, Vinson C. The obesity-cancer link: lessons learned from a fatless mouse. *Cancer Res*. 2007;67:2391–2393.

201. Berndt J, Kovacs P, Ruschke K, et al. Fatty acid synthase gene expression in human adipose tissue: association with obesity and type 2 diabetes. *Diabetologia*. 2007;50:1472–1480.

202. Ogino S, Kawasaki T, Ogawa A, Kirkner GJ, Loda M, Fuchs CS. Fatty acid synthase overexpression in colorectal cancer is associated with microsatellite instability, independent of CpG island methylator phenotype. *Hum Pathol*. 2007;38:842–849.

203. Kinlaw WB, Quinn JL, Wells WA, Roser-Jones C, Moncur JT. Spot 14: a marker of aggressive breast cancer and a potential therapeutic target. *Endocrinology*. 2006;147:4048–4055.

204. Menendez JA, Vellon L, Mehmi I, et al. Inhibition of fatty acid synthase (FAS) suppresses HER2/neu (erbB-2) oncogene overexpression in cancer cells. *Proc Natl Acad Sci U.S.A.* 2004;101:10715–10720.

205. Hardy S, St-Onge GG, Joly E, Langelier Y, Prentki M. Oleate promotes the proliferation of breast cancer cells via the G protein-coupled receptor GPR40. *J Biol Chem*. 2005;280:13285–13291.

206. Kridel SJ, Axelrod F, Rozenkrantz N, Smith JW. Orlistat is a novel inhibitor of fatty acid synthase with antitumor activity. *Cancer Res*. 2004;64:2070–2075.

207. Gonullu G, Ersoy C, Ersoy A, et al. Relation between insulin resistance and serum concentrations of IL-6 and TNF-alpha in overweight or obese women with early stage breast cancer. *Cytokine*. 2005;31:264–269.

208. Cozen W, Gebregziabher M, Conti DV, et al. Interleukin-6-related genotypes, body mass index, and risk of multiple myeloma and plasmacytoma. *Cancer Epidemiol Biomarkers Prev*. 2006;15:2285–2291.

209. Duell EJ, Casella DP, Burk RD, Kelsey KT, Holly EA. Inflammation, genetic polymorphisms in proinflammatory genes TNF-A, RANTES, and CCR5, and risk of pancreatic adenocarcinoma. *Cancer Epidemiol Biomarkers Prev*. 2006;15:726–731.

210. Plaisance I, Morandi C, Murigande C, Brink M. TNF-{alpha} increases protein content in C2C12 and primary myotubes by enhancing protein translation via the TNF-R1, PI3-kinase and MEK. *Am J Physiol Endocrinol Metab*. 2008;294:E241–E250, 00129.2007.

211. Zinman B, Hanley AJG, Harris SB, Kwan J, Fantus IG. Circulating tumor necrosis factor-{alpha} concentrations in a native canadian population with high rates of type 2 diabetes mellitus. *J Clin Endocrinol Metab*. 1999;84:272–278.

212. de Alvaro C, Teruel T, Hernandez R, Lorenzo M. Tumor necrosis factor {alpha} produces insulin resistance in skeletal muscle by activation of inhibitor {kappa}B kinase in a p38 MAPK-dependent manner. *J Biol Chem*. 2004;279:17070–17078.

213. Uysal KT, Wiesbrock SM, Marino MW, Hotamisligil GS. Protection from obesity-induced insulin resistance in mice lacking TNF-[alpha] function. *Nature*. 1997;389:610–614.

214. Zamboni M, Di Francesco V, Garbin U, et al. Adiponectin gene expression and adipocyte NF-[kappa]B transcriptional activity in elderly overweight and obese women: inter-relationships with fat distribution, hs-CRP, leptin and insulin resistance. *Int J Obes*. 2007;31:1104–1109.

215. Wu JT, Kral JG. The NF-[kappa]B/I[kappa]B signaling system: a molecular target in breast cancer therapy. *J Surg Res*. 2005;123:158–169.

216. Biswas DK, Dai S-C, Cruz A, Weiser B, Graner E, Pardee AB. The nuclear factor kappa B (NF-kappa B): A potential therapeutic target for estrogen receptor negative breast cancers. *Proc Natl Acad Sci USA*. 2001;98:10386–10391.

217. Visser M, Bouter LM, McQuillan GM, Wener MH, Harris TB. Elevated C-reactive protein levels in overweight and obese adults. *JAMA*. 1999;282:2131–2135.

218. Erlinger TP, Platz EA, Rifai N, Helzlsouer KJ. C-reactive protein and the risk of incident colorectal cancer. *JAMA*. 2004;291:585–590.

219. McSorley MA, Alberg AJ, Allen DS, et al. C-reactive protein concentrations and subsequent ovarian cancer risk. *Obstet Gynecol*. 2007;109:933–941.

220. Kaaks R, Lukanova A, Kurzer MS. Obesity, endogenous hormones, and endometrial cancer risk: a synthetic review. *Cancer Epidemiol Biomarkers Prev*. 2002;11:1531–1543.

221. Vona-Davis L, Howard-McNatt M, Rose DP. Adiposity, type 2 diabetes and the metabolic syndrome in breast cancer. *Obes Rev*. 2007;8:395–408.

222. Key TJ, Appleby PN, Reeves GK, et al. Endogenous Hormones Breast Cancer Collaborative G. Body mass index, serum sex hormones, and breast cancer risk in postmenopausal women. *J Natl Cancer Inst*. 2003;95:1218–1226.

223. Slattery ML, Potter JD, Curtin K, et al. Estrogens reduce and withdrawal of estrogens increase risk of microsatellite instability-positive colon cancer. *Cancer Res*. 2001;61:126–130.

224. Gann PH, Hennekens CH, Ma J, Longcope C, Stampfer MJ. Prospective study of sex hormone levels and risk of prostate cancer. *J Natl Cancer Inst*. 1996;88:1118–1126.

Chapter 37
Diabetes and Sleep Disorders

Abhijith Hegde and Steve H. Salzman

Introduction

The increasing incidence of both diabetes and sleep apnea coincides with the epidemic of obesity. An increasing body of evidence suggests that the connections between diabetes and obstructive sleep apnea-hypopnea syndrome (OSAH) are not simply due to the common risk factor of obesity. Physiologic derangements that result from OSAH appear to lead to impaired glucose metabolism, increasing the likelihood of diabetes and impairing the efficacy of its treatment.

OSAH is characterized by abnormal breathing patterns during sleep. These abnormal patterns include obstructive apneas, obstructive hypopneas, and respiratory effort related arousals (RERAs). Patients who have sleep apnea typically experience symptoms including excessive daytime sleepiness, fatigue, and neurocognitive dysfunction.

Considerable interest has been focused on the recognized associations between OSAH and organ system dysfunction like systemic hypertension,[1–6] pulmonary artery hypertension,[7–10] myocardial infarction,[11–14] cerebrovascular disease,[15,16] and cardiac arrhythmias.[17–22] Although considerable literature supports a true cause-effect relationship between OSAH and these diseases, the exact mechanisms remain controversial.

This chapter will focus on a brief overview of OSAH and the current literature regarding associations between OSAH and diabetes mellitus (see Fig. 37.1).

Obstructive Sleep Apnea–Hypopnea Syndrome

"Sleep disorders medicine is a clinical specialty which deals with the diagnosis and treatment of patients who complain about disturbed nocturnal sleep, excessive daytime sleepiness, or some other sleep-related problem."[23] Investigations at Stanford University in the 1970s pioneered research in sleep medicine and used respiratory and cardiac sensors combined with electroencephalography, electro-oculography and electromyography in all-night, polygraphic recordings. Holland and colleagues in 1974 named this continuous all-night array of data gathering polysmonography (see Fig. 37.2).[24]

Definitions

Sleep disordered breathing patterns (apnea, hypopnea, and RERA) are defined based on polysomnographic criteria.[25]

S.H. Salzman (✉)
Division of Pulmonary and Critical Care Medicine, Winthrop-University Hospital, Mineola, NY, USA
e-mail: ssalzman@winthrop.org

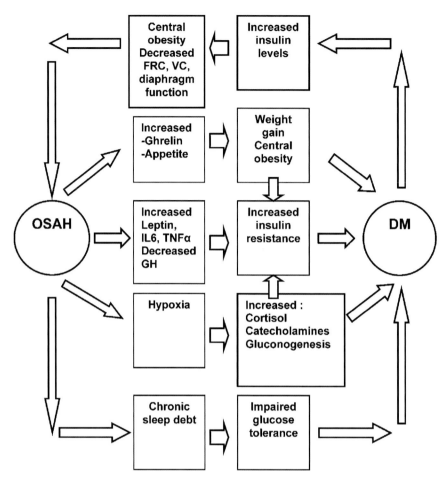

Fig. 37.1 Proven and putative interactions between obstructive sleep apnea–hypopnea syndrome (OSAH) and diabetes (DM). FRC = functional residual capacity, VC = vital capacity, IL6 = interleukin-6, TNFα = tumor necrosis factor alpha, GH = growth hormone

Apnea – A decrease in the airflow to less than 20% of the baseline, lasting at least 10 s, in adults.

Obstructive apnea – Absence of airflow but persistence of ventilatory effort defines obstructive apnea and is caused by the complete or near complete closure of the upper airway (see Fig. 37.2b).

Central apnea – Absence of both airflow and ventilatory effort defines central sleep apnea (see Fig. 37.2a).

Mixed apnea – A combination of both obstructive and central apnea defines a mixed apnea.

Hypopnea – Hypopnea is defined as a decrease in the airflow (to less than 70% of baseline airflow), but not to the extent that is seen with apnea (less than 20% of the baseline), lasting for at least 10 s, and associated with at least a 3% oxyhemoglobin desaturation.

Respiratory effort related arousals (RERAs) – RERAs are defined as a sequence of breaths lasting at least 10 s and characterized by increasing respiratory effort or flattening of the nasal pressure waveform (indicating increased upper airway resistance), leading to arousal from sleep but not meeting the criteria for apnea or hypopnea.

Apnea-hypopnea index (AHI) – the total number of apneas and hypopneas per hour of sleep constitutes the AHI.

Respiratory disturbance index (RDI) – the total number of apneas, hypopneas, and RERAs per hour of sleep constitutes the RDI.

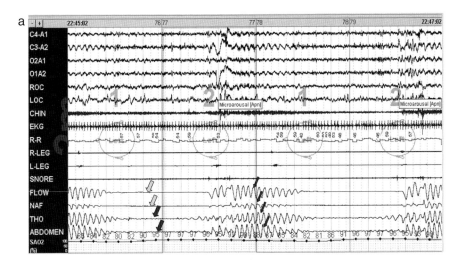

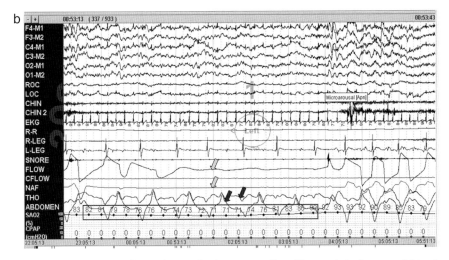

Fig. 37.2a (**a**) Central Sleep Apnea. The figure shows a 2-min segment (four 30-s epochs) of an overnight polysomnogram in a patient with central sleep apnea. The epoch reveals absence of airflow during period of apnea (*light gray wide arrows*) associated with absence of any thoracic or abdominal movement (*dark gray wide arrows*). This combination of absent airflow and absent ventilatory effort (manifested by lack of abdominal/thoracic movement) defines central sleep apnea. The periods of apnea can be seen to alternate with periods of respiration (*narrow dark gray arrows*) and each period of apnea is followed by a microarousal (C4, C3, O2, O1: EEG leads; ROC, LOC: Eye leads; NAF: Nasal air flow; THO: Thorax). The authors acknowledge Mangala Narasimhan, DO, for providing this clinical example. (**b**) Obstructive sleep apnea. The figure shows a 30-s epoch from an overnight polysomnogram of a patient with obstructive sleep apnea. The epoch reveals absence of airflow (*light gray arrows*) with persistence of abdominal and thoracic movements (*dark gray arrows*). This combination of absent airflow with persistent ventilatory effort is characteristic of obstructive sleep apnea. Also noticeable is the oxygen desaturation that is associated with the apnea boxed area in the oxygen saturation channel (SaO2) (F4, F3, C4, C3, O2, O1: EEG leads; ROC, LOC: Eye leads; NAF: Nasal air flow; THO: Thorax). The authors acknowledge Mangala Narasimhan, DO, for providing this clinical example

Obstructive sleep apnea-hypopnea syndrome (OSAH) – OSAH is defined as the presence of an AHI or a RDI >5 events/h in a symptomatic patient or an AHI or a RDI >15 events/h in an asymptomatic patient.[26] The severity of OSAH is defined based on the AHI or the RDI (mild OSAH 5–15 events/h; moderate OSAH 15–40 events/h; severe OSAH > 40 events/h).

Epidemiology

It has become evident that OSAH is a common medical condition and that it remains undiagnosed in many adults. The National Sleep Foundation conducted the Sleep in America 2005 Poll utilizing the Berlin Questionnaire (a validated tool to identify OSAH) via telephone interviews.[27] Of the 1506 respondents, 26% met the Berlin Questionnaire criteria for high risk for OSAH. The poll concluded that as many as one in four American adults could benefit from an evaluation for the presence of sleep disordered breathing.

The prevalence of OSAH is between 3 and 9% using the criteria of an AHI >5 events/h accompanied by at least one symptom, according to one study.[28] However, the reported prevalence of OSAH in the literature is highly variable, due to heterogeneity in the populations studied and the definitions of disease. Prevalence increases with age (two- to threefold by the age of 65 years).[28] Among adults, men have a higher prevalence than women. Among younger adults (under 35 years), African-Americans have a higher prevalence than Caucasians.[29] Asians have a similar prevalence compared to Americans, despite a lower mean body weight.[29]

Pathophysiology of OSAH

Loss of patency of the upper airway during sleep is the primary physiologic change that gives rise to the signs and symptoms of OSAH. In normal subjects, and those with OSAH, during inspiration the intrathoracic pressure becomes subatmospheric, leading to inflow of air. This negative intrathoracic pressure is transmitted to the upper airway, exerting a suction effect on the soft tissues. Before the onset of inspiration, reflexes that stimulate pharyngeal dilator muscles are activated and these dilator muscles keep the upper airway from collapsing in response to the suction effect.

During sleep, the pharyngeal dilator muscles are less active due to diminished neural output from the brainstem nuclei.[30] The caliber of the upper airway is smaller in patients with OSAH, either due to an excess of soft tissue or due to an excessively compliant airway. The combination of these two factors results in either complete or near complete closure of the upper airway in patients with OSAH during sleep. This closure of the upper airway results in obstructive or mixed apnea. With the onset of apnea, the carbon dioxide level in the blood increases, leading to an escalation of the respiratory drive. The patient starts to make progressively stronger inspiratory efforts against a closed upper airway, ultimately leading to arousal from sleep which results in opening of the upper airway. Opening of the airway leads to normalization of the carbon dioxide level, the respiratory drive decreases and the patient resumes sleep. With the onset of sleep, the stage is set for the evolution of the same sequence of events again. This repetitive cycle of sleep, apnea, and arousals from sleep results in fragmentation of sleep and gives rise to the symptoms of sleep apnea. This is a simplified model for the mechanism of OSAH. The true mechanism involves a more complex interplay between cortical, neuromuscular, endocrine, and mechanical components.

Clinical Features

History

Snoring, excessive daytime sleepiness, and fatigue are common symptoms of OSAH. The chronicity and insidious onset of symptoms often leads to unawareness or underestimation of the true severity and significance of these symptoms. The Epworth Sleepiness Scale (ESS) is a simple and quick screening questionnaire which allows the assessment of the severity of subjective sleepiness (Table 37.1).[31] The presence of the patient's bed partner or family member when obtaining the history is very helpful, as the patient's abnormal sleeping patterns are often most reliably reported by them. Some of the other clinical features of OSAH are the following:

- Choking, gasping, or sensation of being smothered, causing arousal from sleep
- Restlessness during sleep

Table 37.1 Epworth sleepiness scale[31]

How likely are you to fall asleep while
- Sitting and reading
- Watching television
- Sitting quietly in a public place
- Riding as a passenger in a car for 1 hour without a break
- Lying down to rest in the afternoon when circumstances permit
- Sitting and talking with someone
- Sitting quietly after lunch without alcohol
- Sitting in a car as the driver, while stopped for a few minutes in traffic

Score:
- 0 = Would never doze
- 1 = Slight chance of dozing
- 2 = Moderate chance of dozing
- 3 = High chance of dozing

A score greater than 10 is consistent with excessive sleepiness

---

Source: Johns.[31]

- Periods of "stopped breathing" (witnessed apneas) terminated by loud snorting or snoring
- Morning headaches, dry mouth
- Daytime cognitive deficits, lack of concentration, changes in mood
- Impaired libido and impotence
- History of gastroesophageal reflux, menstrual irregularities, type 2 diabetes mellitus, hypertension, cardiovascular disease, cerebrovascular disease, renal disease

Physical Exam

The physical exam may be normal but often shows an obese body habitus, large neck circumference (collar size greater than 17), crowded upper airway, and hypertension.

Laboratory

Routine laboratory data are of no value in either establishing or excluding the diagnosis of OSAH.

Diagnosis

Polysomnography

Polysomnography (PSG) is the gold standard for the diagnosis of OSAH. It is an expensive and time-consuming test; therefore, patient selection is important. During the test multiple physiologic variables are measured including sleep stages, respiratory effort and airflow, arterial oxygen saturation, cardiac rate and rhythm, body position, and limb movements (Fig. 37.2). By monitoring these variables, an assessment is made of the total sleep time, sleep efficiency, the different sleep stages, snoring, oxygen desaturation, cardiac rhythm disturbances, abnormal limb movements, and abnormal breathing patterns.

More recently, portable monitors for home sleep studies have become available. However, the information obtained from these devices is more limited as compared to PSG. Overnight pulse oximetry alone is also not a recommended method for the diagnosis or exclusion of OSAH. It can have a high sensitivity or specificity based on the criteria used, but not both.

Treatment

Treatment of OSAH comprises behavioral modification, continuous positive airway pressure (CPAP) by nasal or face mask, oral appliances, medications, and in select cases ENT evaluation for correctable anatomic abnormalities that may be contributing to the OSAH.

Behavioral modifications – Weight loss,[32,33] avoidance of alcohol[34] and drugs that depress the central nervous system and worsen apneas and hypopneas, and education about the risks of driving and using dangerous equipment associated with excessive daytime sleepiness are therapeutic measures that are of benefit and should be recommended to all patients with OSAH.

Continuous Positive Airway Pressure – The cornerstone of treatment for OSAH is CPAP therapy. The positive airway pressure delivered by the CPAP machine functions as a pneumatic splint that keeps the upper airway open while the patient is sleeping. The effectiveness of CPAP is limited by patient compliance, as the device has to be worn nightly, optimally for the entire night. Compliance has been shown to improve with simple interventions like patient education about OSAH and the benefits of CPAP therapy, in-hospital and home care support, and follow-up telephone calls.[35–37]

CPAP when used correctly has been shown to reduce mortality, morbidity, and healthcare costs.[38–41] Therapy also improves subjective and objective sleepiness, quality of life, and cognitive function.[42,43]

Oral Appliances (OA) – A variety of oral appliances are currently in use that have been shown to benefit OSAH patients.[44,45] Some advance the mandible forward while others hold the tongue anteriorly and away from the posterior pharyngeal wall. CPAP is more effective than OA in reducing respiratory disturbances but the subjective outcomes show little difference.[46]

Surgery – Uvulopalatopharyngoplasty is the most common surgery performed for OSAH. Others include genioglossus advancement, maxillary-mandibular advancement, and radiofrequency ablation, alone or in combination. So far, trials have failed to consistently show benefits of surgery. It should be reserved for patients who fail or are not candidates for nonsurgical therapy.

Pharmacologic therapy – Modafinil is the only FDA-approved drug for the treatment of residual hypersomnolence due to OSAH.[47,48] Its role is solely as adjunctive therapy for patients inadequately controlled by CPAP or OA alone and it cannot replace primary therapy. Although several mechanisms appear to be operative, investigation continues as to their relative importance. However, its mechanism of action appears to differ from the traditional adrenergic agents, which probably relates to its low abuse potential. Several mechanisms seem to contribute to its enhancement of wakefulness. There is inhibition of GABA release in the cerebral cortex via serotenergic pathways and augmented dopaminergic effect by blocking its reuptake. In addition, modafinil inhibits the norepinephrine reuptake transporter in the ventrolateral preoptic nucleus.

Sleep Disordered Breathing and Diabetes Mellitus

Obesity has reached epidemic proportions in the United States. It is estimated that more than half of the adult population in this country is overweight or obese. The striking increase in the prevalence of obesity over the last two decades has affected men and women across all ages and in various racial and ethnic groups. Coincident with the increase in obesity has been a dramatic increase in the incidence of cardiovascular disease, cerebrovascular disease, hypertension, and type 2 diabetes mellitus.

The Center for Disease Control and Prevention has noted that the prevalence of diabetes among Americans has risen from 1.5 million to 15.8 million cases per year, from 1980 to 2005. This represents an enormous disease burden and one that is likely to rise further in the years ahead.

As mentioned previously, the reported prevalence of OSAH in the US has varied, depending on the definitions and the population studied. Most experts in the field accept that it remains an underdiagnosed and often untreated malady. As the "epidemic of obesity" worsens, these numbers are likely to increase in the coming years as well.

Phenotypically, the patients with diabetes commonly are hypertensive, overweight or obese, have poor metabolic control, suffer from cardiac disease, and list fatigue and lethargy as common complaints. The typical patient with OSAH has a remarkably similar clinical profile, apart from the hyperglycemia seen in diabetes. The relationship between diabetes and OSAH is controversial because a true causal association has still not been proven. The question of whether diabetes may be a cause or a consequence of sleep disordered breathing, or whether these are just comorbid conditions, still needs to be definitively answered. Obesity as a cause of both insulin resistance and diabetes mellitus is often a confounding factor. Similarly, whether treatment of obstructive sleep apnea with CPAP results in clinical improvement of insulin resistance remains an area of some dispute.

Pathophysiology

Sleep disordered breathing has widespread systemic effects, many of which are underappreciated by those outside of the sleep specialist community. Activation of a multitude of adaptive physiological responses, including endocrine alterations, occurs when cellular gas exchange and acid–base balance are perturbed during apneas, hypopneas, and RERAs. Conversely, manifestation of sleep apnea is critically linked to inputs to the control of breathing. A body of research has established that the control of breathing incorporates both voluntary and involuntary (emotional, metabolic, neural, and endocrine) mechanisms.

Sleep disordered breathing may interact with the endocrine system in several ways (Fig. 37.1). OSAH with recurrent episodes of apnea and hypopnea causes sleep fragmentation and disturbance of the sleep cycle and stages. Frequent arousals from sleep induce stress responses resulting in increased levels of stress hormones.[49] Hypoxia results in alterations in the hypothalamo-pituitary axis and disordered secretion from several endocrine glands.[50] Animal studies using rats and dogs have shown that the levels of ACTH, renin, aldosterone, vasopressin, and corticosteroids increase with acute hypercapnia and hypoxia.[51,52]

Over time, multiple studies have shown an independent association between sleep apnea and insulin resistance.[53–59] Vgontzas et al.[56] showed that the circulating levels of insulin, the adipostatic hormone leptin, and the inflammatory cytokines tumor necrosis factor alpha (TNF-α) and interleukin-6 (IL-6) are increased in patients with sleep apnea, independent of obesity. Both leptin and the two cytokines are released into the interstitial fluid of the adipose tissue and are known to cause marked insulin resistance.[60,61]

A recent study postulated that a possible mechanism for the development of diabetes in patients with sleep disordered breathing is that OSAH contributes to weight gain and obesity, especially central obesity.[62] It is established that central obesity leads to insulin resistance via increased lipolysis and fatty acid availability.[63] Sleep curtailment, as occurs in OSAH, has been shown to increase appetite and ghrelin levels, and to decrease leptin levels, all possibly leading to weight gain.[64]

Studies in animals and humans have shown perturbation in glucose homeostasis as a direct consequence of hypoxia.[65–69] A study by Strohl et al.[53] found that insulin levels increase with the level of apneic activity in patients with a BMI greater than 29. The authors postulated that once a "critical mass" was reached, low oxygen values could trigger release of hormones (catecholamines and cortisol) that would result in gluconeogenesis and/or interfere with insulin action.

A small study of 18 patients with sleep disordered breathing found that the frequency of oxygen desaturations with sleep apnea was associated with abnormalities in glucose tolerance tests and indices of insulin resistance.[70]

In a larger study by Ip et al.,[54] the minimum oxygen saturation in patients with sleep disordered breathing was found to be an independent predictor of fasting insulin levels and insulin resistance.

Punjabi et al.[57] looked at the association of insulin sensitivity and glucose tolerance with hypoxemia secondary to sleep disordered breathing. The investigators included the average drop in oxygen saturation associated with respiratory events as a continuous variable in a multivariable logistic regression model. They found that for every 4% decrease in oxygen saturation, the associated odds ratio for worsening glucose tolerance was 1.99 (95% confidence interval, 1.11–3.56) after adjusting for percent body fat, BMI, and AHI. As with glucose intolerance, insulin resistance also was related to the severity of hypoxemia associated with apneas and hypopneas. The study reported an independent relationship between the minimum oxygen saturation at night and the indices for insulin sensitivity after adjusting for percent body fat. The investigators noted that for a two-point increase in the minimum oxygen saturation during sleep, there was an improvement in the insulin sensitivity suggesting a less insulin-resistant state with less hypoxemia during sleep.

Sleep apnea patients have low growth hormone levels.[58] Growth hormone secretion is decreased in OSAH not only due to obesity but also due to fragmented sleep causing a reduction in the amount of slow wave sleep. Repetitive hypoxemia may, in addition, affect growth hormone secretion. Growth hormone deficiency in adults is associated with impaired psychological well-being, insulin resistance, endothelial dysfunction, increased visceral fat, increased cardiovascular mortality, and accelerated aging.[71]

Spiegel et al.[72] examined the effect of chronic sleep debt on metabolic and endocrine functions. In 11 healthy young men aged between 18 and 27 years, who were restricted to 4 h in bed for 6 nights, there was clear impairment of carbohydrate tolerance. The rate of glucose clearance after injection of an intravenous bolus of glucose (300 mg/kg body weight) was nearly 40% slower compared to when the subjects spent 12 h in bed. Glucose effectiveness (a measure of the ability of glucose to mediate its own disposal independent of insulin) was 30% lower, which is about the same amount of difference observed between normoglycemic white men and patients with non-insulin-dependent diabetes. The acute insulin response to glucose, which has been identified as an early marker for diabetes, was 30% lower, a magnitude similar to that seen in gestational diabetes.

To complete the circle, Strohl et al.[53] hypothesized that hyperinsulinemia causes central fat deposition. Increasing central obesity would result in decreased functional residual capacity (FRC), decreased vital capacity, impaired diaphragm muscle action and, through a coupling of FRC to upper airway size, reduced pharyngeal size. These factors would propagate apneic activity and increase the susceptibility for sleep apnea.

In summary, while there are several putative mechanisms by which OSAH is thought to cause impaired glucose metabolism and insulin sensitivity, a clear and definite answer is still lacking (Fig. 37.1).

Insulin Levels and OSAH

The reported prevalence of OSAH in the United States has varied from 1 to 25%.[57] While many studies that have reported prevalence of OSAH have included patients with moderate to severe obesity (often with BMI in excess of 40 kg/m^2) the prevalence of OSAH in the mildly obese was unknown, until recently. A study conducted by Punjabi et al.[57] examined the prevalence of sleep disordered breathing in 150 otherwise healthy males, who had an average BMI of 30.5 kg/m^2. Using an AHI cutpoint of ≥ 5, ≥ 10, and ≥ 15 events/h as the disease defining cutpoint for sleep disordered breathing, the overall prevalence was 62, 45, and 41%, respectively. The prevalence of sleep disordered breathing with hypersomnolence (defined using the Multiple Sleep Latency Test, which measures the duration in minutes to sleep onset in a darkened room) at the described AHI cutpoints was 27, 24, and 23%, respectively. The Wisconsin Sleep Cohort Study[73] reported a prevalence of 24% in the general adult male population with only 4% self-reported daytime sleepiness. The differences in age of the population studied and methodology may account for some of the differences in the reported prevalence in these two studies.

There were several early studies that reported the association between sleep disordered breathing and insulin resistance. Mondini and Guilleminault[74] reported six cases of sleep apnea syndrome among 19 diabetic patients. Katsumata et al.[75] observed a high prevalence of comorbid sleep apnea with non-insulin-dependent diabetes mellitus in a male hospital-based population. Grunstein et al.[76] reported a strong association between sleep apnea and acromegaly, an insulin-resistant state without an increase in BMI. However, Catterall et al.[77] found no evidence of clinically significant sleep apnea among 16 diabetic patients with severe autonomic neuropathy.

Strohl et al.[53] studied 261 males who were referred to a sleep laboratory for symptoms of sleep disordered breathing. The majority of the patients (>98%) were of Caucasian, non-Hispanic origin. The investigators examined the relationship of levels of apneic activity and BMI to fasting serum insulin and fasting blood glucose concentrations, which were measured the morning after the polysomnography. They found that if BMI remained relatively low (BMI < 29), there is no increase in the fasting insulin levels, regardless of AHI. In patients with BMI >29, an escalation in fasting insulin levels is seen with increasing AHI. The highest levels of insulin were seen in morbidly obese patients (BMI > 33) with an AHI >25. They concluded that fasting insulin levels are directly, significantly, and independently associated with AHI in obese males. There was no statistically significant association between fasting blood glucose and the level of apneic activity in this study. Both fasting insulin levels and fasting blood glucose were independently associated with increase in BMI.

In an effort to find a relationship between sleep apnea, pattern of obesity (central versus generalized), and insulin resistance, Vgontzas et al.[56] conducted a study involving patients with OSAH ($n = 14$), BMI-matched obese control patients without OSAH ($n = 11$), and normal weight control patients ($n = 12$). All the study subjects were male. All the patients with OSAH had an AHI of more than 20. All potential participants in the study underwent PSG for one night and those who met inclusion criteria underwent additional PSG for another three nights. Levels of leptin, interleukin-6, and tumor necrosis factor-α (as markers of insulin resistance) were measured. Computed tomographic (CT) scanning was used to assess and compare the distribution of abdominal fat (intra-abdominal versus subcutaneous) in the sleep apneic individuals and in obese controls. The levels of leptin, tumor necrosis factor-α, and interleukin-6 were highest in the patients with OSAH, lowest in the controls with normal weight, and intermediate in the obese controls without OSAH. The sleep apneic patients had a significantly greater amount of visceral fat compared to obese controls. Visceral but not subcutaneous fat was significantly correlated with AHI and minimum oxygen saturation. In this study, mean fasting blood glucose levels and mean plasma insulin levels were significantly higher in apneics than in obese controls.

In the study by Punjabi et al.[57] the investigators examined the relationship between insulin sensitivity and sleep disordered breathing in mildly obese, otherwise healthy males. They used the oral glucose tolerance test and insulin sensitivity indices derived from the glucose tolerance test to examine this relationship. They found that there was a significant association between the severity of sleep disordered breathing and the 2-h glucose level, the insulin levels and the insulin sensitivity. They did not find a significant association between fasting blood glucose and the AHI.

Ip et al.[54] also looked at a cross-sectional cohort of patients with sleep apnea of varying degrees of intensity. They enrolled 270 subjects in their study and while they had both men and women in the cohort, the majority were male. They used the homeostasis model assessment method for estimation of insulin resistance (HOMA-IR) in their patients. The euglycemic clamp method is considered the gold standard technique for estimation of insulin resistance but the technique is invasive and labor-intensive, hindering its use as a research tool when investigating large numbers of subjects. Many researchers use validated alternatives such as the HOMA-IR and other indices of insulin sensitivity (or insulin resistance). This study also found a significant association between the severity of sleep apnea and fasting insulin levels as well as insulin resistance. Additionally, they also found a significant association between the minimum oxygen saturation and insulin levels and insulin resistance. There was no difference between men and women in terms of these associations.

The prevalence of OSAH in women is reported to be much lower than in men, especially in premenopausal women. In premenopausal women, the prevalence of OSAH has been directly linked to BMI. However, in a study of premenopausal women with polycystic ovary syndrome, OSAH was seen independent of BMI but was significantly associated with indices of insulin resistance.[55] This supported a close independent link between insulin resistance and OSAH in this population.

A hypothesis that was tested recently proposed that diabetes mellitus was associated with central sleep apnea rather than obstructive sleep apnea.[70-78] Participants in this study were part of the Sleep Heart Health Study cohort. The Sleep Heart Health Study was a longitudinal multicenter study designed to determine the cardiovascular and other consequences of sleep disordered breathing. The subjects were an ethnically diverse cohort of men and women aged 40 years and above, who were members of existing parent cohorts. The parent cohorts included the Framingham Heart study, Strong Heart Study, Atherosclerosis Risk in Communities Study and Cardiovascular Health Study among others. Data from 6441 participants constitute the Sleep Heart Health Study cohort. Of these, 4872 participants were without cardiovascular disease at baseline and among these, diabetes was present in 470 individuals. Sleep data in the diabetic individuals ($n = 470$) was compared to the sleep data in the nondiabetic controls ($n = 4402$). Descriptive analyses indicated differences between diabetic and nondiabetic participants in RDI, sleep stages, sleep time with saturation <90%, central sleep apnea index, and periodic breathing (Cheyne–Stokes pattern of respiration). However, multivariable regression analyses eliminated all associations except that between diabetes and periodic breathing as well as diabetes and percentage of sleep time spent in rapid-eye-movement (REM) sleep. There was a nonstatistically significant elevation in the odds of an increased central apnea index. Noteworthy in this report was the lack of association between obstructive sleep apnea and diabetes, once adjustment for BMI was made in the analyses. Based on these results, the study proposed an additional pathway for the development of sleep disordered breathing in diabetes. Instability of breathing during sleep, particularly associated with central breathing abnormalities, may result in part from dysfunction of the autonomic nervous system, a common complication of diabetes.

Although this is one of the largest population studies conducted to date, sleep data were collected by in-home PSG as opposed to the gold standard data collected in a sleep laboratory. As a second counterpoint, the definition of obstructive sleep apnea used in the study is different than the current accepted definition. However, the report adds to the growing body of literature linking abnormalities of glucose metabolism to sleep disordered breathing. It also highlights the fact that obesity is a major confounding factor in such studies. Even more important is the fact that an increased occurrence of sleep disordered breathing in patients with diabetes, even if caused by obesity, may represent a modifiable risk factor for cardiovascular disease.

Similar to the results of the above study, Stoohs and colleagues[79] found that the relationship between worsening insulin sensitivity and sleep disordered breathing in a group of 50 "healthy, normotensive individuals" was completely accounted for by increased BMI.

All the studies involving sleep disordered breathing and diabetes mellitus have been cross-sectional in design and while the preponderance of these show an association between OSAH and indices of insulin sensitivity, a true causal relationship can only be inferred and has never been definitively established. The first longitudinal study of the relationship between sleep disordered breathing and diabetes mellitus was published in 2005.[63] The objective of the study was to determine the prevalence and incidence of diabetes in patients with sleep disordered breathing. The study had 1387 subjects in the cross-sectional analysis. Of this cohort, 978 subjects reported no diagnosis of diabetes on the first visit and these patients were included in the longitudinal analysis. These 978 subjects were followed for 4 years to determine the incidence of diabetes. In the cross-sectional analysis, it was found that self-reported diabetes was three to four times more prevalent in subjects with an AHI of 15 or greater than in those with an AHI of less than 5. An independent relationship existed even after controlling for shared risk factors such as age, gender, and body habitus. A significant independent association was also found when a more inclusive definition for diabetes was used, that included either physician diagnosis or elevated fasting blood glucose. However, the study did not find a statistically significant independent causal effect in the development of type 2 diabetes in the longitudinal analysis. The incidence of diabetes over a 4-year follow-up period was not significantly related to the severity of sleep disordered breathing at the time of initial enrollment in the cohort when shared risk factors were taken into account.

Prospective studies prior to this had used snoring as a surrogate for sleep disordered breathing without the benefit of nocturnal PSG.[80,81] These studies had concluded that snoring is an independent risk factor for the development of diabetes. However, the specificity of snoring for severe sleep disordered breathing is not high.

How does one reconcile the finding of an independent association between sleep disordered breathing and diabetes in multiple cross-sectional studies with the lack of an independent causal effect in the only prospective, longitudinal study to date? Reichmuth et al.,[62] who conducted the longitudinal study, postulate that diabetes is often preceded by a "prediabetic" state including insulin resistance, impaired glucose tolerance, and possibly impaired fasting glucose, but the progression from one of these conditions to diabetes is variable and not well defined. It is possible that sleep disordered breathing impairs glucose metabolism without progression to overt diabetes. A widely accepted theory is that insulin resistance precedes diabetes and in individuals with a genetic predisposition, insulin secretion falters and diabetes ensues. Sleep disordered breathing may not affect this last step independent of other factors such as obesity, age, or genetic predisposition. Other factors that may have affected the results of the longitudinal study are patient selection (selection of a subpopulation of patients who were more resistant to the adverse metabolic effects of sleep apnea, older patients, only 4% of patients with an AHI of more than 30), the type of sleep disordered breathing (pure OSAH versus central apnea or mixed apnea) and the length of follow-up may have been insufficient (the latent period to development of diabetes may extend beyond the duration of the study).

Effect of CPAP Therapy on Insulin Resistance

It is a reasonable hypothesis that if sleep disordered breathing is a cause of diabetes (or insulin resistance), then treatment of the former should result in improvement of the latter. Unfortunately, the data until now have neither definitely supported nor refuted this hypothesis. The effectiveness of any therapy is modified by the compliance with the therapy and use of CPAP, even with the newest, most user-friendly models, is especially beset with noncompliance. There is also the question of the duration of therapy with CPAP required before there is any evidence of improvement in the metabolic profile of the patients with sleep disordered breathing.

Facchini et al.,[82] in a study looking at the effect of 8 weeks of CPAP treatment, did not show any improvement of overnight glucose tolerance in obese patients with OSAH. On the contrary, they found that there was an increase in the levels of plasma glucose and insulin after CPAP treatment. However, this was a small study of four patients. Similarly, in a later study, Smurra et al.[83] found lack of improvement in insulin responsiveness in ten patients (non-obese or moderately overweight with a BMI < 37) after 2 months of CPAP treatment.

Brooks et al.[84] studied insulin responsiveness in ten patients with non-insulin-dependent diabetes mellitus and severe OSAH (mean AHI of 47), both before and after 4 months of CPAP treatment. Insulin responsiveness was measured by the euglycemic clamp method. There was a statistically significant improvement in insulin responsiveness after 4 months of CPAP treatment. However, there was no change in the fasting insulin level, fasting blood glucose level and HbA_{1c}. The authors of the study postulated that this lack of effect may have been due to the fact that the increase in insulin responsiveness was relatively modest, especially in the context of severe insulin resistance in the severely obese patients (mean BMI of 42.7 kg/m^2) in this study. Another possibility was that the patients were at the plateau of the dose-response curve between glycemia and insulin resistance, where improvement in one would not necessarily be paralleled by improvement in the other. Lastly, all three of the above studies (Facchini et al., Smurra et al., and Brooks et al.) may have lacked statistical power due to the small number of patients.

Harsch et al.[85] investigated insulin resistance after CPAP treatment in 40 patients with OSAH (AHI > 20). None of the patients had a diagnosis of diabetes mellitus. The investigators performed studies with the hyperinsulinemic euglycemic clamp method before CPAP treatment was initiated, and then 2 days after, and 3 months after CPAP treatment was initiated. They found that insulin sensitivity improved significantly after 2 days of CPAP treatment and this improvement remained stable after 3 months of treatment. They also noted that the magnitude of improvement was smaller in obese patients as compared to non-obese (BMI < 30) patients, suggesting that in obese individuals insulin sensitivity is mainly determined by obesity and to a smaller extent by sleep apnea. The rapid improvement in insulin sensitivity lends credence to the hypothesis that insulin resistance is mainly induced by increased nocturnal sympathetic drive, mediated by adrenal hormones with short half-lives.

The same group of investigators later published the results of a similar study involving nine patients with overt type 2 diabetes mellitus and OSAH (mean AHI of 43.1).[86] In this study, there was no improvement in insulin sensitivity after 2 days of CPAP treatment but a statistically significant improvement was seen after 3 months of CPAP treatment. The investigators regarded the lack of a quick improvement in insulin sensitivity in the diabetic group as the consequence of a more fixed and genetically determined degree of insulin resistance, which is thus more difficult to reverse in diabetic than in nondiabetic patients. Similar to the study by Brooks et al. this study also did not demonstrate an improvement in HbA_{1c} with CPAP treatment.

Finally, Babu et al.[87] in a study of 25 patients with type 2 diabetes mellitus and OSAH (mean AHI of 56) measured changes in interstitial glucose levels and hemoglobin A_{1c} levels before and after a mean of 83 ± 50 days of CPAP treatment. They observed that mean postprandial glucose values were significantly reduced and that there was a statistically significant reduction in hemoglobin A_{1c} levels after CPAP treatment. Furthermore, in patients who used CPAP for more than 4 h/day, the reduction in HbA1c level was significantly correlated with days of CPAP use.

Summary

In conclusion, sleep disordered breathing is now recognized as being much more prevalent than was originally suspected. The preponderance of cross-sectional studies points toward an independent association between sleep disordered breathing and diabetes mellitus or a "prediabetic" state of insulin resistance. This relationship has not been conclusively shown to be due to a direct causal effect. The data from studies examining the improvement of diabetes with CPAP treatment span the spectrum from no effect, to improvement in insulin sensitivity but not glycemic control, to significant improvement in glycemic control.

Although there is a growing body of literature on this subject, it is clear that the understanding of the complex interactions between diabetes and sleep disordered breathing is still in its infancy. The field remains wide open for further research, especially for the longitudinal analyses and the effects of CPAP treatment.

References

1. Hla KM, Young TB, Bidwell T, et al. Sleep apnea and hypertension. A population-based study. *Ann Intern Med*. 1994;120: 382–388.
2. Lavie P, Herer P, Hoffstein V. Obstructive sleep apnoea syndrome as a risk factor for hypertension: population study. *BMJ*. 2000;320:479–482.
3. Nieto FJ, Young TB, Lind BK, et al. Association of sleep-disordered breathing, sleep apnea, and hypertension in a large community-based study. Sleep Heart Health Study. *JAMA*. 2000;283:1829–1836.
4. Young T, Peppard P, Palta M, et al. Population-based study of sleep-disordered breathing as a risk factor for hypertension. *Arch Intern Med*. 1997;157:1746–1752.
5. Grote L, Ploch T, Heitmann J, et al. Sleep-related breathing disorder is an independent risk factor for systemic hypertension. *Am J Respir Crit Care Med*. 1999;160:1875–1882.
6. Bixler EO, Vgontzas AN, Lin HM, et al. Association of hypertension and sleep-disordered breathing. *Arch Intern Med*. 2000;160:2289–2295.
7. Bradley TD, Rutherford R, Grossman RF, et al. Role of daytime hypoxemia in the pathogenesis of right heart failure in the obstructive sleep apnea syndrome. *Am Rev Respir Dis*. 1985;131:835–839.
8. Sajkov D, Cowie RJ, Thornton AT, et al. Pulmonary hypertension and hypoxemia in obstructive sleep apnea syndrome. *Am J Respir Crit Care Med*. 1994 Feb;149:416–422.
9. Guidry UC, Mendes LA, Evans JC, et al. Echocardiographic features of the right heart in sleep-disordered breathing: the Framingham Heart Study. *Am J Respir Crit Care Med*. 2001;164:933–938.
10. Arias MA, Garcia-Rio F, Alonso-Fernandez A, et al. Pulmonary hypertension in obstructive sleep apnoea: effects of continuous positive airway pressure: A randomized, controlled cross-over study. *Eur Heart J*. 2006;27:1106–1113.
11. Marin JM, Carrizo SJ, Vicente E, et al. Long-term cardiovascular outcomes in men with obstructive sleep apnoea-hypopnoea with or without treatment with continuous positive airway pressure: an observational study. *Lancet*. 2005;365: 1046–1053.
12. Peker Y, Carlson J, Hedner J. Increased incidence of coronary artery disease in sleep apnoea: a long-term follow-up. *Eur Respir J*. 2006;28:596–602.
13. Yumino D, Tsurumi Y, Takagi A, et al. Impact of obstructive sleep apnea on clinical and angiographic outcomes following percutaneous coronary intervention in patients with acute coronary syndrome. *Am J Cardiol*. 2007;99:26–30.
14. Gami AS, Rader S, Svatikova A, et al. Familial premature coronary artery disease mortality and obstructive sleep apnea. *Chest*. 2007;131:118–121.
15. Arzt M, Young T, Finn L, et al. Association of sleep-disordered breathing and the occurrence of stroke. *Am J Respir Crit Care Med*. 2005;172:1447–1451.
16. Yaggi HK, Concato J, Kernan WN, et al. Obstructive sleep apnea as a risk factor for stroke and death. N *Engl J Med*. 2005;353:2034–2041.
17. Mehra R, Benjamin EJ, Shahar E, et al. Association of nocturnal arrhythmias with sleep-disordered breathing: The Sleep Heart Health Study. *Am J Respir Crit Care Med*. 2006;173:910–916.
18. Garrigue S, Pepin JL, Defaye P, et al. High prevalence of sleep apnea syndrome in patients with long-term pacing: the European Multicenter Polysomnographic Study. *Circulation*. 2007;115:1703–1709.
19. Alonso-Fernandez A, Garcia-Rio F, Racionero MA, et al. Cardiac rhythm disturbances and ST-segment depression episodes in patients with obstructive sleep apnea-hypopnea syndrome and its mechanisms. *Chest*. 2005;127:15–22.
20. Zwillich C, Devlin T, White D, et al. Bradycardia during sleep apnea. Characteristics and mechanism. *J Clin Invest*. 1982;69:1286–1292.
21. Miller WP. Cardiac arrhythmias and conduction disturbances in the sleep apnea syndrome. Prevalence and significance. *Am J Med*. 1982;73:317–321.

22. Tilkian AG, Guilleminault C, Schroeder JS, et al. Sleep-induced apnea syndrome. Prevalence of cardiac arrhythmias and their reversal after tracheostomy. *Am J Med.* 1977;63:348–358.

23. Walsh J. *Sleep Disorders Medicine.* Rochester, MN: Association of Professional Sleep Societies; 1986.

24. Holland JV, Dement WC, Raynal DM. *Polysomnography: A Response to a Need for Improved Communication.* Presented at the 14th annual meeting of the association for the psychophysiological study of sleep. Jackson Hole, WY: Association for the pychophysiological study of sleep; 1974:121.

25. Iber C, Ancoli-Israel S, Chesson AL, et al. *The AASM Manual for the Scoring of Sleep and Associated Events.* West Chester, IL: American Academy of Sleep Medicine; 2007.

26. Strohl KP, Redline S. Recognition of obstructive sleep apnea. *Am J Respir Crit Care Med.* 1996;154:279–289.

27. Hiestand DM, Britz P, Goldman M, et al. Prevalence of symptoms and risk of sleep apnea in the US population: Results from the national sleep foundation sleep in America 2005 poll. *Chest.* 2006;130:780–786.

28. Young T, Skatrud J, Peppard PE. Risk factors for obstructive sleep apnea in adults. *JAMA.* 2004;291:2013–2016.

29. Palmer LJ, Redline S. Genomic approaches to understanding obstructive sleep apnea. *Respir Physiol Neurobiol.* 2003;135: 187–205.

30. Strohl KP, Cherniak NS, Gothe B. Physiologic basis of therapy for sleep apnea. *Am Rev Respir Dis.* 1986;134:791.

31. Johns MW. A new method for measuring daytime sleepiness: the Epworth sleepiness scale. *Sleep.* 1991;14:540–545.

32. Browman CP, Sampson MG, Yolles SF, et al. Obstructive sleep apnea and body weight. *Chest.* 1984;85:435–438.

33. Smith PL, Gold AR, Meyers DA, et al. Weight loss in mildly to moderately obese patients with obstructive sleep apnea. *Ann Intern Med.* 1985;103:p850–p855.

34. Issa FG, Sullivan CE. Alcohol, snoring and sleep apnea. *J Neurol Neurosurg Psychiatr.* 1982;45:353–359.

35. Chervin RD, Theut S, Bassetti C, et al. Compliance with nasal CPAP can be improved by simple interventions. *Sleep.* 1997;20:284–289.

36. Pepin JL, Krieger J, Rodenstein D, et al. Effective compliance during the first 3 months of continuous positive airway pressure. A European prospective study of 121 patients. *Am J Respir Crit Care Med.* 1999;160:1124–1129.

37. Aloia MS, Di Dio L, Ilniczky N, et al. Improving compliance with nasal CPAP and vigilance in older adults with OAHS. *Sleep Breath.* 2001;5:13–21.

38. He J, Kryger MH, Zorick FJ, et al. Mortality and apnea index in obstructive sleep apnea. Experience in 385 male patients. *Chest.* 1988;94:9–14.

39. Campos-Rodriguez F, Pena-Grinan N, Reyes-Nunez N, et al. Mortality in obstructive sleep apnea-hypopnea patients treated with positive airway pressure. *Chest.* 2005;128:624–633.

40. Bahammam A, Delaive K, Ronald J, et al. Health care utilization in males with obstructive sleep apnea syndrome two years after diagnosis and treatment. *Sleep.* 1999;22:740–747.

41. Kapur V, Blough DK, Sandblom RE, et al. The medical cost of undiagnosed sleep apnea. *Sleep.* 1999;22:749–755.

42. Giles TL, Lasserson TJ, Smith BJ, et al. Continuous positive airways pressure for obstructive sleep apnoea in adults. *Cochrane Database Syst Rev.* 2006;25(1):CD001106.

43. Patel SR, White DP, Malhotra A, et al. Continuous positive airway pressure therapy for treating sleepiness in a diverse population with obstructive sleep apnea: results of a meta-analysis. *Arch Intern Med.* 2003;163: 565–571.

44. Gotsopoulos H, Chen C, Qian J, et al. Oral appliance therapy improves symptoms in obstructive sleep apnea: a randomized, controlled trial. *Am J Respir Crit Care Med.* 2002;166:743–748.

45. Hoekema A, Stegenga B, De Bont LG. Efficacy and co-morbidity of oral appliances in the treatment of obstructive sleep apnea-hypopnea: a systematic review. *Crit Rev Oral Biol Med.* 2004;15:137–155.

46. Schwartz JR, Hirshkowitz M, Erman MK, et al. Modafinil as adjunct therapy for daytime sleepiness in obstructive sleep apnea: a 12-week, open-label study. *Chest.* 2003;124:2192–2199.

47. Black JE, Hirshkowitz M. Modafinil for treatment of residual excessive sleepiness in nasal continuous positive airway pressure-treated obstructive sleep apnea/hypopnea syndrome. *Sleep.* 2005;28:464–471.

48. Hirshkowitz M, Black JE, Wesnes K, et al. Adjunct armodafinil improves wakefulness and memory in obstructive sleep apnea/hypopnea syndrome. *Respir Med.* 2007;101:616–627.

49. Spath-Schwalbe E, Gofferje M, Kern W, et al. Sleep disruption alters nocturnal ACTH and cortisol secretory patterns. *Biol Psychiatry.* 1991;29:575–584.

50. Semple PD, Beastall GH, Watson WS, et al. Hypothalamic-pituitary dysfunction in respiratory hypoxia. *Thorax.* 1981;36: 605–609.

51. Raff H, Roarty TP. Renin, ACTH and aldosterone during acute hypercapnia and hypoxia in conscious rats. *Am J Physiol.* 1988;254:R431–R435.

52. Raff H, Shinsako J, Keil LC, et al. Vasopressin, ACTH and corticosteroids during hypercapnia and graded hypoxia in dogs. *Am J Physiol.* 1983;244:E453–E458.

53. Strohl KP, Novak RD, Singer W, et al. Insulin levels, blood pressure and sleep apnea. *Sleep.* 1994;17:614–618.

54. Ip MS, Lam B, Ng MM, et al. Obstructive sleep apnea is independently associated with insulin resistance. *Am J Respir Crit Care Med.* 2002;165:670–676.

55. Vgontzas A, Legro RS, Bixler EO, et al. Polycystic Ovary syndrome is associated with obstructive sleep apnea and daytime sleepiness: Role of insulin resistance. *J Clin Endocrinol Metab.* 2001;86:517–520.

56. Vgontzas A, Papanicolaou DA, Bixler EO, et al. Sleep apnea and daytime sleepiness and fatigue: relation to visceral obesity, insulin resistance and hypercytokinemia. *J Clin Endocrinol Metab*. 2000;85:1151–1158.

57. Punjabi NM, Sorkin JD, Katzel LI, et al. Sleep disordered breathing and insulin resistance in middle-aged and overweight men. *Am J Respir Crit Care Med*. 2002;165:677–682.

58. Saaresranta T, Polo O. Sleep-disordered breathing and hormones. *Eur Respir J*. 2003;22:161–172.

59. Saaresranta T, Polo O. Hormones and breathing. *Chest*. 2002;122:2165–2182.

60. Gotamisligil GS, Shargill NS, Spiegelman BM. Adipose expression of tumor necrosis factor-α: direct role in obesity-linked insulin resistance. *Science*. 1993;259:87–91.

61. DeCourten M, Zimmet P, Hodge A, et al. Hyperleptinaemia: the missing link in the metabolic syndrome? *Diabets Med*. 1997;14:200–208.

62. Reichmuth KJ, Austin D, Skatrud JB, et al. Association of sleep apnea and type II diabetes. A population based study. *Am J Respir Crit Care Med*. 2005;172:1590–1595.

63. Rebrin K, Steil GM, Mittelman S, et al. Causal linkage between insulin suppression of lipolysis and suppression of liver glucose output. *J Clin Invest*. 1996;98:741–749.

64. Speigel K, Tasali E, Penev P, et al. Brief communication: sleep curtailment in healthy young men is associated with decreased leptin levels, elevated ghrelin levels, and increased hunger and appetite. *Ann Intern Med*. 2004;141:846–850.

65. Cheng N, Cai W, Jiang M, et al. Effect of hypoxia on blood glucose hormones, and insulin receptor functions in newborn calves. *Pediatr Res*. 1997;41:852–856.

66. Raff H, Bruder ED, Jankowski BM. The effect of hypoxia on plasma leptin and insulin in newborn and juvenile rats. *Endocrine*. 1999;11:37–39.

67. Larsen JJ, Hansen JM, Olsen NV, et al. The effect of altitude hypoxia on glucose homeostasis in men. *J Physiol*. 1997;504: 241–249.

68. Braun B, Rock PB, Zamudio S, et al. Women at altitude: short-term exposure to hypoxia and/or α_1-adrenergic blockade reduces insulin sensitivity. *J Appl Physiol*. 2001;91:623–631.

69. Hjalmarsen A, Aasebo U, Birkeland K, et al. Impaired glucose tolerance in patients with chronic hypoxic pulmonary disease. *Diabetes Metab*. 1996;22:37–42.

70. Tijhonen M, Partinen M, Narvanen S. The severity of obstructive sleep apnoea is associated with insulin resistance. *J Sleep Res*. 1993;2:56–61.

71. Veldhuis JD, Iranmanesh A. Physiological regulation of the human growth hormone (GH)-insulin-like growth factor type I (IGF-I) axis: predominant impact of age, obesity, gonadal function, and sleep. *Sleep*. 1996;19:S221–S224.

72. Speigel K, Leproult R, Van Cauter E. Impact of sleep debt on metabolic and endocrine function. *Lancet*. 1999;354:1435–1439.

73. Young T, Palta M, Dempsey J, et al. The occurrence of sleep-disordered breathing among middle-aged adults. *N Engl J Med*. 1993;328:1230–1235.

74. Mondini S, Guilleminault C. Abnormal breathing patterns during sleep in diabetes. *Ann Neurol*. 1985;17:391–395.

75. Katsumata K, Okada T, Miyao M, et al. High incidence of sleep apnea syndrome in a male diabetic population. *Diabetes Res Clin Pract*. 1991;13:45–51.

76. Grunstein RR, Ho KY, Sullivan CE. Sleep apnea in acromegaly. *Ann Int Med*. 1991;115:527–532.

77. Catterall JR, Calverley PM, Ewing DJ, et al. Breathing, sleep, and diabetic autonomic neuropathy. *Diabetes*. 1984;33: 1025–1027.

78. Resnick H, Redline S, Shahar E, et al. Diabetes and sleep disturbances. Findings from the sleep heart health study. *Diabetes care*. 2003;26:702–709.

79. Stoohs RA, Facchini F, Guilleminault C. Insulin resistance and sleep-disordered breathing in healthy humans. *Am J Respir Crit Care Med*. 1996;154:170–174.

80. Elmasry A, Janson C, Lindberg E, et al. The role of habitual snoring and obesity in the development of diabetes: a 10-year follow-up study in a male population. *J Intern Med*. 2000;248:13–20.

81. Al Delaimy WK, Manson JE, Willett WC, et al. Snoring as a risk factor for type II diabetes mellitus: a prospective study. *Am J Epidemiol*. 2002;155:387–393.

82. Facchini F, Stoohs R, Harter R, et al. Sleep related glucose and insulin plasma concentrations in obese patients with obstructive sleep apnea before and after treatment with nasal CPAP [Abstract]. *J Sleep Res*. 1992;1(suppl 1):71.

83. Smurra M, Philip P, Taillard J, et al. CPAP treatment does not affect glucose-insulin metabolism in sleep apneic patients. *Sleep Medicine*. 2001;2:207–213.

84. Brooks B, Cistulli P, Borkman M, et al. Obstructive sleep apnea in obese on insulin-dependent diabetic patients: effect of continuous positive airway pressure treatment on insulin responsiveness. *J Clin Endocrinol Metab*. 1994;79:1681–1685.

85. Harsch IA, Pour Schahin S, Radespiel-Tröger M, et al. Continuous positive airway pressure treatment rapidly improves insulin sensitivity in patients with obstructive sleep apnea syndrome. *Am J Respir Crit Care Med.* 2004;169:156–162.

86. Harsch IA, Pour Schahin S, Brückner K, et al. The effect of continuous positive airway pressure treatment on insulin sensitivity in patients with obstructive sleep apnoea syndrome and type 2 diabetes. *Respiration.* 2004;71:252–259.

87. Babu AR, Herdegen J, Fogelfeld L, et al. Type 2 diabetes, glycemic control, and continuous positive airway pressure in obstructive sleep apnea. *Arch Intern Med.* 2005;165:447–452.

Chapter 38
HIV Infection and Diabetes

Madhu N. Rao, Kathleen Mulligan, and Morris Schambelan

Introduction

Since the introduction of highly active antiretroviral therapy (HAART) more than a decade ago, there has been a dramatic improvement in the morbidity and mortality associated with human immunodeficiency virus (HIV) infection and AIDS. As survival has improved, a constellation of metabolic and morphologic abnormalities, often referred to as the HIV-associated lipodystrophy syndrome, has become increasingly evident. Features of this syndrome include abnormal glucose metabolism, dyslipidemia, and alterations in body fat distribution including peripheral lipoatrophy and central adiposity. In this chapter, we will focus primarily on the abnormalities of glucose metabolism in patients with HIV/AIDS, including insulin resistance, impaired glucose tolerance, and frank diabetes mellitus. After first considering the effects of HIV infection per se, we will examine the mechanisms by which antiretroviral (ARV) medications are purported to disrupt glucose metabolism. We will then review the impact of the alterations in body fat distribution on carbohydrate homeostasis. Finally, we will briefly discuss the dyslipidemia which often accompanies the disordered glucose metabolism in HIV-infected patients on HAART. We will conclude with a review of treatment options.

Scope of Disease

Initial Reports

Human immunodeficiency virus was first identified as the cause of AIDS in the early 1980s.[1–3] Later in that decade, the era of ARV therapy for HIV began with the introduction of the nucleoside reverse transcriptase inhibitor (NRTI) zidovudine.[4] Soon afterward, the first reports of diabetes emerged beginning with the description of a reversible, drug-induced diabetes in patients receiving the NRTI didanosine in 1993.[5–7] The subsequent development of more potent NRTIs and the introduction of the HIV protease inhibitors (PIs) and non-nucleoside reverse transcriptase inhibitors (NNRTIs), which are typically used in combination with NRTIs, led to the era of highly active antiretroviral therapy (HAART) and to the resultant reduction in the morbidity and mortality of patients with HIV and AIDS.[8] In 1997, soon after the introduction of PIs, a small case series describing seven patients with hyperglycemia was published.[9] Within a year, reports of alterations in body fat distribution appeared, including fat accumulation in the dorsocervical region (buffalo hump)[10] and abdomen,[11,12] and loss of subcutaneous fat in the limbs, face, and buttocks.[13,14] In 1998, the term "HIV lipodystrophy" was first applied to the constellation of abnormalities that included abnormalities of fat distribution, insulin resistance, and dyslipidemia,[13,15] a syndrome with many features in common with the metabolic syndrome in non-HIV-infected individuals.

M. Schambelan (✉)
Division of Endocrinology and Metabolism, University of California, San Francisco, CA, USA
e-mail: morrie@sfghgcrc.ucsf.edu

L. Poretsky (ed.), *Principles of Diabetes Mellitus*, DOI 10.1007/978-0-387-09841-8_38,
© Springer Science+Business Media, LLC 2010

Epidemiology

The reported prevalence of diabetes in patients with HIV infection varies, depending on the population of patients studied. In a 5-year historical cohort study, the cumulative incidence of hyperglycemia (defined as ≥ 2 random blood glucose values of >140 mg/dl) was 5%.[16] A more recent Multicenter AIDS Cohort Study (MACS) in the United States reported a prevalence of diabetes of 7% in HIV-infected patients not using HAART and 14% in HIV-infected patients using HAART, in comparison to a rate of only 5% in HIV-seronegative controls.[17] In the same cohort, the incidence of newly diagnosed diabetes was more than three times higher in HIV-infected subjects using HAART compared to HIV-seronegative controls (4.7 vs. 1.4 events per 100 person-years).[17] In the Swiss HIV Cohort Study, the incidence rate ratio for diabetes was higher in subjects who were male, of older age, obese, of Asian or black ethnicity, and were currently treated with NRTI- or PI-containing regimens.[18]

Recent analyses of data from the Women's Interagency HIV Study (WIHS), a prospective cohort study of women in the United States, showed that longer cumulative exposure to NRTI therapy was associated with an increased incidence of diabetes.[19] In contrast to studies in men, however, the HIV-infected women in this cohort were not found to have a higher incidence or prevalence of diabetes or pre-diabetes[19,20] than did seronegative controls. The majority of both HIV-infected and uninfected women in WIHS were overweight or obese,[21] and increasing BMI was a significant predictor of diabetes and pre-diabetes.[20] Similarly, in another cohort of HIV-infected women, traditional risk factors for diabetes, such as obesity, physical inactivity, first-degree relative with diabetes, and history of delivering a macrosomic infant, have been linked to an increased risk of diabetes in HIV-infected women.[22] In pregnant HIV-infected women, 90% of whom received ARV therapy during pregnancy (and 50% of these were on ARVs prior to pregnancy), 9% developed gestational diabetes mellitus (GDM).[23] All cases of GDM were diagnosed in patients receiving combination ARV therapy.[23] In a study that included oral glucose tolerance testing (OGTT) during pregnancy, impaired glucose tolerance (IGT) and diabetes were noted in 33 and 6% of women on a PI-based regimen, respectively, and 26 and 10% of those using a non-PI-based or no ARV, rates that are higher than those generally seen in the non-HIV-infected population.[24] In a secondary analysis of a large study of prevention of perinatal infection among HIV-infected women treated with ARV therapy, the reported incidence of GDM was highest in the group treated with a PI-based regimen that was started either before pregnancy or early in the first trimester.[25]

The potential impact of body composition abnormalities on the prevalence of abnormal glucose metabolism was suggested by a case–control study in which 7% of HIV-infected patients with altered fat distribution had frank diabetes (defined by 2-h glucose value of >200 mg/dl on OGTT) and 35% had IGT, compared with only 0.5 and 5% in healthy age- and BMI-matched HIV-negative controls, respectively.[26] In the same study, the rates of diabetes and IGT were similar in a group of HIV-infected patients without altered fat distribution and the HIV-negative controls. In another study using OGTT, Carr et al. found rates of diabetes of 7% and impaired glucose tolerance of 16% in HIV-infected patients who were on PIs.[27] Of note, 83% of these patients were described as having some element of lipodystrophy. Similar rates of diabetes and impaired glucose metabolism (IGT or impaired fasting glucose), 6 and 17%, respectively, were evident in a larger cross-sectional study of 614 patients who underwent OGTT;[28] in this study, 62% of patients were diagnosed with lipodystrophy. Patients with traditional risk factors for diabetes who are started on PIs may be at even greater risk for diabetes.[18,29]

Other coexistent conditions may also predispose patients with HIV infection to develop insulin resistance and diabetes. For example, it has been suggested that co-infection with hepatitis C virus worsens insulin sensitivity and hyperglycemia in HIV-infected patients.[30,31]

Effects of HIV Infection on Glucose Metabolism

Determining the effect of HIV infection per se on glucose metabolism has been a difficult task, due to confounding factors such as ARV medication use, alterations in fat distribution, or the presence of a wasting/catabolic state, as well as of traditional risk factors. A study performed in the early 1990s, prior to the advent of HAART, compared glucose metabolism in 10 HIV-infected subjects (50% of whom were on the NRTI zidovudine) and

10 HIV-negative healthy controls.[32] Using a hyperinsulinemic, euglycemic clamp, the investigators found no difference in the total glucose disposal rate (*M*) between these two groups but noted significantly lower circulating insulin (*I*) levels, presumably as a consequence of increased insulin clearance, which yielded a higher calculated peripheral insulin sensitivity (defined as *M/I*) in the patients with HIV. The HIV-infected patients weighed significantly less (by an average of 13 kg) than the control subjects, suggesting that cachexia may have played a role in the observed differences. Another study which assessed non-insulin-mediated glucose uptake (by hypoinsulinemic clamp with somatostatin infusion) found no significant difference between HIV-infected men and HIV-negative controls.[33] Lastly, glucose cycling was reduced by approximately 25% in one study of patients with AIDS (compared to HIV-negative healthy controls), which is consistent with chronic undernutrition.[34] Overall, these data do not suggest that untreated HIV infection contributes significantly to insulin resistance or impaired glucose metabolism.

Effects of ARV Medications

Overview

The effects of ARV medications on glucose metabolism may be mediated by: (1) the decrease in viremia, improved immune function, and restitution to health; (2) a direct impact on peripheral insulin sensitivity and pancreatic β-cell function; (3) the development of lipodystrophy (peripheral lipoatrophy and/or central fat accumulation); or (4) impaired mitochondrial function. In vitro studies using cultured cells and in vivo studies in HIV-negative controls have allowed these potential mechanisms to be assessed separately.

Since the introduction of zidovudine in 1987, the number of ARVs available for the treatment of HIV and AIDS has grown profoundly. There are now five major classes of medications, of which the NRTIs are the oldest and the integrase inhibitors and CCR5 antagonists are the newest (Table 38.1). HAART combines several different classes of ARV medications to attack the virus at different points in its life cycle.[35] Sometimes, due to pharmacokinetic issues, serum levels of certain PIs are "boosted" by the concomitant use of a low dose of the PI ritonavir. For example, lopinavir is always given in conjunction with a low dose of ritonavir (lopinavir/r) to increase circulating drug levels.

Table 38.1 Antiretroviral medications

Nucleoside/tide reverse transcriptase inhibitors	*Protease inhibitors*
Zidovudine	Saquinavir
Didanosine	Ritonavir
Zalcitabine	Indinavir
Stavudine	Nelfinavir
Lamivudine	Amprenavir
Abacavir	Lopinavir/ritonavir
Emtricitabine	Atazanavir
Tenofovir	Fosamprenavir
	Tipranavir
Non-nucleoside reverse transcriptase inhibitors	Darunavir
Delavirdine	*Entry and fusion inhibitors*
Efavirenz	Enfuvirtide
Nevirapine	Maraviroc
Etravirine (available by expanded access)	*Integrase inhibitors*
	Raltegravir

Protease Inhibitors

Overview: Of the ARV medication classes, PIs have been most frequently associated with insulin resistance. However, insulin resistance occurs in the absence of PIs also[17,36,37] (Fig. 38.1). Moreover, as newer medications within this category have been developed, it has become clear that the abnormalities in glucose metabolism are specific to individual agents, rather than a class effect. Earlier studies, performed when a limited number of PIs were available, lumped these agents together in assessing their effect on glucose metabolism. For example, in a cross-sectional study, Walli et al. compared HIV-positive patients on PIs (either indinavir, ritonavir, nelfinavir, or saquinavir) with HIV-positive, therapy-naïve patients and HIV-negative controls.[38,39] Using the intravenous insulin tolerance test (as well as OGTT in a subset of patients), they found a significantly lower median insulin sensitivity in PI-treated patients compared to therapy-naïve, HIV-positive patients and HIV-negative controls. Using paired data, Mulligan et al. noted a significant increase in fasting glucose levels in HIV-infected patients after starting PI-based therapy.[40] Another study that assessed paired data in HIV-infected, therapy-naïve patients before and after 6 months of treatment had similar results:[41] subjects who were placed on a PI-containing regimen had a significantly higher homeostasis model assessment of insulin resistance (HOMA-IR) after 6 months of treatment than subjects placed on a PI-sparing regimen. Subsequent cross-sectional and longitudinal studies, including some randomized trials in treatment-naïve patients, have highlighted the fact that the effects of PIs on glucose metabolism are drug-specific, and not a common trait of all drugs in this class. In the paragraphs that follow, we will review data on the effects of individual PIs on insulin sensitivity and glucose metabolism.

Indinavir: Indinavir was the first PI to come into widespread use, and it is now apparent that it has the most profound effects on glucose metabolism of any PI studied to date. In a prospective, open-label study, Dube et al.[42] evaluated insulin sensitivity in predominantly treatment-naïve, HIV-infected patients before and 2 weeks after starting indinavir monotherapy, and again after 6 weeks on indinavir-based triple therapy. Insulin sensitivity, as determined by the minimal model analysis of the intravenous glucose tolerance test (IVGTT), decreased

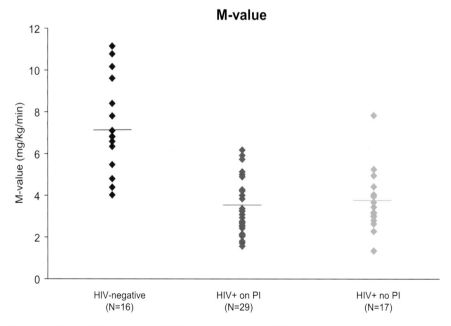

Fig. 38.1 Insulin sensitivity in HIV-positive and HIV-negative subjects. Although there is overlap in the insulin sensitivity of subjects who are HIV infected on PIs, HIV infected not on PIs, and HIV negative, on average, both HIV-infected groups had significantly lower *M* values than HIV-negative controls. Insulin sensitivity was determined using the hyperinsulinemic–euglycemic clamp (unpublished data from K. Mulligan, M. Schambelan, C. Grunfeld; studies were performed at the Clinical Research Center, San Francisco General Hospital)

progressively by 30% over the duration of 8 weeks. Although this decrease could have been an effect of indinavir, confounding factors such as viral suppression, immune system reconstitution, other ARV agents in the regimen, and changes in fat distribution could also have contributed to the induction of insulin resistance. To eliminate these confounding factors, Noor et al.[29] administered indinavir (in therapeutic doses) to HIV-negative healthy volunteers for 4 weeks. Hyperinsulinemic–euglycemic clamps performed before and after showed a significant (20%) decrease in insulin-mediated glucose uptake.[29]

An even greater (30%) decrease in insulin sensitivity was noted after the administration of a single dose of indinavir to healthy adults,[43] suggesting that the effects of indinavir are acute and less likely to be mediated by changes in fat distribution or other confounders. Notably, another study in HIV-negative individuals, which used a threefold higher rate of insulin infusion during a clamp, found no effect of indinavir on insulin-mediated glucose uptake in either skeletal muscle (as assessed by the hyperinsulinemic–euglycemic clamp) or adipose tissue (as assessed by ex vivo adipose tissue glucose uptake).[44] This result is in contrast to those in the aforementioned studies by Noor et al.,[29,43] as well as in vitro studies[45–47] and animal studies[48] in which infusion of indinavir during a glucose clamp in rats rapidly induced insulin resistance that also reversed rapidly when infusion of indinavir was discontinued.

Lopinavir/ritonavir (LPV/r): Studies of insulin sensitivity after treatment with LPV/r have had varying results. In HIV-negative subjects, a single dose of LPV/r acutely decreased insulin sensitivity (measured by a hyperinsulinemic–euglycemic clamp) by 13%, whereas 4 weeks of treatment had no significant effect on insulin sensitivity (measured by the same technique).[49,50] In a separate study in which LPV/r was administered to HIV-negative men for 5 days, a 24% decrease in insulin sensitivity by clamp was noted.[51] Other clinical studies using less sensitive techniques (such as measurements of fasting or random plasma glucose levels) have not shown a significant change in glucose metabolism with LPV/r.[52,53] In a rodent model, therapeutic levels of LPV/r acutely decreased peripheral glucose disposal by 30%; of note, therapeutic levels of ritonavir alone decreased peripheral glucose disposal by more than 50%.[54]

Atazanavir: Atazanavir is one of the more recently developed PIs and, thus far, has not been found to cause changes in glucose metabolism. Two studies in HIV-negative volunteers showed that atazanavir administration for 5 or 10 days (with and without ritonavir boosting) did not change insulin sensitivity (measured by clamp).[51,55] Moreover, HIV-infected men with insulin resistance (as defined by HOMA-IR $\geq$ 3.0) showed a significant improvement in insulin sensitivity (defined by ISI) when switched from a PI-based ARV regimen to an unboosted atazanavir-based regimen.[56] Studies in a rodent model have further confirmed that atazanavir alone does not alter peripheral glucose disposal.[54] Atazanavir is often "boosted" with low-dose ritonavir in order to increase its bioavailability; studies in healthy men have shown that a 10-day course of ritonavir-boosted atazanavir does not significantly alter insulin sensitivity as determined by hyperinsulinemic–euglycemic clamp.[55]

Other protease inhibitors: A single dose of amprenavir did not acutely alter insulin sensitivity (by hyperinsulinemic–euglycemic clamp) in a randomized placebo-controlled study of HIV-negative subjects.[57] HIV-infected patients who were PI naïve before beginning treatment with an amprenavir-based regimen for 48 weeks had a trend ($p = 0.06$) toward worsening insulin sensitivity (by minimal model analysis of IVGTT).[58] Another study showed no change in insulin sensitivity (by HOMA-IR) in subjects treated with nelfinavir.[59] This was confirmed in a subsequent randomized study of PI-naïve, HIV-infected subjects who were treated with nelfinavir for 64 weeks.[60] In a rodent model, amprenavir decreased peripheral glucose disposal moderately (by 18%),[54] whereas tipranavir did not induce an acute change in insulin sensitivity;[61] human studies with this latter agent have not as yet been published.

Mechanisms of PI-induced insulin resistance: Many of the studies cited above, especially those in HIV-negative individuals and those in which the effect is seen after only a single dose, provide strong evidence that specific PIs induce insulin resistance through mechanisms unrelated to the development of lipodystrophy and/or restitution to health. These results in humans are complemented by laboratory-based studies that have identified some of the molecular mechanisms responsible for the impaired insulin-mediated glucose uptake. An in vitro study of glucose transport in rat skeletal muscle showed that 4 h of exposure to indinavir, at various concentrations, had a dose- dependent effect on insulin-mediated glucose uptake.[47] Maximally stimulated insulin-mediated glucose uptake decreased by 40–70%; notably, this included in vitro concentrations of IDV which are equivalent to the peak drug levels achieved in patients in vivo.[45,62] These investigators also found that indinavir caused a decrease in cell-surface GLUT4 translocation which was not due to a disruption of the PI3K or PKB intermediary insulin-signaling pathways. Other studies have shown similar results using 3T3-L1 adipocytes.[46] Based on studies using *Xenopus laevis* oocytes which heterologously expressed either the GLUT1 or the GLUT4 isoforms, it was concluded that the inhibition of insulin-mediated glucose uptake (by ritonavir, indinavir, and amprenavir) is specific to GLUT4,[46] as shown in Fig. 38.2. In conclusion, the results of in vitro studies of insulin-mediated glucose uptake correlate well with the clinical studies regarding the effects of different PIs on insulin sensitivity. Indinavir and ritonavir appear to cause the most significant decrease in insulin-mediated glucose uptake,[54] while atazanavir appears to have either a mild effect[55] or none.[54] (Table 38.2).

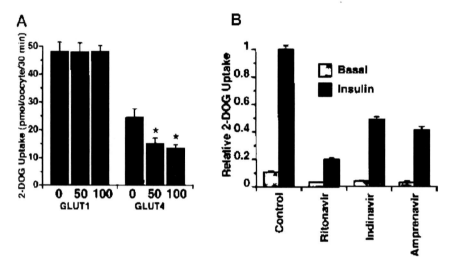

Fig. 38.2 Effects of protease inhibitors on in vitro insulin-mediated glucose uptake. Panel **A** shows that the indinavir (at various concentrations) specifically blocks glucose uptake mediated by the GLUT4 transporter in *X. laevis* oocytes. Panel **B** shows that amprenavir, indinavir, and ritonavir all decrease in vitro glucose uptake (from Murata et al.[46] by permission of American Society for Biochemistry and Molecular Biology)

Table 38.2 Effect of protease inhibitors on insulin resistance

Drug	HIV+ Subjects	HIV– Subjects
Amprenavir	↔ to ↑	↔
Atazanavir	↔	↔
Indinavir	↑↑ to ↑↑↑	↑↑ to ↑↑↑
Lopinavir/r	↔ to ↑↑	↔ to ↑↑
Nelfinavir	↔ to ↑↑	Not done
Ritonavir	↑	↑↑

Other ARV Medication

Non-PI ARV medications, either individually or as a class, have been less intensively studied than PIs with respect to their effect on glucose metabolism.

Nucleoside/tide reverse transcriptase inhibitors: Multiple studies have indicated that ARV regimens that included a thymidine analog NRTI (either zidovudine or stavudine) are associated with increased insulin resistance.[36,63] In the MACS cohort, cumulative exposure to NRTIs was associated with worsening of glucose metabolism [as measured by modified quantitative insulin sensitivity check index (QUICKI) and fasting insulin levels], whereas cumulative exposure to PIs and NNRTIs was not.[63] A small study ($N = 20$) that assessed insulin sensitivity by hyperinsulinemic–euglycemic clamp before and after 3 months of treatment with an NRTI-containing regimen (zidovudine/lamivudine) vs. an NRTI-sparing regimen found that insulin-mediated glucose disposal decreased by 25% with the former.[37] In HIV-negative healthy volunteers, 1 month of stavudine treatment decreased insulin sensitivity modestly (10% from baseline), as determined by clamp.[64] Interestingly, this study also showed a 52% decrease in muscle mitochondrial DNA content. Decreased mitochondrial DNA content has also been noted in adipose tissue biopsies collected from HIV-infected subjects using regimens containing stavudine or zidovudine, compared to HIV-positive subjects on regimens that do not contain these NRTIs and seronegative controls.[65] It has been postulated that decreased mitochondrial function may lead to insulin resistance in non-HIV-infected individuals.[66] Thus, mitochondrial toxicity may be one of the mechanisms by which some NRTIs contribute to insulin resistance.

Other NRTIs: Didanosine was one of the early NRTIs available and, in case reports, has been associated with hyperglycemia,[5–7] presumably mediated by a direct effect on the pancreas. Currently, didanosine is sometimes combined with the NRTI tenofovir, which has been found to boost plasma levels of didanosine and as a consequence increase the risk of hyperglycemia in patients using this combination.[67] At this time, there is little evidence to link other NRTIs (tenofovir, abacavir, lamivudine, emtricitabine) to insulin resistance or diabetes. However, as discussed earlier, these drugs are always used with other agents and, thus, it remains difficult to dissect their individual effects in patients on combination ARV therapy.

Non-nucleoside reverse transcriptase inhibitors (NNRTIs): HIV-infected, ARV therapy-naïve subjects who were treated with nevirapine-based therapy for 6–12 months had no change in insulin sensitivity (by HOMA-IR).[59] This was also true in a randomized study of subjects treated with efavirenz-based therapy for a period of 15 months.[60] A number of "switch studies" (in which patients are switched from a PI-containing regimen to one containing either nevirapine or efavirenz) are also informative with respect to the effects of NNRTIs on glucose metabolism. Patients who were switched from a PI-containing HAART regimen to a regimen containing either efavirenz or nevirapine had a significant improvement in glucose metabolism after 6 months.[68,69] It is important to note that, in these studies of relatively long duration, some of the patients also had an improvement in their fat distribution, making it difficult to separate this effect from that of the change in medication on glucose metabolism.

Another "switch study" which substituted nevirapine for a PI did not find any difference in HOMA-IR after 24 weeks; notably, this study did not select patients based on the presence of insulin resistance or lipodystrophy.[70] Patients selected for the presence of lipoatrophy and insulin resistance who were switched from PIs to efavirenz did not have any improvement in insulin sensitivity after 1 year of treatment, but these patients did not have any significant improvement in lipoatrophy either.[71] Finally, a randomized 24-month trial in which the PI component was replaced with an NNRTI (efavirenz or nevirapine) showed a trend toward improvement in insulin resistance by HOMA-IR.[72] Given the differences among PIs in their effects on insulin resistance as reviewed previously in this chapter, it is likely that the results may have varied depending on the PI which the subjects were receiving at the time of the switch.

Pancreatic β-Cell Effects

In addition to their effects on peripheral insulin sensitivity, ARV medications have been reported to decrease pancreatic insulin secretion. For example, PIs are known to be aspartate endopeptidase inhibitors;[73–75] endopeptidases also convert proinsulin to insulin.[76] Although some studies have shown an increase in the proinsulin:insulin ratio in patients treated with PIs,[77] other studies have not confirmed this presumed inhibition of proinsulin processing.[78,79]

The possibility of abnormal β-cell function in patients on PIs was proposed by Behrens et al.[77] The first report of inadequate insulin secretion was a prospective study of HIV-infected subjects placed on indinavir alone for 2 weeks and subsequently, indinavir-based triple-drug therapy. Subjects were evaluated at baseline, 2 weeks, and 8 weeks by OGTT and IVGTT.[42] Despite a 30% increase in insulin resistance with treatment, the acute insulin response to IV glucose (AIR$_G$) did not increase significantly, suggesting a possible defect in β-cell function. More extensive evaluation of β-cell function using the hyperglycemic clamp technique revealed a significant defect in first-phase insulin secretion in HIV-infected subjects after treatment with PIs.[78] Although second-phase insulin secretion was not changed, the disposition index (which assesses β-cell function in the context of insulin sensitivity) was reduced.[78] In vitro studies have also confirmed that some PIs inhibit insulin secretion by pancreatic β-cells.[80] In one study in HIV-infected patients on HAART, those with lipodystrophy had altered patterns of proinsulin secretion compared to those without lipodystrophy,[81] despite comparable ARV regimens and duration of therapy; these altered patterns of proinsulin secretion may be suggestive of an early defect in β-cell function which occurs in patients with lipodystrophy.

Other Mechanisms

Hepatic insulin sensitivity: In addition to decreasing insulin-mediated glucose uptake in peripheral tissues, PIs may also decrease hepatic insulin sensitivity. In HIV-negative subjects, 4 weeks of indinavir treatment increased fasting endogenous glucose production and glycogenolysis (as determined by stable isotope tracer studies).[82] The ability of insulin to suppress glucose production, measured during a euglycemic–hyperinsulinemic clamp, was also blunted by indinavir and, to a lesser extent, ritonavir.[83] In contrast, amprenavir did not significantly affect insulin-mediated suppression of glucose production.[83] The rank order of these effects of different PIs on endogenous glucose production parallels the magnitude of their effects on whole-body glucose disposal.

Lipolysis, free fatty acids: It has been suggested that an increased rate of lipolysis and increased circulating levels of free fatty acids are a fundamental pathophysiologic mechanism underlying HIV-associated lipodystrophy[84] or insulin resistance in HIV infection.[85] It is possible that this increased release of free fatty acids from adipose tissue contributes to both dyslipidemia (specifically, increased triglyceride levels)[86] and insulin resistance.[85] In this population, administration of the anti-lipolytic drug acipimox (a nicotinic acid analog) decreased free fatty acid levels and improved glucose metabolism[87–89] acutely and after 3 months, suggesting a link between free fatty acids and insulin resistance. In contrast, fasting free fatty acid levels did not increase when indinavir was given to healthy volunteers, and indinavir did not blunt the ability of insulin to suppress free fatty acids during a clamp, arguing against a role for free fatty acids in insulin resistance.[29,43]

Effects of Other Medications

In addition to ARVs, other medications used in patients with HIV and AIDS may cause hyperglycemia. Pentamidine, which was previously used for the treatment and/or the prevention of pneumonia caused by *Pneumocystis jiroveci*, has been reported to cause both initial hypoglycemia as a consequence of insulin release[90] and subsequent hyperglycemia or frank diabetes as a result of β-cell destruction.[91–94] This β-cell injury is similar to the effect of streptozotocin.

Megestrol acetate is a progestational agent which is used in patients with AIDS to stimulate appetite. In addition to binding to the progesterone receptor, megestrol also binds to the glucocorticoid receptor and can cause pseudo-Cushing's syndrome. In the latter context it has been reported to cause a reversible hyperglycemia.[95–97]

Effects of Lipodystrophy on Glucose Metabolism

Overview

The term "lipodystrophy" is non-specific and has been used to describe lipoatrophy alone, fat accumulation alone, or a combination of the two. Most researchers agree that the characteristic feature is subcutaneous

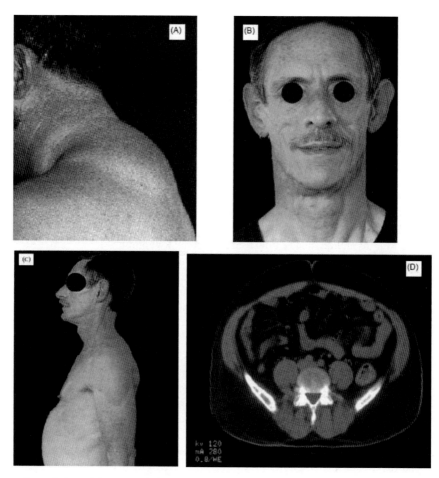

Fig. 38.3 Lipoatrophy and visceral fat accumulation in HIV-infected patients. Panel **A** shows the accumulation of fat in the dorsocervical region (buffalo hump) which can occur as part of the fat redistribution syndrome (reprinted from Lo et al.[10] by permission from Elsevier). Panel **B** shows the loss of subcutaneous fat which can occur in the face, as well as in other regions (reprinted from Carr et al.[13] by permission from Lippincott Williams and Wilkins). Panel **C** shows the accumulation of visceral fat that may occur in HIV-infected patients.[13] Panel **D** depicts the accumulation of visceral adipose tissue as seen by a CT scan at the L4 level (reprinted from Lo et al.[212] by permission of The Endocrine Society)

fat loss, with or without concomitant fat accumulation[98] (Fig. 38.3). The presence of lipodystrophy may affect glucose and lipid metabolism, decrease compliance with ARV medications,[99] and impact quality of life.[100]

Estimates of the prevalence of lipodystrophy in patients on ARV therapy vary widely, from 20 to 83%.[27,101–105] This wide variation is due in part to the lack of established diagnostic criteria. Objective criteria for the definition of lipodystrophy have been proposed,[106] but have not been widely accepted. The various ways in which lipodystrophy is assessed include patient self-report, physical examination/anthropometrics, and DEXA, CT, and MRI scans (for visceral and subcutaneous fat assessment). The severity of lipodystrophy appears to be associated with the duration of PI therapy and of HIV infection.[27] Other factors that have been associated with an increased risk for lipodystrophy (of any kind) include female sex, older age, and increased duration of exposure to ARV medications.[101,107] Although lipodystrophy is generally considered to occur in individuals receiving ARV therapy, one early study suggested that HIV infection per se may alter fat distribution,[108] and one survey reported a prevalence of 4% in treatment-naïve patients with HIV.[27]

Peripheral Lipoatrophy

Transgenic mice engineered to have little or no white adipose tissue have diabetes and/or severe insulin resistance,[109,110] which can be reversed by surgical implantation of adipose tissue[110] or infusion of leptin.[109] In non-HIV-infected individuals, the presence of lipoatrophy in the context of congenital or acquired lipodystrophy has also been associated with insulin resistance and diabetes.[111] In HIV-infected patients, the contribution of lipoatrophy toward the development of insulin resistance is not as clearly established. Although it is reasonable to infer that the progressive loss of subcutaneous fat in these patients may cause some degree of insulin resistance, further studies need to be performed to confirm this mechanism.

Lipoatrophy has been estimated to occur in 21–38% of HIV-infected patients.[104,105,112] Reported estimates of the prevalence and incidence of lipoatrophy vary widely due to ascertainment bias and differences in how the cohorts were assembled. In most studies of fat distribution in which subjects are categorized as having isolated lipoatrophy, isolated visceral adiposity, or mixed syndromes, isolated lipoatrophy is more common than visceral adiposity.[112,104,105] The development of lipoatrophy has been most convincingly associated with the prolonged duration of exposure to a thymidine analog NRTI (stavudine, zidovudine);[60,113,114] other factors that may be associated are older age and increased duration of HIV infection.[101,102,113,115] A prospective study of ARV therapy-naïve patients who were started on combination therapy showed that fat loss was not linked to central fat accumulation in most subjects; over the first 64 weeks of treatment, approximately one-third of the patients gained both trunk and limb fat, one-third lost both trunk and limb fat, and one-fourth gained trunk fat while limb fat decreased.[116]

To characterize the manifestations of lipodystrophy in the adipocyte, 14 patients with HIV who were on HAART and who had features of both lipoatrophy and fat accumulation underwent biopsy of subcutaneous adipose tissue, which revealed pathological atrophy as well as adipocyte apoptosis.[117] More targeted studies of fat morphology in patients with lipoatrophy have shown that their subcutaneous adipose tissue contains smaller adipocytes.[118] Furthermore, there is a decreased expression of specific adipogenic differentiation factors, such as CCAAT-enhancer-binding protein (C/EBP)-β and -α, peroxisome proliferator activator receptor (PPAR)-γ and sterol regulatory element-binding protein 1c (SREBP1c).[118]

In vitro studies have shown that incubation of 3T3-L1 pre-adipocytes with PIs (such as nelfinavir and indinavir) decreases the expression of C/EBP-α, PPAR-γ, and SREBP1 and inhibits the later differentiation of these cells.[119,120] In addition, there may be impaired nuclear localization of SREBP1.[121] PIs also appear to cause apoptosis of fully differentiated adipocytes; of note, this was seen only with nelfinavir but not with indinavir or ritonavir.[119] In vitro studies have also suggested that the PI indinavir induces resistance to insulin for mitogen-activated protein kinase activation.[120]

As opposed to PIs, the mechanism by which NRTIs induce lipoatrophy appears to differ. Like PIs, NRTIs appear to impair the differentiation of adipocytes in vitro.[122] However, NRTIs also cause the depletion of mitochondrial DNA[123] due to the inhibition of DNA polymerase gamma.[124–126] The ARV medications that appear to be most consistently associated with depletion of mitochondrial DNA and lipoatrophy are the thymidine analogue NRTIs stavudine and zidovudine.[14,105,113,127] It has been suggested that the combination of certain PIs and NRTIs may accelerate the development of lipoatrophy.[60,103,113,128]

Adiponectin: Adiponectin is a 30-kDa protein secreted by fat cells that plays an important role in whole-body insulin sensitivity. In rodent models, serum adiponectin levels are decreased in both obese and lipoatrophic mice.[129] In patients with both congenital and acquired generalized lipodystrophies, adiponectin levels are also significantly decreased.[130] Multiple studies have shown that HIV-infected patients on ARV therapy with clinical evidence of altered fat distribution have lower adiponectin levels than those with no alterations in fat distribution.[131,132] However, a large study using objective measurements of fat distribution (whole-body MRI) showed that although there was the expected negative relationship between visceral fat and adiponectin, there was a *positive* relationship between leg subcutaneous fat and adiponectin in HIV-infected patients.[133] The expected positive relationship between adiponectin and insulin sensitivity has been observed in patients with HIV infection.[134] Interestingly, this association became non-significant once the authors adjusted for NRTI use, suggesting that the effect of NRTIs on insulin sensitivity is, in part, mediated through adiponectin. The relationship between adiponectin levels and insulin sensitivity in HIV-infected patients was explored further by Reeds et al.[135]

using the two-stage hyperinsulinemic–euglycemic clamp and stable isotope infusion studies. They found that plasma adiponectin levels were inversely correlated with percent suppression of basal glucose production during low-dose and high-dose insulin infusion.[135]

The direct effects of individual ARV medications or classes of medication on adiponectin have yet to be studied in further detail. Studies in HIV-negative subjects have shown that adiponectin levels increased after 4 weeks of treatment with either indinavir or lopinavir/r;[136] however, there was no change in adiponectin levels in HIV-infected subjects after 3 months of treatment with either an NRTI-containing or an NRTI-sparing regimen.[37] It has been speculated that the increase in adiponectin may be a compensatory response to the induction of insulin resistance with these agents.

Visceral Adiposity

The accumulation of fat in HIV-infected patients can occur in the abdomen, trunk, neck, dorsocervical region, breasts, or as focal lipomatosis.[137] A number of different etiologies for the development of central fat accumulation have been investigated. The "buffalo hump" which some patients develop is reminiscent of that seen in patients with Cushing's syndrome, but comprehensive assessment of cortisol function has ruled out systemic hypercortisolemia in these patients.[10,138] Subjects also have normal glucocorticoid receptor number and affinity.[138] Based on the observation that adipose stromal cells from omental fat, but not subcutaneous fat, can generate active cortisol from inactive cortisone through the expression of 11-β-hydroxysteroid dehydrogenase type 1, it has been postulated that an increased level of cortisol produced locally (i.e., within omental adipose tissue) rather than systemically could cause visceral adiposity in non-HIV-infected patients.[139] However, the single study assessing 11-β-HSD type 1 in HIV-infected patients with lipodystrophy found increased mRNA expression of this enzyme in subcutaneous adipose tissue; levels in omental tissue and enzyme activity levels were not assessed.[140]

A large cohort study found that, over a 5-year period, the increase in waist circumference was correlated with HIV serostatus independent of exposure to ARV therapy.[115] A cross-sectional study also confirmed that ARV medication use is not correlated with increased visceral adiposity.[105] It has been hypothesized that the accumulation of central fat is a separate and distinct process from the loss of fat which occurs at the periphery.[105] For example, it is possible that visceral fat accumulation occurs as a component of the weight gain that occurs frequently with viral suppression, immune reconstitution, and restitution to health.[127] Thus far, a single mechanism unifying the accumulation of central fat and loss of subcutaneous peripheral fat has not been identified.

Overall, central fat accumulation has been reported in 17–40% of HIV-infected men in cross-sectional studies.[104,105,112] Interestingly, the few studies which concomitantly assessed a control group have shown that levels of visceral fat in men are not higher in the HIV population compared with HIV-negative controls matched for age[105] and gender.[105,141] In a cohort study of HIV-infected patients treated with PIs, the incidence of lipodystrophy with central fat accumulation was 77 per 1000 patient years.[101] Studies have indicated that female sex and duration of indinavir use may be additional risk factors for the development of central fat accumulation.[11,101,103]

Disturbances in Lipid Metabolism

Overview

In addition to abnormalities in glucose metabolism and lipodystrophy, HIV-infected patients often develop disturbances in lipid metabolism. The pattern of dyslipidemia observed in these patients is similar to that observed in the metabolic syndrome in non-HIV-infected individuals and consists of elevated serum triglyceride levels and decreased high-density lipoprotein cholesterol (HDL) levels, along with increases in small dense low density lipoprotein cholesterol (LDL). Changes in serum lipids can occur due to either the effects of HIV infection itself, the effects of ARV medications, or the restitution to health.

Because patients with HIV-associated lipodystrophy syndrome often have a constellation of disturbances, it is difficult to separate the individual aspects of this syndrome. For example, a recent report of changes over 5 years after initiation of HAART showed an overall trend to increases in insulin levels and alterations in fat distribution independent of the specific HAART regimen used, with variable effects on triglyceride levels depending on the specific regimen.[142] Although LDL levels tended to decrease after initially increasing, other studies have associated a decrease in LDL with increased use of lipid-lowering agents.[143] Thus, it is important, both in the treatment of this syndrome and in the long-term implications for cardiovascular disease and mortality, to assess both the glucose and the lipid disturbances.

The increased incidence of diabetes in HIV-infected patients may lead to more cardiovascular disease in this population. In addition to diabetes, these patients may also be at increased risk for cardiovascular dysfunction due to other mechanisms. These include endothelial dysfunction from PIs,[144] elevated levels of plasminogen activator inhibitor-1 (PAI-1),[145,146] and increased cholesterol accumulation in macrophages (independent of dyslipidemia).[147]

Retrospective studies that have assessed the occurrence of cardiovascular disease in HIV-infected patients have provided conflicting results; while some have indicated an increased risk,[148,149] others have shown no difference in incidence rates between patients with HIV infection and seronegative controls.[150] The only prospective study (the D:A:D study) found an increased risk of myocardial infarction in patients taking combination ARV therapy;[151] this may be associated with increased exposure to PIs.[152] However, the absolute risk of myocardial infarction in these patients was still quite low (3.5 events per 1000 person-years).

HIV Infection

Studies performed in the era prior to the widespread use of ARV medications indicated that early stages of HIV infection were associated with decreased levels of total, LDL, and HDL cholesterol.[153-156] As HIV infection progressed, patients developed varying degrees of hypertriglyceridemia.[155] With the development of frank AIDS, patients typically had significant triglyceride elevation.[153] Studies using stable isotope tracer techniques indicated that patients with both asymptomatic HIV infection and AIDS have a three- to fourfold increase in the rate of fractional de novo hepatic lipogenesis, which may partially account for the elevated triglyceride levels.[157] Decreased clearance of triglyceride particles[155,158] may also contribute to hypertriglyceridemia. Data in ARV-naïve members of a large HIV cohort study indicate that the prevalence of hypertriglyceridemia is 15%, hypercholesterolemia approximately 8%, and low HDL cholesterol 25%[159,160] (Fig. 38.4).

Given the changes in lipid metabolism that occur with HIV infection, one might ask whether restitution to health in response to effective ARV therapy would reverse these abnormalities. Indeed, in an early study, initiation of zidovudine monotherapy reduced TG levels.[161] However, more recent studies of initiation of HAART have reported increases, rather than decreases, in TG levels.[40,58,114] In contrast, observed increases in total and LDL cholesterol in such studies have been widely attributed to restoration of health. Increases in HDL cholesterol have occurred with some[162,163] but not all[143] HAART regimens. Following is a brief summary of studies examining the effects of ARV therapy on lipids.

Antiretrovirals

PIs: It has been estimated that approximately 28–50% of patients on a PI-based ARV regimen have hypertriglyceridemia and 27–74% have hypercholesterolemia.[77,104,27,160]

As was the case with insulin resistance, PIs differ with regard to the magnitude and nature of their effects on lipids. Ritonavir appears to cause the most profound increase in triglyceride levels,[27,104,164] while newer PIs (such as atazanavir) appear to have minimal effects.[51] Patients with severe hyperlipidemia who were switched

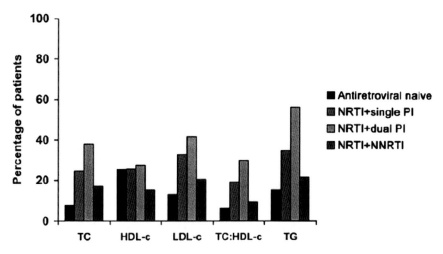

Fig. 38.4 Prevalence of dyslipidemia in HIV-infected subjects. Data from the D:A:D study showing the prevalence of elevated total cholesterol, decreased HDL, elevated LDL, hypertriglyceridemia, and abnormal TC:HDL ratio in HIV-infected subjects who are on various treatment regimens or are ARV naïve (reprinted from Fontas et al.[159] by permission of The University of Chicago Press)

to atazanavir had a 45% improvement in serum triglyceride levels and 18% improvement in total cholesterol.[165] One proposed mechanism by which PIs may cause hypertriglyceridemia is through the inhibition of proteasomal degradation of apolipoprotein B, which is the primary apolipoprotein component of triglyceride and cholesterol-rich particles.[166] In cultured human and rat hepatoma cells, both ritonavir and saquinavir decreased the degradation of apolipoprotein B. Although this mechanism will need to be further validated in human studies, one human study of five patients with dyslipidemia on ARVs showed an increase in the synthesis of apolipoprotein B.[167]

A few studies have assessed changes in LDL cholesterol levels that occur with treatment. LDL cholesterol levels are lower in PI- naïve patients[26,168] and appear to increase after initiation of PI-based therapy.[40,168–171]

In HIV-negative subjects, administration of ritonavir for 2 weeks increased serum triglyceride levels, total cholesterol, and VLDL cholesterol levels while decreasing HDL cholesterol and apolipoprotein A1 levels.[170] In other studies in HIV-negative individuals, indinavir did not change serum lipid values,[29,43] while lopinavir/ritonavir increased serum triglyceride levels.[49]

NNRTIs: A large cohort study reported that, in patients on combination antiviral therapy that included an NNRTI (but no PIs), the prevalence of hypercholesterolemia was 23% and hypertriglyceridemia was 32%.[160] The substitution of NNRTIs (nevirapine and, to a lesser extent, efavirenz) for PIs may help improve triglyceride and total cholesterol levels in patients with dyslipidemia.[69,172] Notably, NNRTIs have been associated with improvement in HDL cholesterol, which occurs rarely with PI-containing regimens.[173,174]

NRTIs: In patients on NRTI therapy alone, the prevalence of hypercholesterolemia was 10% and hypertriglyceridemia 23%.[160] With respect to differences among NRTIs, a randomized study comparing tenofovir and stavudine indicated that tenofovir had a more favorable lipid profile (with less of an elevation of triglyceride and total cholesterol levels).[175] Stavudine has been associated with significant increases in triglyceride levels.[175] Compared with stavudine and zidovudine, abacavir did not significantly affect lipid profiles.[176]

Overall, from epidemiological studies, PIs are associated with the highest occurrence of hypercholesterolemia and hypertriglyceridemia, followed by NNRTIs.[160] However, as is the case with insulin resistance, it is apparent that the effects of ARV medication are drug specific.

Diagnosis

Published guidelines for the management of lipids in patients with HIV recommend that a fasting lipid panel be performed prior to the initiation of ARV treatment and prior to any switches in treatment regimen.[177–179] The lipid panel should be repeated in 3–6 months and, if within the normal range, repeated annually. The diagnosis of dyslipidemia and the goals for lipid reduction should follow the National Cholesterol Education Program (NCEP) guidelines.[180] At this time, the threshold for diagnosis and treatment of lipid abnormalities in HIV-infected patients is the same as that for the non-HIV-infected population.

Diagnosis of Diabetes/Abnormal Glucose Metabolism

Criteria for the diagnosis of abnormal glucose metabolism in HIV-infected patients are the same as those in HIV-seronegative individuals and follow the guidelines of the American Diabetes Association.[181] The assessment of a diabetic patient with HIV infection should include evaluation of both HIV-associated and non-HIV-related risk factors. These include fasting lipid profile, obesity, family history (of premature cardiovascular disease), smoking status, ARV history, and the presence of altered fat distribution.

It is recommended that HIV-infected patients be screened for the presence of diabetes (with a fasting glucose) prior to the initiation of ARV therapy.[177,178] Fasting glucose should subsequently be assessed 3–6 months after starting treatment and then annually. In patients who are at particularly high risk (those with pre-existing risk factors for type 2 diabetes or significant fat redistribution), the use of a 75 g OGTT to screen may be more appropriate.

Treatment

Overview

In ARV-naïve patients who are at high risk for the development of diabetes, or in those with impaired fasting glucose or IGT, initiation of PI-sparing ARV regimens should be considered. Alternatively, based on the apparent lack of effect on glucose metabolism, the PI atazanavir could be tried. Patients on therapy may benefit from having the PI component switched to drugs in other classes, such as the NNRTIs nevirapine and efavirenz or the NRTI abacavir.[177] Patients who continue to have hyperglycemia should be treated according to the standard guidelines established by the American Diabetes Association.[182] These include diet, exercise, weight loss, and medications as needed. Exercise has been shown to reduce abdominal obesity in patients with HIV-associated central fat accumulation,[183,184] but its effect on individuals with lipoatrophy is unknown. Although there have been no studies specifically targeted to reversal of diabetes in HIV-infected patients, several studies have examined the effect of antidiabetic agents in those with insulin resistance and/or altered fat distribution.

Metformin

Metformin is a biguanide which improves glucose metabolism primarily by decreasing hepatic glucose output[185] and can reduce visceral fat. The first randomized study assessing the effects of metformin in HIV-infected patients enrolled subjects who were hyperinsulinemic but not diabetic.[186] Metformin treatment decreased fasting glucose and insulin values and improved insulin levels during an OGTT.[186] Hadigan et al.[187] performed a randomized double-blind, placebo-controlled trial to assess the effects of metformin in HIV-infected patients with lipodystrophy and abnormal glucose metabolism (either impaired glucose tolerance or hyperinsulinemia); 22 of the 25 evaluable subjects were on PIs as part of their ARV regimen. After 3 months, subjects receiving metformin had significant improvement in hyperinsulinemia (as determined by a decrease in insulin AUC on OGTT) but no significant change in glucose AUC. These improvements were sustained at month 6 of treatment.[188]

Other studies have confirmed the improvement in insulin sensitivity that occurs with metformin treatment[189,190] in patients with HIV lipodystrophy. However, the effects of metformin on visceral adipose tissue (VAT) have been inconsistent. Although some studies found a significant decrease in VAT,[186,190] others found

Table 38.3 Trials assessing treatment of insulin resistance in patients with HIV infection

Trial	N	Randomized	Placebo	Blinded	Insulin resistance	VAT	SAT
Metformin							
Saint-Marc and Touraine[186]	N=29	Y	Y	N	↓sum insulin	↓ VAT	↔SAT
Hadigan et al.[187]	N=26	Y	Y	Y	↓insulin AUC	↓ VAT (trend)	↓ SAT
van Wijk et al.[190]	N=39	Y	N	N	↓insulin AUC	↓ VAT	↓ SAT
Mulligan et al.[189]	N=105	Y	N	N	↓insulin AUC	↔VAT	↔SAT
Kohli et al.[191]	N=48	Y	Y	N	↔insulin, glucose AUC	↔VAT	NA
Rosiglitazone							
Gelato et al.[198]	N=8	N	N	N	↑glucose disposal	↓ VAT	↑ SAT
Carr et al.[201]	N=108	Y	Y	Y	↑HOMA-IR	↔VAT	↔SAT
Hadigan et al.[199]	N=28	Y	Y	Y	↓M/I	↔VAT	↓ SAT
van Wijk et al.[190]	N=39	Y	N	N	↓insulin AUC	↔VAT	↑ SAT
Mulligan et al.[189]	N=105	Y	N	N	↓insulin AUC	↔VAT	↔SAT
Cavalcanti et al.[205]	N=96	Y	Y	N	↔insulin AUC	NA	NA
Sutinen et al.[200]	N=30	Y	Y	Y	↔fasting glucose	↔VAT	↔SAT

Note: N=patients enrolled (rather than evaluable); NA=not assessed in study.

either no change[189,191] or only a trend toward decreased VAT[187] (Table 38.3). These reductions in VAT, when they occurred, typically occurred in the presence of general weight loss. The primary side effect of metformin in these studies was gastrointestinal (i.e., nausea and diarrhea). In HIV-infected patients there has also been concern about the potential of metformin to promote lactic acidosis, as hyperlactatemia can occur during treatment with some NRTIs.[192] Although none of the aforementioned studies reported an increase in lactate levels or the occurrence of lactic acidosis, plasma lactate levels should be monitored in HIV-infected patients who are treated with metformin.

In conclusion, metformin has been shown to improve insulin sensitivity in HIV-infected patients who have lipodystrophy, are on ARV treatment, and have insulin resistance. However, the studies are limited by the lack of long-term data (i.e., beyond 6 months) and the fact that patients with a diagnosis of diabetes have not been evaluated.

Peroxisome Proliferator Activated Receptor-γ Agonists

The transcription factor PPAR-γ has been shown to play an important role in adipocyte differentiation and glucose metabolism.[193] The expression of PPAR-γ is decreased in lipoatrophic fat obtained by biopsy from HIV-infected individuals with insulin resistance.[118] In addition, there was a decrease in the expression of SREBP-1, which plays an important role in the PPAR-γ signaling pathway. Other studies have shown that indinavir impairs the intranuclear localization of SREBP-1, induces insulin resistance, and decreases the differentiation of pre-adipocytes.[120]

Treatment with the PPAR-γ agonist troglitazone in non-HIV-infected patients with acquired or congenital lipodystrophy[194] or type 2 diabetes[195–197] increased the amount of subcutaneous adipose tissue and decreased VAT as well as improved insulin resistance and diabetes. Based on these promising results, PPAR-γ agonists such as rosiglitazone and pioglitazone have been evaluated in HIV-infected patients with lipodystrophy, especially those with lipoatrophy. An early pilot study showed that, in eight HIV-infected patients with lipoatrophy and insulin resistance, 6–12 weeks of rosiglitazone therapy significantly improved insulin sensitivity (measured by clamp), increased peripheral subcutaneous fat, and decreased visceral fat.[198] Subsequent randomized studies in larger groups of subjects have confirmed the improvement in insulin sensitivity with rosiglitazone treatment in both subjects who are insulin resistant[189,199] and those who are not.[190,200,201] Pioglitazone also improves insulin sensitivity in HIV-infected patients on HAART who have metabolic abnormalities.[202] Due to the possible increased risk of cardiac ischemia,[203] rosiglitazone is not recommended for use in patients with HIV infection and diabetes. In patients with congestive heart failure, both rosiglitazone and pioglitazone should be used carefully due to the side effects of fluid retention and edema; these agents are contraindicated in patients with class III or IV (New York Heart Association) heart failure.

Adiponectin, an adipocytokine associated with increased insulin sensitivity,[204] has been assessed as a possible factor by which agents that improve insulin action have their salutary effects. Although these studies have been limited, the results available to date suggest that metformin does not alter adiponectin levels,[189,190] even though it improves insulin sensitivity. On the other hand, the thiazolidinedione rosiglitazone increased adiponectin levels[189,190,201] and improved insulin sensitivity in HIV-infected patients with lipodystrophy. Pioglitazone also improved insulin sensitivity and adiponectin levels in HIV-infected patients on HAART, regardless of the presence of fat redistribution.[202]

Sulfonylureas

At this time, there are insufficient published data on the use of sulfonylureas in patients with HIV infection and diabetes to recommend either for or against their use. This is also true of newer insulinotropic agents such as incretin-mimetic agents and DPP-IV inhibitors.

Treatment of Peripheral Lipoatrophy

Given the association between lipoatrophy and insulin resistance/diabetes in non-HIV lipodystrophy, reversal of lipoatrophy may improve glucose metabolism. Therapeutic options for the treatment of lipoatrophy are limited. As mentioned earlier, thiazolidinediones have increased subcutaneous fat in patients with non-HIV-associated lipodystrophy syndromes.[194] However, studies of the effects of rosiglitazone or pioglitazone on subcutaneous adipose tissue in HIV-infected patients have had inconsistent results, with some reporting modest increases[189,190,198,199] and others reporting no effect.[200,201,205]

In view of the limited success with thiazolidinediones, the current recommended strategy for reversing lipoatrophy is to replace the NRTIs most closely associated with lipoatrophy (stavudine and zidovudine) in a patient's HAART regimen with newer NRTIs such as tenofovir or abacavir. Several large randomized studies have demonstrated slow but significant improvements in lipoatrophy using this strategy.[176,206–208] Similarly, patients with lipoatrophy who were switched to an NRTI-sparing regimen that contained the PI lopinavir/ritonavir experienced increases in subcutaneous fat.[209] However, this switch was also associated with an exacerbation of dyslipidemia and a higher rate of virologic failure, illustrating the need to consider all of the potential risks and benefits of such switches. Removal of a PI from the treatment regimen has not been consistently successful in reversing lipoatrophy.[210]

Treatment of Visceral Adiposity

Although switching ARV regimens can reverse lipoatrophy, this strategy has not been as successful in reducing VAT.[211] In addition, as mentioned above, metformin has not consistently reduced VAT in patients with HIV infection,[189,191] and randomized studies of rosiglitazone have consistently shown no effect on VAT.[189,198,201] Treatments that have been used to decrease visceral fat accumulation include growth hormone and growth hormone-releasing hormone. Although pharmacologic doses of growth hormone (GH) have consistently decreased visceral fat, such treatment worsened glucose metabolism.[212–216] Thus, GH is not recommended for patients with impaired glucose tolerance. A recent randomized trial suggested that a synthetic growth hormone-releasing hormone may modestly decrease visceral fat without disrupting glucose metabolism.[217]

Treatment of Lipid Abnormalities

Dyslipidemia and hyperlipidemia in HIV-infected adults should be treated according to the established NCEP guidelines for the general population.[180] In patients who are at particularly high risk for the development of hyperlipidemia, the use of a PI-sparing regimen should be considered at the outset.[177] Alternatively switching to a PI with less of an effect on lipids (such as atazanavir) should be considered, although ritonavir boosting of such PIs may negate much of the benefit of the switch. In patients with lipid disorders, the NCEP dietary guidelines for consumption of fats and cholesterol should be followed.

Lipid-lowering drugs should be considered for the treatment of elevated total cholesterol, LDL cholesterol, or triglycerides. Either hydroxymethylglutaryl-coenzyme A reductase inhibitors (statins) or fibrates may be used, but the former are usually preferred for the treatment of isolated hypercholesterolemia. Since protease inhibitors inhibit the cytochrome P450 3A4 enzyme pathway through which many of the statins are metabolized, the pharmacological interaction of these agents must be carefully considered.[218] Currently, pravastatin and fluvastatin are the preferred statins in HIV-infected individuals.[177,178,219] Low-dose atorvastatin[220] and rosuvastatin may also be used.[221] Simvastatin is contraindicated due to the risk of pharmacokinetic interactions with ARV medications. In small trials of HIV-infected subjects with dyslipidemia, pravastatin decreased LDL cholesterol by 15–20%[222–224] and fluvastatin by 30%.[223] Rosuvastatin decreased TC by 22% and TG by 30% in patients with hyperlipidemia on PI.[221] Atorvastatin decreased total cholesterol and triglyceride by approximately 20%.[225]

Isolated hypertriglyceridemia is generally treated with fibrates. The combination of fibrates and statins, although effective,[226] should be used cautiously. Studies assessing this combination therapy in HIV-infected patients with hyperlipidemia have shown that total cholesterol decreased by 30% and triglycerides by 60%.[225] Calza et al. assessed changes in lipids in patients on HAART therapy and found that fibrates alone decreased triglycerides by 41% and total cholesterol by 22%, compared to a reduction of 35 and 25% with statins alone.[221] Small trials of fenofibrate has shown a decrease in total cholesterol of 14% and triglyceride of 40%;[227] gemfibrozil has shown much more modest effects.[228] Niacin may also improve dyslipidemia in HIV-infected patients but, because it worsens insulin resistance and glucose metabolism, it should be used cautiously.[229,230] A few small studies have shown that omega-3 polyunsaturated fatty acids improve triglyceride levels in HIV-infected patients with hypertriglyceridemia;[231–233] however, this may not be ideal as first-line treatment in HIV-infected patients with hypertriglyceridemia due to insufficient data and the potential for increasing LDL cholesterol.[233] Ezetimibe is a new lipid-lowering agent that blocks the intestinal absorption of cholesterol. Although it has been reported to modestly improve cholesterol levels in HIV-infected patients with hyperlipidemia,[234] a full assessment of its efficacy and safety in HIV-infected individuals is not yet available.

Conclusion

In conclusion, HIV-infected patients are at increased risk for abnormal glucose metabolism, including insulin resistance, diabetes mellitus, and impaired glucose tolerance, due to a number of factors. These include the effect of antiretroviral medications, the effects of HIV infection itself, and associated abnormalities, such as lipodystrophy. ARV medications can contribute to impaired glucose metabolism through their direct effects on peripheral and hepatic insulin sensitivity as well as pancreatic β-cell function. Furthermore, ARV medications can impair glucose metabolism through other mechanisms, such as mitochondrial toxicity and the development of peripheral lipoatrophy and/or visceral fat accumulation. Although PIs have been most commonly associated with abnormal glucose metabolism, individual agents have widely varying effects, ranging from significant (e.g., indinavir) to minimal (e.g., atazanavir). As other classes of medications (NRTIs and NNRTIs) have been increasingly studied, it has become evident that these may also adversely affect glucose metabolism through similar mechanisms.

HIV-infected patients with abnormal glucose metabolism are also at increased risk for dyslipidemia. In conjunction with the morphologic abnormalities (peripheral lipoatrophy and visceral adiposity), these factors may result in increased risk of cardiovascular disease.

References

1. Barre-Sinoussi F, Chermann JC, Rey F, et al. Isolation of a T-lymphotropic retrovirus from a patient at risk for acquired immune deficiency syndrome (AIDS). *Science*. 1983;220(4599):868–871.
2. Gallo RC, Salahuddin SZ, Popovic M, et al. Frequent detection and isolation of cytopathic retroviruses (HTLV-III) from patients with AIDS and at risk for AIDS. *Science*. 1984;224(4648):500–503.
3. Popovic M, Sarngadharan MG, Read E, Gallo RC. Detection, isolation, and continuous production of cytopathic retroviruses (HTLV-III) from patients with AIDS and pre-AIDS. *Science*. 1984;224(4648):497–500.
4. Brook I. Approval of zidovudine (AZT) for acquired immunodeficiency syndrome. A challenge to the medical and pharmaceutical communities. *J Am Med Assoc*. 1987;258(11):1517.
5. Moyle GJ, Nelson MR, Hawkins D, Gazzard BG. The use and toxicity of didanosine (ddI) in HIV antibody-positive individuals intolerant to zidovudine (AZT. *Q J Med*. 1993;86(3):155–163.
6. Munshi MN, Martin RE, Fonseca VA. Hyperosmolar nonketotic diabetic syndrome following treatment of human immunodeficiency virus infection with didanosine. *Diabetes Care*. 1994;17(4):316–317.
7. Vittecoq D, Zucman D, Auperin I, Passeron J. Transient insulin-dependent diabetes mellitus in an HIV-infected patient receiving didanosine. *AIDS*. 1994;8(9):1351.
8. Palella FJ Jr., Delaney KM, Moorman AC, et al. Declining morbidity and mortality among patients with advanced human immunodeficiency virus infection. HIV Outpatient Study Investigators. *N Engl J Med*. 1998;338(13):853–860.
9. Dube MP, Johnson DL, Currier JS, Leedom JM. Protease inhibitor-associated hyperglycaemia. *Lancet*. 1997;350:713–714.
10. Lo JC, Mulligan K, Tai VW, Algren H, Schambelan M. "Buffalo hump" in men with HIV-1 infection. *Lancet*. 1998;351: 867–870.
11. Miller KD, Jones E, Yanovski JA, Shankar R, Feuerstein I, Falloon J. Visceral abdominal-fat accumulation associated with use of indinavir. *Lancet*. 1998;351:871–875.
12. Miller KK, Daly PA, Sentochnik D, et al. Pseudo-Cushing's syndrome in human immunodeficiency virus-infected patients. *Clin Infect Dis*. 1998;27:68–72.
13. Carr A, Samaras K, Burton S, et al. A syndrome of peripheral lipodystrophy, hyperlipidaemia and insulin resistance in patients receiving HIV protease inhibitors. *AIDS*. 1998;12:F51–F58.
14. Saint-Marc T, Partisani M, Poizot-Martin I, et al. A syndrome of peripheral fat wasting (lipodystrophy) in patients receiving long-term nucleoside analogue therapy. *AIDS*. 1999;13:1659–1667.
15. Carr A, Samaras K, Chisholm DJ, Cooper DA. Pathogenesis of HIV-1-protease inhibitor-associated peripheral lipodystrophy, hyperlipidemia, and insulin resistance. *Lancet*. 1998;351:1881–1883.
16. Tsiodras S, Mantzoros C, Hammer S, Samore M. Effects of protease inhibitors on hyperglycemia, hyperlipidemia, and lipodystrophy: A 5-year cohort study. *Arch Intern Med*. 2000;160(13):2050-2056.
17. Brown TT, Cole SR, Li X, et al. Antiretroviral therapy and the prevalence and incidence of diabetes mellitus in the multicenter AIDS cohort study. *Arch Intern Med*. 2005;165(10):1179–1184.
18. Ledergerber B, Furrer H, Rickenbach M, et al. Factors associated with the incidence of type 2 diabetes mellitus in HIV-infected participants in the Swiss HIV Cohort Study. *Clin Infect Dis*. 2007;45(1):111–119.
19. Tien PC, Schneider MF, Cole SR, et al. Antiretroviral therapy exposure and incidence of diabetes mellitus in the Women's Interagency HIV Study. *AIDS*. 2007;21(13):1739–1745.
20. Danoff A, Shi Q, Justman J, et al. Oral glucose tolerance and insulin sensitivity are unaffected by HIV infection or antiretroviral therapy in overweight women. *J Acquir Immune Defic Syndr*. 2005;39(1):55–62.
21. Mulligan K, Anastos K, Justman J, et al. Fat distribution in HIV-infected women in the United States: DEXA substudy in the Women's Interagency HIV Study. *J Acquir Immune Defic Syndr*. 2005;38(1):18–22.
22. Howard AA, Floris-Moore M, Arnsten JH, et al. Disorders of glucose metabolism among HIV-infected women. *Clin Infect Dis*. 2005;40(10):1492–1499.
23. Marti C, Pena JM, Bates I, et al. Obstetric and perinatal complications in HIV-infected women. Analysis of a cohort of 167 pregnancies between 1997 and 2003. *Acta Obstet Gynecol Scand*. 2007;86(4):409–415.
24. Hitti J, Andersen J, McComsey G, et al. Protease inhibitor-based antiretroviral therapy and glucose tolerance in pregnancy: AIDS Clinical Trials Group A5084. *Am J Obstet Gynecol*. 2007;196(4):331–337.
25. Watts DH, Balasubramanian R, Maupin RT Jr., et al. Maternal toxicity and pregnancy complications in human immunodeficiency virus-infected women receiving antiretroviral therapy: PACTG 316. *Am J Obstet Gynecol*. 2004;190(2): 506–516.
26. Hadigan C, Meigs JB, Corcoran C, et al. Metabolic abnormalities and cardiovascular disease risk factors in adults with human immunodeficiency vires infection and lipodystrophy. *Clin Infect Dis*. 2001;32:130–139.
27. Carr A, Samaras K, Thorisdottir A, Kaufmann GR, Chisholm DJ, Cooper DA. Diagnosis, prediction, and natural course of HIV-1 protease-inhibitor-associated lipodystrophy, hyperlipidaemia, and diabetes mellitus: a cohort study. *Lancet*. 1999;353:2093–2099.
28. Saves M, Chene G, Dellamonica P, et al. Incidence of lipodystrophy and glucose and lipid abnormalities during the follow-up of a cohort of HIV-infected patients started on a protease inhibitor (PI)-containing regimen. 9th Conference on Retroviruses and Opportunistic Infections, 302. 2002.

29. Noor MA, Lo JC, Mulligan K, et al. Metabolic effects of indinavir in healthy HIV-seronegative men. *AIDS*. 2001;15(7): F11–F18.

30. Mehta SH, Moore RD, Thomas DL, Chaisson RE, Sulkowski MS. The effect of HAART and HCV infection on the development of hyperglycemia among HIV-infected persons. *J Acquir Immune Defic Syndr*. 2003;33(5):577–584.

31. Howard AA, Lo Y, Floris-Moore M, Klein RS, Fleischer N, Schoenbaum EE. Hepatitis C virus infection is associated with insulin resistance among older adults with or at risk of HIV infection. *AIDS*. 2007;21(5):633–641.

32. Hommes MJT, Romijn JA, Endert E, Eeftinck-Schattenkerk JKM, Sauerwein HP. Insulin sensitivity and insulin clearance in human immunodeficiency virus-infected men. *Metabolism*. 1991;40:651–656.

33. Heyligenberg R, Romijn JA, Hommes MJT, Endert E, Eeftinck Schattenkerk MKM, Sauerwein HP. Non-insulin-mediated glucose uptake in human immunodeficiency virus-infected men. *Clin Sci*. 1993;84:209–216.

34. Stein TP, Nutinsky C, Condoluci D, Schluter MD, Leskiw MJ. Protein and energy substrate metabolism in AIDS patients. *Metabolism*. 1990;39:876–881.

35. U.S. Department of Health and Human Services HIV/AIDS Guidelines, http://aidsinfo.nih.gov. 12-1-2007.

36. Lo JC, Kazemi MR, Hsue PY, et al. The impact of nucleoside reverse transcriptase inhibitor treatment duration and insulin resistance on fasting arterialized lactate levels in patients with HIV infection. *Clin Infect Dis*. 2005;41:1335–1340.

37. Blumer RM, van Vonderen MG, Sutinen J, et al. Zidovudine/lamivudine contributes to insulin resistance within 3 months of starting combination antiretroviral therapy. *AIDS*. 2008;22(2):227–236.

38. Walli R, Herfort O, Michl GM, et al. Treatment with protease inhibitors associated with peripheral insulin resistance and impaired oral glucose tolerance in HIV-1-infected patients. *AIDS*. 1998;12:F167–F173.

39. Walli R, Goebel FD, Demant T. Impaired glucose tolerance and protease inhibitors. *Ann Intern Med*. 1998;129(10): 837–838.

40. Mulligan K, Grunfeld C, Tai VW, et al. Hyperlipidemia and insulin resistance are induced by protease inhibitors independent of changes in body composition in patients with HIV infection. *J Acquir Immune Defic Syndr*. 2000;23:35–43.

41. Visnegarwala F, Darcourt J, Sajja P, et al. Changes in metabolic profile among antiretroviral-naive patients initiating protease inhibitor versus non-protease inhibitor containing HAART regimens. *J Acquir Immune Defic Syndr*. 2003;33(5): 653–655.

42. Dube MP, Edmundson-Melancon H, Qian D, Aqeel R, Johnson D, Buchanan TA. Prospective evaluation of the effect of initiating indinavir-based therapy on insulin sensitivity and B-cell function in HIV-infected patients. *J Acquire Immune Defic Syndr*. 2001;27:130–134.

43. Noor MA, Seneviratne T, Aweeka FT, et al. Indinavir acutely inhibits insulin-stimulated glucose disposal in humans: a randomized, placebo-controlled study. *AIDS*. 2002;16:F1–F8.

44. Shankar SS, Considine RV, Gorski JC, Steinberg HO. Insulin sensitivity is preserved despite disrupted endothelial function. *Am J Physiol Endocrinol Metab*. 2006;291(4):E691–E696.

45. Murata H, Hruz PW, Mueckler M. Indinavir inhibits the glucose transporter isoform Glut4 at physiologic concentrations. *AIDS*. 2002;16(6):859–863.

46. Murata H, Hruz PW, Mueckler M. The mechanism of insulin resistance caused by HIV protease inhibitor therapy. *J Biol Chem*. 2000;275(27):20251–20254.

47. Nolte LA, Yarasheski KE, Kawanaka K, Fisher J, Le N, Holloszy JO. The HIV protease inhibitor indinavir decreases insulin- and contraction- stimulated glucose transport in skeletal muscle. *Diabetes*. 2001;50(6):1397–1401.

48. Hruz PW, Murata H, Qiu H, Mueckler M. Indinavir induces acute and reversible peripheral insulin resistance in rats. *Diabetes*. 2002;51(4):937–942.

49. Lee GA, Seneviratne T, Noor MA, et al. The metabolic effects of lopinavir/ritonavir in HIV-negative men. *AIDS*. 2004;18: 641–649.

50. Lee GA, Lo JC, Aweeka F, et al. Single-dose lopinavir-ritonavir acutely inhibits insulin-mediated glucose disposal in healthy volunteers. *Clin Infect Dis*. 2006;43(5):658–660.

51. Noor MA, Parker RA, O'Mara E, et al. The effects of HIV protease inhibitors atazanavir and lopinavir/ritonavir on insulin sensitivity in HIV-seronegative healthy adults. *AIDS*. 2004;18(16):2137–2144.

52. Martinez E, Domingo P, Galindo MJ, et al. Risk of metabolic abnormalities in patients infected with HIV receiving antiretroviral therapy that contains lopinavir-ritonavir. *Clin Infect Dis*. 2004;38(7):1017–1023.

53. Lafeuillade A, Hittinger G, Philip G, Lambry V, Jolly P, Poggi C. Metabolic evaluation of HIV-infected patients receiving a regimen containing lopinavir/ritonavir (Kaletra). *HIV Clin Trials*. 2004;5(6):392–398.

54. Yan Q, Hruz PW. Direct comparison of the acute in vivo effects of HIV protease inhibitors on peripheral glucose disposal. *J Acquir Immune Defic Syndr*. 2005;40(4):398–403.

55. Noor MA, Flint OP, Maa JF, Parker RA. Effects of atazanavir/ritonavir and lopinavir/ritonavir on glucose uptake and insulin sensitivity: demonstrable differences in vitro and clinically. *AIDS*. 2006;20(14):1813–1821.

56. Guffanti M, Caumo A, Galli L, et al. Switching to unboosted atazanavir improves glucose tolerance in highly pretreated HIV-1 infected subjects. *Eur J Endocrinol*. 2007;156(4):503–509.

57. Lee GA, Rao M, Mulligan K, et al. Effects of ritonavir and amprenavir on insulin sensitivity in healthy volunteers. *AIDS*. 2007;21(16):2183–2190.

58. Dube MP, Qian D, Edmondson-Melancon H, et al. Prospective, intensive study of metabolic changes associated with 48 weeks of amprenavir-based antiretroviral therapy. *Clin Infect Dis*. 2002;35(4):475–481.

59. Fisac C, Virgili N, Ferrer E, et al. A comparison of the effects of nevirapine and nelfinavir on metabolism and body habitus in antiretroviral-naive human immunodeficiency virus-infected patients: a randomized controlled study. *J Clin Endocrinol Metab.* 2003;88(11):5186–5192.

60. Dube MP, Parker RA, Tebas P, et al. Glucose metabolism, lipid, and body fat changes in antiretroviral-naive subjects randomized to nelfinavir or efavirenz plus dual nucleosides. *AIDS.* 2005;19(16):1807–1818.

61. Hruz PW, Yan Q. Tipranavir without ritonavir does not acutely induce peripheral insulin resistance in a rodent model. *J Acquir Immune Defic Syndr.* 2006;43(5):624–625.

62. Anderson PL, Brundage RC, Bushman L, Kakuda TN, Remmel RP, Fletcher CV. Indinavir plasma protein binding in HIV-1-infected adults. *AIDS.* 2000;14(15):2293–2297.

63. Brown TT, Li X, Cole SR, et al. Cumulative exposure to nucleoside analogue reverse transcriptase inhibitors is associated with insulin resistance markers in the Multicenter AIDS Cohort Study. *AIDS.* 2005;19(13):1375–1383.

64. Fleischman A, Johnsen S, Systrom DM, et al. Effects of a nucleoside reverse transcriptase inhibitor, stavudine, on glucose disposal and mitochondrial function in muscle of healthy adults. *Am J Physiol Endocrinol Metab.* 2007;292(6):E1666–E1673.

65. Pace CS, Martin AM, Hammond EL, Mamotte CD, Nolan DA, Mallal SA. Mitochondrial proliferation, DNA depletion and adipocyte differentiation in subcutaneous adipose tissue of HIV-positive HAART recipients. *Antivir Ther.* 2003;8(4):323–331.

66. Petersen KF, Dufour S, Befroy D, Garcia R, Shulman GI. Impaired mitochondrial activity in the insulin-resistant offspring of patients with type 2 diabetes. *N Engl J Med.* 2004;350(7):664–671.

67. Garcia-Benayas T, Rendon AL, Rodriguez-Novoa S, et al. Higher risk of hyperglycemia in HIV-infected patients treated with didanosine plus tenofovir. *AIDS Res Hum Retroviruses.* 2006;22(4):333–337.

68. Martinez E, Garcia-Viejo MA, Blanco JL, et al. Impact of switching from human immunodeficiency virus type 1 protease inhibitors to efavirenz in successfully treated adults with lipodystrophy. *Clin Infect Dis.* 2000;31:1266–1273.

69. Martinez E, Conget I, Lozano L, Casamitjana R, Gatell JM. Reversion of metabolic abnormalities after switching from HIV-1 protease inhibitors to nevirapine. *AIDS.* 1999;13:805–810.

70. Petit JM, Duong M, Masson D, et al. Serum adiponectin and metabolic parameters in HIV-1-infected patients after substitution of nevirapine for protease inhibitors. *Eur J Clin Invest.* 2004;34(8):569–575.

71. Estrada V, De Villar NG, Larrad MT, Lopez AG, Fernandez C, Serrano-Rios M. Long-term metabolic consequences of switching from protease inhibitors to efavirenz in therapy for human immunodeficiency virus-infected patients with lipoatrophy. *Clin Infect Dis.* 2002;35(1):69–76.

72. Fisac C, Fumero E, Crespo M, et al. Metabolic benefits 24 months after replacing a protease inhibitor with abacavir, efavirenz or nevirapine. *AIDS.* 2005;19(9):917–925.

73. Seelmeier S, Schmidt H, Turk V, von der HK. Human immunodeficiency virus has an aspartic-type protease that can be inhibited by pepstatin A. *Proc Natl Acad Sci USA.* 1988;85(18):6612–6616.

74. Kohl NE, Diehl RE, Rands E, et al. Expression of active human immunodeficiency virus type 1 protease by noninfectious chimeric virus particles. *J Virol.* 1991;65(6):3007–3014.

75. DiIanni CL, Davis LJ, Holloway MK, et al. Characterization of an active single polypeptide form of the human immunodeficiency virus type 1 protease. *J Biol Chem.* 1990;265(28):17348–17354.

76. Mackin RB. Proinsulin: recent observations and controversies. *Cell Mol Life Sci.* 1998;54(7):696–702.

77. Behrens G, Dejam A, Schmidt H, et al. Impaired glucose tolerance, beta cell function and lipid metabolism in HIV patients under treatment with protease inhibitors. *AIDS.* 1999;13:F63–F70.

78. Woerle HJ, Mariuz PR, Meyer C, et al. Mechanisms for the deterioration in glucose tolerance associated with HIV protease inhibitor regimens. *Diabetes.* 2003;52:918–925.

79. Danoff A, Ling WL. Protease inhibitors do not interfere with prohormone processing. *Ann Intern Med.* 2000;132(4):330.

80. Koster JC, Remedi MS, Qiu H, Nichols CG, Hruz PW. HIV protease inhibitors acutely impair glucose-stimulated insulin release. *Diabetes.* 2003;52(7):1695–1700.

81. Haugaard SB, Andersen O, Halsall I, Iversen J, Hales CN, Madsbad S. Impaired proinsulin secretion before and during oral glucose stimulation in HIV-infected patients who display fat redistribution. *Metabolism.* 2007;56(7):939–946.

82. Schwarz JM, Lee GA, Park S, et al. Indinavir increases glucose production in healthy HIV-negative men. *AIDS.* 2004;18(13):1852–1854.

83. Lee GA, Schwarz JM, Patzek S, et al. The acute effects of HIV protease inhibitors on glucose production in healthy HIV-negative men. *AntivirTher.* 2007;12(Suppl 2):L46.

84. Sekhar RV, Jahoor F, White AC, et al. Metabolic basis of HIV-lipodystrophy syndrome. *Am J Physiol Endocrinol Metab.* 2002;283(2):E332–E337.

85. Hadigan C, Borgonha S, Rabe J, Young V, Grinspoon S. Increased rates of lipolysis among human immunodeficiency virus-infected men receiving highly active antiretroviral therapy. *Metabolism.* 2002;51(9):1143–1147.

86. Reeds DN, Mittendorfer B, Patterson BW, Powderly WG, Yarasheski KE, Klein S. Alterations in lipid kinetics in men with HIV-dyslipidemia. *Am J Physiol Endocrinol Metab.* 2003;285(3):E490–E497.

87. Hadigan C, Rabe J, Meininger G, Aliabadi N, Breu J, Grinspoon S. Inhibition of lipolysis improves insulin sensitivity in protease inhibitor-treated HIV-infected men with fat redistribution. *Am J Clin Nutr.* 2003;77(2):490–494.

88. Hadigan C, Liebau J, Torriani M, Andersen R, Grinspoon S. Improved triglycerides and insulin sensitivity with 3 months of acipimox in human immunodeficiency virus-infected patients with hypertriglyceridemia. *J Clin Endocrinol Metab.* 2006;91(11):4438–4444.

89. Lindegaard B, Frosig C, Petersen AM, et al. Inhibition of lipolysis stimulates peripheral glucose uptake but has no effect on endogenous glucose production in HIV lipodystrophy. *Diabetes.* 2007;56(8):2070–2077.

90. Seltzer HS. Drug-induced hypoglycemia. A review of 1418 cases. *Endocrinol Metab Clin North Am.* 1989;18(1):163-183.

91. Abourizk NN, Lyons RW, Madden GM. Transient state of NIDDM in a patient with AIDS. *Diabetes Care.* 1993;16(6): 931–933.

92. Nasti G, Zanette G, Inchiostro S, Donadon V, Tirelli U. Diabetes mellitus following intravenous pentamidine administration in a patient with HIV infection. *Arch Intern Med.* 1995;155(6):645–646.

93. Coyle P, Carr AD, Depczynski BB, Chisholm DJ. Diabetes mellitus associated with pentamidine use in HIV-infected patients. *Med J Aust.* 1996;165(10):587–588.

94. Uzzan B, Bentata M, Campos J, et al. Effects of aerosolized pentamidine on glucose homeostasis and insulin secretion in HIV-positive patients: a controlled study. *AIDS.* 1995;9:901–907.

95. Jain P, Girardi L, Sherman L, Berelowicz M, Smith L. Insulin resistance and development of diabetes mellitus associated with megestrol acetate therapy. *Postgrad Med J.* 1996;72:365–367.

96. Kilby JM, Tabereaux PB. Severe hyperglycemia in an HIV clinic: preexisting versus drug-associated diabetes mellitus. *J Acquir Immune Defic Syndr Hum Retrovirol.* 1998;17(1):46–50.

97. Gonzalezd V, Herrero AA, Martinez HP, Garcia DB, Jimenez CE. Hyperglycemia induced by megestrol acetate in a patient with AIDS. *Ann Pharmacother.* 1996;30(10):1113–1114.

98. Grinspoon S, Carr A. Cardiovascular risk and body-fat abnormalities in HIV-infected adults. *N Engl J Med.* 2005;352(1): 48–62.

99. Blanch J, Rousaud A, Martinez E, et al. Factors associated with severe impact of lipodystrophy on the quality of life of patients infected with HIV-1. *Clin Infect Dis.* 2004;38(10):1464–1470.

100. Ammassari A, Antinori A, Cozzi-Lepri A, et al. Relationship between HAART adherence and adipose tissue alterations. *J Acquir Immune Defic Syndr.* 2002;31(Suppl 3):S140–S144.

101. Martinez E, Mocroft A, Garcia-Viejo MA, et al. Risk of lipodystrophy in HIV-1-infected patients treated with protease inhibitors: a prospective cohort study. *Lancet.* 2001;357(9256):592–598.

102. Heath KV, Singer J, O'Shaughnessy MV, Montaner JS, Hogg RS. Intentional nonadherence due to adverse symptoms associated with antiretroviral therapy. *J Acquir Immune Defic Syndr.* 2002;31(2):211–217.

103. Galli M, Cozzi-Lepri A, Ridolfo AL, et al. Incidence of adipose tissue alterations in first-line antiretroviral therapy: the LipoICoNa Study. *Arch Intern Med.* 2002;162(22):2621–2628.

104. Saves M, Raffi F, Capeau J, et al. Factors related to lipodystrophy and metabolic alterations in patients with human immunodeficiency virus infection receiving highly active antiretroviral therapy. *Clin Infect Dis.* 2002;34(10): 1396–1405.

105. Bacchetti P, Gripshover B, Grunfeld C, et al. Fat distribution in men with HIV infection. *J Acquir Immune Defic Syndr.* 2005;40(2):121–131.

106. Carr A, Emery S, Law M, Puls R, Lundgren JD, Powderly WG. An objective case definition of lipodystrophy in HIV-infected adults: a case-control study. *Lancet.* 2003;361(9359):726–735.

107. Lichtenstein KA, Ward DJ, Moorman AC, et al. Clinical assessment of HIV-associated lipodystrophy in an ambulatory population. *AIDS.* 2001;15:1389–1398.

108. Kotler DP, Rosenbaum K, Wang J, Pierson RN. Studies of body composition and fat distribution in HIV-infected and control subjects. *J Acquir Immune Defic Syndr Hum Retrovirol.* 1999;20:228–237.

109. Shimomura I, Hammer RE, Ikemoto S, Brown MS, Goldstein JL. Leptin reverses insulin resistance and diabetes mellitus in mice with congenital lipodystrophy. *Nature.* 1999;401:73–76.

110. Gavrilova O, Marcus-Samuels B, Graham D, et al. Surgical implantation of adipose tissue reverses diabetes in lipoatrophic mice. *J Clin Invest.* 2000;105(3):271–278.

111. Garg A. Acquired and inherited lipodystrophies. *N Engl J Med.* 2004;350(12):1220–1234.

112. Heath KV, Hogg RS, Singer J, Chan KJ, O'Shaughnessy MV, Montaner JS. Antiretroviral treatment patterns and incident HIV-associated morphologic and lipid abnormalities in a population-based chort. *J Acquir Immune Defic Syndr.* 2002;30(4): 440–447.

113. Mallal SA, John M, Moore CB, James IR, McKinnon EJ. Contribution of nucleoside analogue reverse transcriptase inhibitors to subcutaneous fat wasting in patients with HIV infection. *AIDS.* 2000;14(10):1309–1316.

114. Shlay JC, Visnegarwala F, Bartsch G, et al. Body composition and metabolic changes in antiretroviral-naive patients randomized to didanosine and stavudine vs. abacavir and lamivudine. *J Acquir Immune Defic Syndr.* 2005;38(2):147–155.

115. Brown TT, Chu H, Wang Z, et al. Longitudinal increases in waist circumference are associated with HIV-serostatus, independent of antiretroviral therapy. *AIDS.* 2007;21(13):1731–1738.

116. Mulligan K, Parker RA, Komarow L, et al. Mixed patterns of changes in central and peripheral fat following initiation of antiretroviral therapy in a randomized trial. *J Acquir Immune Defic Syndr.* 2006;41(5):590–597.

117. Domingo P, Matias-Guiu X, Pujol RM, et al. Subcutaneous adipocyte apoptosis in HIV-1 protease inhibitor-associated lipodystrophy. *AIDS.* 1999;13:2261–2267.

118. Bastard JP, Caron M, Vidal H, et al. Association between altered expression of adipogenic factor SREBP1 in lipoatrophic adipose tissue from HIV-1-infected patients and abnormal adipocyte differentiation and insulin resistance. *Lancet.* 2002;359(9311):1026–1031.

119. Dowell P, Flexner C, Kwiterovich PO, Lane MD. Suppression of preadipocyte differentiation and promotion of adipocyte death by HIV protease inhibitors. *J Biol Chem.* 2000;275(52):41325–41332.

120. Caron M, Auclair M, Vigouroux C, Glorian M, Forest C, Capeau J. The HIV protease inhibitor indinavir impairs sterol regulatory element- binding protein-1 intranuclear localization, inhibits preadipocyte differentiation, and induces insulin resistance. *Diabetes.* 2001;50(6):1378–1388.

121. Caron M, Auclair M, Sterlingot H, Kornprobst M, Capeau J. Some HIV protease inhibitors alter lamin A/C maturation and stability, SREBP-1 nuclear localization and adipocyte differentiation. *AIDS.* 2003;17(17):2437–2444.

122. Roche R, Poizot-Martin I, Yazidi CM, et al. Effects of antiretroviral drug combinations on the differentiation of adipocytes. *AIDS.* 2002;16(1):13–20.

123. Nolan D, Hammond E, Martin A, et al. Mitochondrial DNA depletion and morphologic changes in adipocytes associated with nucleoside reverse transcriptase inhibitor therapy. *AIDS.* 2003;17(9):1329–1338.

124. Lewis W, Dalakas MC. Mitochondrial toxicity of antiviral drugs. *Nat Med.* 1995;1(5):417–422.

125. Dalakas MC, Illa I, Pezeshkpour GH, Laukaitis JP, Cohen B, Griffin JL. Mitochondrial myopathy caused by long-term zidovudine therapy. *N Engl J Med.* 1990;322(16):1098–1105.

126. Lewis W, Simpson JF, Meyer RR. Cardiac mitochondrial DNA polymerase-gamma is inhibited competitively and noncompetitively by phosphorylated zidovudine. *Circ Res.* 1994;74(2):344–348.

127. Mallon PW, Miller J, Cooper DA, Carr A. Prospective evaluation of the effects of antiretroviral therapy on body composition in HIV-1-infected men starting therapy. *AIDS.* 2003;17(7):971–979.

128. van Der Valk M, Gisolf EH, Reiss P, et al. Increased risk of lipodystrophy when nucleoside analogue reverse transcriptase inhibitors are included with protease inhibitors in the treatment of HIV-1 infection. *AIDS.* 2001;15(7): 847–855.

129. Yamauchi T, Kamon J, Waki H, et al. The fat-derived hormone adiponectin reverses insulin resistance associated with both lipoatrophy and obesity. *Nat Med.* 2001;7(8):941–946.

130. Haque WA, Shimomura I, Matsuzawa Y, Garg A. Serum adiponectin and leptin levels in patients with lipodystrophies. *J Clin Endocrinol Metab.* 2002;87(5):2395.

131. Estrada V, Martinez-Larrad MT, Gonzalez-Sanchez JL, et al. Lipodystrophy and metabolic syndrome in HIV-infected patients treated with antiretroviral therapy. *Metabolism.* 2006;55(7):940–945.

132. Verkauskiene R, Dollfus C, Levine M, et al. Serum adiponectin and leptin concentrations in HIV-infected children with fat redistribution syndrome. *Pediatr Res.* 2006;60(2):225–230.

133. Kosmiski LA, Bacchetti P, Kotler DP, et al. Relationship of fat distribution with adipokines in human immunodeficiency virus infection. *J Clin Endocrinol Metab.* 2008;93(1):216–224.

134. Addy CL, Gavrila A, Tsiodras S, Brodovicz K, Karchmer AW, Mantzoros CS. Hypoadiponectinemia is associated with insulin resistance, hypertriglyceridemia, and fat redistribution in human immunodeficiency virus-infected patients treated with highly active antiretroviral therapy. *J Clin Endocrinol Metab.* 2003;88(2):627–636.

135. Reeds DN, Yarasheski KE, Fontana L, et al. Alterations in liver, muscle, and adipose tissue insulin sensitivity in men with HIV infection and dyslipidemia. *Am J Physiol Endocrinol Metab.* 2006;290(1):E47–E53.

136. Lee GA, Mafong DD, Noor MA, et al. HIV protease inhibitors increase adiponectin levels in HIV-negative men. *J Acquir Immune Defic Syndr.* 2004;36(1):645–647.

137. Chen D, Misra A, Garg A. Clinical review 153: lipodystrophy in human immunodeficiency virus-infected patients. *J Clin Endocrinol Metab.* 2002;87(11):4845–4856.

138. Yanovski JA, Miller KD, Kino T, et al. Endocrine and metabolic evaluation of human immunodeficiency virus-infected patients with evidence of protease inhibitor-associated lipodystrophy. *J Clin Endocrinol Metab.* 1999;84:1925–1931.

139. Bujalska IJ, Kumar S, Stewart PM. Does central obesity reflect "Cushing's" disease of the omentum? *Lancet.* 1997;349: 1210–1213.

140. Sutinen J, Kannisto K, Korsheninnikova E, et al. In the lipodystrophy associated with highly active antiretroviral therapy, pseudo-Cushing's syndrome is associated with increased regeneration of cortisol by 11beta-hydroxysteroid dehydrogenase type 1 in adipose tissue. *Diabetologia.* 2004;47(10):1668–1671.

141. Palella FJ Jr., Cole SR, Chmiel JS, et al. Anthropometrics and examiner-reported body habitus abnormalities in the multicenter AIDS cohort study. *Clin Infect Dis.* 2004;38(6):903–907.

142. Shlay JC, Bartsch G, Peng G, et al. Long-term body composition and metabolic changes in antiretroviral naive persons randomized to protease inhibitor-, nonnucleoside reverse transcriptase inhibitor-, or protease inhibitor plus nonnucleoside reverse transcriptase inhibitor-based strategy. *J Acquir Immune Defic Syndr.* 2007;44(5): 506–517.

143. Riddler SA, Li X, Chu H, et al. Longitudinal changes in serum lipids among HIV-infected men on highly active antiretroviral therapy. *HIV Med.* 2007;8(5):280–287.

144. Stein JH, Klein MA, Bellehumeur JL, et al. Use of human immunodeficiency virus-1 protease inhibitors is associated with atherogenic lipoprotein changes and endothelial dysfunction. *Circulation.* 2001;104(3):257–262.

145. Yki-Jarvinen H, Sutinen J, Silveira A, et al. Regulation of plasma PAI-1 concentrations in HAART-associated lipodystrophy during rosiglitazone therapy. *Arterioscler Thromb Vasc Biol.* 2003;23(4):688–694.

146. Hadigan C, Meigs JB, Rabe J, et al. Increased PAI-1 and tPA antigen levels are reduced with metformin therapy in HIV-infected patients with fat redistribution and insulin resistance. *J Clin Endocrinol Metab.* 2001;86(2):939–943.

147. Dressman J, Kincer J, Matveev SV, et al. HIV protease inhibitors promote atherosclerotic lesion formation independent of dyslipidemia by increasing CD36-dependent cholesteryl ester accumulation in macrophages. *J Clin Invest*. 2003;111(3): 389–397.
148. Mary-Krause M, Cotte L, Simon A, Partisani M, Costagliola D. Increased risk of myocardial infarction with duration of protease inhibitor therapy in HIV-infected men. *AIDS*. 2003;17(17):2479–2486.
149. Triant VA, Lee H, Hadigan C, Grinspoon SK. Increased acute myocardial infarction rates and cardiovascular risk factors among patients with human immunodeficiency virus disease. *J Clin Endocrinol Metab*. 2007;92(7):2506–2512.
150. Bozzette SA, Ake CF, Tam HK, Chang SW, Louis TA. Cardiovascular and cerebrovascular events in patients treated for human immunodeficiency virus infection. *N Engl J Med*. 2003;348(8):702–710.
151. Friis-Moller N, Sabin CA, Weber R, et al. Combination antiretroviral therapy and the risk of myocardial infarction. *N Engl J Med*. 2003;349(21):1993–2003.
152. Friis-Moller N, Reiss P, Sabin CA, et al. Class of antiretroviral drugs and the risk of myocardial infarction. *N Engl J Med*. 2007;356(17):1723–1735.
153. Grunfeld C, Kotler DP, Hamadeh R, Tierney A, Wang J, Pierson RN Jr. Hypertriglyceridemia in the acquired immunodeficiency syndrome. *Am J Med*. 1989;86:27–31.
154. Shor-Posner G, Basit A, Lu Y, et al. Hypocholesterolemia ia associated with immune dysfunction in early human immunodeficiency virus-1 infection. *Am J Med*. 1993;94:515–519.
155. Grunfeld C, Pang M, Doerrler W, Shigenaga JK, Jensen P, Feingold KR. Lipids, lipoproteins, triglyceride clearance, and cytokines in human immunodeficiency virus infection and the acquired immunodeficiency syndrome. *J Clin Endocrinol Metab*. 1992;74:1045–1052.
156. Zangerle R, Sarcletti M, Gallati H, Reibnegger G, Wachter H, Fuchs D. Decreased plasma concentrations of HDL cholesterol in HIV-infected individuals are associated with immune activation. *J Acquir Defic Syndr*. 1994;7:1149–1156.
157. Hellerstein MK, Grunfeld C, Wu K, et al. Increased de novo hepatic lipogenesis in human immunodeficiency virus infection. *J Clin Endocrinol Metab*. 1993;76:559–565.
158. Sekhar RV, Jahoor F, Pownall HJ, et al. Severely dysregulated disposal of postprandial triacylglycerols exacerbates hypertriacylglycerolemia in HIV lipodystrophy syndrome. *Am J Clin Nutr*. 2005;81(6):1405–1410.
159. Fontas E, van Leth F, Sabin CA, et al. Lipid profiles in HIV-infected patients receiving combination antiretroviral therapy: are different antiretroviral drugs associated with different lipid profiles? *J Infect Dis*. 2004;189(6):1056–1074.
160. Friis-Moller N, Weber R, Reiss P, et al. Cardiovascular disease risk factors in HIV patients – association with antiretroviral therapy. Results from the DAD study. *AIDS*. 2003;17:1179–1193.
161. Mildvan D, Machado SG, Wilets I, Grossberg SE. Endogenous interferon and triglyceride concentrations to assess response to zidovudine in AIDS and advanced AIDS-related complex. *Lancet*. 1992;339:453–456.
162. Anastos K, Lu D, Shi Q, et al. Association of serum lipid levels with HIV serostatus, specific antiretroviral agents, and treatment regimens. *J Acquir Immune Defic Syndr*. 2007;45(1):34–42.
163. Sterne JA, May M, Bucher HC, et al. HAART and the heart: changes in coronary risk factors and implications for coronary risk in men starting antiretroviral therapy. *J Intern Med*. 2007;261(3):255–267.
164. Cameron DW, Heath-Chiozzi M, Danner S, et al. Randomised placebo-controlled trial of ritonavir in advanced HIV-1 disease. The Advanced HIV Disease Ritonavir Study Group. *Lancet*. 1998;351(9102):543–549.
165. Mobius U, Lubach-Ruitman M, Castro-Frenzel B, et al. Switching to atazanavir improves metabolic disorders in antiretroviral-experienced patients with severe hyperlipidemia. *J Acquir Immune Defic Syndr*. 2005;39(2):174–180.
166. Liang JS, Distler O, Cooper DA, et al. HIV protease inhibitors protect apolipoprotein B from degradation by the proteasome: a potential mechanism for protease inhibitor-induced hyperlipidemia. *Nat Med*. 2001;7(12):1327–1331.
167. Schmitz M, Michl GM, Walli R, et al. Alterations of apolipoprotein B metabolism in HIV-infected patients with antiretroviral combination therapy. *J Acquir Immune Defic Syndr*. 2001;26(3):225–235.
168. Riddler SA, Smit E, Cole SR, et al. Impact of HIV infection and HAART on serum lipids in men. *J Am Med Assoc*. 2003;289(22):2978–2982.
169. Domingo P, Sambeat MA, Perez A, Ordonez J. Effect of protease inhibitors on apolipoprotein B levels and plasma lipid profile in HIV-1-infected patients on highly active antiretroviral therapy. *J Acquir Immune Defic Syndr*. 2003;33(1): 114–116.
170. Purnell JQ, Zambon A, Knopp RH, et al. Effect of ritonavir on lipids and post-heparin lipase activities in normal subjects. *AIDS*. 2000;14:51–57.
171. Periard D, Telenti A, Sudre P, et al. Atherogenic dyslipidemia in HIV-infected individuals treated with protease inhibitors. The Swiss HIV Cohort Study. *Circulation*. 1999;100(7):700–705.
172. Calza L, Manfredi R, Colangeli V, et al. Substitution of nevirapine or efavirenz for protease inhibitor versus lipid-lowering therapy for the management of dyslipidaemia. *AIDS*. 2005;19(10):1051–1058.
173. Negredo E, Ribalta J, Paredes R, et al. Reversal of atherogenic lipoprotein profile in HIV-1 infected patients with lipodystrophy after replacing protease inhibitors by nevirapine. *AIDS*. 2002;16(10):1383–1389.
174. van Der Valk M, Kastelein JJ, Murphy RL, et al. Nevirapine-containing antiretroviral therapy in HIV-1 infected patients results in an anti-atherogenic lipid profile. *AIDS*. 2001;15(18):2407–2414.
175. Gallant JE, Staszewski S, Pozniak AL, et al. Efficacy and safety of tenofovir DF vs stavudine in combination therapy in antiretroviral-naive patients: a 3-year randomized trial. *J Am Med Assoc*. 2004;292(2):191–201.

176. Carr A, Workman C, Smith DE, et al. Abacavir substitution for nucleoside analogs in patients with HIV lipoatrophy: a randomized trial. *J Am Med Assoc.* 2002;288(2):207–215.

177. Schambelan M, Benson CA, Carr A, et al. Management of metabolic complications associated with antiretroviral therapy for HIV-1 infection: recommendations of an International AIDS Society-USA panel. *J Acquir Immune Defic Syndr.* 2002;31(3):257–275.

178. Wohl DA, McComsey G, Tebas P, et al. Current concepts in the diagnosis and management of metabolic complications of HIV infection and its therapy. *Clin Infect Dis.* 2006;43(5):645–653.

179. Dube MP, Stein JH, Aberg JA, et al. Guidelines for the evaluation and management of dyslipidemia in human immunodeficiency virus (HIV)-infected adults receiving antiretroviral therapy: recommendations of the HIV Medical Association of the Infectious Disease Society of America and the Adult AIDS Clinical Trials Group. *Clin Infect Dis.* 2003;37(5):613–627.

180. Executive Summary of The Third Report of The National Cholesterol Education Program (NCEP) Expert Panel on Detection, Evaluation, And Treatment of High Blood Cholesterol In Adults (Adult Treatment Panel III). *J Am Med Assoc.* 2001;285(19):2486–2497.

181. Report of the Expert Committee on the Diagnosis and Classification of Diabetes Mellitus. *Diabetes Care.* 2002;25(Suppl 1):S5–S20.

182. Standards of Medical Care for Patients With Diabetes Mellitus; American Diabetes Association. *Diabetes Care.* 2002;25(Suppl 1):S33–S49.

183. Roubenoff R, Schmitz H, Bairos L, et al. Reduction of abdominal obesity in lipodystrophy associated with human immunodeficiency virus infection by means of diet and exercise: case report and proof of principle. *Clin Infect Dis.* 2002;34(3):390–393.

184. Jones SP, Doran DA, Leatt PB, Maher B, Pirmohamed M. Short-term exercise training improves body composition and hyperlipidaemia in HIV-positive individuals with lipodystrophy. *AIDS.* 2001;15(15):2049–2051.

185. Stumvoll M, Nurjhan N, Perriello G, Dailey G, Gerich JE. Metabolic effects of metformin in non-insulin-dependent diabetes mellitus. *N Engl J Med.* 1995;333:550–554.

186. Saint-Marc T, Touraine JL. Effects of metformin on insulin resistance and central adiposity in patients receiving effective protease inhibitor therapy. *AIDS.* 1999;13:1000–1002.

187. Hadigan C, Corcoran C, Basgoz N, Davis B, Sax P, Grinspoon S. Metformin in the treatment of HIV lipodystrophy syndrome: A randomized controlled trial. *J Am Med Assoc.* 2000;284(4):472–477.

188. Hadigan C, Rabe J, Grinspoon S. Sustained benefits of metformin therapy on markers of cardiovascular risk in human immunodeficiency virus-infected patients with fat redistribution and insulin resistance. *J Clin Endocrinol Metab.* 2002;87(10): 4611–4615.

189. Mulligan K, Yang Y, Wininger DA, et al. Effects of metformin and rosiglitazone in HIV-infected patients with hyperinsulinemia and elevated waist/hip ratio. *AIDS.* 2007;21(1):47–57.

190. van Wijk JP, de Koning EJ, Cabezas MC, et al. Comparison of rosiglitazone and metformin for treating HIV lipodystrophy: a randomized trial. *Ann Intern Med.* 2005;143(5):337–346.

191. Kohli R, Shevitz A, Gorbach S, Wanke C. A randomized placebo-controlled trial of metformin for the treatment of HIV lipodystrophy. *HIV Med.* 2007;8(7):420–426.

192. Vrouenraets SM, Treskes M, Regez RM, et al. Hyperlactataemia in HIV-infected patients: the role of NRTI-treatment. *Antivir Ther.* 2002;7(4):239–244.

193. Yki-Jarvinen H. Thiazolidinediones. *N Engl J Med.* 2004;351(11):1106–1118.

194. Arioglu E, Duncan-Morin J, Sebring N, et al. Efficacy and safety of troglitazone in the treatment of lipodystrophy syndromes. *Ann Intern Med.* 2000;133(4):263–274.

195. Mori Y, Murakawa Y, Okada K, et al. Effect of troglitazone on body fat distribution in type 2 diabetic patients. *Diabetes Care.* 1999;22:908–912.

196. Kawai T, Takei I, Oguma Y, et al. Effects of troglitazone on fat distribution in the treatment of male type 2 diabetes. *Metabolism.* 1999;48(9):1102–1107.

197. Kelly IE, Han TS, Walsh K, Lean MEJ. Effects of a thiazolidinedione compound on body fat and fat distribution of patiens with type 2 diabetes. *Diabetes Care.* 1999;22:288–293.

198. Gelato MC, Mynarcik DC, Quick JL, et al. Improved insulin sensitivity and body fat distribution in HIV-infected patients treated with rosiglitazone: a pilot study. *J Acquir Immune Defic Syndr.* 2002;31(2):163–170.

199. Hadigan C, Yawetz S, Thomas A, Havers F, Sax PE, Grinspoon S. Metabolic effects of rosiglitazone in HIV lipodystrophy: a randomized, controlled trial. *Ann Intern Med.* 2004;140(10):786–794.

200. Sutinen J, Hakkinen AM, Westerbacka J, et al. Rosiglitazone in the treatment of HAART-associated lipodystrophy – a randomized double-blind placebo-controlled study. *Antivir Ther.* 2003;8(3):199–207.

201. Carr A, Workman C, Carey D, et al. No effect of rosiglitazone for treatment of HIV-1 lipoatrophy: randomised, double-blind, placebo-controlled trial. *Lancet.* 2004;363(9407):429–438.

202. Gavrila A, Hsu W, Tsiodras S, et al. Improvement in highly active antiretroviral therapy-induced metabolic syndrome by treatment with pioglitazone but not with fenofibrate: a 2 × 2 factorial, randomized, double-blinded, placebo-controlled trial. *Clin Infect Dis.* 2005;40(5):745–749.

203. Nissen SE, Wolski K. Effect of rosiglitazone on the risk of myocardial infarction and death from cardiovascular causes. *N Engl J Med.* 2007;356(24):2457–2471.

204. Cnop M, Havel PJ, Utzschneider KM, et al. Relationship of adiponectin to body fat distribution, insulin sensitivity and plasma lipoproteins: evidence for independent roles of age and sex. *Diabetologia.* 2003;46(4):459–469.

205. Cavalcanti RB, Raboud J, Shen S, Kain KC, Cheung A, Walmsley S. A randomized, placebo-controlled trial of rosiglitazone for HIV-related lipoatrophy. *J Infect Dis.* 2007;195(12):1754–1761.

206. McComsey GA, Ward DJ, Hessenthaler SM, et al. Improvement in lipoatrophy associated with highly active antiretroviral therapy in human immunodeficiency virus-infected patients switched from stavudine to abacavir or zidovudine: the results of the TARHEEL study. *Clin Infect Dis.* 2004;38(2):263–270.

207. John M, McKinnon EJ, James IR, et al. Randomized, controlled, 48-week study of switching stavudine and/or protease inhibitors to combivir/abacavir to prevent or reverse lipoatrophy in HIV-infected patients. *J Acquir Immune Defic Syndr.* 2003;33(1):29–33.

208. Martin A, Smith DE, Carr A, et al. Reversibility of lipoatrophy in HIV-infected patients 2 years after switching from a thymidine analogue to abacavir: the MITOX Extension Study. *AIDS.* 2004;18(7):1029–1036.

209. Tebas P, Zhang J, Yarasheski K, et al. Switching to a protease inhibitor-containing, nucleoside-sparing regimen (lopinavir/ritonavir plus efavirenz) increases limb fat but raises serum lipid levels: results of a prospective randomized trial (AIDS clinical trial group 5125s). *J Acquir Immune Defic Syndr.* 2007;45(2):193–200.

210. Carr A, Hudson JCJ, Law M, et al. HIV protease inhibitor substitution in patients with lipodystrophy: a randomized, controlled, open-label, multicentre study. *AIDS.* 2001;15:1811–1822.

211. Moyle GJ, Sabin CA, Cartledge J, et al. A randomized comparative trial of tenofovir DF or abacavir as replacement for a thymidine analogue in persons with lipoatrophy. *AIDS.* 2006;20(16):2043–2050.

212. Lo JC, Mulligan K, Noor M, et al. The effects of recombinant human growth hormone on body composition and glucose metabolism in HIV-infected patients with fat accumulation. *J Clin Endocrinol Metab.* 2001;86:3480–3487.

213. Lo JC, Mulligan K, Noor MA, et al. The effects of low dose growth hormone in HIV-infected men with fat accumulation: a pilot study. *Clin Infect Dis.* 2004;39:732–735.

214. Schwarz JM, Mulligan K, Lee J, et al. Effects of recombinant human growth hormone on hepatic lipid and carbohydrate metabolism in HIV-infected patients with fat accumulation. *J Clin Endocrinol Metab.* 2002;87:942–945.

215. Kotler DP, Muurahainen N, Grunfeld C, et al. Effects of growth hormone on abnormal visceral adipose tissue accumulation and dyslipidemia in HIV-infected patients. *J Acquir Immune Defic Syndr.* 2004;35(3):239–252.

216. Grunfeld C, Thompson M, Brown SJ, et al. Recombinant human growth hormone to treat HIV-associated adipose redistribution syndrome: 12 week induction and 24-week maintenance therapy. *J Acquir Immune Defic Syndr.* 2007;45(3):286–297.

217. Falutz J, Allas S, Blot K, et al. Metabolic effects of a growth hormone-releasing factor in patients with HIV. *N Engl J Med.* 2007;357(23):2359–2370.

218. Neuvonen PJ, Niemi M, Backman JT. Drug interactions with lipid-lowering drugs: mechanisms and clinical relevance. *Clin Pharmacol Ther.* 2006;80(6):565–581.

219. Fichtenbaum CJ, Gerber JG, Rosenkranz SL, et al. Pharmacokinetic interactions between protease inhibitors and statins in HIV seronegative volunteers: ACTG Study A5047. *AIDS.* 2002;16(4):569–577.

220. Palacios R, Santos J, Gonzalez M, et al. Efficacy and safety of atorvastatin in the treatment of hypercholesterolemia associated with antiretroviral therapy. *J Acquir Immune Defic Syndr.* 2002;30(5):536–537.

221. Calza L, Colangeli V, Manfredi R, et al. Rosuvastatin for the treatment of hyperlipidaemia in HIV-infected patients receiving protease inhibitors: a pilot study. *AIDS.* 2005;19(10):1103–1105.

222. Boccara F, Simon T, Lacombe K, et al. Influence of pravastatin on carotid artery structure and function in dyslipidemic HIV-infected patients receiving antiretroviral therapy. *AIDS.* 2006;20(18):2395–2398.

223. Benesic A, Zilly M, Kluge F, et al. Lipid lowering therapy with fluvastatin and pravastatin in patients with HIV infection and antiretroviral therapy: comparison of efficacy and interaction with indinavir. *Infection.* 2004;32(4):229–233.

224. Moyle GJ, Lloyd M, Reynolds B, Baldwin C, Mandalia S, Gazzard BG. Dietary advice with or without pravastatin for the management of hypercholesterolaemia associated with protease inhibitor therapy. *AIDS.* 2001;15(12):1503–1508.

225. Henry K, Melroe H, Huebesch J, Hermundson J, Simpson J. Atorvastatin and gemfibrozil for protease-inhibitor-related lipid abnormalities. *Lancet.* 1998;352(9133):1031–1032.

226. Aberg JA, Zackin RA, Brobst SW, et al. A randomized trial of the efficacy and safety of fenofibrate versus pravastatin in HIV-infected subjects with lipid abnormalities: AIDS Clinical Trials Group Study 5087. *AIDS Res Hum Retroviruses.* 2005;21(9):757–767.

227. Badiou S, Merle DB, Dupuy AM, Baillat V, Cristol JP, Reynes J. Fenofibrate improves the atherogenic lipid profile and enhances LDL resistance to oxidation in HIV-positive adults. *Atherosclerosis.* 2004;172(2):273–279.

228. Miller J, Brown D, Amin J, et al. A randomized, double-blind study of gemfibrozil for the treatment of protease inhibitor-associated hypertriglyceridaemia. *AIDS.* 2002;16(16):2195–2200.

229. Gerber MT, Mondy KE, Yarasheski KE, et al. Niacin in HIV-infected individuals with hyperlipidemia receiving potent antiretroviral therapy. *Clin Infect Dis.* 2004;39(3):419–425.

230. Dube MP, Wu JW, Aberg JA, et al. Safety and efficacy of extended-release niacin for the treatment of dyslipidaemia in patients with HIV infection: AIDS Clinical Trials Group Study A5148. *Antivir Ther.* 2006;11(8):1081–1089.

231. de Truchis P, Kirstetter M, Perier A, et al. Reduction in triglyceride level with N-3 polyunsaturated fatty acids in HIV-infected patients taking potent antiretroviral therapy: a randomized prospective study. *J Acquir Immune Defic Syndr.* 2007;44(3): 278–285.

232. Gerber JG, Kitch DW, Fichtenbaum CJ, et al. Fish Oil and Fenofibrate for the Treatment of Hypertriglyceridemia in HIV-Infected Subjects on Antiretroviral Therapy: Results of ACTG A5186. *J Acquir Immune Defic Syndr*. 2008;47:459–466.

233. Wohl DA, Tien HC, Busby M, et al. Randomized study of the safety and efficacy of fish oil (omega-3 fatty acid) supplementation with dietary and exercise counseling for the treatment of antiretroviral therapy-associated hypertriglyceridemia. *Clin Infect Dis*. 2005;41(10):1498–1504.

234. Negredo E, Molto J, Puig J, et al. Ezetimibe, a promising lipid-lowering agent for the treatment of dyslipidaemia in HIV-infected patients with poor response to statins. *AIDS*. 2006;20(17):2159–2164.

Part VIII
Therapy of Diabetes Mellitus – General Principles

Chapter 39
Glycemic Goals

David J. Brillon

Introduction

Both type 1 and type 2 diabetes are accompanied by microvascular and macrovascular complications. For decades the association between chronic hyperglycemia and the development of long-term eye, kidney, and nerve disease was suspected based on animal models of diabetes[1-3] and the long-term observations of clinicians.[4] Nonetheless, the belief that normalization of blood glucose would prevent end organ damage was not universally accepted.[5]

By the 1980s several small prospective multicenter randomized trials were conducted to address this question. These studies were of short duration[6] or had conflicting results regarding the benefits of glycemic control on microvascular disease.[6-8] Indeed, achieving lower blood glucose levels appeared to worsen established retinopathy for the initial 8 months.[6]

Microvascular Disease

To definitively address the question of glycemic control and the development of diabetic microvascular disease, a large randomized interventional trial, which would eventually involve 29 centers in the US and Canada, was begun. A total of 1441 patients with type 1 diabetes were recruited from 1983 to 1989 to comprise the cohorts of the Diabetes Control and Complications Trial or DCCT.[9] Two cohorts were studied – a primary prevention cohort, to determine if intensive glycemic control would prevent the development of diabetic retinopathy, and a secondary intervention cohort to determine if intensive glycemic control would ameliorate the progression of early diabetic retinal disease. For the primary prevention cohort subjects had to have 1–5 years duration of diabetes, absence of retinopathy by fundus photography, and urinary albumin excretion <40 mg/24 h. The secondary intervention cohort criteria were 5–15 years duration of diabetes, mild (one microaneurysm) to moderate nonproliferative retinopathy, and urinary albumin excretion <200 mg/24 h. Patients were randomized to either conventional or intensive glycemic control. Intensive therapy included multiple (three or more) daily insulin injections (MDI) or continuous subcutaneous insulin injection (CSII) via an insulin pump. Insulin doses were adjusted according to fingerstick blood glucose (BG) values (obtained at least four times a day), dietary intake, and level of physical activity. The goal of intensive therapy included premeal BG levels 70–120 mg/dl, postprandial levels under 180 mg/dl, and hemoglobin A1c (HbA1c) levels within the nondiabetic range (<6.05%). To help achieve the goals, subjects met monthly with the physician, nurse educator, and dietician of the study and were contacted by telephone to review and adjust their regimen as necessary. Subjects randomized to conventional therapy received the usual diabetes treatment of the time, 1–2 insulin injections a day. The goals were to avoid symptomatic hypo- or hyperglycemia but not to achieve specific target glucose levels. Although subjects in the

D.J. Brillon (✉)
Division of Endocrinology, Diabetes and Metabolism, Weill Cornell Medical College, New York, NY, USA
e-mail: djbrillo@med.cornell.edu

L. Poretsky (ed.), *Principles of Diabetes Mellitus*, DOI 10.1007/978-0-387-09841-8_39,
© Springer Science+Business Media, LLC 2010

conventional arm also received diet and exercise education, they only performed once daily glucose monitoring and met with the study team on a once every 3 month basis.

Both cohorts (a total of 1441 patients) were followed for a mean of 6.5 years. During this time seven field stereoscopic fundus photos, 24 h urine albumin excretion, clinical neuropathy assessment, peripheral nerve conduction studies, and autonomic nerve testing were performed. About 99% of the participants completed the study. From an initially statistically identical HbA1c at the beginning of the study, the intensively treated group reached a nadir of 6.9% at 6 months. Throughout the subsequent 6 years a statistically significant HbA1c separation (approximately 7.2% vs. 9.1%) between intensive and conventional therapy was maintained.

The trial was ended prematurely due to significant outcome differences between intensively and conventionally treated subjects. Outcome curves for retinopathy were initially similar but separated after 3 years. Intensive therapy decreased the mean risk of progression of retinopathy by 76% in the primary prevention and by 54% in the secondary intervention cohorts. In addition, the adjusted risk of proliferative or severe nonproliferative retinopathy was reduced by 47% and the need for photocoagulation by 56% in the secondary intervention group. Similarly, with regard to diabetic renal disease, intensive therapy resulted in significant reductions in risk of microalbuminuria of 34% (primary cohort) and 43% (secondary cohort). In the secondary intervention cohort, approximately 10% of whom had microalbuminuria at onset, the risk of albuminuria >300 mg/24 h was reduced by 56%. The appearance of clinical neuropathy (defined as the presence of signs or symptoms of peripheral neuropathy accompanied by either abnormal nerve conduction in at least two peripheral nerves or abnormal autonomic testing) was reduced with intensive therapy by 69% in the primary cohort and by 57% in the secondary intervention cohort. The reductions were significant for both peripheral and autonomic neuropathy.[10,11]

The positive reductions in cumulative incidence of microvascular complications were also analyzed within subgroups of the DCCT subjects defined on the basis of several baseline covariates to ensure consistency of results. These included age (adolescents versus adults), gender, duration of diabetes, baseline HbA1c, and mean blood pressure. The effect of intensive treatment was consistently maintained in all subgroups in both the primary and secondary cohorts. Thus the DCCT conclusively demonstrated that intensive glycemic control therapy delays the onset and slows the progression of diabetic retinopathy, nephropathy, and neuropathy in individuals with type 1 diabetes.

The DCCT was the largest and longest duration study of glycemic control in type 1 diabetes. Several months prior to its publication a study involving 102 subjects with type 1 diabetes in Sweden was published. As with the DCCT, subjects participating in the Stockholm Diabetes Intervention Study (SDIS) were randomized to intensive versus standard therapy and followed for 7.5 years.[12] Mean HbA1c levels were reduced from 9.4 to 8.5% in the standard treatment group and from 9.5 to 7.1% in the intensive treatment group. After 7.5 years both progression of nonproliferative retinopathy and the need for laser photocoagulation was less in the group receiving intensive control. There were more patients in the standard group with albumin excretion of at least 300 mg/24 h and with nephropathy as defined by subnormal glomerular filtration rates. Peripheral nerve conduction velocities deteriorated more in the standard treatment group. These results were the first to describe the beneficial effects of intensive therapy on retarding the development and progression of microvascular complications in patients with type 1 diabetes.

Based on the DCCT and SDIS studies published in 1993, most diabetes organizations advocated the use of intensive glycemic control therapy for all individuals with type 1 and type 2 diabetes.[13] The latter group was not studied in either trial. However, as the microvascular complications were all too similar in both types of diabetes[14,15] the extrapolation was applied. This recommendation was not universally accepted.[16,17] It was felt that the use of intensive insulin therapy in type 2 diabetes may lead to an increase in cardiovascular morbidity and/or mortality due to increased hypoglycemia, higher insulin levels, and/or greater weight gain. This concern had some basis in prior epidemiologic studies demonstrating that coronary artery disease (CAD) occurs with greater frequency in type 2 than in type 1 diabetes, a difference attributable not only to the older age of onset of type 2 diabetes but also to the dysmetabolic state that accompanies the disease.[18-20]

A group of investigators at Kumamoto University in Japan replicated the design of the DCCT, but in individuals with type 2 diabetes.[21] Fifty-five subjects with no retinopathy and urine albumin excretion <30 mg/24 h composed the primary prevention group and 55 patients with mild retinopathy and albumin excretion<300 mg/24 h comprised the secondary intervention group. All subjects were then randomized to intensive

(>2 insulin injections per day) or conventional (1–2 insulin injections per day) therapy. The goal of the conventional group was the absence of symptomatic hyper- or hypoglycemia. The numeric targets for the intensive group were fasting glucose <140 mg/dl, 2 h postprandial glucose <200 mg/dl, and HbA1c <7%. Follow-up data were obtained at 3 months and then every 6 months for 6 years. Separation of HbA1c (9.4% in the conventional subjects and 7.1% in those receiving intensive treatment) was maintained through the study. Risk reduction for progression of retinopathy in the combined cohorts was 69%, a result similar to the DCCT (see Table 39.1). Intensive therapy also reduced the average risk of worsening in retinopathy by 70%. After 6 years, nerve conduction velocities were significantly improved in the intensively treated subjects while median nerve conduction velocities deteriorated in the subjects receiving conventional therapy. Intensive glycemic control by MDI delayed the onset and slowed the progression of diabetic retinopathy, nephropathy, and neuropathy compared to conventional treatment. This study extended the confirmation of beneficial effects of intensive glycemic therapy seen in the DCCT and in the SDIS to individuals with type 2 diabetes.

Table 39.1 Risk reductions in microvascular disease

Study	Retinopathy		Microalbuminuria	
	Primary (%)	Secondary (%)	Primary (%)	Secondary (%)
DCCT	76	54	34	43
Kumamoto	76	56	62	52

The DCCT was designed as an intervention trial to compare two treatment modalities and not to determine complication risk at various levels of glycemic control. Nonetheless, the data were analyzed and presented in a subsequent paper, which examined the relationship between glycemic levels, as reflected by HbA1c, and the risk of retinopathy progression.[22] There was a continuously increasing risk of retinopathy progression with increasing mean HbA1c levels. Some prior retrospective studies had not found such a relationship for microalbuminuria[23] and retinopathy progression[24] for HbA1c levels below 8%. Analysis of the DCCT data, comprising over 9000 patient-years of observation, found a similar and significant reduction in retinal, renal, and neurological complication rates associated with decline in HbA1c. This relationship was consistent over the entire range of HbA1c in the study, even for levels less than 8% (see Fig. 39.1). Thus for a 10% reduction in HbA1c there is a constant

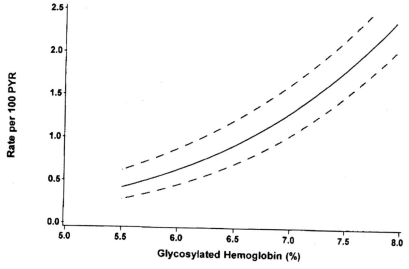

Fig. 39.1 The absolute risk of sustained retinopathy progression (hazard rate per 100 patient-years) in the combined treatment groups as a function of the updated mean HbA1c during follow-up in the DCCT estimated from a Poisson progression model with 95% confidence bands (from DCCT Research Group[25], with permission)

39% decrease in retinopathy progression. As the rate of events per 100 patient-years is greater at higher HbA1c values, the absolute reduction in risk is greater with reduction in HbA1c at higher values. Nonetheless, there exists no threshold HbA1c value below which a reduction in HbA1c is not accompanied by a reduction in risk for retinopathy and for nephropathy. When the risk of progression of retinopathy is extrapolated over the 9 years of follow-up in the DCCT the cumulative incidence of progression is lowered from 20% at a HbA1c of 8% to an incidence of 5.5% at a HbA1c of 6%.[25]

Another question regarding the extrapolation of the DCCT, SDIS, and Kumamoto studies was whether the motivated volunteers screened and selected for enrollment were representative of the general diabetes patient population. In order to address the comparability of the DCCT cohort and the validity of generalizing the DCCT results, a contemporaneous population based cohort was necessary. The Wisconsin Epidemiologic Study of Diabetic Retinopathy (WESDR) was a large population based incidence study of people with both type 1 and type 2 diabetes conducted concurrently with the DCCT.[26] The measurement of the main endpoint, diabetic retinopathy, was determined using similar methods of classification. Of the patients with type 1 diabetes being followed in the WESDR, 891 subjects underwent baseline and 4-year follow-up assessment. Of these, 39 and 111 met the DCCT inclusion criteria for the primary and secondary cohorts, respectively. The DCCT study cohorts were comparable to the WESDR type 1 population with regard to age, gender, BMI, blood pressure, and insulin dose. Because of the DCCT baseline eligibility criteria, retinopathy severity was higher in the WESDR group. Thus, the comparison supports the extrapolation of the DCCT results to the general type 1 diabetes population.

At the close of the DCCT in 1993, subjects who were in the conventional group were offered intensive treatment and as part of the study closeout were instructed in intensive therapy. Those subjects in both the former intensive and conventional groups were also offered participation in an observational study to continue following the DCCT cohorts. The Epidemiology of Diabetes Intervention and Complications (EDIC) is a follow-up observational study of the DCCT cohort to continue to monitor the long-term micro- and macrovascular complications of type 1 diabetes.[27] One of the study objectives is to compare the effects of the prior intensive or conventional treatments administered during the DCCT on the subsequent development and progression of more advanced retinopathy and nephropathy. About 1375 of the 1421 surviving DCCT subjects participated in the EDIC study. During the study all subjects received their diabetes care from their own physicians but were seen yearly for evaluation by the research team. Annual retinal fundus photography was obtained based on year of enrollment in the DCCT, with 1208 (605 in the intensive DCCT group) subjects undergoing evaluation at year 4 of EDIC.

By the end of the first year of EDIC, the HbA1c levels in the 1208 subjects had begun to merge (8.1% in the conventional and 7.7% in the intensive group). During the first 4 years of EDIC, the median HbA1c values were 8.2% for the conventional and 7.9% for the former intensive groups; a smaller but still statistically significant difference. The year-4 fundus photography results revealed that 49% of the subjects from the conventional group had progression of retinopathy from the DCCT baseline, while only 18% of the intensive group had progression. To assess the change in retinopathy during the EDIC years, the level of retinopathy was evaluated for fundus photographs obtained at years 1–4 of EDIC and retinopathy progression was compared to the level of retinopathy at the end of the DCCT (see Fig. 39.2). By EDIC year 4 the cumulative incidence of further progression of retinopathy was 70% lower in the intensive than in the conventional treatment group.[28] The significant reduction in retinopathy from end of the DCCT to year 4 of EDIC was similar regardless of the level of retinopathy at the end of the DCCT. Severe nonproliferative retinopathy, or worse, occurred in 10% of the conventional group but only 2% of the intensive group. This 76% reduction was significant even when adjusting for the level of retinopathy at the end of the DCCT. In addition, the risk of progression of retinopathy was highly associated with the mean HbA1c level during both the DCCT and EDIC studies.

Similar results were detected for progression of nephropathy during EDIC. At years 3 and 4, the onset of microalbuminuria was reduced 53%, from 11% in the conventional treatment group to 5% in the intensive group. The risk of new albuminuria was decreased by 86% in the intensive group.

Fundus photography and urine albumin measurements continued to be collected throughout the EDIC study. Despite statistically nonsignificant Hb1Ac differences between the former intensive and conventional groups by year 5 of EDIC, the cumulative incidence of further 3-step progression of retinopathy as well as development of

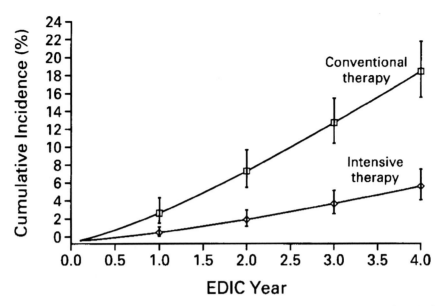

Fig. 39.2 Cumulative incidence of further progression of retinopathy (an increase of at least three steps from the level at the end of the DCCT) in the former conventional therapy and intensive therapy groups. The data are based on regression analysis adjusted for the level of retinopathy at the end of the DCCT, whether patients received therapy as primary prevention or secondary intervention, and both the duration of diabetes and the glycosylated hemoglobin value on enrollment in the DCCT. Patients who underwent scatter photocoagulation during the DCCT were excluded from the analysis (22 in the conventional group and 9 in the intensive therapy group). Bars denote 95% confidence intervals (from DCCT/EDIC Research Group[28], with permission. Copyright © 2000 Massachusetts Medical Society. All rights reserved)

microalbuminuria and albuminuria at EDIC year 8 continued to be less in the former DCCT intensive treatment group.[29,30]

During the 8 years of EDIC, with an increase in the HbA1c of the intensive group and a reduction in the separation of HbA1c levels between the intensive and conventional DCCT groups, it would be expected, based on the relationship of glycemic control to microvascular disease,[22] that the effects of intensive therapy during the DCCT would be reduced. In contrast, the benefits of intensive control on retinopathy and on nephropathy persist for at least 8 years after termination of separate intensive and conventional treatment and despite rising HbA1c levels. The positive effects of glycemic control appear to be long lasting. These results could be attributed to the effects of chronic hyperglycemia on advanced glycation end products accumulation in end organs, leading to microvascular disease,[31] but the exact reason for the persistence of the effects of past glycemic exposure is not known.

Thus, intensive glycemic control will delay the onset and slow the progression of diabetic microvascular disease in individuals with both type 1 and in type 2 diabetes. From the DCCT and EDIC study results, the positive benefits of intensive over conventional therapy will be greater the earlier they are implemented and can persist for up to 8 years after cessation of intensive treatment.

Macrovascular Disease

Although microvascular disease can lead to substantial morbidity, the major cause of mortality in both type 1 and type 2 diabetes is cardiovascular disease.[32–35] As was the case with microvascular disease, clinicians had long recognized an association of poor glycemic control with the development of macrovascular outcomes in patients with diabetes. Several prospective studies have confirmed that hyperglycemia is a predictor for cardiovascular disease.[36-39] Nonetheless, the belief that reduction of hyperglycemia decreases cardiovascular disease is not universally accepted.[40,41]

In the DCCT, the number of combined major macrovascular events (cardiac, cerebrovascular, and peripheral vascular) was twice as high in the conventional treatment (40 events) group than in the intensive treatment group (23 events), but this difference was not statistically significant.[42] Lipid risk factors associated with cardiovascular disease such as increased total and LDL cholesterol and elevated triglyceride levels were all significantly reduced in the intensive treatment group. As mentioned above, the DCCT cohorts were of young age at entry (13–39 years). In addition, the inclusion criteria eliminated patients with hypertension, hypercholesterolemia, and known cardiovascular disease. Such baseline demographics made it likely that few cardiovascular events would occur by DCCT study end.

One of the objectives of the EDIC study was to continue to monitor CV outcomes in the DCCT cohort. In addition, surrogate measures of cardiovascular disease were added to the microvascular assessments. B-mode ultrasonography was used to measure carotid intima-media wall thickness (IMT), an established index of atherosclerosis,[43] at years 1 and 6 of EDIC.[44] Increased IMT was significantly associated with HbA1c both at the time of measurement and during the 6.5 years of the DCCT. Subjects receiving conventional treatment during the DCCT developed greater age related increases in IMT than the intensively treated subjects.

The DDCT/EDIC Research Group had decided in 1996 not to perform any between treatment group analyses of cardiovascular events until a set target of 50 participants in the DCCT conventional group had experienced a CV event. This would ensure 85% power to detect a 50% reduction in the risk of CV events between the DCCT intensive and conventional treatment groups. Cardiovascular events were nonfatal myocardial infarction; nonfatal stroke; death judged to be due to CV disease; subclinical myocardial infarction (identified on annual EKG); angina; or the need for revascularization with angioplasty or coronary-artery bypass. The target number of conventional group participants was reached at the beginning of 2005 and the analyzed results were announced in June of that year. Among the 1375 DCCT/EDIC participants who remained in the study at the time of analysis, those in the former intensive treatment group had a 42% decrease (95% confidence interval, 9–63%; $p = 0.02$) in the risk of any CV disease and a 57% reduction (95% confidence interval 12–79%; $p = 0.02$) in the risk of nonfatal myocardial infarction or stroke or death from CV disease.[45] The mean HbA1c during the DCCT accounted for most of the effects of intensive treatment on reducing the risk of cardiovascular disease. This study was the first to show that intensive insulin therapy reduces the incidence of cardiovascular disease in individuals with diabetes.

Several studies looked at the effect of glycemic control on cardiovascular disease in type 2 diabetes. As mentioned above, the Kumamoto study evaluated a cohort of 110 individuals with type 2 diabetes. The total number of combined cardiovascular events in the conventional treatment group was twice that of the intensive treatment group, but was not statistically significant due to the small number of patients in the trial.

A much larger group of patients were studied in the United Kingdom Prospective Diabetes Study. The UKPDS was a multicenter intervention trial of over 5000 patients with newly diagnosed type 2 diabetes. The objective of the UKPDS was to determine if intensive glycemic control reduces the risk of diabetic complications in individuals with type 2 diabetes and, as a secondary aim, to compare various treatment modalities.[46] The study was conducted by general practitioners in 23 centers throughout the UK between 1977 and 1991. Patients with type 2 diabetes, 25–65 years of age, with FBG >6 mmol/L on two occasions were enrolled. All subjects were initially treated with diet modification alone for a 3-month period. At the end of 3 months, those patients who failed to achieve glycemic control (FBG >6.0 mmol/L) were randomized to various pharmacologic treatment modalities. Patients with BMI over 120% ($N = 2187$) were randomized to diet alone, sulfonylurea (SU) agent (chloropramide or glibenclamide), insulin, or metformin. Non-overweight patients ($N = 2022$) were randomly assigned to diet alone, sulfonylurea therapy (chlorpropramide or glibenclamide/glipizide) or insulin.

The conventional or diet alone subjects received dietary education every 3 months with goals to attain normal body weight, eliminate hyperglycemic symptoms, and maintain HbA1c levels <15 mmol/L. If either symptoms of hyperglycemia or FBG > 15 mmol/L occurred then the subject was again randomized to one of the pharmacologic agents with the aim once more to avoid hyperglycemic symptoms and keep FBG <15 mmol/L. The goal of intensive therapy was to attain near-normal FBG values (<6 mmol/L). As with the conventional cohort, a second drug was added if the FBG exceeded 15 mmol/L. Median follow-up was 10.7 years.

Unlike the DCCT, SDIS, and Kumamoto studies, the level of glycemia and HbA1c in the diet and pharmacologic groups was not maintained throughout the trial. Addition of drugs to the initial designated monotherapy was often necessary. HbA1c levels increased in all groups over the duration of the study so that, at the end of 10 years, the intensive treatment group median HbA1c level was 7.0% as compared to a 7.9% value for the conventional treatment group. Despite this modest difference, intensive glycemic control with either sulfonylurea or insulin resulted in a significant 21% risk reduction in the progression of retinopathy and a 33% risk reduction in albuminuria.[46] There was no evidence of any glycemic threshold for the effects of intensive glucose control on reducing microvascular complication rates. Thus the results of the UKPDS reaffirm the positive effect of intensive glucose therapy with insulin (and/or sulfonylurea) on reducing the development of microvascular complications in persons with type 2 diabetes.

The results for macrovascular endpoints in the UKPDS were not as definitive. The 16% risk reduction for combined fatal or nonfatal myocardial infarction and sudden death was just above statistical significance ($p = 0.052$). Epidemiologic analysis, however, revealed a continuous association between the risk of cardiovascular complications and the level of glycemia.[47] When overweight subjects treated with metformin were compared to the conventional diet-treated overweight group, there were significant risk reductions for diabetes-related death and diabetes-related endpoint, including fatal or nonfatal myocardial infarction.[48] These results occurred with only a 0.6% HbA1c separation between intensive (7.4%) and conventional (8%) groups, suggesting that the beneficial effects of metformin could have also been due to the drug's ability to improve lipid levels and decrease levels of plasminogen-activator inhibitor type 1. In contrast to the findings with metformin alone, there appeared to be an increase in diabetes-related death when metformin was added to SU to improve glycemic control. Explanations for these disparate results are lacking and a definitive conclusion regarding the effect of intensive glycemic control on CV outcomes based on the UKPDS study results cannot be reached.

In a later study, the effects of intensive glycemic control were evaluated in patients admitted to the coronary care units of 19 Swedish hospitals with suspected acute myocardial infarction and hyperglycemia (admission glucose levels at or above 198 mg/dl). In the Diabetes Mellitus, Insulin Glucose Infusion in Acute Myocardial Infarction (DIGAMI) study,[49] 620 patients were randomized to a control or infusion group. Those 306 patients in the infusion group received intravenous insulin infusion while in the coronary care unit (CCU) followed by four times daily subcutaneous insulin for 3 or more months to maintain glucose levels in a stable normoglycemic range. The control group of 314 patients was treated according to standard CCU practice and did not receive insulin unless clinically indicated. The primary aim of the DIGAMI study was to test whether early and rapid metabolic control in diabetic patients with acute myocardial infarction would reduce 3-month mortality rate. At 3 months, although HbA1c was $7.5 \pm 1.8\%$ in the control group and $7.0 \pm 1.6\%$ in the infusion group, the mortality rates were not significantly different. At 1 year, HbA1c levels in the infusion were lower than in the control group (7.0% vs. 7.5%). There was also a 31% lower 1-year mortality rate in the infusion group (18.6% vs. 26.1%, $p = 0.0273$). A larger study of 1253 patients (DIGAMI 2)[50] was designed to discern whether the insulin infusion alone or the combination of insulin infusion followed by intensive subcutaneous insulin administration was responsible for the reduced 1-year mortality rates seen in the initial DIGAMI study. Unfortunately, the study not only was unable to answer this question but also was unable to replicate the initial DIGAMI reduction in mortality rates, as the HbA1c levels in all groups were essentially identical (approximately 6.8%).

A smaller earlier intervention trial of 153 male subjects with type 2 diabetes also evaluated intensive versus conventional glycemic control. The Veterans Affairs Cooperative Study in Glycemia Control was a feasibility study for a larger trial.[51] Subjects were randomized to intensive therapy, using a stepped multiple insulin injection algorithm plus glipizide, or conventional treatment, using 1 or 2 insulin injections a day. The two groups achieved a HbA1c difference of 2.1% (9.2% vs. 7.1%) for 27 (range 18–35) months. The percentage of subjects experiencing a cardiovascular (CV) event was higher, though not statistically so, in the intensive (21.3%) than in the conventional group (11.5%).

The large clinical trials showing beneficial effects of intensive therapy on microvascular disease in individuals with type 2 diabetes fail to show a consistent statistically significant benefit on macrovascular disease. In the case of the UKPDS, the largest of the trials, the fact that patients were selected for the presence of newly diagnosed diabetes and for the absence of known CV disease could have resulted in the inability of the study to reach a significant difference in myocardial infarction rates. In addition, the continually rising glucose levels during the study, resulting in both an intensive group HbA1c above 8.0% and a modest HbA1c separation during the last 5 years of the trial, may have contributed to the lack of significant reduction in CV disease. It has long been recognized that an increase in CV risk occurs prior to the development of overt type 2 diabetes, at a time when HbA1c may be within the normal range and impaired glucose intolerance is present.[52–54] Much of this increased risk may be related to the lipid, blood pressure, and other metabolic abnormalities that often occur in individuals with impaired glucose tolerance. On the other hand, the ability of intensive glycemic control to decrease CV disease may require achieving lower glucose levels than those resulting in improvement in microvascular complications.

In order to determine whether achieving such lower glucose levels would indeed result in a reduction in CV events in individuals with type 2 diabetes mellitus, the NIH has sponsored the Action to Control Cardiovascular Risk in Diabetes (ACCORD) Trial.[55] Over 10,000 middle-aged and older patients with type 2 diabetes at high risk for CV disease were randomized into the ACCORD trial at 77 centers in the United States and Canada. The ACCORD study is also, using a double 2×2 factorial design, evaluating the effects on CV events of treatment to increase high-density lipoprotein cholesterol and lower triglyceride (in the context of optimal LDL cholesterol and good glycemic control) and of intensive blood pressure control (in the context of good glycemic control). Primary outcome is the first occurrence of a major CV event, defined as nonfatal MI, nonfatal stroke, or cardiovascular death. The glycemic arm of the trial tests whether a therapeutic strategy that targets a HbA1c level of <6.0% will reduce the occurrence of major CV events more than a strategy that targets a HbA1c in the 7.0–7.9% range. The ACCORD trial is scheduled to conclude on June 30th, 2009, at which time the participants will have been followed for 4–8 (mean 5.6) years.

In summary, based on currently completed clinical trials, intensive glycemic therapy will reduce the incidence of cardiovascular disease and events in individuals with type 1 diabetes. Whether intensive glycemic control has the same effect in type 2 diabetes remains to be proven. It is important to keep in mind that control of blood pressure and correction of lipid abnormalities will result in substantial reductions in cardiovascular disease in individuals with type 2 diabetes[56–58] and such therapy should be instituted.

Adverse Effects of Intensive Glycemic Control

Intensive glycemic control is not without possible side effects. These include weight gain, drug-specific side effects, costs in both time and money, and hypoglycemia. The occurrence of low blood glucose level carries the greatest risk, including significant morbidity and death. Several fold increases in mild to moderate hypoglycemia occur in all trials utilizing intensive glycemic control.[59] In the DCCT, the incidence of severe hypoglycemia (documented BG <50 mg/dl requiring the assistance of another person for correction) was increased threefold in the intensive treatment group (61.2 episodes/100 patient-years) compared to the conventional group (18.7 episodes/100 patient-years).[60] The intensive group did not have an increase in deaths, myocardial infarctions, or strokes attributable to hypoglycemia. There was also no difference in cognitive function, as assessed by a battery of cognitive testing, in the intensive treatment group at the close of the DCCT[61] or at follow-up testing 18 years from the onset of the study.[62] Similar results regarding the incidence of hypoglycemia were found in the Stockholm Diabetes Intervention Study. The incidence of hypoglycemia, including recurrent episodes, during the DCCT was found to have greater association with the most recent HbA1c than with past values or the average HbA1c during the DCCT trial.[25] There was a 26% (95% CI 22–29) increase in the risk of severe hypoglycemia for each 10% reduction in current HbA1c in the intensive group. The increased risk per 10% lower HbA1c was 54% (95% CI 49–60) in the conventionally treated subjects. For both treatment groups, the risk gradient for HbA1c <8% was lower than for values >8%.[25] Over the 6.5 years of the DCCT, 65% of the patients in the intensive group had at least one episode of severe hypoglycemia vs. 35% of the conventionally treated subjects. The number of prior episodes of hypoglycemia was the strongest predictor of future episodes.[60]

In type 2 diabetes, the risk of hypoglycemia and severe hypoglycemia is an order of magnitude less than that in type 1 diabetes. In the UKPDS, the rate of hypoglycemic episodes increases over time in the insulin treated patients but decreases over time in patients treated with oral agents. The percentage of patients with any hypoglycemia was 15.2% for patients on chlorpropramide, for glibenclamide – 20.5%, for insulin – 25.5%, for metformin – 8.3%, and for diet alone – 7.9%. Severe hypoglycemic episodes occurred in 1.8–2% of patients on insulin, 1.0–1.4% on glibenclamide, 1–1.2% on chlorpropramide, 0.6% on metformin and 0.7% on diet alone.[46,48]

Intensive glycemic control also lowers the threshold for hormonal response to hypoglycemia, leading to impaired glucose counter-regulation.[63,64] Patients with type 2 diabetes release counter-regulatory hormones at a higher plasma glucose level and in higher amounts for a similar degree of overall glycemic control.[65] This may account for the lower incidence of hypoglycemia in type 2 diabetes.

Weight gain will also accompany intensive glycemic control, with the exception of patients treated with metformin. In the DCCT, after 6.5 years, the prevalence of being overweight (BMI >27.8 kg/m^2 for men and >27.3 kg/m^2 for women) was 33.1% in the intensive treatment group compared to 19.1% in the conventional treatment group.[66,67] Intensive group subjects with a family history of type 2 diabetes experienced greater central weight gain than subjects with no such family history.[68] Weight gain is especially troubling in individuals with type 2 diabetes, given the high incidence of associated obesity. In the UKPDS, subjects treated with SUs gained 1.7 and 2.6 kg, while patients on insulin gained an average of 4.0 kg.[46]

Side effects, besides hypoglycemia and weight gain, of the oral agents used to achieve glycemic control in individuals with type 2 diabetes include gastrointestinal symptoms, lactic acidosis, edema, and fluid retention and, in the case of the thiazolidenedione class, congestive heart failure and possible increase in myocardial infarction rates.[69–71] The possible adverse effects of high insulin levels in the setting of insulin resistance on vascular smooth muscle cell migration/proliferation and the development of atherosclerosis remain controversial.[72,73]

Glycemic Control Target Levels

Hemoglobin A1c levels are used as a measurement to both determine recent mean plasma glucose levels and to predict future risk of developing diabetes complications. Recently, the concept of glucose variability, particularly postprandial glucose levels, as an additional independent predictor of complications has been proposed.

Several epidemiological studies have shown that plasma glucose levels 2 h after an oral glucose challenge is an independent predictor of cardiovascular disease risk.[74–76] Post-challenge absolute and incremental glucose levels were more strongly associated with B-mode ultrasonography carotid artery intima–media thickness than fasting glucose levels or HbA1c.[77] The majority of the patients in these studies, however, had impaired glucose tolerance(IGT) or mild diabetes and HbA1c levels that were within the nondiabetic reference ranges.

The effect of postprandial glucose lowering agents on macrovascular disease has been looked at in interventional studies of individuals with IGT and type 2 diabetes. The STOP-NIDDM research study[78] evaluated whether the alpha-glucosidase inhibitor acarbose, a compound that specifically reduces postprandial hyperglycemia, would reduce the risk of progression to diabetes, development of hypertension, and cardiovascular disease. In this international, multicenter placebo-controlled trial, 1429 patients with impaired glucose tolerance were randomized to placebo or acarbose and followed for a mean of 3.3 years. Acarbose use was associated with a 49% relative risk reduction in CVD events (hazard ratio of 0.51; 95% confidence interval 0.28–0.95, $p = 0.03$). Esposito et al.[79] compared the effects of the insulin secretagogues repaglinide and glyburide in 175 patients with type 2 diabetes. Following a 6–8 week titration period, subjects were randomized to one of the two medications for 12 months. Carotid B-mode ultrasound intima–media thickness (CIMT) measurements and serum samples for inflammatory markers were obtained at baseline and at study end. Despite similar declines in HbA1c levels of approximately 0.9%, postprandial glucose was 148 ± 28 mg/dl in the repaglinide group and 180 ± 32 mg/dl in the glyburide group ($p < 0.01$). CIMT regression was observed in 52% of patients in the repaglinide group but only 18% of the patients receiving glyburide ($p < 0.01$). Inerleukin-6 and c-reactive protein also decreased more in the repaglinide group ($p = 0.04$ and 0.02, respectively).

Proposed mechanisms through which postprandial hyperglycemia may impact endothelial function include increased production of inflammatory markers and free radicals.[80] Monier et al.[81] assessed the relative contributions of sustained hyperglycemia and acute glucose fluctuations on measures of oxidative stress in 21 patients with type 2 diabetes and 21 age and sex matched controls. Urinary 8-iso prostaglandin F 2 alpha, an indicator of total body free radical production, was associated with both the mean amplitude of glycemic excursions (MAGE) ($r = 0.86$, $p < 0.001$) and postprandial incremental area under the curve ($r = 0.55$, $p < 0.009$). There was no significant correlation between free radical production and 24 h glucose production, fasting glucose concentration, or HbA1c.

Despite the correlations of surrogate measures of atherosclerosis with postprandial glucose elevations seen in the above small studies, there has been no confirmatory evidence from the large clinical trials of an independent effect of glycemic variability on complications of diabetes. Several analyses of the DCCT data set have found that glycemic variability does not independently predict the risk of complications beyond that of HbA1c level.[82–84] In 2001, an ADA consensus panel did not recommend the routine use of postprandial blood glucose testing.[85]

Clinical target levels for intensive glycemic control are based on consensus committees reviewing the available study data. Unfortunately, as presented in the sections above, none of the large randomized trials evaluating the effects of glycemic control on micro and macrovascular complications have attained mean HbA1c levels in the nondiabetes range. Thus, a difference of opinion exists among diabetologists and professional organizations regarding specific glycemic targets, with no hard evidence supporting one over the other. The two most cited glycemic target levels from United States organizations are the American Diabetes Association (ADA) recommendations[86] and the American Association of Clinical Endocrinologists (AACE) Medical Guidelines.[87]

Clearly, patients with both type 1 and type 2 diabetes must be given appropriate dietary and pharmacologic therapy to eliminate the symptoms of hyperglycemia and prevent the consequences of extreme uncontrolled diabetes, i.e., ketoacidosis and hyperosmotic state. The positive effects of intensive glycemic control on the development and the progression of microvascular disease in the clinical trials of patients with both type 1 and type 2 diabetes form the basis for the ADA target glucose and HbA1c levels as outlined in Table 39.2 below. A case could be made to attempt to achieve glucose levels as close to normal as possible as, in secondary clinical trial analyses, there is no threshold of HbA1c level below which further reduction in microvascular disease does not occur. Thus, the AACE glycemic HbA1c target of less than 6.5% is lower than that of the ADA.

Table 39.2 Recommended glycemic goals

	Nondiabetes glycemic levels	Diabetes treatment targets
A1C	<6	<7
FBG (plasma)	<100 mg/dl	70–130 mg/dl
	<5.6 mmol/l	3.9–7.2 mmol/l
2 h	<140 mg/dl	<180 mg/dl
postmeal BG (plasma)	<7.8 mmol/l	<10 mmol/l

Source: Data from American Diabetes Association.[86]

Concurrent chronic illness does not limit the achievement of glycemic control.[88] This must be tempered by the fact that the incidence of hypoglycemia will be increased threefold for near-normal glucose levels. For individuals with other diseases where the consequences of severe hypoglycemia may result in morbidity or death, the attainment of normal glucose levels with insulin or SU therapy would not be advisable. If the patient has a disease which significantly shortens life expectancy, then the need to prevent long-term complications is absent. Treatment goals must be individualized to account for concomitant disease, the presence of hypoglycemic awareness, and the ability of the patient to monitor glucose levels and follow an intensive treatment plan. For patients with type 2 diabetes, it is also important to focus on the concomitant dysmetabolic state and to address any abnormalities in lipids and blood pressure. The ultimate goal of glycemic control is to attain the lowest HbA1c level that will not adversely affect patient safety. Although the recommended goal is a HbA1c <7% or <6.5%, for most patients without other medical illnesses one can attempt to reach a value of 6.0%, providing no treatment side effects occur. For patients with mild or early onset diabetes, on diet alone or on pharmacologic agents that cannot cause hypoglycemia, HbA1c levels within the normal range should be readily achievable.

Summary

Intensive glycemic control effectively prevents the occurrence and delays the progression of microvascular complications in both type 1 and type 2 diabetes. Intensive therapy will also reduce the incidence of cardiovascular disease in type 1 diabetes. Demonstration of beneficial effects of glycemic control on decreasing CV events in type 2 diabetes is lacking. Attention to blood pressure and lipid control is also important in both types of diabetes.[89] The incidence of hypoglycemia is increased threefold with intensive glycemic control. Current recommendations advocate attaining near-normal glucose levels when safely feasible.

Helpful internet source for additional information on glycemic goals:

- ADA clinical practice guidelines
  (http://www.diabetes.org/diabetescare)

References

1. Engerman R, Bloodworth JM, et al. Relationship of microvascular disease in diabetes to metabolic control. *Diabetes.* 1977;26:760–769.
2. Engerman RL, Kern TS. Progression of incipient diabetic retinopathy during good glycemic control. *Diabetes.* 1987;36: 808–812.
3. Cohen AJ, McGill PD, Rosetti RG, Guberski DL, Like AA. Glomerulopathy in spontaneously diabetic rat: impact of glycemic control. *Diabetes.* 1987;36:944–951.
4. Pirart J. Diabetes mellitus and its degenerative complications: a prospective study of 4,400 patients observed between 1947 and 1973. *Diabetes Care.* 1978;38:252–261.
5. Ingelfinger FJ. Debates in diabetes. *N Engl J Med.* 1977;296:1228–1230.
6. Kroc Collaborative Study Group. Blood glucose control and the evolution of diabetic retinopathy and albuminuria. *N Engl J Med.* 1984;311:365–372.
7. Dahl-Jorgensen K, Hanssen KF, Kierulf P, Bjoro T, Sandvik L, Aagenaes O. Reduction of urinary albumin excretion after 4 years of continuous subcutaneous insulin-infusion in insulin-dependent diabetes mellitus. *Acta Endocrinologica.* 1988;117:19–25.
8. Lauritzen T, Frost-Larsen K, Larsen H-W, Deckert T. Steno Study Group. Effect of 1 year of near- normal blood glucose levels on retinopathy in insulin- dependent diabetes. *Lancet.* 1983;1:200–204.
9. DCCT Research Group. The effect of intensive treatment of diabetes on the development and progression of long-term complications in insulin-dependent diabetes mellitus. *N Engl J Med.* 1993;329:977–986.
10. DCCT Research Group. The effects of intensive treatment of diabetes therapy on the development and progression of neuropathy. *Ann Int Med.* 1995;122:561–568.
11. DCCT Research Group. The effect of intensive diabetes therapy on measures of autonomic nervous system function in the DCCT. *Diabetologia.* 1998;41:416–423.
12. Reichard P, Nilsson BY, Rosenquist U. The effect of long term intensified treatment on the development of microvascular complications of diabetes mellitus. *N Engl J Med.* 1993;329:304–309.
13. Implications of the Diabetes Control and Complications Trial. American Diabetes Association Position Statement. *Diabetes Spectrum.* 1993;6:225–227.
14. Klein R, Klein BEK, Moss SE, Davis MD, DeMets DL. Glycosylated hemoglobin predicts the incidence and progression of diabetic retinopathy. *JAMA.* 1988;260:2864–2871.
15. Klein R, Klein BEK, Moss SE, Davis MD, DeMets DL. The Wisconsin Epidemiologic Study of Diabetic Retinopathy: X. Four year incidence and progression of diabetic retinopathy when age at diagnosis is 30 years or more. *Arch Opthalmol.* 1989;107:244–249.
16. Lasker RD. DCCT: implications for policy and practice. *N Engl J Med.* 1993;329:1035–1036.
17. Nathan DM. Inferences and implications. Do results from the DCCT apply in NIDDM? *Diabetes Care.* 1995;18:251–257.
18. Reaven GM. Pathophysiology of insulin resistance in human disease. *Physiol Rev.* 1995;75:473–486.
19. Balkau B, Eschwege E, Papoz L, et al. Risk factors for early death in non-insulin-dependent diabetes and men with known glucose tolerance status. *Br Med J.* 1993;307:295–298.
20. Hsueh WA, Law RE. Cardiovascular risk continuum: implications of insulin resistance and diabetes. *Am J Med.* 1998;105(1A):4S-14S.
21. Ohkubo Y, Kishikawa H, Araki E, et al. Intensive insulin therapy prevents the progression of diabetic microvascular complications in Japanese patients with non-insulin-dependent diabetes mellitus. *Diab Res Clin Prac.* 1995;28:103–117.

22. DCCT Research Group. The relationship of glycemic exposure (HbA1c) to the risk of development and progression of retinopathy in the DCCT. *Diabetes*. 1995;44:968–983.

23. Krolewski AS, Laffel LMB, Krolewski M, Quinn M, Warram JH. Glycosylated hemoglobin and the risk of microalbuminuria inpatients with insulin-dependent diabetes mellitus. *N Engl J Med*. 1995;332:1251–1255.

24. Warram JH, Manson JE, Krolewski AS. Glycosylated hemoglobin and the risk of retinopathy in insulin-dependent diabetes. *N Engl J Med*. 1995;332:1305–1306.

25. DCCT Research Group. The absence of a glycemic threshold for the development of long- term complications: The perspective of the DCCT. *Diabetes*. 1996;45:1289–1298.

26. DCCT Research Group, Klein R, Moss S. A comparison of the study populations in the DCCT and the WESDR. *Arch Int Med*. 1995;155:745–754.

27. EDIC Research Group. EDIC: design, implementation and preliminary results of a long-term follow-up of the DCCT cohort. *Diabetes Care*. 1999;22:99–111.

28. DCCT/EDIC Research Group. Retinopathy and nephropathy in patients with type 1 diabetes four years after a trial of intensive therapy. *N Engl J Med*. 2000;342:381–389.

29. DCCT/EDIC Research Group. Effect of intensive therapy on the microvascular complications of type 1 diabetes. *JAMA*. 2002;287:2563–2569.

30. DCCT/EDIC Research Group. Sustained effect of intensive treatment of type 1 diabetes mellitus on development and progression of diabetic nephropathy. *JAMA*. 2003;290:2159–2167.

31. Genuth S, Sun W, Cleary P, et al. Glycation and carboxymethyllysine levels in skin collagen predict the risk of future 10-year progression of diabetic retinopathy and nephropathy in the Diabetes Control and Complications Trial and Epidemiology of Diabetes Intervention and Complications participants with type 1 diabetes. *Diabetes*. 2005;54:3103–3111.

32. Geiss S, Herman WH, Smith PJ. Mortality in non-insulin-dependent diabetes. In: Harris M, ed. *Diabetes in America*. 2nd ed. Bethesda, MD: National Institutes of Health (NIH publ.No 95-1468); 1995:133–155.

33. Krolewski AS, Kosinski EJ, Warram JH, et al. Magnitude and determinants of coronary artery disease in juvenile-onset, insulin-dependent diabetes mellitus. *Am J Cardiol*. 1987;59:750–755.

34. Laing SP, Swerdlow AJ, Slater SD, et al. Mortality from heart disease in a cohort of 23,000 patients with insulin-treated diabetes. *Diabetologia*. 2003;46:760–765.

35. Thom T, Haase N, Rosamond W, et al. for the American Heart Association Statistics Committee and Stroke Statistics Subcommittee. Heart disease and stroke statistics-2006 update: a report from the American Heart Association Statistics Committee and Stroke Statistics Subcommittee. Circulation 113: e85–e151; 2006

36. Niskanen L, Turpeinen A, Pentilla I, Uusitupa MI. Hyperglycemia and compositional lipoprotein abnormalities as predictors of cardiovascular mortality in type 2 diabetes: a 15 year follow-up from the time of diagnosis. *Diabetes Care*. 1998;21:1861–1869.

37. Wei M, Gaskill SP, Haffner SM, Stern MP. Effects of diabetes and level of glycemia on all cause and cardiovascular mortality. The San Antonio Heart Study. *Diabetes Care*. 1998;21:1167–1172.

38. Lehto S, Ronnemma T, Pyorala K, Laakso M. Poor glycemic control predicts coronary heart disease events in patients with type 1 diabetes without nephropathy. *Arterioscler Thromb Vasc Biol*. 1999;19:1014–1019.

39. Selvin E, Marinopoulos S, Berkenblit G, et al. Met-analysis: glycosylated hemoglobin and cardiovascular disease in diabetes mellitus. *Ann Int Med*. 2004;141:421–431.

40. Barrett-Connor E. Does hyperglycemia really cause coronary heart disease? *Diabetes Care*. 1997;20:1620–1622.

41. Orchard TJ, Olson JC, Erbey JR, et al. Insulin resistance-related factors, but not glycemia, predict coronary artery disease in type 1 diabetes: 10 year follow-up data from the Pittsburgh Epidemiology of Diabetes Complications Study. *Diabetes Care*. 2003;26:1374–1379.

42. DCCT Research Group. Effect of intensive diabetes management on macrovascular events and risk factors in the DCCT. *Am J Cardiol*. 1995;75:894–903.

43. Burke GL, Evans GW, Riley WA, et al. Arterial wall thickness is associated with prevalent cardiovascular disease in middle-aged adults: the Atherosclerosis Risk in Communities (ARIC) Study. *Stroke*. 1995;26:386–391.

44. DCCT/EDIC Research Group. Intensive diabetes therapy and carotid intima-media thickness in type 1 diabetes mellitus. *N Engl J Med*. 2003;348:2294–2303.

45. DCCT/EDIC Research Group. Intensive diabetes treatment and cardiovascular disease in patients with type 1 diabetes. *N Engl J Med*. 2005;355:2643–2652.

46. UKPDS Group. Intensive blood glucose control with sulfonylureas or insulin compared with conventional treatment and risk of complications in patients with type 2 diabetes (UKPDS 33). *Lancet*. 1998;352:837–853.

47. Stratton IM, Adler AI, Neil HA, et al. Association of glycemia with macrovascular and microvascular complications of type 2 diabetes (UKPDS 35): Prospective observational study. *BMJ*. 2000;321:405–412.

48. UKPDS Group. Effect of intensive blood glucose control with metformin complications on in overweight patients with type 2 diabetes (UKPDS 34). *Lancet*. 1998;352:854–865.

49. Malmberg K, Ryden L, Efendic S, et al. Randomized trial of insulin-glucose infusion followed by subcutaneous insulin treatment in diabetic patients with acute myocardial infarction (DIGAMI study): effects on mortality at 1 year. *J Am Coll Cardiol*. 1995;26:57–65.

50. Malmberg K, Ryden L, Wedel H, et al. for the DIGAMI 2 investigators. Intense metabolic control by means of insulin in patients with diabetes mellitus and acute myocardial infarction (DIGAMI 2): effects on mortality and morbidity. *Eur Heart J.* 2005;26:650–661.

51. Abraira C, Colwell J, Nuttall F, et al. Cardiovascular events and correlates in the veterans affairs diabetes feasibility trial. *Arch Int Med.* 1997;157:181–188.

52. Balkau B, Shipley M, Jarrett RJ, Pyorala M, Forhan A, Eschwege E. High blood glucose concentration is a risk factor for mortality in middle-aged nondiabetic men: 20 year follow-up in the Whitehall Study, the Paris Prospective Study, and the Helsinki Policemen Study. *Diabetes Care.* 1998;21:360–367.

53. Coutinho M, Gerstein HC, Wang Y, Yusuf S. The relationship between glucose and incident cardiovascular events: a meta-regression analysis of published data form 20 studies of 95,783 individuals followed for 12.4 years. *Diabetes Care.* 1999;22:233–240.

54. Khaw KT, Wareham N, Bingham S, Luben R, Welch A, Day N. Association of hemoglobin A1c with cardiovascular disease and mortality in adults: the European prospective investigation into cancer in Norfolk. *Ann Int Med.* 2004;141: 413–420.

55. The ACCORD Study Group. Action to control cardiovascular risk in diabetes (ACCORD) trial: design and methods. *Am J Cardiol.* 2007;99:21i-33i.

56. Bakris GL. The importance of blood pressure control in the patient with diabetes. *Am J Med.* 2004;116(S5A):S30–S38.

57. Heart Protection Study Collaborative Group. MRC/BHF Heart Protection Study of cholesterol lowering with simvastatin in 5963 people with diabetes: a randomized placebo-controlled trial. *Lancet.* 2003;361:2005–2016.

58. Colhoun HM, Betteridge DJ, Durrington PM, et al. for the CARDS investigators. Primary prevention of cardiovascular disease with atorvastatin in type 2 diabetes in the Collaborative Atorvastatin Diabetes Study (CARDS): multi-centre randomized placebo-controlled trial. *Lancet.* 2004;364:685–696.

59. Cryer P. Hypoglycemia: the rate limiting factor in the glycaemic management of type I and type II diabetes. *Diabetologia.* 2002;456:937–948.

60. DCCT Research Group. Hypoglycemia in the DCCT. *Diabetes.* 1997;46:271–286.

61. DCCT Research Group. Effects of intensive diabetes therapy in neuropsychological function in adults in the DCCT. *Ann Int Med.* 1996;124:379–388.

62. Jacobson AM, Musen G, Ryan CM, et al. Long-term effect of diabetes and its treatment on cognitive function. *N Engl J Med.* 2007;356:1842–1852.

63. Amiel SA, Tamborlane WV, Simonson DC, Sherwin RS. Defective glucose counterregulation after strict glycemic control of insulin-independent diabetes mellitus. *N Engl J Med.* 1987;316:1376–1383.

64. Kinsley BT, Windom B, Simonson DS. Differential regulation of counter-regulatory hormone secretion and symptoms during hypoglycemia in IDDM. *Diabetes Care.* 1995;18:17–26.

65. Levy CJ, Kinsley BT, Bajaj M, Simonson DS. Effect of glycemic control on glucose counter-regulation during hypoglycemia in NIDDM. *Diabetes Care.* 1998;21:1330–1338.

66. DCCT Research Group. Adverse events and their association with treatment regimens in the diabetes control and complications trial. *Diabetes Care.* 1995;18:1415–1427.

67. DCCT Research Group. Influence of intensive diabetes treatment on body weight and composition of adults with type 1 diabetes in the diabetes control and complications trial. *Diabetes Care.* 2001;24:1711–1721.

68. Purnell JQ, Dev RK, Steffes MW, et al. Relationship of family history of type 2 diabetes, hypoglycemia and autoantibodies to weight gain and lipids with intensive and conventional therapy in the diabetes control and complications trial. *Diabetes.* 2003;52:2623–2629.

69. DeFronzo RA. Pharmacologic therapy for type 2 diabetes mellitus. *Ann Intern Med.* 1999;131:281–303.

70. Nissen SE, Wolski K. Effect of rosiglitazone on the risk of myocardial infarction and death from cardiovascular causes. *N Engl J Med.* 2007;356:2425–2471.

71. Singh S, Loke YK, Furberg CD. Thiazolidinediones and heart failure: a teleo-analysis. *Diabetes Care.* 2007;30:2148–2153 May 29, 2007 Epub.

72. Abraira C, Maki KC. Does insulin treatment increase cardiovascular risk in NIDDM? *Clin Diabetes.* 1995;13:29–31.

73. Nigro J, Osman N, Dart AM, Little PJ. Insulin resistance and atherosclerosis. *Endocrine Rev.* 2006;27:242–259.

74. The DECODE Study Group, the European Diabetes Epidemiology Group. Glucose intolerance and mortality: comparison of WHO and American Diabetes Association diagnostic criteria. *Lancet.* 1999;354:617–621.

75. Balkau B, Shipley M, Jarrett RJ, et al. High blood glucose concentration is a risk factor for mortality in middle-aged nondiabetic men: 20-year follow-up in the Whitehall Study, the Paris Prospective Study, and the Helsinki Policemen Study. *Diabetes Care.* 1998;22:360–367.

76. Hanefeld M, Fischer S, Julius U, et al. the DIS Group. Risk factors for myocardial infarction and death in newly detected NIDDM: the diabetes intervention study, 11 year follow-up. *Diabetologia.* 1996;39:1577–1583.

77. Temelkova-Kurktschiev TS, Koehler C, Henkel E, Leonhardt W, Fueker K, Hanefeld M. Post challenge plasma glucose and glycemic spikes are more strongly associated with atherosclerosis than fasting glucose or HbA1c level. *Diabetes Care.* 2000;23:1830–1834.

78. Chiasson J-L, Josse RG, Gomis R, Hanefeld M, Karasik A, Laasko M. The Stop NIDDM Trial. Acarbose treatment and the risk of cardiovascular disease and hypertension in patients with impaired glucose tolerance. *JAMA.* 2003;290:486–494.

79. Esposito K, Giugliano D, Nappo F, Marfella R. the Campanian Postprandial Hyperglycemia Study Group. Regression of carotid atherosclerosis by control of postprandial hyperglycemia in type 2 diabetes mellitus. *Circulation*. 2004;110:214–219.

80. Ceriello A. Postprandial hyperglycemia and diabetes complications. *Diabetes*. 2005;54:1–7.

81. Monnier L, Mas E, Ginet C, et al. Activation of oxidative stress by acute glucose fluctuations compared with sustained chronic hyperglycemia in patients with type 2 diabetes. *JAMA*. 2006;295:1681–1687.

82. Service FJ, O'Brien PC. The relation of glycemia to the risk of development and progression of retinopathy in the diabetes control and complications trial. *Diabetologia*. 2001;44:1215–1220.

83. McCarter RJ, Hempe JM, Chalew SA. Mean blood glucose and biological variation have greater influence on HbA1c levels than glucose instability. *Diabetes Care*. 2006;29:352–355.

84. Kilpatrick ES, Rigby A, Atkin SL. The effect of glucose variability on the risk of microvascular complications in type 1 diabetes. *Diabetes Care*. 2006;29:1486–1490.

85. American Diabetes Association. Postprandial blood glucose. *Diabetes Care*. 2001;24:775–778.

86. American Diabetes Association. Standards of medical care in diabetes-2008. *Diabetes Care*. 2008;31(S1):S16–S24.

87. American Association of Clinical Endocrinologists. Medical guidelines for clinical practice for the management of diabetes mellitus. *Endocrine Practice*. 2007;13(S1):16.

88. El-Kebbi IM, Zeimer DC, Cook C, Miller CD, Gallina DL, Phillips LS. Comorbidity and glycemic control in patients with type 2 diabetes. *Arch Int Med*. 2001;161:1295–1300.

89. Gaede P, Veldel P, Larsen N, Jensen GVH, Parving H-H, Pederson O. Multifactorial intervention and cardiovascular disease in patients with type 2 diabetes. *N Engl J Med*. 2003;348:383–393.

Chapter 40
Behavioral and Educational Approaches to Diabetes Self-Management

Maria A. Mendoza, Monique Welbeck, and Grishma Parikh

Introduction

Diabetes is a life-long disease managed primarily by the individual.[1] The key to successful self-management of this chronic disease is to provide the individual with knowledge, psychomotor skills, and effective psychological coping to facilitate lifestyle modifications.[2] The process of adult learning is not an exact science. It is highly individualized. Oftentimes, the clinician would find that strategies successful for one person might not be successful for others.

Adult learning within the process of diabetes self-management education does not occur in a vacuum. Indeed, the medical system, health-care providers, and most especially the individual with diabetes must be prepared and motivated to manage this chronic disease in order to prevent its acute and chronic complications. A model for the improvement of chronic illness management was developed by Wagner[3] to highlight a collaborative approach to chronic illness care. In this model the providers are not thinking that it is only the patient's responsibility for diabetes self-management and patients are not assuming that it is the providers' responsibility to take care of their chronic disease. Productive interactions between the "informed, activated" patient and the "prepared, proactive" practice team in the context of a supportive system and surrounding community are the focus of this model.[3,4] We (patients and providers) are all in this together.

The Diabetes Prevention Program study in 2002 showed that individuals at increased risk of developing type 2 diabetes who made lifestyle changes reduced their risk of getting type 2 diabetes by 58%.[5] It is estimated that at least 10 million Americans at high risk for type 2 diabetes can sharply decrease their chances of getting the disease with diet and exercise.[5] This study expanded the role of the diabetes educator in the primary prevention of diabetes.

Adult learning is a continuous and complex process that involves an interaction between the learner and the material to be learned, usually facilitated by an educator/team.[6] In many instances motivated adults learn through their own efforts. In the traditional sense learning involves an acquisition of knowledge and skills through a variety of media.[7] From the perspective of the diabetes self-management education, learning encompasses a much greater objective. It includes the dimension of behavior change by the individual as a result of the improvement in knowledge.[8]

This chapter addresses practical aspects in diabetes self-management education. It discusses how to evaluate the readiness of the individual to enter the learning process. It describes strategies on how to motivate adults to learn diabetes self-management. The chapter also provides practical recommendations on how a physician can facilitate adult learning in a clinical setting. It addresses the issue of adherence to the self-management regimen. It also explores the role of the diabetes team. At the end of the chapter is a sampling of resources for patient teaching.

M.A. Mendoza (✉)
Jacobi Medical Center, City University of New York, New York, NY, USA
e-mail: mariaa.mendoza@nbhn.net

L. Poretsky (ed.), *Principles of Diabetes Mellitus*, DOI 10.1007/978-0-387-09841-8_40,
© Springer Science+Business Media, LLC 2010

How Adults Learn

The learning process in adults is very different from children.[9] Major differences exist in their motivation, self-direction, orientation, participation, and experiences they bring to learning. Table 40.1 summarizes the characteristics of the adult learners.

Table 40.1 Characteristics of adult learners

- Self-directed
- Internally motivated
- Problem oriented
- Active participant in learning
- Experienced

Adults are very *self-directed*.[10,11,15] They want to be active participants in their own learning. Self-learning is very common among adults. They want to choose instructional media that would be comfortable to them. For example, they would rather read materials about diabetes care instead of attending classes if they do not have the time to do so or they feel threatened in a group setting. Some may prefer to watch a video on how to do a fingerstick rather than do it with an educator, because they want the flexibility of watching the film at any time and as many times as they need. Some want the interaction in a classroom situation rather than self-instruction because they enjoy the group dynamics.

Adults are *internally motivated* to learn.[9] This means that the individual recognizes a need and perceives the learning program as a way of meeting this need. This need is derived from something that the individual perceives as important.[12] It is usually problem oriented. For example, the reason why a person with diabetes would come to a class is to learn a specific skill relevant to meeting a need or goal. It could be as practical as injecting insulin or doing a fingerstick. Or, it could be a desire to solve a problem such as treating or preventing hypoglycemia or how to adjust insulin doses.

Learning among adults is best accomplished through *active participation*.[13] In general, adults want to be involved in all the stages of learning toward goal accomplishment. It is important for the facilitator and the adult learner to discuss learning needs and goals. These needs and goals should be *learner centered*,[9–12] i.e., determined by the learner, not the educator or team. The ways to acquire the knowledge and skills have to be individualized to the learner's preference. Hands-on learning and group process with active interaction are preferred over passive lecturing. Adults want to ask questions specific to their personal needs; provision for this type of interaction is a good teaching technique.

Adults come into the learning situation with *lots of experience*.[9,11,13,14,15] They want to share these experiences with others. The educator must encourage learners to discuss their experiences and provide instructions based on these. Many times sharing experiences would also be a good way to learn. For example, a person who modified the technique of glucose monitoring to deal with decreased sensation in the fingertips should be encouraged to share this with others. Also, having the personal experience provides credibility that is important to adult learners. An instructor who has no diabetes and has not done fingersticks five times a day would not be able to share the pain and apprehension of the person with diabetes going through this experience.

Diabetes Self-Management Training/Education

Diabetes self-management training (DSMT) or diabetes self-management education (DSME) is an interactive, collaborative, ongoing process involving the learner with diabetes and the educator/team.[7] This process involves (1) assessment of the learner and specific education needs, (2) identification by the patient/learner of self-management goals, (3) provision of education and behavioral interventions to achieve goals, and (4) evaluation of the learning process and outcomes, i.e., attainment of goals.[7] Education does not necessarily translate into behavior change.[8,16] The ultimate goal of DSMT is to change behavior. Although knowledge is a necessary component to achieve learning and behavior change, it is not sufficient by itself. Thus, DSME involves not only the provision of knowledge and skills but also psychological counseling, if needed, to facilitate lifestyle modification.[7,16]

The American Association of Diabetes Educators (AADE) recommends that all educators should measure the AADE 7 self-care behaviors that include the following:[17]

- Healthy eating
- Being active
- Monitoring
- Taking medications
- Problem solving
- Healthy coping
- Reducing risks

The above list is comprehensive and it is not practical or possible for a busy physician to cover everything. This is where the team approach to teaching becomes important. The physician should at least discuss with the patient and the family, as appropriate, the diabetes disease process and treatment options.

DSMT can be provided in a variety of settings depending on availability of resources. Some physicians may be comfortable in providing survival skill instructions to their patients. Physicians in a large group practice may hire a certified diabetes educator who may be a nurse, dietitian, or psychologist to provide patient teaching onsite. Those in small practice my have to refer patients to other facilities such as hospital-based or free-standing privately owned programs. There has to be some mechanism in place for this type of referrals. Knowledge of third-party reimbursement for diabetes education would be helpful to determine where patients could be referred. In some regions, education of patients with diabetes is part of the general medical care and therefore could not be billed separately.[18] Some city or municipal hospitals may offer free educational services to the community for patients with diabetes and their families. This would be a good resource for patients who do not have insurance coverage.

Recognizing the importance of training/education in providing a comprehensive diabetes management, in 2004 Medicare included DSMT and medical nutrition training (MNT) as reimbursable services provided to patients with diabetes both for initial and follow-up training.[19,20] This is a major step in offsetting the cost of diabetes training which is one of the barriers for providing comprehensive care. For further information about the specifics of the regulations and benefit coverage the reader is referred to the following website: http://www.cms.hhs.gov/manuals/102_policy/bp102index.asp.

When patients are referred to another institution for patient education, the physician should be aware of the quality of service provided by the agency.[21] The physician should know the general philosophy of the education program, the curriculum, length and frequency of classes, teaching methodologies used, the credentials of the staff in the program, and the procedure for patient follow-up. Collaborative relationship between the physician and the diabetes education staff is essential for continuity of patient management.[22] Communication, through verbal and written reports, has to be maintained for documentation purposes.[20]

The Diabetes Education Team

The composition of the diabetes education team varies from one institution to another depending on its size and financial resources. The team may be comprised of a nurse, physicians, dietitians, psychologists, social workers, pharmacists, exercise physiologists, ophthalmologist, optometrist, podiatrist, and other related disciplines. Coordinating patient education can be a problem in large, complex organizations.[21] The team approach provides the patient with expert perspective on different aspects of diabetes self-care management. For example, the dietitian provides expertise on diet therapy while an exercise physiologist provides an expert perspective on exercise and physical activities. However, like any situation where a variety of people provide patient education, consistency in message conveyed is an important issue to address.[23] Patients get confused if they hear different opinions from a variety of experts. Having a written curriculum and agreeing on the content to be delivered prior to conducting learning sessions can prevent this problem. Regular staff meetings are good channels to resolve conflicting opinions among staff.

All American Diabetes Association (ADA)-recognized DSME programs have at least a registered nurse and a registered dietitian. These staff members must be certified diabetes educators or have recent experience in diabetes education and management. They are credentialed by the National Certification Board for Diabetes Educators after fulfilling all the criteria for experience in diabetes teaching and mastery of specific body of knowledge in diabetes and adult teaching demonstrated by passing a written examination (Fig. 40.1).[17]

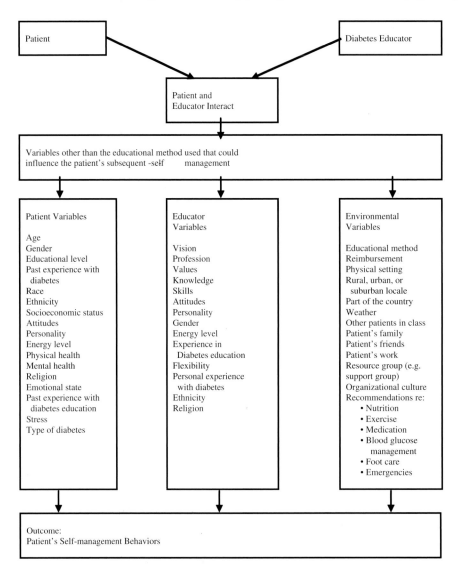

Fig. 40.1 A model depicting the complexity of variables that can influence diabetes management. Reprinted with permission from Anderson and Funnell[2]

Assessment of Learning Needs

Because adult learners come to the educational experience with a variety of personal, family, and cultural factors there is not one standard for teaching content. Assessment of the individual needs is the first step to facilitate learning. Various factors (physical, psychological, social, and cognitive) that may hinder learning should

Table 40.2 Barriers to learning

Physical barriers	Psychological barriers	Social barriers	Cognitive barriers
Pain	Fear	Lack of family support	Low-literacy skills
Blindness	Denial	Language barrier	Memory impairment
Hard of hearing	Anxiety	Limited financial resources	
Poor manual dexterity	Depression	Poor access to care	
Fatigue	Lack of motivation	Beliefs and values	
Physical symptoms of hyperglycemia or hypoglycemia	Dependency		

be assessed (see Table 40.2). Having the diagnosis of diabetes poses and additional stressor to the learning situation.[24] Many may have learned bits and pieces about diabetes self-management over a period of time and experiences and they may be asked to unlearn some things. Furthermore, since learning encompasses more than knowledge acquisition, these patients are also asked to modify their behavior toward a healthier lifestyle.

The different factors that need to be considered in this assessment process are discussed below. This section only includes the assessment of the adult learner. For information about diabetes teaching in children and adolescents we refer the reader to the end of the chapter for a listing of resources.

Adult Literacy

With increasing complexity of the health-care system, the subject of health literacy has been the focus of much attention lately. A report by the Institute of Medicine and Agency for Healthcare Research and Quality stated that there are about 90 million adults in the United States who are unable to maneuver the health-care system and fully benefit from it.[25] Functional health literacy means the ability to read, comprehend, and use information to make decisions pertaining to health issues. To be considered health literate the person needs to be able to do tasks such as reading and understanding written health instructions, medicine labels, consent forms, and appointment schedules; understanding written and oral information from health-care providers; and act on these information.[26]

The 2003 National Assessment of Adult Literacy by the National Center for Education Statistics survey found that about 14% (30 million) have "below basic" level of prose literacy (the ability to use printed and written information to function in the society toward achievement of goals and developing knowledge and potential).[27] These skills may include reading and understanding a bus or train schedules, appointments, medication or food labels, and the like.

The cost of health care among persons with inadequate health literacy is higher than those who have adequate health literacy. It is estimated that about $50–$73 billion could be saved each year by improving health literacy.[28–30] These savings can be realized mostly by reducing unnecessary hospitalizations, delays in treatment, and problems with prescriptions.

Health literacy is an issue in diabetes self-management education.[31] The individual with diabetes needs to be able to understand and process the information and then act on it. In a study of 2659 low-income patients in an ambulatory center at two public hospitals, it was found that about 42% did not understand the instruction "to take medicine on empty stomach."[32] Diabetes instructions are far more complex than this. For example, when learning insulin dose adjustment according to fingersticks and carbohydrate intake, the individual has to be able to do the mechanical aspect of the task, understand the interaction between blood glucose, carbohydrate intake, physical activity, and insulin, and use this information making a decision about dose adjustment. This is not a simple task for a patient with low literacy and instructions must be tailored to the individual.

Assessing functional health literacy is not very straightforward. Routine screening is actually controversial because of the possibility of stigmatizing those with low literacy.[33] There is always a possibility that physicians might refrain from taking low literacy patients because they are more difficult to treat. Many adults would not volunteer the information regarding their inability to read and write because of shame.[34] Unfortunately, the person's years of schooling do not always predict level of health literacy.[33] Educational and literacy levels are important factors that influence learning. They determine how people learn and the amount of complexity they can tolerate in a learning situation.[35] Some learn best by listening versus reading, while others prefer viewing a video.

There are several methods for measuring literacy, but probably none is practical for use in clinical practice. Physical appearance is an unreliable measure of literacy skills. Patient's educational level and ability to communicate do not measure literacy level. Many patients have average IQ and can be very articulate. Estimating patient's reading level in a clinical setting is neither practical nor reliable since it does not necessarily translate to comprehension. A simple and practical way to assess literacy by a general internist is to ask patient to read a medicine label and ask them to tell how they would take that medication.[33] This can be a useful screening tool to rule out the possibility of low health literacy. Patients will attempt to conceal their inability to read and write through avoidance of the situation.[35] These are some red flags that should alert the physician to possible low literacy problem.

- *Problem with eyesight*: "I forgot my eyeglasses." "My eyes are tired, could you read this for me?"
- *Lack of interest in reading instructions*: "I'd let my wife read it first." "I don't need these papers. Just show me how."
- *Unable to figure out written instructions*: "Could you please tell me which one of these papers is for the eye doctor?" "Could you please mark the paper for the eye doctor."
- *Inability to tell you the name of their medicine*: "I take one red pill and two white pills."
- *Not taking their medications as prescribed*: This may not be related to low literacy in many instances. However, inability to read medication labels should be ruled out when patients do not take their medications properly.
- *Missing appointments*: Again this may not mean low literacy but a patient who misses many appointments may actually have difficulty reading and following written instructions given by the physician.
- *Refuses to fill out forms*: "It takes too much time." "I'll take it home and let my daughter do it."
- *Underutilization of the health-care services*: Many patients may have other reasons for doing this but those with low literacy almost always underutilize health-care services.

Many patients with low literacy have developed coping mechanisms to deal with their learning disability. Many are able to learn diabetes self-management if taught at a level they can comprehend.[36] The physician should be sensitive to the patient's needs by asking questions to verify understanding of the verbal or written instructions. One should never assume that the patient understands. There are a variety of methods to evaluate learning initially and periodically in future visits. Methods used to decrease literacy demands and to evaluate learning are expanded upon below.

Psychosocial Factors

Fear, anxiety, denial, depression, and other psychological states can interfere with readiness to learn. The physician and educator should be aware of these problems and refer the patient to the psychiatrist, psychologist, or social worker as appropriate. Social stressors such as lack of insurance and lack of social support may also interfere with learning and should be part of the routine assessment prior to the learning encounters (see Chapter 46).

Cultural Patterns

The prevalence of diabetes is highest among the ethnic minority populations such as African Americans, Hispanic Americans, and Native Americans.[37] However, in big cities like New York other minority groups may also be prevalent. According to a study carried out by the New York City Department of Health and Mental Hygiene, diabetes is prevalent among the South Asians who comprise people from Bangladesh, Pakistan, India, and Sri Lanka.[38] The study indicates that "more than half of the New Yorkers whose families are from the

Indian subcontinent have either diabetes or prediabetes." Unfortunately, this community has historically been underrepresented within the health-care system.

Generally, ethnic groups also have a lower health status than the majority of the population.[37] The values, beliefs, rules of behavior, and lifestyle practices of the person guide their thinking and actions in particular ways.[39] The shortage or lack of culturally appropriate diabetes education materials and skilled educators has a negative and therefore nonproductive impact on an individual's self-management and understanding of diabetes. Therefore, physicians need to address the needs of ethnic groups by providing culturally competent and relevant diabetes self-management approach. This can help strengthen the effectiveness of diabetes self-management and control. The educational material and tools must speak to cultural relevance in order to be fully utilized by the patient. Teaching must encompass behaviors, attitudes, and policies that are reflective in the ethnic/cultural group. Assumptions should be avoided based on an individual's ethnic identification. Thus, physician education that includes cultural competence as a component of disease management strategy is essential in deploying the highest standards in the chronic management of diabetes if the community is to reap the benefits of the improvements in diabetes management and education.

Culture greatly influences the way the person makes decision regarding health care. When facilitating learning for a patient who belongs to a particular ethnic group, a cultural assessment needs to be done. This assessment is focused on elements relevant to the medical problem and interventions as well as the evaluation of the effectiveness of treatment.[40,41]

- What language does the patient speak?
- What role does the family play in patient's illness?
- What is the patient's status within the family structure? What are the patient's role/responsibilities/obligations within the family?
- Where does the patient live? With whom? Type of neighborhood (health-care resources, environmental stressors)?
- Who does the patient go to for health advice or treatment of diabetes?
- Does the patient use folk medicines? If so, what are they?
- What does the patient expect from diabetes treatment?
- What is the patient's perception about the health-care system?
- Who makes decisions for patients in terms of health care?
- What values does the patient have regarding foods?
- What are the patient's religious or spiritual beliefs and values?
- What are the patient's routine daily activities?

Effective communication, both verbal and nonverbal, is the first step used to engaging the patient from a different culture in a meaningful interaction.[42] Awareness of the ethnic groups' rules of conversation such as social introduction, demonstrating respect, and lack of hurried behavior is one of the key communication skills. The medical practitioners must have knowledge about when to choose a personalized or more detached mode of communication; when to select direct or indirect approaches; and when and how to use silence or touch to interact with different ethnic groups is very important.[41]

Whenever possible, the patient should be referred to an educator with knowledge and skills in dealing with the specific culture. This person has to be able to adapt communication and interaction patterns, make relevant cultural assessment, and modify the diabetes education program to suit the patient's needs. Patient's cultural beliefs and values should be considered when facilitating the patient to learn diabetes self-management practices. A common mistake is to do nutritional counseling without taking into consideration the patient's values about food, meal preparation, the type of ethnic food he or she eats, dietary patters, and religious practices involving fasting or feasting.

Special Needs of the Elderly

Diabetes affects the elderly population at a high rate and incidence of cognitive impairment increases with age.[37] Diabetes is associated with decline in cognitive function which is often undiagnosed and related to poorer diabetes control.[43–50] This group has special needs that have to be considered when providing diabetes self-management education. When assessing the needs of the elderly, one has to keep in mind that there are several factors that may affect their learning. These factors[34–37] are outlined in Table 40.3

Table 40.3 Factors that may affect learning in the elderly

- Sensory impairment: vision, hearing
- Psychomotor abilities (opening pill bottles, drawing up insulin, testing blood glucose)
- Coexisting medical conditions
- Memory and learning abilities
- Financial issues (fixed income)
- Family and social support
- Access to care (transportation)

In dealing with the elderly with diabetes, it is important not to make assumptions about the patient's mental competence, cognitive function, and physical abilities based on age. These have to be assessed individually since the person can learn at any age.[12] Negative attitudes of the health-care professionals toward the elderly can affect their behavior and management of diabetes. Stereotypes about the elderly may lead to withholding treatment choices and educational opportunities.

A multidisciplinary approach is essential in caring for the elderly and cognitively impaired. DSME for these individuals should be done on a one-to-one basis using slow paced stepwise method of teaching and involving memory aids. Some simple strategies to use with elderly and cognitively impaired for DSME are as follows:[48,49]

- Suggest glucose meter with large display and simple to use
- Simplify medication, especially insulin regimen; if possible, avoid sliding scale
- Emphasize symptoms of hypoglycemia and give specific instructions for its treatment
- Involve care giver during educational sessions
- Give clear simple written instructions for patients to take home

Adolescents

Knowledge of the adolescents' attention span and developmental and cognitive maturity levels are important considerations in teaching adolescent groups.[50] Developmental delays or learning disabilities may hamper understanding of diabetes self-management; therefore necessary accommodations should be made to facilitate learning. Moreover, diabetes management may not be a priority of a teenager and this can result in poor control. To complicate matters, changing hormones can mean more problems with glycemic control.[50]

At this stage of development, adolescents search for self-identity and independence. They are becoming more aware of their body image and how their peer group perceives them.[50] They want to be independent and this can conflict with their parents who feel overprotective and responsible for their child's diabetes care. A diagnosis of diabetes may cause or worsen feelings of low self-esteem, eating disorders, distorted body image, and depression. Adolescents are at an age where formal operational thinking and abstract reasoning are beginning to develop.[50] Therefore, they can comprehend the importance of diabetes self-management but environmental factors can and will impede their efforts to do so.

The adolescent is focused on short-term rather than long-term goals.[9] Explaining the relevance of their choices for glucose control rather than on long-term complications of diabetes might be more effective in motivating them toward self-management. Use of innovative and interactive modalities of learning can be very useful in teaching adolescents. For example, use of computers, videos, games, camp experiences, and peer support groups that focus on decision making are more effective than a structured group class. The teen must be encouraged freedom of choice and self-direction.[51] Involving the family or caregiver throughout the educational and psychosocial processes is imperative. Several discussion boards and support groups for teens and parents of children with diabetes exist and might be very helpful in coping and supporting adaptive strategies.

Persons with Disabilities

The American with Disabilities Act requires that diabetes educators provide reasonable accommodations to people with disabilities in response to their particular individual needs.[52] The educator must acknowledge the needs assessment and plan appropriately to accommodate the patient's learning needs. Diabetes educators must provide patients with a comprehensive, individualized education program that takes into consideration the patient's disability and its impact on the learning process.[53] The educational content should be consistent and equal to the information provided to those without any disabilities or functional limitations. The only variance will be the teaching methods, tools, and/or mode of delivery. In addition, the educational materials should incorporate disability-specific factors in all phases of diabetes education.[52] For example, patients with limited or no sight may need to have instructions in Braille or special talking books. There are a variety of adaptive devices for the visually impaired available in the market such as talking glucometers, insulin pen devices, and others. There are also agencies for the blind and visually impaired where patients can be referred to for assistance.

Deaf and hard of hearing individuals experience communication barriers that impact on their processing of health-related educational information or the ability to carry out necessary tasks.[52] Providers should be somewhat knowledgeable about deaf culture and barriers to communication and refer patients to an educator who is readily accessible and qualified to meet the needs of deaf and hard of hearing patients. This includes obtaining an interpreter fluent in American Sign Language to provide translation at the time of patient encounter. Other forms of visual communication should also be used such as reading materials and pamphlets, if the patients are literate to the English language. In a Harvard medical school study, participants who were deaf or hearing impaired suggested that clinicians ask patients about their preferred communication approach (e.g., lip-reading, sign language, writing notes).[54]

In an attempt to assess understanding of education provided, the educator should have the patient use their form of communication to either repeat the key information and/or perform return demonstration.[55] At the end of the chapter is a list of websites for persons with disabilities.

Behavioral Aspect of SMBG Monitoring

At present, self-monitoring of blood glucose (SMBG) is recommended for all patients with diabetes, especially those who use insulin.[56] It is recognized as being useful in sensitizing the patient to the advantages of diet control and physical exercise, determining and adjusting the dosage of medication at the beginning of treatment or during a dosage change, and monitoring glucose control during acute illness.[57]

Most important, glycemic target goals should be set by both patient and provider. This goal has to be clearly spelled out and assessed periodically. Patients may be empowered by teaching them how to interpret the results of SMBG. The immediate feedback of the effect of diet and exercise on blood glucose can help motivate patients to continue to improve their behavior.[58,59]

Major obstacles to regular use of SMBG are financial constraints, physical discomfort, lack of motivation, depression, and inability to interpret and respond to results. Oftentimes, patients do not see the importance of monitoring, so the educator should review the results with them and provide positive reinforcement at every encounter.[59] Giving the patient clear instructions, providing them with the necessary skills to perform the task, and exploring with them how to incorporate this to fit their daily life may help to improve adherence to SMBG.

Learning Styles

The individual's preference for teaching–learning experiences in diabetes self-management is a major consideration in planning the diabetes education sessions.[8] Sessions may be conducted in a group, individual settings, or may even be self-directed. Learning styles vary from one person to another.[14] A combination of different modalities is frequently used to enhance the learning process. Learning styles may be didactic (lecture) or participatory (group discussion), or a combination of both. To present materials the educator may use a variety of media or techniques such as audio/visual materials, high tech interactive or noninteractive computer programs, Internet, games and simulations, case studies, or vignettes, as appropriate.

The Internet is the fastest growing information medium with potentially great impact on health education.[60] The demographics of a typical Internet user are believed to closely resemble an average American.[61] As more people take greater initiative in their health care, many use the Internet to explore options and learn about new developments and research about diseases. Although research[60] suggests that there is a slightly greater interest in use of Internet in younger population it was also found that many other patients with diabetes without population it was also found that many older patients without previous Internet experience are willing to take part in Internet-based self-management programs if barriers to participation are minimized.

There are a number of advantages of the Internet[60] as a medium of support in diabetes self-management education. It is accessible and can potentially reach a great majority of patients with diabetes. It is low cost compared to individual or small group classes. It provides flexibility since it can be done at home at any time as many times as desired. Many Internet sites provide information (some interactive), linkages with other related sites, and forum for people to interact with one another and share experiences. It is not a remote occurrence for a physician to have patients coming in to their office with printed materials about diabetes collected over the Internet. The role of the physicians and diabetes educators in such a situation is to provide the person seeking knowledge through the Worldwide Net the ability to sift through massive amount of information. A list of Internet sites providing diabetes health information is found at the end of this chapter.

Methods to Decrease Literacy Demands

People who have low-literacy skills are able to learn diabetes self-management skills. Teaching strategies need to be adjusted to enhance learning. The atmosphere has to be nonthreatening for the patient. There are certain things to remember when dealing with patients with low literacy.

- Do not overload patient with information. Provide only the essential information the patient needs to do self-management.
- Make instructions brief and simple. Use simple layman words. Avoid medical terms.
- Introduce one concept at a time. Use common analogies to explain concepts. Provide examples to enhance explanation.
- Avoid distractions and interruptions as much as possible during the learning session.
- Introduce one change at a time. Make sure that patient understands and is comfortable with the change before introducing another.
- Use a variety of media to present information. Enhance instructions with use of pictures, charts, models, audiovisual aids, etc.
- Remember to evaluate patient's understanding frequently. Encourage patient to ask questions or seek clarification as needed.
- Reinforce learning through use of drills, practice exercises, and experiential learning. Use patient's real-life problems to facilitate application of concepts learned.

Evaluation

Paraphrasing is one of the earliest methods to evaluate patient understanding.[62] The patient is asked to explain his/her understanding of the information. This method allows both the patient and the physician to have an interaction about the material taught. The patient is able to clarify the information as needed. The physician is able to assess any gaps in information or areas of misconceptions and provides immediate feedback.

Skills demonstration such as insulin injections, blood glucose testing, meal planning, etc., provides knowledge to the physician about patient's use of the proper techniques. More importantly, the physician is made aware of the patient's psychomotor impairments that may interfere with the proper performance of the skill. For example, a patient with rheumatoid arthritis may have difficulty in handling the syringe or the glucometer; a patient with poor eyesight may not be able to accurately draw up the proper dose of insulin. This would provide the opportunity for the physician to recommend some adaptations to ensure safety and accuracy or refer the patient to the educator for further counseling. There are a variety of adaptive devices available to help patient cope with their disabilities.

The physician should ask for frequent *feedback* from the patient to assess understanding of information. The patient is encouraged to ask questions to enhance his/her knowledge. The physician also asks questions to verify patient comprehension. Questions answerable by yes or no should be avoided. The examples include questions such as "Do you understand?" or "Do you know how to do this now?" Most patients would answer these questions affirmatively because they may be embarrassed to admit lack of understanding or they do not want "to bother the busy physician." Examples of questions that yield more information about patient comprehension are "Explain to me why…" or "show me how…." Patients who do not know the answer to these questions would feel free to tell the physician to repeat the instruction or procedure if they do not understand.

In this age of electronic communication, feedback may be done through other means such as e-mails, text mails, chat lines, etc. These formats facilitate communication among patients and between patients and their care team at any time and place. Patients can e-mail their provider or team for questions, comments, or feedback about their diabetes management. They can network with other patients to learn through their experiences. It is reassuring for many to feel that their team or partners in care are just an e-mail or phone call away.

Because learning diabetes self-management encompasses more than knowledge acquisition *evaluating behavior change* leading to a health lifestyle is the ultimate measure of success. There are several methods to measure behavior change. A direct measure is actually observing change in behavior such as self-monitoring of blood glucose, engaging in physical activities regularly, and consuming healthy diet. In some instances, the physician or educator may have to rely on self-report, which decreases the reliability and validity of measurement. Indirectly, the effects of behavior change can be measured in terms of metabolic outcomes such as improvement in HbA_{1c}, blood glucose, blood pressure, lipid levels, weight loss, etc.

Patient Resources on the Internet

Additional internet resources can be found at the end of Chapter 51

American Diabetes Association
http://www.diabetes.org
It offers information for medical providers and patients including news, nutrition, and exercise guidelines.

Center for Current Research
http://www.lifestages.com/health/diabetes.html
It offers summaries of recent medical research derived from articles from medical journals. Users may request information on unlisted topics for a fee.

Children with Diabetes
http://www.childrenwithdiabetes.com
It provides support and information for children and families affected by diabetes. It includes up-to-date headlines related to clinical, nutritional, and research reviews about juvenile diabetes. It provides links to news and patient advocacy sites.

Diabetes Action Research and Educational Foundation
http://www.daref.org
It offers information about education and program services including a Native American program, an international program, public service, a diabetes camp for children, and a diabetes university program and information about research projects and upcoming events. It includes a recipe and tip of the week and links to related sites.

Diabetes Digest

http://www.diabetesdigest.com

It provides general information for patients with diabetes such as an overview of the disease, types of diabetes, symptoms, treatment, care, and prevalence. It includes information on oral medications, insulin, glucometers, and nutrition. It also includes an online newsletter and links to popular articles from diabetes digest.

Diabetes News

http://www.diabetesnews.com

Home page of the diabetes news which offers information on new diabetes products and islet cell transplantation as well as reports on current research in related areas. It provides access to current and past issues of Diabetes Forecast, a health and wellness magazine of the ADA.

Diabetes Research and Wellness Foundation

http://www.diabeteswellness.net

It provides information on research grants and wellness programs sponsored by the foundation and information on how to develop self-management skills for people with diabetes. It includes articles on weight loss, aspirin, and exercise.

Diabetes Research Institute

http://www.drinet.org/html/the_diabetes_research_institute.htm

It provides patient articles on a variety of topics such as islet cell transplantation, encapsulation, genetic engineering, xenotransplantation, immunogenetics, molecular biology, research lipids, and cardiovascular research. It also provides information about current clinical trials.

Hypoglycemia Support Foundation, Inc.

http://www.hypoglycemia.org

It offers information and support to patients about hypoglycemia, causes, diagnosis, and treatment. It provides information on how to contact the association to receive a packet of materials with reference lists and useful information. It also provides links to related sites.

Joslin Diabetes Center

http://www.joslin.harvard.edu

It offers news, information, education, and programs for patients with diabetes. It also provides links to articles on diabetes, monitoring, insulin, oral medications, nutrition, exercise, and complications.

National Eye Institute: Diabetic Eye Disease

http://www.nei.nih.gov

It offers patients and consumers program materials on diabetic eye disease through brochures, fact sheets, public service announcements, and press releases.

NIDDK: National Diabetes Clearinghouse: Diabetes Diagnosis

http://diabetes.niddk.nih.gov/dm/pubs/diagnosis/index.htm

It provides an overview of diagnostic criteria for type 1 and type 2 diabetes mainly for consumers and patients. It also provides a link to the Combined Health Information Database (CHID) for additional resources.

NIDDK: Diabetic Neuropathy

http://diabetes.niddk.nih.gov/dm/pubs/neuropathies/index.htm

It offers consumer information on diabetic neuropathy including an overview of the condition, incidence, causes, symptoms, types, diagnosis, treatment, foot care, and experimental treatments. It also includes a list of organizations providing support and a suggested list of reading materials.

Exercise

American Diabetes Association (ADA): Exercise: Just the FAQs

http://www.diabetes.org/exercise

It provides general information on the importance of exercise for people with diabetes. It includes a diabetes quiz, fact sheets, and related Diabetes Forecast articles.

Diabetes Exercise and Sports Association (DESA)*formerly known as* **International Diabetic Athletes Association (IDAA)**

http://www.diabetes-exercise.org It

It provides support to patients with diabetes who participate in fitness activities. It offers membership details and information about regional chapters and support groups as well as product catalog and a calendar of upcoming events. It also provides a link to related sites.

Self-Monitoring

Diabetes Monitor: Devices for Glucose Monitoring

http://diabetesmonitor.com/other-3a.htm

It presents a wide variety of monitoring system and product Web sites. It provides connections to sites offering new noninvasive and minimally invasive glucometers as well as software for patients with diabetes to monitor blood readings and maintain overall control.

Annual Guide to Diabetes Products and Services

http://www.diabetes.org/diabetes-forecast/resource-guide.jsp

It provides a comprehensive guide to diabetes products and services. It includes a review of the current technology and system limitations of various glucose meters. It provides a list of diabetes medications and booklet of information on medicine for people with diabetes. It includes a review of a variety of insulin delivery devices such as insulin syringes, insulin pens, automatic injectors, jet injectors, and pumps.

Medications

Insulin Pumpers

http://www.insulinpumpers.org

It provides support and educational materials on insulin pump therapy to patients with diabetes of all age groups. It provides answers to frequently asked questions about insulin pumps, instructions on how to use pumps, printable log sheets, a directory of physicians who prescribe pumps, and chart forums. It provides links to the home pages of several insulin pump manufacturers, information on carbohydrate content of various foods, and other information on diabetes and insulin pumps.

Medicines for People with Diabetes

http://diabetes.niddk.nih.gov/dm/pubs/medicines_ez/index.htm

It provides a list of diabetes medications and booklet of information on medicine for people with diabetes. It provides information on types of diabetes, treatments, low blood sugar, and help with recognizing whether or not prescribed medicines are working.

Nutrition

American Diabetes Association (ADA): Dietary Recommendations for Persons with Diabetes

http://www.diabetes.org/nutrition-and-recipes/nutrition/healthyfoodchoices.jsp

It reviews the dietary recommendations from the ADA. It includes information on specific nutrients, sugar substitute, sodium, and alcohol.

American Dietetic Association

http://www.eatright.org

It provides patients with diabetes daily nutritional tips, a catalog of publications, a reading list, featured articles, nutrition fact sheets, and information on the food guide pyramid. It also includes a list of dietitian, information of government affairs, and links to related sites.

American Heart Association (AHA): Hyperlipidemia

http://www.americanheart.org

It offers a patient guide to hyperlipidemia and a discussion about the various types of this disorder. It includes a list of related AHA publications and access to online guides regarding specific syndromes, treatments, and diets.

American Obesity Association (AOA)

http://www.obesity.org

It offers information about the mission of the organization, facts, statistics about obesity, health insurance and treatment of adult obesity, and contact details. It includes a discussion of health problems associated with obesity.

NIDDK: I Have Diabetes: What I Need to Know About Eating and Diabetes

http://diabetes.niddk.nih.gov/dm/pubs/eating_ez/index.htm

It offers nutritional guidelines and details on maintaining good eating habits. It contains a patient education pamphlet for newly diagnosed patients. It presents an overview of use of diet in controlling diabetes. It includes a section on food groups and food pyramids.

Support Groups

NIDDK: Financial Help for Diabetes Care

http://diabetes.niddk.nih.gov/dm/pubs/financialhelp/

It provides information on financial help for diabetes care such as Medicaid programs, the Department of Veterans Affairs, the Hill-Burton Program, the Bureau of Primary health care, Health care Financing Administration Office of Beneficiary Relations, and local public health departments

Suggested Resources for People with Disabilities

National Center for Learning Disabilities

http://www.ncld.org

NCLD provides essential information to parents, professionals, and individuals with learning disabilities, promotes research and programs to foster effective learning, and advocates for policies to protect and strengthen educational rights and opportunities.

CHADD (Children and Adults with Attention Deficit Disorders)

http://www.chadd.org

It provides education, advocacy, and support for individuals with AD/HD; provide a support network for parents and caregivers; to provide a forum for continuing education; to be a community resource and disseminate accurate, evidence-based information about AD/HD to parents, educators, adults, professionals, and the media; to promote ongoing research; and to be an advocate on behalf of the AD/HD community. CHADD also publishes a variety of printed materials to keep members and professionals current on research advances, medications, and treatments affecting individuals with AD/HD.

Hearing Exchange

http://www.hearingexchange.com

It provides chats and message boards for people with hearing loss, parents, and professionals. It has books, magazines, and other products related to hearing loss.

National Alliance for the Mentally Ill

http://www.nami.org

NAMI is dedicated to the eradication of mental illnesses and to the improvement of the quality of life of all whose lives are affected by these diseases. NAMI has organizations in every state and in over 1100 local communities across the country who join together to meet the NAMI mission through advocacy, research, support, and education.

National Institute of Mental Health

http://www.nimh.nih.gov

The National Institute of Mental Health (NIMH) is the largest scientific organization in the world dedicated to research focused on the understanding, treatment, and prevention of mental disorders and the promotion of mental health.

American Foundation for the Blind

http://www.afb.org

AFB is a national nonprofit group that expands possibilities for people with vision loss. AFBs priorities include broadening access to technology; elevating the quality of information and tools for the professionals who serve people with vision loss; and promoting independent and healthy living for people with vision loss by providing them and their families with relevant and timely resources.

Lighthouse International

http://www.lighthouse.org

A nonprofit organization dedicated to preserving vision and to providing critically needed vision and rehabilitation services to help people of all ages overcome the challenges of vision loss. Through clinical services, education, research, and advocacy, the Lighthouse enables people with low vision and blindness to enjoy safe, independent, and productive lives.

NIDDK: Kidney Disease of Diabetes

http://kidney.niddk.nih.gov/kudiseases/pubs/kdd/index.htm

It provides consumer information on diabetic nephropathy including an overview of the condition, incidence in type I and type II, causes, symptoms, course of disease, diagnosis, medications, treatment, and dialysis and transplantation. It also includes a list of organizations providing support and a suggested list of reading materials.

National Kidney Foundation

http://www.kidney.org

Voluntary organization that seeks to prevent kidney and urinary tract diseases, improve the health and well-being of individuals and families affected by these diseases, and increase the availability of all organs for transplantation. Goals include supporting research and research training, continuing education of health-care professionals, expanding patient services and community resources, educating the public, shaping health policy, and fund raising.

References

1. Anderson RM, Funnell MM. Theory is the cart, vision is the horse: reflections on research in diabetes patient education. *Diabetes Educ*. 1999;25:43–51.
2. Anderson RM, Funnell MM. *The Art of Empowerment: Stories and Strategies for Diabetes Educators*. Alexandria, VA: American Diabetes Association; 2000:27.
3. Wagner EH. Chronic disease management: what will it take to improve care for chronic illness? *Effect Clin Pract*. 1998;1:2–4.
4. Wagner EH, Austin B, Von Korff M. Improving outcomes in chronic illness. *Manag Care Q*. 1996;4:12–25.
5. Diabetes Prevention Program Research Group. Reduction in the evidence of type 2 diabetes with life-style intervention or metformin. *N Engl J Med*. 2002;346:393–403.
6. Redman BK. *The Process of Patient Education*. 7th ed. St. Louis: Mosby; 1993.
7. Mensing C, Boucher J, Cypress M, et al. National standards for diabetes self-management education. *Diabetes Care Suppl*. 2007;30:S96–S103.
8. Walker EA. Characteristics of the adult learner. *Diabetes Educ*. 1999;25:16–24.
9. Knowles M. *The Adult Learner: A Neglected Species*. 4th ed. Houston, TX: Gulf Publishing Co.; 1990.
10. Knowles M. *Self-Directed Learning*. Chicago: Follett; 1975.
11. Tough A. How adults learn and change. *Diabetes Educ*. 1985;11:21–25.
12. Brookfield SD. *The Skillful Teacher: On Techniques Trust, and Responsiveness in the Classroom*. San Francisco, CA: Jossey-Bass; 1990.
13. Darkenwald GG, Merriam SB. *Adult Education Foundation of Practice*. New York: Harper Collins Publishing, Inc; 1982.
14. Brookfield SD. *Understanding and Facilitating Adult Learning: A Comprehensive Analysis of Principles and Effective Practices*. San Francisco, CA: Jossey-Bass; 1986.
15. Mezirow J. *Transformative Learning: A Guide for Educators of Adults*. San Francisco, CA: Jossey-Bass; 1991.

16. Peyrot M. Behavior change in diabetes education. *Diabetes Educ.* 1999;25:62–73.
17. Martin C, Daly A, McWhorter LS, et al. The scope of practice, standards of practice, and standards of professional performance for diabetes educators. *Diabetes Educ.* 2005;31:487–512.
18. Walker EA, Wylie-Rosett J, Shamoon H. Health education for diabetes self-management. In: Porte D, Sherwin R, Rifkin H eds. *Ellenberg and Rifkin's Diabetes Mellitus.* 5th ed. Stanford, CT: Appleton & Lange; 1997:1341–1351.
19. Medicare Benefit Policy manual, accessed 11/07 from CMS' Web page at: http://www.cms.hhs.gov/manuals/102_policy/bp102 index.asp
20. MNT Services for Beneficiaries with Diabetes or Renal Disease-Correction, CMS Transmittal A-03-009, accessed 11/07 from CMS' Web page at: http://www.cms.hhs.gov/manuals/pm_trans/A03009.pdf
21. Prospect Associates. Final Report; Survey of physician practice behaviors related to the treatment of people with diabetes mellitus (endocrinologists). Doc#NO1DK82233, NIDDK, NIH. 1991.
22. Anderson RM, Funnell MM. The role of the physician in patient education. *Practical Diabetol.* 1990;9:10–12.
23. Brown SA. Interventions to promote diabetes self-management: state of the science. *Diabetes Educ.* 1999; 26(6 suppl):52–61.
24. Walker EA. Health behavior: from paradox to paradigm. *Diabetes Spectrum.* 2001; 14(1):6–8.
25. Berkman ND, DeWalt DA, Pignone MP, et al. *Literacy and Health Outcomes.* Rockville, MD: Agency for Healthcare Research and Quality: AHQR publication 04-E007-2 Evidence report/technology assessment No 87 2004.
26. Kirsch I, Jungeblut A, Jenkins L, Kolstad A. *Adult Literacy in America: A First Look at the Findings of the National Adult Literacy Survey.* Washington, DC: National Center for Education Statistics, US Department of Education; 1993.
27. Kutner M, Greenber E, Baer J. *A First Look at the Literacy of America's Adults in the 21st Century.* Washington, DC: National Center for Education Statistics, Department of Education; December 2005
28. Baker DW, Gazmararian JA, Willimas MW, et al. Functional health literacy and the risk of hospital admission among Medicare managed care enrollees. *Am J Public Health.* 2002;92:1278–1283.
29. Howard DH, Gazmararian J, Parker RM. The impact of low health literacy on the medical costs of Medicare managed care enrollees. *Am J of med.* 2005;118:371–377.
30. Hartsell Z. Health care illiteracy: Implications for providers. JAAPA, 2005. (Access 11/27/07 @ http://www.jaapa.com/issues/ j20050501/articles/illiteracy0505.htm)
31. Overland JE, Hoskins PL, McGill MJ, Yue DK. Low literacy: a problem in diabetes education. *Diabetic Med.* 1993;10:847–850.
32. Williams MV, Parker RM, Baker DW, et al. Inadequate functional health literacy among patients at 2 public hospitals. *JAMA.* 1995;274:1677–1682.
33. Marcus EN. The silent epidemic – the health effects of illiteracy. *New Engl J of Med.* 2006;355:339–341.
34. Mendoza MA. A study to compare inner city black men and women completers and non-attenders of diabetes self-care classes. Doctoral Dissertation. Teachers College, Columbia University, 1999.
35. Stanley K. Low-literacy materials for diabetes nutrition education. *Practical Diabetol.* 1999:36–44.
36. Walker EA, Mendoza MA. The strength of many voices: a review of the Johns Hopkins guide to diabetes. *Diabetes Spectrum.* 1998;11:192–193.
37. Cowie CC, Byrd-Holt DD, Flegal KM, et al. Prevalence of diabetes and impaired fasting glucose in adults in the US population. *Diabetes Care.* 2006;29:1263–1268.
38. The New York City Department of Health and mental Hygiene press release: More than 100,000 New Yorkers face complications due to seriously out-of-control diabetes. Accesses 11/07 at http://www.nyc.gov/html/doh/pr2007/pr002-07.shtml.
39. United States Department of Health and Human Services. Secretary's Task Force on Black and Minority Health, Vol I–VIII. Washington, DC, US Government Printing Office, 1985–1986.
40. Leininger M. Leininger's acculturation health care assessment tool for cultural patterns in traditional and nontraditional pathways. *J Transcultural Nurs.* 1991; 2(2):40–42.
41. Tripp-Reimer T. *Cultural Assessment in Nursing Assessment: A Mutidimentsional Approach.* Bellack J, Bamford P, eds. Monterey, CA: Wadsworth health Services; 1984:226–246.
42. Tripp-Reimer T, Choi E, Kelley S, Enslein JC. Cultural barriers to care: Inventing the problem. *Diabetes Spectrum.* 2001;14(1):13–22. Winter.
43. Suhl E, Bonsignore P. Diabetes self-management education for older adults: general principles and practical application. *Diabetes Spectrum.* 2006;19:234–240.
44. Gregg EW, Yaffe K, Cauley JA, et al. Is diabetes associated with cognitive impairment and cognitive decline among older women? *Arch Intern Med.* 2000;160:174–180.
45. Kanaya AM, Barrett-Connor E, Gildengorin G, Yaffe K. Change in cognitive function by glucose tolerance status in older adults: a 4-year study of the Rancho Bernardo Study Cohort. *Arch Intern Med.* 2004;28:1327–1333.
46. Arvanitakis Z, Smith WR, Aggarwal NT, Bennett DA. Diabetes and function in different cognitive systems in older individuals without dementia. *Diabetes Care.* 2006;29:560–565.
47. Munshi M, Grande L, Hayes M, et al. Cognitive dysfunction is associated with poor diabetes control in older adults. *Diabetes Care.* 2006;29;1794–1799.
48. American Association of Diabetes Educators. Special considerations for the education and management of older adults with diabetes. *Diabetes Educ.* 2000;26:37–39.
49. Glasgow RE, Toodert DJ, Hampson SE, et al. Improving self-care among older patients with type II diabetes: the "sixty-something. . ." study. *Patient Educ Counseling.* 1992;19:16–24.

50. Roemer JB, McGee T. Type I diabetes in youth. In: Franz MJ ed. *A Core Curriculum for Diabetes Education*. 5th ed. Diabetes in the life cycle and research. Chicago: American Association of Diabetes Educators:2003.

51. Channon SJ, Huws-Thomas MV, Rollnick S, et al. A multicenter, randomized, controlled trial of motivational interviewing in teenagers with diabetes. *Diabetes Care*. 2007;30:1390–1395.

52. Margello-Anast H, Estarziau M, Kaufman G. Cardiovascular disease knowledge among culturally deaf patient in Chicago. *Preventative Med*. 2006;42:235–239.

53. American Association of Diabetes Educators. Position statement on diabetes education for people with diabetes. *Diabetes Educ*. 2006;32:835–847.

54. Zagaria M. Low health literacy, a safety concern among the elderly. *US Pharm*. 2006;10:28–34.

55. American Association of Diabetes Educators. Position statement on self-monitoring of blood glucose: benefits and utilization. *Diabetes Educ*. 2006;32:835–847.

56. Goldstein DE, Little RR, Lorenz RA, et al. Tests of glycemia in diabetes. *Diabetes Care*. 2004;27:1761–1773.

57. Le Devehat C. Self-monitoring of blood glucose and type 2 diabetes mellitus. *Diabetes Metab*. 2006; 32(2):17–20.

58. Mancuso M, Ingegnosi C, Caruso-Nicoletti M. Self monitoring blood glucose and quality of care. *ACTA Biomed*. 2005; 76(3):56–58.

59. American Association of Diabetes Educators. Position statement on effective utilization of blood glucose monitoring. *Diabetes Educ*. 32;2006:835–847.

60. Feil EG, Glasgow RE, Boles S, McKay G. Who participates in internet-based self-management programs? A study among novice computer users in primary care setting. *Diabetes Educ*. 2000; 26(5):806–811.

61. IntelliQuest, Worldwide Internet/online Tracking Service (WWITS). 1998. Available at http://www.intelliquest.com/

62. Doak CC, Doak LG, Root J. *Teaching Patients with Low Literacy Skills*. 2nd ed. Philadelphia, PA: JB Lippincott Co; 1996.

Chapter 41
Dietary Therapy of Diabetes Mellitus

Gladys Witt Strain, Rosalia Doyle, and Faith Ebel

When a new diagnosis of diabetes is established, among the first stressful thoughts experienced by patients are concerns that they will not be able to eat foods they prefer and that their way of living will be compromised. If certain dietary changes do not occur, the individual may not be able to control his/her blood glucose and may find himself/herself at risk for the host of complications associated with poorly controlled diabetes. However, it is seldom acknowledged that a person with diabetes should be eating the diet which is basically similar to that of nondiabetic individuals, according to the recommendations of the *Dietary Guidelines for Americans*, 2005.[1] These guidelines do not impose a foreboding protocol but advise how everyone should be eating to consume the nutrients the human body requires and avoid the weight-related illnesses. "Healthy eating" and working toward an optimal lifestyle, including physical activity, are of primary importance. No longer should a "diabetic diet" or an American Diabetes Association diet (ADA diet) be prescribed by a physician. Rather, it is recommended that a diet prescription be based on careful assessment of food preferences, eating habits, and other lifestyle factors. This may require certain expertise that is often beyond the nutrition training of the medical practitioner and can also consume costly medical practice time. In consultation with the patient, a registered dietitian can develop recommendations that are attainable and consistent with reasonable treatment goals.

A review of the most recent food pyramid provides healthy eating choices and also incorporates the importance of physical activity for the development of an optimal lifestyle.[1] However, a more specific Diabetes Food Guide Pyramid has been developed which moves the starchy vegetables and the high-protein beans/legumes from their respective vegetable and meat groups to the starch group. For purposes of dietary planning, The Diabetes Pyramid (Fig. 41.1) makes it possible to visualize the number of servings of the various food groups recommended and the size of those servings. The serving sizes have been adjusted so that the servings are relatively similar, between 80 and 100 cal for approximately 15 g of carbohydrate. (The low-calorie vegetables are an exception.) This allows for more flexibility in meal planning. The American Diabetes Association encourages those with diabetes to follow an individualized meal plan and lifestyle regimen as a vital part of their diabetes management to control blood glucose levels and body weight.[2]

In addition to near-normal blood glucose levels, patients with diabetes should achieve normal blood pressure levels and lipid profiles. Normalized metabolic homeostasis is directed toward the prevention and/or the delay of complications associated with diabetes. This is done by balancing carbohydrate intake and caloric expenditure with medications that modify glucose metabolism. Medical nutrition therapy (MNT) has demonstrated improvement in HbA1c levels by ~1–2%.[3–5] However, the most recent analysis Cochrane Collaboration reviewing 36 articles involving 18 trials following 1467 participants emphasized that the data on the efficacy of dietary treatment of type 2 diabetes were not of high quality and that well-designed studies were urgently needed.[6]

Developing a deficit in energy intake is a primary focus of treatment plans for patients with type 2 diabetes. Adequate calories should be provided to achieve and/or maintain a reasonable weight. This may not be the acceptable weight as defined by a body mass index (weight/height^2) of 18–25.[7] Rather, a reasonable weight

R. Doyle (✉)
Division of Endocrinology, Department of Medicine, Friedman Diabetes Institute, Beth Israel Medical Center, New York, NY, USA
e-mail: rdoyle@chpnet.org

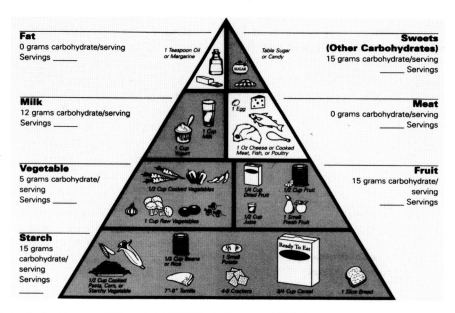

Fig. 41.1 Diabetes food guide pyramid (Copyright© Eli Lilly & Company, All Rights Reserved. Used with permission)

may be that weight which is achievable and can be maintained over the long term to provide glycemic control with the incorporation of a modified food and exercise program.[8,9] The Diabetes Prevention Program (DPP) examined 3234 adults at high risk for developing type 2 diabetes. The lifestyle intervention group reduced their risk of developing type 2 diabetes by 58% as compared to the control (placebo). This risk reduction was seen in individuals with a 7% weight reduction and physical activity of 150 min/week.[3] This is exactly the current recommendation of the American Diabetes Association for appropriate intervention to improve blood glucose utilization in individuals with type 2 diabetes.[2]

For the patient with type 1 diabetes who is dependent on exogenous insulin, the meal plan should respect the food preferences of the patient as much as possible. Carbohydrate content of meals and snacks is coordinated with insulin administration and the exercise program. If blood sugars become unexpectedly high or low, reviewing the actual grams of carbohydrate consumed at the previous meal may offer an explanation for the blood sugar aberration. When carbohydrate intake and/or the intensity and duration of exercise are modified, the patient is taught to modify the type and/or dosage of insulin. Some patients prefer extra carbohydrate snacks to balance an increase in exercise; however, modification of their medication dosage is preferred. As for all persons with diabetes, a reasonable body weight with normalized blood sugars, blood pressure, and lipid levels is the treatment goals.

Another group of patients who frequently are managed with the insulin and carefully monitored blood sugar control are the patients who develop gestational diabetes as discussed in Chapter 15. The careful regulation of carbohydrate intake and its distribution throughout the day in multiple meals and snacks are the hallmarks of this treatment which seldom presents compliance problems for these well-motivated patients.[10,11] A minimum of 175 g/day of carbohydrate is encouraged.[2] One recent study reports that infants had lower birth weights when their mothers were consuming less than 40% carbohydrate in their diets.[11,12] Daily caloric needs are generally adjusted in the second half of pregnancy for women of normal weight to 30–32 kcal/kg. For overweight women a moderate caloric restriction to 25 kcal/kg is advised.

For most persons with type 2 diabetes the importance of caloric deficit in implementing weight change should be emphasized, since at least 80% of such patients are overweight.[13] Increased body weight (BMI > 25) in combination with elevated visceral body fat stores, estimated by waist circumference ≥35 in. in women and ≥40 in. in men, can increase risk for cardiovascular disease.[14] However, it is important to notice that some Asian populations have an increased risk of type 2 diabetes and cardiovascular disease at a body mass index (BMI)

>23 in combination with increased visceral stores, estimated by waist circumference of ≥31 in. in women and ≥35 in. in men.[2]

Weight change is best accomplished with a combination of both diet and exercise. If the control of caloric intake is not stressed in the treatment plan, little weight change generally results.[15] Exercise for the person with diabetes will be discussed in Chapter 33 of this volume. Extreme strategies of starvation and very low calorie diets seldom achieve long-term weight change.[16] A moderate caloric deficit of 500 cal will produce an average 1 lb a week decrease in weight, and blood sugars generally normalize if the patient achieves a consistent caloric deficit. It is acknowledged that food records are inaccurate and generally underreport food intake and overreport energy expenditure.[17,18] To estimate energy needs resting, energy requirements (basal needs) can be calculated using a nomogram developed by and available in the Mayo Clinic Diet Manual, 1994,[19] or various equations including the generally accepted Harris and Benedict equations.[20]

$$\text{For men: BEE} = 66.4 + 13.7(W) + 5(H) - 6.8(A)$$

$$\text{For women: BEE} = 65.5 + 9.6(W) + 1.8(H) - 4.7(A)$$

BEE is basal energy, A is age in years, W is weight in kilograms, and H in height in centimeters.

Atthe current time the American Dietetics Association has reported the increased accuracy of the Mifflin St Joer equation.[21,22] The Dietetics Association is encouraging its use in estimating energy needs for patients; however, our own work in morbid obesity and that of Das et al. support the usefulness of the Harris Benedict equation.[23,24] Since clinical equipment may already be programmed with the Harris Benedict equation to determine resting energy expenditure, the continued use of such equipment does not seem inappropriate or unwise.

With height, weight, age, and sex, basal needs can be approximated and modified by a factor for activity and the thermic effect of food (energy needed to process food intake, 7%). Usually total daily energy expenditure is approximately 40% above basal for light activity. After an assessment of the level of daily activity, a range of 30–50% above basal is commonly used. From these estimations a potential energy intake can be calculated to achieve the desired rate of weight loss. This should be shared with the patient, so that they can better understand the amount of change necessary to produce the agreed upon energy deficit and diet modifications required to produce a modest weight loss and blood glucose normalization.

Even with all their known inaccuracies, food records do remain an integral part of the treatment protocol. They provide important qualitative information on the individuals' *perception* of what they are consuming and their food preferences. In developing a food plan, such records are essential. However, if perfect 1200 calorie food intake records are provided by the weight stable 100 kg patient as representative, then basic problems with perception exist and must be explored. It should be understood that such patients are not necessarily withholding or actually distorting what they consume. The interpretation of what constitutes a portion can vary greatly. Perhaps between meal eating was not remembered or recorded. Other patients may discount calories from alcohol, juices, or other calorie-containing beverages. For such patients foods of high volume and low-energy value (low caloric density) can be particularly helpful.[25] The use of lower fat foods which are less energy dense is achieving more popular support, but the labels of such foods must be reviewed for one cannot assume that all such foods are reduced in calories. Increased sugar may be added to help maintain the texture of lower fat products. This increase in carbohydrate certainly may not be helpful to the diabetic patient trying to control his blood glucose. For these reasons many of the foods labeled as reduced in fat or sugars must be carefully evaluated and may not be appropriate.

Currently the controversy concerning the macronutrient composition of the diet has been in the foreground. Four common weight loss diets were compared for efficacy.[26] Low carbohydrate intake and metabolic changes have been carefully reviewed.[27] The current recommendation of the American Diabetes Association does not encourage diets with <130 g of carbohydrate.[2] For most persons with type 2 diabetes a modest weight loss of 5–10% substantially improves glycemic control, but many patients are unwilling to accept such goals.[9] The 200 lb woman is not satisfied weighing 180 lb and may persist in food restriction efforts until relapse and regain occur. Setting reasonable, maintainable goals in collaboration with the patient is an obligation of the health care provider. For some, blood glucose levels may normalize with moderate, consistent caloric deficit even before much weight loss occurs.[28]

However, for many overweight and obese persons weight loss has remained an elusive goal. Most overweight individuals will not be able to achieve and maintain the standard that has been set for a normalized body weight. Although a 10% weight change can substantially improve blood glucose control, for those unable to sustain energy restriction, polypharmacy including medications that help produce a caloric deficit may be tried. Currently the choices are limited to the two medications, sibutramine and orlistat, approved for long-term usage. Sibutramineis a centrally acting norepinephrine, dopamine, and serotonin reuptake inhibitor, and Orlistat acts in the gut to decrease fat absorption by inhibiting pancreatic lipase. These medications are generally used only as part of a comprehensive program including behavior modification, diet instruction, and increased physical activity.[29]

For those with diabetes and refractory obesity with a BMI over 35, surgery for weight loss is now a viable option.[30,31] Long-term follow-up has impressively demonstrated the normalization of blood glucose achieved with an acceptable risk–benefit ratio.[32,33]

It is of importance to note that type 2 diabetes may also occur and be diagnosed with a normal body mass index of 25 or below.[34] When this occurs factors of body fat distribution, genetics, medications, physical activity, and diet composition (high carbohydrate and low fiber) may play an important role and should be evaluated.

Thus weight status, its modification, and maintenance have an important role in type 2 diabetes management. It should be noted that treatment protocols to effectively sustain a reasonable body weight are acknowledged as time consuming, costly, and not frequently followed over the long term. However, the costs of the complications of poorly controlled diabetes far outweigh the cost of the MNT intervention.[5,35,36] It is also of note that only a limited number of sufficiently trained persons are available to help with the implementation of needed weight change. Another obstacle that contributes to the problem is the frequent lack of third-party reimbursement for nutrition services. The necessary changes in perception and behavior will most often not occur with only the handout of a diet sheet in the doctor's office.

The nutrition recommendations for all persons with diabetes have recently been reviewed by the American Diabetes Association and are discussed below.[2]

Macronutrients

Carbohydrate

Carbohydrate intake is the dietary focus of blood sugar control. Based on the individual's glucose needs, weight status, lipid profile, and eating habits, carbohydrate intake should be individualized. For years free sugars were banned in the diets of those with diabetes, probably because it was assumed that their quick absorption might contribute to elevated blood sugars. Starches were encouraged as substitutes. Scientific evidence is limited to support this common practice. Fruits and milk have been shown to have lower glycemic responses than most starches.[37] Sucrose produces a response similar to common starches like rice, potato, and bread.[38] Although various starches per gram of carbohydrate do have different effects on blood sugar, for purposes of dietary planning it is the total amount of carbohydrate consumed rather than the source that merits primary consideration. However, it should be mentioned that the effects of pizza and Chinese food on elevating blood sugars seem to far surpass the effects of their measured carbohydrate concentration.[39] The variation in responses to different carbohydrates stresses the importance of the patient performing self glucose monitoring to determine the quantities of specific foods that can be tolerated and allow to maintain glycemic control. In dietary planning, the frequency and choice of using sucrose-containing foods and/or concentrated sweets must be carefully weighed in the light of their low nutrient density and carbohydrate concentration. Making gram for gram carbohydrate substitutions will work, but frequently such substitutions become additions and then have a negative effect. Fruit is among the most maligned of the carbohydrates, and sometimes patients are forbidden fruit even by diabetologists. With fruits, portion sizes and total grams of carbohydrate merit strict attention. For many fruits the defined portion sizes for 15 g of carbohydrate are much smaller than generally consumed by most people.

Another dietary sugar, fructose, produces a smaller blood glucose increase than sucrose and has been proposed as a "natural" sweetener. The moderate consumption of fructose-containing foods has presented no problem, but when fructose is consumed in large amounts, up to 20% of the calories, it is known to adversely effect blood lipids.[40] The sweeteners that have calories from carbohydrate like fruit juice concentrate, molasses, honey, and corn syrup have direct effects on blood sugar similar to sucrose and offer no advantage to persons with diabetes. Foods are also frequently flavored with the sugar alcohols: sorbitol, mannitol, and xylitol. The sugar alcohols have about one-half the calories of table sugar and a reduced glycemic response. Individuals do have different sensitivities to the sugar alcohols, and they are known to have a laxative effect in many persons. Nonnutritive sweeteners are encouraged for people with diabetes to add increased variety to their food choices. Nonnutritive sweeteners (acesulfame potassium, saccharin, aspartame, sucralose, and neotame) are approved for use in the United States according to the Food and Drug Administration (FDA). One cannot help but question if indeed they have any effect on weight status. However, no adverse effects of nonnutritive sweeteners have been demonstrated in humans after many years of usage over a wide range of dosages.

Postprandial blood glucose responses are mainly affected by the quantity of carbohydrate consumed. However, the type of carbohydrate ingested also is a factor. Significant details to review when looking at post-prandial blood glucose levels are the type of food, type of starch, preparation methods used, ripeness, and amount of processing.

Low glycemic diets have been a focus of much recent research, but at the current time there is not sufficient, consistent information to conclude that such diets lower the risk for diabetes or are effective in weight reduction to improve glycemic control.[2] Such diets are generally rich in fiber and other important nutrients so that they can be encouraged as a component of the "healthy eating plan." The recent meeting of the Dietary Carbohydrate Task Force of the International Life Sciences Institute concluded that many studies purporting to investigate lower glycemic index (GI) interventions actually studied lower glycemic loads (GL) that unavailable carbohydrate (e.g., dietary fiber), independent of GI, seems to have at least as big an effect on health outcome as GI itself. Lower GI and GL diets are beneficial for health in persons with impaired glucose metabolism, but it is as yet unclear what they mean for healthy persons. The larger the divergence of glucose metabolism from the norm, the larger the effect of lower GI and GL interventions.[41]

Fiber

For years fiber has received much attention for its disease prevention effects in the general population. Recently the literature is replete with articles demonstrating improved blood glucose management in both type 1 and type 2 diabetes with high-fiber diets.[42–44] Fiber-rich foods such as beans or cereals with 5 or more grams of fiber per serving and fruits and vegetables are emphasized due to their nutrient content.[45] Both soluble and insoluble fibers are encouraged in amounts similar to the recommendations for the general population (20–35 g or 14 g/1000 cal). However, it is the soluble vegetable fibers that are touted for their capacity to slow the absorption of food, inhibit glucose absorption, and bind cholesterol.

Protein

At the current time no data are available to indicate that the protein needs of persons with diabetes are different from the dietary reference intake (DRI) for the general population, 0.8 g/kg of body weight. According to the Kidney Disease Outcomes Quality Initiative, 2007, for an individual with diabetes and chronic kidney disease (stages 1–4), 0.8 g/kg of body weight protein is recommended.[46] It is acknowledged that most individuals consume above this recommended allowance. The American Diabetes Association suggests 10–20% of the total caloric intake from protein sources. Since nephropathy is one of the complications of diabetes as discussed in Chapter 22, special attention may be given to the protein concentration of the diet. Data are available to indicate that with protein restriction the rate of fall in glomerular filtration rate (GFR) can be retarded.[47] However, other studies have contradictory results, possibly due to factors of patient selection and/or compliance with the protocol.[48] As kidney disease progresses further restriction to 0.6 g/kg is sometimes advised in an attempt to slow the decline in GFR. Recent research has focused on the type of protein and its effect on the kidney. Diets using soy protein have been shown to reduce hyperfiltration of the kidneys in diabetic individuals.[49] On this basis the substitution of vegetable proteins for animal protein has been suggested as a measure to help prevent the development and/or treatment of kidney disease. However, MNT for diabetic kidney disease may be required to focus on other macro and micronutrients as well as protein.[46]

Fats

For individuals with diabetes, less than 7% of the total calories consumed should come from saturated fat. Recommendations on total fat must be left to a matter of individualization depending on weight, lipid status, and treatment goals. People who are at a healthy weight and have normal lipid levels are recommended by the American Diabetes Association to follow the National Cholesterol Education Program (NCEP) and slowly, over an extended time frame of 2 years, reduce their fat intake to <25–35%: saturated fat <7%, polyunsaturated <10%, and monounsaturated <20%. Less than 200 mg of dietary cholesterol daily and negligible *trans*-fatty acid intake is recommended. Omega 3 fatty acids from fish and other seafood are encouraged two times per week. However, it must be emphasized that most individuals with type 2 diabetes are not at a healthy weight. If weight loss is to be implemented, then total fat reduction may be advised. Fats can easily be identified by patients and decreased to lower energy intake. Even in reduced fat diets the use of fatty fish is encouraged for the benefits of their omega 3 content. Monounsaturated fats like olive oil and canola oil have been shown not to increase the LDL cholesterol and may improve glycemic control and triglyceride and HDL cholesterol levels. However, in type 2 diabetes efforts directed toward weight loss to decrease insulin resistance may be thwarted by these energy-dense oils. Plant sterols and stanol esters, also known as phytosterols, may lower blood cholesterol (total and LDL cholesterol) levels by decreasing its absorption in the intestine. These effects may be seen in amounts of ~2 g/day.[50]

For many the texture and flavor of fat are important to eating satisfaction, but as a means of implementing weight loss and improving dyslipidemia, a decrease in total fat is suggested and specifically saturated fats are discouraged. This has resulted in the development of many calories reduced, low fat and/or fat-free products. Are such foods helpful in the achievement of weight loss and the improvement of blood glucose control? The use of foods reduced in fat or produced with a nonabsorbable fat substitute may or may not alter the composition and total calories of the diet. Alternative foods may be consumed in such quantities that can compensate for the changes in fat intake so that total energy is not reduced. To make possible the reduction of fat in certain foods, carbohydrate may be added, but this could affect glycemic control. Fat-free baked products are a common example of foods that may not be reduced in total calories since carbohydrate if often added. Therefore, the "sugar-free" products may not be reduced in either fat or calories. Modified foods can be helpful to increase the variety of food choices, but patients with diabetes must be taught to use them wisely as an aid to calorie, fat, and carbohydrate control in order to foster compliance with their meal plans.

Alcohol

Alcohol is metabolized differently than the other macronutrients, and for people with diabetes a few words of caution are important. The general recommendations from the Dietary Guidelines for Americans[1] advise two drinks per day for men and no more than one drink for women. It is of note that alcohol is not metabolized to glucose and can inhibit gluconeogenesis. If alcohol is not consumed with food and the patient is taking medication to lower blood glucose, hypoglycemia can result. Alcohol, if taken, should be taken with food. To make a caloric adjustment for alcohol intake, each beverage (12 oz beer, 5 oz wine, or $1\frac{1}{2}$ oz distilled spirits) is best equated to two fat exchanges from the diabetic meal plan. Caution should be used when combining alcohol with other beverages that contain carbohydrates (juice, soda, etc.) for it may raise blood glucose levels. In addition, excessive use of alcohol, consisting of three or more alcoholic beverages daily, may lead to elevations in blood glucose. Alcohol is not advised for pregnant women, those with a history of alcohol abuse, and the elderly who may have problems with balance and coordination. For people with diabetes and other medical problems like pancreatitis, elevated triglycerides, or neuropathy, the consumption of alcohol is discouraged. The use of alcohol is also contraindicated with certain medications, particularly metformin which is frequently prescribed for type 2 diabetes, since alcohol can increase the effects of metformin on lactate metabolism which increases the risk of lactic acidosis. The effect of alcohol consumption on diabetes has recently been reviewed. [51]

Micronutrients: Vitamins and Minerals

As the general population, persons with diabetes have no need for vitamin and mineral supplementation when the dietary intake is adequate. However, the assessment of an adequate dietary intake requires training and consumes professional time. Many physicians prescribe a pill containing the reference dietary intake (RDI) of the established vitamins as an "insurance policy." For the elderly with reduced energy intake, a multivitamin supplement is commonly given. With the increased risk for heart disease and its adverse outcome in persons with diabetes, antioxidants may be prescribed, but there is little evidence that this practice is beneficial.[52,53] Routine supplementation with C, E, and carotene is not advised because of the lack of evidence of efficacy and safety concerns when used on a long-term basis.

Of the minerals, calcium supplementation is frequently advised, particularly after menopause for women, since dietary calcium may not be sufficient, but as for all the other vitamins and minerals the recommendations are similar to those for the general population.

Chromium has been encouraged because of its positive metabolic role particularly in type 2 diabetes. However, its use remains a topic for research and the American Diabetes Association does not support its use as beneficial to glycemic control.[2] Most people with diabetes have not been found to be chromium deficient unless they have been receiving chromium-deficient parenteral nutrition. Magnesium is acknowledged for its role in insulin sensitivity and its deficiency can contribute to carbohydrate intolerance; however, only when low serum magnesium levels can be established is repletion with magnesium appropriate. The use of diuretics may result in potassium loss that requires supplementation. Hyperkalemia may occur in patients taking angiotensin converting enzyme (ACE) inhibitors, with renal insufficiency or hyporeninemic hypoaldosteronism.

Sodium is the mineral that receives much attention by both the medical profession and the general public. Dietary recommendations regarding sodium use precipitate frequent medical debate.[54] Recommendations for people with diabetes are no different than for the general population. While the average sodium intake in this country exceeds 3000 mg/day suggested by some health authorities, with hypertension alone 2300 mg/day or with hypertension, symptoms of heart failure, and nephropathy <2000 mg/day is recommended.

There is not sufficient information available to justify the recommendation of herbs and supplements for diabetes care. As with the general population, caution should be advised on the use of supplements due to their lack of standardized ingredients and possible drug interactions.[2]

Implementation

The above guidelines are simple and straightforward, but their implementation remains complex. Adhering to these guidelines is a challenge not only in diabetes management but for the population in general. From the government's continuing survey of food intake it is reported that approximately one-third of the population eat at least some food from all the food groups daily, but only 1–3% of the population eat the recommended number of servings from all the food groups on any given day. If as a people we are all doing so poorly, can we expect those with diabetes to do that much better? Strategies to improve compliance with dietary protocols are under continuous development. However, as with the problem of producing a sustained weight change, patients revert to previous patterns over time and require long-term monitoring. Third-party payers remain reluctant to cover the needed extended duration of nutrition services.

To approach the development of a workable dietary strategy, first data must be gathered on the food intake pattern that produces the current level of control with a defined exercise program (or lack of it) and the medications prescribed for the management of blood glucose. Blood glucose monitoring is advised with the recording of food intake to identify problems even for those who are managing their diabetes with "diet" only. Many patients fail to identify many sources of carbohydrate other than the free sugars and starches as affecting blood sugars. To distribute carbohydrate throughout the day attention must also be paid to the milk products, fruits, and starchy vegetables that are consumed. If improved blood glucose control is the treatment focus, then the possible interchange of food groups with carbohydrate to increase variety and help enhance dietary compliance needs thorough review with the patient. This must be coordinated with the individual's blood glucose responsiveness to certain foods as ascertained from the food records and blood glucose data. This will help individually determine the portion sizes of certain foods to maintain more normalized blood glucose control. However, such expansion of personal knowledge alone may not result in long-term dietary behavior change. Food choices are the result of a complex interplay of environment, social, familial, and behavioral factors. To modify food choices, the mediating variables that have been important in the development of food preferences require identification. With an understanding of the usual eating habits and the factors that influence them, efforts to promote more "healthy eating" have a greater potential for being sustained. Designing dietary protocols to improve diabetes management and blood sugar control is, indeed, complicated. The nutritionist has little published literature to approach the problem. What should be eaten can be defined clearly and succinctly, as above, but motivating the patient sufficiently to activate such an eating plan is the challenge. Techniques incorporating motivational interviewing and cognitive behavioral principles in treatment protocols have shown promise but remain in the testing phase as to their efficacy in promoting the needed long-term dietary changes.[55,56] Very little work has been done in regard to changing preferences and effective prevention in the ethnic minorities who are rapidly increasing not only in numbers but in their body size which in turn impacts upon their incidence of type 2 diabetes.

Summary

Exogenous insulin was the magic tool developed for the treatment of type 1 diabetes, but even with this tool, the dietary component of treatment for diabetes remains at the forefront of both effective intervention and the prevention of disease progression for all patients. Diabetes remains a dreaded disease for its feared restrictions on the total life of an individual and the modifications of lifestyle required for glycemic control and to prevent disease progression. It must be stressed that the foods recommended for a person with diabetes are those advised for all Americans to be in good health and to avoid the weight-related illnesses. Food selections have been clearly defined in the consensus statement of the American Diabetes Association. The challenge remains to assist patients to comply with these recommendations by modifying their food choices and behaviors regarding food consumption and exercise.

Web Sites for Additional Information

National Diabetes Education Program
   hhtp://ndep.nih.gov
National Institute of Diabetes and Digestive Diseases
   www.niddk.nih.gov
Food and Nutrition Information
   www.fns.usda.gov/fns

American Diabetes Association
www.diabetes.org
American Dietetic Association
www.eatright.org
Center for Nutrition Policy and Promotion
www.usda.gov/cnpp

References

1. U.S. Department of Health and Human Services and U.S. Department of Agriculture. *Dietary Guidelines for Americans.* 6th ed. Washington, DC: U.S. Government Printing Office; January 2005: 1–19.
2. American Diabetes Assn. Nutrition recommendations and principles for people with diabetes mellitus. *Diabetes Care.* 2008;31(Suppl 1):S61–S77.
3. Knowler WC, Barrett-Connor E, Fowler SE, et al. Diabetes Prevention Program Research Group. Reduction in the incidence of type 2 diabetes with lifestyle intervention or Metformin. *N Engl J Med.* 2002;346:393–403.
4. Pastors JG, Franz MJ, Warshaw H, Daly A, Arnold MS. How effective is medical nutrition therapy in diabetes care?. *J Am Dietetic Assn.* 2003;103(7):827–831.
5. Look AHEAD Research Group. Pi-Sunyer X, Blackburn G, Brancati FL, et al. Reduction in weight and cardiovascular disease risk factors in individuals with type 2 diabetes: one-year results of the look AHEAD trial. *Diabetes Care.* 2007;30:1374–1383.
6. Nield L, Moore HJ, Hooper I, et al. Dietary advice for treatment of type 2 diabetes mellitus in adults. *Cochrane Data Base Syst Rev.* 2007;CD004097:1–75, (on line).
7. National Institutes of Health, Heart, Lung, and Blood Institute. Clinical Guidelines on the Identification, Evaluation, and Treatment of Overweight and Obesity in Adults—The Evidence Report. NIH Publication no. 98-4083 Sept 1998 p xvii.
8. Willett WC, Dietz WH, Colditz GA. Primary care: guidelines for a healthy weight. *N Engl J M.* 1999;341:427–434.
9. Foster GD, Wadden TA, Vogt RA, Brewer G. What is a reasonable weight loss? Patients' expectations and evaluation of obesity treatment outcome. *J Consult Clin Psychol.* 1998;65:79–85.
10. Reader DM. Medical nutrition therapy and lifestyle interventions. *Diabetes Care.* 2007;30:S188–S193.
11. Crowther CA, Hiller JE, Moss JR, McPhee AJ, Jeffries WS, Robinson JS. for the Australian Carbohydrate Intolerance Study in Pregnant Women (ACHOIS) Trial Group. Effect of treatment of gestational diabetes mellitus on pregnancy outcomes. *N Engl J Med.* 2005;352:2477–2486.
12. Major CA, Henry MJ, Veciana M, Morgan MA. The effects of carbohydrate restriction in patients with diet controlled gestational diabetes. *Obstet Gynecol.* 1998;91:600–604.
13. Kuczmarski RJ, Flegal KM, Campbell SM, Johnson CL. Increasing prevalence of overweight among US adults: National Health and Nutrition Examination Surveys 1960–1991. *JAMA.* 1994;272:205–211.
14. Katzel LI, Bleeker ER, Coleman EG, Rogus EM, Sorkin JD, Goldberg AP. Effects of weight loss vs aerobic exercise training on risk factors for coronary disease in healthy, obese, middle-aged and older men. A randomized controlled trial. *JAMA.* 1995;274:1915–1921.
15. Gordon NF, Scott CB, Levine BD. Comparison of single versus multiple lifestyle interventions: are the antihypertensive effects of exercise training and diet-induced weight loss additive?. *Am J Cardiol.* 1997;79:763–767.
16. National Task Force on the Prevention and Treatment of Obesity, NIH. Very low calorie diets. *JAMA.* 1993;270:967–974.
17. Lavienja AJ, Braam LA, Ocke MC, Bueon-de-Mesquita HB, Seidell JC. Determinants of obesity-related underreporting of energy intake. *Am J Epidemiol.* 1998;147:1081–1086.
18. Lichtman SW, Pisarska K, Berman ER, et al. Discrepancy between self-reported and actual caloric intake and exercise on obese subjects. *New Engl J Med.* 1992;327:1893–1896.
19. Nelson JK, Moxness KE, Jensen MD, Gastineau CF. *Mayo Clinic Diet Manual.* 7th ed. St. Louis, MO: Mosby-Year Book Inc.; 1994: 656.
20. Schofield WN, Schofield C, James WPT. Basal metabolic rate. *Human Nutr: Clin Nutr.* 1985;39c(Suppl 1):1–96.
21. Mifflin MD, St Jeor ST, Hill LA, Scott BJ, Daugherty SA, Koh YO. A new predictive equation for resting energy expenditure in healthy individuals. *Am J Clin Nutr.* 1990;51:241–247.
22. Frankenfield D, Roth-Yousey L, Compher C. Evidence Analysis Working Group. Comparison of predictive equations for resting metabolic rate in healthy nonobese and obese adults: a systematic review. *Am Dietet Assn.* 2005;105:775–789.
23. Das SK, Saltzman E, McCrory MA, et al. Energy expenditure is very high in extremely obese women. *J Nutr.* 2004;134: 1412–1416.
24. Strain GW, Wang J, Gagner M, Pomp A, Inabnet WB, Heymsfield SB. Bioimpedance for severe obesity: comparing research methods for total body water & resting energy expenditure. *Obesity.* 2008;16:1953–1956.
25. Bell EA, Rolls BJ. Energy density of foods affects energy intake across multiple levels of fat content in lean and obese women. *Am J Clin Nutr.* 2001;73:1010–1018.
26. Gardner CD, Klazand A, Alhassan S, et al. Comparison of Atkins, Zone, Ornish, and LEARN diets for change in weight and related risk factors among overweight premenopausal women. *JAMA.* 2007;297:969–977.

27. Westman EC, Feinman RD, Mavropoulas JC, et al. Low carbohydrate nutrition and metabolism. *Am J Clin Nutr*. 2007;86: 276–284.

28. National Institutes of Health, Heart, Lung, and Blood Institute. Clinical guidelines on the identification, evaluation, and treatment of overweight and obesity in adults—the evidence based report. *Obes Res*. 1998;6(suppl 2):110S.

29. National Institutes of Health, Heart, Lung, and Blood Institute. Clinical guidelines on the identification, evaluation, and treatment of overweight and obesity in adults—the evidence based report. *Obes Res*. 1998;6(suppl 2):100S.

30. Colquitt J, Clegg A, Lovemen E, Royle P, Sidhu MK. Surgery for morbid obesity. *Cochrane Data Base Syst Rev*. 2005; 4:CD003641 [online accessed 1-8-08].

31. Buchwald H, Avidor Y, Brunwald E, et al. Bariatric surgery: a systematic review and meta-analysis. *JAMA*. 2004;292: 1724–1737.

32. Sjostrom L, Narbo K, Sjostrom D, et al. Effects of bariatric surgery on mortality in Swedish obese subjects. *N Engl J Med*. 2007;357:741–752.

33. Adams TD, Gress RE, Smith SC, et al. Long-term mortality after gastric bypass surgery. *N Engl J Med*. 2007;357:753–761.

34. WHO Expert Consultation. Appropriate body-mass index for Asian populations and its implications for policy and intervention strategies. *Lancet*. 2004;363:157–163.

35. Flechtner-Mors M, Ditschuneit HH, Johnson TD, Suchard MA. Adler Metabolic and weight loss effects of long-term dietary intervention in obese patients: four year results. *Obes Res*. 2000;8:399–402.

36. UK Prospective Diabetes Study Group. Intensive blood glucose control with sulphonylureas or insulin compared with conventional treatment and risk complications in patients with type 2 diabetes (UKPDS 33). *Lancet*. 1998;352:837–853.

37. Hollenbeck CB, Coulston A, Donner C, et al. The effects of variation in percent of naturally occurring complex and simple carbohydrates on plasma glucose and insulin response in individuals with non-insulin-dependent diabetes mellitus. *Diabetes*. 1985;34:151–155.

38. Jenkins DAJ, Wolever TMS, Jenkins AL, et al. The glycemic response to carbohydrate foods. *Lancet*. 1984;2:388–391.

39. Nuttall FQ, Mooradian AD, DeMarais R, Parker S. The glycemic effect of different meals approximately isocaloric and similar in protein, carbohydrate, and fat content as calculated using the ADA exchange lists. *Diabetes Care*. 1983;6:432–435.

40. Franz MJ, Horton ES, Bantle JP, et al. Nutrition principles for the management of diabetes and related complications (technical review). *Diabetes Care*. 1994;17:490–518.

41. Howlett J, Ashwell M. Glycemic response and health: summary of a workshop. *Am J Clin Nutr*. 2008;87:212s–216s.

42. Chandalia M, Garg A, Lutjohann D, et al. Beneficial effects of high fiber intake in patients with type 2 diabetes mellitus. *N Engl J Med*. 2000;342:1392–1398.

43. Wylie-Rosett J, Segal-Isaacson CJ, Segal-Isaacson A. Carbohydrates and increases on obesity: does the type of carbohydrate make a difference?. *Obes Res*. 2004;12:124S–129S.

44. Brand-Miller J, Hayne S, Petocz P, Colagiuri S. Low-glycemic index diets in the management of diabetes: a meta-analysis of randomized controlled trials. *Diabetes Care*. 2003;26:2261–2267.

45. Liese AD, Schulz M, Fang F, et al. Dietary glycemic index and glycemic load, carbohydrate and fiber intake, and measures of insulin sensitivity, secretion, and adiposity in the Insulin Resistance Atherosclerosis Study. *Diabetes Care*. 2005;28:2832–2838.

46. Clinical Practice Guidelines and Clinical Practice Recommendations for Diabetes and Chronic Kidney Disease. *Am J Kidney Dis*. 2007;49(suppl 2):S95–S105.

47. Robertson L, Waugh N, Robertson A. Protein restriction for diabetic renal disease. *Cochrane Data Base Syst Rev*. 2007; (4):CD002181.

48. Dussol B, Iovanna C, Raccah D, et al. A randomized trial of low-protein diet in type 1 and in type 2 diabetes mellitus patients with incipient and overt nephropathy. *J Ren Nutr*. 2005;15:398–406.

49. Fanti P, Asmis R, Stephenson TJ, Sawaya BP, Franke AA. Positive effect of dietary soy in ESRD patients with systemic inflammation–correlation between blood levels of the soy isoflavones and the acute-phase reactants. *Nephrol Dial Transplant*. 2006;Aug;21(8):2239–2246.

50. Lichtenstein AH, Deckelbaum RJ. Stanol/sterol ester-containing foods and blood cholesterol levels. American Heart Assn. *Circulation*. 2001;103:1177–1179.

51. Howard AA, Arnsten JH, Gourevitch MN. Effect of alcohol consumption on diabetes mellitus: a systemic review. *Ann Internal Med*. 2004;140:211–219.

52. Yusuf S, Dagenais G, Pogue J, et al. Vitamin E supplementation and cardiovascular events in high risk patients. Heart outcomes prevention evaluation study investigators. *N Engl J Med*. 2000;342:154–160.

53. GISSI-Prevention Investigators. Dietary supplementation with n-3 polyunsaturated fatty acids and vitamin E after myocardial infarction: results of the GSSI-prevention trial. *Lancet*. 1999;354:447–455.

54. Loria CM, Obarzanek E, Ernst N. Choose and prepare foods with less salt: dietary advice for all Americans. *J Nutr*. 2001;131:536S–551S.

55. Di Lillo V, Siegfried NJ, West DS. Incorporating motivational interviewing into behavior obesity treatment. *Cogn Behav Pract*. 2003;10:120–130.

56. Wadden TA, Butryn ML, Wilson C. Lifestyle modification for the management of obesity. *Gastroenterology*. 2007;132: 2226–2238.

Chapter 42
Exercise in the Therapy of Diabetes Mellitus

Sefton Vergano, Rajiv Bhambri, and Stephen H. Schneider

Introduction

Exercise has been advocated for patients with diabetes for centuries, but it was only in 1990 that the American Diabetes Association (ADA) felt there was enough evidence of benefit to recommend exercise as a routine part of the treatment of type 2 diabetes mellitus. Since that time, the use of exercise in the treatment of type 2 diabetes has become well accepted, although its place in the treatment of type 1 diabetes remains less clear. In recent years, the role of exercise in the prevention of type 2 diabetes and in the treatment of the metabolic syndrome has proven to be of particular interest. Indeed, current research seems to confirm a role for both aerobic exercise as well as resistance training in both the treatment and the prevention of the disease. Nevertheless, our understanding of the complex interactions of exercise with diabetes is still incomplete, and the most effective ways to use exercise in the treatment of the disease are still under investigation.

During exercise major cardiorespiratory and circulatory responses help to efficiently supply the increased oxygen and energy needs of the working muscles. Whole body oxygen consumption and glucose turnover may increase more than tenfold and even greater increases may occur in the skeletal muscles.[1] In healthy individuals, a complex hierarchy of hormonal responses regulates the alterations in fuel metabolism necessary to maintain normal plasma glucose levels during prolonged activity.[2] This metabolic response to exercise may be severely disordered in patients with diabetes mellitus. In order to understand the effects of diabetes on fuel metabolism during exercise, it is important to first review the normal physiology.

Metabolic Changes During Exercise in Normal Individuals

As exercise intensity increases there is a linear relationship between heart rate, oxygen consumption, and workload. Eventually, however, oxygen consumption plateaus in the face of increasing exercise intensity. The point at which oxygen uptake plateaus is known as the maximal aerobic exercise capacity, or VO_2max. Exercise above this point can only be sustained for a short time because it represents non-aerobic metabolism and is limited by lactic acid accumulation. The VO_2max is important for a number of reasons. It is a useful tool to express the degree of aerobic fitness of an individual. In general, a higher VO_2max predicts better performance in endurance-type activity. It also allows comparison of individuals of widely varying fitness levels. For example, at the same percentage of any individuals VO_2max, a roughly similar metabolic response will occur. In addition, the VO_2max has been useful in communicating recommendations for exercise in various groups of individuals. Because the VO_2max is rarely directly measured in individual patients, indirect techniques for estimating workloads as a percent of the VO_2max have been developed and are discussed later in the chapter.

S.H. Schneider (✉)
Division of Endocrinology, Metabolism and Nutrition, UMDNJ-Robert Wood Johnson Medical School, New Brunswick, NJ, USA
e-mail: schneide@umdnj.edu

L. Poretsky (ed.), *Principles of Diabetes Mellitus*, DOI 10.1007/978-0-387-09841-8_42,
© Springer Science+Business Media, LLC 2010

Moderate Intensity Exercise (50–75% VO₂max)

In the initial stages of exercise muscle glycogen is the chief source of energy.[3] As continued exercise depletes muscle glycogen, the working muscles must take up glucose and nonesterified fatty acids (NEFA) from the circulation.[4] Recent evidence suggests that utilization of local triglyceride stores, both intra-myocellular and extra-myocellular, in skeletal muscle may also be an important source of free fatty acid for oxidation during physical activity. In the postprandial state glucose is derived from an increased hepatic production that closely matches peripheral glucose utilization and can maintain euglycemia during moderate intensity exercise for long periods of time. However, during prolonged exercise glucose utilization may exceed splanchnic glucose output and hypoglycemia may develop.

The role of neurohormonal adaptation during exercise is twofold:

(a) to supply the exercising muscles with their increased fuel and oxygen requirements and
(b) to maintain whole body glucose homeostasis to supply the brain with adequate substrate.

It is not clear what triggers the endocrine response to exercise; it may result from the stimulation of afferent nerves from the working muscles or from subtle deviations in the blood glucose and/or from feed forward mechanisms originating within the hypothalamus.[5] At the start of exercise, a fall in the circulating insulin levels occurs due to an increased alpha adrenergic input to the beta cells.[6] This physiologic decrease in insulin levels promotes peripheral lipolysis and removes the inhibiting effects of insulin on hepatic glycogenolysis and gluconeogenesis. As exercise continues, an increase in the level of the counterregulatory hormone glucagon facilitates liver glycogenolysis and later gluconeogenesis, further enhancing hepatic glucose output.[4] Figure 42.1 illustrates the hormonal response to exercise.

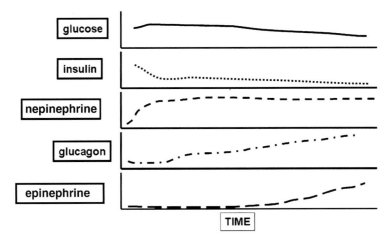

Fig. 42.1 The hormonal response to exercise

With more prolonged exercise insulin secretion continues to fall and there is a further release of counterregulatory hormones. A rise in circulating epinephrine levels and falling insulin levels lead to an increase in blood NEFA levels[7] due to both increased lipolysis and decreased NEFA re-esterification in the liver. The liver utilizes the glycerol released during triglyceride breakdown as a substrate for gluconeogenesis and the NEFA are delivered to the working muscles as an energy source. The increased availability of NEFA for muscle metabolism helps restrain the rate of muscle glucose utilization and therefore helps to limit the fall in glucose during prolonged exercise. In fact, the major role of catecholamines during prolonged exercise is to stimulate lipolysis. Their main impact on hepatic gluconeogenesis is probably via the mobilization of gluconeogenic precursors from peripheral sites and the provision of free fatty acids as an energy source for gluconeogenesis.[8] Catecholamines also stimulate glycogenolysis in inactive muscles during the later stages of prolonged exercise.[9] In this situation the glycogen is metabolized to lactate in non-exercising muscle. Lactate can then be delivered to exercising muscle where it can be oxidized as fuel, as well as to the liver for gluconeogenesis. This complex and redundant series of hormonal responses regulate blood glucose during exercise with remarkable efficiency and the redundancy of the system insures that glucose homeostasis is robust.

High Intensity Exercise (>75% VO$_2$max)

During very high intensity exercise the relationship between peripheral glucose utilization and hepatic glucose production may be reversed. Because virtually all of the fuel for high intensity activity is provided by local energy stores of muscle glycogen, hepatic glucose production often significantly exceeds peripheral glucose utilization leading to hyperglycemia that persists into the postexercise state. The added glucose production most likely originates from hepatic glycogenolysis[5] and epinephrine may be involved in its regulation.[10] There may also be a brief period of relative insulin resistance following very intense exercise causing elevated blood glucose. When postexercise hyperglycemia occurs in normal individuals, it is transient and self-correcting.

Muscle Glucose Uptake During Exercise

The increased muscle glucose uptake during exercise is related to the intensity of the exercise once a steady state has been achieved.[5] In general, the greater the exercise intensity, the greater the relative utilization of carbohydrate as an energy source. For example, at exercise of roughly 50% of an individual's VO$_2$max, half of the energy requirement is supplied by carbohydrate while 80% of energy requirements may be supplied by carbohydrate at exercise approaching 80% of the VO$_2$max. Since plasma insulin levels fall during exercise, the increased muscle glucose uptake must be mediated by insulin-independent mechanisms or via an increased insulin action on muscle. Exercise probably acts in both ways[5] but the insulin-independent mechanism predominates. During exercise there is an insulin-independent increase in the concentration of the main glucose transporter protein GLUT 4 on the muscle membrane.[11] This is thought to be due to the translocation of the GLUT 4 from the cytoplasm to the sarcolemma.[12] This increase in the number of GLUT 4 on the surface of the cell leads to an increase in the glucose uptake from the circulation into the muscle cell. In addition to changes within the muscle itself, enhanced muscle perfusion during exercise improves glucose uptake through increased delivery of insulin and glucose to working muscle.

Postexercise State

In the postexercise period the hormones return to basal levels and glycogen and triglyceride stores are repleted. If exercise is of sufficient intensity and duration to deplete muscle glycogen and adequate carbohydrate is made available, the amount of glycogen will rebound to well above pre-exercise levels, a phenomenon called supercompensation. Of great therapeutic importance is the observation that muscle insulin sensitivity is enhanced for prolonged periods of time following a single bout of moderately intense activity. Insulin sensitivity is typically enhanced for 12–24 h, but after sufficient exercise, alterations lasting up to 72 h have been noted. This results in a sustained improvement of insulin sensitivity in individuals who exercise every other day or more. The mechanisms by which exercise results in these sustained benefits are unclear. A relationship to muscle glycogen levels is suggested by the observation that exercise of intensity and duration sufficient for glycogen depletion is generally required for this effect to occur. In addition, athletes who take in large amounts of glucose following exercise and achieve glycogen levels above basal have been reported to have impaired insulin sensitivity. On the other hand, the increase in insulin sensitivity that follows exercise clearly persists at a time when glycogen stores have returned to normal. Another mechanism for improved carbohydrate utilization following exercise may relate to

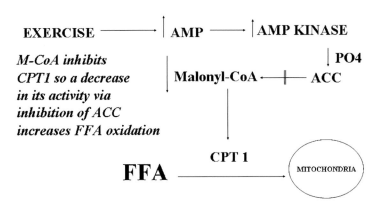

Fig. 42.2 The role of AMP kinase in enhancing free fatty acid utilization during exercise. During exercise, ATP is broken down to AMP which activates the enzyme AMP kinase. AMP kinase causes a downstream decrease in the inhibition of CPT1 allowing increased free fatty acid oxidation in the mitochondria. AMP = adenosine monophosphate, PO4 = phosphate group, ACC = acetyl-CoA carboxylase, M-CoA = malonyl-CoA, CPT1 = carnitine palmitoyltransferase, FFA = free fatty acids

the activation of the enzyme AMPK (AMP-activated protein kinase) (see Fig. 42.2). During exercise, ATP is broken down to AMP to release energy. As AMP builds up, it increases the activity of the enzyme AMPK. This enzyme is activated during exercise of the intensity required to lead to improved postexercise glucose uptake. In addition to shifting fuel utilization acutely toward the oxidation of FFA it may also stimulate subsequent glucose utilization by mechanisms independent of insulin action, possibly involving the nitrous oxide system.

Recently, attention has turned to the role of intra-myocellular triglyceride metabolism as a regulator of insulin sensitivity. In general, states of increased triglyceride accumulation in skeletal muscle and liver are associated with insulin resistance. Breakdown products of the metabolism of free fatty acids (FFA), the building blocks of triglycerides, can activate serine kinases and suppress the activity of the insulin receptor and insulin receptor substrates. Reduction of fat stores in skeletal muscle during exercise could be a mechanism enhancing subsequent insulin sensitivity. Nevertheless, when highly trained endurance athletes are studied, levels of triglyceride in skeletal muscle are actually increased in between exercise bouts. Despite this increase in myocellular fat stores, such athletes are characterized by a high degree of insulin sensitivity. This has been called the "athlete's paradox." New information suggesting that the breakdown products of FFA metabolism and not the storage triglyceride themselves may induce insulin insensitivity helps to clarify this apparent problem. In the postexercise period rapid restoration of triglyceride stores may actually result in a decrease in these metabolically active intermediates, thus improving insulin sensitivity.[13]

Adaptations to Physical Training

Exercise performed on a regular basis with an intensity, duration, and frequency sufficient to improve cardiorespiratory fitness, strength, and flexibility is called physical training. Alterations in cardiac and respiratory efficiency and in the neurologic coordination of motor activity are an important factor in improved performance. In addition, there are important cellular adaptations of skeletal muscles with physical training (see Table 42.1). This response differs during aerobic training (i.e., low to moderate intensity) as compared to resistance training. The changes associated with aerobic training include the following:

(a) An increase of the oxidative capacity of the type I slow twitch fibers as well as a change in the type II fast twitch fibers toward the so-called type IIa fiber type with a greater oxidative capacity.[14]
(b) An increase in the number of capillaries around muscle fibers[15] which allows for more efficient exchange of nutrients and waste products.

Table 42.1 Adaptations to aerobic training

– Transformation of the glycolytic type IIb muscle fibers to type IIa muscle fibers with a greater oxidative capacity
– Increased number of muscle capillaries and muscle perfusion
– Increased size, number, and metabolic capacity of mitochondria
– Increased availability of muscle glucose transporter GLUT 4
– Increased activity of the enzymes hexokinase and glycogen synthase
– Increased adiponectin receptors (adiponectin is a hormone produced by adipose tissue that is a major mediator of insulin sensitivity)
– Decreased inflammatory cytokines

(c) An increase in the size, number, and metabolic activity of mitochondria[16] with a greater capacity for ATP production and oxidative phosphorylation. (This may be mediated in part through the activation of AMPK.)
(d) An increase in the number of GLUT 4 transporters available for translocation to the cell surface.[17]
(e) An increase in the activity of the enzymes hexokinase and glycogen synthase with an improved capacity for increased glucose uptake, glucose phosphorylation, and storage, respectively.
(f) An increase in the expression of adiponectin receptors,[18] as well as a decrease in inflammatory cytokines known to be associated with insulin resistance.[19]

These changes occur in the face of little or no muscle hypertrophy and are most obvious in the type 1 and type 2a oxidative fibers.

The adaptive response to resistance training results predominantly in the hypertrophy of type 2b fast twitch fibers with minimal changes in oxidative capacity or vascularization. In addition to hypertrophy, much of the early improvement in strength during resistance training is related to more efficient neurologic regulation of fiber recruitment within the muscle.

These changes in muscle function along with the cardiorespiratory and circulatory adaptations to physical training lead to a more efficient use of energy and improvements in aerobic endurance. There is no evidence that the adaptations to exercise in patients with diabetes differ substantially from those of normal individuals.

Exercise Capacity of Patients with Diabetes

Patients with type 1 diabetes appear to have a normal exercise capacity when metabolic derangements are well controlled. In chronically under-insulinized patients, an inability to store glycogen and a tendency to dehydration can result in poor endurance capacity. In patients with autonomic dysfunction the cardiovascular response to exercise can be further impaired. The situation in patients with type 2 diabetes is more complex. A number of studies suggest that these patients may have a mild impairment of aerobic exercise capacity. Many studies show a VO_2max roughly 15% lower than controls with apparently similar levels of physical activity. Interestingly, preliminary studies suggest that this difference may be present prior to the onset of overt disease and can even be found in first-degree relatives (see Fig. 42.3). This is associated with a relatively high percentage of fast twitch fibers, which are less insulin sensitive as well as a decrease in mitochondrial and capillary density. It appears that the decrease in VO_2max in patients with diabetes could be related, at least in part, to acquired or genetic alterations in mitochondrial function.[20] Skeletal muscle mitochondria in individuals with type 2 diabetes have been shown to be reduced in size and may have a reduced oxidative phosphorylation capacity via decreased enzyme activity. These defects have also been demonstrated in preliminary studies in nondiabetic but insulin-resistant relatives of those with diabetes. In addition, impaired activation of AMPK has been found in insulin-resistant, obese, and diabetic individuals.[21] Nevertheless, patients with type 2 diabetes do respond to physical training with an increase in oxidative capacity, and it is important to note that the *relative* ability of these patients

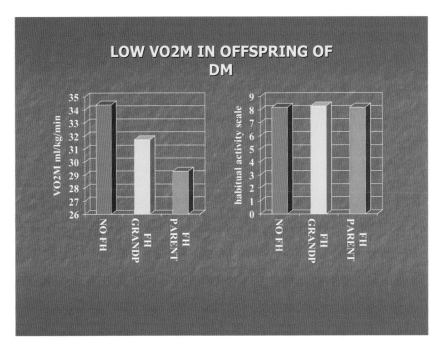

Fig. 42.3 Impaired aerobic exercise capacity in close relatives of individuals with type 2 diabetes mellitus. In subjects with equivalent baseline activity levels, there is a significant decrease in VO2max in those with a first- or second-degree relative with type 2 diabetes as compared to those with no family history. NO FH, no family history of diabetes; FH GRANDP, second-degree relative with diabetes; FH PARENT, first-degree relative with diabetes (from Thamer et al.[20])

to improve aerobic exercise capacity during training appears to be normal. There is no evidence that resistance training elicits a unique response in patients with diabetes.

Fuel Metabolism During Exercise in Patients with Diabetes

Type 1 Diabetes

A number of factors influence the metabolic response to exercise in patients with type 1 diabetes mellitus. These include the adequacy of insulinization, metabolic control, the presence or absence of complications, exercise intensity, duration, type, and recent food intake.[1] The ability of the body to maintain glucose levels in the face of intense exercise is remarkable. In trained athletes moderate activity of many hours duration may be associated with minimal changes in plasma glucose. Nevertheless, inadequate regulation of plasma glucose levels is common in patients with type 1 diabetes. Similar problems often occur in patients with long-standing type 2 diabetes mellitus who have reached a point of absolute insulin deficiency and are dependent upon exogenous insulin.

One of the major reasons for the sometimes disappointing results of exercise as a means of improving glucose control in type 1 diabetes is hypoglycemia. Hypoglycemia is common in patients with type 1 diabetes during exercise and may require increased carbohydrate intake and a decreased insulin dose which limits potential improvements in glucose control. While the various causes of hypoglycemia during exercise in patients with type 1 diabetes are not always clear there are a number of factors which contribute (see Table 42.2) to it:

(a) Relative hyperinsulinemia: Exercise is normally associated with a fall in circulating insulin. Subcutaneously injected insulin prior to exercise cannot be shut off and this can lead to a state of relative hyperinsulinemia.

Table 42.2   Contributing factors toward exercise-related hypoglycemia in insulin treated patients

1. Lack of physiologic suppression of plasma insulin levels
2. Enhanced absorption of insulin injected over exercising muscle
3. Impaired counterregulatory responses of glucagon and epinephrine
4. Increased insulin sensitivity
5. Medications (i.e., beta-adrenergic blockers) in those with impaired glucagon response

A dose of insulin appropriate at rest may be excessive during exercise. Also, if insulin is injected directly over the exercising muscle its absorption can be accelerated.[22,23] This effect is particularly important for regular insulin and when exercise occurs within 1–2 h after injection. The absorption of insulin is increased even further if the insulin is injected accidentally directly into the exercising muscle. In addition to the early hypoglycemia, rapid depletion of the insulin depot can actually result in insulin deficiency later in the day and contribute to hyperglycemia and erratic glucose control.

(b) Impaired counterregulatory response: Patients with type 1 diabetes and relatively long-standing disease (>5 years) may have a blunted glucagon and epinephrine response to hypoglycemia.[24] This may occur in the absence of overt autonomic neuropathy. When combined with the lack of physiological insulin suppression this may be an important contributor to hypoglycemia during exercise.

(c) Increased insulin sensitivity: Hypoglycemia can occur not only during exercise but also as long as 6–10 h after a brisk exercise bout. This is because of an exercise-induced increase in insulin action that may take some time to manifest and that can persist for hours.[25,26] Such clinically important episodes can be severe, and if exercise is performed in the evening, hypoglycemia may occur in the early morning hours while the patient is asleep.

(d) Drugs: Beta-adrenergic blockers may aggravate insulin-induced hypoglycemia. However, because of the redundancy of the hormonal system regulating plasma glucose, this problem is generally confined to patients who already have an impaired glucagon response. This is especially true for patients with long-standing type 1 diabetes where glucagon secretion is often impaired but is less common in the larger group of patients with type 2 diabetes.[27] Ethanol may also predispose the patient with type 1 diabetes to exercise-induced hypoglycemia by inhibiting gluconeogenesis and decreasing hepatic glycogen stores.

In contrast to the more common hypoglycemia, some patients in poor metabolic control may experience a paradoxical rise in blood glucose with exercise as a result of absolute insulin deficiency. The deficiency leads to hyperglycemia (fasting blood glucose >300 mg/dl), frequent ketosis, and dehydration (see Fig. 42.4).[28,29] This is probably because the insulin deficiency and the associated excess of counterregulatory hormones cause an increased hepatic glucose and ketone body production that exceeds peripheral utilization. For practical purposes

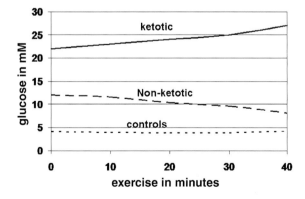

Fig. 42.4   Effects of exercise in severely insulin-deficient patients with type 1 diabetes mellitus – paradoxical hyperglycemia. Blood glucose in ketotic diabetic patients paradoxically increased with greater duration of exercise, unlike the control group and the non-ketotic diabetic group

patients with a *fasting* blood glucose >300 mg/dl or who have evidence of ketones are those at risk for paradoxical hyperglycemia. In these patients adequate insulinization needs to be achieved before exercise can exert beneficial effects.

Another situation where significant hyperglycemia may occur in patients with type 1 diabetes is following very high intensity exercise.[30] This is usually transient and results from brisk hepatic glycogenolysis at a time when peripheral tissues are relatively insulin resistant and are primarily using stored glycogen as an energy source. Unlike the situation in healthy individuals the hyperglycemia may be prolonged in patients with type 1 diabetes because increased endogenous insulin fails to compensate.

Type 2 Diabetes

The metabolic response to exercise in most patients with type 2 diabetes is similar to healthy individuals, and as noted above it will be modified by a number of factors including drug therapy and exercise intensity.

Patients with type 2 diabetes mellitus have a relatively low incidence of exercise-induced hypoglycemia. This is probably related to intact glucagon and epinephrine responses. However, hypoglycemia can occur in patients with type 2 diabetes treated with insulin or insulin secretagogues.

Benefits of Exercise Training

The potential benefits of regular physical activity in patients with diabetes are numerous and include improvements in insulin sensitivity and glycemic control, reduction in cardiovascular risk, improvements in blood pressure, lipid profile and coagulation factors, and weight loss (see Table 42.3).[31,32]

Table 42.3 Benefits of regular exercise in diabetes

– Improved insulin sensitivity
– Improved glycemic control in type 2 diabetes
– Decreased triglycerides
– Decreased numbers of small, dense LDL cholesterol particles
– Increased HDL cholesterol (with intensive exercise regimens)
– Decreased blood pressure
– Increased fibrinolytic activity
– Weight loss
– Decreased visceral adiposity
– Increased lean body mass
– Reduced cardiovascular risk
– Positive behavior modification
– Improved self-esteem and sense of well-being

Insulin Sensitivity

A number of studies have shown an improvement in glucose tolerance following a single exercise bout in normal individuals and patients with type 1 and 2 diabetes.[33–36] A single episode of exercise in patients with type 2 diabetes can typically improve insulin sensitivity at the liver and muscle for up to 16 h or longer.[37] Individuals undergoing long-term physical training regimens with an exercise frequency of three or more sessions per week have improved insulin-stimulated muscle glucose uptake and glucose tolerance and decreased insulin levels.[35,38–40] In most studies it is not clear to what extent these improvements are due to the summed effects of acute exercise bouts vs. the trained state per se. In one study after 6 months of physical training insulin sensitivity dramatically improved 12 h after the last exercise bout but had returned to baseline within a week of subjects becoming sedentary, suggesting that acute exercise effects may predominate.[41] Certainly, more prolonged improvements in metabolic control could result indirectly through changes in body composition that occur during physical training such as decreased visceral fat and increased muscle mass.

The mechanisms underlying possible beneficial effects of the trained state include the following:

(a) Increased insulin-stimulated glucose disposal owing to increased skeletal muscle blood flow.[38]
(b) Increased insulin-responsive GLUT 4 glucose transporter availability in skeletal muscle with physical training.[12]
(c) Increased activity of mitochondrial enzymes involved in oxidation and storage of glucose in skeletal muscle.
(d) Increased conversion of type IIb to type IIa muscle fibers. (Type IIa fibers have higher concentration of glucose transporters, greater capillary density, and are more insulin responsive.)
(e) Decreased intra-abdominal and intramuscular fat stores.
(f) Increased muscle mass during programs of resistance training which may partially compensate for insulin insensitivity through the availability of an increased glucose storage space.[42]

Exercise and Glycemic Control

Type 2 Diabetes

There is substantial evidence that exercise training improves insulin sensitivity and decreases elevated blood glucose in patients with type 2 diabetes mellitus. Exercise programs performed at 50–70% VO_2max for 30–40 min, 3–4 times/week consistently show about a 10–20% drop in the HgA1c from baseline. Long-term studies have shown a sustained effect over as long as 5 years of regular exercise.[43,44] The maximum benefit is seen in patients with impaired glucose tolerance, mild type 2 diabetes, and those who are the most insulin resistant.[35,45] This is consistent with the effect of exercise training on insulin sensitivity. While the accumulated effects of individual exercise bouts are clearly a major contributor to improved overall blood glucose control, other factors such as changes in body composition, decreased visceral fat, and behavioral changes promoted by regular physical activity should not be underestimated.

Type 1 Diabetes

The beneficial effect of exercise on glycemic control in type 1 diabetic patients is less clear. Despite improvements in insulin sensitivity with decreased exogenous insulin requirements,[46] studies showing improved glucose control with regular exercise in large patient populations are lacking. One study noted a mild initial improvement in glucose control in 25 type 1 diabetic patients trained for >3 months that was lost by the third month of observation despite continued adherence to the exercise regimen.[47] The relatively high incidence of hypoglycemia during exercise in type 1 diabetic patients with resultant increased carbohydrate intake and decreased insulin dose probably offsets the benefit of the enhanced glucose disposal. Nevertheless, some patients with type 1 diabetes can achieve improved glucose control with exercise, although intensive self-monitoring and a predictable training regimen are usually required. More importantly, potential beneficial effects of physical training on body composition, psychological state, and cardiovascular risk factors can often be achieved along with a decrease in insulin requirements even in the absence of improvements in HgA1c. Hence exercise should not be discouraged but instead promoted in appropriate patients.

Exercise and Dyslipidemia

Type 2 diabetes is associated with a characteristic dyslipidemia related to an increased risk of premature atherosclerosis. Most often this consists of hypertriglyceridemia, low levels of HDL cholesterol, and normal or only modestly elevated levels of LDL cholesterol. Additional changes in the composition of LDL cholesterol may also contribute to increased atherogenesis. The mechanisms by which exercise affects lipid metabolism are complex, but activation of lipoprotein lipase, changes in hepatic lipase activity, altered caloric balance, and changes in body composition and fat distribution may contribute.

Studies have shown that the most consistent effect of exercise training is a reduction in the plasma triglyceride levels, which fall up to 30% from baseline.[48–50] Some of the decrease in triglycerides seen with exercise may be transient and related to individual exercise bouts mirroring the effects of exercise on carbohydrate metabolism.[45]

Changes in LDL cholesterol with regular exercise have been less consistently demonstrated. There may be a decrease in the concentration of the small dense LDL particles, which are thought to be more atherogenic.[51] The effects are more pronounced in the patients who are more insulin resistant and have higher initial triglyceride levels. Many studies have not shown an increase in the HDL cholesterol with exercise even when the plasma triglyceride levels decrease. This could be due to the moderate intensity of the exercise regimens in the studies. In nondiabetic individuals, HDL cholesterol increases are seen only with high intensity exercise performed over a long period of time; many patients with type 2 diabetes are unable or unwilling to exercise to this intensity.

Patients with type 1 diabetes often have a lipid profile that differs from their counterparts with type 2 diabetes. When in good metabolic control HDL cholesterol levels may actually be elevated and major abnormalities of cholesterol and triglyceride measurements are unimpressive. Nevertheless, a very high incidence of premature CAD is found in these patients. Regular exercise has a favorable effect on the lipid profile in patients with type 1 diabetes similar to that seen in nondiabetic individuals.[5]

Exercise and Hypertension

Hypertension has been associated with the insulin resistance syndrome in patients with impaired glucose tolerance and type 2 diabetes. In trained subjects, both the resting pressure and the blood pressure response to exercise are reduced. Regular exercise in patients with type 2 diabetes may help improve hypertension especially in insulin-resistant/hyperinsulinemic patients.[45,47,52,53] Decreases of 5–10 mmHg of both systolic and diastolic pressure are typically found with exercise training in appropriate subgroups of patients.

Exercise and Fibrinolysis

Many patients with type 2 diabetes have an impaired fibrinolytic system with increased levels of plasminogen activator inhibitor-1 (PAI-1), the major inhibitor of tissue plasminogen activator. An acute exercise bout activates the fibrinolytic system, and there is an association of aerobic fitness with enhanced fibrinolytic activity. Some of this effect may be mediated indirectly through decreased levels of insulin and triglycerides.[41] Recent studies confirm that these improvements persist after years of regular exercise. Results from the Diabetes Prevention Program show modest but significant reductions in markers of coagulation and inflammation in those who exercised over an almost 3-year follow-up period.[54]

Exercise and Obesity

Weight loss has been shown to improve glucose control and insulin sensitivity, reduce blood pressure, and decrease cardiovascular risk. Even moderate weight loss (7–10% from baseline) is generally sufficient to improve glucose tolerance and reduce cardiovascular risk in patients with type 2 diabetes mellitus. Evidence suggests that in order to achieve weight loss, a combination of diet, exercise, and behavior modification is essential.[55,56] Exercise alone without dietary restriction is often not effective because of a compensatory increase in appetite and decrease in spontaneous activity. The combination of exercise and moderate caloric restriction is more effective than diet alone.[53,54,57,58] Exercise is also one of the strongest predictors of maintenance of weight loss.[53,54,56]

The beneficial effects of exercise in a weight-reducing program are often underestimated. Exercise increases lean body mass, which can obscure the loss of body fat when body weight is the criterion of success. In addition, exercise may cause a disproportionate loss of intra-abdominal fat, which has been most closely associated with the metabolic abnormalities in the insulin resistance syndrome. For weight reduction, an exercise frequency of at least 5–6 times a week, which burns 250–300 cal/session, is generally required. Initially this is difficult in most patients with type 2 diabetes because of their poor metabolic fitness. Studies from Blair et al. on the so-called obese fit individual suggest that overweight patients who maintain a substantial program of regular exercise have a risk factor profile and risk of cardiovascular events similar to that of normal weight individuals.[59]

In the last few years there has been heightened interest in resistance exercise as a weight loss tool. Greater muscle mass produced by resistance exercise results in an increased resting metabolic rate which could help with weight maintenance. Recent studies also suggest that the addition of resistance exercise to an aerobic exercise program potentiates the beneficial metabolic effects of the latter on insulin sensitivity.[77]

Exercise and Cardiovascular Disease

Insulin resistance is thought to be an important risk factor for premature atherosclerosis in most type 2 diabetic patients. Studies have shown that these patients are more sedentary compared with controls and have an unfavorable cardiovascular risk factor profile. The beneficial effects of physical training on those cardiovascular risk factors which are most common in patients with type 2 diabetes suggest that regular exercise might play an important role in diminishing their very high incidence of premature coronary artery disease.

Although there are no completed randomized controlled trials assessing reduction in cardiovascular events induced by physical activity in type 2 diabetes, available evidence supports the concept that physical activity may play an important role in reducing cardiovascular risk in type 2 diabetes (see Fig. 42.5).[60] Large nonrandomized studies of both men and women with type 2 diabetes and impaired glucose tolerance have found that physical activity is associated with a decreased risk for cardiovascular disease.[58] It also appears that the amount of physical activity is inversely associated with coronary events.[61,62]

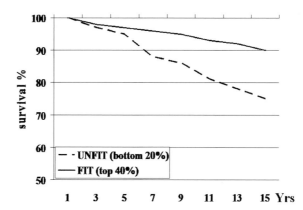

Fig. 42.5 Effects of fitness on cardiovascular mortality in patients with type 2 diabetes mellitus. Of 1263 men with type 2 diabetes, patients who scored in the lowest 20% (UNFIT) on a maximal exercise test had significantly greater mortality than those who scored in the top 40% (FIT) over the course of the study with average follow-up of 11.7 years (from Wei et al.[60])

The ongoing Look AHEAD trial, a large, randomized controlled study, aims to evaluate the long-term morbidity and mortality effects of intense lifestyle intervention in over 5000 patients with type 2 diabetes. It is scheduled to last over 11 years, and it will look specifically at changes in cardiovascular morbidity and mortality due to weight loss through physical activity, decreased caloric intake, and behavior modification. Although it is too soon for meaningful results in its primary outcomes, preliminary results show significant improvements in metabolic and disease markers.[63]

Table 42.4 Risks of exercise in diabetic patients

1. Metabolic
   (a) Paradoxical hyperglycemia
   (b) Hypoglycemia
2. Vascular
   (a) Vitreous hemorrhage and traction retinal detachment
   (b) Proteinuria
3. Neurologic
   (a) Foot injury
   (b) Excessive increases in blood pressure
   (c) Postexercise hypotension
   (d) Musculoskeletal injuries and degenerative joint disease

Risk of Exercise in Patients with Diabetes

The risks associated with exercise can be divided into metabolic, vascular, neurologic, and musculoskeletal and are summarized in Table 42.4.

Metabolic Derangements

Both hypoglycemia and paradoxical hyperglycemia are important complications of physical activity in patients with type 1 diabetes mellitus and in a smaller group of patients with type 2 disease. The mechanisms responsible for the surprisingly high incidence of hypoglycemia in these patients are discussed above. A number of options are available to avoid hypoglycemia in patients with type 1 diabetes and are summarized in Table 42.5. These should be individualized for each patient based on his/her response to exercise. Similar guidelines to avoid hypoglycemia have been advised for patients with type 2 diabetes taking insulin and some patients on sulfonylureas. Some of the measures recommended are as follows:

Table 42.5 Recommendations to avoid exercise-related hypoglycemia in patients with diabetes

1. Decrease dose of insulin prior to exercise (usually about 30–50%)
2. Avoid injecting short-acting insulin 1–2 h prior to exercise
3. Avoid injecting insulin directly over the exercising muscle
4. Ingest rapidly absorbable carbohydrates (about 15–30 g every 30 min) during exercise to avoid hypoglycemia during exercise
5. Ingest slowly absorbable carbohydrates and proteins to avoid delayed hypoglycemia

(a) Decreasing the dose of insulin taken prior to exercise. In general, reduction of about 30–50% in the insulin dose can be anticipated with moderate intensity exercise of >30-min duration. Greater reductions will be needed for more prolonged exercise. Because of their rapid onset and short duration of action, the newer very short-acting analogs of insulin are less likely to cause hypoglycemia.
(b) Avoiding injection of short-acting insulin into an area where the underlying muscles will be used during exercise within the next 1–2 h. For example, avoid injecting into the thigh if bicycling is planned.
(c) Consuming snacks of rapidly absorbable carbohydrates in the event that exercise is spontaneous and a dose of insulin has already been injected. About 15–30 g of carbohydrates ingested every 30 min is generally adequate for moderate intensity exercise. Larger amounts of carbohydrate are unlikely to be absorbed quickly and will only result in greater hyperglycemia later on.
(d) Exercising in the morning prior to the breakfast insulin dose, a time which appears to have the lowest risk of hypoglycemia. If possible, exercise should be avoided in the late evening, as this increases the risk of hypoglycemia in the early morning hours due to increased insulin sensitivity. Large meals preceding an

exercise session should be avoided as they place an additional stress on the cardiovascular system. Delayed hypoglycemia may be avoided by ingesting slowly absorbable carbohydrates and proteins at bedtime.[64] A high carbohydrate bedtime snack along with an agent which slows its absorption such as an intestinal sucrase inhibitor may also be useful. Use of the shorter acting insulin analogs, such as lispro, with evening food intake may also be helpful.

(e) Performing a brief burst of very high intensity exercise, which has a paradoxical hyperglycemic effect, in the event hypoglycemia develops during an exercise bout or at a time when carbohydrate is not readily available. For example, a 10 s maximal sprint can sometimes be used to temporarily restore glucose levels toward normal.[65]

The variability of the individual's response to physical activity in patients with type 1 diabetes cannot be overemphasized. As a result, self-monitoring of blood glucose (SMBG) by the patient done before, during, and after exercise is an essential step in developing personalized exercise recommendations.

When the *fasting* blood glucose is >250 mg/dl with ketones or >300 mg/dl with or without ketones, exercise should be delayed and such patients should be first adequately insulinized.

Microvascular Risks

While controlled studies are not available, observational evidence suggests that physical activity commonly precedes retinal hemorrhage in patients with advanced proliferative retinopathy. Most commonly, this is associated with hypoglycemia, rapid head movements which would increase shear forces, direct trauma to the eyes, or large swings in blood pressure. There is no evidence that regular exercise increases the risks of developing retinopathy or causes retinal hemorrhage in individuals with mild diabetic eye disease. In patients with more advanced retinopathy it is particularly important to avoid exercises that result in Valsalva maneuvers or levels of physical activity that cause a rise in the systolic blood pressure to >200 mmHg.

High intensity exercise increases the quantity of protein in the urine for hours after the exercise is completed. In as many as 30% of patients with diabetes whose baseline urine protein is normal, intense exercise creates a transient proteinuria. Assessments of quantitative urine protein excretion should be done at least 24 h after the last bout of exercise. Exercises that result in large increases in systolic blood pressure should probably also be avoided in patients with established nephropathy. Although no long-term studies of the effects of exercise on the progression of nephropathy are available, observational studies suggest that athletes do not have an increased risk of developing diabetic renal disease.

Neurological Risks

Patients with diabetes can be plagued by both peripheral and autonomic neuropathy. It is prudent to limit weight-bearing exercises in patients with significant peripheral neuropathy as repetitive exercise on insensitive feet will increase the risk for ulcerations and fractures. In addition, loss of proprioception can make some exercises dangerous, such as those involving free weights. Diabetic patients with autonomic neuropathy are at increased risk for excessive increases in blood pressure during exercise, postexercise hypotension, and sudden cardiac death. General measures to reduce the risks from exercise include maintaining adequate hydration during and after exercise and avoiding exercise in extremely hot or cold environments.

Exercise Recommendations

Compliance with exercise programs is a major problem. In a study of 255 diabetic patients in a diabetes education program that emphasized exercise, compliance with exercise fell from 80% at 6 weeks to <50% at 3 months and <20% at 1 year.[45] To improve adherence to exercise programs, the activity should be enjoyable and convenient and the patient should be educated about the physiology of physical activity, its potential benefits, and risks. Quantitative indices of progress to provide feedback should be utilized, e.g., measurements of heart rate during submaximal exercise and measurements of body composition.[66] Also, the goals should be realistic. The guidelines and recommendations for exercise in diabetic patients are summarized in Table 42.7.[67,68]

Pre-exercise Evaluation

Prior to starting an exercise program all patients with diabetes should undergo a detailed history, physical examination, and appropriate studies with the focus on complications of diabetes affecting the eyes, heart, blood vessels, kidneys, and nervous system.[41] The goal of evaluating diabetic patients prior to starting a more intensive exercise program is to identify those patients who are at increased risk of having a serious adverse event with strenuous activity. As noted before, the response to exercise will be influenced by the type and intensity of exercise as well as the presence or absence of complications.

The most feared adverse effect of exercise in diabetic patients is sudden death due to arrhythmias or ischemia. Fortunately this is an extremely rare event. Cardiovascular risk prediction models based on the Framingham[69] or UKPDS studies,[70] or the risk assessment tool Diabetes PHD available at the American Diabetes Association (ADA) website, may be helpful in assessing a patient's risk. It has been suggested that any individual whose risk of cardiovascular disease exceeds 10% should undergo some form of formal cardiac exercise testing prior to initiating an exercise program. However, using a 10% cutoff would include an extremely high percentage of the population with type 2 diabetes mellitus. It therefore seems reasonable that individuals who will be exercising at an intensity similar to that which they experience during their activities of daily living probably do not need extensive formal cardiac evaluation. In contrast, in line with the updated 2002 guidelines from the American Heart Association/American College of Cardiology, a stress test evaluation is now more strongly recommended for those diabetic patients about to embark on a more vigorous exercise regimen.[71] Specific evidence-based studies evaluating risk stratification of diabetic patients prior to initiating an exercise regimen are lacking. Most completed and ongoing studies examine the broader categories of symptomatic patients (i.e., those with angina, anginal equivalents, shortness of breath, dyspnea on exertion, etc.) and asymptomatic patients. Unfortunately, the approach initially proposed by the ADA in its 1998 consensus position focusing heavily on the number of established cardiac risk factors has yet to be validated. The DIAD (Detection of Ischemia in Asymptomatic Diabetics) study found that the strongest predictors of abnormal adenosine stress SPECT myocardial perfusion imaging in asymptomatic patients were cardiac autonomic dysfunction (i.e., abnormal Valsalva), male sex, and diabetes duration.[72]

There are a number of noninvasive approaches to evaluate a patient for underlying cardiovascular disease. Exercise electrocardiography, stress myocardial perfusion imaging, and stress echocardiography can detect myocardial ischemia. The sensitivity, specificity, and positive and negative predictive values for the diagnosis of coronary artery disease in symptomatic diabetic patients is presented in Table 42.6; there is limited data for

Table 42.6 Sensitivity, specificity, and predictive values for the diagnosis of coronary artery disease in symptomatic patients with diabetes

Type of test	Sensitivity (%)	Specificity (%)	PPV (%)	NPV (%)
Exercise ECG stress test[a]	47	81	85	41
Dobutamine stress echocardiography[b]	82	54	84	50
Nuclear stress test[c]	86	56	n/a	n/a

[a]Lee et al.[97]
[b]Hennessy et al.[98]
[c]Kang et al.[99]

Table 42.7 Guidelines and recommendations for exercise in diabetic patients

1. Pre-exercise evaluation
   A. Detailed history, physical examination, and appropriate studies with focus on complications of diabetes affecting eyes, heart, blood vessels, kidneys, and nervous system
   B. Exercise stress test: for those starting a moderate to high intensity exercise program and those judged to have an increased risk for ischemic heart disease including
      (a) Type 2 diabetes of >10 years duration
      (b) Type 1 diabetes >15 years duration
      (c) Presence of peripheral vascular disease
      (d) Autonomic neuropathy
      (e) Nephropathy
      (f) Presence of multiple traditional risk factors

2. Aerobic exercise involving large muscle groups
   A. Frequency: minimum 3–5 times a week
   B. Intensity: 40–60% VO_2max
   C. Duration: >10 min/session; >150 min cumulatively per week

3. Resistance exercise, in those without contraindication, targeting all major muscle groups
   A. Frequency: three times a week
   B. Intensity: a resistance that can be overcome for 15 repetitions
   C. Duration: three sets of 8–10 repetitions

asymptomatic diabetic patients. Although the recently completed DIAD study mentioned above failed to show any morbidity or mortality benefit to routine screening of asymptomatic diabetic patients with myocardial perfusion imaging, there was a lower than expected event rate and therefore further investigation is still required. Newer imaging studies like CT angiography, cardiac magnetic resonance imaging, and coronary artery calcium scoring are also being studied to assist in the risk stratification of diabetic patients, although data on these techniques are more limited. Because currently there is not enough information available to support a specific evidence-based approach to identify potential significant cardiovascular disease, the general guidelines proposed by the ADA in a 2007 Consensus Statement are based on clinical judgment. Patients whom a clinician may judge to be most likely at risk for cardiovascular disease may include those with cerebrovascular or peripheral vascular disease, renal disease, autonomic neuropathy, an abnormal ECG, and traditional cardiovascular disease risk burden. The role, if any, for a cardiac CT to obtain a coronary artery calcium score is still controversial, and further research is needed to clarify the use of newer technologies in evaluating diabetic patients for cardiovascular risk and to identify the benefits, if any, of earlier intervention.[73]

Type of Exercise

Recommendations for the type, intensity, and duration of exercise depend on the risks for the individual patient and the desired benefit/outcome such as athletic training, improvements in insulin sensitivity, weight loss, and changes in body composition or enhancing muscle strength and flexibility.

The ADA recommends repetitive aerobic exercise involving large muscle groups that can be maintained for a prolonged period in patients with diabetes mellitus.[41] Examples of such exercise include brisk walking, jogging, swimming, rowing, dancing, cycling, and other endurance activities. The benefits of exercise for a given level of energy expenditure are not dependent on the mode of exercise. Hence, the type of aerobic activity should be determined by patient preference and risks based on complications of diabetes. For example, a patient with severe peripheral neuropathy would be wise to avoid jogging and instead consider exercises such as swimming or cycling.

In addition to aerobic exercise recent research has suggested the benefit of resistance training of a sufficient intensity to build and maintain muscle strength, endurance, and fat-free mass in healthy individuals.[74] In patients with diabetes, resistance training has been shown to improve insulin sensitivity in the absence of changes in maximal oxygen uptake (VO$_2$max).[40,75,76] A number of recent randomized, controlled trials have consistently demonstrated a decrease in the HgA1c ranging from 0.5 to 1.2% with resistance training. Recent studies also indicate that resistance training is likely to potentiate the beneficial effects of aerobic exercise.[77] Well-designed resistance training programs with careful monitoring are safe[40,78] and light weights with high repetitions can be used to enhance upper body muscle strength in almost all patients including healthy older individuals. However, resistance exercise may not be advisable for some patients with long-standing diabetes and increased risk for ischemic heart disease and patients with diabetic nephropathy and proliferative retinopathy.

Frequency

Because much of the improvement in insulin sensitivity following a bout of exercise is transient, it is recommended that patients with diabetes engage in aerobic exercises at least every other day or 3–5 days each week. There should not be more than two consecutive days without physical activity. It is not yet clear if multiple shorter bouts of activity throughout the day will result in similar improvements in glucose control. The optimal training regimen to achieve glycemic and cardiovascular improvements will vary depending on a patient's baseline fitness, pre-existing risk factors, and desired goals of therapy. Several organizations including the AHA, American College of Sports Medicine (ACSM), and the ADA have advocated inclusion of both moderate to vigorous intensity aerobic exercises most days of the week and resistance training at least 2–3 times/week to a regular schedule of physical activity.

Intensity

The intensity of exercise is usually given to the patient in the form of a recommendation for a specific target heart rate during activity. Most of the studies that show metabolic benefit, i.e., improved glucose disposal and insulin sensitivity, are seen with an exercise intensity of 50–75% of an individual's VO$_2$max. Also, the AHA recommends engaging in activities that use between 700 and 2000 cal/week.[79] Lower intensity exercise (<50% VO$_2$max), which may be associated with improved patient adherence, may also have beneficial cardiorespiratory and circulatory effects, but beneficial effects on insulin sensitivity may not occur.[80,81] On the other hand, higher intensity exercise (>75% VO$_2$max) may be associated with increased cardiovascular risk, musculoskeletal injuries, and decreased patient adherence. While most programs emphasize exercises that improve fitness as demonstrated by an increased maximal oxygen uptake, recent studies suggest that regular participation in low to moderate intensity physical activity may reduce the risk of type 2 diabetes, hypertension, and coronary artery disease despite suboptimal effects on the VO$_2$max.[55,82,83]

Heart rate during exercise is linearly related to exercise intensity. If one knows the basal and maximal heart rate, it is possible to estimate a percent of VO$_2$max based on an individual's heart rate during a given activity. Most exercise prescriptions are given as a recommended exercise heart rate. Most patients can learn to measure their own heart rate and for those who cannot, inexpensive devices are available for use during exercise. The HR$_{max}$ should ideally be determined during formal exercise testing. If the true HR$_{max}$ is not known then one can estimate it from the following equation: HR$_{max}$ = 220 − patient age (years).

Fifty percentage of a maximum heart rate can be estimated by the following equation:

$$0.5(HR_{max} - HR_{rest}) + HR_{rest}$$

where HR$_{rest}$ is the basal heart rate which is determined before arising in the morning. Another commonly used approach to prescribing exercise makes use of the rating of perceived exertion. This analog scale can be used by patients to estimate their relative workload with acceptable accuracy after some training. Resistance exercise programs emphasize what is called high volume resistance exercise. Patients perform a series of activities involving different muscle groups with a short rest period between each set. One approach is to determine a level of resistance which can be performed 15 times without significant discomfort. The patient is then instructed to perform 8–12 repetitions of this activity two to three times with a brief rest period (less than 90 s) between each set. Resistance exercise of this intensity results in changes of pulse and blood pressure similar to the aerobic exercise recommended above and appears to be equally safe for most patients with diabetes.

To reduce the risk of musculoskeletal injuries and prepare the cardiorespiratory system and skeletal muscles for the progressive increase in exercise intensity, a warm up of 5–10 min is recommended. The warm-up period involves low intensity aerobic exercise such as walking. Stretching exercises (but not with breath holding) are quite useful in patients with diabetes who often complain of decreased flexibility. Stretching should be done following a brief aerobic warm up to avoid muscle injury. A cooldown period similar to the warm up should be done at the end of the exercise session. This usually involves 10 min of activity at an intensity of 30–40% of that done during the exercise session. This will help gradually reduce the heart rate down to the pre-exercise level and may reduce the risk of postexercise hypotension and arrhythmias.

Duration

Depending on the intensity of the exercise regimen, the duration of each session will vary in order to provide the optimal benefit. Exercise done at 40–60% VO_2max, 3–5 times per week, should last at least 20 min/session and cumulatively at least 150 min/week. In addition to, or instead of, this regimen a patient may perform at least 90 min/week of vigorous intensity exercise at >60% VO_2max. Approaches using two or more short exercise sessions of, for example, 10 min may be beneficial, but the effectiveness of this approach for improving metabolic control is still unclear.

Exercise and the Prevention of Type 2 Diabetes Mellitus

Decreased physical activity, independent of obesity, is a well-established risk factor for the development of type 2 diabetes in high-risk individuals. Insulin resistance and visceral adiposity play an important role in the development of impaired glucose tolerance and frank type 2 diabetes. Therefore, physical activity, by decreasing insulin resistance and visceral adiposity in these high-risk patients, is likely to be useful to prevent or delay the development of type 2 diabetes.

Individuals at high risk for the development of type 2 diabetes mellitus include those with a family history, members of high-risk ethnic groups such as Native Americans and individuals from the Indian subcontinent, a history of gestational diabetes,[84,85] patients with the polycystic ovary syndrome, and any individual with android-type obesity and the cluster of risk factors that make up the metabolic syndrome (see below). Various types of studies have supported the hypothesis that regular physical activity may prevent or substantially delay the onset of type 2 diabetes. These include cross-cultural, migrant, and other observational studies[86–88] and prospective studies in subjects at high risk for developing type 2 diabetes.[89–91] Recently, large interventional trials have reinforced the benefits of exercise in reducing the risk for type 2 diabetes. These include the Malmo study from Sweden,[48] the Da Quing study from China[92], and the Finnish Diabetes Prevention Study.[93] These prospective but not randomized studies show a reduction in the risk of type 2 diabetes of between 15 and 60% with similar benefits for older and younger individuals and for men and women.

The results of the Diabetes Prevention Program, a large randomized controlled trial in the United States, confirmed the benefit of exercise in the prevention or delay in onset of type 2 diabetes. Over 3000 nondiabetic patients at risk for developing diabetes underwent either intense lifestyle modification including 150 h of moderate intensity exercise with diet training and a goal of 7% weight loss, metformin treatment twice daily, or placebo. After an average 2.8-year follow-up, intense lifestyle modification reduced the incidence of diabetes by 58%, significantly greater than the 31% reduction by metformin therapy.[94] Significant improvements were also noted in insulin sensitivity, markers of inflammation (i.e., C-reactive protein), and coagulation. There is some concern regarding the sustainability of the intervention in light of the fact that only 58% continued to achieve the goal activity level by the end of the study. In addition, some analyses suggest that the cost of implementing the program may be prohibitively high.[95]

Exercise and the Metabolic Syndrome

The metabolic syndrome is a constellation of metabolic abnormalities that predicts an increased risk for type 2 diabetes and/or cardiovascular disease. Current theories attempting to explain the underlying pathophysiology highlight a combination of insulin resistance, fat repartitioning, and a pro-inflammatory state. Although the specific criteria for the syndrome have been debated by several organizations such as the World Health Organization and the International Diabetes Foundation, the general components are similar. These include abdominal obesity, glucose intolerance (impaired fasting glucose, impaired glucose tolerance, or overt type 2 diabetes), dyslipidemia (both hypertriglyceridemia and low HDL cholesterol), and hypertension. As the role for regularly scheduled, moderate to severe intensity exercise has become more established for the treatment and prevention of diabetes, guidelines for the treatment of the metabolic syndrome also have come to include regular routines of moderate physical activity. The Look AHEAD study mentioned above will also have important ramifications for both the consequences and the treatment of the metabolic syndrome.[96]

Summary

Exercise has been shown to be a useful tool in the treatment of diabetes mellitus. Improvements of HgA1c levels of 1–2% are generally found in patients with type 2 diabetes mellitus undergoing a modest exercise program three to five times per week. In addition, exercise has beneficial effects on body composition and a variety of cardiovascular risk factors and is associated with a decreased risk of premature coronary artery disease. The benefits of exercise on glucose control are more difficult to attain in patients with type 1 diabetes, but beneficial effects on cardiovascular risk factors are likely to be valuable. Aerobic exercises of moderate intensity are generally recommended for patients with diabetes but high volume resistance exercises are also of benefit and should be included for appropriate patients. While the mechanisms remain incompletely understood it is clear that exercise on a regular basis acts through improved insulin sensitivity in liver and skeletal muscle as well as changes in body composition. The risks of initiating a moderate intensity exercise program for most patients with diabetes are minimal. Patients with neurologic and vascular complications of diabetes may need to limit certain activities. Patients treated with insulin and some oral agents are at risk of hypoglycemia related to exercise. These patients require special education and a regimen based on frequent home blood glucose monitoring. In addition to improving the clinical status of patients with established diabetes, exercise may play an even more important role in prevention of type 2 diabetes in high-risk populations. A safe and effective exercise program can be devised for the great majority of patients with diabetes mellitus and should be a part of every comprehensive treatment regimen.

Internet Resources

http://www.diabetes.org/diabetesphd/default.jsp
http://www.mayoclinic.com/health/diabetes/DA00123
http://www.dtu.ox.ac.uk/index.php?maindoc=/riskengine/
http://hp2010.nhlbihin.net/atpiii/calculator.asp?usertype=prof

References

1. Vitug A, Schneider SH, Ruderman NB. Exercise and type 1 diabetes mellitus. In: *Exerc Sport Sci Rev.* 1988;16:285–304.
2. Wahren J. Glucose turnover during exercise in healthy man and in patients with diabetes mellitus. *Diabetes.* 1979;28(suppl 1):82–88.

3. Wahren J, Felig P, Ahlborg G, et al. Glucose metabolism during leg exercise in man. *J Clin Invest*. 1971;50:2715–2725.

4. Ahlborg G, Felig P, Hagenfeldt L, et al. Substrate turnover during prolonged exercise in man. *J Clin Invest*. 1974;53:1080–1090.

5. Wasserman DH, Zinman B. Exercise in individuals with IDDM (Technical Review). *Diabetes Care*. 1994;17:924–937.

6. Galbo H, Christensen NJ, Holst JJ. Catecholamines and pancreatic hormones during autonomic blockade in exercising man. *Acta Physiol Scand*. 1977;101:428–437.

7. Wasserman DH, Lacy DB, Goldstein RE, et al. Exercise-induced fall in insulin and the increase in fat metabolism during prolonged exercise. *Diabetes*. 1989;38:484–490.

8. Moates JM, Lacy DB, Cherrington AD, et al. The metabolic role of the exercise-induced increment in epinephrine. *Am J Physiol*. 1988;255:E428–E436.

9. Ahlborg G. Mechanism for glycogenolysis in nonexercising human muscle during and after exercise. *Am J Physiol*. 1985;248:E540–E545.

10. Marliss EB, Simantirakis E, Purdon C, et al. Glucoregulatory and hormonal responses to repeated bouts of intense exercise in normal male subjects. *J Appl Physiol*. 1991;71:924–933.

11. Goodyear LJ, King PA, Hirshman MF, et al. Contractile activity increases plasma membrane glucose transporters in absence of insulin. *Am J Physiol*. 1990;258:E667–E672.

12. Kennedy JW, Hirshman MF, Gervino EV, et al. Acute exercise induces GLUT4 translocation in skeletal muscle of normal human subjects and subjects with type 2 diabetes. *Diabetes*. 1999;48:1192–1197.

13. Schenk S, Horowitz J. Acute exercise increases triglyceride synthesis in skeletal muscle and prevents fatty acid-induced insulin resistance. *J Clin Invest*. 2007;117(6):1690–1698.

14. Saltin B, Henriksson J, Nyaard E, et al. Fiber types and metabolic potentials of skeletal muscles in sedentary man and endurance runners. In: Milvy P, ed. *The Marathon: Physiological, Medical, Epidemiological, and Psychological Studies*. New York, NY: Annals of the New York Academy of Sciences; 1977: vol 301, 3–29.

15. Saltin B, Rowell LB. Functional adaptations to physical activity and inactivity. *Fed Proc*. 1980;39:1506–1513.

16. Holloszy JO. Biochemical adaptations to exercise. Aerobic metabolism. In: Wilmore JH, ed. *Exercise and Sport Sciences Reviews*. New York, NY: New York Academic Press; 1973: vol 1, 4471.

17. Hayashi T, Wojtaszewski JF, Goodyear LJ. Exercise regulation of glucose transport in skeletal muscle. *Am J Physiol*. 1997;273:E1039–E1051.

18. Bluher M, Williams CJ, Kloting N, et al. Gene expression of adiponectin receptors in human visceral and subcutaneous adipose tissue is related to insulin resistance and metabolic parameters and is altered in response to physical training. *Diabetes Care*. 2007;30(12):3110–3115.

19. Kadoglou NP, Iliadis F, Angelopoulou N, et al. The anti-inflammatory effects of exercise training in patients with type 2 diabetes mellitus. *Euro J Cardiovasc Prev Rehab*. 2007;14(6):837–843.

20. Thamer C, Stumvoll M, Niess A, et al. Reduced skeletal muscle oxygen uptake and reduced beta-cell function: two early abnormalities in normal glucose-tolerant offspring of patients with type 2 diabetes. *Diabetes Care*. 2003;26(7): 2126–2132.

21. Sriwijitkamol A, Coletta DK, Wajcberg E, et al. Effect of acute exercise on AMPK signaling in skeletal muscle of subjects with type 2 diabetes: a time-course and dose-response study. *Diabetes*. 2007;56(3):836–848.

22. Zinman B, Murray FT, Vranic M, et al. Glucoregulation during moderate exercise in insulin treated diabetics. *J Clin Endocrinol Metab*. 1977;45:641–647.

23. Koivisto VA, Felig P. Effect of leg exercise on insulin absorption in diabetic patients. *N Engl J Med*. 1978;298:79–83.

24. Schneider SH, Vitug A, Mertz MAL, et al. Abnormal hormonal response to prolonged exercise in type 1 diabetes. *Diabetes*. 1987;36(suppl I):16A, (Abstract).

25. Wojtaszewski JF, Hansen BF, Kiens B, et al. Insulin signaling in human skeletal muscle: time course and effect of exercise. *Diabetes*. 1997;46:1775–1781.

26. Richter EA, Mikines KJ, Galbo H, et al. Effect of exercise on insulin action in human skeletal muscle. *J Appl Physiol*. 1989;66:876–885.

27. Bolli G, DeFeo P, Compagnucci P, et al. Important role of adrenergic mechanism in acute glucose counterregulation following insulin-induced hypoglycemia in type 1 diabetes. *Diabetes*. 1982;31:641–647.

28. Berger M, Berchtold P, Cupper HJ, et al. Metabolic and hormonal effects of muscular exercise on juvenile type diabetes. *Diabetologia*. 1977;13:355–365.

29. Hagenfeldt L. Metabolism of free fatty acids and ketone bodies during exercise in normal and diabetic man. *Diabetes*. 1979;28(suppl 1):66–70.

30. Mitchell TH, Abraham G, Schiffrin A, et al. Hyperglycemia after intense exercise in IDDM subjects during continuous subcutaneous insulin infusion. *Diabetes Care*. 1988;11:311–317.

31. Kriska AM, Blair SN, Pereira MA. The potential role of physical activity in the prevention of non-insulin dependent diabetes mellitus: The epidemiological evidence. In: Holloszy JO, ed. *Exercise and Sports Sciences Reviews*. Baltimore, MD: Williams and Wilkins; 1994:vol 22, 121–143.

32. Wallberg-Henriksson H. Exercise and diabetes mellitus. In: Holloszy JO, ed. *Exercise and Sport Sciences Reviews*. Baltimore, MD: Williams and Wilkins; 1992:vol 20, 339–368.

33. Minuk HL, Vranic M, Hanna AK, Abisser AM, Zinman B. Glucoregulatory and metabolic response to exercise in obese noninsulin-dependent diabetes. *Am J Physiol*. 1981;240:E458–E464.

34. Giacca A, Groenewoud Y, Tsui E, et al. Glucose production, utilization, and cycling in response to moderate exercise in obese patients with Type 2 diabetes and mild hyperglycemia. *Diabetes*. 1998;47:1763–1770.
35. Martin IK, Katz A, Wahren J. Splanchnic and muscle metabolism during exercise in NIDDM patients. *Am J Physiol*. 1995;269:E583–E590.
36. Wallberg-Henriksson H, Gunnarsson R, Henriksson J, et al. Increased peripheral insulin sensitivity and Muscle mito-chondrial enzymes but unchanged blood glucose control in type 1 diabetics after physical training. *Diabetes*. 1982;31: 1044–1050.
37. Schneider SH, Amorosa LF, Khachadurian AK, et al. Studies on the mechanism of improved glucose control during exercise in type 2 (non-insulin dependent) diabetes. *Diabetologist*. 1984;26:355–360.
38. Hollszy JO, Schultz J, Kusnierkiewic J, et al. Effects of exercise on glucose tolerance and insulin resistance. *Acta Med Scand Suppl*. 1986;711:55–65.
39. Reitman JS, Vasquez B, Dimes I, et al. Improvement of glucose homeostasis after exercise-training in non-insulin-dependent diabetes. *Diabetes Care*. 1984;7:434–441.
40. Dela F, Larsen JJ, Mikines KJ, Ploug T, Petersen LN, Galbo H. Insulin-stimulated muscle glucose clearance in patients with NIDDM: effects of one-legged physical training. *Diabetes*. 1995;44:1010–1020.
41. Burstein R, Polychronakos C, Toews CJ, MacDoughall JD, Guyda HJ, Posner BI. Acute reversal of enhanced insulin action in trained athletes. *Diabetes*. 1985;34:750–760.
42. Miller WJ, Sherman WM, Ivy JL. Effects of strength training on glucose tolerance and post-glucose insulin response. *Med Sci Sports Exerc*. 1984;16:539–543.
43. Diabetes mellitus and exercise (ADA position statement). *Diabetes Care*. 2001;24(suppl 1):S51–S55.
44. Schneider SH. Long-term exercise programs. In: Ruderman N, Devlin JT, eds. *The Health Professional's Guide to Diabetes and Exercise*. Alexandria, VA: American Diabetes Association; 1995: 123–132.
45. Krottkiewski M, Lonnroth P, Manrwoukas K, et al. Effects on physical training of insulin secretion and effectiveness and glucose metabolism in obesity and type 2 (non-insulin dependent) diabetes mellitus. *Diabetologia*. 1985;28:881–890.
46. Yki-Jarvinen H, DeFronzo RA, Koivisto VA. Normalization of insulin sensitivity in type I diabetic subjects by physical training during insulin pump therapy. *Diabetes Care*. 1984;7:520–527.
47. Schneider SH, Khachadurian AK, Amorosa LF. Ten-year experience with exercise-based outpatient life-style modification program in the treatment of diabetes mellitus. *Diabetes Care*. 1992;15:1800–1810.
48. Ruderman NE, Ganda OP, Johansen K. The effect of physical training on glucose tolerance and plasma lipids in maturity onset diabetes. *Diabetes*. 1979;28:89–91.
49. Schneider SH, Vitug A, Ruderman NB. Atherosclerosis and physical activity. *Diab Metab Rev*. 1986;1:513–553.
50. Eriksson KF, Lindgarde F. Prevention of type II (noninsulin dependent) diabetes mellitus by diet and physical exercise: the six year Malmo feasibility study. *Diabetologia*. 1991;34:891–898.
51. Houmard JA, Bruno NJ, Bruner RK, et al. Effects of exercise training on chemical composition of plasma LDL. *Atheroscler Thromb*. 1994;14:325–330.
52. Krotkiewski M, Mandrousask K, Sjostrom L, et al. Effects of long term physical training on body fat, metabolism and BP in obesity. *Metabolism*. 1979;28:650–658.
53. Rocchini AP, Katch V, Schork A, et al. Insulin and blood pressure during weight loss in obese adolescents. *Hypertension*. 1987;10:267–273.
54. Diabetes Prevention Program Research Group. Intensive lifestyle intervention or metformin on inflammation and coagulation in participants with impaired glucose tolerance. *Diabetes*. 2005;54:1566–1572.
55. NHLBI Obesity Education Initiative expert panel on the identification, evaluation, and treatment of overweight and obesity in adults. Clinical guidelines on the identification, evaluation, and treatment of overweight and obesity in adults- the evidence report. *Obes Res*. 1998;6:51S-310S.
56. Wing RR. Physical activity in the treatment of the adulthood overweight and obesity: current evidence and research issues. *Med Sci Sports Exerc*. 1999;31:S547–S552.
57. Helmirch SP, Ragland DR, Leung RW, et al. Physical activity and reduced occurrence of non-insulin-dependent diabetes mellitus. *N Engl J Med*. 1991;325:147–152.
58. Wing RR. Behavioral Strategies for weight reduction in obese type II diabetic patients. *Diabetes Care*. 1989;12:139–144.
59. Lee C, Blair S, Jackson A. Cardiorespiratory fitness, body composition, and all-cause and cardiovascular disease mortality in men. *Amer J of Clin Nutr*. 1999;69(3):373–380.
60. Wei M, Gibbons L, Kampert J, et al. Low cardiorespiratory fitness and physical inactivity as predictors of mortality in men with type 2 diabetes. *Ann Int Med*. 2000;132(8):605–611.
61. Kohn HW, Gordon NF, Villegas JA, et al. Cardiorespiratory fitness, glycemic status, and mortality risk in men. *Diabetes Care*. 1992;15:184–192.
62. Hu FB, Stampfer MJ, Solomon C, et al. Physical activity and risk for cardiovascular events in diabetic women. *Ann Intern Med*. 2001;134:96–105.
63. Look AHEAD Research Group. Reduction in weight and cardiovascular disease risk factors in individuals with type 2 diabetes: one-year results of the look AHEAD trial. *Diabetes Care*. 2007;30(6):1374–1383.
64. Nathan DM, Madnek SF, Dellahanty L. Programming pre-exercise snacks to prevent postexercise hypoglycemia in intensively treated insulin-dependent diabetics. *Ann Intern Med*. 1985;102:483–486.

65. Bussau VA, Ferreira LD, Jones TW, et al. The 10-s maximal sprint: a novel approach to counter an exercise-mediated fall in glycemia in individuals with type 1 diabetes. *Diabetes Care*. 2006;29(3):601–606.

66. Schneider SH, Ruderman NB. Exercise and NIDDM (Technical Review). *Diabetes Care*. 1990;13:785–789.

67. Sigal R, Kenny GP, Wasserman DH, et al. Physical activity/exercise and type 2 diabetes. *Diabetes Care*. 2006;29: 1433–1438.

68. Eves N, Plotnikoff R. Resistance training and type 2 diabetes. *Diabetes Care*. 2006;29:1933–1941.

69. Anderson KM, Odell PM, Wilson PW, et al. Cardiovascular disease risk profiles. *Am Heart J*. 1991;121:293–298.

70. Stevens R, Kothari V, Adler AI, et al. The UKPDS risk engine: a model for the risk of coronary heart disease in Type 2 diabetes (UKPDS 56). *Clin Sci*. 2001;101:671–679.

71. ACC/AHA. Guideline update for exercise testing: summary article. *Circulation*. 2002;106:1883–1892.

72. Wackers FJT, Young LH, Inzucchi SE, et al. Detection of silent myocardial ischemia in asymptomatic diabetic subjects: the DIAD study. *Diabetes Care*. 2004;27:1954–1961.

73. Bax JJ, Young LH, Frye RL, et al. Screening for coronary artery disease in patients with diabetes. *Diabetes Care*. 2007;30: 2729–2736.

74. American College of Sports Medicine. The recommended quantity and quality of exercise for developing and maintaining cardiorespiratory and muscular fitness, and flexibility in healthy adults (Position Stand). *Med Sci Sports Exerc*. 1998;30:975–991.

75. Szczypaczewska M, Nazar K, Kaciwba-Uscilko H. Glucose tolerance and insulin response to glucose load in body builders. *Int J Sports Med*. 1989;10:34–37.

76. Smutok MA, Reece A, Goldberg AP, et al. Strength training improves glucose tolerance similar to jogging in middle-aged men (letter). *Med Sci Sports Exerc*. 1989;21(suppl 2):S33.

77. Sigal R, Kenny G, Boule N, et al. Effects of aerobic training, resistance training, or both on glycemic control in type 2 diabetes: a randomized trial. *Ann Int Med*. 2007;147(6):357–369.

78. Durak EP, Jovanovic-Peterson L, Peterson CM. Randomized crossover study of effect of resistance training on glycemic control, muscular strength and cholesterol in type 1 diabetic men. *Diabetes Care*. 1990;13:1039–1043.

79. Fletcher GF, Balady G, Froelicher VF, et al. A statement for health professionals from the American Heart Association (Exercise Standards). *Circulation*. 1995;91:580–612.

80. King AC, Haskell WL, Taylor CB, et al. Home based exercise training in healthy older men and women. *JAMA*. 1991;266:1535–1542.

81. Paffenberger RS, Wing AL, Hyde RT. Physical activity as an index of heart attack risk in college alumni. *An J Epidemiol*. 1978;108:161–175.

82. Fletcher GF, Balady G, Blair SN, et al. Benefits and recommendations for physical activity programs for all Americans (Statement on Exercise). *Circulation*. 1996;94:857–862.

83. American College of Sports Medicine. Physical activity, physical fitness and hypertension (Position Stand). *Med Sci Sports Exerc*. 1993;25:i–x.

84. Ruderman NB, Schneider SH, Berchtold P. The metabolically-obese, normal weight individual. *Am J Clin Nutr*. 1981;34:1617–1621.

85. Ruderman NB, Berchtold P, Schneider SH. Obesity associated disorders in normal weight individuals: some speculations. *Int J Obesity*. 1982;6:151–157.

86. Taylor R. Physical activity and prevalence of diabetes in Melanesian and Indian men in Fiji. *Diabetologia*. 1984;27:578–582.

87. Dowse GK, Zimmet PZ, Gareeboo H, et al. Abdominal obesity and physical activity are risk factors for NIDDM and impaired glucose tolerance in Indian, Creole, and Chinese Mauritians. *Diabetes Care*. 1991;14:271–282.

88. Kawate R, Yamakido M, Nishimoto Y, et al. Diabetes mellitus and its vascular complications in Japanese migrants on the Island of Hawaii. *Diabetes Care*. 1979;2:161–170.

89. Kriska AM, Blair SN, Pereira MA. The potential role of physical activity in the prevention of non-insulin dependent diabetes mellitus: The epidemiological evidence. *Exerc Sports Sci Rev*. 1991;22:121–143.

90. Hu FB, Sibal RJ, Rich-Edwards JW, et al. Walking compared with vigorous physical activity and risk of type 2 diabetes in women: a prospective study. *JAMA*. 1999;282:1433–1439.

91. Manson JE, Nathan DM, Krolewski AS, Stampfer MJ, Willett WC, Hennekens CH. A prospective study of exercise and incidence of diabetes among U.S. male physicians. *JAMA*. 1992;268:63–67.

92. Pan X, Li G, Hu YH. Effects of diet and exercise in preventing NIDDM in people with impaired glucose tolerance. The Da Quing IGT and Diabetes Study. *Diabetes Care*. 1997;20:537–544.

93. Tuomilehto J, Lindstrom J, Eriksson JG, et al. Prevention of type 2 diabetes mellitus by changes in lifestyle among subjects with impaired glucose tolerance. The Finnish Diabetes Prevention Study Group. *N Engl J Med*. 2001;344:1343–1350.

94. Knowler WC, Barrett-Connor E, Fowler SE, et al. Reduction in the incidence of type 2 diabetes mellitus with lifestyle intervention or metformin. *N Engl J Med*. 2002;346:393–403.

95. Eddy D, Schlessinger L, Kahn R. Clinical outcomes and cost-effectiveness of strategies for managing people at high risk for diabetes. *Ann Int Med*. 2005;143:251–264.

96. Eckel RH, Grundy SM, Zimmet P. The metabolic syndrome. *Lancet*. 2005;365:1415–1428.

97. Lee DP, Fearon WF, Froelicher VF. Clinical utility of the exercise ECG in patients with diabetes and chest pain. *Chest*. 2001;119:1576–1581.

98. Hennessy TG, Codd MB, Kane G, et al. Evaluation of patients with diabetes mellitus for coronary artery disease using dobutamine stress echocardiography. *Coron Artery Dis.* 1997;8:171–174.
99. Kang X, Berman DS, Lewin H, et al. Comparative ability of myocardial perfusion single-photon emission computed tomography to detect coronary artery disease in patients with and without diabetes mellitus. *Am Heart J.* 1999;137:949–957.

Chapter 43
Therapy of Type 1 Diabetes Mellitus

Pejman Cohan and Anne L. Peters

The treatment of type 1 diabetes is simple in theory: replace the missing endogenous production of insulin with exogenous insulin in a manner that mimics normal physiology. The difficulties in doing this are myriad, however, in part stemming from the fact that endogenous insulin is delivered in intricate pulses to the portal circulation whereas exogenous insulin is provided subcutaneously through the peripheral circulation. Additionally, the beta cells in the pancreas sense minute changes in blood sugar levels and secrete insulin, glucagon, amylin, incretins, and other hormones to balance blood sugar levels. The traditional monitoring of blood sugar levels four times per day with two to three injections of insulin does not come close even approximately to what should be happening with regards to insulin regulation.

Newer insulin production technology that has led to the development of insulin analogues has made insulins easier to use, with less hypoglycemia. Insulin delivery devices, from pens to pumps, provide more options for patients. Monitoring technology, with easy to use glucose meters and continuing glucose sensing, makes it easier to follow blood sugar levels and react to trends. None of this approaches the functionality of the human beta cell, however, and it will be our ability to restore and maintain beta cell mass that will truly treat (and potentially cure) type 1 diabetes. This review will focus on the treatments that are currently available, the evolving area of continuous glucose monitoring and possible cures for type 1 diabetes.

Insulin

Prior to the discovery of the therapeutic role for animal insulin in the treatment of human diabetes by Banting and Best in 1922 type 1 diabetes was a fatal disease.[1] In parts of the world where access to insulin is limited, people with type 1 diabetes continue to suffer from poor outcomes.[2] In most of the developed world, however, insulin is readily available.

Characteristics of Insulin Preparations

Increasing numbers of various insulin types are becoming available, ranging from the traditional insulins to insulin analogues.[3,4] This diversity of choice in terms of onset and duration of action allows use of exogenous insulin to mimic normal physiology more closely, thereby allowing for improvements in glycemic control with less hypoglycemia. However, insulin is not a simple drug to prescribe, since inappropriate doses can result in severe hypoglycemia. In people with type 1 diabetes integrating the carbohydrate content of the meal and other factors such as exercise and illness is necessary to determine the required insulin dose.[5,6] Patients need access to a health-care team, with education on diabetes self-management and nutrition.

A.L. Peters (✉)
University of Southern California Keck School of Medicine, Los Angeles, CA, USA
e-mail: momofmax@mac.com

L. Poretsky (ed.), *Principles of Diabetes Mellitus*, DOI 10.1007/978-0-387-09841-8_43,
© Springer Science+Business Media, LLC 2010

Knowledge of the pharmacology of each of the various insulin preparations is required, coupled with observation of individual patient reactions. Historically four properties characterized insulin preparations used for injection: concentration, species source, purity, and type.[7] Issues regarding species source and purity have become moot, since most insulin preparations are now based on highly purified human insulin.

As for concentration, insulin is generally marketed in 10-ml vials at a concentration of 100 units/ml (units-100). Thus, an injection of 0.5 ml delivers 50 units of insulin. Fortunately, calculations by the patient are obviated by the use of syringes with the number of units marked directly on the barrel. In Europe, other concentrations of insulin can be obtained (such as units-40). Additionally, a more concentrated form of insulin known as units-500 can be purchased by special order in the United States for use in patients who require large amounts of insulin due to severe insulin resistance.[8] Care must be taken when using insulins that are other than units-100 since errors in dosing can occur if insulin syringes meant for the units-100 concentration of insulin are used.

Types of Insulin

From a therapeutic point of view, three characteristics of the time course of action of the different types of insulin preparations are important: onset of action, time of peak activity, and duration of action. These depend on the rate of absorption after the subcutaneous injection. Table 43.1 summarizes the data on the insulin preparations currently on the market. These are general guidelines and may not pertain exactly to the clinical situation in which patients' physical activity and eating patterns differ from conditions imposed by a research study setting. The ranges are also only approximations because of the great intrinsic variability among patients and because the response of an occasional patient may differ considerably from the values listed.

Table 43.1 Time course of action of insulin preparations (times are approximations and may vary in different individuals)

Type	Onset (min)	Peak (h)	Duration (h)
Rapid acting • Lispro • Aspart • Glulisine	5–15	0.5–2.0	3.0–5.0
Short acting • Regular	0.50–1.0	2.0–4.0	6.0–8.0
Intermediate acting • NPH	2.0–4.0 h	4.0–10.0	10.0–16.0
Long acting • Glargine • Detemir	2–4 3–8	None None	~24 6–23*

*Duration depends on dose given (modified from AACE Diabetes Mellitus Guidelines, *Endocr Pract.* 2007;13(Suppl 1):17)

Variability of Insulin

There are many reasons that insulin has a variable action in a given individual. Insulin analogues tend to be less variable (that is, they have the least intra-subject variability when injected in the same individual and their activity is measured on different days) than the older insulins, particularly those of the lente series (lente and ultralente) which are the most variable.[9–11] The volume of a dose of insulin may alter its absorption, although this may be less true with the newer analogues. The site of injection can influence rate of absorption of the insulin as well as the depth of injection (intramuscular versus subcutaneous versus intradermal).[12–15] Once again, the analogue insulins tend to be less impacted by the site of injection than older insulin preparations.[16] Finally, regional blood flow can alter the absorption of insulin with factors such as exercise, skin temperature, and hydration status impacting absorption.[17] Patients with type 1 diabetes are often able to recognize variability in insulin activity and use this knowledge to inject insulin at different sites for different purposes (e.g., inject in a site that yields faster activity when the blood glucose level is high).

Species/Source

The initial insulins were purified from actual animal pancreases.[1] They were named for the species they came from pork, beef, and beef/pork. In 1986 the first recombinant human insulin was released onto the market. Because it is human insulin, produced in *Escherichia coli*, it is less immunogenic than the older animal insulin and has largely replaced use of the older animal insulins.

Comparing Regular Versus Analogue Insulins

The first type of insulin to be produced was regular insulin. It has no modifying agent and currently is the only one that should be administered intravenously. Figure 43.1 shows the structure of the insulin molecule, with its α and β chains, and region for self-aggregation and modification. When regular insulin is injected there is a delay in its absorption due to self-aggregation that occurs between insulin molecules.[18] Regular insulin forms a hexamer in subcutaneous tissue and must dissociate into a monomeric form to be absorbed. To overcome this problem insulin analogues have been created based on the knowledge that the related hormone insulin-like growth factor I (IGF-1) acts similarly to insulin but does not self-aggregate due to differences in the C-terminal portion of the β chain.[3] An analogue is regular human insulin that has been altered through a modification in its structure (usually in its amino acid composition, but other modifications are possible) that changes its tendency for self-aggregation and thus its absorption, but not its binding to the insulin receptor.[4] Table 43.2 compares all available insulin analogues and describes the modifications of each. In summary, rapid-acting insulin analogues tend to reduce postprandial hyperglycemia and reduce rates of hypoglycemia compared to regular insulin and long-acting analogues reduce nocturnal hypoglycemia and weight gain.[9] These findings are most evident in individuals with type 1 diabetes when all-analogue regimens are compared with all-human insulin regimens (early studies tended to compare a hybrid of analogue rapid-acting insulin with NPH as the bolus insulin).[9] Finally, analogue insulins reduce intra- and inter-subject variability in blood sugar response, which is related to the reduction in rates of hypoglycemia.

Rapid-Acting Insulin Analogues

Approved by the US FDA in 1996, insulin lispro (Humalog) was the first insulin analogue to enter the market. It is produced through recombinant DNA methods using *E. coli*. Lispro differs from regular insulin by inversion of the amino acids lysine and proline in the C-terminus of the β chain. This inversion reduces the formation of dimers and hexamers (which typically occurs with regular insulin) and thereby significantly facilitates the rate of absorption of lispro.[19–21] This increases both the onset of action and the time to peak concentration and decreases the time of return to baseline, more closely mimicking normal physiology. Insulin aspart (Novolog) was the second rapid-acting insulin to be introduced. Aspart differs from regular insulin by replacement of proline at position 28 of the β chain with the negatively charged aspartic acid.[22,23] It is produced by recombinant DNA technology using a modified strain of the yeast *Saccharomyces cerevisiae* (baker's yeast) as the production organism. The newest rapid-acting analogue is insulin glulisine (Apidra), which is produced from nonpathogenic *E. coli*. Insulin glulisine differs from human insulin in that the amino acid asparagine at position B3 is replaced by lysine and the lysine in position B29 is replaced by glutamic acid.[24,25] All three rapid-acting analogues are approved for treatment of type 1 and type 2 diabetes mellitus. Lispro and aspart have a Category B designation in pregnancy (presumed safety based on animal studies); glulisine is Category C (uncertain safety).

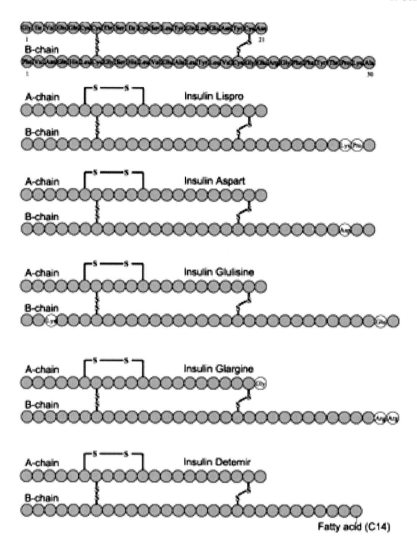

Fig. 43.1 Structure of the insulin molecule and alterations for various insulin analogues

Table 43.2 Differences in amino acid sequence of different insulin analogues

Type	Chain	Alteration
Lispro	β chain	Proline (b28)/lysine (b29) switched to lysine (b28)/proline (b29)
Aspart	β chain	Proline (b28) replaced by aspartic acid (b28)
Glulisine	β chain	Asparagine (b3) replaced by lysine (b3) lysine (b29) replaced by glutamic acid (b29)
Glargine	β chain	Two arginines added to end (b30) of β chain
	α chain	Asparagine (a21) replaced by glycine (a21)
Detemir	β chain	C-14 fatty acid side chain (myristic acid attached to lysine (b29). Threonine (b30) removed

The amino acid modifications in lispro, aspart, and glulisine result in subcutaneous absorption rates that are twice as fast and peak levels that are higher than those of regular insulin. More importantly, peak insulin action occurs approximately twice as fast with the rapid-acting analogues as compared to regular insulin and the levels return to baseline more rapidly than with regular insulin. These pharmacokinetic and pharmacodynamic properties more closely resemble physiologic meal-induced insulin secretion and provide greater flexibility and convenience to the patient since the analogues may be injected immediately before a meal or even after eating (as opposed to 30 min prior to meals for regular insulin).[26] Reviews of published clinical studies that compare the rapid-acting insulin analogues to regular insulin reveal the following generalizations:[3,4,9] (1) All three rapid-acting insulin analogues are superior to regular insulin in controlling postprandial hyperglycemia; (2) inter- and intra-patient variability tends to be reduced with the insulin analogues; (3) rapid-acting insulin analogues usually result in less hypoglycemia (a finding that is more pronounced in studies comparing all-analogue insulin to human insulin versus studies in which rapid-acting insulin is added to NPH as a basal insulin where rates of hypoglycemia may not be different[9]); and (4) rapid-acting insulin analogues are usually comparable to regular insulin at lowering HbA1c levels, although occasionally there is a greater improvement with the analogues.[27]

Long-Acting Insulin

Two long-acting insulin analogues are currently available. The first insulin glargine (Lantus) was approved by the US FDA in April 2000 and is produced by replacement of asparagine at position 21 of the α chain of regular insulin with glycine and addition of two arginine molecules to the C-terminus of the β chain. These modifications shift the isoelectric point leading to formation of microprecipitates in the subcutaneous tissue from which small amounts of insulin glargine are slowly released, resulting in a relatively constant concentration over 24 h.[28,29] In pharmacodynamic studies, insulin glargine was found to have a mean duration of action of 22 ± 4 h, without a pronounced peak. This profile allows glargine to be dosed once daily as basal insulin. In contrast, NPH insulin reaches a peak between 4 and 8 h, with a duration of action between 12 and 16 h. The fluctuations in diurnal serum insulin levels are significantly less in patients treated with glargine, compared to NPH or ultralente.[30]

The vast majority of clinical studies involving glargine have compared its efficacy and tolerability to NPH insulin. From these studies one common theme emerges:[31,32] once-daily glargine appears to be similar if not more efficacious than NPH in glycemic control and is associated with a significantly lower rate of hypoglycemia (particularly at night) as well as less glucose fluctuation.

Approved in June 2005, insulin detemir (Levemir) constitutes the other long-acting insulin analogue. Whereas all of the other insulin analogues are produced by either amino acid addition, inversion, or substitution of regular insulin, insulin detemir is produced by deletion of the final C-terminal amino acid molecule of regular insulin and addition of a 14-carbon fatty acid chain to lysine in position 29 of the β chain. These modifications allow insulin detemir to self-associate into hexamers and to also bind to albumin, both of which slowdown its systemic absorption.[33,34] Pharmacodynamic studies indicate that insulin detemir has a relatively flat action profile with a duration of action that appears dose dependent (mean duration of action ranging from 6 to 23 h). At higher doses (>0.4 units/kg), the duration of action is approximately 20 h. At lower dose (<0.4 units/kg), the duration of action is shorter and twice-daily dosing may be necessary.[35] Multiple studies suggest that intra-patient variability in insulin action is less with detemir compared with NPH and glargine.[36,37] The rates of hypoglycemia and weight gain are lower when detemir is compared to NPH.[33,38,39]

Both glargine and detemir are approved for the treatment of adult and pediatric patients with type 1 diabetes mellitus or adult patients with type 2 diabetes mellitus who require basal (long-acting) insulin. Because of their chemical properties, glargine and detemir cannot be mixed in the same syringe with other insulin preparations. Both have a category C designation in pregnancy. Detemir, because of its somewhat shorter duration of action, is often used as a twice a day drug, compared to glargine which is often used once a day in patients with type 1 diabetes.[35,40] However, individual patients may differ, with some needing only once-daily detemir and others needing twice a day glargine.

Premixed Insulins

Premixed insulin preparations should not be routinely used for the treatment of most patients with type 1 diabetes, due to the lack of flexibility, fixed ratios of rapid acting to longer acting insulin, and lack of data on achieving and maintaining tight control. However, in patients where reaching and maintaining near euglycemia is not possible and/or where this is the only insulin available, premixed insulin can be used to avoid the acute complications of diabetes and maintain control that is as close to target as possible.

Clinical Use of Insulin Analogues

In the treatment of type 1 diabetes, use of insulin analogues has become increasingly common. This is in part due to the clearly recognized need for achieving near euglycemia in people with type 1 diabetes and the marked increase in risk for severe hypoglycemia seen in studies using non-analogue insulin.[41] In patients followed at one DCCT center HbA1c levels fell with an increase in the rate of hypoglycemia on non-analogue insulin.[42] Once lispro was introduced, HbA1c levels continued to fall *without* a further increase in hypoglycemia. Reducing the variability of insulin activity and lessening weight gain make insulin analogues easier use in type 1 diabetes.

An important concept in using premeal insulin, and adequately lowering postprandial blood glucose levels, is the concept of "lag time." This is the ideal period of time during which a short or rapid-acting insulin should be injected before a meal in order to optimally control the postprandial blood glucose level.[43] The higher the blood sugar, the longer the lag time between insulin injection and eating. Although it is often easiest to inject insulin immediately prior to eating, use of continuous glucose monitoring makes the lag in onset of rapid-acting insulin more apparent in some individuals.

Intensive Insulin Therapy

The goal of insulin therapy is to provide insulin replacement in as physiologic a fashion as possible. Figure 43.2 shows the time course of action for the available insulin preparation – rapid-, short-, intermediate-, and long-acting. Ideally, for patients with type 1 diabetes, the most physiologic regimen is the use of a basal insulin combined with premeal boluses (Figs. 43.3 and 43.4). This can be accomplished either with a long-acting insulin such as glargine or with a detemir and premeal rapid-acting insulin (called multiple daily insulin injection or MDI therapy), or by using continuous subcutaneous insulin infusion (CSII) therapy. These approaches offer the most flexibility in lifestyle. However, these types of regimens require that patients either give 4–6 injections of insulin per day or master the use of an insulin pump plus learn how to do carbohydrate counting and test blood sugar levels before each insulin injection. Generally this requires self-monitoring of blood glucose levels more than three times per day [44,45] since an increased frequency of self-monitoring of blood glucose (SMBG) in people

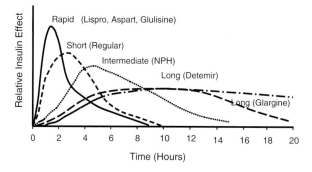

Fig. 43.2 Duration of action of various injected insulin preparations

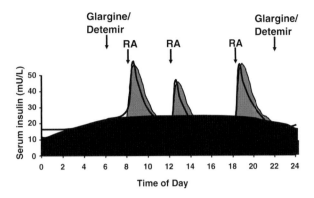

Fig. 43.3 Idealized insulin secretion and insulin replacement

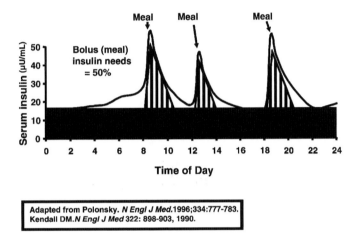

Fig. 43.4 Basal bolus insulin therapy

with type 1 diabetes on intensified regimens is associated with an improved HbA1c.[45] On non-analogue insulins patients on intensive regimens gain more weight and experience more hypoglycemia, as shown in the Diabetes Control and Complications Trial (DCCT).[46]

Less intensive regimens, such as twice a day NPH and regular insulin, may require less testing by the patient, but because the patient is taking an intermediate-acting insulin (NPH) they have much less flexibility in lifestyle. The insulin will peak 6–12 h after injection and the patient will need to eat at that time. To avoid hypoglycemia patients will often keep their blood sugar levels above target. No matter what the regimen, the goal for every patient is to keep their HbA1c level as close to normal as possible with a minimum number of hypoglycemic reactions, particularly avoiding severe reactions (that is, insulin reactions that require assistance of another person for treatment).

CSII Versus MDI

Continuous subcutaneous insulin infusion therapy was first used in the late 1970s. Its use has gradually increased since. Initial models were large and bulky, while current insulin pumps are available from a wide range of manufacturers with many features, including technology that helps calculate insulin doses. Early benefits were a reduction in episodes of hypoglycemia and a lowering of the fasting blood sugar level (by increasing insulin delivery to overcome the dawn phenomenon). Risks include diabetic ketoacidosis and infusion site infections.[47]

Benefits of CSII have been hard to quantitate, in part because studies are small and technology advances quickly. In earlier studies, comparing CSII to NPH-based MDI regimens, CSII was associated with improvements in outcomes, such as a reduction in rates of severe hypoglycemia.[48] The five-Nations Study Group, assessing 272 patients using CSII versus MDI, revealed less hypoglycemia and lower HbA1c levels in patients in CSII therapy. However, MDI therapy was NPH based, rather than based on a long-acting insulin analogue.[49] More recent studies comparing CSII to MDI regimens using rapid and long-acting insulin analogues show fewer differences.[50] In a pilot study involving 21 people with type 1 diabetes who had hypoglycemia unawareness and recurrent episodes of severe hypoglycemia, CSII, MDI, and intensive education alone were compared over 24 weeks. In both the analogue and the CSII groups there was a restoration of hypoglycemia awareness and a reduction in severe hypoglycemia. In both groups there was a reduction in HbA1c, although it did not reach significance in the CSII group.[51] A short-term (5 weeks in each arm) randomized cross-over study in 100 people with type 1 diabetes showed a reduction in glycemic exposure (as measured by fructosamine levels and continuous glucose monitoring) in patients on CSII compared to MDI with aspart and glargine insulin. The biggest improvement in glucose control was in the overnight/early morning blood sugar levels.[52]

A retrospective study from Sweden, comparing patients who chose CSII ($n = 563$) versus MDI therapy with glargine ($n = 513$), showed a greater reduction in HbA1c with CSII therapy (-0.59% versus -0.2%, $P < 0.001$), especially in those with a higher initial HbA1c level.[53] A retrospective study of the use of CSII in Spain revealed that patients followed on CSII for 2 years had greater improvements in HbA1c and greater reduction in the number of hypoglycemic episodes (mild and severe) compared to baseline therapy with MDI. Rates of diabetic ketoacidosis were not increased.[54] None of these studies are well randomized or include use of newer insulin pump features, such as bolus delivery calculators.

There is no well-studied approach to determining insulin to carbohydrate ratios (I:C) or correction ratios, and differing recommendations exist as to how to calculate these factors.[55–57] In many cases an initial dose is calculated based on what the patient appears to be doing on his/her initial insulin regimen or estimated based on the patient's weight. The dose is then adjusted based on pre- and 2 h postprandial blood sugar levels. In the American Diabetes Association guide for treating type 1 diabetes, the algorithm for determining the I:C is to multiply the body weight (lbs) by 2.8 and dividing this product by the total daily dose of insulin.[55] Another recommendation [56] suggests calculating the amount of carbohydrate for one unit of rapid-acting insulin by dividing 500 by the total daily insulin dose. Thus using the former method, in a 145-pound patient using 38 units of insulin per day, the I:C ratio is 1:11 and with the latter method it is 1:13. Use of pump bolus calculators can be effective [57] but requires accurately setting the target blood sugar level, the I:C, the insulin sensitivity (IS), and insulin on board factor, as self as accurate carbohydrate counting and a premeal blood sugar measurement.

In a study using a hyperinsulinemic euglycemic clamp technique, individual carbohydrate ratios were determined in patients with type 1 diabetes. Patients undergoing a glucose clamp were fed a meal and their exact insulin to carbohydrate ratio was determined. The average carbohydrate ratio was 1:9.3.[58] Additionally the investigators found that the peak postprandial blood sugar level occurred approximately 70 min (68.5 ± 8.8 min) after a meal. This finding is quite similar to a recent study using continuous glucose monitoring in which the time to peak postprandial blood glucose was 72 ± 23 min.[59]

Much of the literature involving CSII is in children, where management is somewhat different than in adults.[60] In a study comparing MDI with glargine and aspart versus CSII with aspart in 32 adolescents (average age of 13 years) with type 1 diabetes over 16 weeks the HbA1c was unchanged in the glargine group (8.2% versus 8.1%) and improved in the CSII group [61] (8.1–7.2%, $P < 0.05$ versus glargine group). Another pilot study showed that early use of CSII (within 1 month of diagnosis) in children ($n = 28$, mean age 12.1 ± 6 years) with new-onset type 1 diabetes led to a reduction in HbA1c from $10.5 \pm 2.4\%$ to between 6.5 and 7.4% over the next 18 months, with stable C-peptide levels over the first year of treatment.[62]

CSII offers the most flexibility with regards to reducing and adjusting the basal insulin levels and can calculate and deliver doses of insulin with greater accuracy than giving insulin by injection (the smallest increment on a syringe is 0.5 units, whereas pumps can deliver much smaller doses). In addition, pumps can make an estimation of how much insulin is still active, reducing correction doses to avoid overcorrection.

Whether or not to use CSII versus MDI is often a personal decision, and patients may change from one therapy to another and then back again. Quality of life is similar with either approach.[63] The greatest risk of CSII is an increased risk for diabetic ketoacidosis (DKA) because of the lack of available long-acting depot insulin. Therefore, some patients benefit from a hybrid of a once-daily dose of long-acting insulin to prevent DKA and CSII dosing for premeal and correction doses.[64] It is important to have a health-care team knowledgeable in the use of CSII and the necessary troubleshooting.

Side Effects of Insulin Therapy

The side effects of insulin therapy include delayed local skin reactions to injected insulin, true or systemic insulin allergy, insulin resistance, insulin-induced lipoatrophy, and insulin-induced lipohypertrophy. Three other possible sequelae of insulin administration are considered therapeutic effects, not side effects. The most common effect is hypoglycemia.[41] The other two are weight gain and the development of insulin edema. Weight gain often occurs as high blood sugars become normalized, with a subsequent reduction of glycosuria. The calories once lost in the urine can account for 70–100% of the weight gained.[65,66] Insulin edema occurs when a patient who was generally in very poor glycemic control begins to use insulin regularly, which, through its salt-retaining properties, causes the accumulation of fluid and an increase in plasma volume. This can lead to localized or even generalized edema.[67]

Local Reaction at the Site of Injection

Localized reactions at the site of insulin injection have become much less frequent with the advent of more pure human insulin preparations. However, local reactions do still occur[68] and have been associated with a hypersensitivity to non-insulin components, such as the latex in the insulin needle.[69] Patients should be referred to an allergist for testing, so that the offending antigens can be avoided. Generally it is possible to switch from one type of insulin to another or to find products that do not cause the allergy.

Systemic Insulin Allergy

True allergy to insulin, also called systemic insulin allergy, is rare, occurring in approximately 0.1% of diabetic patients receiving insulin.[7] The same sort of a reaction can occur to protamine, which is found in NPH insulin. It is much more common in patients with a history of interrupted insulin therapy than in those whose therapy has been continuous and in those who have received protamine in large doses previously (for instance to reverse anticoagulation following coronary artery bypass surgery). The manifestations of insulin allergy are usually seen within 1 or 2 weeks of the resumption of interrupted insulin therapy. The hallmark of true insulin allergy is an immediate local reaction (within 30–60 min) that gradually increases until large areas surrounding the injection site are involved.[7] In approximately one half of the patients, the reaction soon spreads into a generalized urticarial pattern and is occasionally associated with angioneurotic edema or even anaphylactic shock.[70,71] These systemic reactions are often preceded by gradual increases in the severity of an immediate local reaction, which may serve as a warning that serious difficulties lie ahead unless desensitization occurs.

  These immediate reactions seem to be allergic responses to the insulin molecule itself. They are rarely alleviated by the use of extremely pure insulin preparations. The clinical similarity to penicillin allergy is striking and the immunologic characteristics of true insulin allergy are almost identical to those of penicillin allergy. Both types of allergy involve [1] exquisite sensitivity to minute amounts of the antigen on conjunctival or intradermal testing, [2] passive transfer of an antibody (identified as IgE) that is capable of sensitizing normal skin to a subsequent challenge by the antigen, [3] high titers (as measured by direct assays) of IgE antibodies to the particular antigen in question, and [4] successful treatment by desensitization in almost all cases.[7] Although true insulin allergy is mediated by the same antibody (IgE) that causes atopic disease (asthma, allergic rhinitis, and urticaria), patients allergic to insulin apparently have no greater predisposition to atopy than do other patients. On the other hand, one-third of patients with true insulin allergy had a history of penicillin allergy.[71]

Treatment of Insulin Allergy

Skin testing by an allergist can be helpful – a variety of different types and species of insulin can be tested to determine if there are any that can be tolerated by the patient. To desensitize a patient, very small but gradually increasing amounts of insulin are injected after relatively short periods. These minute doses of the antigen bind to IgE, but the amount of histamine and other chemical mediators of inflammation released by the IgE–mast cell combination is too small to cause clinical symptoms. As the dose of injected insulin is gradually increased, the amount of insulin bound to IgE is thought to increase at a slow enough pace that the resultant mast cell degranulation causes no symptoms. Eventually, all of the IgE affixed to mast cells are bound to the increasing doses in insulin and the patient can tolerate the usual therapeutic doses of insulin.[7] This desensitization should be undertaken by an allergist or someone experienced in performing the procedure.

Insulin-Induced Lipoatrophy

Insulin-induced lipoatrophy is characterized by a loss of subcutaneous fat at the sites of insulin injections. Although this condition has become much less common with the introduction of more pure insulins, it still occurs.[72] Even though this form of local lipoatrophy is a benign condition, the cosmetic effect can be disturbing. Although the cause of this reaction is not certain, an immune response to contaminants in the administered insulin preparation may be involved.[73] Often injection of pure preparations of insulin into the affected sites leads to resolution of the problem.[74] However, lipoatrophy has occurred with nearly all type of insulin and means of delivery.[75]

Insulin-Induced Lipohypertrophy

Many patients receiving insulin manifest lipohypertrophy of subcutaneous fat tissue at the site of injection. This condition is likely due to a local lipogenic effect of insulin. Lipohypertrophy is a common problem: In one study it was found in approximately half of individuals using insulin.[76] Duration of insulin use, frequency of changing injection sites, and how often the needles were changed – all correlated with the development of lipohypertrophy.[76] Lipohypertrophy is also common at the abdominal sites of needle placement in patients using insulin pumps. One factor that predisposes to this reaction is repeated injections in the same place.[77] Once lipohypertrophy develops, patients may tend to continue injecting at this site because there may be less pain than at other sites. In addition to cosmetic considerations, continued injection into these areas is probably not wise because absorption of insulin from such sites is delayed and erratic.[78] Avoidance of lipohypertrophic areas for future insulin injections sometimes results in a gradual disappearance of hypertrophied areas. Severe insulin-induced lipohypertrophy has been successfully treated with liposuction.[79] In addition to lipohypertrophy, the development of fibrocollagenous nodules has been described at injection sites.[80] Injecting repeatedly into these areas leads to a marked deterioration of glycemic control which returned to normal once alternative sites were used.

Non-insulin Therapy: Pramlintide

Pramlintide (Symlin) is an analogue of amylin, a neuroendocrine hormone that is co-secreted from the beta cell along with insulin.[81,82] Pramlintide is injected prior to a meal, along with insulin, and it acts to reduce the postprandial blood glucose rise.[83] It does this both by causing a delay in gastric emptying as well as reducing postprandial glucagon levels. Additionally, it has an effect on satiety reducing the number of calories consumed with resultant weight loss.[84]

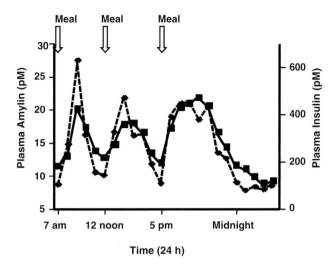

Fig. 43.5 Effects of pramlintide in subjects with type 1 diabetes

When pramlintide is added to the treatment regimen of a patient with type 1 diabetes there is generally a fall in HbA1c of ~0.3–0.5% with a reduction in weight of ~0.4–0.6 kg over 30–52 weeks [85,86] (Fig. 43.5). Additionally, patients often note an enhanced sense of well-being. In one study, patients taking pramlintide had a greater sense of treatment satisfaction, compared to placebo, with similar levels of glycemic control. This was true whether the patient was using CSII or MDI.[87]

The major serious side effect noted in the original clinical trials was an increase in the rate of severe hypo-glycemia.[88] This was predominantly due to the fact that the pramlintide was added to a fixed dose of premeal insulin. When patients took the pramlintide they ate less and became hypoglycemic. Subsequent studies in which insulin doses were reduced and the pramlintide titrated to effect showed no difference in rates of severe hypo-glycemia between the pramlintide-treated and the control groups.[85,86] Therefore, when starting pramlintide the dose of premeal insulin should be reduced by 50%. When using CSII a square wave bolus over 2–3 h is often most effective (to mesh with the delay in food absorption) and with MDI, a switch to premeal regular insulin (with its longer duration of action) can be useful. Finally, in patients who perform carbohydrate counting, pram-lintide can be started before the meal with the rapid-acting insulin injected after the meal, the dose based on the amount of carbohydrate consumed.

Devices

Insulin Pens

Insulin pens were first introduced in the 1980s, in an attempt to make insulin delivery more convenient and possibly less fear-inducing.[89,90] By definition they contain some form of insulin, although there are also pens prefilled with pramlintide to administer along with insulin. Pens tend to be preferred by patients when compared to vials and syringes.[91] Insulin pens may also be more accurate.[92,93] However, pens are devices and must be used appropriately. Some require reusable cartridges, others are prefilled. Each time a new needle is attached; it must be primed with a flush of two to four units of insulin so that a full dose is delivered. Occasionally pens malfunction and do not deliver the desired amount of insulin.[94] If a patient using an insulin pen has unexplained high blood sugars, the use of a new pen and reinforcement of the need for priming should be considered. The patient should see a stream of insulin flow from the tip of the pen needle before assuming the pen is ready for use. All patients should know how to use a vial and syringe, in case pens are not available. Most insulin preparations are now available in pen form.

Continuous Glucose Monitoring

Short of a cure for type 1 diabetes, technology that can continuously monitor blood glucose levels, particularly if coupled to a pump to create a closed loop system, has long been sought. Initial, less successful attempts at continuous glucose monitoring included a 3-day Minimed Continuous Glucose Monitoring System (CGMS) and the GlucoWatch G2 Biographer.[95] The former did not provide real-time data to patients and was not widely used, although it did provide a 3-day retrospective report of blood glucose levels and trends.[96] The GlucoWatch Biographer was a large wristwatch-like device that drew up interstitial fluid through the skin and measured glucose levels every 10 min for up to 13 h.[97] Alarms alerted the user to high, low, and falling glucose levels. Neither device was reliable for detecting hypoglycemia and the GlucoWatch had a high rate of false alarms.[98] It did not improve control beyond what is possible with standard SMBG.[99]

Current devices have been shown to be more useful. The Medtronic Minimed Continuous Glucose Monitor (CGM), the Dexcom STS, and the Navigator (not FDA approved at the time of this writing) provide near-continuous monitoring of interstitial glucose levels every 1–5 min and a continuous readout of glucose values and trends. These devices can be set to alarm when reaching a high or low targets as well as when glucose levels are rising or falling rapidly. However, because they read interstitial fluid rather than blood glucose concentration, there is a physiologic lag between meter reading and the corresponding blood glucose levels. This lag is greatest during periods of rapid glucose change and can be up to 20 min. Due to this lag, and the lack of large clinical trials assessing the accuracy of these devices in clinical use, CGM systems are approved for adjunctive use, not as replacement for SMBG.[95,100]

Traditional models for assessing the accuracy of single point-in-time blood glucose testing, such as the traditional Clarke error grid, do not accurately assess the functionality of CGM because they do not factor in the benefits of knowing the direction and rate of glucose change. Therefore, the continuous glucose-error grid analysis (CG-EGA) was developed to measure these dynamic properties.[101] The CG-EGA works by analyzing pairs of reference and sensor readings as a process in time, with point and rate comparisons combined into a single accuracy analysis for each of three blood glucose ranges hypoglycemia (<70 mg/dl), euglycemia (70–180 mg/dl), and hyperglycemia (>180 mg/dl). Results are then plotted on a grid subdivided into five zones representing the clinical outcome that might occur if the patient acted on the CGM data. Values in zones A and B represent accurate or benign error readings; values in zone C may result in unnecessary corrections; values in zone D signify a dangerous failure to detect and treat; and values in zone E denote erroneous treatment.[101]

In a study to assess the accuracy of the FreeStyle Navigator CGM 58 subjects with type 1 diabetes wore two sensors simultaneously and had frequent venous measurements taken while residing for 5 days in a clinical research center.[102] Comparison of the 20,362 FreeStyle Navigator measurements with the laboratory reference method gave mean and median absolute relative differences (ARDs) of 12.8 and 9.3%, respectively. The percentage in the Clarke error grid zone A was 81.7% and in zone B was 16.7%. Readings were similar on days 1 and 5 of sensor use.

Sensors last from 3 to 7 days, with the Dexcom system marketing the longest-lasting sensor.[103] Each system is somewhat different and requires training on its features. In all there is a physiologic lag between the interstitial and the capillary glucose levels, which is most pronounced when the blood sugar levels are falling or increasing rapidly.[104] Calibration of the CGM system is best done during periods of relative glucose stability.[105]

Small studies have been done to assess the utility of CGM. These studies produced largely positive results, although changes in HbA1c levels were small. In a small study ($n = 24$) of adults with type 1 diabetes over 3 months there was a significant decrease in HbA1c level of $0.4 \pm 0.5\%$ from baseline (starting HbA1c = $7.43 \pm 1.0\%$). This difference was significant when compared to a control group who did not wear the CGM. Although there was a difference in the time spent within the target range, there was not a significant reduction in rates of hypoglycemia.[106] In a larger home use study, 140 adults with diabetes were followed in a 12-week observational study using the Dexcom 3-day CGM device.[107] Overall, a reduction in HbA1c of $0.4 \pm 0.05\%$ (least squares mean $\pm$ SE, $P < 0.0001$) was found. The greatest HbA1c reductions were found in patients with the highest initial HbA1c values as well as in those who used the CGM device most frequently.

A multicenter study evaluated the safety and effectiveness of the 7-day Dexcom CGM in 86 subjects.[108] Subjects wore a sensor for 7 days during each of three consecutive periods. During the first period subjects were blinded to the data and were unblinded for the second two periods. Overall, 97.2% of the 6811 matched (CGM to SMBG) data points fell in the Clarke error grid zones A and B, with an 11% median absolute relative difference. After unblinding, subjects reduced the time spent in hypoglycemic range (<55 mg/dl) by 0.3 h/day, reduced the time spent in hyperglycemic range (>240 mg/dl) by 1.5 h/day, and increased time in the target zone (81–140 mg/dl) by 1.4 h/day. This study was not designed to assess the change in HbA1c levels.

In another randomized controlled study of insulin-requiring patients using the DexCom STS sensor, those given access to continuous glucose readings and alerts/alarms managed episodes of hyperglycemia and hypoglycemia more effectively than control subjects blinded to this information.[109] On average, the unblinded group spent 21% ($P < 0.0001$) less time in hypoglycemic (<55 mg/dl), 23% ($P < 0.0001$) less time in hyperglycemic (>240 mg/dl), and 26% ($P < 0.0001$) more time in the target glycemic range (81–140 mg/dl).

The application of the CGM systems to help people with type 1 diabetes when performing exercise or doing other strenuous activity has been studied. In one study, patients with type 1 diabetes performing vigorous physical activity were studied with a Guardian RT CGM.[110] Five subjects with type 1 diabetes were monitored before, during, and after a 60-min vigorous spinning class using the Guardian RT CGM. Three of the subjects were found to have late-onset hypoglycemia which was identified with the CGM technique, suggesting that CGM could be a useful tool in monitoring the response to exercise. CGM has been found to be helpful in marathon runners.[111] Another application for CGM has been to assess glycemic control following islet cell transplantation.[112] In a study of eight subjects with type 1 diabetes following islet cell transplantation, CGM revealed that less glycemic variability and hypoglycemia were present in C-peptide-positive patients after transplantation.

Many of the studies on CGM have been performed in children. DirecNet is a consortium of investigators who are examining the utility of CGM and other treatment modalities in children with type 1 diabetes.[113] DirecNet studies should help define the benefits and limitations of CGM in this population.

In summary, the benefits of CGM could be multiple, although large clinical trials have not been performed to prove these benefits. Potential advantages of CGM include its ability to alarm when patients fall below a certain threshold blood sugar as well as when the blood sugar is trending toward hypoglycemia. This could allow for earlier treatment or even avoidance of hypoglycemia. Real-time data can provide the user with the knowledge of whether glucose levels are rising or falling before a snack or meal and insulin dose and carbohydrate load consumed can be adjusted. High alarms can alert users to significant hyperglycemia. Finally, the stored data can be used for retrospective analysis by the health-care provider, with a focus on adjusting basal rates, overnight blood sugars and correction boluses, and carbohydrate ratios. Drawbacks include the high cost, the inaccuracies of measurement, the risk for insulin stacking (giving insulin too often when the blood sugar level is high), and technical difficulties with the devices.

The Future

Closed Loop Systems

A closed loop system would provide seamless blood glucose management, with the sensor feeding information to a pump, which in turn delivers insulin based on a series of algorithms. Although not yet available, such systems are being developed.[114] A pilot study was performed using two Minimed CGMS sensors and a Minimed pump which communicated via radiofrequency to a laptop computer containing algorithms that provided closed loop control of insulin delivery.[115] The closed loop use of the system was compared to its open loop use. Although the mean glucose levels were the same with both type of use, 75% of the time during closed loop treatment patients were between 70 and 180 mg/dl compared to 63% of the time for the open loop approach. As part of the Long-term Sensor System Project ten individuals with type 1 diabetes were implanted with a pump (Medical Research Group, Minimed Medtronic) for peritoneal insulin delivery and a central intravenous glucose sensor was implanted close to the right atrium. The pump and the sensor were connected by a subcutaneous lead. Over 9 months of use, the glucose levels by the intravenous sensors correlated fairly well with meter values ($r = 0.83$–0.93). Glucose control was similar to that seen with CSII and standard CGM. The lag in the response of the intravenous sensors to the change in glucose levels was the major limitation to mimicking nondiabetic physiology.[116]

Attempts to further develop and refine insulin infusion algorithms should help overcome some of the existing barriers to closing the loop,[117,118] although the lag-time issues with the sensors still need to be resolved.

Replacing Beta Cells

Pancreas Transplantation

Whole pancreas transplantation, most commonly in conjunction with a kidney transplant, although occasionally done alone, has been available for over 20 years. It can offer patients with type 1 diabetes varying degrees of insulin independence over time.[119] Traditionally pancreas transplants were difficult to perform due to the inherent fragility of the organ during surgical manipulation and the need to manage the pancreatic exocrine secretions. Techniques have improved over time, with the use of bladder drainage (which allows the measurement of urinary amylase to assess exocrine function) and improved matching between donor and recipient. Introduction of new immunosuppressive agents, such as tacrolimus and mycophenolate mofetil, and reduction of corticosteroid doses have reduced rates of acute rejection and improved graft survival. In a study of early transplant recipients (1982–1993) and more recent transplant recipients rates of at least one rejection episode in the first year after transplant were 76 and 33%, respectively.[120]

Pancreas graft survival has increased over time. With current immunosuppressive regimens the 3-year graft survival approaches 80%.[121] Simultaneous pancreas kidney (SPK) transplants have had better outcomes than pancreas transplant alone (PTA), although rates for PTA survival have improved markedly. Twenty-five percent of pancreas transplants are PTA in the United States,[122] with a small percentage as living donor pancreas transplantation. Due to the risks associated with surgery and immunosuppression this procedure is reserved for those who are unable to safely use insulin or those already requiring immunosuppression for a kidney transplant. The leading cause of death in patients following pancreas transplant is cardiovascular disease.[121]

Islet Cell Transplantation

Islet cell transplantation has been explored as a method for treating type 1 diabetes.[123] Early efforts were limited by the technical difficulties inherent in isolating sufficient numbers of islets from the donor pancreas. From 1990 to 1998, 267 islet allotransplantations were performed, with insulin independence of only 8% at 1 year.[124] Success with seven patients following the Edmonton Protocol (which consists of a glucocorticoid-free combination of daclizumab, tacrolimus, and sirolimus as well as specialized procedures for isolation of islets) leads to hope that this procedure could be beneficial to many with type 1 diabetes.

Unfortunately, many hurdles need to be overcome exist until this therapy (or a modification of it) can benefit a large number of individuals with type 1 diabetes. For instance, when Edmonton Protocol was replicated at additional institutions, the insulin-free success rate was center dependent, ranging from 23 to 90% depending on the institution.[127,128] Additionally, islet cells from more than one donor are usually required to obtain enough cells for a functional transplant, making supply of islet cells a significant hurdle. Further, such approach also exposes the recipient to the risk of multiple donors. Side effects associated with the infusion of the islets into the liver through the portal vein include bleeding, portal vein thrombosis, and portal hypertension.[124] The immunosuppressive agents can cause mouth ulcerations, edema, proteinuria, hypercholesterolemia, and hypertension among other complications.[126]

Finally, islets fail over time, making improvement relatively short-lived.[125] Only 10% of patients are insulin free at 5 years, although the majority (83%) from Edmonton retain some islet cell function (as measured by C-peptide secretion) at 5 years.[129] The reasons for the islet cell loss are unknown, although many theories are under investigation. The causes of islet cell loss likely involve some form of acute and/or chronic rejection as well as possible thrombotic and inflammatory reactions.[130] Thus, current candidates for islet cell transplantation are those with hypoglycemia unawareness with recurrent, severe episodes of hypoglycemia in spite of maximal medical therapy – patients who are not able to safely survive on exogenous insulin regimens.

To overcome some of these barriers, safer immunosuppressive regimens are being studied[131] and new methods for producing islet cells are being explored. Islet cells encased in a biodegradable scaffolds might improve survival.[132] Stem cell research may help with both embryonic and adult stem cells showing promise for providing sources of islet cells for transplantation.[133,134] Encapsulation technologies might help enhance the immunosuppression-free survival of transplanted islet cells.[135]

Immunologic Modification

Type 1 diabetes is an autoimmune disease, and treatments involving "turning off" or creating tolerance to the autoimmune response to the beta cell could cure type 1 diabetes (and would eliminate the problem associated with rejection of transplanted beta cells). Much animal research has been done in this area, and small clinical trials have been begun. The autoimmunity appears to be due to alterations in both T- and B-cell activity, although the full details of the disorder are far from fully elucidated.[136] Researchers have studied various approaches to the treatment of early type 1 diabetes with the hope of stopping process of beta cell destruction and possibly preventing the development of the autoimmune process altogether.

Use of existing markers of islet cell autoimmunity (anti-GAD, anti-islet cell, and anti-insulin antibodies) can help predict who is most likely to progress to type 1 diabetes.[137] In the Diabetes Prevention Trial, relatives of patients with type 1 diabetes who were at high risk for developing the disease were started on low-dose insulin therapy. This was, however, shown not to be effective in slowing the progression to type 1 diabetes.[138] Another approach is to use insulin as an autoantigen in an attempt to delete insulin-reactive T cells and target T-cell receptors through use of vaccines.[139] Other forms of therapy to induce tolerance are under investigation.[140] Clinical Trials Database studies include those investigating the effects of rituximab, polyclonal anti-T-lymphocyte globulin (ATG), mycophenolate mofetil–daclizumab, proleukin, and rapamune and study of thymoglobulin, TRX4, monoclonal antibody, hOKT3gamma1 (Ala–Ala).[141] Additionally, TrialNet is a consortium of investigators around the world who are studying the prevention and early treatment of type 1 diabetes. Their website lists opportunities to join ongoing clinical research trials.[142]

Microencapsulation

Another approach to the restoration of beta cell function is to inject human or porcine islets that are protected with microcapsules. This would allow for implantation without need for immunosuppression. Microcapsules have to be biocompatible and permselective, in order for them to function as fully regulated islet cells. Early human studies are underway to assess the safety and viability of these techniques.[143,144]

Treatment of Macrovascular Risk

Patients with type 1 diabetes have an increased risk of cardiovascular disease when compared to people without diabetes.[145] When 173 subjects with type 1 diabetes, 834 participants with type 2 diabetes, and 1294 participants without diabetes were compared during an 18-year follow-up, cardiovascular mortality rates per 1000 person-years were 23.1 in subjects with type 1 diabetes, 35.3 in participants with type 2 diabetes, and 4.6 in those without diabetes. Risk of cardiovascular disease (CVD) was related to glycemic control, with an increment of 1% in HbA1c increasing CVD mortality by 52.5% in people with type 1 diabetes and by 7.5% in subjects with type 2 diabetes.

Data from the Epidemiology of Diabetes Interventions and Complications (EDIC) Trial, which is the follow-up to the DCCT, showed that over a mean of 17 years of follow-up (DCCT + EDIC), intensive treatment reduced the risk of any cardiovascular disease event by 42% ($P = 0.02$) and the risk of nonfatal myocardial infarction, stroke, or death from cardiovascular disease by 57% ($P = 0.02$).[146] The decrease in HbA1c levels during the DCCT was significantly associated with a reduction in the risk of CVD. Microalbuminuria and albuminuria were associated with a significant increase in the risk of cardiovascular disease, but differences between treatment groups remained significant after adjusting for these factors. Subjects in the intensively controlled groups also had lower geometric mean coronary artery calcium scores than did those in the conventionally treated group, and the amount of coronary calcium was associated with the HbA1c level.[147]

In addition, individuals with type 1 diabetes and the metabolic syndrome appear to have the greatest risk for developing CVD. In one study people with type 1 diabetes and the metabolic syndrome, as defined by the WHO, had a significantly higher macrovascular composite end point (OR = 3.3, $P = 0.02$), compared to individuals with type 1 diabetes without the metabolic syndrome. Therefore, these individuals are at higher risk for CVD and should receive aggressive risk factor modification.[148]

Summary

Type 1 diabetes is a treatable but not curable disease. Improvements in the treatment of type 1 diabetes have occurred through the development of insulin analogues and technologies that make living with type 1 diabetes easier. In most cases, adequate treatment of type 1 diabetes requires intensive patient education, with a team consisting of a dietitian, diabetes educator, endocrinologist, and others. A focus needs to be directed at reaching glycemic and CVD risk modifying targets and maintaining near-normal values over time. A cure for type 1 diabetes remains elusive, but promising research both in new approaches to islet cell transplantation and in immunomodulation may ultimately lead to elimination of this manageable yet problematic disease.

References

1. Heller S, Kozlovski P, Kurtzhals P. Insulin's 85th anniversary—an enduring medical miracle. *Diabetes Res Clin Pract.* 2007;78:149–158.
2. Otieno CF, Kayima JK, Omonge EO, Oyoo GO. Diabetic ketoacidosis: risk factors, mechanisms and management strategies in sub-Saharan Africa: a review. *East Afr Med J.* 2005;82(12 Suppl):S197–S203.
3. Hirsch I. Insulin Analogues. *N Engl J Med.* 2005;352:174–183.
4. Vazquez-Carrera M, Silvestre JS. Insulin analogues in the management of diabetes. *Methods Find Exp Clin Pharm.* 2004;26:445–461.
5. Kelley DE. Sugars and starch in the nutritional management of diabetes mellitus. *Am J Clin Nutr.* 2003;78:858S–864S.
6. ADA Insulin Administration. *Diabetes Care.* 2004;27:S.
7. Harmel ALP, Mathur R. *Davidson Diabetes Mellitus.* 5th ed. Philadelphia, PA: WB Saunders Company; 2004.
8. Cochran E, Musso C, Gorden P. The use of U500 insulin in patients with extreme insulin resistance. *Diabetes Care.* 2005;28:1240–1244.
9. Gough SCL. A review of human and analogue insulin trials. *Diab Res Clin Pract.* 2007;77:1–15.
10. Galloway JA, Spradlin CT, Nelson RL, Wentworth SM, Davidson JA, Swarner JL. Factors influencing the absorption, serum insulin concentration, and blood glucose responses after injections of regular insulin and various insulin mixtures. *Diabetes Care.* 1981;4:366–376.
11. Binder C, Lauritzen T, Faber O, Pramming S. Insulin pharmacokinetics. *Diabetes Care.* 1984;7:188–199.
12. Sindelka G, Heinemann L, Berger M, et al. Effect of insulin concentration, subcutaneous fat thickness and skin temperature on subcutaneous insulin absorption in healthy subjects. *Diabetologia.* 1994;37:377.
13. Thow J, Home P. Insulin injection technique: depth of injection is important. *Brit Med J.* 1990;301:3–4.
14. Bantle JP, Neal L, Frankamp LM. Effects of the anatomical region used for insulin injections in type 1 diabetic subjects. *Diabetes Care.* 1993;12:1592–1597.
15. Guerra SM, Kitabchi AE. Comparison of the effectiveness of various routes of insulin injection: insulin levels and glucose response in normal subjects. *J Clin Endocrinol Metab.* 1976;42:869–874.
16. Guerci B, Sauvanet JP. Subcutaneous insulin: pharmacokinetic variability and glycemic variability. *Diabetes Met.* 2005;31(4 Pt 2):4S7–4S24.
17. Koivisto VA, Felig P. Alterations in insulin absorption and in blood glucose control associated with varying insulin injection sites in diabetic patients. *Ann Intern Med.* 1980;92:59.
18. Blundell TL, Cutfield JF, Cutfield SM, et al. Three-dimensional atomic structure of insulin and its relationship to activity. *Diabetes.* 1972;21(suppl 2):492–505.
19. Howey DC, Bowsher RR, Brunelle RL, Woodworth JR. Lys(B28), Pro(B29)-human insulin. A rapidly absorbed analogue of human insulin. *Diabetes.* 1994;43:396–402.

20. Jacobs MA, Keulen ET, Kanc K, et al. Metabolic efficacy of preprandial administration of Lys(B28), Pro(B29) human insulin analog in IDDM patients: a comparison with human regular insulin during a three-meal test period. *Diabetes Care*. 1997;20:1279–1286.

21. Howey DC, Bowsher RR, Brunell RL, et al. [Lys(B28), Pro(B29)]-human insulin: effect of injection time on postprandial glycemia. *Clin Pharm Ther*. 1995;58:459–469.

22. Raskin P, Guthrie RA, Leiter L, Riis A, Jovanovic L. Use of insulin aspart, a fast-acting insulin analog, as the mealtime insulin in the management of patients with type 1 diabetes. *Diabetes Care*. 2000;23:583–588.

23. Home PD, Lindholm A, Riis A. Insulin aspart vs human insulin in the management of long-term blood glucose control in type 1 diabetes mellitus: a randomized controlled trial: European Insulin Aspart Study Group. *Diabet Med*. 2000;17:762–770.

24. Becker RH, Frick AD, Nosek L, Heinemann L, Rave K. Dose-response relationship of insulin glulisine in subjects with type 1 diabetes. *Diabetes Care*. 2007;30:2506–2507.

25. Becker RH, Frick AD. Clinical pharmacokinetics and pharmacodynamics of insulin glulisine. *Clin Pharmacokinetics*. 2008;47:7–20.

26. Rave K, Klelin O, Frick AD, Becker RH. Advantage of premeal-injected insulin glulisine compared with regular human insulin in subjects with type 1 diabetes. *Diabetes Care*. 2006;29:1812–1817.

27. Garg SK, Rosenstock J, Ways K. Optimized basal-bolus insulin regimens in type 1 diabetes: insulin glulisine versus regular human insulin in combination with basal insulin glargine. *Endocr Pract*. 2005;11:11–17.

28. Heinemann L, Linkeschova R, Rave K, Hompesch B, Sedlak M, Heise T. Time-action profile of the long-acting insulin analog glargine (HOE901) in comparison with those of NPH insulin and placebo. *Diabetes Care*. 2000;23:644–649.

29. Pieber TR, Eugene-Jolchine I, Derobert E. Efficacy and safety of HOE 901 versus NPH insulin in patients with type 1 diabetes. The European Study Group of HOE 901 in type 1 diabetes. *Diabetes Care*. 2000;23:157–162.

30. Gerich J, Becker RHA, Zhu R, Bolli GA. Fluctuation of serum basal insulin levels following single and multiple dosing of insulin glargine. *Diabetes Technol Ther*. 2006;8:237–243.

31. Ratner RE, Hirsch IB, Neifing JL, Garg SK, Mecca TE, Wilson CA. Less hypoglycemia with insulin glargine in intensive insulin therapy for type 1 diabetes. US Study Group of Insulin Glargine in Type 1 Diabetes. *Diabetes Care*. 2000;23:639–643.

32. Porcellati F, Rossetti P, Pampanelli S, et al. Better long-term glycaemic control with the basal insulin glargine as compared with NPH in patients with type 1 diabetes mellitus given meal-time lispro insulin. *Diabetic Med*. 2004;21:1213–1220.

33. Raskin P. Efficacy and safety of insulin detemir. *Endo Met Clin North Am*. 2007;36(suppl 1):21–32.

34. Brunner GA, Sendlhofer G, Wutte A, et al. Pharmacokinetic and pharmacodynamic properties of long-acting insulin analogue NN304 in comparison to NPH insulin in humans. *Exp Clin Endo Diab*. 2000;108:100–106.

35. Porcellati F, Rossetti P, Busciantella MR, et al. Comparison of pharmacokinetics and dynamics of the long-acting insulin analogs glargine and detemir at steady state in type 1 diabetes: a double-blind randomized, crossover study. *Diabetes Care*. 2007;30:2447–2452.

36. Axelson M, Madsbad S, Perrild H, Kristensen A, Axelson M. More predictable fasting blood glucose with the new soluble basal insulin analogue, insulin detemir: a comparison with NPH in type 1 diabetic patients. *Diabetes Res Clin Pract*. 2000;50(Suppl 1):S79–S82.

37. Kurtzhals P. Pharmacology of insulin detemir. *Endo Met Clin North Am*. 2007;36(suppl 1):14–20.

38. Hermansen K, Lund P, Clemmensen K, et al. 3-month results from Denmark within the globally prospective and observational study to evaluate insulin detemir treatment in type 1 and type 2 diabetes: The PREDICTIVE Study. *Rev Diabet Stud*. 2007;4:89–97.

39. Hermansen K, Madsbad S, Perrild H, Kristensen A, Axelsen M. Comparison of the soluble basal insulin analog insulin detemir with NPH randomized open crossover trial in type 1 diabetic subjects on basal-bolus. *Diabetes Care*. 2001;24:296–301.

40. Pieber TR, Treichel H-C, Hompesch B, et al. Comparison of insulin detemir and insulin glargine in subjects with type 1 diabetes using intensive therapy. *Diabetic Med*. 2007;24:635–642.

41. The Diabetes Control and Complications Trial (DCCT) Research Group. The effect of intensive treatment of diabetes on the development and progression of long-term complications in insulin-dependent diabetes mellitus. *N Engl J Med*. 1993;329:977–986.

42. Chase HP, Lockspeiser T, Perry B, et al. The impact of the DCCT and Humalog insulin on glycohemoglobin levels and severe hypoglycemia in type 1 diabetes. *Diabetes Care*. 2001;24:430–434.

43. DeWitt DE, Hirsch IB. Outpatient insulin therapy in type 1 and type 2 diabetes mellitus: scientific review. *JAMA*. 2003;289:2254–2264.

44. American Diabetes Association. Standards of medical care in diabetes—2008. *Diabetes Care*. 2008;31(Suppl 1):S12–S54.

45. Schutt M, Kern W, Krause U, et al. Is the frequency of self-monitoring of blood glucose related to long-term metabolic control? Multicenter analysis including 24,500 patients from 191 centers in Germany and Austria. *Exp Clin Endo Diab*. 2006;114:383–388.

46. Purnell JQ, Hokanson JE, Marcovina SM, Steffes MW, Cleary PA, Brunzell JD. Effect of excessive weight gain with intensive therapy of type 1 diabetes on lipid levels and blood pressure: results from the DCCT. *JAMA*. 1998;280:140–146.

47. American Diabetes Association. Continuous subcutaneous insulin infusion (position statement). *Diabetes Care*. 2004;27:S110.

48. Bode BW, Steed RD, Davidson PC. Reduction in severe hypoglycemia with long-term continuous subcutaneous insulin infusion in type 1 diabetes. *Diabetes Care*. 1996;19:324–327.

49. Hoogma RP, Hammond PJ, Gomis R, et al. Comparison of the effects of continuous subcutaneous insulin infusion (CSII) and NPH-based multiple daily insulin injections (MDI) on glycaemic control and quality of life: results of the 5-nations trial. *Diabet Med.* 2006;23:141–147.

50. Lepore G, Dodesini AR, Nosari I, Trevisan R. Both continuous subcutaneous insulin infusion and a multiple daily insulin injection regimen with glargine as basal insulin are equally better than traditional multiple daily insulin injection treatment. *Diabetes Care.* 2003;26:1321–1322.

51. Thomas RM, Aldibbiat A, Griffin W, Cox MAA, Leech NJ, Shaw JAM. A randomized pilot study in type 1 diabetes complicated by severe hypoglycemia, comparing rigorous hypoglycemia avoidance with insulin analogue therapy, CSII or education alone. *Diabetic Med.* 2007;24:778–783.

52. Hirsch IB, Bode BW, Garg S, et al. Continuous subcutaneous insulin infusion (CSII) of insulin aspart versus multiple daily injection of insulin aspart/insulin glargine in type 1 diabetic patients previously treated with CSII. *Diabetes Care.* 2005;28:533–538.

53. Fahlen M, Eliasson B, Oden A. Optimization of basal insulin delivery in type 1 diabetes: a retrospective study on the use of continuous subcutaneous insulin infusion and insulin glargine. *Diabetic Med.* 2005;22:382–386.

54. Gimenez M, Conget I, Jansa M, Vidal M, Chiganer G, Levy I. Efficacy of continuous subcutaneous insulin infusion in type 1 diabetes: a 2-year perspective using the established criteria for funding from a National Health Service. *Diabet Med.* 2007;24:1419–1423.

55. Davidson PC, Hebblewhite HR, Bode BW, et al. Statistically based CSII parameters: correction factor, CF (1700 rule), carbohydrate-insulin ratio, CIR (2.8 rule), and basal-to-total ratio. *Diabetes Technol Ther.* 2003;5:237.

56. Walsh J, Roberts R. *Pumping Insulin.* San Diego, CA: Torrey Pines Press; 2006: 139–141.

57. Gross TM, Kayne D, King A, Rother C, Juth S. A bolus calculator is an effective means of controlling postprandial glycemia in patients on insulin pump therapy. *Diabetes Technol Ther.* 2003;5:365–369.

58. Bevier WC, Zisser H, Palerm CC, et al. Calculating the insulin to carbohydrate ratio using the hyperinsulinaemic-euglycaemic clamp-a novel use for a proven technique. *Diabetes/Metabolism Res Rev.* 2007;23:472–478.

59. Manuel-y-Keenoy B, Vertommen J, Abrams P, Van Gaal L, De Leeuw I, Messeri D, Poscia A. Postprandial glucose monitoring in type 1 diabetes mellitus: use of a continuous subcutaneous monitoring device. *Diabetes Metab Res Rev.* 2004 Nov-Dec;20 (2):S24–S31.

60. Silverstein J, Klingensmith G, Copeland K, et al. Care of children and adolescents with type 1 diabetes. *Diabetes Care.* 2005;28:186–212.

61. Doyle EA, Weinzimer SA, Steffen AT, et al. A randomized, prospective trial comparing the efficacy of CSII with MDI using glargine. *Diabetes Care.* 2004;27:1554–1558.

62. Ramachandani N, Ten S, Anhalt H, et al. Insulin pump therapy from the time of diagnosis of type 1 diabetes. *Diabetes Technol Ther.* 2006;8:663–669.

63. Hoogma RP, Spijker AJ, van Doorn-Scheele M, et al. Quality of life and metabolic control in patients with diabetes mellitus type 1 treated by CSII or MDI injections. *Neth J Med.* 2004;62:383–387.

64. Alemzadeh R, Parton EA, Holzum MK. Feasibility of continuous subcutaneous insulin infusion and daily supplemental insulin glargine injection in children with type 1 diabetes. *Diabetes Technol Ther.* 2009 Aug;11(8): 481–486.

65. Shank ML, Del Prato S, DeFronzo RA. Bedtime insulin/daytime glipizide: effective therapy for sulfonylurea failures in NIDDM. *Diabetes.* 1995;44:165.

66. Carlson MG, Campbell PJ. Intensive insulin therapy and weight gain in IDDM. *Diabetes.* 1993;42:1700.

67. Lee P, Kinsella J, Borkman M, Carter J. Bilateral pleural effusions, ascites, and facial an peripheral oedema in a 19-year-old woman 2 weeks following commencement of insulin lispro and detemir—an unusual presentation of insulin oedema. *Diabetic Med.* 2007;24:1282–1285.

68. Radermecker RP, Scheen AJ. Allergy reactions to insulin: effects of continuous subcutaneous insulin infusion and insulin analogues. *Diabetes/Met Res Rev.* 2007;23:348–355.

69. Towse A, O'Brien M, Twaroj FJ, Braimon J, Moses AC. Local secondary reaction to insulin injection. A potential role for latex antigens in insulin vials and syringes. *Diabetes Care.* 1995;18:1195–1197.

70. Scheer BG, Sitz KV. Suspected insulin anaphylaxis and literature review. *J Ark Med Soc.* 2001;97:311–313.

71. Kaya A, Gungor K, Karakose S. Severe anaphylactic reaction to human insulin in a diabetic patient. *J Diabetes Complicat.* 2007; Mar-Apr21(2):124–127.

72. Radermecker RP, Pierard GE, Scheen AJ. Lipodystrophy reactions to insulin: effects of continuous insulin infusion and new insulin analogs. *Am J Clin Dermatol.* 2007;8:21–28.

73. Wilson RM, Douglas CA, Tattersall RB, et al. Immunogenicity of highly purified bovine insulin: a comparison with conventional bovine and highly purified human insulins. *Diabetologia.* 1985;28:667.

74. Valenta LJ, Elias AN. Insulin-induced lipodystrophy in diabetic patients resolved by treatment with human insulin. *Ann Intern Med.* 1985;102:790.

75. Al-Khenaizan S, Al Thubaiti M, Al Alwan I. Lispro insulin-induced lipoatrophy: a new case. *Pediatr Diabetes.* 2007;8: 393–396.

76. Vardar B, Kizilci S. Incidence of lipohypertrophy in diabetic patients and a study of influencing factors. *Diabetes Res Clin Pract.* 2007;77:231–236.

77. Young RJ, Steel JM, Frier BM, et al. Insulin injection sites in diabetes—a neglected area?. *BMJ*. 1981;283:349.
78. Chowdhury TA, Escudier V. Poor glycaemic control caused by insulin induced lipohypertrophy. *BMJ*. 2003;327: 383–384.
79. Hardy KJ, Gill GV, Bryson JR. Severe insulin-induced lipohypertrophy successfully treated by liposuction. *Diabetes Care*. 1993;16:929.
80. Wallymahmed ME, Littler P, Clegg C, Haggani MT, MacFarlane IA. Nodules of fibrocollagenous scar tissue induced by subcutaneous insulin injections: a cause of poor diabetic control. *Postgrad Med J*. 2004;80:732–733.
81. Koda JE, Fineman M, Rink TJ, Dailey GE, Muchmore DB, Linarelli LG. Amylin concentrations and glucose control. *Lancet*. 1992;339:1179–1180.
82. Singh-Franco D, Robles G, Gazze D. Pramlintide acetate injection for the treatment of type 1 and type 2 diabetes mellitus. *Clin Therapeutics*. 2007;29:535–562.
83. Weyer C, Gottlieb A, Kim DD, et al. Pramlintide reduces postprandial glucose excursions when added to regular insulin or insulin lispro in subjects with type 1 diabetes: a dose-timing study. *Diabetes Care*. 2003;26:3074–3079.
84. Chapman I, Parker B, Doran S, et al. Low-dose pramlintide reduced food intake and meal duration in healthy, normal-weight subjects. *Obesity*. 2007;15:1179–1186.
85. Ratner RE, Dickey R, Fineman M, et al. Amylin replacement with pramlintide as an adjunct to insulin therapy improves long-term glycaemic and weight control in type 1 diabetes mellitus: a 1-year, randomized controlled trial. *Diabetic Med*. 2004;21:1204–1212.
86. Whitehouse F, Kruger DF, Fineman M, et al. A randomized study and open-label extension evaluating the long-term efficacy of pramlintide as an adjunct to insulin therapy in type 1 diabetes. *Diabetes Care*. 2002;25:724–730.
87. Marrero DG, Crean J, Zhang B, et al. Effect of adjunctive pramlintide treatment on treatment satisfaction in patients with type 1 diabetes. *Diabetes Care*. 2007;30:210–216.
88. www.symlin.com
89. Da Costa S, Brackenridge B, Hicks D. A comparison of pen use in the United States and the United Kingdom. *Diabetes Educ*. 2002;28:52–59.
90. Rex J, Jensen KH, Lawton SA. A review of 20 years' experience with the NovoPen family of insulin injection devices. *Clin Drug Invest*. 2006;26:367–401.
91. Graff MR, McClanahan MA. Assessment by patients with diabe mellitus of two insulin pen delivery systems versus vial and syringe. *Clin Ther*. 1998;20:486–496.
92. Ltief AN, Schwenk WF. Accuracy of pen injectors in children with type 1 diabetes. *Diabetes Care*. 1999;22:137–140.
93. Ginsberg BH, Parkes JL, Soaracino C. The kinetics of insulin administration by insulin pens. *Horm Metab Res*. 1994;26:584–587.
94. Albareda M, Balmes L, Wagner A, Corcoy R. Insulin pens and acute deterioration in blood glucose control. *Arch Int Med*. 1999;159:100–102.
95. Klonoff DC. Continuous glucose monitoring: roadmap for 21st century diabetes therapy. *Diabetes Care*. 2005;28:1231–1239.
96. Gross TM, Bode BW, Einhorn D, et al. Performance evaluation of the MiniMed continuous glucose monitoring system during patient home use. *Diabetes Technol Ther*. 2000;2:49–56.
97. Dunn TC, Eastman RC, Tamada JA. The GlucoWatch biographer: a frequent automatic and noninvasive glucose monitor. *Ann Med*. 2000;32:632–641.
98. The Diabetes Research in Children Network (DirecNet) Study Group. Accuracy of the GlucoWatch G2 Biographer and the continuous glucose monitoring system during hypoglycemia. experience of the diabetes research in children network. *Diabetes Care*. 2004;27:722–726.
99. Chase HP, Beck R, Tamborlane W, et al. A randomized multicenter trial comparing the GlucoWatch Biographer with standard glucose monitoring in children with type 1 diabetes. *Diabetes Care*. 2005;28:1101–1106.
100. Metzger M, Leibowitz G, Wainstein J, Glaser B, Itamar R. Reproducibility of Glucose Measurements Using the Glucose Sensor. *Diabetes Care*. 2002;25:1185–1191.
101. Kovatchev BP, Gonder-Frederick LA, Cox DJ, Clarke WL. Evaluating the accuracy of continuous glucose-monitoring sensors: continuous glucose-error grid analysis illustrated by TheraSense Freestyle Navigator data. *Diabetes Care*. 2004;27: 1922–1928.
102. Weinstein RL, Schwartz SL, Brazg RL, Bugler JR, Peyser TA, McGarraugh GV. Accuracy of the 5-day FreeStyle navigator continuous glucose monitoring system: comparison with frequent laboratory reference measurements. *Diabetes Care*. 2007;30:1125–1130.
103. Garg S, Jovanovic L. Relationship of fasting and hourly blood glucose levels to HbA1c values: safety, accuracy, and improvements in glucose profiles obtained using a 7-day continuous glucose sensor. *Diabetes Care*. 2006;29:2644–2649.
104. Buckingham B, Caswell K, Wilson DM. Real-time continuous glucose monitoring. *Curr Opin Endocrinol Diabetes Obes*. 2007;14:288–295.
105. DirecNet Study Group. Evaluation of factors affecting CGMS calibration. *Diabetes Technol Ther*. 2006;8:318–325.
106. Garg SK, Kelly WC, Voelmle MK, et al. Continuous home monitoring of glucose. Improved glycemia control with real-life use of continuous glucose sensors in adult subjects with type 1 diabetes. *Diabetes Care*. 2007;30:3023–3025.
107. Bailey TS, Zisser HC, Garg SK. Reduction in hemoglobin A1C with real-time continuous glucose monitoring: results from a 12-week observational study. *Diabetes Technol Ther*. 2007;9:203–210.

108. Garg S, Jovanovic L. Relationship of fasting and hourly blood glucose levels to HbA1c values: safety, accuracy, and improvements in glucose profiles obtained using a 7-day continuous glucose sensor. *Diabetes Care*. 2006;29:2644–2649.

109. Garg S, Zisser H, Schwartz S, et al. Improvement in glycemic excursions with a transcutaneous, real-time continuous glucose sensor: a randomized controlled trial. *Diabetes Care*. 2006;29:44–50.

110. Wilson DM, Beck RW, Tamborlane WV, et al. Efficacy of continuous real-time blood glucose monitoring during and after prolonged high-intensity cycling exercise: spinning with a continuous glucose monitoring system. *Diabetes Technol Ther*. 2006;8:627–635.

111. Cauza E, Hanusch-Enserer U, Strasser B, et al. Continuous glucose monitoring in diabetic long distance runners. *Int J Sports Med*. 2005;26:774–780.

112. Paty BW, Senior PA, Lakey JR, Shapiro AM, Ryan EA. Assessment of glycemic control after islet transplantation using the continuous glucose monitor in insulin-independent versus insulin-requiring type 1 diabetes subjects. *Diabetes Technol Ther*. 2006;8:165–173.

113. Direct Net Diabetes Research in Children Network (DirecNet) Study Group. Buckingham B, Beck RW, Tamborlane WV, et al. Continuous glucose monitoring in children with type 1 diabetes. *J Pediatrics*. 2007;151:388–393.

114. Clarke WL, Kovatchev B. The artificial pancreas: how close are we to closing the loop?. *Pediatr Endocrinol Rev*. 2007;4:314–316.

115. Steil GM, Rebrin K, Darwin C, Hariri F, Saad M. Feasibility of automating insulin delivery for the treatment of type 1 diabetes. *Diabetes*. 2006;55:3344–3350.

116. Renard E, Costalat G, Chevassus H, Bringer J. Artificial beta-cell: clinical experience toward an implantable closed-loop insulin delivery system. *Diabetes Metab*. 2006;32:497–502.

117. Hovorka R, Chassin LJ, Wilinska ME. Closing the loop: the ADICOL experience. *Diabetes Technol Ther*. 2004;6:307–318.

118. Grant P. A new approach to diabetic control: fuzzy logic and insulin pump technology. *Med Eng Phys*. 2007;29:824–827.

119. Burke GW, Ciancio G, Sollinger HW. Advances in pancreas transplantation. *Transplantation*. 2004;77(Suppl):S62–S67.

120. Odorico JS, Becker YT, Groshek M, et al. Improved solitary pancreas transplant graft survival in the modern immunosuppressive era. *Cell Transplant*. 2000;9:919.

121. Mai M, Ahsan N, Gonwa T. The long-term management of pancreas transplantation. *Transplantation*. 2006;82:991–1003.

122. Stratta RJ, Lo A, Shokouh-Amiri MH, et al. Improving results in solitary pancreas transplantation with portal-enteric drainige, thymoglobulin induction, and tacrolimus/mycopehnolate mofetil-based immunosuppression. *Transpl In*. 2003;16:154.

123. Sharpiro AM, Lakey JR, Ryan EA, et al. Islet transplantation in seven patients with type 1 diabetes mellitus using a glucocorticoid-free immunosuppressive regimen. *N Engl J Med*. 2000;343:230–238.

124. Srinivasan P, Huang GC, Amiel SA, Heaton ND. Islet cell transplantation. *Postgrad Med J*. 2007;83:224–229.

125. Ryan EA, Lakey JR, Rajotte RV, et al. Clinical outcomes and insulin secretion after islet transplantation with the edmonton protocol. *Diabetes*. 2001;50:710–719.

126. Foud T, Ricordi C, Baidal DA, et al. Islet transplantation in type 1 diabetes mellitus using cultured islets and steroid-free immunopsuppression: Miami experience. *Am J Transplant*. 2005;5:2037–2046.

127. Ault A. Edmonton's islet success tough to duplicate elsewhere. *Lancet*. 2003;361:2054.

128. Shapiro AM, Ricordi C, Haring B. Edmonton's islet success has indeed been replicated elsewhere. *Lancet*. 2003;9391:1242.

129. Ryan EA, Paty BW, Senior PA, et al. Five-year follow-up after clinical islet transplantation. *Diabetes*. 2005;54:2060–2069.

130. Balamurugan AN, Bottino R, Giannoukakis N. Prospective and challenges of islet transplantation for the therapy of autoimmune diabetes. *Pancreas*. 2006;32:231–243.

131. Shaprio AM, Lakey JR, Paty BW, et al. Strategic opportunities in clinical islet tranpslantation. *Transplantation*. 2005;79:1304–1307.

132. Dufour JM, Rajotte RV, Zimmerman M, et al. Development of an ectopic site for islet transplantation, using biodegradable scaffolds. *Tissue Eng*. 2005;11:1323–1331.

133. Palma CA, Lindeman R, Tuch BE. Blood into beta-cells: can adult stem cells be used as a therapy for type 1 diabetes?. *Regen Med*. 2008;3:33–47.

134. Miszta-Lane H, Mirbolooki M, James Shapiro AM, Lakey JR. Stem cell sources for clinical islet transplantation in type 1 diabetes: embryonic and adult stem cells. *Med Hypotheses*. 2006;67:909–913.

135. Beck J, Angus R, Madsen B, Britt D, Vernon B, Nguyen KT. Islet encapsulation: strategies to enhance islet cell functions. *Tissue Eng*. 2007;13:589–599.

136. Bour-Jordan H, Bluestone JA. B cell depletion: a novel therapy for autoimmune disorders?. *JCI*. 2007;117:3642–3644.

137. Bingley PJ, Gale EA. European Nicotinamide Diabetes Intervention Trial (ENDIT) Group. Progression to type 1 diabetes in islet cell antibody-positive relatives in the European nicotinamide diabetes intervention trial: the role of additional immune, genetic and metabolic markers of risk. *Diabetologia*. 2006;49:881–890.

138. Diabetes Prevention Trial – Type 1 Diabetes Study Group. Effects of insulin in relatives of patients with type 1 diabetes mellitus. *N Engl J Med*. 2002;346:1685–1691.

139. Liu E, Li M, Jasinski J, et al. Deleting islet autoimmunity. *Cell Biochem Biophys*. 2007;48:177–182.

140. Matthews JB, Ramos E, Bluestone JA. Clinical trials of transplant tolerance: slow but steady progress. *Am J Transplant*. 2003;3:794–803.

141. Clinical Trials Database http://clinicaltrials.gov/ct2/results?term=type+1+diabetes&show_flds=Y . Accessed 1/23/2008.

142. Trial Net. http://www2.diabetestrialnet.org /. Accessed 1/23/2008.

143. Calafiore R, Basta G, Luca G, et al. Standard technical procedures for microencapsulation of human islets for graft into nonimmunosuppressed patients with type 1 diabetes mellitus. *Transplant Proc.* 2006;38:1156–1157.

144. Calafiore R, Basta G. Artificial pancreas to treat type 1 diabetes mellitus. *Methods Mol Med.* 2007;140:197–236.

145. Juutilainen A, Lehto S, Rönnemaa T, Pyörälä K, Laakso M. Similarity of the impact of type 1 and type 2 diabetes on cardiovascular mortality in middle-aged subjects. *Diabetes Care.* 2008;31:714–719.

146. Nathan DM, Cleary PA, Backlund JY, et al. Intensive diabetes treatment and cardiovascular disease in patients with type 1 diabetes. *N Engl J Med.* 2005;353:2643–2653.

147. Cleary PA, Orchard TJ, Genuth S, et al. The effect of intensive glycemic treatment on coronary artery calcification in type 1 diabetic participants of the diabetes control and complications trial/epidemiology of diabetes interventions and complications (DCCT/EDIC) study. *Diabetes.* 2006;55:3556–3565.

148. McGill M, Molyneaux L, Twigg SM, Yue DK. The metabolic syndrome in type 1 diabetes: does it exist and does it matter?. *J Diabetes Complicat.* 2008;22:18–23.

Chapter 44
Treating Type 2 Diabetes Mellitus

Susan Herzlinger and Martin J. Abrahamson

Prevalence of DM2

Diabetes currently affects 23.6 million people in the United States, or 7.8% of the population, and 246 million people worldwide.[1,2] Approximately 90–95% of those affected have type 2 diabetes (DM2). Diabetes is the fifth leading cause of death by disease in the United States and was estimated to cost $174 billion in direct and indirect expenditures in 2007.[3] Clearly this is an enormous burden in terms of both human suffering and economic cost.

Rationale for Therapy

Current consensus treatment guidelines from both the American Diabetes association and the European Association for the Study of Diabetes are to lower the A1C to <7% and to get the A1C as close to normal as possible. Glycemic control has been shown to reduce the microvascular and macrovascular complications of the disease. Older adults who are functional, cognitively intact, and have significant life expectancy should be treated to these same goals. Reduction of the A1C to levels closer to normal, as in the ADVANCE trial which targeted an A1C of 6.5% and the ACCORD trial which targeted an A1C of 6%, has not been shown to reduce cardiovascular mortality in those subjects with established cardiovascular disease or those at high risk for cardiovascular disease.[4] In fact, the glucose-lowering arm of the ACCORD trial was stopped because of excess mortality in those participants who were randomized to very tight glucose control – the precise etiology of these deaths is unclear.[5] Despite the fact that intensive glucose control with the goal of achieving an A1C of <6.5% did not reduce risk for cardiovascular events in subjects with established CAD or those at risk for CAD in either the ADVANCE, ACCORD, or VA Diabetes Studies, subjects treated intensively in the ADVANCE trial demonstrated a significant 21% reduction in new or worsening diabetic nephropathy.

One study supporting early intensive therapy for newly diagnosed patients with type 2 diabetes mellitus was the United Kingdom Prospective Diabetes Study or UKPDS. The UKPDS was a randomized multicenter trial that randomized 5102 patients to either conventional dietary management or intensive therapy with either sulfonylurea, insulin, or, if overweight, metformin. The UKPDS showed that early intensive therapy in patients with newly diagnosed DM2 reduced risk of clinically evident microvascular complications by 25%. There was a nonsignificant reduction of 16% in the risk of myocardial infarction.[6] At 10-year follow-up of the UKPDS cohort, there was a significant effect of early intensive therapy on both microvascular and macrovascular disease. In the sulfonylurea–insulin group, microvascular disease risk was reduced by 24% and risks of myocardial infarction and death from any cause were reduced by 15 and 13%, respectively. In the metformin treatment group, there were sustained risk reductions in several key categories: 21% for any diabetes-related end point, 33% for myocardial infarction, and 27% for death from any cause.[7] This study is the first to show that early

M.J. Abrahamson (✉)
Joslin Diabetes Center, Harvard Medical School, Boston, MA, USA
e-mail: martin.abrahamson@joslin.harvard.edu

L. Poretsky (ed.), *Principles of Diabetes Mellitus*, DOI 10.1007/978-0-387-09841-8_44,
© Springer Science+Business Media, LLC 2010

glycemic control can reduce the incidence of macrovascular as well as microvascular complications in subjects with type 2 diabetes.

According to the Centers for Disease Control and Prevention's National Health and Nutrition Examination Survey, approximately 55% of people with diabetes do not achieve their target blood sugar levels with their current treatment regimen – despite increasing evidence that glycemic control decreases the incidence of microvascular and macrovascular complications.[8] In addition, two-thirds of adult men and women in the United States with DM2 have a BMI of 27 or greater.[9] Data support that weight loss (even a modest amount) supports patients in their efforts to achieve and sustain glycemic control.[10]

Choice of Initial Therapy

It is important to consider the pathophysiologic defects present in people with type 2 diabetes when considering how to initiate and advance pharmacologic treatment of the disease. Patients with DM2 usually have two major defects contributing to hyperglycemia – insulin resistance and impaired beta cell function. Insulin resistance is often the first "hit": obesity (particularly abdominal and visceral fat) and physical inactivity contribute to this. Nearly all groups at risk for DM2 – Native Americans, African Americans, Mexican Americans – have high rates of insulin resistance and obesity.[11] Insulin resistance causes impaired glucose use and uptake as well as glycogen storage by muscle.[12] Insulin resistance in the liver leads to increased basal hepatic glucose output, as insulin is less efficacious at suppressing gluconeogenesis.[13,14] Initially pancreatic insulin production increases to maintain normoglycemia. With time, the severity of the disease increases with impaired beta cell function which leads to progressive hyperglycemia. Decreased insulin response to both glucose and amino acids leads to postprandial hyperglycemia.[15] The liver also starts to produce more glucose, as the inhibitory effect of insulin declines. Hyperglycemia begets higher blood glucose, as "glucose toxicity" further impairs insulin secretion and action.[16]

Lifestyle Modification

Lifestyle modification is an essential component of any treatment regimen for people with type 2 diabetes. This includes reduction of intake of total calories, saturated and trans fatty acids, cholesterol, and sodium and increased physical activity to improve glycemic control, blood pressure, and dyslipidemia.[17] While this approach alone fails to achieve glycemic targets in the vast majority of patients, change in diet and exercise patterns should be the cornerstone of any treatment plan. Individualized medical nutrition therapy is recommended as needed to achieve weight loss goals and may be helpful in preventing those at risk for the development of type 2 diabetes. The goal of nutrition therapy in people who have diabetes is to use this approach to lower glucose levels as much as possible.[17] An important caveat to the ADA recommendations is that the pleasure of eating should be maintained by limiting food choices only when indicated by scientific evidence.

Physicians should emphasize the necessity for weight loss and strategies for optimizing glycemia through diet modification. These include decreasing dietary fat, increasing whole grain, and dietary fiber intake. There is some suggestion that change in dietary composition alone, independent of energy intake, can improve glucose control. Dietary fat modification, for example, has been shown to improve insulin sensitivity. In one Swedish study, 162 healthy subjects were chosen at random to receive a controlled, isoenergetic diet for 3 months containing either a high proportion of saturated or monounsaturated fatty acids. The study found that decreasing saturated fat and increasing monounsaturated fat improved insulin sensitivity but had no effect on insulin secretion.[18]

In terms of carbohydrate choices, there is a suggestion that a higher intake of dietary fiber decreases risk of developing diabetes and may then be useful in controlling glycemia. From the Nurses Health Study II, one paper examined the association between glycemic index, glycemic load, and dietary fiber and the risk of type 2 diabetes. A subset of 91,249 young women were followed for 8 years for development of DM2. Glycemic index of food intake was significantly associated with an increased risk of diabetes, while cereal fiber intake was associated with a decreased risk of diabetes. Glycemic load was not significantly associated with risk.[19] In the

Insulin Resistance Atherosclerosis Study, 978 middle-aged adults with normal (67%) or impaired (33%) glucose tolerance had improved insulin sensitivity and decreased fasting insulin levels associated with increased whole grain intake.[20] A follow-up study found that no association of glycemic index, glycemic load, or carbohydrate intake associated with insulin sensitivity or with fasting insulin levels after adjusting for total energy intake. Fiber intake, however, was positively associated with improved insulin sensitivity and inversely with adiposity.[21]

In practice, MNT can be remarkably effective in reducing the A1C. There are several randomized trials demonstrating benefit. In the UK Prospective Diabetes Study (UKPDS) 30,444 newly diagnosed patients with type 2 diabetes were randomized to intensive or conventional therapy after 3 months of nutrition counseling from a dietitian. During the initial period of nutritional counseling, the mean HbA1C decreased by 1.9% (from ~9 to ~7%), fasting plasma glucose was reduced by 46 mg/dl, and there were average weight losses of ~5 kg after 3 months.[22]

Another study of 179 individuals with DM2 compared usual nutrition care consisting of only one visit with a more intensive nutrition intervention, which included at least three visits with a dietitian. With the more intensive nutrition intervention, changes in lifestyle significantly improved glucose control. The fasting plasma glucose level decreased by 50–100 mg/dl and the A1C dropped by 1–2%. The average duration of diabetes for all subjects was 4 years and the decrease in A1C was 0.9% (from 8.3 to 7.4%). In the subgroup of subjects with a duration of diabetes <1 year, the decrease in A1C was 1.9% (from 8.8 to 6.9%).[23]

Randomized controlled nutrition therapy outcome studies have documented decreases in A1C of ~1% in newly diagnosed type 1 diabetes, 2% in newly diagnosed type 2 diabetes, and 1% in type 2 diabetes with an average duration of 4 years. MNT should be considered as monotherapy, along with physical activity, in the initial treatment of type 2 diabetes, provided the person has a fasting plasma glucose <200 mg/dl. Individuals with DM2 diabetes who cannot achieve optimal control with MNT and whose disease may be progressing due to beta cell failure should be prescribed blood glucose-lowering medication, along with additional encouragement to achieve goals of MNT and physical activity.[24]

In overweight and obese individuals, weight loss has been shown to decrease insulin resistance. For weight loss, either low-carbohydrate or low-fat diets may be effective in the short term (up to 1 year). It is not established whether the benefits of a high-protein diet are durable, nor what the long-term effects on kidney function are.

Two studies that established the efficacy of lifestyle measures in preventing diabetes include the Finnish Diabetes Prevention Study and the Diabetes Prevention Program or DPP. In the Finnish study, 522 overweight subjects with impaired glucose tolerance were randomly assigned to an intervention or control group. The intervention group received individualized counseling to lose weight and reduce intake of total and saturated fat and to increase intake of fiber and physical activity. Subjects were followed for 3.2 years and received an oral glucose tolerance test annually. Results at the end of 1 year showed a weight loss of 4.2 and 0.8 kg for the intervention and control groups, respectively. The cumulative incidence of diabetes after 4 years was 11% in the intervention group and 23% in the control group. Thus the risk of diabetes was reduced by 58% in the intervention group by lifestyle changes.[25]

The DPP, a multicenter National Institutes of Health study, was a randomized trial involving more than 3200 adults who were >25 years of age and who were at increased risk of developing type 2 diabetes due to impaired glucose tolerance, being overweight and having a family history of type 2 diabetes. The study involved a control group (standard care plus a placebo pill) and two intervention groups: one that received an intensive lifestyle modification (healthy diet and moderate physical activity of 30 min/day for 5 days/week) and one that received standard care plus metformin. Participants in the intensive lifestyle modification group had reduced their risk of developing diabetes by 58% compared with the medication intervention group who reduced their risk by 31%. Even more dramatic was the finding that individuals over 60 years of age in the intensive lifestyle modification group decrease their incidence of developing type 2 diabetes by 71%.[26]

Initiating a Medication

When diet and exercise are not sufficient to control blood glucose, initiation of a medication is indicated. There has been a marked increase in the number of oral and injectable antihyperglycemic agents available over the last

5 years. Currently, there are numerous classes of drugs that can be used to initiate or intensify treatment. These include insulin sensitizers, insulin secretagogues, and agents that delay the absorption of carbohydrate from the bowel. Insulin sensitizers include the biguanide metformin and thiazolidinediones. Insulin secretagogues include sulfonylureas, non-sulfonylurea secretagogues, (GLP-1) agonists, and DPP4 inhibitors. Alpha glucosidase inhibitors delay the absorption of carbohydrate from the GI tract. Finally there is an analogue of amylin, a peptide co-secreted with insulin from the beta cell, pramlintide, which is indicated for use with insulin in patients with both type 1 and type 2 diabetes. Both the American Diabetes Association and the European Association for the Study of Diabetes recommend starting treatment with metformin and continuing to augment therapy with additional agents to maintain recommended glycemic control (i.e., A1C < 7%) in most patients at the time of diagnosis of type 2 diabetes.[27]

Metformin

Metformin is the only biguanide currently in use.[11] Although available internationally for decades, metformin was not approved for clinical use in the United States until 1995. Metformin is the only available medication of this class in the United States, as its predecessor phenformin was discontinued due to its high association with lactic acidosis in 1976. Metformin improves insulin sensitivity and decreases insulin resistance, targeting a primary defect in type 2 diabetes. Metformin suppresses hepatic glucose production and increases glucose utilization, which only occurs in the presence of insulin as metformin enhances insulin action at the postreceptor level in peripheral tissues. The principal site of action of metformin is the liver where it inhibits hepatic glucose production. This drug also enhances glycogen formation and glucose oxidation in muscle.[28] This occurs without increased insulin secretion, thus limiting the risk of hypoglycemia. In fact, insulin levels are stable to decrease with metformin therapy. Metformin also increases glucose utilization by the intestine. This reduction of hepatic glucose production reduces fasting plasma glucose, while the increase in insulin-mediated glucose utilization principally affects postprandial glycemia.

Efficacy

The effect of metformin on glucose control is equal to or superior to other oral agents. Metformin lowers fasting blood glucose by approximately 20% and A1C by about 1.5%. The Metformin Multicenter Study Group compared 143 patients treated with metformin with 146 patients treated with placebo. The metformin group had lower mean fasting plasma glucose (189 ± 5 vs. 244 ± 6 mg/dl) and A1Cs (7.1±0.1 vs. 8.6±0.2%).[29] Metformin also has a favorable effect on metabolism and weight, which is of considerable importance in the typical diabetes type 2 population.

One major benefit of starting with metformin is that it is one of the few medications (other than exenatide and sitagliptin) that does not cause weight gain and is actually associated with mild weight loss. The weight loss is on the order of 2–3 kg, 88% of which is adipose tissue.[30] Metformin does not cause hypoglycemia when used as monotherapy and does not increase plasma insulin levels. In the ADOPT study in patients with recently diagnosed type 2 diabetes, metformin was more effective than glyburide and provided more durable glycemic control with less hypoglycemia and weight gain.[31]

Metformin also has modest benefits on lipid profile. This includes small drop in LDL and triglycerides and a small increase in HDL. The drops in LDL and triglycerides are likely due to reduced hepatic production of VLDL.[32] There may be cardiovascular and mortality benefit beyond these mild improvements in lipid profiles. In the UKPDS, patients' whose body weight was more than 120% of their ideal weight and who used metformin as monotherapy demonstrated a reduction in risk of MI by 39%, and risk of death from any cause was reduced by 36%. At 10-year follow-up, significant risk reductions persisted.

Side effects of metformin are primarily gastrointestinal and may be dose limiting in some patients. Anorexia, metallic taste, nausea, diarrhea, and vomiting may ensue with initiation of therapy. These side effects are usually mild and transient and may abate with extended release preparations or dose reductions. These side effects may also ameliorate the weight loss effects of metformin if tolerable to the patient. In the clinical trials of metformin, 5% discontinued use of the drug due to gastrointestinal side effects.

Vitamin B_{12} deficiency is more common in patients treated with metformin, with a greater than twofold increased likelihood of vitamin B_{12} deficiency in one study.[33] Metformin may disrupt calcium-dependent vitamin B_{12} intrinsic factor complex in the terminal ileum. This effect is rarely significant enough to cause anemia.

Metformin also causes a small increase in basal and postprandial lactate, likely due to the increased conversion of glucose to lactate by the intestinal mucosa. Lactate then enters the portal circulation, where it can become a substrate for gluconeogenesis or be cleared by the liver.[11] Lactic acidosis is a rare, serious adverse event linked to metformin therapy. The perceived risk is much higher than empiric risk data, likely due to the association with the other biguanide, phenformin. The incidence of lactic acidosis with phenformin was 10–20 times that of metformin. The reported incidence of lactic acidosis with metformin is 3 per 100,000 patient-years. The majority of cases occur in patients with renal insufficiency or illnesses that impair renal function, both of which are contraindications to metformin use. Most cases occur when a condition increasing blood lactate is present, such as hypoxia, hypotension, liver disease, or alcoholism. If metformin is the cause of the lactic acidosis, the medication can be removed by hemodialysis.[34] Metformin should also be stopped in any serious medical condition, particularly when hypotension, impaired tissue perfusion, or increased blood lactate is present or expected.

Contraindications to metformin therapy

Decreased renal function: Plasma creatinine ≥ 1.5 mg/dl for men and ≥ 1.4 mg/dl for women or a creatinine clearance <60 ml/min
Age >80 unless creatinine clearance is ≥ 60 ml/min
Liver disease
Alcohol abuse
Sepsis, myocardial infarction, or acute illness with decreased tissue perfusion
Acute or chronic metabolic acidosis, including diabetic ketoacidosis
During IV radiographic contrast administration

Adapted from the Glucophage XR Prescribing Information, Bristol-Myers Squibb Company, Princeton, NJ 08543, USA, October, 2000.

In summary, metformin reduces the A1C by approximately 1.5%, is generally well tolerated, and is not associated with either weight gain or hypoglycemia. Metformin is an appropriate choice for initial therapy of DM2 in most patients. Over time, patients may have progressive hyperglycemia due to progressive beta cell failure. At this point, other medications must be added to achieve target glycemia. Metformin can be combined with sulfonylureas, TZDs, exenatide, sitagliptin, or insulin.

Thiazolidinediones

Thiazolidinediones or TZDs are an attractive therapy for diabetes in that these drugs target the "first hit" in the natural history of diabetes: insulin resistance. TZDs principally work by increasing insulin sensitivity. TZDs bind to and activate one or more peroxisome proliferator-activated receptors (PPARs), which regulate gene expression. Through PPARs, TZDs act on muscle, liver, and adipose tissue to increase glucose utilization and decrease glucose production, but the mechanism through which this occurs is not entirely clear. TZDs lower fasting and postprandial glucose and result in a 1.0–1.6% decrement in the A1C.[35,36]

TZDs initially attracted interest as improvement in insulin sensitivity was thought to modify cardiac risk. TZDs are also associated with numerous vascular benefits, including reducing carotid intima–media thickness, endothelial dysfunction, and restenosis after angioplasty.[37] Pioglitazone, but not rosiglitazone, is also associated with LDL stability and reduction in triglycerides. In a review of six randomized trials, low-density lipoprotein

(LDL) cholesterol levels typically remained constant when monotherapy or combination therapy with pioglitazone was used, while increases in LDL cholesterol levels ranging from 8 to 16% were noted in studies of rosiglitazone.[38] High-density lipoprotein (HDL) cholesterol levels increased by approximately 10% with both drugs. Decreases in triglyceride levels were observed more often with pioglitazone than with rosiglitazone.

There are two TZDs available in the United States, rosiglitazone and pioglitazone, both of which were approved in 1999. Rosiglitazone and pioglitazone are used as monotherapy or with a sulfonylurea, metformin, or insulin. However, there are concerns with combined thiazolidinedione and insulin therapy because of an increased incidence of heart failure.

TZDs are also associated with weight gain, which can be significant. Weight gain is proportional to the dose and duration of therapy. There may be a small increase in appetite and fluid retention is a part of this weight gain. The principal driver of weight gain, however, is thought to be fat cell proliferation with a redistribution of adipose tissue from the viscera to subcutaneous depots.[39] This redistribution from visceral to subcutaneous fat is part of the reason that insulin sensitivity increases while weight increases.[40]

Use of TZDs has declined for several reasons. In addition to associated weight gain and edema, there is recent concern that TZDs increase the incidence of heart failure and cardiac death. One meta-analysis found that while patients given TZDs had increased risk for development of congestive heart failure across a wide background of cardiac risk the risk of cardiovascular death was not increased with either of the two TZDs.[41] Another meta-analysis that received widespread attention reported that the incidence of cardiac events with pioglitazone therapy was significantly less than with rosiglitazone therapy.[42] While the conclusions of this study remain controversial, concerns of cardiotoxic effects of TZDs persist pending the results of additional trials currently underway.

TZDs can be used in combination with metformin, insulin, sulfonylureas, exenatide, and sitagliptin but is not often selected for add-on therapy due to the associated fluid retention, weight gain, and ambiguity regarding cardiovascular effects described above. Rosiglitazone carries an FDA black box warning against potential increased risk of heart attack, and both drugs have black box warnings regarding increased risk of congestive heart failure. Nevertheless, these drugs are quite efficacious in controlling glycemia.

Sulfonylureas

Sulfonylureas (SUs) are a class of commonly prescribed antidiabetic drugs used to increase insulin secretion. All secretagogues have the following mechanism of action as they all bind to the SU receptor. SUs stimulate insulin secretion by causing the closure of the adenosine triphosphate (ATP)-dependent potassium channel (K_{ATP}) in the plasma membrane of the beta cell. When a sulfonylurea binds to the sulfonylurea receptor, or when plasma glucose levels are elevated, the K_{ATP} channel closes. When the K_{ATP} channel closes, potassium accumulates at the plasma membrane causing the depolarization of the membrane. When the membrane depolarizes, voltage-dependent calcium channels open and Ca^{2+} enters the intracellular compartment. The increase in Ca^{2+} stimulates migration and exocytosis of insulin granules. SUs also increase responsiveness of beta cells to both glucose and non-glucose secretagogues such as amino acids, resulting in more insulin secretion.

Clinical use of SUs in the United States dates back to 1954, when the first generation of these drugs was introduced. Second-generation SUs are more potent, allowing lower doses, and safer due to shorter duration of action than the first-generation agents. There are three so-called second-generation sulfonylureas on the market in the United States: glyburide, glipizide, and glimepiride. SUs are fairly efficacious, resulting in an average 1–2% decrement in A1C when used as monotherapy.[43,44] The duration of action of second-generation SUs ranges from 12 to 24 h and they are generally given in once-a-day or divided doses. The longer acting agents (for example, glyburide) better suppress morning hepatic glucose production and thus result in lower fasting blood glucose. However, this longer duration of action also results in more hypoglycemic episodes.

The principal side effects from SUs are the weight gain and risk of hypoglycemia that often accompany their use. Weight gain is typically on the order of 2–5 kg, which is counterproductive in this group of patients.[16,6] Sulfonylurea therapy eventually fails to provide adequate glycemic control in the majority of patients with type 2 diabetes; the durability of efficacy is a known issue but may be related to the natural history of diabetes rather than the mechanism of action of the drugs.

There is also a controversy regarding a potential association between SUs and cardiovascular morbidity.[16] The first suggestion regarding this link came from the University Group Diabetes project, which found an increased cardiovascular mortality in the group randomized to treatment with SUs versus insulin.[45] Because of questions related to methodology, several studies attempted to replicate these results. A retrospective cohort study of 5795 newly diagnosed type 2 diabetic patients from Canada, for example, compared levels of exposure to monotherapy with first- and second-generation sulfonylureas and metformin to determine whether increased mortality was associated with increased drug exposure. Risk of death increased twofold with higher daily doses of the first-generation sulfonylureas and 40% with glyburide, but not metformin. Similar associations were observed for death caused by an acute ischemic event.[46] The mechanism of this association with cardiovascular events is unclear. One thought is that because there are sulfonylurea receptors in the heart, use of SUs at the time of a myocardial infarction prevents adequate cardiac vasodilatation and resulting in more myocardial damage. Glimepiride, a second-generation agent, preferentially binds to the pancreatic beta cell SU receptors versus other agents and may not have the same cardiac risks, although this has not been proven. SUs carry a black box warning as mandated by the FDA that these agents may increase risk of cardiovascular disease. Despite this there is no clear evidence that SU use is associated with any increase in cardiovascular mortality – this was demonstrated in the UKPDS which showed no increase in cardiovascular mortality in subjects taking SUs when compared to those taking metformin or insulin.

SUs are typically metabolized by the liver and cleared by the kidney, limiting their use in patients with liver or kidney disease. SUs can be used as monotherapy or combined with all of the other oral therapies, exenatide and insulin.

The Meglitinide Analogues: Non-sulfonylurea Secretagogues

The rationale for development of non-SU secretagogues was to target a principal defect in DM2: inadequate prandial insulin response or so-called early-phase insulin response. In DM2, mealtime insulin response is delayed and blunted, whereas normal prandial insulin increases rapidly and peaks within 1 h.[47] The loss or attenuation of early-phase insulin secretion in type 2 diabetes results in inadequate insulin suppression of hepatic glucose production.[48] The aim of the non-SU secretagogues is to increase mealtime insulin secretion and reduce risk of hypoglycemia in the postabsorptive phase after the meal.

There are two non-SU insulin secretagogues available in the United States, repaglinide and nateglinide. These medications spur rapid and short-lived secretion of insulin from the pancreas. The mechanism of action of these medications is similar to that of SUs, as they bind to the SU receptor, but the duration of action is much shorter. This results in increased insulin secretion right after the meal, as well as less risk of hypoglycemia.[49] The non-SU secretagogues are rapidly absorbed, metabolized primarily by the liver, and more than 90% excreted in bile.

In terms of efficacy, the secretagogues are similar to metformin, but only repaglinide is comparable to the SUs. Repaglinide reduces A1C by about 0.7[50] to 1.5%.[51] In a head-to-head trial, repaglinide was similar to SUs with regard to glucose-lowering effects.[52] The major advantage of non-SU secretagogues over SUs is their shorter duration of action. Because the medication is cleared within 4 h and insulin levels return to baseline within 2 h, the risk of hypoglycemia when skipping a meal (and thus a dose) is low.[53] One study of 6000 patients with DM2 showed that before switching to repaglinide, 38% of patients ate when not hungry due to fear of hypoglycemia. This figure was reduced to 10% when repaglinide replaced usual therapy.[54] An added benefit of these short-acting agents is that patients do not need to eat when not hungry due to fear of hypoglycemia and do not gain as much weight as a result.

Another advantage of repaglinide over sulfonylureas is predominately hepatic clearance, with less than 10% renally excreted. This allows mealtime dosing in patients with renal disease who have a higher risk of hypoglycemia with sulfonylureas. The plasma half-life of repaglinide is extended in patients with severe renal impairment (from 1.5 to 3.6 h) but can be used without any special precautions in patients with mild-to-moderate renal impairment. Nateglinide is hepatically metabolized, with renal excretion of active metabolites. With decreased renal function, active metabolites can accumulate and cause hypoglycemia.

Both repaglinide and nateglinide are dosed before meals and can be used in combination with metformin or a TZD.

α-Glucosidase Inhibitors

Two α-glucosidase (AG) inhibitors, acarbose and miglitol, are available in the United States. AG inhibitors are a distinct class of antihyperglycemic agents that does not target a pathologic defect in DM2 but instead targets the enzyme α-glucosidase. α-Glucosidase is an enzyme that acts in the brush border of the proximal intestine to metabolize disaccharides and complex carbohydrates. Inhibition of the enzyme results in delayed carbohydrate absorption and blunted postprandial glucose excursions. This is coupled with a small reduction in postprandial insulin secretion, likely owing to the smaller rise in blood glucose. The overall efficacy of AG inhibitors is not as pronounced as some of the other oral agents, with average reduction in A1C by approximately 0.5–1.0%.[55] But there is no weight gain or hypoglycemia associated with the medication, a considerable advantage.[56] Many patients have trouble tolerating the primary side effects of flatulence, diarrhea, and abdominal discomfort. In one study of 893 patients treated with *acarbose*, only 16–20% were still taking the drug after 1 year and half of them stopped the drug during year 2.[57] Slow dosage increases minimize gastrointestinal side effects. The usual initial dose is 50 mg before meals. With higher doses the occurrence of side effects increases without improved effect on glycemia.[58]

There is conflicting data as to whether AG inhibitors favorably alter serum lipids. One study found that LDL cholesterol decreased and HDL cholesterol increased in response to therapy,[59] but a larger meta-analysis found no significant effect. That meta-analysis found no association with morbidity or mortality with use.[60] There may be a small decrement in body weight associated with use.

The Incretin System

With the exception of metformin, one frustration for both patient and physician with the available therapies is that they cause weight gain – in addition to other adverse effects including edema and risk of hypoglycemia. This led to considerable interest in a novel approach to treating diabetes type 2 by employing so-called incretin hormones. Eating triggers the secretion of numerous gut hormones that regulate motility and secretion of pancreatic enzymes, bile and stomach acid. These gut hormones also stimulate insulin secretion. The observation that enteral nutrition stimulates more insulin release than parenteral nutrition led to the development of the "incretin concept."[61] The incretin effect is the increase of glucose-stimulated insulin release in the presence of nutrients in the gut. Subsequently, several gut-derived hormones involved in glucose homeostasis were identified. The principal of these incretin hormones are glucose-dependent insulinotropic polypeptide (GIP) and glucagon-like peptide 1 (GLP-1). GLP-1 is the only incretin hormone used clinically.

GLP-1 is synthesized in the enteroendocrine L cells in the distal ileum and colon, but GLP-1 secretion is likely triggered by endocrine and neural signals when food is sensed more proximally in the small intestine or stomach.[62] GLP-1 levels are low in the fasting state and increase soon after eating. Incretin hormone levels decline rapidly, though as they are rapidly degraded by the enzyme dipeptidyl peptidase 4 (DPP4) resulting in a half-life on the order of minutes. GLP-1 receptors are present on myriad tissues; most relevant are the beta islet cells of the pancreas, central nervous system (including the hypothalamus), and adipose tissue. But GLP-1 receptors are also present in the peripheral nervous system, heart, lung, liver, kidney, and gastrointestinal tract. In the pancreas, GLP-1 causes increased insulin secretion. Sustained levels increase insulin synthesis and beta cell proliferation. The effect of incretins is glucose dependent; blood glucose must be >55 mg/dl to produce an effect.[63] There is also some promising evidence that GLP-1 enhances beta cell survival, which may delay the progression of DM2.[64] GLP-1 also helps to control blood glucose by inhibiting glucagon secretion, slowing gastric emptying, and actually decreasing food ingestion. This last effect is important in addressing the central cause of most type 2 diabetes mellitus: obesity.

The evidence for the anorexigenic effects of GLP-1 comes from both human and animal testing. Intracerebroventricular administration of GLP-1 reduces calorie intake in animal models, while the GLP-1 receptor antagonist exendin 9–39 increases food intake.[65] Obese people have less GLP-1 secretion in response to eating than lean people, and weight loss improves GLP-1 levels.[66] Patients with DM2 also have reduced GLP-1 secretion with meals. Reduced GLP-1 secretion could, therefore, contribute to obesity, and replacement may restore satiety. This effect is thought to be primarily due to delayed gastric emptying, but the CNS studies in animals also suggest that GLP-1 may suppress appetite centrally. Central administration is not necessary of course: obese subjects receiving subcutaneous GLP-1 for 5 days, just before each meal, reduced their calorie intake by 15% and lost 0.5 kg in weight.[67]

Actions of incretin hormones
Increased insulin secretion, especially at meals (incretin effect)
Suppression of glucagon secretion, except during hypoglycemia
Increased synthesis of proinsulin
Increase in pancreatic islet cell mass
Inhibition of beta cell apoptosis
Slowed gastric emptying
Increased satiety
Weight loss

Adapted from Drucker and Nauck.[62]

There are currently only two FDA-approved medications that manipulate the incretin system to modulate blood glucose. These are exenatide, a GLP-1 analogue, and sitagliptin, a DPP4 inhibitor. Other GLP-1 analogues, including a one-weekly formulation, as well as alternative DPP4 inhibitors are currently in development.

GLP-1 Analogues

The FDA approved the first incretin mimetic, exenatide, in April 2005. Exenatide is a synthetic form of exendin-4, which was discovered during an investigation for active peptides in lizard venom.[68] Exendin-4 has approximately 50% homology to mammalian GLP-1 and thus binds to the GLP-1 receptor and has the distinct advantage of being DDP4 degradation resistant. GLP-1 analogues require injection, however, and each injection lasts approximately 4–6 h in plasma circulation. The starting dose of exenatide is 5 μg twice daily – generally before breakfast and dinner – for the first 4 weeks, followed by a dose increase to 10 μg twice daily. Exenatide reduces A1C by about 0.8–1.0% over 30 weeks and is associated with modest weight loss of approximately 1.5–3 kg. The open-label extension demonstrated continued weight loss of 4–5 kg after 80 weeks.[69] There has been no difference demonstrated between exenatide and insulins glargine or biphasic aspart in open-label noninferiority studies, but these agents are associated with weight gain and risk of hypoglycemia.[70,71]

Liraglutide, a partially DPP4-resistant GLP-1 analogue, is in phase 3 clinical trials and is being reviewed by the FDA at the time of writing. Liraglutide has a longer half-life than exenatide and can be given as a once-daily injection but is otherwise quite similar in mechanism of action. Liraglutide reduces A1C by up to 1.75% with concomitant weight loss and transient nausea, vomiting, and diarrhea.[72]

There is also a long-acting exenatide in phase 3 clinical trials which has not yet been approved for clinical use. Exenatide long-acting release (LAR) formula is injected weekly instead of twice daily – clearly advantageous from the patient perspective. Preliminary data suggest that exenatide LAR is more potent, with greater decreases in mean A1C over 30 weeks with no increased risk of hypoglycemia and similar reductions in body weight.[73] This effect is likely due to increased suppression of glucagon and resultant decrease in fasting glucose with essentially continuous GLP-1 analogue. The twice-daily formula is more effective for control of postprandial hyperglycemia.

There is a risk of hypoglycemia with GLP-1 analogues but mostly when used in conjunction with sulfonylureas.[74,75] Off-label usage with insulins would clearly increase this risk. Side effects are generally gastrointestinal, principally nausea plus/minus vomiting. Nausea peaked in clinical trials in the first 8 weeks of therapy and then waned. Incidence of severe nausea was 5–6%, but overall incidence of gastrointestinal side effects of any kind was common – approximately 15–40% depending on the compound and trial – but rarely severe enough to spur trial withdrawal.

In addition, there may be an association between exenatide and pancreatitis. The FDA reviewed 30 postmarketing reports of acute pancreatitis and an additional six of hemorrhagic pancreatitis in patients taking exenatide (Byetta®). An association between Byetta® and acute pancreatitis was suspected in some of these cases. There are no known patient characteristics that determine when pancreatitis associated with Byetta will be complicated by the hemorrhagic or necrotizing forms of this condition. If pancreatitis is confirmed, exenatide should be stopped and not restarted. The FDA recommends that other antidiabetic therapies be considered in patients with a history of pancreatitis. The FDA asked the maker of Byetta, Amylin Pharmaceuticals, Inc., to include information about acute pancreatitis in the "Precautions" section of the product label.

Exenatide is approved for use in the United States with sulfonylurea, metformin, and/or a TZD; insulin is a notable exception to this list. Several other GLP-1 agonists and formulations are in development.

DPP-4 Inhibitors

Because the GLP-1 analogues are injectable, there is considerable interest on oral incretin therapy. DPP-4 degrades endogenous GLP-1, resulting in a short half-life. The DPP-4 inhibitors block degradation, resulting in prolonged action of GLP1. While DPP-4 inhibitors are not associated with weight loss, these agents are "weight neutral" and are associated with few side effects. The risk of hypoglycemia is increased only due to combination therapy, such as with insulin and sulfonylureas.

Not surprisingly, the DPP-4 inhibitors decrease glycemia by a similar mechanism to GLP-1. They augment insulin secretion and inhibit glucagon release, leading to enhanced suppression of endogenous glucose production.[76] The only DPP-4 inhibitor available in the United States is sitagliptin, which was approved by the Food and Drug Administration in October 2006 for use as monotherapy or in combination with metformin, TZDs, or SUs. Another DPP-4 inhibitor, vildagliptin, was approved in Europe in February 2008, and several other compounds are under development. In clinical trials performed to date, DPP4 inhibitors lower HbA1C levels by 0.6–0.9% points are weight neutral and relatively well tolerated without significant gastrointestinal upset.[77,78] In combination with metformin, the decrement in A1C is approximately 2%. Markers of insulin secretion and beta cell function were also significantly improved with sitagliptin.

GLP-1 agonists and DPP-4 inhibitors both effectively increase GLP-1. Exenatide can be added to one or more oral therapies when those therapies are inadequate, often as an alternative to insulin. Sitagliptin can be used as monotherapy or add-on therapy to other oral agents. DPP-4 inhibitors are not associated with weight loss but do not cause weight gain. There is no associated nausea, vomiting, or delayed gastric emptying.

DPP-4 inhibitors have not been associated with characteristic infections, but the incidence of upper respiratory and urinary tract infections is increased in clinical trials. Because DPP-4 is present in cell membranes, including those of lymphocytes, there are some theoretical concerns regarding impaired immune function. There was also increased risk of headache seen in meta-analysis of DPP-4 inhibitor trials.[63]

Amylin Agonists (Pramlintide)

Pramlintide is a synthetic analogue of the beta cell hormone amylin, which is co-secreted with insulin from the pancreatic beta cell and which is deficient in diabetes. It is administered subcutaneously before meals and slows gastric emptying, inhibits glucagon production in a glucose-dependent fashion, and predominantly decreases postprandial glucose excursions.[79] In terms of glycemic control, pramlintide is moderately effective with A1C decrements of 0.5–0.7% in clinical trials. Adverse effects include nausea and hypoglycemia.[80] Approximately 30% of treated participants in the clinical trials have developed nausea, but this side effect tends to abate with time on therapy. Weight loss associated with this medication is ~1–1.5 kg over 6 months, some of which may be due to gastrointestinal side effects and increased satiety due to slowed gastric transit. Pramlintide is approved for use only with insulin, but trials as a weight loss medication, both alone and in combination with leptin, are underway.

Insulin

Because of the decline in beta cell function over time,[81] many patients with type 2 diabetes eventually require insulin therapy. Oral hypoglycemic agents lose efficacy over time in part due to loss of insulin secretory capacity of the beta cell. In the UKPDS, for example, 50% of the participants originally controlled with monotherapy needed the addition of another agent after 3 years and 75% needed multiple therapies at 9 years.[82] Insulin therapy is indicated when adequate glycemic control is not achieved using diet, exercise, and one or more oral agents. Although insulin is both the most physiologic and the effective medication to lower blood glucose, most patients are reluctant to proceed to insulin and many physicians are loathe to start insulin therapy for a variety of reason. Many patients view the need for insulin as a personal failure or a harbinger of doom. Other reasons why patients and physicians are often reluctant to start insulin include concerns about weight gain and hypoglycemia. The progressive nature of type 2 diabetes should be reviewed with patients early in the course of disease management so that they understand why insulin treatment may be necessary. In addition the issues of weight gain and risk of hypoglycemia need to be addressed with patients, in particular the risk of hypoglycemia which is very low in patients with type 2 diabetes taking insulin.

Under normal, nondiabetic circumstances, insulin is secreted in a pulsatile manner under basal, unstimulated conditions and in response to meals.[83] In 24 h, approximately 50% of insulin production is basal and 50% is prandial. Basal insulin is secreted overnight and between meals to suppress hepatic glucose production. These proportions should guide exogenous insulin therapy. There are many types of insulin available, and the differing pharmacokinetics of these agents can be used to mimic pulsatile physiologic insulin release via multiple daily injections. The details of the onset and duration of actions of these insulins are detailed elsewhere in this book (Chapter 43). Generally, insulins can be grouped by pharmacokinetics: rapid-, short-, intermediate-, and long-acting. Longer acting insulins are used as basal insulin one or two times daily, while short- and rapid-acting insulins are used for mealtime coverage. Premixed insulins combine basal and prandial insulin, generally comprised of short- and intermediate-acting insulins in a wide range of ratios (90:10 to 50:50). The regimen that best mimics normal pancreatic function is the so-called basal-bolus regimen. Once or twice per day basal (long- or intermediate-acting) insulin is employed to mimic the fasting and postabsorptive state, and bolus (rapid- or short-acting) insulin is used at mealtime. The rapid-acting insulins produce less postprandial hypoglycemia than short-acting insulins,[84] largely related to duration of action. Long-acting insulin analogues are associated with less hypoglycemia due to a less pronounced peak in insulin action compared to NPH.[85]

Premixed insulins, which combine a rapid-acting with intermediate-acting insulin, generally provide good but not excellent control. These insulins are generally given twice daily but are occasionally given three times daily before all meals. Certainly premixed insulin have a significant advantage over basal insulin alone, given the rapid-acting prandial control and result in a significantly better reduction in HbA1C.[86] Premixing avoids errors from mixing by the patient in a syringe and reduces the numbers of injections, which is advantageous in the elderly, those with visual or fine-motor impairment.[87] But premixed insulins are in a fixed ratio, which limits flexibility to titrate the mealtime and basal components because dose increases may predispose to early or late hypoglycemia.

For most patients with type 2 diabetes who are not achieving therapeutic goals on oral medications, initial therapy with insulin usually consists of the addition of basal insulin to the regimen of oral hypoglycemics. Addition of basal insulin can lower the A1C by up to 1.6%. One study showed that the impact of postprandial hyperglycemia on HbA1C increases with improved control. Postprandial glycemic control was found to account for 70% of overall glycemic control when the HbA1C is less than 7.3% but 50% when the HbA1C is between 7.3 and 8.4%.[88] In various "Treat-to-Target" trial, once-daily basal insulin targeting fasting plasma glucose levels allowed the majority of patients to achieve a HbA1C of less than 7%.[89] In these studies, once-daily NPH and detemir or NPH and glargine were equally efficacious, but NPH was associated with significantly more episodes of hypoglycemia than either of these basal analogues, in particular nocturnal hypoglycemia. Insulin can be combined with metformin, sulfonylureas, meglitinides, and thiazolidinediones. Of note, despite a theoretic synergy of basal insulin with prandial incretin therapy, these combinations are not yet approved. We do not recommend discontinuing oral antidiabetes medications when insulin is initiated, since there is synergy and an "insulin-sparing" effect when insulin sensitizers,[90] including metformin, are continued. Limiting insulin doses may be helpful in minimizing insulin-related weight gain.

The ADA and EASD recommend starting with a bedtime intermediate-acting insulin or morning or evening long-acting insulin at 10 units or 0.2 U/kg. This dose should be titrated upward by 2–3 units every 3 days until the fasting morning glucose is at goal (70–130 mg/dl).[27] While more physicians are using long duration insulin analogues that have a more "flat" profile of action, NPH may be a more appropriate choice in patients who have significant increases in blood glucose over the course of the early morning.

If the HbA1C is still above goal 2–3 months after initiating basal insulin, preprandial blood glucose patterns should be examined. If the prelunch is elevated, then rapid-acting insulin should be added at breakfast. If the predinner value is elevated, then NPH could be added at breakfast or rapid-acting insulin at lunch. If prebedtime glucose is elevated, rapid-acting insulin is needed at dinner. The addition of presupper prandial insulin to a bedtime basal insulin can be achieved sometimes by substituting a premixed insulin analogue at supper and stopping the bedtime basal insulin analogue or NPH. If this fails to get the A1C to goal, then it is likely that prandial insulin at breakfast and lunch will be needed – this can be achieved by using prandial insulin alone at the meal or using premixed insulin once, twice, or sometimes three times daily. There is no true "maximal dose" of insulin, although variability of insulin absorption increases with higher doses.[91] In type 2 diabetes, insulin requirements are typically greater than in type 1 due to insulin resistance. Doses often exceed 1 U/kg to achieve normoglycemia in type 2 diabetes.

Side effects of insulin include weight gain and hypoglycemia. The weight gain associated with insulin can be marked and create a circle of increasing insulin requirements due to increased body size, leading to further weight gain. In the DCCT, mean weight gain after the first year was 3.6 ± 4.8 kg and 3.0 ± 4.1 kg for men and women, respectively, with intensive therapy.[92] Weight gain varied at 9-year follow-up. Less than 5% of men and 15% of women in the conventional treatment group had major weight gain (20% of baseline or approximately 14 kg), compared with about 35% of women and <30% of men in the intensive treatment group. In the UKPDS, mean weight gain after 10 years of insulin therapy was about 7 kg for subjects with type 2 diabetes on intensive treatment with sulfonylureas or insulin, with the most rapid weight gain occurring when insulin was first initiated.[93] Intensive therapy with insulin in the DCCT also caused a relatively high rate of hypoglycemia of 61 per 100 patient-years.[94] However studies of insulin use in type 2 diabetes have shown significantly less hypoglycemia than that observed in patients with type 1 diabetes. Insulin analogues with longer durations of actions may decrease the risk of hypoglycemia compared with NPH. Rapid-acting insulin analogues, called rapid-acting insulins, may reduce the risk of hypoglycemia compared with regular insulin,[27,95] due to pharmacokinetics that are more closely matched to postprandial glycemic patterns.

With intensive basal-bolus regimens, excellent glycemic control can be achieved, but patients need to test glucose levels more frequently: hypoglycemia. Premixed insulins may be more convenient for some patients but provide patients with less "flexible" lifestyle options in that ideally they should follow more consistent carbohydrate intake at meals and have meals at roughly similar times each day. With the variety of preparations of insulin with different pharmacokinetics, patient regimens can be individualized to meet the metabolic and lifestyle needs of the patients. Age, patient motivation, general health, and goals of treatment should all be considered in choosing an appropriate regimen.

Conclusions

There are numerous medications available to achieve glycemic targets. While many organizations recommend use of metformin at the time of diagnosis of type 2 diabetes, lifestyle modification remains an essential component of any treatment regimen. If this alone is recommended as initial treatment, then medications should be started within 3 months if A1C targets are not achieved. In the absence of contraindications, metformin should be the initial choice of therapy. Sulfonylureas are usually the next logical choice due to their long safety profile and low cost. But in an elderly patient or patient with renal impairment, where the risk of hypoglycemia may be increased, another medication like a DPP4 inhibitor or non-SU secretagogue may make more sense. In an obese patient, a trial with exenatide should be considered despite frequent GI side effects and lack of long-term data. The following is a summary of available therapies as recommended by the ADA and EASD:

Summary of Glucose-Lowering Interventions

Intervention	Expected decrease in HbA1C (%) with monotherapy	Advantages	Disadvantages
Tier 1: Well-validated core			
Step 1: Initial therapy			
Lifestyle to decrease weight and increase activity	1.0–2.0	Broad benefits	Insufficient for most within first year
Metformin	1.0–2.0	Weight neutral	GI side effects, contraindicated with renal insufficiency
Step 2: Additional therapy			
Insulin	1.5–3.5	No dose limit, rapidly effective, improved lipid profile	One to four injections daily, monitoring, weight gain, hypoglycemia, analogues are expensive
Sulfonylurea	1.0–2.0	Rapidly effective	Weight gain, hypoglycemia (especially with glibenclamide or chlorpropamide)
Tier 2: Less well validated			
Thiazolidinedione	0.5–1.4	Improved lipid profile (pioglitazone), potential decrease in MI (pioglitazone)	Fluid retention, CHF, weight gain, bone fractures, expensive, potential increase in MI (rosiglitazone)
GLP-1 agonist	0.5–1.0	Weight loss	Two injections daily, frequent GI side effects, long-term safety not established, expensive
Other therapy			
α-Glucosidase inhibitor	0.5–0.8	Weight neutral	Frequent GI side effects, three times/day dosing, expensive
Glinide	0.5–1.5[a]	Rapidly effective	Weight gain, three times/day dosing, hypoglycemia, expensive
Pramlintide	0.5–1.0	Weight loss	Three injections daily, frequent GI side effects, long-term safety not established, expensive
DPP-4 inhibitor	0.5–0.8	Weight neutral	Long-term safety not established, expensive

[a]Repaglinide more effective in lowering HbA1C than nateglinide.
Reproduced from Nathan et al.[96]

References

1. "All about diabetes." American Diabetes Association. http://www.diabetes.org/about-diabetes.jsp (Accessed November 2008)
2. The International Diabetes Federation Diabetes Atlas. Available at: http://www.idf.org/home/index.cfm?unode=3B96906B-C026-2FD3-87B73F80BC22682A . Accessed November, 2008.
3. "Direct and indirect costs of diabetes." American Diabetes Association. http://www.diabetes.org/diabetes-statistics/cost-of-diabetes-in-us.jsp (Accessed November 2008)
4. ADVANCE Collaborative Group. Patel A, MacMahon S, Chalmers J, et al. Intensive blood glucose control and vascular outcomes in patients with type 2 diabetes. *NEJM.* 2008;358:2560–2572.
5. Action to Control Cardiovascular Risk in Diabetes Study Group. Gerstein HC, Miller ME, Byington RP, et al. Effects of intensive glucose lowering in type 2 diabetes. *NEJM.* 2008;358:2545–2559.
6. UKPDS Group. Intensive blood-glucose control with sulphonylureas or insulin compared with conventional treatment and risk of complications in patients with type 2 diabetes. *Lancet.* 1998;352:837–853.
7. Holman RR, Paul SK, Bethel MA, Matthews DR, Neil HA. 10-year follow-up of intensive glucose control in type 2 diabetes. *NEJM.* 2008;359:1577–1589.
8. Saydah SH, Fradkin J, Cowie CC. Poor control of risk factors for vascular disease among adults with previously diagnosed diabetes. *JAMA.* 2004;291:335–342.
9. "Fact sheet Diabetes and obesity." International Diabetes Federation. http://www.idf.org/home/index.cfm?unode=5EBAF6D9-127B-43B5-8BE1-48D33AB7DE77#facts ./ Accessed November 2008.
10. Look AHEAD Research Group. Pi-Sunyer X, Blackburn G, Brancati FL, et al. Reduction in weight and cardiovascular disease risk factors in individuals with type 2 diabetes: one-year results of the look AHEAD trial. *Diabetes Care.* 2007;30:1374–1383.
11. Bailey CJ, Turner RC. Metformin. *NEJM.* 1996;334:574–579.
12. Shulman GI, Rothman DL, Jue T, Stein P, DeFronzo RA, Shulman RG. Quantitation of muscle glycogen synthesis in normal subjects and subjects with non-insulin-dependent diabetes by 13C nuclear magnetic resonance spectroscopy. *NEJM.* 1990;322:223–228.
13. Consoli A, Nurijan M, Capani F, Gerich J. Predominant role of gluconeogenesis in hepatic glucose production in NIDDM. *Diabetes.* 1989;38:550–557.
14. Hosker JP, Rudenski AS, Burnett MA, Matthrews DR, Turner RC. Similar reduction in first and second phase B-cell responses at different glucose levels in type II diabetes and effect of gliclazide therapy. *Metabolism.* 1989;38:767–772.
15. Porte D Jr. Beta-cells in type II diabetes mellitus. *Diabetes.* 1991;40:166–180.
16. Inzucchi SE. Oral antihyperglycemic therapy for type 2 diabetes. *JAMA.* 2002;287:360–372.
17. ADA. Nutrition recommendations and interventions for diabetes. *Diabetes Care.* 2008;31:S61–S78.
18. Vessby B, Unsitupa M, Hermansen K, et al. Substituting dietary saturated for monounsaturated fat impairs insulin sensitivity in healthy men and women: The KANWU Study. *Diabetologia.* 2001;44:312–319.
19. Schulze MB, Liu S, Rimm EB, Manson JE, Willett WC, Hu FB. Glycemic index, glycemic load, and dietary fiber intake and incidence of type 2 diabetes in younger and middle-aged women. *Am J Clin Nutr.* 2004;80:348–356.
20. Liese AD, Roach AK, Sparks KC, Marquart L, D'Agostino RB Jr, Mayer-Davis EJ. Whole-grain intake and insulin sensitivity: the insulin resistance atherosclerosis study. *Am J Clin Nutr.* 2003;78:965–971.
21. Liese AD, Schulz M, Fang F, et al. Dietary glycemic index and glycemic load, carbohydrate and fiber intake, and measures of insulin sensitivity, secretion, and adiposity in the insulin resistance atherosclerosis study. *Diabetes Care.* 2005;28:2832–2838.
22. UK Prospective Diabetes Study 7. Response of fasting plasma glucose to diet therapy in newly presenting type II diabetic patients. *Metabolism.* 1990;39:905–912.
23. Franz MJ, Monk A, Barry B, et al. Effectiveness of medical nutrition therapy provided by dietitians in the management of non-insulin-dependent diabetes mellitus: a randomized, controlled clinical trial. *J Am Diet Assoc.* 1995;95:1009–1017.
24. Pastors JG, Warshaw H, Daly A, Kulkarni A. The evidence for the effectiveness of medical nutrition therapy in diabetes management. *Diabetes Care.* 2002;25:608–613.
25. Tuomilehto J, Lindstrom J, Erikksson JG, et al. Prevention of type 2 diabetes mellitus by changes in lifestyle among subjects with impaired glucose tolerance. *N Engl J Med.* 2001;344:1343–1350.
26. Knowler WC, Barrett-Connor E, Fowler SE, et al. Diabetes Prevention Program Research Group. Reduction in the incidence of type 2 diabetes with lifestyle intervention or metformin. *NEJM.* 2002;346:393–403.
27. Nathan DM, Buse JB, Davidson MB, et al. Management of hyperglycemia in type 2 diabetes: a consensus algorithm for the initiation and adjustment of therapy: a consensus statement from the American Diabetes Association and the European Association for the Study of Diabetes. *Diabetes Care.* 2006;29:1963–1972.
28. Bailey CJ, Puah JA. Effect of metformin on glucose metabolism in the mouse soleus muscle. *Diabetes Metab.* 1986;12:212–218.
29. DeFronzo RA, Goodman AM. Efficacy of metformin in patients with non-insulin-dependent diabetes mellitus. The Multicenter Metformin Study Group. *NEJM.* 1995;333:541–549.
30. Stumvoll M, Nurjhan N, Perriello G, Dailey G, Gerich JE. Metabolic effects of metformin in non-insulin-dependent diabetes mellitus. *NEJM.* 1995;333:550–554.
31. Herman WH, Hafner SM, Kahn SE, et al. ADOPT: The effectiveness of metformin versus glyburide in type 2 diabetes. *Diabetologia.* 2007;50:S362.

32. Bailey CJ. Biguanides and NIDDM. *Diabetes Care.* 1992;15:755–772.

33. Ting RZ, Szeto CC, Chan MH, Ma KK, Chow KM. Risk factors of vitamin B(12) deficiency in patients receiving metformin. *Arch Intern Med.* 2006;166:1975–1979.

34. Gan SC, Barr J, Arieff AI, Pearl RG. Biguanide-associated lactic acidosis. Case report and review of the literature. *Arch Intern Med.* 1992;152:2333–2336.

35. Lebovitz HE, Dole JF, Patwardhan R, Rappaport EB, Freed MI. Rosiglitazone monotherapy is effective in patients with type 2 diabetes. *J Clin Endocrinol Metab.* 2001;86:280–288.

36. Aronoff S, Rosenblatt S, Braithwaite S, Egan JW, Mathisen AL, Schneider RL. Pioglitazone hydrochloride monotherapy improves glycemic control in the treatment of patients with type 2 diabetes: a 6-month randomized placebo-controlled dose-response study. The Pioglitazone 001 Study Group. *Diabetes Care.* 2000;23:1605–1611.

37. Fonseca V. Rationale for the use of insulin sensitizers to prevent cardiovascular events in type 2 diabetes mellitus. *Am J Med.* 2007;120:S18–S25.

38. Yki-Järvinen H. Thiazolidinediones. *NEJM.* 2004;351:1106–1118.

39. Fonseca V. Effect of thiazolidinediones on body weight in patients with diabetes mellitus. *Am J Med.* 2003;115:42S–48S.

40. Miyazaki A, Mahankali M, Matsuda M, et al. Effect of pioglitazone on abdominal fat distribution and insulin sensitivity in type 2 diabetic patients. *J Clin Endocrinol Metab.* 2002;87:2784–2791.

41. Lago RM, Singh PP, Nesto RW. Congestive heart failure and cardiovascular death in patients with prediabetes and type 2 diabetes given thiazolidinediones: a meta-analysis of randomised clinical trials. *Lancet.* 2007;370:1129–1136.

42. Lincoff AM, Wolski K, Nicholls SJ, Nissen SE. Pioglitazone and risk of cardiovascular events in patients with type 2 diabetes mellitus: a meta-analysis of randomized trials. *JAMA.* 2007;298:1180–1188.

43. Rosenstock J, Samols E, Muchmore DB, Schneider J. Glimepiride, a new once-daily sulfonylurea. A double-blind placebo-controlled study of NIDDM patients. Glimepiride Study Group. *Diabetes Care.* 1996;19:1194–1199.

44. Schade DS, Jovanovic L, Schneider J. A placebo-controlled, randomized study of glimepiride in patients with type 2 diabetes mellitus for whom diet therapy is unsuccessful. *J Clin Pharmacol.* 1998;38:636–641.

45. Goldner MG, Knatterud GL, Prout TE. Effects of hypoglycemic agents on vascular complications in patients with adult-onset diabetes. Clinical implications of UGDP results. *JAMA.* 1971;218:1400–1410.

46. Simpson SH, Majumdar SR, Tsuyuki RT, et al. Dose-response relation between sulfonylurea drugs and mortality in type 2 diabetes mellitus: a population-based cohort study. *CMAJ.* 2006;174:169–174.

47. Owens DR. Repaglinide–prandial glucose regulator: a new class of oral antidiabetic drugs. *Diabetes Med.* 1998;15:S28–S36.

48. Gerich JE. Metabolic abnormalities in impaired glucose tolerance. *Metabolism.* 1997;46(12 S1):40–43.

49. Black C, Donnelly P, McIntyre L, Royle PL, Shepherd JP, Thomas S. Meglitinide analogues for type 2 diabetes mellitus. *Cochrane Database Syst Rev.* 2007;2:CD004654.

50. Goldberg RB, Einhorn D, Lucas CP, et al. A randomized placebo-controlled trial of repaglinide in the treatment of type 2 diabetes. *Diabetes Care.* 1998;21:1897–1903.

51. Madsbad S, Kilhovd B, Lager I, Mustajoki P, Dejgaard A. Scandinavian Repaglinide Group. Comparison between repaglinide and glipizide in Type 2 diabetes mellitus: a 1-year multicentre study. *Diabet Med.* 2001;18:395–401.

52. Wolffenbuttel BH, Landgraf R. A 1-year multicenter randomized double-blind comparison of repaglinide and glyburide for the treatment of type 2 diabetes. Dutch and German Repaglinide Study Group. *Diabetes Care.* 1999;22:463–467.

53. Dornhorst A. Insulinotropic meglitinide analogues. *Lancet.* 2001;358:1709–1716.

54. Landgraf R, Frank M, Bauer C, Dieken ML. Prandial glucose regulation with repaglinide: its clinical and lifestyle impact in a large cohort of patients with type 2 diabetes. *Int J Obes Relat Metab Disord.* 2000;24(suppl 3):38–44.

55. Chiasson JL, Josse RG, Hunt JA, et al. The efficacy of acarbose in the treatment of patients with non-insulin-dependent diabetes mellitus. A multicenter controlled clinical trial. *Ann Intern Med.* 1994;121:928–935.

56. Johnston PS, Lebovitz HE, Coniff RF, Simonson DC, Raskin P, Munera CL. Advantages of alpha-glucosidase inhibition as monotherapy in elderly type 2 diabetic patients. *J Clin Endocrinol Metab.* 1998;83(5):1515–1522.

57. Catalan VS, Couture JA, LeLorier J. Predictors of persistence of use of the novel antidiabetic agent acarbose. *Arch Intern Med.* 2001;161:1106–1112.

58. Van de Laar FA, Lucassen PL, Akkermans RP, van de Lisdonk EH, Rutten GE, van Weel C. Alpha-glucosidase inhibitors for patients with type 2 diabetes: results from a Cochrane systematic review and meta-analysis. *Diabetes Care.* 2005;28:154–163.

59. Hoffmann J, Spengler M. Efficacy of 24-week monotherapy with acarbose, metformin, or placebo in dietary-treated NIDDM patients: the Essen-II Study. *Am J Med.* 1997;103:483–490.

60. Van de Laar FA, Lucassen PL, Akkermans RP, van de Lisdonk EH, Rutten GE, van Weel C. Alpha-glucosidase inhibitors for patients with type 2 diabetes: results from a cochrane systematic review and meta-analysis. *Diabetes Care.* 2005;28:154–163.

61. Elrick H, Stimmler L, Hlad CJ, Arai Y. Plasma insulin response to oral and intravenous glucose administration. *J Clin Endocrinol Metab.* 1964;24:1076–1082.

62. Drucker DJ, Nauck MA. The incretin system: glucagon-like peptide-1 receptor agonists and dipedyl peptiinase-4 inhibitors in type 2 diabetes. *Lancet.* 2006;368:1696–1704.

63. Amori RE, Lau J, Pittas AG. Efficacy and safety of incretin therapy in type 2 diabetes: systematic review and meta analysis. *JAMA.* 2007;298:194–206.

64. Farilla L, Bulotta A, Hirshberg B, et al. Glucagon-like peptide 1 inhibits cell apoptosis and improves glucose responsiveness of freshly isolated human islets. *Endocrinology.* 2003;144:5149–5158.

65. Turton MD, O'Shea D, Gunn I, et al. A role for glucagon-like peptide-1 in the central regulation of feeding. *Nature*. 1996;379:69–72.

66. Verdich C, Toubro S, Buemann B, Lysgård Madsen J, Juul Holst J, Astrup A. The role of postprandial releases of insulin and incretin hormones in meal-induced satiety¾effect of obesity and weight reduction. *Int J Obes Relat Metab Disord*. 2001;25:1206–1214.

67. Naslund E, King N, Mansten S, et al. *Br J Nutr*. 2004;91:439–446.

68. Drucker DJ, Nauck MA. The incretin system:g glucagons-like peptide-1 receptor agonists and dipedyl peptidase-4 inhibitors in type 2 diabetes. *Lancet*. 2006;368:1696–1704.

69. Riddle MC, Henry RR, Poon TH, et al. Exendin elicits sustained glycaemic control and progressive reduction of body weight in patients with type 2 diabetes inadequately controlled by sulphonylureas with or without metformin. *Diabetes Metab Res Rev*. 2006;22:483–491.

70. Heine RJ, Van Gaal LF, Johns D, Mihm MJ, Widel MJ, Brodows RG. Exenatide versus insulin glargine in patients with suboptimally controlled type 2 diabetes: a randomized trial. *Ann Intern Med*. 2005;143:559–569.

71. Nauck MA, Duran S, Kim D, et al. A comparison of twice-daily exenatide and biphasic aspart in patients with type 2 diabetes who were suboptimally controlled with sulfonylurea and metformin: a non-inferiority study. *Diabetologia*. 2007;50:259–267.

72. Vilsbøll T, Zdravkovic M, Le-Thi T, et al. Liraglutide, a long-acting human glucagon-like peptide-1 analog, given as monotherapy significantly improves glycemic control and lowers body weight without risk of hypoglycemia in patients with type 2 diabetes. *Diabetes Care*. 2007;30:1608–1610.

73. Drucker DJ, Buse JB, Taylor K, et al. for the DURATION-1 Study Group. Exenatide once weekly versus twice daily for the treatment of type 2 diabetes: a randomised, open-label, non-inferiority study. *Lancet*. 2008;372:10.

74. Buse JB, Henry RR, Han J, Kim DD, Fineman MS, Baron AD. Exenatide-113 Clinical Study Group. Effects of Exenatide (Exendin-4) on Glycemic Control Over 30 Weeks in Sulfonylurea-Treated Patients With Type 2 Diabetes. *Diabetes Care*. 2004;27:2628–2635.

75. Kendall DM, Riddle MC, Rosenstock J, et al. Effects of exenatide (exendin-4) on glycemic control over 30 weeks in patients with type 2 diabetes treated with metformin and a sulfonylurea. *Diabetes Care*. 2005;28:1083–1091.

76. Balas B, Baig MR, Watson C, et al. The dipeptidyl peptidase IV inhibitor vildagliptin suppresses endogenous glucose production and enhances islet function after single-dose administration in type 2 diabetic patients. *J Clin Endocrinol Metab*. 2007;92(4):1249–1255.

77. Goldstein B, Feinglos M, Lunceford J, Johnson J, Williams-Herman D. Sitagliptin 036 Study Group. Effect of initial combination therapy with sitagliptin, a dipeptidyl peptidase-4 inhibitor, and metformin on glycemic control in patients with type 2 diabetes. *Diabetes Care*. 2007;30:1979–1987.

78. Raz I, Hanefeld M, Xu L, Caria C, Davies M, Williams-Herman D. Sitagliptin Study 023 Group. Efficacy and safety of the dipeptidyl peptidase-4 inhibitor sitagliptin as monotherapy in patients with type 2 diabetes mellitus. *Diabetologia*. 2006;49:2564–2571.

79. Schmitz O, Brock B, Rungby J. Amylin agonists: a novel approach in the treatment of diabetes. *Diabetes*. 2004;5:S233–S238.

80. Riddle M, Frias J, Zhang B, et al. Pramlintide improved glycemic control and reduced weight in patients with type 2 diabetes using basal insulin. *Diabetes Care*. 2007;30:2794–2799.

81. UKPDS Group. UK Prospective Diabetes Study 16: overview of six years' therapy of type 2 diabetes—a progressive disease. *Diabetes*. 1995;44:1249–1258.

82. Turner RC, Cull CA, Frighi V, Holman RR. for the UKPDS Study Group. Glycemic control with diet, sulfonylurea, metformin or insulin in patients with type 2 diabetes. Progressive requirement for multiple therapies. *JAMA*. 1999;281:2005–2012.

83. Polonsky KS, Given BD, Van Cauter E. 24-hour profiles and patterns of insulin secretion in normal and obese subjects. *J Clin Invest*. 1988;81:442.

84. Brunelle R, Llewelyn J, Anderson JH, et al. Meta-analysis of the effect of insulin lispro on severe hypoglycemia in patients with type 1 diabetes. *Diabetes Care*. 1998;21:1726–1731.

85. Rosskamp RH, Park G. Long-acting insulin analogs. *Diabetes Care*. 1999;22:B109–B113.

86. Raskin P, Allen E, et al. Initiating insulin in type 2 diabetes. *Diabetes Care*. 2005;28:260–265.

87. Coscelli C, Clabrese G, Fedel D, et al. Use of premixed insulin among the elderly. *Diabetes Care*. 1992;15:1628–1630.

88. Monnier L, Lapinski H, Colette C. Contributions of fasting and postprandial plasma glucose to overall diurnal hyperglycemia in type 2 diabetic patients. *Diabetes Care*. 2003;26:881–885.

89. Riddle MC, Rosenstock J, Gerich J. The Treat-to-Target Trial: Randomized addition of glargine or human NPH insulin to oral therapy of type 2 diabetic patient. *Diabetes Care*. 2003;26:3080–3086.

90. Yki-Jarvinen H, Kauppinen-Maklein R, et al. Insulin glargine or NPH combined with metformin in type 2 diabetes: the LanMET study. *Diabetologia*. 2006;49:442–451.

91. Binder C, Lauritzen T, Faber O, Pramming S. Insulin pharmacokinetics. *Diabetes Care*. 1984;7:188–199.

92. Diabetes Control and Complications Trial Research Group. Influence of intensive diabetes treatment on body weight and composition of adults with type 1 diabetes in the diabetes control and complications trial. *Diabetes Care*. 2001;24:1711–1721.

93. UK Prospective Diabetes Study (UKPDS) Group. Intensive blood glucose control with sulphonylureas or insulin compared with conventional treatment and risk of complications in patients with type 2 diabetes (UKPDS 33). *Lancet*. 1998;352:837–853.

94. Diabetes Control and Complications Trial Research Group. The effect of intensive diabetes treatment on the development and progression of long-term complications in insulin-dependent diabetes mellitus: the diabetes control and complications trial. *N Engl J Med*. 1993;329:978–986.

95. Dailey G, Rosenstock J, Moses RG, Ways K. Insulin glulisine provides improved glycemic control in patients with type 2 diabetes. *Diabetes Care*. 2004;27:2363–2368.

96. Nathan DM, Buse JB, Davidson MB et al. Medical management of hyperglycaemia in type 2 diabetes mellitus: a consensus algorithm for the initiation and adjustment of therapy: A consensus statement from the American Diabetes Association and the European Association for the Study of Diabetes. *Diabetologia*. 2008;51:8.

Chapter 45
Prevention of Microvascular Complications of Diabetes – General Overview

Vincent Yen

Hyperglycemia in both type 1 and type 2 diabetes appears to set off a complex network of intracellular signaling mechanisms that lead to the characteristic microvascular complications of diabetes – retinopathy, nephropathy, and neuropathy. Chronic hyperglycemia (as measured by Hgb A1c) is clearly the main common etiologic factor behind these complications, and thus treatment methods aimed toward maintaining euglycemia are the most effective means of preventing microvascular complications.[1,2] The actual mechanisms by which hyperglycemia can lead to these changes are under study; theories center around interconnected pathways being abnormally activated in the setting of excess glucose in the system. Experimental evidence aimed at inhibition of components of these signaling pathways provides data regarding both pathogenesis as well as prevention of complications, separate from the standard, albeit difficult, approach of maintenance of euglycemia. This brief summary outlines some possible final common pathways that might account for the findings regarding the otherwise very diverse presentation of these pathologies.

Pathophysiologic findings that are seen in common across the spectrum include[3]

(1) accumulation of periodic acid Schiff (PAS) positive deposits for CHO-containing plasma proteins that have extravasated because of increased vascular permeability; these proteins are tightly cross-linked into vessel wall matrix components by collagen-linked advanced glycosylated proteins;
(2) expanded extracellular matrix production (e.g., glomerular mesangial cells or retinal basement membrane)
(3) cellular hypertrophy and hyperplasia (e.g., retinal endothelial cells and arterial smooth muscle cells).

One overall theory regarding vascular pathology is that of reactive oxygen species (ROS)/oxidative stress[4] and inflammation. Reactive oxygen species, or oxidants, are produced as intermediates in redox reactions leading from O_2 to H_2O_2; free radicals (capable of independent existence) such as superoxide O_2^- appear to be important ROS in microvascular biology. These molecules, through effects on cell growth regulation, cell differentiation, modulation of extracellular matrix, inactivation of nitric oxide, and stimulation of kinases and proinflammatory genes trigger endothelial dysfunction, activation of growth factors (such as vascular endothelial growth factor [VEGF], and transforming growth factor beta [TGF beta]), and eventually, characteristic dysfunctional changes in extracellular matrix, as well as in vessel walls, which exhibit abnormal permeability to proteins.[5,6] Type 1 patients with known microvascular disease show increased markers of inflammation – C-reactive protein, nitrotyrosine, vascular cell adhesion molecule, monocyte superoxide anion release, tumor necrosis factor, interleukin-6 (IL-6), interleukin-1beta release, with activation of MAP kinase (involved in cell growth), and NFκB (involved in apoptosis) – as compared to patients without microvascular disease.[6,7] Impaired endothelial function has been demonstrated in both type 1 and type 2 diabetes, as well as in insulin-resistant states.[8] Some theories regarding how oxidative stress can be enhanced and might then lead to the aforementioned pathologic findings include[9]

V. Yen (✉)
Saint Vincent's Medical Center, New York Medical College, New York, NY, USA
e-mail: vinyen@mindspring.com

L. Poretsky (ed.), *Principles of Diabetes Mellitus*, DOI 10.1007/978-0-387-09841-8_45,
© Springer Science+Business Media, LLC 2010

(1) via *advanced glycosylated end product* (AGE) formation;

(2) via *accumulated sorbitol* and other polyols from overflow of glucose from a saturated hexokinase pathway to the alternative *aldose reductase* pathway, leading to neural myoinositol depletion and reduced Na/K ATPase activity;

(3) increased flux through the *hexosamine* pathway, from fructose 6-phosphate

(4) from *protein kinase C* activation, via hyperglycemia-related increased synthesis of a major activator, diacylglycerol,[10] but also secondarily via the previous pathways, such as from AGEs or VEGF. (Protein kinase activity, which encompasses a large family of enzymes that catalyze the highly regulated transfers of phosphate from ATP to a wide variety of specific proteins in the process of most cellular activities,[5] is a critical regulator of intracellular signaling/gene expression and therefore, when abnormal, a key source of postreceptor metabolic derangements).

The pathways have many links, and many of the identified growth factors are seen to be increased by all of the above four processes. Additionally, AGEs, for instance, can increase reactive oxygen species themselves.[11] There are likely to be differing effects or predominance locally, depending on the organ system. For example, PK C inhibition, using ruboxistaurin, appears to delay macular edema via antipermeability effects, but proliferation-related pathology is not affected;[12] in the kidney this antipermeability effect appears to reduce proteinuria.[13] Regarding neuropathy, there seem to be some differences from nephropathy and retinopathy, in terms of correlations to other metabolic syndrome markers in some studies,[14] as well as with occasional spontaneous improvement.[15] In neuropathy, PK C inhibition with ruboxistaurin plus antioxidants such as tocopherol given to diabetic rats improved nerve conduction velocities.[16] Interestingly, when looking at a microvascular pathologic condition such as neuropathy, which can occur at relatively normal Hgb A1c levels and can present with acute episodes, an implication has been raised regarding the incidence of complications related to acute glucose fluctuations – postprandial and otherwise – as compared to chronic hyperglycemia, as measured by Hgb A1c. Some data[17] suggest a higher level of oxidative stress, as estimated from 24 h urinary excretion of free 8-iso-prostaglandin F2alpha, in patients that had higher mean amplitude of glycemic excursions as measured by continuous glucose monitoring systems.

Importantly, there are likely genetic components to an individual's predisposition to developing complications, as there are patients with long-standing type 1 diabetes that do not develop any complications. One study described 405 patients from the Joslin clinic, average age 69.5 years with average onset of type 1 at 12.6 years of age, who responded to a questionnaire. Out of which 46.8% described no clinical microvascular complications; HgA1C did not appear to correlate with risk in this cohort. Importantly, the mean age of death in the parents of these patients was almost 30 years higher than their birth cohort of the time, suggesting that genetic factors predisposing to longevity may have also protected these patients from diabetic complications.[18] Additionally, diabetic nephropathy has been shown to cluster in families and in specific ethnic groups; a cross-sectional study[19] showed an association of diabetic nephropathy in a type 1 diabetic patient with parental hypertension, cardiovascular disease, diabetes, and (paternal) cardiovascular mortality. Similar clustering and increased risk based on family history have been seen with retinopathy.[20] Thus, one might speculate that a diabetic individual's response to hyperglycemia, perhaps, for example, at the level of the cytokine response of that patient's AGE receptors to AGE binding, may be one of the types of genetic determinants that would predispose an individual to the development of microvascular complications from hyperglycemia.

At the cellular level, oxidative stress (imbalance between the relative rates of oxidant generation and levels of antioxidants that metabolize those reactive species) can be shown to induce many of the forms of diabetic vascular pathology, including endothelial dysfunction (impaired endothelium-dependent vasodilation, especially in regard to nitric oxide/cGMP pathways, which itself causes oxidative stress), vascular leakage, leukocyte adhesion, and cellular apoptosis. Hyperglycemia, as well as free fatty acids, can induce increased formation of reactive oxygen species and subsequent oxidative stress. Involved mechanisms may include mitochondrial-originated superoxide anions, which accelerate NO degradation;[4,6,7] alteration of cellular redox secondary to increased flux through the polyol pathway; AGE formation, which leads to tissue factor generation through the activation of NADP (nicotinamide adenine dinucleotide phosphate) oxidase, an enzyme involved in the formation of reactive oxygen species;[21] and finally, activation of protein kinase C, which seems to occupy a central role.

As mentioned earlier, PKC is a family of related serine/threonine kinases expressed in the vasculature (especially the beta form). It has been postulated that hyperglycemia can lead to de novo synthesis of DAG (diacyl glycerol), which will activate PKC; also hyperglycemia-related overexpression and activity of growth factors and vasoactive materials such as VEGF will activate PKC; and hyperglycemia-related formation of AGEs will also activate PKC.[5] Note that oxidative stress itself can activate PKC, which in turn will create further oxidative stress. In endothelial cell cultures where mitochondrial superoxide formation is suppressed, AGE formation, PKC activation, and sorbitol formation are seen to be reduced.[22] Pathologic changes induced by PKC include inhibition of nitric oxide production, altered gene expression for extracellular matrix proteins, fibronectin, type IV collagen, VEGF, TGF beta, CTGF (connective tissue growth factor), and adhesion molecules; infusion of these substances in experimental animal models leads to the characteristic blood vessel leakage, cell proliferation and apoptosis, tissue fibrosis, and production and deposition of extracellular matrix (ECM) proteins. Inhibition of PKC has beneficial effects on retinopathy and nephropathy, including endothelial cell permeability, in experimental models.[3]

Briefly, regarding the other pathways:

(1) *The formation of AGEs:*[23] a process that links diabetes to a state of accelerated aging, involves hyperglycemia-related irreversible, nonenzymatic covalent Amadori modification and cross-linking of proteins (including collagen, extracellular matrix/basement membrane proteins, nucleic acids, and lipoproteins) into large structures, such as carboxymethyllysine, pentosidine, and pyralline; such glycated molecules have altered function affecting vascular wall homeostasis and interactions with cytokines, macrophages, platelets, and lipoproteins. Deposited AGEs can be identified in diabetic tissues, and experimental infusion of AGEs can result in characteristic pathologic changes such as vascular leakage and reduced NO-mediated vasodilation.[24] Receptors for AGE (RAGE) in endothelial cells and macrophages, and their mRNA products from AGE binding, can lead to further stimulation of growth factors. Serum levels of AGEs correlate with glycemia, albeit within a much more prolonged time period compared with the more commonly known glycated product, Hgb A1c. Diabetic renal tissue samples show higher levels of RAGE/RAGE mRNA compared to nondiabetic controls.[25] Notably, activation of PPAR gamma by thiazolidinedione has been shown to downregulate RAGE and inhibit smooth muscle cell proliferation in rat carotid artery models,[26] potentially providing an additional mechanism for prevention of microvascular complications. Additionally, agents such as aminoguanidine, which block AGE formation can prevent microvascular pathologies in animal models.[27–30]

(2) Overburden of the glycolysis pathway with increased flux through the *hexosamine* pathway from fructose 6-phosphate can lead to excess O-linked glycosylation of target proteins, which in turn, can lead to downstream activation of gene expression for PAI-1, fibroblast growth factors, TGF alpha and beta, as well as effects on eNO synthase activity.[5]

(3) Activation of the *polyol pathway* to reduce glucose to sorbitol, mediated by aldose reductase, has been postulated to lead to reduced intracellular myoinositol and altered NADP potential and generation of reactive species and thus oxidative stress and vascular damage. Clinical trials using aldose reductase inhibitors have not been shown to be of significant benefit regarding microvascular complications.[31]

Growth factors in common that are involved in the development of various microvascular complications, include vascular endothelial growth factor (VEGF), seen to be increased in proliferative retinopathy, and TGF beta, which is increased in diabetic nephropathy and which has been shown to stimulate the changes of mesangial expansion and basement membrane hypertrophy.[4,5]

At the tissue level, these types of pathologies translate into some of the findings of the organ-specific complications. In neuropathy, findings include (1) slowing of nerve conduction velocities, perhaps related to depletion of sodium/potassium adenosine triphosphatase (possibly related to increased glycol through the activated aldose reductase system); (2) mulitfocal loss of axons perhaps, secondary to endoneural hypoxia/ischemic microvascular damage/endothelial dysfunction; (3) advanced glycation of nerve proteins leading to pathology diverted to expansion and away from remodeling and waste removal, with nerve microvascular basement membrane thickening, pericyte degeneration, and endothelial cell hyperplasia.[32] In early nephropathy, increased glomerular volume and glomerular capillary pressure lead to increased GFR and kidney size. With progression of diabetes, the basement membranes of the glomerulus, tubules, and the Bowman capsule thicken. This is followed by mesangial expansion and accelerated damage of arterioles as well as reduced filtration rate. This process progresses to diffuse glomerular sclerosis.[33] In the retina,[34] proliferative retinopathy and macular edema are the main causes of functional loss. Loss of pericytes (apoptotic?) from retinal capillaries with a subsequent loss of blood flow autoregulation followed by loss of capillary endothelial cells with resultant hypoxia is seen. Neovascularization and glial proliferation may result in hemorrhage, macular distortion, and retinal detachment.

Summary

Molecular, cellular, and tissue pathologies seen in the microvascular complications of chronic hyperglycemia – nephropathy, retinopathy, and neuropathy – have some findings in common, such as expanded extracellular matrix/basement membrane thickening, altered proliferation and death of vascular cells, vascular leakage, angiogenesis, endothelial dysfunction, and evidence of oxidative stress. Important etiologic players which act in concert as a result of hyperglycemia to cause the above findings include reactive oxygen species/superoxide, protein kinase C, advanced glycosylated end products, diacylglycerol, aldose reductase/sorbitol, transcription factor NFκB, and growth factors such as VEGF (angiogenesis) and TGF beta (profibrotic). Manipulation of some of these pathways, via protein kinase C inhibition (or blocking the expression of PKC regulated genes), or blockage of formation of AGEs (or disruption of currently formed ones), for example, may provide further benefit toward preventing microvascular complications, beyond the standard approach of maintenance of euglycemia, since not all diabetic patients are able to meet their metabolic goals.[35,36]

References

1. The Diabetes Control and Complications Trial Research Group. The effect of intensive treatment of diabetes on the development and progression of long-term complications in insulin dependent diabetes mellitus. *N Engl J Med*. 1993;329:977–986.
2. The UK Prospective Diabetes Study (UKPDS) Group. Intensive blood-glucose control with sulphonylureas or insulin compared with conventional treatment and risk of complications in patients with type 2 diabetes (UKPDS 33). *Lancet*. 1998;352:837–853.
3. Brownlee M. Biochemistry and molecular cell biology of diabetic complications. *Nature*. 2001;414:813–820.
4. Brownlee M. The pathophysiology of diabetic complications: a unifying mechanism. *Diabetes*. 2005;54:1615–1625.
5. He Z. King GL Microvascular complications of diabetes. *Endocrinol Metab Clin N Am*. 2004;33:215–238.
6. Pennathur S Heinecke JW. Oxidative stress and endothelial dysfunction in vascular disease. *Curr Diabetes Rep*. 2007;7: 257–264.
7. Schram MT, Chaturvedi N, Schalkwijk C, et al. The EURODIAB prospective complications study group: vascular risk factors and markers of endothelial dysfunction as determinants of inflammatory markers in type 1 diabetes. *Diabetes Care*. 2003;26:2165–2173.
8. Rask-Madsen C. King GL Mechansims of disease: endothelial dysfunction in insulin resistance and diabetes. *Nat Clin Pract Endocrinol Metab*. 2007;3:4656.
9. Powers AC. Diabetes mellitus. In: *Harrison's Endocrinology*. New York, USA: McGraw-Hill; 2006, Ch 17: pp. 299–300.
10. Xia P, Inoguchi T, Kern TS, Engerman RL, Oates PJ, King GL. Characterization of the mechanism for the chronic activation of diacylglycerol-protein kinase C pathway in diabetes and hypergalactosemia. *Diabetes*. 1994;43:1122–1129.
11. Wolf G. New insights into the pathophysiology of diabetic nephropathy: from hemodynamics to molecular pathology. *Eur J Clin Invest*. 2004;34:785.
12. The PKC-DRS Study Group. The effect of ruboxistaurin on visual loss in patients with moderate to severe to very severe nonproliferative diabetic retinopathy: initial results of the PK C beta inhibitor DR study multicenter randomized clinical trial. *Diabetes*. 2005;54:2188–2197.
13. Tuttle KR, Bakris GL, Toto RD, McGill JB, Hu K, Anderson PW. The effect of ruboxistaruin on neprhopathy in type 2 diabetes. *Diabetes Care*. 2005;28:2686–2690.
14. Tesfaye S, Chaturvedi N, Eaton SE, et al. Vascular risk factors and diabetic neuropathy. *N Engl J Med*. 2005;352:341–350.
15. Young RJ, Ewing DJ, Clarke BF. Chronic and remitting painful diabetic polyneuropathy: correlations with clinical features and subsequent changes in neurophysiology. *Diabetes Care*. 1988;11:34.
16. Cameron NE, Cotter MA. Effects of protein kinase C beta inhibition on neurovascular dysfunction in diabetic rats: interaction with oxidative stress and essential fatty acid dysmetabolism. *Diabetes Metab Res Rev*. 2002;18:315.

17. Monnier L, Mas E, Gine C, et al. Activation of oxidative stress by acute glucose fluctuations compared with sustained chronic hyperglycemia in patients with Type 2 diabetes. *JAMA*. 2006;295:1681–1687.
18. Keenan HA, Costacou T, Sun JK, et al. Clinical factors associated with resistance to microvascular complications of in diabetic patients of extreme disease duration. *Diabetes Care*. 2007;30:1995–1997.
19. Thorn LM, Forsblom C, Fagerudd J, et al. Clustering of risk factors in parents of patients with type 1 diabetes and nephropathy. *Diabetes Care*. 2007;30:1162–1167.
20. The Diabetes Control and Complications Research Group. Clustering of long term complications in families with diabetes in the diabetes control and complciations trial. *Diabetes*. 1997;46:1829.
21. Cai H. NAD(P)H oxidase-dependent self propagation of hydrogen peroxide and vascular disease. *Circ Res*. 2005;96:818–822.
22. Nishikawa T, Edelstein D, Du XL, et al. Normalizing mitochondrial superoxide formation blocks three pathways of hyperglycemic damage. *Nature*. 2000;404:787–790.
23. Brownlee M, Cerami A, Vlassara H. Advanced glycation end products in tissue and the biochemeical basis of diabetic complications. *N Engl J Med*. 1988;318:1315–1321.
24. Vlassara H, Striker LJ, Teichberg S, et al. Advanced glycation end products induce glomerular sclerosis and albuminuria in normal rats. *Proc Natl Acad Sci USA*. 1994;22:11704–11708.
25. Tanji N. Markowitz GS et al Expression of advanced glycation end products and their cellular receptor RAGE in diabetic nepropathy and nondiabetic renal disease. *J Am Soc Nephrol*. 2000;11:1656–1666.
26. Wang K, Zhou Z. Zhang M et al Peroxisome Proliferator Activator receptor gamma down regulates receptor for advanced glycation end products and inhibits smooth muscle cell proliferation in diabetic and non diabetic rat carotid artery injury model. *J Pharmacol Exp Ther*. 2006;317:37–43.
27. Hammes HP, Mariatn S, et al. Aminoguanidine treatment inhibits the development of experimental diabetic retinopathy. *Proc Natl Acad Sci USA*. 1991;88:11555–11558.
28. Ellis E, Good BH. Prevention of glomerular basement membrane thickening by aminoguanidine in experimental diabetes mellitus. *Metabolism*. 1991;40:1016–1019.
29. Li YM, Steffes M. Donnely T et al Prevention of cardiovascular and renal pathology of aging by the advanced glycation inhibitor aminoguanidine. *Proc Natl Acad Sci USA*. 1996;93:3902–3907.
30. Singh R, Barden A, Mori T, Beilin L. Advanced glycation end products: a review. *Diabetologia*. 2001;44:129–146.
31. Clark CM, Lee DA. Prevention and treatment of complications of diabetes mellitus. *N Engl J Med*. 1995;332:1210–1217.
32. Cameron NE, Eaton SE, Cotter MA. Tesfaye S Vascular factors and metabolic interactions in the pathogenesis of diabetic neuropathy. *Diabetologia*. 2001;44:1973–1988.
33. Fioretto P, Steffes MW, Brown DM, Mauer SM. An overview of renal pathology in insulin dependent diabetes mellitus in relation to altered glomerular hemodynamics. *Am J Kidney Dis*. 1992;20:549–558.
34. Frank RN. Diabetic retinopathy. *N Engl J Med*. 2004;350:48–58.
35. Resnick HE, Bardsley J Foster GL et al. Achievement of American Diabetes Association clinical practice recommendations among U.S. adults with diabetes, 1999–2002. The national health and nutrition examination survey. *Diabetes Care*. 2006;29:531–537.
36. Devaraj S, Cheung AT, Jialal I, et al. Evidence of increased inflammation and microcirculatory abnormalities in patients with type 1 diabetes and their role in microvascular complications. *Diabetes*. 2007;56:2790–2796.

Chapter 46
Psychiatric Care of the Patient with Diabetes

Jennifer L. Kraker and Stephen J. Ferrando

Introduction

Diabetes mellitus (DM) is an increasingly prevalent and complex chronic illness with significant psychosocial and psychiatric ramifications. Stress and psychiatric illness can contribute to the development of the disease itself,[1] via neurohormonal pathways and the side effects of psychiatric medication treatment, and psychiatric symptoms and disorders are prevalent and can have profound effects on the disease course of diabetes.[2] Thus, there is a pressing need for integration of general medical care and psychiatric care for the diabetic patient in order to improve quality of life and illness outcomes.

This chapter will provide a background to appreciate the interplay between mental health and diabetes by distilling the current literature. We review the epidemiology of psychiatric disorders in diabetes, the effects of psychiatric symptoms and disorders on the course of diabetes, psychiatric and neurocognitive comorbidities caused by diabetes, and psychiatric treatment of the diabetic patient. With this summary, we hope to offer the clinician an appreciation for how to recognize and treat psychiatric aspects of diabetes and when a referral for psychiatric or other mental health consultation is likely warranted.

Psychiatric Symptoms and Disorders and the Risk for Diabetes

There is now abundant literature to suggest that psychiatric symptoms and disorders often precede the onset of diabetes and may in fact comprise independent risk factors.[3] Large epidemiological studies have documented that the presence of depressive and anxiety symptoms at a baseline measurement predicts the later onset of metabolic syndrome and diabetes. In a prospective population-based Norwegian study, Engum[4] found that individuals reporting symptoms of depression and anxiety at baseline had increased risk for onset of type 2 diabetes at 10-year follow-up, after controlling for established diabetes risk factors. Interestingly, baseline diabetes was not associated with the presence of depressive or anxiety symptoms at follow-up (see next section). In a Swedish cohort of approximately 5200 individuals followed for 8–10 years, Eriksson et al.[1] found that the presence of distress symptoms at baseline (anxiety, apathy, depression, fatigue, and insomnia) predicted the onset of abnormal glucose tolerance and diabetes for men and abnormal glucose tolerance for women. The potential etiological mechanisms mediating the relationships between depression/anxiety/distress and diabetes are speculative, complex, and involve both neurohormonal and behavioral mechanisms. Depression/anxiety and prolonged stress affect the entire neuroendocrine system via activation of the central sympathetic nervous system

S.J. Ferrando (✉)
Division of Psychosomatic Medicine, Department of Psychiatry, Payne Whitney Clinic, New York-Presbyterian Hospital, Weill Cornell Medical College, New York, NY, USA
e-mail: sjferran@med.cornell.edu

and hypothalamus–pituitary–adrenal (HPA) axis. Activation of the HPA axis causes excessive cortisol production that induces insulin resistance, dyslipidemia, visceral obesity, and type 2 diabetes.[3,5,6] Also, depression may diminish healthy dietary and physical activity, leading to cardiovascular and diabetes risk.[3]

In addition to depression and anxiety, there is now a growing literature linking other forms of mental illness including schizophrenia, schizoaffective disorder, and bipolar disorder to the risk for diabetes. This relationship has been found to exist independently of the known effects of antipsychotic medications (particularly the second-generation atypical antipsychotics) on weight gain and glucose homeostasis (see below). Patients with schizophrenia, independent of antipsychotic medication use, are two to three times more likely than the general population to have type 2 diabetes.[7] In one hospital-based sample, 50% of bipolar and 26% of schizoaffective disorder patients were found to have type 2 diabetes.[8] In addition to the disorders themselves, newer generation atypical antipsychotic medications, particularly clozapine and olanzapine (and to a lesser degree and more inconsistently, risperidone, quetiapine, ziprasidone, aripiprazole) have been associated with dyslipidemia, insulin resistance, and hyperglycemia.[9] In general, the risk associated with these medications is proportional to weight gain; however, clozapine and olanzapine may have direct effects on glucose regulation independent of adiposity.

A synthesis of the above data would support the notion that primary care patients be regularly screened for chronic distress and psychiatric disorders. Further, patients with significant symptoms should be referred for mental health treatment as indicated but should also be counseled regarding the effects of psychotropic medication, diet, and exercise on diabetes risk and should be monitored regularly for the development of metabolic complications, including dyslipidemia, insulin resistance, and diabetes. For patients treated with second-generation antipsychotics, The American Diabetes Association in conjunction with the American Psychiatric Association have published consensus guidelines for the monitoring of patients taking these medications (Table 46.1).

Table 46.1 Consensus guidelines for monitoring patients taking second-generation antipsychotic medications (SGAs)*

	Baseline	4 weeks	8 weeks	12 weeks	Quarterly	Annually	Every 5 years
Personal/family history	X					X	
Weight (BMI)	X	X	X	X	X		
Waist circumference	X					X	
Blood pressure	X			X		X	
Fasting plasma glucose	X			X		X	
Fasting lipid profile	X			X			X

*More frequent assessments may be warranted based on clinical status

Epidemiology of Psychiatric Disorders in Patients Who Have Diabetes

It has long been recognized that depression and other forms of pathological distress are more common in patients with diabetes compared to individuals without the illness. Early studies focused on psychopathology in children with type 1 diabetes from clinical populations, documenting higher rates of psychopathology, particularly depression, compared to nondiabetic children. Psychiatric disorders were generally found in 20–50% of patients. However, these studies were limited due to use of nonstandardized diagnostic instruments, the confounding of somatic depressive symptoms with those of diabetes, and the rates which tended to be inflated due to over-selection for patients in specialty clinics with increased diabetes illness severity and complications.[10]

Since the late 1980s, studies employing representative samples of persons with both type 1 and type 2 diabetes and nondiabetic comparisons, using standardized psychiatric diagnostic instruments, have appeared in the literature. A sampling of such epidemiological studies from the USA and Europe is presented in Table 46.2. The Epidemiological Catchment Area Study (ECA) is the first such study (USA; $N = 2552$) comparing rates of psychiatric disorders in individuals with diabetes (as well as arthritis, heart disease, hypertension, or chronic lung disease) to rates in persons with no medical illness.[11] Findings from the ECA were largely reflective of

Table 46.2 Population-based prevalence rates of psychiatric disorders in diabetic compared to nondiabetic individuals, the USA, the UK, and Germany

References	Sample	N	Type 1/ type 2	Prevalence of psychiatric disorder, diabetic individuals	Prevalence of psychiatric disorder, nondiabetic individuals
Wells et al.[11]	US/Los Angeles; NIMH epidemiologic catchment area	2552	Both	Diabetic $N = 154$ Depression: 14.4% Substance use: 21.6% Anxiety: 26.2%	Depression: 6.9% Substance use: 17.3% Anxiety: 10.5%
Kruse, Shmitz & Thefeld (2003)[12]	Germany; cross-sectional national	4169	Both	Diabetic $N = 141$ Depression: 10.2% Substance use: 9.0% Anxiety: 15.6%	Depression: 6.2% Substance use: 12.6% Anxiety: 8.8%
Das-Munshi et al. (2007)[13]	UK; cross-sectional, national	8580	Both	Diabetic $N = 239$ Depression: 1.6% Anxiety: 6.9% Mixed anxiety/depression: 11.5% Comorbid anxiety/depression: 1.6% Any common mental disorder: 21.6%	Depression: 1.1% Anxiety: 5.0% Mixed anxiety/depression: 8.8% Comorbid anxiety/depression: 1.5% Any common mental disorder: 16.3%

subsequent studies. Individuals with history of diabetes were found to have a prevalence of 26% lifetime and 16% current anxiety disorders, 14% lifetime, and 10% current depressive disorders, both twice the rate of these disorders in medically healthy participants. Substance use disorders (22% lifetime and 6% current) were not significantly more frequent than the nonmedical population (17% lifetime and 6% current). Studies from the UK and Germany reflect a similar pattern for increased rates of overall psychiatric illness, particularly depression, anxiety, and their combination in patients with diabetes compared to the general population.

It is important to note that subclinical depressive and anxiety symptoms are also prevalent in patients with diabetes and may have considerable association with illness burden, particularly physical symptoms and disability. For example, in a clinic population of patients with type 1 and type 2 diabetes screened with the Hospital Anxiety and Depression Scale, 28% reported moderate-to-severe anxiety and/or depressive symptoms, which were associated with increased physical symptom burden.[14] Similarly, in a study of 581 African-American patients with diabetes, 27% reported significant depressive symptoms (Beck Depression Inventory [BDI] score > 14). Those with BDI scores >14 had more proliferative retinopathy and were more likely to be on disability.[15]

Differential Diagnosis of Psychiatric and Neuropsychiatric Symptoms in Diabetes

There are a number of important differential diagnostic considerations regarding psychopathology in diabetes, which are outlined in Table 46.3 and discussed in more detail throughout this chapter. First, patients should be assessed for prior history of psychiatric disorder, including mood (depression and mania), anxiety, psychotic, and substance use disorders. The presence of premorbid psychopathology is a predictor of recurrence of these illnesses during the course of diabetes. Second, when applicable, the neuroendocrine effects of atypical antipsychotic medications and other psychotropic medications should be considered in terms of their effect on diabetes management. Third, the acute and chronic/recurrent neuropsychiatric effects of hyper- and hypoglycemia must be considered regarding their effects on mood and cognition. Fourth, cognitive impairment is prevalent in diabetes and should always be considered as an etiological factor in neuropsychiatric symptomatology. Fifth, common medical complications, comorbidities, and their treatments in diabetes, particularly cardiovascular, cerebrovascular, and renal disease, may cause or exacerbate neuropsychiatric symptoms, including more extreme manifestations such as delirium.

Table 46.3 Differential diagnostic considerations for psychiatric and neuropsychiatric symptoms in diabetes

- Premorbid history of psychiatric disorder, including mood (depression and mania), anxiety, psychotic, and substance use disorders
- Acute and chronic neuropsychiatric effects of hyperglycemia
- Acute and chronic neuropsychiatric effects of hypoglycemia
- Neuroendocrine adverse effects of psychotropic drugs, particularly second-generation antipsychotics, mood stabilizers, and tricyclic antidepressants
- Neurocognitive impairment secondary to microvascular ischemic disease
- Neuropsychiatric complications of common medical comorbidities and their treatments (e.g., cardiovascular, cerebrovascular, and renal disease)

Psychosocial Approach to the Diabetic Patient May Improve Disease Burden

A new diagnosis of a chronic illness is inherently stressful. It is common to mourn the loss of healthy life potential to face challenges in adapting to the management of a chronic illness and to cope with associated disabilities. Jacobson[16] described the stages of adaptation specific to diabetes, which include (1) adjustment to the onset of diabetes, (2) adherence to treatment – both behavioral and pharmacological, and (3) intensifying treatment and diabetic complications. Understanding the stress response that occurs at each stage of the diabetes offers clinicians opportunities to screen for and treat distress and psychiatric comorbidities.

A New Diagnosis: The Onset of Diabetes

Type 1

The diagnosis of type 1 diabetes (T1DM) is associated with increased psychiatric morbidity.[16–18] The onset of type 1 diabetes is abrupt and often requires hospitalization, which can precipitate an acute stress or adjustment reaction in children and their caretakers. Maladjustment to type 1 diabetes may include denial, anxiety, sadness, irritability, exaggerated dependency, and mourning of the loss of one's healthy potential.[8] Cohort studies show that over 30% of children develop a clinically significant adjustment disorder within 3 months of their diagnosis.[19] Despite near full recovery rates at 1-year follow-up, children with difficulty initially adapting are more likely to experience future psychiatric complications.[6,7,20,21] Screening for and treating behavioral complications and maladjustment may improve long-term prognosis and should begin at the onset of diagnosis. The Behavior Assessment System for Children (BASC) or the Child Health Questionnaire (CHQ) are considered reliable measures.[22]

In addition to assessment of the child, clinicians should also assess the psychosocial status of primary caregivers (usually parents) and the family. Parents of children newly diagnosed with type 1 diabetes are at risk for experiencing anxiety and depression related to heightened experiences of parenting stress and poor self-efficacy, which is their perceived ability to manage diabetes in their child.[23] Key questions for caregivers are outlined in Table 46.4

Table 46.4 Questions to ask parents and caregivers of children diagnosed with diabetes

- What is nature of their relationship to the patient?
- How much care are they responsible for?
- Do they feel personally equipped to deliver that care?
- What degree of stress they are under?
- Do they have a history of psychiatric illness?
- What type and amount of help is available and how much would they accept?
- What expectations do they have from medical services?
- Are they aware of available support from voluntary organizations?

Type 2

While the onset of type 2 diabetes is distinct from that of type 1, as it is often a gradual process occurring in an adult, adjustment is equally complex. Adjustment varies greatly depending on the circumstances of diagnosis (i.e., anticipated vs. unanticipated) and sociodemographic characteristics such as gender and ethnicity. Patients who have no prior diabetes risk factors or active medical symptoms and who are not "primed" to expect the diagnosis are the most vulnerable to distress, which includes shock, sadness, anger, guilt, loneliness, and fear.[24] These responses and prior history of depression and/or anxiety may portend future stress, depression, and anxiety. Addressing a difficult adjustment early in the course of the disease may delay progression to complications. Early intervention should include psychiatric and cognitive assessment and treatment as necessary, coupled with diabetes education and skills training to enhance self-efficacy regarding diabetes treatment and lifestyle adjustments (e.g., diet, exercise, smoking cessation). In addition, it is necessary to incorporate social supports and a favorable doctor–patient relationship.

Treatment Adherence

Good diabetes self-care requires both emotional and practical social support and motivation to adhere to behavioral (dietary, exercise, and smoking cessation programs) and medical management (monitoring of blood glucose, medications, and follow-up with health-care providers). In a recent meta-analysis of 33 studies, low social support was robustly associated with poor diabetes control.[25] Further, psychiatric symptoms, particularly depression, profoundly interfere with adherence to medication and behavior changes necessary to prevent metabolic complications. Repeat assessment for symptoms of distress and social support and the impact of these on treatment adherence should be an integral component of routine follow-up.

Type 1

The mental health of youth with diabetes is highly dependent on the attitudes and well-being of their families or caregivers. This is often complicated by the significant burden to parents and caregivers of diabetic individuals. Well-established factors associated with good treatment adherence in youth include good communication (namely child and parent agreement), positive family attributes (warmth, support, and cohesion), and parental psychological well-being.[26–28] Cross-sectional and longitudinal data support that tight metabolic control is associated with the psychological well-being of the child.[29–31] Other longitudinal data support the notion that adolescents who have perceived negative responses from their friends are less likely to adhere to treatment.[32] A longitudinal study of 111 individuals with type 1 diabetes stratified patients by low, medium, and high levels of resilience (a combination of high self-esteem, self-efficacy, mastery, and optimism).[22] Low resilience at baseline was associated with rising distress and fewer self-care behaviors when faced with increasing distress and worsening HgbA1c across time.

Effective interventions that can be delivered or facilitated by diabetes providers and which can improve adherence and quality of life include peer-driven psychoeducational/empowerment approaches[33] and short-term coping skills training.[34] In the former intervention, patients acquire what they regard to be trustworthy information and coping skills accompanied by regular contact with other people with type 1 diabetes, giving them an increased sense of control in their lives and empowerment to change. The latter consists of a series of small group efforts designed to teach adolescents the coping skills of social problem solving, social skills training, cognitive behavior modification, and conflict resolution. The most effective interventions appear to provide skills and enhance social support. A recent meta-analysis showed strong social support to be a more sensitive correlate of glycemic control than stress management interventions.[16]

Type 2

Self-care behaviors (defined as attending appointments, diet, exercise, and adherence to medications) are fundamental to diabetes treatment and are established determinants of disease prognosis. Psychosocial factors are associated with these behaviors and ultimately affect treatment adherence.

Several cross-sectional studies show that stressful life events and perceived daily burden of diabetes are associated with poor treatment adherence.[35] Conversely, self-efficacy,[36] social support, and problem-focused coping skills were associated with improved blood glucose control.[25] Character traits followed in a longitudinal study ($N = 105$) found that high levels of neuroticism (anxiety, self-consciousness, vulnerability, depression, and hostility) predicted lower levels of blood glucose control.[37] In a study of 367 diabetic individuals, those who characterized their providers as "dismissive" were less likely to adhere to their treatment regimen compared to patients with more favorable characterizations.[38,39]

Accumulating evidence from clinical studies indicates that major depression in diabetic patients is linked with obesity, poor adherence to antidiabetic regimens, and consequently poor glycemic control, thus increasing risk for complications.[40,41] A clinical study by Ciechanowski et al. ($N = 367$) showed that depression symptom severity was associated with poor treatment adherence.[42] The relationship may be bidirectional, as poor glycemic control may adversely affect mood and thereby reinforce the relationship between diabetes and depression.

It is important to mention the relationship between alcohol use and treatment adherence. A large ($N = 65,996$) cross-sectional study of diabetes registrants from the Kaiser Permanente database showed that increasing use of alcohol was associated with poor self-care.[43]

Intensifying Treatment and Complications

Type 1

The increased need for insulin and the development of early complications is a time of increased risk for the reoccurrence or development of psychiatric comorbidities.

Insulin therapy is the only treatment option for type 1 diabetes, whose very treatment may create fear of its primary side effect, hypoglycemia. Hypoglycemia can cause sweating, tremors, slowed reaction time, and cognitive deterioration. At an extreme, severe hypoglycemia may precipitate seizures and even induce a coma. Patients can become confused and incapacitated so that they require the assistance of others in treating the hypoglycemia.

Type 2

A large international study involving 13 countries, known as the Diabetes Attitudes Wishes and Needs (DAWN) trial, found that nearly 50% of all type 2 diabetic patients not yet taking insulin interpreted the initiation of insulin therapy as a personal failure of their own self-care regimen, while less than 25% believed that insulin would help control their diabetes.[44] Other concerns about including insulin in therapy of type 2 diabetes were that diabetes was progressing and that insulin treatment may cause diabetes complications. A longitudinal study in Germany ($N = 420$) showed a higher rate of affective disorders in type 2 individuals with diabetes compared to type 1. It could be hypothesized, as subjects feared, that this may indicate a more chronic stage of the disease with longer duration, older age, and increase in complications.[45]

Psychiatric Comorbidities in Diabetic Patients

Depression

Depression in diabetes is associated with adverse psychosocial and medical outcomes, including poor adherence to dietary and medication treatment, functional impairment, poor glycemic control, increased risk of diabetic complications such as micro- and macrovascular disease, increased medical costs, and mortality.[46–50] Cross-sectional, correlational associations between depression and hyperglycemia and between depression and diabetes complications have been established. In one meta-analysis of 24 cross-sectional studies, Lustman et al.[46] found consistent small-to-moderate effect size relationships between depression and hyperglycemia. In another meta-analysis of 27 cross-sectional studies, DeGroot et al.[47] found a significant overall association between depression and diabetes complications, with individual small-to-moderate effect size ($r = 0.17$–0.32) associations between depression and retinopathy, nephropathy, neuropathy, macrovascular complications, and sexual dysfunction. The causal relationships among these associations are clearly important, but, based on the current literature, they are not precisely clear. It would be particularly important to establish whether depression leads to hyperglycemia which in turn leads to increased diabetic complications, and in turn, whether treatment of depression would reverse these effects.

In terms of physical symptom burden, studies have found that depressive symptoms are consistently correlated with subjective reports of both hyperglycemic (e.g., thirst, polyuria) and hypoglycemic (e.g., trembling, faintness) diabetic symptoms, as well as with symptoms commonly associated with depression, such as fatigue and confused thoughts.[51] Like the associations between hyperglycemia and diabetes complications, the etiological nature of the relationship of depression and diabetes symptoms is unclear. On one hand, diabetes and its complications may cause somatic symptoms. On the other hand, depression has multiple somatic symptoms and, further, may reduce the threshold for reporting diabetic symptoms ("symptom amplification").[31]

Diagnosis of Depression in Diabetes

Given the overlap of somatic symptoms of depression with symptoms of diabetes, the clinical diagnosis of depression in diabetic patients may be confounded. For example, whether or not to attribute complaints of fatigue to depression, hyperglycemia, hypoglycemia, or to some combination of these is a common clinical dilemma. One solution is to exclude somatic symptoms such as fatigue, appetite changes, sleep disturbance, and poor concentration in making a diagnosis of depression in diabetic patients, instead focusing on symptoms such as depressed mood, loss of interest, hopelessness, and guilt. However, previous studies suggest that the symptom characteristics of depression are similar in diabetic and nondiabetic psychiatric outpatients.[52] Further, in studies utilizing the Beck Depression Inventory as a screening tool, rates of depression are similar whether or not the somatic subscale items are included.[53] These findings suggest that an inclusive approach can be used, utilizing both somatic and mood symptoms in making a depression diagnosis as long as one or both of the cardinal symptoms of depressed mood and loss of interest are present.

Screening for Depression in Diabetes

Given the prevalence of depression in diabetes, routine screening is critical in order to identify patients at risk and to initiate treatment. The Beck Depression Inventory (BDI), a 20-item self-report measure of depressive symptoms, is the most frequently employed measure.[54] BDI score of ≥ 10 has a positive predictive value (PPV) of 0.45 and a score of ≥ 16 has a PPV of 0.71 for identifying major depression in diabetes.[55] It is translated into many languages and is an accepted measure to monitor effects of treatment. The Center for Epidemiological Studies – Depression Scale (CES-D) –[56] is also an extensively utilized 20-item self-report measure where a score of ≥ 16 differentiates depressed from nondepressed adults. McHale and colleagues[57] found the CES-D to be the most sensitive of several measures (the BDI was not included) in detecting depression in diabetes. The Hospital Anxiety and Depression Scale (HADS) is a 14-item self-report scale that was designed to screen for both depressive and anxiety symptoms in the medically ill.[58] Finally, the Patient Health Questionnaire 9-item depression screening module is now widely used to screen for depression in primary care. It is a 9-item self-report measure that mirrors the Diagnostic and Statistical Manual for Mental Disorders, Fourth Edition, criteria for major depression. Because of this design it requires less than 5 min of patient and provider time. It can be utilized as a categorical diagnostic measure or a continuous measure of depression severity and can be utilized to track treatment response. Lamers and colleagues[59] found that a cutoff score of ≥ 6 on the PHQ-9 had a sensitivity of 0.96 and a specificity of 0.81 for a depression diagnosis in elderly diabetic patients.

Antidepressant Medication Treatment of Depression in Diabetes

Despite the relatively high prevalence of depression in diabetes, there have been only two randomized controlled trials (RCTs) of antidepressant medication treatment of depression in this population, both conducted by the same group of investigators. In the first such study, Lustman et al.[60] compared nortriptyline (mean dose 60 mg/day: mean blood level approximately 75 ng/ml, therapeutic range 50–150 ng/ml) to placebo on their effects on change in depressive symptoms and glycemic control, as measured by HgbA1c, in an 8-week study of 68 type 1 or 2 diabetic patients with poor glycemic control (HgbA1c $\geq$ 9%), with or without major depression. In the subset of 28 patients with major depression, nortriptyline was statistically superior to placebo in reducing depressive symptoms as measured by the BDI (nortriptyline -10.2 vs. placebo -5.5, $p < 0.02$) and showed a numerically greater percentage in remission (BDI < 10; nortriptyline 57% vs. placebo 36%, $p = 0.45$), the nonsignificance of the latter finding likely being related to the small sample size. While dropout did not differ between groups, nortriptyline-treated patients compared to placebo-treated patients reported more dry mouth and, of particular concern, nortriptyline was found to have an independent adverse effect of glycemic control (discussed in next section).

Because of the latter finding regarding nortriptyline and glycemic control, and because of the generally better safety profile of the selective serotonin reuptake inhibitors (SSRIs), Lustman et al.[28] conducted an 8-week RCT comparing fluoxetine (up to 40 mg/day) to placebo in 60 type 1 or 2 diabetic individuals with major depression. Reduction in depressive symptoms was significantly greater in fluoxetine-treated patients than placebo-treated patients (BDI, -14.0 vs. -8.8, $p < 0.03$; HAM-D -10.7 vs. -5.2, $p < 0.01$) and more patients achieved clinical response in the fluoxetine-treated group (HAM-D, 66% vs. 37%, $p = 0.03$; BDI, 48% vs. 29%, $p = 0.09$). Further, a trend toward greater reduction in HgA1C was found in the fluoxetine vs. the placebo group (-0.40% vs. -0.07%, $p = 0.13$) (discussed further in next section). There was no difference in attrition or adverse events in the fluoxetine vs. the placebo groups.

Lustman and colleagues[61] noted that as few as 40% of patients with depression remained well after treatment, approximately 15% had chronic treatment resistant depression, and depression recurrence was associated with decline in glycemic control. Thus, they conducted a multisite randomized trial to determine whether maintenance treatment with sertraline was superior to placebo in prevention of depression recurrence. Depressed diabetic patients were treated openly with 16 weeks of sertraline (mean dose 118 mg) and those who achieved remission were randomized to continued sertraline or placebo and followed for up to 1 year. Sertraline was superior to placebo in prophylaxis against depression (hazard ratio 0.51, $p = 0.02$), with elapsed time before recurrence in one-third of the patients increasing from 57 days with placebo to 226 days with sertraline. Improvements in glycemic control seen during open-label treatment were maintained in those whose depression remained in remission. These findings underscore the importance of the maintenance of antidepressant treatment for depressed diabetic patients.

Given that the vast majority of diabetes care is delivered to patients in the primary care setting, Katon and colleagues[62] conducted a randomized trial (The Pathways Study) to determine whether enhancing quality of care for depression improves both depression and diabetes outcomes. Patients with diabetes and major depression and/or dysthymia from nine primary care clinics were randomly assigned to a stepped case management intervention ($N = 164$) or usual care ($N = 165$). The intervention provided enhanced education and support of antidepressant medication treatment prescribed by the primary care physician or problem-solving therapy delivered in primary care. After 1 year, when compared with usual care patients, intervention patients showed greater improvement in adequacy of dosage of antidepressant medication treatment, less depression severity, a higher rating of patient-rated global improvement, and higher satisfaction with care. Glycemic control did not differ between the two groups despite the superior depression outcome in the intervention group.

Psychotherapeutic Treatments of Depression in Diabetes

There have been numerous randomized controlled trials of psychological interventions to reduce depression/distress and improve glycemic control in diabetes, which have been reviewed extensively elsewhere.[63] Interventions studied vary greatly with the most prevalent being supportive counseling by physician or diabetes nurse, group cognitive behavioral therapy, and motivation enhancement. While interventions are generally effective in reducing depression/distress compared to control conditions, more intensive therapies such as cognitive behavioral therapy (CBT) and motivation enhancement produce the greatest benefits.

Effect of Depression Treatment on Glycemic Control in Depressed Diabetic Patients

Given the relationship between the presence of depression and poor glycemic control, it stands to reason that investigators have studied whether or not treatment of depression is associated with improved glycemic control. The mechanisms of such improvement might be hypothesized due to improvement in adherence to diabetes treatment, to reversal of depression-induced physiological changes associated with hyperglycemia, and to the potential direct euglycemic effects of antidepressant medication, or some combination of these. In general, depression treatment studies in diabetes have only begun to address these issues and, given that they are largely limited to measurement of HgA1c levels before and after 8 weeks of treatment, are insufficient to address individual or additive effects of these putative factors.

Regarding antidepressants, early uncontrolled studies suggested that treatment with tricyclic and monoamine oxidase inhibitor antidepressants might have beneficial effects on glucose control in diabetic individuals; however, there were case reports of severe hyperglycemia associated with these agents. As mentioned in the previous section, Lustman et al.,[60] in their RCT of nortriptyline vs. placebo found that nortriptyline treatment of non-depressed diabetic patients with baseline mean HgA1c 12.7% was associated with a significant decrease in glycosylated hemoglobin levels relative to placebo-treated patients. This effect was not associated with increases in weight or with poor medication or glucometer adherence patterns in the nortriptyline group. However, in the depressed subgroup, there was no differential change in glycosylated hemoglobin levels between the nortriptyline and the placebo groups, suggesting that depression improvement might at least offset the adverse nortriptyline effect. Indeed, a path analysis revealed that nortriptyline was associated with beneficial change in BDI-depressive symptoms (path coefficient 0.43) which was in turn associated with change in glycosylated hemoglobin (path coefficient 0.20), which offset the direct deleterious effect of nortriptyline on glycosylated hemoglobin (path coefficient −0.36) (see Figure p. 217 of Ref.[60])

In their study of fluoxetine vs. placebo in depressed diabetic patients with baseline HgA1c of 8.4%, Lustman et al.[28] found that fluoxetine was associated with a trend toward greater reduction in HgbA1c compared to placebo. This effect was unrelated to depression response, changes in weight, or baseline HgbA1c, leading these investigators to postulate a fluoxetine-specific effect. This is consistent with findings from studies of fluoxetine in obese type 2 diabetic patients, in which fluoxetine was associated with improvements in glycemic control, reductions in required insulin levels, and improved peripheral and hepatic insulin action, unrelated to changes in weight.[64–67]

In terms of the effect of psychotherapy on glycemic control, Lustman et al.,[68] in a 10-week RCT with 6-month follow-up of cognitive behavioral psychotherapy (CBT) plus diabetes education vs. diabetes education alone in depressed diabetic patients with mean baseline HgA1c of 10.2%, found that depressed diabetic patients who achieved remission of depression, regardless of treatment assignment, had lower glycosylated hemoglobin levels at study completion than those who did not achieve remission. While CBT was more effective in treating depression over 10 weeks and 6 months, the CBT group only had significantly better glycosylated hemoglobin levels at 6 months.[68] These findings also suggested independent benefits of depression improvement based on glycemic control. In a meta-analysis conducted by Ismail et al.,[63] intensive psychological therapies including CBT and motivation enhancement therapy were associated with a reduction of 1% in glycosylated hemoglobin, effects large enough to reduce the risk of development and progression of diabetic microvascular complications.

In sum, findings of improved glycemic control in RCTs of depression treatment in diabetes suggest beneficial effects of depression improvement independent of treatment as well as both deleterious (nortriptyline) and beneficial (fluoxetine and sertraline) independent effects of antidepressant medication. Nonetheless, the biological, psychological, and or social mechanism(s) of the observed benefits of depression improvement on glycemic control remain to be elucidated.

Anxiety

The association between diabetes and anxiety has been studied less thoroughly than depression, even though anxiety symptoms and disorders may be more prevalent. Anxiety is an exaggerated emotional response to fear, out of proportion to what non-anxious people experience. People with diabetes are subject to disease-specific fears such as hyper- and hypoglycemia, long-term complications of the disease, and day-to-day stresses of disease management. Specific fear of hypoglycemia is particularly prevalent among patients with prior hypoglycemic events, greater fluctuations in blood glucose levels, and long-term insulin treatment. This fear may have a significant negative impact on diabetes management, metabolic control, and subsequent health outcomes.[69] Several studies suggest that generalized anxiety disorder (GAD) is associated with poor glucose control and an increase in the reporting of symptoms.[70,71] A recent review of 18 studies ($N = 4076$) found that individuals with diabetes had a 27% prevalence for an anxiety disorder and 40% reported subclinical anxiety symptoms. Female diabetic individuals were more likely than males to develop anxiety, and there seems to be an equal distribution of anxiety spectrum disorders in type 1 and type 2 diabetes.[72] Large multinational studies show prevalence rates of moderate-to-severe anxiety in type 1 diabetes between 5 and 17%, though some cultural differences may effect the rates.[73] A cross-sectional cohort study of 600 women with type 2 diabetes found the prevalence of anxiety to be as frequent as depression. Anxiety was associated with African-American race, less education, and the presence of two or more long-term diabetes-related complications.[74]

Treatment of Anxiety in Diabetes

Treatment of anxiety in diabetes is understudied and is generally coupled with depression treatment, since the two are often comorbid. Wild et al. reviewed the literature on psychotherapeutic treatment of hypoglycemia fear and found that interventions including blood glucose awareness training and cognitive behavioral therapy can reduce levels of fear and improve disease management.[42] Others have found that, in addition to improving glycemic control, group-based diabetes management training can reduce anxiety.[75] There is accumulating evidence for efficacy of biofeedback and mindfulness-based stress reduction interventions, with similar results over short-term follow-up, though studies are limited by small numbers of participants and long-term outcome measures.[76,77]

In terms of medication intervention, a randomized controlled trial of short-term treatment of generalized anxiety disorder (GAD) with alprazolam showed reduction in anxiety symptoms and decrease of more than 1% in HgbA1c levels over the course of 3 months.[78] Otherwise, antidepressant medication treatments, particularly SSRIs, are indicated for the treatment of chronic anxiety disorders (GAD, panic disorder, social anxiety disorder, posttraumatic stress disorder, and obsessive compulsive disorder) and have been shown to be safe and effective for depressed patients with diabetes (see "Depression" section).

Cognitive Dysfunction

Dysregulated blood glucose and its metabolic sequelae have well-established cognitive effects. The effects of diabetes seem to be most clinically relevant at critical time periods, namely when the brain undergoes developmental change during childhood and during neurodegenerative processes of old age.[79] Cognitive dysfunction is associated with poor diabetes self-care, therefore requiring greater dependency on others for practical support.[80]

Type 1 Diabetes

Impairments in intelligence, attention, learning, memory, problem solving, and mental and motor speed are more common in type 1 diabetic patients than in the general population.[81,82,83] The magnitude of these deficits varies across studies. Early onset of diabetes is a reliable predictor of poor cognition in children. Longitudinal studies have found lower intelligence quotients (IQ), reduced mental efficiency, and poor academic performance in children with type 1 diabetes. A meta-analysis of 33 neuropsychological studies in adults with type 1 diabetes showed a consistent slowing of mental speed and a decreased ability to flexibly apply acquired knowledge in a new situation.[84] Though the effect size was relatively small, 0.5 standard deviation away from the norm, the daily intellectual effects and the effects on global functioning across the life span were pronounced. The neurocognitive abnormalities may be an effect of the disease itself, the result of hyperglycemia, hypoglycemia, insulin therapy, or some combination of these factors.

Type 2 Diabetes

Several longitudinal studies provide compelling evidence for the increased risk of cognitive impairment in type 2 diabetes. One cohort ($N = 529$) found 10.8–17.5% (36) of elderly patients with type 2 diabetes to have cognitive impairment or dementia.[85] As previously discussed, depression is often comorbid in diabetes, which may confound the assessment of cognitive function because of associated cognitive symptomatology. Further, elderly patients with diabetes may have "vascular depression," characterized by depressive symptoms and executive dysfunction produced by microvascular injury affecting subcortical–frontal circuitry.[86]

Thirteen aggregated longitudinal studies showed individuals with type 2 diabetes to have an overall relative risk of 1.5–2.0 of developing Alzheimer's disease (AD) and 2.0–2.5 relative risk of developing vascular dementia;[87] key determinants for dementia were dysregulated amyloid, insulin, and glucose metabolism. A recent prospective study from the Cardiovascular Health Cohort ($N = 2547$) points to an association between the apolipoprotein E epsilon 4 allele (APOE) and risk for developing anxiety disorder or mixed anxiety disorder and vascular dementia in individuals with diabetes.[88] Several cross-sectional studies and nationwide prospective studies link increased insulin secretion,[89] assessed by C-peptide,[90,91] or increased fasting insulin[92] to cognitive impairment in diabetes.

Other cross-sectional studies underscore the associations of age >65 years[93,94] duration of diabetes and use of insulin therapy[95] with cognitive impairment. Overall clinical determinants of cognitive decline are summarized in Table 46.5.

Table 46.5 Risk factors for cognitive impairment in diabetes

- HgbA1c > 7%
- Age >65
- Long duration of DM
- Insulin-treated DM
- APOE 4 allele
- Increased insulin secretion

Pathophysiology of Cognitive Dysfunction in Diabetes

The etiological mechanisms of cognitive dysfunction in diabetes have not yet been entirely elucidated. However, multiple contributors have been identified.

Acute and recurrent hypoglycemia are associated with cognitive dysfunction.[96,97] Acute hypoglycemia impairs cognitive performance at a blood glucose level of 2.2–3.0 mmol/l in healthy subjects. Generally, complex functions (psychomotor speed, executive function, and verbal memory) are most sensitive to hypoglycemia. Onset of hypoglycemic cognitive dysfunction is immediate, but recovery may be delayed. Adaptation to hypoglycemia, partly due to increased brain glucose uptake capacity, may occur. Chronic effects of recurrent hypoglycemia remain controversial. On one hand, patients with severe recurrent hypoglycemia tested in a euglycemic state had significant impairment in verbal learning and lexical memory compared to diabetic individuals with only mild hypoglycemia and nondiabetic controls.[98] However, major prospective studies, including the Diabetes Control and Complications Trial,[99] have not found greater degrees of cognitive dysfunction in patients with repeated episodes of hypoglycemia. Structural and functional brain changes are not only associated with recurrent severe hypoglycemia but also with hyperglycemia and early disease onset and may in part be due to hyperglycemic microvascular disease.

Interestingly, while diabetic ketoacidosis is often accompanied by global cognitive impairment and delirium, more moderate levels of acute hyperglycemia have not been found to significantly alter performance on cognitive tasks. Experimentally induced acute hyperglycemia at levels of 14.4 or 21.1 mmol/l was not associated with impairment in tests of associative learning, attention, or mental flexibility. However, chronic hyperglycemia is associated with microvascular changes in the brain that are responsible for chronic cognitive decline.[100]

Structural and functional neuroimaging can also shed light on brain pathology in diabetes. Notably, cross-sectional neuroimaging data have shown individuals with type 2 diabetes to have a more permeable blood–brain barrier (BBB),[101] an increase in subcortical lacunar infarcts, cerebral atrophy[65,102], and periventricular white matter hyperintensity.[103]

Single photon emission computed tomography (SPECT 217) in elderly diabetic patients found that 31.4% of subjects showed parieto-temporal hypoperfusion and 34.2% had fronto-temporal hypoperfusion patterns of abnormalities, while 11.4% displayed unclassifiable findings and 8.5% showed no detectable abnormalities.[104]

On a physiological level, CNS abnormalities of glucose and energy metabolism suggest that insulin and insulin-like growth factor type I and II (IGF-I and IGF-II) signaling mechanisms may play a role in cognitive decline in diabetes and in the development of Alzheimer's disease.[105] In addition, impaired dorsomedial striatum N-methyl-D-aspartate (NMDA) receptor signaling in diabetes may contribute to learning deficits,[106] and such deficits have been improved in animal models via administration of D-cycloserine, a modulator of NMDA receptor function.[107]

Further, increased acetylcholinesterase activity, oxidative-nitrosative stress, and inflammation have been documented in the brains of diabetic rats and reversed by chronic administration of lycopene, an antioxidant and an anti-inflammatory agent.[108]

Decreased acetylcholine, serotonin turnover, and decreased dopamine activity have also been shown. Of note, all of these deficits were reversed with insulin. Insulin receptors are found throughout the brain, with high concentration in the hippocampus, a region associated with learning and memory.

Cognitive Function Assessment

All individuals with type 2 diabetes, particularly patients with long-term disease, recurrent hypoglycemia, prolonged hyperglycemia, children, and the elderly, warrant a cognitive assessment. Commonly utilized screening

Table 46.6 Domains of cognitive impairment in diabetes and examples of associated neuropsychological tests	
	General cognitive deficits Mini mental status exam (MMSE)
	Verbal learning and memory Word list recall (Rey Auditory Verbal Learning test, California Verbal learning test) Verbal recognition Paragraph recall
	Processing speed Digit symbol coding test Trail making test Part A and B
	Executive function Stroop tasks Trail making test Part B Wisconsin card sorting test Clock drawing test

and assessment measures are outlined in Table 46.6. Cognitive screening using a bedside Mini Mental State Examination (MMSE) is most useful for detecting early to later stages of dementia in diabetes (a score of <23 out of 30 is considered suggestive of dementia).[96] Patients with scores less than 23 on the MMSE were less likely to participate in their activities of daily living (ADLs), self-care, and were more likely to require hospitalization. However, the MMSE is not able to detect deficits in key cognitive domains affected early in diabetes, notably psychomotor processing speed and executive dysfunction. Another bedside test, the Clock Drawing Test (CDT), is useful for detecting deficits in executive function and has been linked to everyday functional decline.[109]

For patients with suspected deficits not adequately characterized by MMSE and/or CDT, formal neuropsychological assessment is suggested. There are a wide range of neurocognitive batteries in the literature that target global cognitive functioning, verbal learning and memory, psychomotor processing speed, and executive function. These tests must be interpreted by a licensed neuropsychologist, merely characterize deficits, and do not clarify underlying etiopathology. Nonetheless, such assessment can be immensely helpful in estimating cognitive disability and tracking the effects of treatment.

Does Diabetes Treatment Improve Function?

There is a considerable literature documenting the benefit of improved glycemic control on existing cognitive dysfunction. Ryan et al.[110] found that improved glycemic control led to better working memory in individuals with type 2 diabetes. In this study, patients who were treated with either rosiglitazone or glyburide added onto to metformin monotherapy underwent cognitive improvement as measured by the Paired Associates Learning Test. This change was significantly correlated with improved glycemic control. Meneilly et al.[111] reported improvement on selective cognitive tasks with increased glycemic control in a small study of 16 elderly diabetic patients.

Conclusion

Diabetes, distress, and psychiatric disorders are intimately intertwined. Optimal diabetes care should integrate a firm knowledge of associated psychiatric and neuropsychiatric symptoms in diabetes, ongoing screening of all patients for distress and cognitive impairment, enhanced services in the primary care setting (e.g., group and individual diabetes education, skill building and support, as well as enhanced depression care delivered by trained nursing and other staff), and linkage with mental health services for patients with complicated presentations and who are refractory to first-line treatments. Such interventions have been well documented to improve both quality of life and diabetes management.

Acknowledgments The authors would like to thank Charles Gross, M.A., for his editorial assistance on this chapter.

References

1. Eriksson AK, Ekbom A, Granath F, Hilding A, Efendic S, Ostenson CG. Psychological distress and risk of pre-diabetes and Type 2 diabetes in a prospective study of Swedish middle-aged men and women. *Diabet Med*. 2008;25(7):834–842.
2. Lustman PJ, Griffith LS, Clouse RE, Cryer PE. Psychiatric illness in diabetes mellitus. Relationship to symptoms and glucose control. *J Nervous Mental Disease*. 1986;174(12):736–742.
3. Fenton WS, Stover ES. Mood disorders: cardiovascular and diabetes comorbidity. *Curr Opin Psychiatr*. 2006;19:421–427.
4. Engum A. The role of depression and anxiety in onset of diabetes in a large population-based study. *J Psychosom Res*. 2007;62:31–38.
5. Bjorntorp P. Heart and soul: stress and the metabolic syndrome. *Scand Cardiovasc J*. 2001;**35**:172–177.
6. Rosmond R. Stress-induced disturbances of the HPA axis: a pathway to type 2 diabetes? *Med Sci Monit*. 2003;**9**:RA35–RA39.
7. Smith M, Hopkins D, Peveler RC, Holt RI, Woodward M, Ismail K. First- v. second-generation antipsychotics and risk for diabetes in schizophrenia: systematic review and meta-analysis. *Br J Psychiatry*. 2008 Jun;192(6):406–411.

8. Regenold WT, Thapar RK, Marano C, Gavirneni S, Kondapavuluru PV. Increased prevalence of type 2 diabetes mellitus among psychiatric inpatients with bipolar I affective and schizoaffective disorders independent of psychotropic drug use. *J Affect Disord*. 2003 Feb;73:301–302.

9. Newcomer JW. Second-generation (atypical) antipsychotics and metabolic effects: a comprehensive literature review. *CNS Drugs*. 2005;19(Suppl 1):1–93.

10. Lustman PJ, Amado H, Wetzell RD. Depression in diabetics: a critical appraisal. *Compr Psychiatry*. 1983;24:65–73.

11. Wells KB, Golding JM, Burnam MA. Affective, substance use and anxiety disorders in persons with arthritis, diabetes, heart disease, high blood pressure and chronic lung conditions. *Gen Hosp Psychiatr*. 1989;11(5):320–327.

12. Kruse J, Schmitz N, Thefeld W. On the association between diabetes and mental disorders in a community sample: results from the German National Health Interview and Examination Survey. *Diabetes Care*. 2003;26(6):1841–1846.

13. Das-Munshi J, Stewart R, Ismail K, Bebbington PE, Jenkins R, Prince MJ. Diabetes, common mental disorders and disability; findings from the UK National Psychiatric Morbidity Survey. *Psychosom Med*. 2007;69:543–550.

14. Lloyd CE, Dyer PH, Barnett AH. Prevalence of symptoms of depression and anxiety in a diabetes clinic population. *Diabet Med*. 2000;17:198–202.

15. Roy A, Roy M. Depressive symptoms in African-American type 1 diabetics. *Depress Anxiety*. 2001;13:28–31.

16. Jacobson AM. The psychological care of patients with insulin-dependent diabetes mellitus. *N Engl J Med*. 1996;334(19):1249–1253.

17. Kovacs M, Obrosky DS, Goldston D, Drash A. Major depressive disorder in youths with IDDM. A controlled prospective study of course and outcome. *Diabetes Care*. 1997;20(1):45–51.

18. Northam EA, Matthews LK, Anderson PJ, Cameron FJ, Werther GA. Psychiatric morbidity and health outcome in Type 1 diabetes – perspectives from a prospective longitudinal study. *Diabet Med*. 2005;22(2):152–157.

19. Kovacs M, Feinberg TL, Paulauskas S, Finkelstein R, Pollock M, Crouse-Novak M. Initial coping responses and psychosocial characteristics of children with insulin-dependent diabetes mellitus. *J Pediatr*. 1985;106(5):827–834.

20. Kovacs M, Ho V, Pollock MH. Criterion and predictive validity of the diagnosis of adjustment disorder: a prospective study of youths with new-onset insulin-dependent diabetes mellitus. *Am J Psychiatr*. 1995;152(4):523–528.

21. Grey M, Cameron ME, Lipman TH, Thurber FW. Psychosocial status of children with diabetes in the first 2 years after diagnosis. *Diabetes Care*. 1995;18(10):1330–1336.

22. Cameron FJ, Smidts D, Hesketh K, Wake M, Northam EA. Early detection of emotional and behavioural problems in children with diabetes: the validity of the child health questionnaire as a screening instrument. *Diabet Med*. 2003;20(8):646–650.

23. Streisand R, Mackey ER, Elliot BM, et al. Parental anxiety and depression associated with caring for a child newly diagnosed with type 1 diabetes: opportunities for education and counseling. *Patient Educ Couns*. 2008;73(2):333–338.

24. Peel E, Parry O, Douglas M, Lawton J. Diagnosis of type 2 diabetes: a qualitative analysis of patients' emotional reactions and views about information provision. *Patient Educ Couns*. 2004;53:269–275.

25. Chida Y, Hamer M. An association of adverse psychosocial factors with diabetes mellitus: a meta-analytic review of longitudinal cohort studies. *Diabetologia*. 2008;51(12):2168–2178.

26. Liakopoulou M, Alifieraki T, Katideniou A, et al. Maternal expressed emotion and metabolic control of children and adolescents with diabetes mellitus. *Psychother Psychosom*. 2001;70(2):78–85.

27. Viner R, McGrath M, Trudinger P. Family stress and metabolic control in diabetes. *Arch Disease Childhood*. 1996;74(5):418–421.

28. Auslander WF, Bubb J, Rogge M, Santiago JV. Family stress and resources: potential areas of intervention in children recently diagnosed with diabetes [erratum appears in Health Soc Work 1993 Aug;18(3):194]. *Health Social Work*. 1993;18(2):101–113.

29. Kovacs M, Mukerji P, Drash A, Iyengar S. Biomedical and psychiatric risk factors for retinopathy among children with IDDM. *Diabetes Care*. 1995;18(12):1592–1599.

30. Leonard BJ, Jang Y-P, Savik K, Plumbo PM, Christensen R. Psychosocial factors associated with levels of metabolic control in youth with type 1 diabetes. *J Pediatr Nurs*. 2002;17(1):28–37.

31. Yi JP, Vitaliano PP, Smith RE, Yi JC, Weinger K. The role of resilience on psychological adjustment and physical health in patients with diabetes. *Br J Health Psychol*. 2008;13(Pt 2):311–325.

32. Hains AA, Berlin KS, Davies WH, Parton EA, Alemzadeh R. Attributions of adolescents with type 1 diabetes in social situations: relationship with expected adherence, diabetes stress, and metabolic control. *Diabetes Care*. 2006;29(4):818–822.

33. Booker S, Morris M, Johnson A. Empowered to change: evidence from a qualitative exploration of a user-informed psycho-educational programme for people with type 1 diabetes. *Chronic Illness*. 2008;4(1):41–53.

34. Grey M, Boland EA, Davidson M, Yu C, Sullivan-Bolyai S, Tamborlane WV. Short-term effects of coping skills training as adjunct to intensive therapy in adolescents. [see comment]. *Diabetes Care*. 1998;21(6):902–908.

35. Eriksson AK, Ekbom A, Granath F, Hilding A, Efendic S, Ostenson CG. Psychological distress and risk of pre-diabetes and Type 2 diabetes in a prospective study of Swedish middle-aged men and women. *Diabet Med*. 2008;25:834–842.

36. Nakahara R, Yoshiuchi K, Kumano H, Hara Y, Suematsu H, Kuboki T. Prospective study on influence of psychosocial factors on glycemic control in Japanese patients with type 2 diabetes. *Psychosomatics*. 2006;47:240–246.

37. Lane JD, McCaskill CC, Williams PG, Parekh PI, Feinglos MN, Surwit RS. Personality correlates of glycemic control in type 2 diabetes. *Diabetes Care*. 2000;23:1321–1325.

38. Ciechanowski PS, Katon WJ, Russo JE, Walker EA. The patient-provider relationship: attachment theory and adherence to treatment in diabetes. *Am J Psychiatr*. 2001;158:29–35.

39. Golin CE, DiMatteo MR, Gelberg L. The role of patient participation in the doctor visit. Implications for adherence to diabetes care. *Diabetes Care*. 1996;19:1153–1164.

40. McKellar JD, Humphreys K, Piette JD. Depression increases diabetes symptoms by complicating patients' self-care adherence. *Diabetes Educ*. 2004;30:485–492.

41. Lustman PJ, Griffith LS, Clouse RE. Depression in adults with diabetes. Results of 5-year follow-up study. *Diabetes Care*. 1988;11:605–612.

42. Ciechanowski PS, Katon WJ, Russo JE. Depression and diabetes: impact of depressive symptoms on adherence, function, and costs. *Arch Intern Med*. 2000;160:3278–3285.

43. Ahmed AT, Karter AJ, Liu J. Alcohol consumption is inversely associated with adherence to diabetes self-care behaviours. *Diabet Med*. 2006;23:795–802.

44. Peyrot M, Rubin RR, Lauritzen T, et al. The international DAP: Resistance to insulin therapy among patients and providers: results of the cross-national Diabetes Attitudes, Wishes, and Needs (DAWN) study. [see comment]. *Diabetes Care*. 2005;28(11):2673–2679.

45. Hermanns N, Kulzer B, Krichbaum M, Kubiak T, Haak T. Affective and anxiety disorders in a German sample of diabetic patients: prevalence, comorbidity and risk factors. *Diabet Med*. 2005 Mar;22(3):293–300.

46. Lustman PJ, Griffith LS, Freedland KE, Clouse RE. Fluoxetine for depression in diabetes: a randomized double-blind placebo-controlled trial. *Diabetes Care*. 2000;23:618–623.

47. De Groot M, Anderson R, Freedlan KE, Clouse RE, Lustman PJ. Association of depression and diabetes complications: A meta-analysis. *Psychosomatic Med*. 2001;63:619–630.

48. Chiechanowski PS, Katon WJ, Russo JE. Depression and diabetes: Impact of depressive symptoms on adherence, function and costs. *Arch Intern Med*. 2000;160:3278–3285.

49. Musselman DL, Betan E, Larsen H, Phillips LS. Relationship of depression to diabetes types 1 and 2: epidemiology, biology and treatment. *Biol Psychiatry*. 2003;54:317–329.

50. Katon WJ, Rutter C, Simon G, et al. The association of comorbid depression with mortality in patients with type 2 diabetes. *Diabetes Care*. 2005;28:2668–2672.

51. Chiechanowski PS, Katon WJ, Russo JE. The relationship of depressive symptoms to symptom reporting, self-care and glucose control in diabetes. *Diab Care*. 2002;25:731–736.

52. Lustman PJ, Freedland KE, Carney RM, Hong BA. Similarity of depression in diabetic and psychiatric patients. *Psychosom Med*. 1992;54:602–611.

53. Lustman PJ, Griffith LS, Clouse RE. Depression in adults with diabetes. *Semin Clin Neuropsychiatry*. 1997;2:15–23.

54. Beck AT, Beamesderfer A. Assessment of depression: the depression inventory. *Mod Probl Pharmacopsychiatry*. 1974;7:151–169.

55. Lustman PJ, Clouse RE, Griffith LS, Carney RM, Freedland KE. Screening for depression in diabetics using the Beck Depression Inventory. *Psychosom Med*. 1997;59:24–31.

56. Radloff LS. The CES -D scale: a self-report depression scale for research in the general population. *Appl Psychol Meas*. 1977;1:385–401.

57. McHale M, Hendrikz J, Dann F, Kenardy J. Screening for depression in patients with diabetes mellitus. *Psychosom Med*. 2008;70:869–874, Epub 2008 Oct 8.

58. Zigmond AS, Snaith RP. The hospital anxiety and depression scale. *Acta Psychiatr Scand*. 1983;67:361–370.

59. Lamers F, Jonkers CC, Bosma H, Penninx BW, Knottnerus JA, van Eijk JT. Summed score of the Patient Health Questionnaire-9 was a reliable and valid method for depression screening in chronically ill elderly patients. *J Clin Epidemiol*. 2008;61:679–687.

60. Lustman PJ, Griffith LS, Clouse RE, et al. Effects of nortriptyline on depression and glycemic control in diabetes: results of a double-blind, placebo-controlled trial. *Psychosomatic Medicine*. 1997;59:241–250.

61. Lustman PJ, Clouse RE, Nix BD, et al. Sertraline for prevention of depression recurrence in diabetes mellitus: a randomized, double-blind, placebo-controlled trial. *Arch Gen Psychiatr*. 2006;63:521–529.

62. Katon WJ, Von Korff M, Lin EH, et al. The pathways study: a randomized trial of collaborative care in patients with diabetes and depression. *Arch Gen Psychiatr*. 2004;61:1042–1049.

63. Ismail K, Winkley K, Rabe-Hesketh S. Systematic review and meta-analysis of randomised controlled trials of psychological interventions to improve glycaemic control in patients with type 2 diabetes. *Lancet*. 2004;363:1589–1597.

64. Gray DS, Fujioka K, Devine W, Bray GA. Fluoxetine treatment of the obese diabetic. *Int J Obes*. 1992;16:193–198.

65. Daubressse J-C, Kalanowski J, Krezentowski G, Kutnowski M, Scheen A, Van Gaal L. Usefulness of fluoxetine in obese non-insulin-dependent diabetics: a multicenter study. *Obes Res*. 1996;4:391–396.

66. Maheux P, Ducros F, Bourque J, Garon J, Chaisson J-L. Fluoxetine improves insulin sensitivity in obese patients with non-insulin-dependent diabetes mellitus independently of weight loss. *Int J Obes*. 1997;21:97–102.

67. Potter van Loon BJ, Radder JK, Frolich M, Krans HMJ, Zwinderman AH, Meinders AE. Fluoxetine increases insulin action in obese nondiabetic and in obese non-insulin-dependent diabetic individuals. *Int J Obes*. 1992;16:79–85.

68. Lustman PJ, Griffith LS, Freedland KE, Kissel SS, Clouse RE. Cognitive behavior therapy for depression in type 2 diabetes mellitus: a randomized, controlled trial. *Ann Intern Med*. 1998;120:613–621.

69. Wild D, von Maltzahn R, Brohan E, Christensen T, Clauson P, Gonder-Frederick L. A critical review of the literature on fear of hypoglycemia in diabetes: Implications for diabetes management and patient education. *Patient Educ Couns.* 2007 68(1):10–15, Epub 2007 Jun 19.Sep.

70. Lustman PJ. Anxiety disorders in adults with diabetes mellitus. *Psychiatr Clin N Am.* 1988;11(2):419–432.

71. Anderson RJ, Grigsby AB, Freedland KE, et al. Anxiety and poor glycemic control: a meta-analytic review of the literature. *Int J Psychiatr Med.* 2002;32(3):235–247.

72. Grigsby AB, Anderson RJ, Freedland KE, Clouse RE, Lustman PJ. Prevalence of anxiety in adults with diabetes: a systematic review. *J Psychosom Res.* 2002;53(6):1053–1060.

73. Lloyd CE, Zgibor J, Wilson RR, Barnett AH, Dyer PH, Orchard TJ. Cross-cultural comparisons of anxiety and depression in adults with type 1 diabetes. *Diabetes/Metabolism Res Rev.* 2003;19(5):401–407.

74. Peyrot M, Rubin RR. Levels and risks of depression and anxiety symptomatology among diabetic adults. [see comment]. *Diabetes Care.* 1997;20(4):585–590.

75. Kulzer B, Hermanns N, Reinecker H, Haak T. Effects of self-management training in Type 2 diabetes: a randomized, prospective trial. *Diabet Med.* 2007;24:415–423.

76. McGinnis RA, McGrady A, Cox SA, Grower-Dowling KA. Biofeedback-assisted relaxation in type 2 diabetes. *Diabetes Care.* 2005;28(9):2145–2149.

77. Rosenzweig S, Reibel DK, Greeson JM, et al. Mindfulness-based stress reduction is associated with improved glycemic control in type 2 diabetes mellitus: a pilot study. *Altern Ther Health Med.* 2007;13:36–38.

78. Lustman PJ, Griffith LS, Clouse RE, et al. Effects of alprazolam on glucose regulation in diabetes. Results of double-blind, placebo-controlled trial. *Diabetes Care.* 1995;18(8):1133–1139.

79. Biessels GJ, Deary IJ, Ryan CM. Cognition and diabetes: a lifespan perspective. *Lancet Neurol.* 2008;7(2):184–190.

80. Sinclair AJ, Girling AJ, Bayer AJ. Cognitive dysfunction in older subjects with diabetes mellitus: impact on diabetes self-management and use of care services. All Wales Research into Elderly (AWARE) Study. *Diabetes Res Clin Pract.* 2000;50(3):203–212.

81. Schoenle EJ, Schoenle D, Molinari L, Largo RH. Impaired intellectual development in children with Type I diabetes: association with HbA(1c), age at diagnosis and sex. *Diabetologia.* 2002;45(1):108–114.

82. Northam EA, Anderson PJ, Jacobs R, Hughes M, Warne GL, Werther GA. Neuropsychological profiles of children with type 1 diabetes 6 years after disease onset. *Diabetes Care.* 2001;24(9):1541–1546.

83. Northam EA, Anderson PJ, Werther GA, Warne GL, Andrewes D. Predictors of change in the neuropsychological profiles of children with type 1 diabetes 2 years after disease onset. *Diabetes Care.* 1999;22(9):1438–1444.

84. Brands AMA, Biessels GJ, de Haan EHF, Kappelle LJ, Kessels RPC. The effects of type 1 diabetes on cognitive performance: a meta-analysis [see comment]. *Diabetes Care.* 2005;28(3):726–735.

85. Bruce DG, Casey GP, Grange V, et al. Fremantle Cognition in Diabetes S: Cognitive impairment, physical disability and depressive symptoms in older diabetic patients: the Fremantle Cognition in Diabetes Study. *Diabetes Res Clin Pract.* 2003;61(1):59–67.

86. Alexopoulos GS, Meyers BS, Young RC, Campbell S, Silbersweig D, Charlson M. 'Vascular depression' hypothesis. *Arch Gen Psychiatr.* 1997;54:915–922.

87. Biessels GJ, Staekenborg S, Brunner E, Brayne C, Scheltens P. Risk of dementia in diabetes mellitus: a systematic review. [erratum appears in Lancet Neurol. 2006 Feb;5(2):113]. *Lancet Neurology.* 2006;5(1):64–74.

88. Irie F, Fitzpatrick AL, Lopez OL, et al. Enhanced risk for Alzheimer disease in persons with type 2 diabetes and APOE epsilon4: the Cardiovascular Health Study Cognition Study. *Arch Neurol.* 2008;65(1):89–93.

89. Dominguez RO, Marschoff ER, Guareschi EM, et al. Collaborative group for the study of the oxidative stress and related a: insulin, glucose and glycated hemoglobin in Alzheimer's and vascular dementia with and without superimposed Type II diabetes mellitus condition. *J Neural Transmission.* 2008;115(1):77–84.

90. Okereke O, Kang JH, Gaziano JM, Ma J, Stampfer MJ, Grodstein F. Plasma C-peptide and cognitive performance in older men without diabetes. *Am J Geriatric Psychiatr.* 2006;14(12):1041–1050.

91. Okereke OI, Pollak MN, Hu FB, Hankinson SE, Selkoe DJ, Grodstein F. Plasma C-peptide levels and rates of cognitive decline in older, community-dwelling women without diabetes. *Psychoneuroendocrinology.* 2008;33:455–461.

92. van Oijen M, Okereke OI, Kang JH, et al. Fasting insulin levels and cognitive decline in older women without diabetes. *Neuroepidemiology.* 2008;30:174–179.

93. Stewart R, Liolitsa D. Type 2 diabetes mellitus, cognitive impairment and dementia. *Diabet Med.* 1999;16:93–112.

94. Awad N, Gagnon M, Messier C. The relationship between impaired glucose tolerance, type 2 diabetes, and cognitive function. *J Clin Exp Neuropsychol.* 2004;26:1044–1080.

95. Korf ESC, White LR, Scheltens P, Launer LJ. Brain aging in very old men with type 2 diabetes: the Honolulu-Asia Aging Study. *Diabetes Care.* 2006;29:2268–2274.

96. Warren RE, Frier BM. Hypoglycemia and cognitive function. *Diabetes Obes Metab.* 2005 Sep;7(5):493–503.

97. Draelos MT, Jacobson AM, Weinger K, et al. Cognitive function in patients with insulin-dependent diabetes mellitus during hyperglycemia and hypoglycemia. *Am J Med.* 1995;98:135–144.

98. Sachon C, Grimaldi A, Digy JP, Pillon B, Dubois B, Thervet F. Cognitive function, insulin-dependent diabetes and hypoglycaemia. *J Int Med.* 1992;231:471–475.

99. Austin EJ, Deary IJ. Effects of repeated hypoglycemia on cognitive function. A psychometrically validated reanalysis of the diabetes control and complications trial data. *Diabetes Care*. 1999;22:1273–1277.

100. Wessels AM, Scheltens P, Barkhof F, Heine RJ. Hyperglycaemia as a determinant of cognitive decline in patients with type 1 diabetes. *Eur J Pharmacol*. 2008;585:88–96, Epub 2008 Mar 4.

101. Starr JM, Wardlaw J, Ferguson K, MacLullich A, Deary IJ, Marshall I. Increased blood-brain barrier permeability in type II diabetes demonstrated by gadolinium magnetic resonance imaging [see comment]. *J Neurol Neurosurg Psychiatr*. 2003;74(1):70–76.

102. Tiehuis AM, van der Graaf Y, Visseren FL, et al. Diabetes increases atrophy and vascular lesions on brain MRI in patients with symptomatic arterial disease. *Stroke*. 2008;39:1600–1603.

103. van Harten B, Oosterman JM. Potter van Loon B-J, Scheltens P, Weinstein HC: Brain lesions on MRI in elderly patients with type 2 diabetes mellitus. *Euro Neurol*. 2007;57:70–74.

104. Niwa H, Koumoto C, Shiga T, et al. Clinical analysis of cognitive function in diabetic patients by MMSE and SPECT. *Diabetes Res Clin Pract*. May; 2006 72(2):142–147, Epub 2005 Dec 1.

105. Steen E, Terry BM, Rivera EJ, et al. Impaired insulin and insulin-like growth factor expression and signaling mechanisms in Alzheimer's disease – is this type 3 diabetes? *J Alzheimers Dis*. 2005;7(1):63–80.

106. Palencia CA, Ragozzino ME. The influence of NMDA receptors in the dorsomedial striatum on response reversal learning. *Neurobiol Learn Mem*. 2004;82:81–89.

107. Monahan JB, Handelmann GE, Hood WF, et al. D-cycloserine, a positive modulator of the N-methyl-D-aspartate receptor, enhances performance of learning tasks in rats. *Pharmacol Biochem Behav*. 1989;34:649–653.

108. Kuhad A, Sethi R, Chopra K. Lycopene attenuates diabetes-associated cognitive decline in rats. *Life Sci*. 2008;83:128–134, Epub 2008 Jun 8.

109. Samton JB, Ferrando SJ, Sanelli P, Karimi S, Raiteri V, Barnhill JW. The clock drawing test: diagnostic, functional, and neuroimaging correlates in older medically ill adults. *J Neuropsychiatry Clin Neurosci*. 2005;17:533–540.

110. Ryan CM, Freed MI, Rood JA, Cobitz AR, Waterhouse BR, Strachan MW. Improving metabolic control leads to better working memory in adults with type 2 diabetes. *Diabetes Care*. 2006;29:345–351.

111. Meneilly GS, Cheung E, Tessier D, Yakura C, Tuokko H. The effect of improved glycemic control on cognitive functions in the elderly patient with diabetes. *J Gerontol*. 1993;48:M117–M121.

Chapter 47
Management of Diabetes and Hyperglycemia in the Hospital Setting

Samantha DeMauro-Jablonski and Silvio E. Inzucchi

Introduction

Diabetes mellitus and hyperglycemia are frequently encountered in hospitalized patients and present complex management problems. This issue will continue to stress the health-care system in the United States as an increase in the overall diabetes prevalence is anticipated over the coming decades.[1] Since diabetic patients are hospitalized more often than their non-diabetic peers, hyperglycemia in the hospital will become an increasingly common scenario. Hospitalizations can relate directly to uncontrolled diabetes, such as diabetic ketoacidosis (DKA), hyperosmotic hyperglycemic syndrome (HHS), or severe hypoglycemia; or to the complications of diabetes including cardiac disease, stroke, foot infections, amputations, and kidney disease; or to the variety of general medical conditions to which the diabetic patient is predisposed (community acquired pneumonia, influenza, etc.). National hospital discharge data from 2004 estimate that 609,000 admissions to the hospital involved a primary diagnosis of diabetes, while 5.2 million admissions carried a non-diabetic principal diagnostic code (i.e., diabetes as a "secondary diagnosis").[2] Trends toward monitoring patients more closely in an outpatient setting, with adherence to new practice guidelines concerning glucose management, may potentially decrease hospitalization rates related to metabolic control. A recent study at the Veterans Administration confirms that, with increasing emphasis shifted toward improved outpatient access care for diabetic patients, admissions for uncontrolled diabetes have, in fact, decreased.[3] However, the overall disease burden of the diabetic patient, especially in regard to the myriad of cardiovascular complications of the disease, continues unabated. As a result, managing diabetic inpatients will become increasingly important, as will the development of evidence-based strategies aimed at improving their clinical outcomes.

Chronic complications of diabetes and how they relate to long-term control of blood glucose, as reflected by glycosylated hemoglobin concentrations, are now widely recognized. In the late 1990s, the *United Kingdom Prospective Study Group (UKPDS)* demonstrated that intensive glucose control in patients with type 2 diabetes reduced microvascular complications by approximately 25%, leading practitioners to aim for tighter long-term glycemic management.[4] This had already been illustrated in type 1 diabetes in the *Diabetes Control and Complication Trial (DDCT)*, which clearly established that the duration and degree of hyperglycemia directly related to microvascular complications including retinopathy, nephropathy, and neuropathy. In addition, when DCCT patients were subsequently followed in the Epidemiology of Diabetes Interventions and Complications (EDIC) study, the benefits of cardiovascular outcomes of early intensive treatment of blood glucose were reaffirmed despite little ultimate difference in terminal HbA1c among the treatment groups.[5] Thus, intensive management of both type 1 and type 2 diabetes in the outpatient setting has emerged as a major public health priority over the past decade, with increasingly aggressive international guidelines endorsed by professional organizations and societies. In contrast, the management of comparatively brief episodes of hyperglycemia in

S.E. Inzucchi (✉)
Section of Endocrinology, Yale University School of Medicine, Yale Diabetes Center, Yale-New Haven Hospital, New Haven, CT, USA
e-mail: silvio.inzucchi@yale.edu

L. Poretsky (ed.), *Principles of Diabetes Mellitus*, DOI 10.1007/978-0-387-09841-8_47,
© Springer Science+Business Media, LLC 2010

the inpatient setting has, until recently, been largely ignored. Indeed, the role of careful monitoring and tight glucose control among hospitalized diabetic patients is less clear and certainly not as well studied. The available data from which we need to make management decisions are derived from several retrospective studies and a handful of prospective investigations, most of which have their limitations.

The needs of the hospitalized patient with diabetes are complex. The management of hyperglycemic emergencies, DKA and HHS, will be discussed in Chapter 18. When diabetes accompanies (but does not directly cause) hospitalization, glucose management is still often very challenging, due to the stress hyperglycemia, which results from the effects of circulating counter-regulatory factors, especially epinephrine and cortisol. In addition, parenteral nutrition, glucocorticoids, and catecholamine-derived pressor agents are frequently used, further exacerbating the tendency for elevated blood glucose levels. These effects may be counterbalanced by frequent deviation from the patient's typical nutritional intake. As a result, both severe hyperglycemic excursions and episodes of hypoglycemia may emerge. Notably, there is convincing experimental evidence to suggest that the hyperglycemic milieu itself may have deleterious short-term effects on hemodynamic status, oxidative stress, endothelial and immune function, and wound healing (Fig. 47.1).[6] Accordingly, tight glucose control in the short term, to reverse these processes, may improve clinical outcomes. In this light, treatment goals and strategies for the inpatient management of diabetes have evolved significantly over the past decade, as retrospective data emerged correlating in-hospital hyperglycemia with increased morbidity and mortality and as prospective trials began to suggest a major short-term benefit on morbidity and mortality from stringent inpatient glycemic management. In the following pages, we will review the published literature in this area, while pointing out the accompanying controversies.

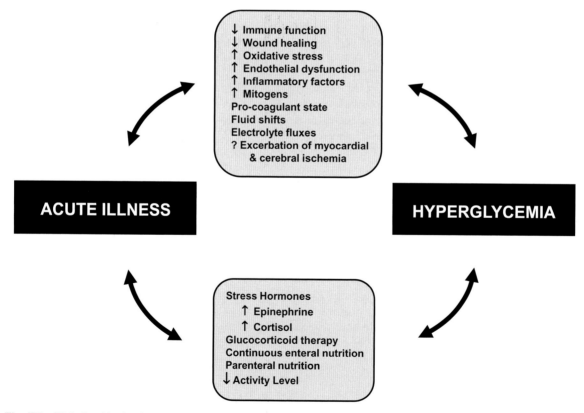

Fig. 47.1 Clinical and basic science studies suggest a complex, bidirectional relationship between acute illness and hyperglycemia. With permission from Inzucchi[6]

Retrospective Data

Patients with diabetes have increased lengths of stay, in-hospital complication rates, and mortality as compared to non-diabetic patients receiving similar care. A prospective cohort study of 2178 patients with type 2 diabetes demonstrated a significant increase in total operative mortality following coronary artery bypass graft surgery.[7] A large retrospective subgroup analysis of the Thrombolysis In Myocardial Infarction (TIMI) trial compared mortality in diabetic versus non-diabetic patients with acute coronary syndrome. After adjusting for baseline characteristics, patients with diabetes demonstrated increased death rates at both 30 days and 1 year.[8] Increased morbidity and mortality in diabetes is not unique to cardiac diseases. Another prospective study followed patients with an admission to the hospital for an acute exacerbation of chronic obstructive pulmonary disease (COPD) and demonstrated a significantly higher 2-year mortality rate among those with diabetes.[9] A retrospective analysis of admissions to the intensive care unit for trauma demonstrated that patients with diabetes had increased need for ventilator support and number of intensive care days compared to non-diabetic individuals, matched for trauma severity score. Clearly, the diabetic patient is at increased risk of adverse outcomes following a variety of other systemic illnesses and surgical procedures. Not surprisingly, this risk appears to be inversely correlated with the quality of long-term glycemic control,[10] likely reflecting the increased burden of vascular diseases, the impaired ability to fight infection, and altered wound healing which is well characterized in this population. But is there any evidence that control of blood glucose in the short term – i.e., during acute hospitalizations – exerts any effect on patient outcomes?[6]

Retrospective data have widely confirmed an association between hyperglycemia during hospitalizations and mortality – a relationship that, paradoxically, appears to be stronger in those without an established history of diabetes.[9,6,11,12] Several studies have shown a positive relationship between hospital hyperglycemia and mortality in critical care patients, irrespective of a prior diabetes history[13,14] (Fig. 47.2). In one retrospective study, non-diabetic patients with hyperglycemia at admission in the neurosurgical, cardiac, and cardiothoracic intensive care units (ICUs) experienced increased mortality, although this relationship did not hold true for diabetic patients.[15] In another retrospective analysis of elderly patients with acute myocardial infarction, a graded increase in 30-day and 1-year mortality was observed with increasing admission blood glucose concentrations, primarily driven by those not recognized as having diabetes on admission. In the diabetic subgroup, mortality was increased, but only in those whose admission glucose exceeded 240 mg/dL[16] (Fig. 47.3). Another retrospective study examined patients with diabetes and unstable angina or non-ST elevation MI. Admission glucose as a

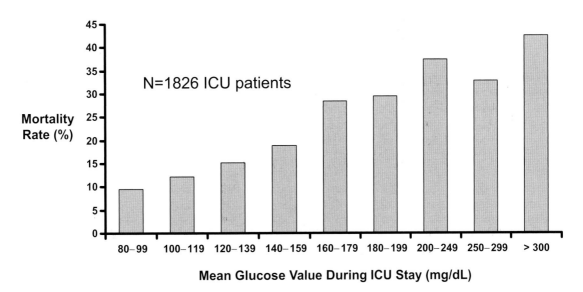

Fig. 47.2 Hospital mortality and glucose control in a medical–surgical ICU. With permission from Krinsley[14]

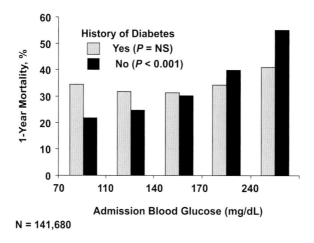

Fig. 47.3 Admission blood glucose and 1-year mortality in elderly AMI patients. Adapted from Kosiborod et al.[16]

continuous variable was positively correlated with 2-year all-cause mortality. When the glucose concentrations were divided into quartiles, the highest (≥275 mg/dL) had an unadjusted hazard ratio of 2.66 (95% confidence interval 1.83–3.86) when compared to the lowest quartile (≤153 mg/dl). Of note, however, those patients with any in-hospital hypoglycemia (≤55 mg/dL) had a higher 2-year all-cause mortality when compared to the referent group (all glucose measurements between 56 and 119 mg/dL).[17] Several retrospective studies have also investigated admission hyperglycemia as it relates to cerebral ischemia. A meta-analysis strongly suggests that elevated glucose in non-diabetic individuals during acute stroke predicts increased in-hospital mortality (relative risk of 3.07 as compared to euglycemic patients) as well as poorer functional recovery.[11] Observational studies in hospitalized patients with community acquired pneumonia,[18] COPD,[19] or those undergoing general surgical procedures[20] also indicate similar relationships between elevated in-hospital blood glucose concentrations and adverse clinical outcomes.

A large retrospective study of hospitalized patients confirmed hyperglycemia to be a predictor of poor outcomes in patients with no established history of diabetes. Among 1886 study patients, 12% had "new hyperglycemia." These patients were more likely to be admitted to an intensive care unit (ICU) and had a 16% total in-hospital mortality compared to 3% among diabetic patients and 1.7% among patients with normal blood glucoses. In a corresponding group admitted to the ICU, the mortality rate approached one out of three patients, which was threefold higher than in the other two groups. Newly hyperglycemic patients also experienced longer hospital stays and required transfers more frequently to chronic care facilities.[12] Whether such individuals actually have undiagnosed diabetes or are simply manifesting stress hyperglycemia due to the severity of their illness remains unclear. Swedish investigators have further explored this issue by examining patients admitted with acute myocardial infarction but no prior history of diabetes. Fasting glucose and glycosylated hemoglobin were measured and oral glucose tolerance testing was conducted. Of this cohort, 35% had impaired glucose tolerance and 31% had newly discovered diabetes upon discharge. Three months after discharge, 40% had impaired glucose tolerance and 25% had diabetes,[21] suggesting that the glucose abnormalities discovered during cardiovascular hospitalizations may reflect underlying metabolic derangements and are not simply due to a stress response.

Despite these mainly retrospective data, whether hyperglycemia is a marker of severe injury or illness or whether it represents a treatable consequence that affects patient outcomes remains unclear. Interesting prospective data on the treatment of hyperglycemia in hospitalized patients now offer some direction for clinicians.

Prospective Clinical Trials

Treatment of diabetes and hyperglycemia in the inpatient setting has evolved significantly over the past decade as data have emerged from several prospective, randomized clinical trials, suggesting improved patient outcomes, primarily in the critical care setting, when glucose is managed intensively. The Diabetes Mellitus Insulin–Glucose Infusion in Acute Myocardial Infarction (DIGAMI) study examined the treatment of hyperglycemia in the coronary care unit during acute myocardial infarction. Patients with known diabetes or a blood glucose >198 mg/dL within 24 h of a myocardial infarction were randomly assigned to two treatment groups. The intervention group was administered intravenous insulin with 5% dextrose infusion, adjusted according to blood glucose concentrations, targeting a level of 126–196 mg/dl and then switched to a four injection insulin regimen for at least 3 months as outpatients. The control group was treated according to standard care. Intensive glucose management was associated with a 29% reduction in 1-year mortality ($p=0.027$). Moreover, a predetermined low-risk subgroup, which had never been treated with insulin previously, benefited even further, with an impressive 52% mortality reduction. Although there was more hypoglycemia in the intensive treatment group, there was no evidence that these patients experienced any adverse clinical outcomes.[22] This profound decrease in mortality with intensive insulin treatment suggested that aggressive management of diabetes in the setting of acute coronary syndrome may be warranted. However, the mechanism of how and why insulin improved outcomes remained unclear. In addition, due to the DIGAMI study's design, it was difficult to sort out the effects of the insulin infusion versus the more intensive discharge antihyperglycemic regimen on mortality.

A follow-up study from this group, DIGAMI-2, looked again at intensive insulin treatment during acute myocardial infarction. In contrast to the original DIGAMI investigation, this randomized controlled trial contained a third arm in which subjects were treated with an insulin–dextrose infusion (titrated to maintain blood glucose 126–180 mg/dl); however, no intensive subcutaneous insulin program was prescribed upon discharge, in an attempt to decipher the individual roles of stringent inpatient versus outpatient glucose management. DIGAMI-2 did not find any significant differences in mortality among the three groups. However, the study was ultimately underpowered due to sluggish subject recruitment, little difference in overall blood glucose control between the treatment groups, and an overall low post-MI event rate among all participants. DIGAMI-2 therefore could not provide a clear answer as to whether or not intensive insulin therapy improves outcomes following acute cardiac hospitalizations.[23] A more recent prospective study addressed this same issue [hyperglycemia: Intensive Insulin in Infarction (HI-5) study]. Patients with hyperglycemia (>140 mg/dL), with or without a prior history of diabetes, and acute myocardial infarction were randomized to receive either intensive intravenous insulin or conventional insulin therapy. The intravenous insulin was administered in conjunction with 5% dextrose using a protocol targeting a blood glucose of 72–180 mg/dL for at least 24 h. There were no differences between the groups in the primary outcomes of in-hospital, 3- and 6-month mortality. A significant reduction, however, was observed in intensively treated patients, in congestive heart failure during both the inpatient period and the incidence of reinfarction at 3 months. Although this was a negative study, similar to DIGAMI-2, the overall mortality in HI-5 was lower than expected, reducing the power to detect any difference in mortality, and there was no significant difference in nonfasting glucose between the groups.[24] Both of these studies, therefore, add little to the evidence base at this time.

A large, nonrandomized study in the cardiothoracic ICU examined intravenous versus subcutaneous insulin therapy in the perioperative period in patients undergoing coronary artery bypass grafting (CABG). Patients from 1987 to 1991 were treated conventionally with subcutaneous insulin by adjusted "sliding scale" to maintain blood glucose <200 mg/dL if they had a history of diabetes or post-operative glucose >200 mg/dL. Patients enrolled from 1992 to 2001 were instead treated with intravenous insulin. The intravenous insulin was administered, with a target of 150–200 mg/dL between 1992 and 1998, 125–175 mg/dL during the period 1999–2000, and 100–150 mg/dL from 2001. The intensive insulin group had a significantly lower blood glucose, less deep sternal wound infections (relative risk = 0.34, $p = 0.005$),[25] and, ultimately, reduced mortality (2.5% versus 5.3%, $p<0.0001$) compared to the conventional group. Specifically, cardiovascular mortality, which comprised most of the events, was significantly lower in intensively treated patients. This study suggested that intensive insulin therapy, resulting in better glucose control, reduces cardiac mortality in CABG patients. However, its design had serious flaws in that patients were not randomized and the original control group was treated 10 years prior to the conclusion of the study. Other advances in cardiac surgery and anesthetic techniques were likely to have contributed to the reduced morbidity and mortality rates[13]

A related prospective study has examined the role of *intraoperative* insulin infusion during cardiothoracic surgery. In this prospective, randomized trial, 199 patients with and without diabetes received intravenous insulin in the operating room to maintain blood glucose between 80 and 100 mg/dL. The conventionally treated group received insulin in the operating room only if the blood glucose was >200 mg/dL. Both groups were treated with insulin infusion after surgery. There were no differences in the primary clinical composite outcome between the groups, although an increase in stroke events was noted in the intensive treatment group (4% versus 1% with conventional therapy; p=0.020). This study, although small, is concerning, and intraoperative insulin infusion with such rigid targets cannot be recommended at this time.[26]

The most widely cited prospective and randomized trial in this area examined the impact of intensive glucose control with intensive insulin infusion in a surgical ICU. Mechanically ventilated patients were randomized by Van den Berghe et al. to receive intravenous insulin if glucose exceeded 110 mg/dL with an aggressive goal of 80–110 mg/dL or conventional therapy, where insulin was infused only if glucose reached 215 mg/dL, with a more conservative target of 180–200 mg/dL. The difference in mean ICU glycemia between the groups was marked (103 versus 153 mg/dl). A significant 42% relative decrease in ICU mortality as well as a 34% relative reduction of in-hospital mortality was detected in the patients assigned to intensive insulin therapy (Fig. 47.4).[27] A 46% reduction in septicemia was also demonstrated with intensive insulin therapy. The intensive insulin therapy group also had significantly less renal impairment, required fewer blood transfusions, and demonstrated less ventilator dependency.[27] Most of the benefit was observed in patients who remained in the ICU for at least 5 days. This was a provocative study that has had a major impact on the standard of care in the intensive care unit. However, the data have often been inappropriately extrapolated to other inpatient settings.

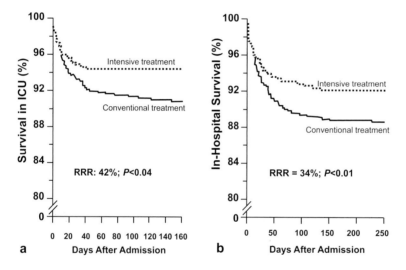

Fig. 47.4 The effect of intensive insulin therapy in the surgical intensive care unit on mortality. Adapted with permission from Van Den Berghe et al.[27]

A similar study by the same group was conducted in their medical ICU, where patients tend to be older and more chronically ill than are in surgical units. The study's design was identical to the surgical ICU study. Patients admitted to the MICU with an anticipated stay of at least 3 days were randomized to receive intensive versus conventional insulin therapy. In this study, both ICU and hospital mortality were reduced (RRR = −18%) in those patients who did require ICU care for 3 days or more. However, in the intention to treat analysis, there were no significant differences in mortality rates, although significant reductions in renal impairment and decreased ventilator time in the intensively treated group were observed.[28] Insulin infusion was associated with more hypoglycemia (as expected and as found in any intensive insulin therapy trial). Moreover, there was a trend toward worse outcomes in any patient who developed hypoglycemia. In addition, patients randomized to intensive treatment who stayed in the ICU for less than 3 days appeared to have increased mortality, although of only borderline statistical significance. The questions raised by these data led the authors to pool their data from both units to assess for any harm from intensive glucose lowering. Once again a significant increase in hypoglycemia in the intensively treated groups, in both the medical and surgical ICUs, was revealed. However, the mortality among those individuals in the intensively treated group with hypoglycemia did not significantly differ from the corresponding group of conventionally treated patients. Interestingly, there was a non-significant increase in mortality in patients with a prior history of diabetes and a mean daily blood glucose <110 mg/dL.[29] The discrepancy between the impressive findings in the SICU study and the mixed results in the MICU has resulted in significant controversy, with some authorities proposing that rigid glucose control in all ICU settings may not be warranted, that glucose targets should be different in diabetic versus non-diabetic patients, or that insulin infusion should be initiated only after 3 days in the ICU have elapsed.

A more recent randomized multicenter study assessed intensive insulin therapy with a goal glucose of 80–110 mg/dL in patients with sepsis [Volume Substitution and Insulin Therapy in Severe Sepsis (VISEP) study] but was terminated early because of a significant increase in hypoglycemia in the active therapy group (17% versus 4% with conventional care).[30] Despite a significant difference in the mean blood glucose concentration in the two treatment groups (112 versus 151 mg/dl), there was no difference in the co-primary outcomes of death from any cause at 1 month and morbidity, as assessed by a standardized organ failure score. Another insulin infusion study [Glucontrol (yet to be published)] from the medical intensive care unit compared a glucose target of 80–110 to 140–180 mg/dL and was similarly terminated prematurely as there was no apparent mortality benefit and significantly more hypoglycemic episodes in the intensively treated patients were observed.[31]

Finally, the NICE-SUGAR study reported its important findings in 2009. In this large, multicenter investigation, ICU patients (mixed medical and surgical) were randomized to intensive therapy with intravenous insulin infusion (using a uniform, web-based protocol) and a blood glucose target of 81–108 mg/dl versus "conventional" care with an insulin infusion beginning only at a glucose threshold of 180 mg/dl and a target of 140–180 mg/dl. A total of 6104 patients were randomized, and the two groups had similar baseline characteristics. Surprisingly, 829 patients (27.5%) in the intensive group and 751 (24.9%) in the conventional group reached the primary outcome of mortality at 90 days (OR, 1.14; 95% CI, 1.02 to 1.28; $p=0.02$). Treatment effect did not differ significantly between operative (surgical) patients and nonoperative (medical) patients (ORs, 1.31 and 1.07, respectively; $p=0.10$). Severe hypoglycemia, defined as a blood glucose <40 mg/dl was much more common in intensively managed patients (6.8% versus 0.5%, $p<0.001$). No difference was observed between the two groups, however, in hospitalization and ICU length of stay, or the need for mechanical ventilation or renal replacement therapy. These data suggest that the more stringent blood glucose target <110 mg/dl may not be necessary to optimize patient outcomes – that achieving a blood glucose in the 140 mg/dl range may be sufficient. Indeed, lowering blood glucose levels too low may place patients at some risk. It is important to note, however, that this trial compared extremely tight to reasonably good glucose control. Accordingly, its findings do not necessarily refute those of earlier trials – in which the treatment objective in the control groups was to not address hyperglycemia until it reached well above the 200 mg/dl range.

We also believe that the finding of greater mortality in NICE SUGAR's intensively-treated group requires further analysis, especially since 10% of that cohort's patients were considered "early withdrawls," and never received the insulin infusion protocol. Despite this, their outcomes were assessed in the classical intent-to-treat analysis. The specific mortality in this subset of patients has as of yet not been reported; to what extent this may have driven the difference in overall mortality between the randomized groups is not yet clear. Moreover, a precise explanation for the increased mortality in the intensive group has not yet been demonstrated, but was not obviously related to hypoglycemic events.

Nonetheless, based on the totality of the evidence from now multiple randomized clinical trials, it appears that the results from the original Van den Berghe et al. investigation in a single surgical ICU stand apart from virtually all other studies. Accordingly, the attainment of euglycemia with intravenous insulin is no longer considered the standard of care in critically ill patients (see below).

Treatment of hyperglycemia in the non-critically ill hospitalized patient has not been well studied. There are essentially no trials examining anything but short-term metabolic outcomes. Conventional strategies, such as regular insulin "sliding scales," often result in significant hyperglycemia and hypoglycemia in diabetic patients.[32] A prospective randomized multicenter trial in hospitalized, but not critically ill, patients with type 2 diabetes investigated the glycemic control achieved using sliding scale versus a "basal–bolus" (or basal–prandial) insulin regimen with glargine and glulisine insulin analogues. There was a significant improvement in glycemic control, defined as a mean glucose <140 mg/dL, among the basal–bolus group compared to the sliding scale group, with two-thirds of the former achieving this target compared to one-third of the latter. It should be noted, however, that the mean daily dose of insulin in the basal–bolus group was more than threefold higher than with sliding scales. Rates of hypoglycemia were the same at 3%, with no severe hypoglycemia occurring in either group and no difference in the length of stay.[33] This study takes a major step toward establishing basal–bolus insulin regimen as safe and effective; however, a larger study is required to see if this may translate to an impact on inpatient morbidity and mortality.

Treatment Recommendations

Intensive Care Units

The American Association of Clinical Endocrinologists and the American Diabetes Association have recently published a consensus statement with revised glucose targets for hospitalized patients (Table 47.1).[34] For patients in the ICU, intravenous insulin remains the preferred method to achieve and maintain blood glucose control. The targets recently proposed by ACE and ADA (140–180 mg/dl) are reasonable. At our own institution, the target had originally been 100–140 mg/dl, soon after publication of the first Van den Berghe paper. We subsequently lowered it slightly to 90–120 mg/dl (as seen in Fig. 47.5), in the context of mounting enthusiasm for tight blood glucose control in the ICU. With both protocols, our hypoglycemia rates were very low. In light of the NICE – SUGAR data and the recently revised national guidelines, however, we have decided to pilot a modified version of our original protocol, with a 120–160 mg/dl target. We chose this so that our mean blood glucose achieved would be approximately 140 mg/dl - close to the actual level attained (145 mg/dl) by the control group in NICE – SUGAR.

Table 47.1 AACE–ADA Consensus Statement on Inpatient Glycemic Control: Main Recommendations

ICU Setting	Non–ICU Setting

• Intravenous insulin infusion is preferred.
• Starting threshold should be no higher than 180 mg/dl.
• Maintain BG 140–180 mg/dl, with greater benefit likely toward the lower end of this range.
• Lower targets (110–140 mg/dl) are not evidence-based, but may be appropriate in selected patients if a hospital is already successfully achieving them.
• Targets <110 mg/dl are not recommended because of safety concerns.
	• For most patients:
	  - pre-meal BG <140 mg/dL
	  - random BG <180 mg/dL
	• *More* stringent targets may be appropriate in stable patients under previously tight control before hospitalization.
	• *Less* stringent targets are appropriate in patients with severe comorbidities.
	• Scheduled subcutaneous insulin with basal, nutritional (prandial), and correction doses is preferred. Prolonged use of regular insulin sliding scales is discouraged.

Source: Moghissi ES, Korytkowski MT, DiNardo M, Einhorn D, Hellman R, Hirsch IB, Inzucchi SE, Ismail-Beigi F, Kirkman MS, Umpierrez GE; American Association of Clinical Endocrinologists; American Diabetes Association. American Association of Clinical Endocrinologists and American Diabetes Association consensus statement on inpatient glycemic control. Diabetes Care. 2009 Jun;32(6):1119–31.

When used, an insulin infusion should be administered only by a validated written or computerized protocol. Blood glucose should be monitored hourly at least until stable. The best protocols involve detailed algorithms which incorporate not only the current glucose value but also its rate of change and the current insulin infusion rate.[35] Protocols that do not take these variables into account inevitably result in higher hypoglycemia rates. The insulin infusion protocol used at our institution is validated and has been implemented/adapted by many other

YALE INSULIN INFUSION PROTOCOL (2008)

The following insulin infusion protocol is intended for use in hyperglycemic adult patients in an <u>ICU setting</u>, but is not specifically tailored for those individuals with diabetic emergencies, such as diabetic ketoacidosis (DKA) or hyperglycemic hyperosmolar states (HHS). When these diagnoses are being considered, or if BG ≥ 500 mg/dL, the responsible physician should be consulted for specific orders. Also, <u>notify the responsible physician immediately</u> if the response to the insulin infusion is unusual or unexpected, or if any situation arises that is not adequately addressed by these guidelines. Any patient on an insulin infusion should have frequent measurement of serum electrolyte concentrations, especially potassium.

Initiating the Insulin Infusion

1.) INSULIN INFUSION: Mix 1 unit Regular Human Insulin per 1 cc 0.9 % NaCl. Administer via infusion pump (in increments of 0.5 unit/hr.)
2.) PRIMING: Flush 20 cc of infusion through all IV tubing before infusion begins (to saturate the insulin binding sites in the tubing.)
3.) THRESHOLD: IV insulin is indicated in any critically ill patient with persistent BG ≥ 140 mg/dl; *consider* use if BG ≥ 120 mg/dL.
4.) TARGET BLOOD GLUCOSE (BG) LEVEL: **90-120 mg/dL**
5.) BOLUS & INITIAL INSULIN INFUSION RATE: <u>If initial BG ≥ 150 mg/dL</u>, divide by 70, then round to nearest 0.5 units for bolus AND initial drip rate. <u>If initial BG < 150 mg/dL</u>, divide by 70 for initial drip rate only (i.e., NO bolus.)
   Examples: 1.) Initial BG = 335 mg/dL: 335 ÷ 70 = 4.78, round ↑ to 5: 5 units IV bolus + start infusion @ 5 units/hr.
                2.) Initial BG = 148 mg/dL: 148 ÷ 70 = 2.11, round ↓ to 2: start drip @ 2 units/hr (<u>NO</u> bolus.)

Blood Glucose (BG) Monitoring

1.) Check BG hourly until stable (3 consecutive values within target range). In hypotensive patients, capillary blood glucose (i.e., fingersticks) may be inaccurate and obtaining blood sample from an indwelling vascular catheter may be preferable.
2.) Then check BG Q2 hours; once stable x 12-24 hours. BG checks can then be spaced to Q4 hours IF:
   a.) no significant change in clinical condition   AND   b.) no significant change in nutritional intake.
3.) If any of the following occur, consider the temporary resumption of hourly BG monitoring, until BG is again stable (2-3 consecutive BG values within target range):
   a.) any change in insulin infusion rate (i.e., BG out of target range)
   b.) significant changes in clinical condition
   c.) initiation or cessation of steroid or pressor therapy
   d.) initiation or cessation of renal replacement therapy (dialysis, CVVH, etc.)
   e.) initiation, cessation, or rate change of nutritional support (TPN, PPN, tube feedings, etc.)

Changing the Insulin Infusion Rate

If BG < 50 mg/dL:
HOLD INSULIN INFUSION   Give 1 amp (25 g) D50 IV; recheck BG Q15 minutes.
                                             ⇒ When BG ≥ 90 mg/dL, wait 1 hour, recheck BG. If still ≥ 90 mg/dL, restart infusion at 50% of most recent rate.

If BG 50-69 mg/dL:
HOLD INSULIN INFUSION   If <u>symptomatic</u> (or unable to assess), give 1 amp (25 g) D50 IV; recheck BG Q15 minutes.
                                             If <u>asymptomatic</u>, give 1/2 Amp (12.5 g) D50 IV or 8 ounces juice; recheck BG Q15-30 minutes.
                                             ⇒ When BG ≥ 90 mg/dL, wait 1 hour, recheck BG. If still ≥ 90 mg/dL, restart infusion at 75% of most recent rate.

If BG ≥ 70 mg/dL:
STEP 1: Determine the <u>CURRENT BG LEVEL</u> - identifies a <u>COLUMN</u> in the table:

BG 70-89 mg/dL	BG 90-119 mg/dL	BG 120-179 mg/dL	BG ≥ 180 mg/dL

STEP 2: Determine the <u>RATE OF CHANGE</u> from the prior BG level - identifies a <u>CELL</u> in the table - Then move right for INSTRUCTIONS:
[Note: If the last BG was measured 2-4 hours before the current BG, calculate the hourly rate of change. Example: If the BG at 2PM was 150 mg/dL and the BG at 4PM is now 120 mg/dL, the total change over 2 hours is –30 mg/dL; however, the hourly change is –30 mg/dL ÷ 2 hours = -15 mg/dL/hr.]

BG 70-89 mg/dL	BG 90-119 mg/dL	BG 120-179 mg/dL	BG ≥ 180 mg/dL	INSTRUCTIONS*
		BG ↑ by > 40 mg/dL/hr	BG ↑	INCREASE INFUSION by "2Δ"
	BG ↑ by > 20 mg/dL/hr	BG ↑ by 1-40 mg/dL/hr *OR* BG UNCHANGED	BG UNCHANGED *OR* BG ↓ by 1-40 mg/dL/hr	INCREASE INFUSION by "Δ"
BG ↑	BG ↑ by 1-20 mg/dL/hr, BG UNCHANGED, *OR* BG ↓ by 1-20 mg/dL/hr	BG ↓ by 1-40 mg/dL/hr	BG ↓ by 41-80 mg/dL/hr	NO INFUSION CHANGE
BG UNCHANGED *OR* BG ↓ by 1-20 mg/dL/hr	BG ↓ by 21-40 mg/dL/hr	BG ↓ by 41-80 mg/dL/hr	BG ↓ by 81-120 mg/dL/hr	DECREASE INFUSION by "Δ"
BG ↓ by > 20 mg/dL/hr *see below†*	BG ↓ by > 40 mg/dL/hr	BG ↓ by > 80 mg/dL/hr	BG ↓ by > 120 mg/dL/hr	HOLD INFUSION for 30min, then DECREASE by "2Δ"

†HOLD INSULIN INFUSION; check BG Q15-30 min; when ≥90 mg/dL, restart infusion at 75% of most recent rate.

*CHANGES IN INFUSION RATE ("Δ") are determined by the current rate:

Current Rate (units/hr)	Δ = Rate Change (units/hr)	2Δ = 2X Rate Change (units/hr)
< 3	0.5	1
3 – 6	1	2
6.5 – 9.5	1.5	3
10 – 14.5	2	4
15 – 19.5	3*	6*
20 – 24.5*	4*	8*
≥ 25*	5*	10*

* Depending on the clinical circumstances, infusion rates typically range between 2 and 10 units/hour. Doses in excess of 20 units/hour are unusual, and if required, the responsible physician should be notified to explore other potential contributing factors (including technical problems, such as a dilutional error, etc.)

Fig. 47.5 Yale Insulin Infusion Protocol with target glucose of 90–120 mg/dL. Adapted from: Goldberg et al.[37]

hospitals[36, 37] Once the patient's clinical status improves and transfer to the general ward is imminent, a proper transition protocol to insulin injections should be used. This protocol should incorporate the most recent insulin infusion rate. In addition, some degree of overlap between intravenous and subcutaneous insulin regimen should be ensured so as to prevent recurrent hyperglycemia.[38]

General Medical–Surgical Wards

For non-critically ill patients, the AACE-ADA guidelines recommend a fasting glucose <140 mg/dL and a non-fasting glucose <180 mg/dL. These professional organizations further recommend that each diabetic patient (and, moreover, those with new hyperglycemia) has a HbA1c measured upon admission, has access to diabetes education, and has proper discharge planning for appropriate follow-up. Furthermore, the routine use of an insulin sliding scale is discouraged in patients who are eating, with a more proactive and anticipatory insulin regimen advised, typically involving some form of basal insulin with superimposed prandial or nutritional insulin before meals ("bolus"), ideally in the form of a short-acting insulin analogue (e.g., lispro, aspart, glulisine).[39] These boluses can be adjusted with additional "correction insulin" (same type) if pre-meal hyperglycemia is present.

It should be noted that the non-ICU targets are largely extrapolated from clinical trial data from the ICU setting, as well as from outpatient standards of care. They are therefore not evidence based for this patient subgroup. Our current protocol for managing the non-critically ill patient with diabetes or hyperglycemia is shown in Fig. 47.6.[6] Once a patient is admitted to the hospital and diabetes and/or hyperglycemia is established or suspected, blood glucose should be monitored by finger stick regularly. The fasting patient should have blood glucose monitored every 6 h. The nonfasting patient should be monitored prior to each meal and at bedtime. Occasionally patients suffering from hypoglycemia and severe hyperglycemia may benefit from more frequent monitoring. Measuring HbA1c is important in those with established diabetes to discern the quality of blood glucose control prior to admission. This may effect decisions regarding changes in therapy both during and after hospitalization. In those with newly recognized hyperglycemia, a HbA1c may help determine the presence of diabetes prior to admission.

Non-critically ill patients with type 1 diabetes who are fasting (or in whom nutritional intake is doubtful) should have an insulin drip strongly considered to optimally control glucose and prevent ketosis. Admittedly, most hospitals find it challenging to administer insulin infusions outside of the ICU setting, but safe and effective glucose control can be achieved with proper staffing and education. When an insulin infusion is not possible, fasting patients with type 1 diabetes or insulin-requiring type 2 diabetes should receive their usual long-acting insulin dose, but a modest dosage reduction should be considered, especially in the latter group. Small doses of short- or rapid-acting insulin are added and adjusted to the glucose concentration, every 6 h, to maintain glycemic control. While fasting, to prevent catabolism, an infusion of 5% dextrose is reasonable (75–125 ml/h) as long as the patient is not hyperglycemic.

Type 2 diabetic patients on oral agents (or other non-insulin injectables) who are not eating should have their antihyperglycemic medications stopped. Oral agents, which may have been resulting in adequate glucose control in the outpatient arena, usually require discontinuation for a variety of reasons. Metformin, for example, is appropriately held in the setting of dehydration, vascular collapse, renal insufficiency, acidosis, altered hepatic function, or when intravenous contrast is used for diagnostic imaging procedures. Sulfonylureas are also appropriately held when any decrease in caloric intake is anticipated. Thiazolidinediones are now contraindicated in the setting of heart failure. α-Glucosidase inhibitors, dipeptidyl peptidase-4 inhibitors, and glucagon-like peptide-1 mimetics at present have little or no role in glucose management in the hospitalized diabetic patient, given their predominate effect in the post-prandial setting. As a result, most hospitalized patients with type 2 diabetes are reliant on insulin therapy and the requisite close glucose monitoring, until the clinical picture is clarified. Adjusted doses of rapid-/short-acting insulin can be considered if glucose remains elevated. We prefer Regular insulin Q 6-h, although the rapid analogues can also be used, but they may need to be dosed more frequently. If adequate control is not achieved, the addition of a basal insulin should be considered. Once food is reinitiated,

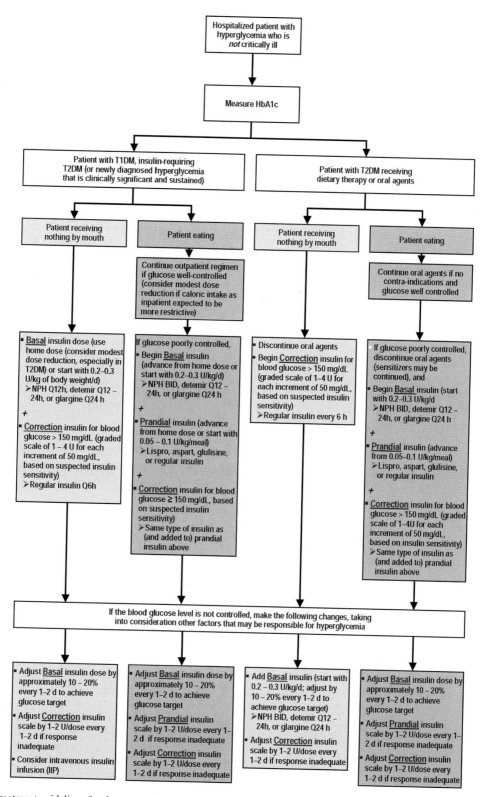

Fig. 47.6 Treatment guidelines for the non-critical inpatient with diabetes. With permission from Inzucchi[6]

and if renal, cardiac, and hepatic functions remain stable, oral agents can be restarted, as long as the outpatient regimen is adequately controlling the blood glucose prior to admission. One might consider a reduction in dose because of the imposed dietary compliance within the hospital.

Type 2 diabetic patients on oral agents who are eating and stable may have their medications continued during their hospital stays, as long as the regimen is effective and well tolerated prior to admission. However, very often, insulin therapy will be necessary to properly control glucose in the setting of the stress of illness. Insulin not only allows for more precise control but also is more flexible than oral therapies and can be rapidly advanced if severe hyperglycemia develops. Accordingly, the decision to continue oral agents during hospitalization must be carefully considered.

Patients with type 1 or insulin-requiring type 2 diabetes who are eating may be continued on their outpatient regimen if it had been previously successful, although modest dosage reductions (especially in type 2 diabetes) should be considered to compensate for more restrictive diets in the hospital. Those not well controlled should have their regimens advanced to an aggressive basal–bolus program, which allows the greatest flexibility during hospitalizations, which are frequently marked by periodic interruptions in the meal schedule due to tests and procedures. In all patients, close monitoring and careful, frequent insulin dosing adjustments are necessary to maintain glucose control. Obviously, it is fruitless to initiate major changes in the antihyperglycemic regimen in patients in the hospital for brief periods of time.

Since observational data suggest that hyperglycemia in non-diabetic patients may carry with it even greater risk than that in diabetic patients, those with "new hyperglycemia" should generally be intensively managed as above.

Although aggressive insulin strategies have their advantages in the hospital, the patient's ability to measure glucose and adjust insulin must be assessed prior to discharge so that the regimen can be implemented at home safely. Many patients without known diabetes who manifest hyperglycemia during hospitalization may not require treatment upon discharge. However, they should have their hemoglobin A1c and fasting glucose rechecked after recovery from illness. Appropriate follow-up with a primary care provider, an endocrinologist, or a diabetes educator/nurse practitioner should be ensured prior to discharge.

Finally, we would emphasize that, in the more stable patients, the hospital may be an appropriate setting to reassess and improve self-management skills, which are critically important for long-term successful treatment. Accordingly, ready access to diabetes education either during the hospital stay or soon thereafter should be ensured by all institutions.

Summary

Developments over the past decade have significantly influenced the treatment of diabetes in the hospital setting. Although the precise treatment targets remain somewhat controversial, quality glycemic management has become a top priority at most centers. A growing research base, including large randomized clinical trials, have led to the development of rational practice guidelines which serve to standardize our previously disparate approaches to care. The most recent studies in critically ill patients suggest that good, but perhaps not extremely tight glucose control, may be sufficient to optimize patient outcomes. Less is known about the best strategies in non-critically ill patients. Future studies should focus on determining which hospitalized patients benefit the most (or the least) from intensive glucose control; the preferred glycemic management strategies on general medical–surgical wards; and important operational issues concerning discharge planning, especially in those patients with newly detected hyperglycemia.

References

1. Mainous AG III, Baker R, Koopman RJ, et al. Impact of the population at risk of diabetes on projections of diabetes burden in the United States: an epidemic on the way. *Diabetologia*. 2007;50:934–940.
2. Sunny K. Burden of hospitalizations primarily due to uncontrolled diabetes. *Diabetes Care*. 2007;30:1281–1282.

3. Maciejewski ML, Maynard C. Diabetes-related utilization and costs for inpatient and outpatient services in the veterans administration. *Diabetes Care*. 2004;27:B69–B73.

4. UKPDS Group. Intensive blood-glucose control with sulphonylureas or insulin compared with conventional treatment and risk of complications in patients with type 2 diabetes (UKPDS 33. *Lancet*. 1998;352:837–853.

5. The DCCT Reasearch Group. Effect of intensive therapy on the microvascular complications of type 1 diabetes mellitus. *JAMA*. 2002;287:2563–2569.

6. Inzucchi SE. Management of hyperglycemia in the hospital setting. *N Engl J Med*. 2006;355:1903–1911.

7. Woods SE, Smith MJ, Sohail S, et al. The influence of type 2 diabetes mellitus in patients undergoing coronary artery bypass graft surgery: An 8-year prospective cohort study. *Chest*. 2004;126:1789–1795.

8. Donahoe SM, Stewart GC, McCabe CH, et al. Diabetes and mortality following acute coronary syndromes. *JAMA*. 2007;298:765–775.

9. Gudmundsson G, Gislason T, Lindberg E, et al. Mortality in COPD patients discharged from hospital: the role of treatment and co-morbidity. *Respir Res*. 2006;7:109–117.

10. Dronge AS, Perkal MF, Kancir S, et al. Long-term glycemic control and postoperative infectious complications. *Arch Surg*. 2006;141:375–380.

11. Capes SE, Hunt D, Malmberg K, et al. Stress hyperglycemia and prognosis of stroke in nondiabetic and diabetic patients: A systematic overview. *Stroke*. 2001;32:2426–2432.

12. Umpierrez GE, Isaacs SD, Bazargan N, et al. Hyperglycemia: An independent marker of in-hospital mortality in patients with undiagnosed diabetes. *J Clin Endocrinol Metab*. 2002;87:978–982.

13. Furnary AP, Gao G, Grunkemeier GL, et al. Continuous insulin infusion reduces mortality in patients with diabetes undergoing coronary artery bypass grafting. *J Thorac Cardiovasc Surg*. 2003;125:1007–1021.

14. Krinsley JS. Association between hyperglycemia and increased hospital mortality in a heterogeneous population of critically ill patients. *Mayo Clin Proc*. 2003;78:1471–1478.

15. Whitcomb BW, Pradhan EK, Pittas AG, et al. Impact of admission hyperglycemia on hospital mortality in various intensive care unit populations. *Crit Care Med*. 2005;33:2772–2777.

16. Kosiborod M, Rathore SS, Inzucchi SE, et al. Admission glucose and mortality in elderly patients hospitalized with acute myocardial infarction :Implications for patients with and without recognized diabetes. *Circulation*. 2005;111:3078–3086.

17. Svensson AM, McGuire DK, Abrahamsson P, et al. Association between hyper- and hypoglycaemia and 2 year all-cause mortality risk in diabetic patients with acute coronary events. *Euro Heart J*. 2005;26:1255–1261.

18. McAlister FA, Majumdar AR, Blitz S, et al. The relation between hyperglycemia and outcomes in 2,471 patients admitted to the hospital with community-acquired pneumonia. *Diabetes Care*. 2005;28:810–815.

19. Baker EH, Janaway CJ, Philips BJ, et al. Hyperglycemia is associated with poor outcomes in patients admitted to hospital with acute exacerbations of chronic obstructive pulmonary disease. *Thorax*. 2006;61:284–289.

20. Pomposelli JJ, Baxter JK 3rd, Babineau TJ, et al. Early postoperative glucose control predicts nosocomial infection rate in diabetic patients. *J Parenter Enteral Nutr*. 1998;22:77–81.

21. Norhammar A, Tenerz A, Nilsson G, et al. Glucose metabolism in patients with acute myocardial infarction and no previous diagnosis of diabetes mellitus: A prospective study. *Lancet*. 2002;359:2140–2144.

22. Malmberg K, Ryden L, Efendic S, et al. Randomized trial of insulin-glucose infusion followed by subcutaneous insulin treatment in diabetic patients with acute myocardial infarction (DIGAMI Study): Effects on mortality at 1 year. *J Am Coll Cardiol*. 1995;26:57–65.

23. Malmberg K, Ryden L, Wedel H, et al. Intense metabolic control by means of insulin in patients with diabetes mellitus and acute myocardial infarction (DIGAMI 2): effects on mortality and morbidity. *Euro Heart J*. 2005;26:650–661.

24. Cheung NW, Wong VW, McLean M. The Hyperglycemia: Intensive insulin infusion in infarction (HI-5) study. *Diabetes Care*. 2006;29:765–770.

25. Furnary AP, Zerr KJ, Grunkemeier GL, et al. Continuous intravenous insulin infusion reduces the incidence of deep sternal wound infection in diabetic patients after cardiac surgical procedures. *Ann Thorac Surg*. 1999;67:352–362.

26. Gandhi GY, Nuttall GA, Abel MD, et al. Intensive intraoperative insulin therapy versus conventional glucose management during cardiac surgery. *Ann Intern Med*. 2007;146:233–243.

27. Van den Berghe G, Wouters P, Weekers F, et al. Intensive insulin therapy in critically ill patients. *N Engl J Med*. 2001;345: 1359–1367.

28. Van den Berghe G, Wilmer A, Hermans G, et al. Intensive insulin therapy in the medical ICU. *N Engl J Med*. 2006;354:449–461.

29. Van den Berghe G, Wilmer A, Milants I, et al. Intensive insulin therapy in mixed medical/surgical intensive care units. *Diabetes*. 2006;55:3151–3159.

30. Brunkhorst FM, Engel C, Bloos F. Intensive insulin therapy and pentastarch resuscitation in severe sepsis. *N Engl J Med*. 2008;358:125–139.

31. Preiser JC, Devos P, Ruiz-Santana S, et al. A prospective randomised multi-centre controlled trial on tight glucose control by intensive insulin therapy in adult intensive care units: the Glucontrol study. *Intensive Care Med*. 2009;35(10):1738–1748.

32. Queale WS, Seidler AJ, Brancati FL, et al. Glycemic control and sliding scale insulin use in medical inpatients with diabetes mellitus. *Arch Intern Med*. 1997;157:545–552.

33. Umpierrez GE, Smiley D, Zisman A, et al. Randomized study of basal bolus insulin therapy in the inpatient management of patients with type 2 diabetes (RABBIT 2 Trial. *Diabetes Care*. 2007;30:2181–2186.

34. Moghissi ES, Korytkowski MT, Di Nardo M, et al. American Association of Clinical Endocrinologists; American Diabetes Association. American Association of Clinical Endocrinologists and American Diabetes Association consensus statement on inpatient glycemic control. *Diabetes Care*. 2009;32(6):1119–1131.

35. Meigering S, Corstjens AM, Tulleken JE, et al. Towards a feasible algorithm for tight glycaemic control in critically ill patients: a systematic review of the literature. *Critical Care*. 2006;10(R19):1–7.

36. Goldberg PA, Siegel MD, Sherwin RS, et al. Implementation of a safe and effective insulin infusion protocol in a medical intensive care unit. *Diabetes Care*. 2004;27:461–467.

37. Goldberg PA, Roussel MG, Inzucchi SE. Clinical results of an updated insulin infusion protocol in critically ill patients. *Diabetes Spect*. 2005;18:188–191.

38. Schmeltz LR, DeSantis AJ, Schmidt K, et al. Conversion of intravenous insulin infusions to subcutaneously administered insulin glargine in patients with hyperglycemia. *Endocr Pract*. 2006;12:641–650.

39. ADA. Standards of medical care in diabetes. *Diabetes Care*. 2007;31:S12–S54.

Chapter 48
The Future of Diabetes Therapy

Graham T. McMahon

Introduction

The epidemic of diabetes shows no signs of abating.[1] Diabetes is already having an enormous impact on the health and well-being of more than 150 million people, a number that is predicted to grow in the United States and throughout the globe, creating substantial strain on health-care systems.[1] Diabetes mellitus causes resource-intensive complications,[2] and while preventive care is effective in reducing overall utilization and improving outcome,[3] it too is expensive and requires teams of care providers at a time when the United States is facing a shortage of endocrinologists.[4] The future of diabetes therapy must include preventive efforts and improvements in therapeutics incorporating oral and injectable therapies, and will also need to embrace improvements in technology and care efficiency if targets are to be met (Table 48.1). This chapter examines some of the ongoing work in preventing and treating diabetes and outlines some of the approaches that will form part of future armamentaria.

Prevention of Type 2 Diabetes

The diabetes prevention program demonstrated the efficacy of weight loss and exercise in reducing the incidence of diabetes in people with impaired glucose tolerance.[5] Medical management of obesity is an ongoing challenge, but new developments offer some hope that insights into the neurohormonal mechanisms of appetite regulation and peripheral fat metabolism can lead to novel therapeutics. Surgical developments may also have an emerging role in the prevention of diabetes.

Anorectic Drugs

Several companies are pursuing discrete cannabinoid receptor antagonists to induce weight loss among patients with or at high risk for diabetes. Patients with a body mass index greater than 30 who were randomized to receive 20 mg of rimonabant daily weighed approximately 4.7 kg less than patients treated with placebo after 1 year.[6] Unfortunately all of the weight was regained in patients who discontinued the drug. Rimonabant appears to have a modest effect on atheroma burden.[7] Nevertheless, the drug is not approved in the United States owing to concerns for psychiatric effects.[8] Other manufacturers are developing similar cannabinoid receptor type 1 (CB-1) antagonists, including taranabant,[9] surinabant,[10] SLV319,[11] and CP-945598.

Serotonergic 5-HT2C and 5-HT1B receptors mediate inhibitory controls of eating. A number of serotonergic drugs, including selective serotonin reuptake inhibitors, dexfenfluramine, and 5-HT2C receptor agonists such as

G.T. McMahon (✉)

Division of Endocrinology, Diabetes and Hypertension, Brigham and Women's Hospital, Boston, MA 02115, USA

e-mail: gmcmahon@partners.org

Table 48.1 Future diabetes therapeutics

Drugs to normalize glucose
  – GLP-1 analogues
  – DPP-IV inhibitors
  – SGLT-2 inhibitors
  – Dual PPAR alpha-gamma agonists
  – Protein tyrosine kinase inhibitors
  – Glucokinase activators
  – Glucagon receptor antisense therapy
  – Rexinoids
Drugs to reduce the impact of hyperglycemia
  – Ruboxistaurin
  – Sulodexide
Novel insulins
  – Inhaled insulin
  – Oral insulin
Transplantation
  – Islet transplantation
  – Stem cell therapy
Advanced diabetes technology
  – Insulin pumps
  – Continuous glucose monitors
  – Pen devices
  – Online care management

lorcaserin[12] and WAY-161503, have been shown to significantly attenuate rodent body weight gain.[13] This effect is strongly associated with marked hypophagia and is probably mediated by the hypothalamic melanocortin system.[14]

Peptide YY (PYY) is a naturally occurring human hormone produced by specialized endocrine cells (L cells) in the gut in proportion to the calorie content of a meal. Research has demonstrated the role of PYY in regulating appetite control. Intranasal PYY is among the targets under development for the treatment of obesity, and early studies have demonstrated reduction in caloric intake and a moderating effect on appetite and weight loss in human subjects in some,[15] but not in all,[16] studies.

Drugs Affecting Peripheral Metabolism

Antiobesity drugs that influence metabolic targets rather than the central anorectic pathways are also being explored. Some thermogenic approaches include the activation of adrenergic, thyroid hormone, or growth hormone receptors and the inhibition of glucocorticoid receptors. If drugs that address peripheral metabolism cause weight loss by increasing fat oxidation, they not only address a cause of obesity but also should promote loss of fat rather than lean tissue and improve insulin sensitivity.

Beta-3-adrenergic agonists induce weight loss thermogenically and improve insulin sensitivity in rodents. Their main sites of action are white and brown adipose tissue and muscle. Beta-3-adrenergic agonists have a more rapid insulin sensitizing than antiobesity effect but have been as yet minimally explored in humans. Compounds CL-316243 and TAK-677 are in development, but results have been disappointing thus far: in the one reported human study, TAK-677 had minimal effect on energy metabolism, even at the highest dose. There was little or no change in 24-h respiratory quotient and no change in fasting concentrations of glucose, free fatty acids, and insulin.[17]

Bariatric Surgery

Bariatric surgery is likely to become more widespread as average weight continues to climb in the United States and around the world. As compared with conventional therapy, bariatric surgery appears to be a viable option for the treatment of severe obesity, resulting in long-term weight loss, reduced mortality, improved lifestyle, and improvement in risk factors that were present preoperatively.[18,19] Results from Sweden indicate that the greatest weight loss is achieved with gastric bypass, followed by vertical-banded gastroplasty and banding.[19] Among patients who are not yet diabetic, bariatric surgery can significantly delay or prevent the onset of diabetes.[18] There is evidence that hormonal changes following surgery may contribute to the degree of weight loss – recent data show that postprandial levels of PYY and glucagon-like peptide (GLP)-1 rise following bariatric surgery, a change that enhances satiety.[20]

Treatment of Hyperglycemia

Hyperglycemia is a cardinal manifestation of diabetes mellitus, and normalizing glucose levels has been shown to reduce the incidence of microvascular complications[21] and may play a role in abating some of the macrovascular complications of diabetes.[22]

Future developments must continue to examine strategies to expand the appropriate use of the currently available oral hypoglycemic agents and insulin. However the future holds the promise of more efficacious drugs with potentially fewer adverse events.

DPP-IV Inhibitors

Inhibitors of the dipeptidyl peptidase-IV (DPP-IV) enzyme are becoming increasingly available for the treatment of diabetes. Inhibition of this enzyme increases the GLP-1 concentration and improves periprandial insulin secretion and glucagon suppression. Agents such as sitagliptin, saxagliptin,[23] vildagliptin,[24] and alogliptin[25] provide moderate reductions in HbA1c (ranging from 0.4 to 0.8% above placebo for patients starting at an HbA1c of less than 9%), minimal risk of hypoglycemia, and weight neutrality.[26] Medications from this class have been studied for use as single agents, in combination with other oral agents or in combination with insulin.[27] Their long-term safety is not yet established, they remain expensive, and their place in the diabetic treatment algorithm remains to be defined. However, inhibition of the DPP-IV enzyme is an example of how novel discoveries in medicine can translate into an expanded pharmaceutical armamentarium.

GLP-1 Analogues

Exenatide LAR

A once-weekly formulation of exenatide (exenatide LAR) has been developed and studied in initial clinical trials. Early data suggest that the LAR formulation is more efficacious at reducing HbA1c and weight than the twice-daily formulation of exenatide and is also associated with a lower incidence of gastrointestinal adverse events. In a trial of 45 subjects with type 2 diabetes with a mean hemoglobin A1c (HbA1c) of 8.5% on oral agents, administration of 2 mg of exenatide LAR once weekly for 15 weeks was associated with a mean reduction in HbA1c of 1.7% and a mean weight loss of 3.8 kg as compared to placebo.[28] Early data from a comparison study between twice-daily exenatide and once-weekly exenatide suggest the superiority of the long-acting formulation.[29]

Liraglutide

Liraglutide is a glucagon-like peptide-1 receptor analogue, which is obtained by derivatizing glucagon-like peptide-1 with a fatty acid, providing a compound with pharmacokinetic properties that are suitable for once-daily dosing.[30]

Liraglutide has demonstrated improvement in HbA1c levels. Among patients with an initial HbA1c of 8.5% treated for 14 weeks, the mean reduction was 1.7%. A mean placebo-adjusted weight loss of 1.3 kg over 3 months was observed.[31] In addition, there are indications of improved beta cell function in patients with type 2 diabetes treated with liraglutide.[32] Liraglutide is well tolerated; the adverse events that are most frequently reported include nausea and diarrhea.

Most intriguingly, a series of studies have indicated that the GLP-1 analogues can increase beta cell mass by stimulating beta cell proliferation and neogenesis.[33] If such improvements in beta cell function and longevity can be duplicated in humans, there may be a compelling reason to prescribe these drugs more frequently.

CJC-1131

CJC-1131 is a GLP-1 analogue that consists of a DPP-IV-resistant form of GLP-1 joined to a reactive chemical linker group that allows GLP-1 to form a covalent and irreversible bond with serum albumin following subcutaneous (SC) injection.[34] In humans, CJC-1131 has a half-life of approximately 10 days.[35]

A 12-week, randomized, double-blind, placebo-controlled, multicenter study looked at the effects of a combination of CJC-1131 and metformin on glycemic control and body weight in type 2 diabetic patients not achieving adequate glycemic control on oral agents and found that CJC-1131 at a dose of ~2.6 µg/kg improved HbA1c values by 1.1% from a starting mean of 8%. There were no indications of local intolerance or immunogenicity.[36]

Other GLP1 Analogues

Taspoglutide is a matrix-free sustained release formation GLP-1 receptor agonist which is expected to be administered subcutaneously weekly or biweekly.[37] Albiglutide is a recombinant albumin-GLP-1 fusion protein that mimics GLP-1 action. Albiglutide appears to have less potent anorectic effects than exenatide and liraglutide. In contrast, LY548806 is an intravenously delivered GLP-1 analogue that was investigated for use in the acute care setting and may help control stress-induced hyperglycemia, but has been halted in phase II development.[38]

Protein Tyrosine Phosphatase Inhibitors

Insulin receptor signaling is mediated by tyrosine phosphorylation. Mounting evidence indicates that protein tyrosine phosphatase (PTP)1B negatively regulates insulin signaling making it a prime target for enhancing insulin sensitivity. PTP1b-deficient mice have enhanced insulin sensitivity without the weight gain seen with other insulin sensitizers such as peroxisome proliferator-activated receptor (PPAR)-gamma agonists, probably due to a second action of PTP1B as a negative regulator of leptin signaling. Isis 113715, PTP-3848 and trodusquemine are all in development.[39]

Glucokinase Activators

Glucokinase catalyzes the first step in glycolysis, phosphorylation of glucose to glucose-6-phosphate, and is an ideal sensor of physiologic changes in blood glucose levels. In pancreatic beta cells, glucokinase is the rate-limiting enzyme in glucose metabolism and determines the rate of glucose-induced insulin secretion.[40] Several manufacturers are examining the potential of glucokinase agonists. Early studies indicated that LY2121260, a glucokinase activator, augmented insulin secretion in an animal model.[41] Other investigators have expressed concern that activation of glucokinase could exacerbate hepatic fat accumulation.[42] AZD1656, AZD6370, LY2599506, and NN9101, R1511 are all in active development.

Interfering with the Glucagon Receptor

Antisense technology is used to diminish the production of proteins that have been implicated in a disease. The binding of an antisense drug to its target mRNA results in degradation of the mRNA which is therefore not translated by the ribosome into a functional protein. A glucagon receptor antisense therapeutic that has been developed in rodent models of type 2 diabetes decreased glucagon receptor expression, normalized blood glucose, improved glucose tolerance, and preserved insulin secretion. In addition to decreasing expression of cAMP-regulated genes in liver and preventing glucagon-mediated hepatic glucose production, glucagon receptor inhibition increased serum concentrations of active GLP-1 and insulin levels in pancreatic islets in rodents.[43]

Dual PPAR Alpha-Gamma Agonists

PPARs are ligand-activated transcription factors of nuclear hormone receptor superfamily composed of three subtypes, including PPAR-alpha, PPAR-delta, and PPAR-gamma. Activation of PPAR-alpha with medications such as fenofibrate and gemfibrozil reduces triglycerides and increases HDL concentration. PPAR-delta agonists, acting predominantly in skeletal muscle, have been shown to reduce triglyceride levels and small, dense low-density lipoproteins, as well as to significantly increase HDL levels, but may also be linked to carcinogenesis.[44] PPAR-gamma is expressed predominantly in adipose tissue, and to a lesser extent in macrophages, muscle, and liver. PPAR-gamma has received considerable attention since the mid-1990s, when it was found to be the molecular target of insulin-sensitizing, antidiabetic drugs known as thiazolidinediones.

Multimodal drugs which can reduce hyperglycemia and concomitantly inhibit the progression of secondary cardiovascular complications may offer valuable therapeutic option by combining aspects of each of these effects. Several basic and clinical studies have exemplified the beneficial effects of PPAR-alpha and PPAR-gamma ligands in reducing intermediary measures of cardiovascular risk, resulting in the development of PPAR-alpha/gamma dual agonists such as muraglitazar, tesaglitazar, and ragaglitazar. However, these have been noted to produce several cardiovascular risks and carcinogenicity.[45] A study that randomized 1159 subjects with type 2 diabetes to receive either 5 mg of muraglitazar with metformin daily or 30 mg of pioglitazone with metformin daily demonstrated a greater lowering of HbA1c with muraglitazar (-1.1%) as compared with the submaximal dose of pioglitazone (-0.9%). Similarly, tesaglitazar improved lipid and glucose measures in a 24-week study.[46] Improvements in HDL and reductions in triglycerides have been noteworthy with these drugs.

Development of this class of agents was largely suspended when reports emerged that, as compared with placebo or pioglitazone, muraglitazar was associated with an excess incidence of major adverse cardiovascular events, attributed in part to their imbalanced and supra-therapeutic activity on their target receptors.[47,48]

Rexinoids

Agonists for the nuclear receptor PPAR-gamma and its heterodimeric partner, retinoid X receptor (RXR), are effective agents for the treatment of type 2 diabetes. RXR agonists can be effective in lowering blood glucose by a mechanism that is likely independent of PPAR-gamma/RXR transactivation. However, hypertriglyceridemia is a recognized side effect of RXR agonist therapy and can be a limitation in the development of these compounds.[49]

Sodium–Glucose Cotransporter Type 2 Inhibitors

The inhibition of renal glucose reabsorption is a novel approach to the treatment of diabetes. In normal individuals, glucose present in the plasma is filtered by the kidneys, but virtually all of it is reabsorbed, such that less than 1% of filtered glucose appears in the urine.[50] Increasing the renal excretion of glucose by inhibition renal reabsorption has been demonstrated to reduce plasma glucose levels independently of insulin action. Glucose reabsorption is mediated through sodium–glucose cotransporters (SGLTs). SGLTs exist in two isoforms. SGLT1 transports dietary glucose from the gastrointestinal epithelium and is also expressed in the liver, lung, and kidney; mutations in SGLT1 result in severe diarrhea and dehydration that can be fatal unless glucose and galactose are removed from the diet. In contrast, SGLT2 is selectively expressed in the kidney.[51] A mutation in SGLT2 results in familial renal glycosuria.[52] Familial renal glycosuria is a surprisingly benign syndrome and has not been reported to be associated with an increased predilection to urinary tract infections or dehydration.

Consequently a number of pharmaceutical companies are developing inhibitors of SGLT2. A number of compounds show promise including dapagliflozin,[53] sergliflozin,[54] JNJ-28431754, GSK-189075 (each of which is in at least one clinical trial as of mid-2008), AVE-2268, YM-543, TA-7284, and Roche-7201. In a rat study, once-daily dapagliflozin treatment over 2 weeks significantly lowered fasting and postprandial glucose levels at doses ranging from 0.1 to 1.0 mg/kg and resulted in a significant increase in glucose utilization rate accompanied by a significant reduction in glucose production.[53] Clinical trials will demonstrate whether the anticipated risk of dehydration and genitourinary infections will be problematic.

Preventing Diabetes-Related Complications

Preventing diabetes-related complications requires an integrated approach addressing hyperlipidemia, hypertension, hypercoagulability, and hyperglycemia. As trials supporting the utility of managing these risks emerge, researchers continue to pursue targeted strategies to reduce the pathologic impact of chronic hyperglycemia.

Ruboxistaurin

Although numerous studies have shown that good control of blood glucose levels helps reduce the incidence of microvascular complications associated with diabetes, there is still a need for adjunctive medications and treatments to stop or slow the processes once they begin. Ruboxistaurin is a drug that is designed to reduce microvascular complications by selectively inhibiting the function of protein kinase C (PKC)-beta, which may have a role in the treatment of diabetic microvascular disease. Studies in patients with microalbuminuria and diabetic retinopathy have shown mild-to-moderate efficacy in secondary end points, but the overall efficacy of the drug has so far been disappointing. In a study of 252 subjects with moderate-to-severe nonproliferative diabetic retinopathy, 32 mg daily of ruboxistaurin did not have any significant effect on the progression of diabetic retinopathy, but treated patients had a delayed occurrence of moderate visual loss and sustained moderate visual loss.[55] Among patients with diabetic peripheral neuropathy, treatment for 6 months with 32 mg daily of ruboxistaurin resulted in reduced sensory symptoms and quality of life, but no objective improvements in nerve conduction studies.[56] Unfortunately there has been little evidence of any consistent effect of protein kinase C inhibition on microalbuminuria or glomerular filtration rate,[57,58] though an early study suggested differential preservation of existing renal function in treated patients.[57]

Sulodexide

Sulodexide, a mixture of heparan and dermatan sulfate (80/20%), targets metabolic defects in matrix and basement membrane synthesis as well as endothelial cell function. Sulodexide apparently alters glomerular permeability and reduces proteinuria by a non-blood pressure, non-renin–angiotensin–aldosterone system (RAAS)-related mechanism. As a result, sulodexide could effectively increase therapeutic options in those patients who fail to respond to RAAS inhibition. Sulodexide is absorbed orally and has been shown to reduce proteinuria in animal models of diabetic nephropathy. Human studies (including the SUN-micro and SUN-macro trials) examining the effect of sulodexide on renal function are in their early stages, but early data suggest moderate effects on the albumin excretion rate.[59]

Improvements in Insulin Therapy and Glucose Monitoring

Glucose Monitoring and Glucose Sensors

Fingerstick glucose monitoring is often the most frustrating component of insulin therapy; patients being treated with multi-dose insulin often have to check their glucose levels up to seven times daily. Plasma glucose levels are most accurately reflected in samples drawn from arterialized beds such as the fingertips. Other sources for glucose measurement include tear fluid[60] and interstitial fluid.[61] Thermal, raman, impedence, and infrared spectroscopy, optical coherence tomography, temperature-modulated localized reflectance, ultrasound, and electromagnetic sensing have all shown promise in facilitating less-invasive glucose testing.[62]

A number of manufacturers (including Minimed, Abott and Dexcom) have produced continuous glucose sensors with greater accuracy and reliability than ever before, and can be used for upto 7 continuous days. Mean absolute relative differences in glucose measurements approximate 15%, with excellent performance during hypoglycemia.[63] These devices are readily portable and appear to result in sustained HbA1c improvements in patients who wear them.[64]

Insulin Pump Therapy

Continuous subcutaneous insulin infusion offers a system for achieving treatment targets with a lower incidence of severe hypoglycemia. Patients with type 1 diabetes who require insulin therapy generally prefer the flexibility, convenience, and physiologic glycemic control of continuous subcutaneous insulin infusion.[65] A pump system controlled by a hand-held remote (Omnipod[TM]) was launched and appears to have great potential as unique approach to managing diabetes.[66]

Insulin pump therapy continues to advance and now incorporates semi-closed devices that include subcutaneous glucose sensors with a subcutaneous insulin delivery system. The ultimate goal of continuous insulin infusion is to create an "artificial pancreas," where ambient glucose levels automatically trigger appropriate insulin release from an insulin reservoir. Plasma glucose concentrations can change dramatically within minutes, but these changes are only slowly reflected in subcutaneous tissue, making subcutaneous monitors insufficiently reliable to guide rapid changes in insulin delivery. Achievement of such a closed loop system of sensing and delivery has been limited by the inability to create a reliable intravascular glucose sensor with sufficient longevity. Predictive algorithms for determining insulin need are in development.

Future insulin pumps may be internally implanted. Experience with internally implanted pumps has been variable to date. Insulin precipitation, short battery life, pocket infections, and catheter obstructions have been challenging.[67,68] However, for patients with severe and frequent hypoglycemia, the pumps are largely successful. Prototypes in development are smaller, have larger screens, and provide more intuitive navigation and feedback to users.

Inhaled Insulin

Optimism for the potential utility of inhaled insulin has given way to disappointment as the first inhaled insulin product was withdrawn from the market in 2008. The market failure of Exubera[TM] illustrated the importance of portability, linear dosimetry, dose consistency, and safety.[69] Development of the other inhaled insulin formulations (including liquid-based insulin) has now largely ceased, partly on the basis of reports of increased frequency of lung cancer among users of inhaled therapy as compared to control patients.[70] Nasal[71] and transdermal insulin delivery systems[72] continue to hold promise.

Oral and Buccal Insulin

The bioavailability of insulin administered orally is low since the oral mucosae form an effective mechanical barrier to proteins, and the protein's enteral absorption is limited by its susceptibility to proteases. A liquid aerosol formulation of insulin is in development and aims to introduce fine aerosolized insulin droplets at high velocity into the mouth for buccal and oropharyngeal absorption. This formulation requires approximately 20 sprays at each meal to generate glucose lowering.[73] To date the studies have been shorter than 1 week and have involved less than 100 participants in total but have shown modest glycemic responses.[73,74,75]

Improved Pen Devices

Insulin pen devices are an important component of insulin delivery since they are convenient, discrete, attractive, and portable. Their combination with microfine needles make insulin delivery almost painless.[76] Modern plastic syringes are disposable and lightweight. More than 80% of insulin-treated patients with diabetes in Europe are using an insulin pen. Insulin pens for long-term use incorporate more sophisticated functions such as memory functions and insulin dose calculators.[77] Physicians play a critical role in presenting pen devices as an option to patients[78] and providing appropriate training;[79] use of pens can contribute to improved outcomes in diabetes. Future years will bring continued advances in ease of use, stability, and reliability.[80]

Together these technologies could enhance the ease and convenience of glucose testing, provide a more accurate picture of each patient's glucose profile, and allow clinicians to provide the most timely and appropriate interventions to improve quality of care.

Transplantation for Diabetes

Islet Transplants

Islet transplantation has been aggressively pursued for the treatment of type 1 diabetes. Since there are risks associated with immunosuppression, the most suitable candidates for islet transplants are patients with unstable type 1 diabetes and hypoglycemic unawareness.[81] Islet transplantation has afforded this patient population with better metabolic control, normalization of HbA1c, prevention of severe hypoglycemia, and substantial improvement in quality of life. The intrahepatic infusion procedure necessitates only a short hospital stay and has been well tolerated – bleeding and portal vein thrombosis have been the most common adverse effects. Many patients require more than one infusion. Islet preparation protocols have matured but islet availability is an ongoing limitation. The rate of insulin independence 1 year after transplantation continues to rise,[82] though remains low, approximating 50% at 1 year and 33% at 2 years.[83] Ongoing work continues to improve the specificity of the immunosuppressive protocols and the engraftment of islets (including the use of incretins). Alternative sites (including omentum and subcutaneous sites) are being explored. Xenogeneic islets obtained from porcine or other animal sources hold promise to improve the availability of islets, but current hurdles include potential transmission of porcine endogenous retroviruses to immunosuppressed recipients and immunogenicity.[84]

Stem Cell Therapy

Great progress has been made in creating beta cells from a wide variety of embryonic or adult stem cell sources. Mesenchymal, hematopoietic and pancreatic ductal cell progenitors can be differentiated into beta cells.[85,86] Hepatocytes can be transdifferentiated.[87] Intra-islet precursors can be harvested and matured in vivo.[88] Most encouraging are the data showing that human embryonic stem cells can generate glucose-responsive insulin-secreting cells in vivo.[89] Each of these developments provides new avenues for discovery and offers great potential not only to provide a reliable source for islet transplants but also for auto-transplantation.

Whole-Pancreas Transplantation

Whole-pancreas transplantation results in sustained euglycemia but is associated with significant surgical and postoperative complications – largely related to the venous or enteric drainage systems and pancreatitis.[83] Pancreas transplantation is performed as a simultaneous pancreas and kidney transplant, a pancreas after kidney transplant, or a pancreas transplant alone. Each form of transplant is characterized by its own indications, risks, and outcomes. Ongoing experiments will continue to refine the surgical techniques and immunosuppressive regimens to further improve outcomes, though it is unlikely that this approach to diabetes treatment will very significantly expand given the constraint on the supply of whole pancreata and the relatively narrow indications for the procedure.

Systems to Improve the Quality of Diabetes Care

Several guidelines and diabetes management programs have been developed nationally and locally to improve diabetes care in the community. However, empirical data suggest that compliance with diabetes clinical practice recommendations is inadequate in primary care and that a large proportion of patients with diabetes remain at high risk.[90] Over recent years, there have been encouraging improvements in several processes and some intermediate outcomes of diabetes quality of care in the United States. Although the level of care continues to fall short of what is recommended, annual lipid testing, dilated eye and foot examinations, self-monitoring of blood glucose level, and adoption of aspirin use and pneumococcal and influenza vaccinations have sizably improved. Impressive improvements in lipid control and some improvement in glycemic control have occurred, but blood pressure control has not improved.[91]

Improving Compliance

Approximately half of the medicines prescribed in the treatment of chronic diseases such as diabetes are not taken, which is costly on personal, economic, and societal levels.[92] Simplifying treatment regimens can sometimes improve adherence and treatment outcomes for both short- and long-term treatments.[93] More complex strategies, including combinations of more thorough patient instructions and counseling, reminders, close follow-up, supervised self-monitoring, rewards for success, family therapy, psychological therapy, crisis intervention, and manual telephone follow-up, have been each demonstrated to improve adherence and treatment outcomes.[92] In general, the results of studies on adherence suggest that more frequent interaction with patients improves adherence. However, these complex strategies for improving adherence with long-term medication prescriptions are not very effective despite the amount of effort and resources they consume.

A variety of simple and technological strategies have been designed to improve patient compliance. The Bang and Olufsen C-cap[94] is an electronic cap for pen injection systems and uses visual and acoustic reminder signals to help patients remember to take their medications. A similar compliance system for dispensing tablets, the "Helping hand" is also in development.[95]

Communications and Home Monitoring

It has become clear that if new technology can be made both relevant and valuable, patients will use it. Some 70% of the US population access the Internet[96] which makes web-based technology a particularly attractive mechanism to engage patients with chronic diseases. Increasingly, patients express willingness to engage with their provider using secure communications,[96] and many systems now provide patients the opportunity to review results of investigations and read their clinicians' notes online.[97] Moreover, the widespread acceptance of wireless communication technologies indicates that future care models incorporating extensive home monitoring and tailored feedback have potential for broad adoption by patients with type 2 diabetes.[96] How these new systems will fit with current clinical workflow and reimbursement mechanisms remains to be established.

Home monitoring can facilitate engagement of patients in their care and may improve adherence.[98] Home glucose monitoring has not been shown to have a significant impact on overall control outside of its use in a structured feedback care management program.[99,100] Home blood pressure monitoring improves the proportion of patients achieving blood pressure targets[101] and is generally easy and reliable for patients. Increasingly such information can be uploaded to a central data repository for interpretation by a clinician.[102,103] As the use of electronic medical records advances, it is likely that these will increasingly incorporate the facility to upload glucometer or home blood pressure readings.

Care Management

Of systems approaches to improving diabetes care, combining patient education, a nurse, or both with arrangements for follow-up or multiple professional intervention have most consistently led to improvements in patient outcomes as well as the process of care.[104] Nurses can communicate with the patient and the physician, help facilitate patient and practitioner adherence, provide patient education, and, if they are trained and if detailed management protocols are available, assume some of the responsibilities for direct care. Patient education is important for involving patients in their own diabetes management and for improving self-management and compliance to therapy. Moreover, it can encourage patients to change their lifestyle with regard to diet, smoking habit, and physical exercise, all of which help to achieve good glycemic control and to postpone or prevent the development of complications.

More comprehensive approaches to integrating care including follow-up, phone contact, and the use of Internet-based feedback and communication have demonstrated significant efficacy[103] but can be expensive.

Summary

Though prevention of diabetes is a critical objective in improving the health of the population, it is difficult to achieve. As the prevalence of diabetes continues to rise, future practitioners will have a series of elegant pharmacologic tools and a suite of technological supports that aim to facilitate the provision of high-quality care. Patients will be able to care for themselves with convenient, perhaps painless glucose sensing and medications with fewer adverse events. A broader supply of beta cells and superior immunosuppression will enhance the utility of islet transplantation for patients with type 1 diabetes. Closed loop systems may offer the potential for smoother glycemic control in patients requiring insulin. All patients will be assisted when functional care teams are not only created but supported. When patients and their clinicians can be provided with the best tools to prevent, monitor, and treat diabetes, everyone benefits. New therapies in diabetes will help to achieve that universal goal.

References

1. Green A, Christian Hirsch N, Pramming SK. The changing world demography of type 2 diabetes. *Diabetes Metab Res Rev*. Jan–Feb 2003;19(1):3–7.
2. Clarke P, Gray A, Legood R, Briggs A, Holman R. The impact of diabetes-related complications on healthcare costs: results from the United Kingdom Prospective Diabetes Study (UKPDS Study No. 65). *Diabet Med*. Jun 2003;20(6):442–450.
3. Gaede P, Lund-Andersen H, Parving HH, Pedersen O. Effect of a multifactorial intervention on mortality in type 2 diabetes. *N Engl J Med*. Feb 7 2008;358(6):580–591.
4. Rizza RA, Vigersky RA, Rodbard HW, et al. A model to determine workforce needs for endocrinologists in the United States until 2020. *Endocr Pract*. May–Jun 2003;9(3):210–219.
5. Knowler WC, Barrett-Connor E, Fowler SE, et al. Reduction in the incidence of type 2 diabetes with lifestyle intervention or metformin. *N Engl J Med*. Feb 7 2002;346(6):393–403.

6. Pi-Sunyer FX, Aronne LJ, Heshmati HM, Devin J, Rosenstock J. Effect of rimonabant, a cannabinoid-1 receptor blocker, on weight and cardiometabolic risk factors in overweight or obese patients: RIO-North America: a randomized controlled trial. *JAMA*. Feb 15 2006;295(7):761–775.

7. Nissen SE, Nicholls SJ, Wolski K, et al. Effect of rimonabant on progression of atherosclerosis in patients with abdominal obesity and coronary artery disease: the STRADIVARIUS randomized controlled trial. *JAMA*. Apr 2 2008;299(13): 1547–1560.

8. Steinberg BA, Cannon CP. Cannabinoid-1 receptor blockade in cardiometabolic risk reduction: safety, tolerability, and therapeutic potential. *Am J Cardiol*. Dec 17 2007;100(12A):27P–32P.

9. Addy C, Li S, Agrawal N, et al. Safety, tolerability, pharmacokinetics, and pharmacodynamic properties of taranabant, a novel selective cannabinoid-1 receptor inverse agonist, for the treatment of obesity: results from a double-blind, placebo-controlled, single oral dose study in healthy volunteers. *J Clin Pharmacol*. Apr 2008;48(4):418–427.

10. Lamota L, Bermudez-Silva FJ, Marco EM, et al. Effects of adolescent nicotine and SR 147778 (Surinabant) administration on food intake, somatic growth and metabolic parameters in rats. *Neuropharmacology*. Jan 2008;54(1):194–205.

11. Lange JH, Coolen HK, van Stuivenberg HH, et al. Synthesis, biological properties, and molecular modeling investigations of novel 3,4-diarylpyrazolines as potent and selective CB(1) cannabinoid receptor antagonists. *J Med Chem*. Jan 29 2004;47(3):627–643.

12. Thomsen WJ, Grottick AJ, Menzaghi F, et al. Lorcaserin, a novel selective human 5-HT2C agonist: in vitro and in vivo pharmacological characterization. *J Pharmacol Exp Ther*. Feb 5 2008;325(2):577–587.

13. Rosenzweig-Lipson S, Zhang J, Mazandarani H, et al. Antiobesity-like effects of the 5-HT2C receptor agonist WAY-161503. *Brain Res*. Feb 16 2006;1073–1074:240–251.

14. Halford JC, Harrold JA, Boyland EJ, Lawton CL, Blundell JE. Serotonergic drugs : effects on appetite expression and use for the treatment of obesity. *Drugs*. 2007;67(1):27–55.

15. Degen L, Oesch S, Casanova M, et al. Effect of peptide YY3–36 on food intake in humans. *Gastroenterology*. Nov 2005;129(5):1430–1436.

16. le Roux CW, Borg CM, Murphy KG, Vincent RP, Ghatei MA, Bloom SR. Supraphysiological doses of intravenous PYY3-36 cause nausea, but no additional reduction in food intake. *Ann Clin Biochem*. Jan 2008;45(Pt 1):93–95.

17. Redman LM, de Jonge L, Fang X, et al. Lack of an effect of a novel beta3-adrenoceptor agonist, TAK-677, on energy metabolism in obese individuals: a double-blind, placebo-controlled randomized study. *J Clin Endocrinol Metab*. Feb 2007;92(2):527–531.

18. Sjostrom L, Lindroos AK, Peltonen M, et al. Lifestyle, diabetes, and cardiovascular risk factors 10 years after bariatric surgery. *N Engl J Med*. Dec 23 2004;351(26):2683–2693.

19. Sjostrom L, Narbro K, Sjostrom CD, et al. Effects of bariatric surgery on mortality in Swedish obese subjects. *N Engl J Med*. Aug 23 2007;357(8):741–752.

20. le Roux CW, Aylwin SJ, Batterham RL, et al. Gut hormone profiles following bariatric surgery favor an anorectic state, facilitate weight loss, and improve metabolic parameters. *Ann Surg*. Jan 2006;243(1):108–114.

21. UK Prospective Diabetes Study (UKPDS) Group. Intensive blood-glucose control with sulphonylureas or insulin compared with conventional treatment and risk of complications in patients with type 2 diabetes (UKPDS 33). *Lancet*. Sep 12 1998;352(9131):837–853.

22. Nathan DM, Cleary PA, Backlund JY, et al. Intensive diabetes treatment and cardiovascular disease in patients with type 1 diabetes. *N Engl J Med*. Dec 22 2005;353(25):2643–2653.

23. Rosenstock J, Sankoh S, List JF. Glucose-lowering activity of the dipeptidyl peptidase-4 inhibitor saxagliptin in drug-naive patients with type 2 diabetes. *Diabetes Obes Metab*. Mar 18 2008;10(5):376-386.

24. Garber AJ, Sharma MD. Update: vildagliptin for the treatment of Type 2 diabetes. *Expert Opin Investig Drugs*. Jan 2008;17(1):105–113.

25. Deacon CF. Alogliptin, a potent and selective dipeptidyl peptidase-IV inhibitor for the treatment of type 2 diabetes. *Curr Opin Investig Drugs*. Apr 2008;9(4):402–413.

26. Chahal H, Chowdhury TA. Gliptins: a new class of oral hypoglycaemic agent. *QJM*. Nov 2007;100(11):671–677.

27. Fonseca V, Baron M, Shao Q, Dejager S. Sustained efficacy and reduced hypoglycemia during one year of treatment with vildagliptin added to insulin in patients with type 2 diabetes mellitus. *Horm Metab Res*. Mar 11 2008;40(6):427-430.

28. Kim D, MacConell L, Zhuang D, et al. Effects of once-weekly dosing of a long-acting release formulation of exenatide on glucose control and body weight in subjects with type 2 diabetes. *Diabetes Care*. Jun 2007;30(6):1487–1493.

29. Drucker DJ, Buse JB, Taylor K, Kendall DM, Trautmann M, Zhuang D, Porter L. Exenatide once weekly versus twice daily for the treatment of type 2 diabetes: a randomised, open-label, non-inferiority study. *Lancet*. Oct 4 2008;372(9645):1240–1250.

30. Agerso H, Jensen LB, Elbrond B, Rolan P, Zdravkovic M. The pharmacokinetics, pharmacodynamics, safety and tolerability of NN2211, a new long-acting GLP-1 derivative, in healthy men. *Diabetologia*. Feb 2002;45(2):195–202.

31. Vilsboll T, Zdravkovic M, Le-Thi T, et al. Liraglutide, a long-acting human glucagon-like peptide-1 analog, given as monotherapy significantly improves glycemic control and lowers body weight without risk of hypoglycemia in patients with type 2 diabetes. *Diabetes Care*. Jun 2007;30(6):1608–1610.

32. Vilsboll T, Brock B, Perrild H, et al. Liraglutide, a once-daily human GLP-1 analogue, improves pancreatic B-cell function and arginine-stimulated insulin secretion during hyperglycaemia in patients with Type 2 diabetes mellitus. *Diabet Med*. Feb 2008;25(2):152–156.

33. Rolin B, Larsen MO, Gotfredsen CF, et al. The long-acting GLP-1 derivative NN2211 ameliorates glycemia and increases beta-cell mass in diabetic mice. *Am J Physiol Endocrinol Metab.* Oct 2002;283(4):E745–E752.

34. Kim JG, Baggio LL, Bridon DP, et al. Development and characterization of a glucagon-like peptide 1-albumin conjugate: the ability to activate the glucagon-like peptide 1 receptor in vivo. *Diabetes.* Mar 2003;52(3):751–759.

35. Giannoukakis N. CJC-1131. ConjuChem. *Curr Opin Investig Drugs.* Oct 2003;4(10):1245–1249.

36. Ratner R, Dreyfus J, Castaigne J. Effects of DAC-GLP-1 (CJC-1131) on glycemic control and weight over 12 weeks in metformin-treated patients with type 2 diabetes. *65th Scientific Sessions of the American Diabetes Association.* San Diego, CA; 2005.

37. Giannoukakis N. BIM-51077, a dipeptidyl peptidase-IV-resistant glucagon-like peptide-1 analog. *Curr Opin Investig Drugs.* Oct 2007;8(10):842–848.

38. Millican R, Myers S, Koester A, et al. A soluble DPP-4 protected GLP-1 analog (LY548806) with potential for treatment of hyperglycemia in acute care settings. 1504-P. Paper presented at: 65th Session of the American Diabetes Association, 2005; San Diego, CA.

39. Koren S, Fantus IG. Inhibition of the protein tyrosine phosphatase PTP1B: potential therapy for obesity, insulin resistance and type-2 diabetes mellitus. *Best Pract Res Clin Endocrinol Metab.* Dec 2007;21(4):621–640.

40. Liang Y, Najafi H, Smith RM, et al. Concordant glucose induction of glucokinase, glucose usage, and glucose-stimulated insulin release in pancreatic islets maintained in organ culture. *Diabetes.* Jul 1992;41(7): 792–806.

41. Efanov AM, Barrett DG, Brenner MB, et al. A novel glucokinase activator modulates pancreatic islet and hepatocyte function. *Endocrinology.* Sep 2005;146(9):3696–3701.

42. Couzin J. Medicine. Drug deals diabetes a one-two punch. *Science.* Jul 18 2003;301(5631):290.

43. Sloop KW, Cao JX, Siesky AM, et al. Hepatic and glucagon-like peptide-1-mediated reversal of diabetes by glucagon receptor antisense oligonucleotide inhibitors. *J Clin Invest.* Jun 2004;113(11):1571–1581.

44. Barish GD, Narkar VA, Evans RM. PPAR delta: a dagger in the heart of the metabolic syndrome. *J Clin Invest.* Mar 2006;116(3):590–597.

45. Tannehill-Gregg SH, Sanderson TP, Minnema D, et al. Rodent carcinogenicity profile of the antidiabetic dual PPAR alpha and gamma agonist muraglitazar. *Toxicol Sci.* Jul 2007;98(1):258–270.

46. Ratner RE, Parikh S, Tou C. Efficacy, safety and tolerability of tesaglitazar when added to the therapeutic regimen of poorly controlled insulin-treated patients with type 2 diabetes. *Diab Vasc Dis Res.* Sep 2007;4(3):214–221.

47. Nissen SE, Wolski K, Topol EJ. Effect of muraglitazar on death and major adverse cardiovascular events in patients with type 2 diabetes mellitus. *JAMA.* Nov 23 2005;294(20):2581–2586.

48. Balakumar P, Rose M, Ganti SS, Krishan P, Singh M. PPAR dual agonists: are they opening Pandora's Box? . *Pharmacol Res.* Aug 2007;56(2):91–98.

49. Li X, Hansen PA, Xi L, Chandraratna RA, Burant CF. Distinct mechanisms of glucose lowering by specific agonists for peroxisomal proliferator activated receptor gamma and retinoic acid X receptors. *J Biol Chem.* Nov 18 2005;280(46): 38317–38327.

50. Moe O, Berry C, Rector FJ. Renal transport of glucose, amino acids, sodium, chloride and water. In: Brenner B, ed. *Brenner and Rector's the Kidney.* Philadelphia, PA: WB Saunders;1996:375–415.

51. Wells RG, Pajor AM, Kanai Y, Turk E, Wright EM, Hediger MA. Cloning of a human kidney cDNA with similarity to the sodium-glucose cotransporter. *Am J Physiol.* Sep 1992;263(3 Pt 2):F459–F465.

52. van den Heuvel LP, Assink K, Willemsen M, Monnens L. Autosomal recessive renal glycosuria attributable to a mutation in the sodium glucose cotransporter (SGLT2). *Hum Genet.* Dec 2002;111(6):544–547.

53. Han S, Hagan DL, Taylor JR, et al. Dapagliflozin, a selective SGLT2 inhibitor, improves glucose homeostasis in normal and diabetic rats. *Diabetes.* Mar 20 2008;57(6):1723-1729.

54. Katsuno K, Fujimori Y, Takemura Y, et al. Sergliflozin, a novel selective inhibitor of low-affinity sodium glucose cotransporter (SGLT2), validates the critical role of SGLT2 in renal glucose reabsorption and modulates plasma glucose level. *J Pharmacol Exp Ther.* Jan 2007;320(1):323–330.

55. The effect of ruboxistaurin on visual loss in patients with moderately severe to very severe nonproliferative diabetic retinopathy: initial results of the Protein Kinase C beta Inhibitor Diabetic Retinopathy Study (PKC-DRS) multicenter randomized clinical trial. *Diabetes.* Jul 2005;54(7):2188–2197.

56. Casellini CM, Barlow PM, Rice AL, et al. A 6-month, randomized, double-masked, placebo-controlled study evaluating the effects of the protein kinase C-beta inhibitor ruboxistaurin on skin microvascular blood flow and other measures of diabetic peripheral neuropathy. *Diabetes Care.* Apr 2007;30(4):896–902.

57. Tuttle KR, Bakris GL, Toto RD, McGill JB, Hu K, Anderson PW. The effect of ruboxistaurin on nephropathy in type 2 diabetes. *Diabetes Care.* Nov 2005;28(11):2686–2690.

58. Tuttle KR, McGill JB, Haney DJ, Lin TE, Anderson PW. Kidney outcomes in long-term studies of ruboxistaurin for diabetic eye disease. *Clin J Am Soc Nephrol.* Jul 2007;2(4):631–636.

59. Heerspink HL, Greene T, Lewis JB, et al. Effects of sulodexide in patients with type 2 diabetes and persistent albuminuria. *Nephrol Dial Transplant.* Dec 18 2007;23:1946–1954.

60. Yang X, Pan X, Blyth J, Lowe CR. Towards the real-time monitoring of glucose in tear fluid: holographic glucose sensors with reduced interference from lactate and pH. *Biosens Bioelectron.* Jan 18 2008;23(6):899–905.

61. Kost J, Mitragotri S, Gabbay RA, Pishko M, Langer R. Transdermal monitoring of glucose and other analytes using ultrasound. *Nat Med*. Mar 2000;6(3):347–350.

62. Tura A, Maran A, Pacini G. Non-invasive glucose monitoring: assessment of technologies and devices according to quantitative criteria. *Diabetes Res Clin Pract*. Jul 2007;77(1):16–40.

63. Kovatchev B, Anderson S, Heinemann L, Clarke W. Comparison of the numerical and clinical accuracy of four continuous glucose monitors. *Diabetes Care*. Mar 13 2008;31:1160–1164.

64. Bailey TS, Zisser HC, Garg SK. Reduction in hemoglobin A1C with real-time continuous glucose monitoring: results from a 12-week observational study. *Diabetes Technol Ther*. Jun 2007;9(3):203–210.

65. White RD. Insulin pump therapy (continuous subcutaneous insulin infusion). *Prim Care*. Dec 2007;34(4):845–871.

66. Zisser H, Jovanovic L. OmniPod Insulin Management System: patient perceptions, preference, and glycemic control. *Diabetes Care*. Sep 2006;29(9):2175.

67. Selam JL, Micossi P, Dunn FL, Nathan DM. Clinical trial of programmable implantable insulin pump for type I diabetes. *Diabetes Care*. Jul 1992;15(7):877–885.

68. Gin H, Renard E, Melki V, et al. Combined improvements in implantable pump technology and insulin stability allow safe and effective long term intraperitoneal insulin delivery in type 1 diabetic patients: the EVADIAC experience. *Diabetes Metab*. Dec 2003;29(6):602–607.

69. McMahon GT, Arky RA. Inhaled insulin for diabetes mellitus. *N Engl J Med*. Feb 1 2007;356(5):497–502.

70. Food and Drug Administration. Exubera (insulin human [rDNA origin]) Inhalation Powder September 2008. http://www.fda.gov/Safety/MedWatch/SafetyInformation/Safety-RelatedDrugLabelingChanges/ucm122978.htm. Accessed Nov 25th 2009.

71. Jain AK, Khar RK, Ahmed FJ, Diwan PV. Effective insulin delivery using starch nanoparticles as a potential trans-nasal mucoadhesive carrier. *Eur J Pharm Biopharm*. Dec 8 2007;69(2):426-435.

72. Roxhed N, Samel B, Nordquist L, Griss P, Stemme G. Painless drug delivery through microneedle-based transdermal patches featuring active infusion. *IEEE Trans Biomed Eng*. Mar 2008;55(3):1063–1071.

73. Guevara-Aguirre J, Guevara-Aguirre M, Saavedra J, Bernstein G, Rosenbloom AL. Comparison of oral insulin spray and subcutaneous regular insulin at mealtime in type 1 diabetes. *Diabetes Technol Ther*. Aug 2007;9(4):372–376.

74. Guevara-Aguirre J, Guevara M, Saavedra J, Mihic M, Modi P. Oral spray insulin in treatment of type 2 diabetes: a comparison of efficacy of the oral spray insulin (Oralin) with subcutaneous (SC) insulin injection, a proof of concept study. *Diabetes Metab Res Rev*. Nov-Dec 2004;20(6):472–478.

75. Guevara-Aguirre J, Guevara M, Saavedra J, Mihic M, Modi P. Beneficial effects of addition of oral spray insulin (Oralin) on insulin secretion and metabolic control in subjects with type 2 diabetes mellitus suboptimally controlled on oral hypoglycemic agents. *Diabetes Technol Ther*. Feb 2004;6(1):1–8.

76. Schwartz S, Hassman D, Shelmet J, et al. A multicenter, open-label, randomized, two-period crossover trial comparing glycemic control, satisfaction, and preference achieved with a 31 gauge x 6 mm needle versus a 29 gauge x 12.7 mm needle in obese patients with diabetes mellitus. *Clin Ther*. Oct 2004;26(10):1663–1678.

77. Ignaut DA, Venekamp WJ. HumaPen Memoir: a novel insulin-injecting pen with a dose-memory feature. *Expert Rev Med Devices*. Nov 2007;4(6):793–802.

78. Rubin RR, Peyrot M. Factors affecting use of insulin pens by patients with type 2 diabetes. *Diabetes Care*. Mar 2008;31(3):430–432.

79. Thurman JE. Insulin pen injection devices for management of patients with type 2 diabetes: considerations based on an endocrinologist's practical experience in the United States. *Endocr Pract*. Oct 2007;13(6):672–678.

80. Da Costa S, Brackenridge B, Hicks D. A comparison of insulin pen use in the United States and the United Kingdom. *Diabetes Educ*. Jan–Feb 2002;28(1):52–56.

81. Hogan A, Pileggi A, Ricordi C. Transplantation: current developments and future directions; the future of clinical islet transplantation as a cure for diabetes. *Front Biosci*. 2008;13:1192–1205.

82. Fiorina P, Secchi A. Pancreatic islet cell transplant for treatment of diabetes. *Endocrinol Metab Clin North Am*. Dec 2007;36(4):999–1013.

83. Meloche RM. Transplantation for the treatment of type 1 diabetes. *World J Gastroenterol*. Dec 21 2007;13(47):6347–6355.

84. Rood PP, Buhler LH, Bottino R, Trucco M, Cooper DK. Pig-to-nonhuman primate islet xenotransplantation: a review of current problems. *Cell Transplant*. 2006;15(2):89–104.

85. D'Ippolito G, Diabira S, Howard GA, Menei P, Roos BA, Schiller PC. Marrow-isolated adult multilineage inducible (MIAMI) cells, a unique population of postnatal young and old human cells with extensive expansion and differentiation potential. *J Cell Sci*. Jun 15 2004;117(Pt 14):2971–2981.

86. Gmyr V, Kerr-Conte J, Vandewalle B, Proye C, Lefebvre J, Pattou F. Human pancreatic ductal cells: large-scale isolation and expansion. *Cell Transplant*. Jan-Feb 2001;10(1):109–121.

87. Yang LJ. Liver stem cell-derived beta-cell surrogates for treatment of type 1 diabetes. *Autoimmun Rev*. Jul 2006;5(6): 409–413.

88. Dor Y, Brown J, Martinez OI, Melton DA. Adult pancreatic beta-cells are formed by self-duplication rather than stem-cell differentiation. *Nature*. May 6 2004;429(6987):41–46.

89. Kroon E, Martinson LA, Kadoya K, et al. Pancreatic endoderm derived from human embryonic stem cells generates glucose-responsive insulin-secreting cells in vivo. *Nat Biotechnol*. Apr 2008;26(4):443–452.

90. Beckles GL, Engelgau MM, Narayan KM, Herman WH, Aubert RE, Williamson DF. Population-based assessment of the level of care among adults with diabetes in the U.S. *Diabetes Care*. Sep 1998;21(9):1432–1438.

91. Saaddine JB, Cadwell B, Gregg EW, et al. Improvements in diabetes processes of care and intermediate outcomes: United States, 1988–2002. *Ann Intern Med*. Apr 4 2006;144(7):465–474.

92. Haynes RB, Yao X, Degani A, Kripalani S, Garg A, McDonald HP. Interventions to enhance medication adherence. *Cochrane Database Syst Rev*. 2005;4:CD000011.

93. Odegard PS, Capoccia K. Medication taking and diabetes: a systematic review of the literature. *Diabetes Educ*. 2007;33(6):1014–1029, discussion 1030–1011.Nov-Dec.

94. Bang and Olufsen Medicom. Intelligent pen cap top nominee for INDEX: Award. http://www.medicom.bang-olufsen.com/sw6059.asp. Accessed Nov 25th 2009.

95. Bang and Olufsen Medicom. The Helping Hand. http://www.medicom.bang-olufsen.com/sw431.asp. Accessed Nov 25th 2009.

96. Watson AJ, Bell AG, Kvedar JC, Grant RW. Reevaluating the digital divide: current lack of internet use is not a barrier to adoption of novel health information technology. *Diabetes Care*. Mar 2008;31(3):433–435.

97. Kimmel Z, Greenes RA, Liederman E. Personal health records. *J Med Pract Manage*. Nov-Dec 2005;21(3):147–152.

98. Taylor JR, Campbell KM. Home monitoring of glucose and blood pressure. *Am Fam Physician*. Jul 15 2007;76(2):255–260.

99. Harris MI. Frequency of blood glucose monitoring in relation to glycemic control in patients with type 2 diabetes. *Diabetes Care*. Jun 2001;24(6):979–982.

100. Murata GH, Shah JH, Hoffman RM, et al. Intensified blood glucose monitoring improves glycemic control in stable, insulin-treated veterans with type 2 diabetes: the Diabetes Outcomes in Veterans Study (DOVES). *Diabetes Care*. Jun 2003;26(6):1759–1763.

101. Cappuccio FP, Kerry SM, Forbes L, Donald A. Blood pressure control by home monitoring: meta-analysis of randomised trials. *BMJ*. Jul 17 2004;329(7458):145.

102. Montori VM, Helgemoe PK, Guyatt GH, et al. Telecare for patients with type 1 diabetes and inadequate glycemic control: a randomized controlled trial and meta-analysis. *Diabetes Care*. May 2004;27(5):1088–1094.

103. McMahon GT, Gomes HE, Hickson Hohne S, Hu TM, Levine BA, Conlin PR. Web-based care management in patients with poorly controlled diabetes. *Diabetes Care*. Jul 2005;28(7):1624–1629.

104. Renders CM, Valk GD, Griffin SJ, Wagner EH, Eijk Van JT, Assendelft WJ. Interventions to improve the management of diabetes in primary care, outpatient, and community settings: a systematic review. *Diabetes Care*. Oct 2001;24(10):1821–1833.

Part IX
Diabetes Prevention

Chapter 49
Prevention of Type 1 Diabetes Mellitus

Paolo Pozzilli and Chiara Guglielmi

Introduction

Type 1 diabetes (T1D) results from the autoimmune destruction of insulin-producing beta cells in the pancreas. Genetic, metabolic, and environmental factors act together to precipitate the onset of the disease. The excess mortality associated with complications of T1D and the increasing incidence of childhood T1D emphasize the importance of therapeutic strategies to prevent this chronic metabolic disorder.

Clinical T1D represents the end stage of a process resulting from the progressive beta cell destruction following an asymptomatic period that may last for years. This knowledge, together with recent advances in the ability to identify individuals at increased risk for clinical disease, has paved the way for trials aimed at preventing or delaying the clinical onset of T1D. Individuals at risk for T1D can be identified by a positive family history, or by genetic, immunological, or metabolic markers. These markers can be combined to achieve a higher positive predictive value for T1D and to identify those individuals to be selected for intervention trials.

T1D is one of the most widespread chronic disease of childhood affecting children, adolescents, and young adults. In 1985 people with diabetes (all types included) were 30 millions worldwide, in 1995 135 million, and in 2001 approximately 177 million.[1]

The global incidence of T1D in children and adolescents is rising with an estimated overall annual increase of approximately 3%. The increase in incidence of T1D has been shown in countries having both high- and low-prevalence figures, with an indication of a steeper increase in some of the low-prevalence countries.[2] Several European studies have suggested that, in relative terms, the increase is more pronounced in young children. Although T1D usually accounts for only a minority of the total burden of diabetes in a population, it is the predominant form of the disease in younger age groups in most developed countries.

T1D accounts for about 10% of all cases of diabetes, occurs most commonly in people of European descent, and affects 2 million people in Europe and North America. The lowest incidence has been found in Asia and Oceania, the highest in Europe. In particular for western Europe an increase of cases of T1D of 18.3% from 1994 to 2000 has been observed.[3] There is also a marked geographic variation in incidence, with a child in Finland being about 400 times more likely than a child in Venezuela to acquire the disease. The current global increase in incidence of 3% per year is well reported, and it is predicted that the incidence of T1D will be 40% higher in 2010 than in 1998.[4] This rapid rise strongly suggests a promoting effect of the environment on susceptibility genes in the evolving epidemiology of T1D.

P. Pozzilli (✉)
Department of Endocrinology and Diabetes, University Campus Bio-Medico, Rome, Italy
e-mail: p.pozzilli@unicampus.it

L. Poretsky (ed.), *Principles of Diabetes Mellitus*, DOI 10.1007/978-0-387-09841-8_49,
© Springer Science+Business Media, LLC 2010

Pathogenesis of T1D: An Update in View of Defining Preventive Tools

There are three main categories of factors involved in the pathogenesis of T1D. These are including genetic, immunological, and environmental factors. Genetic studies have been completed in families with multiple members affected by this disease and in monozygotic twins. These studies indicate that in T1D the genetic factors are highly relevant but complex and cannot be classified within a specific model of inheritance.[5]

Like other organ-specific autoimmune diseases, T1D has human leukocyte antigen (HLA) associations. The HLA complex on chromosome 6 comprises the first gene shown to be associated with the disease which is considered to contribute about half of the familial basis of T1D. Two combinations of HLA haplotypes are of particular importance. They are DR4-DQ8 and DR3-DQ2 which are present in 90% of children with T1D.[6] A third haplotype, DR15-DQ6, is found in less than 1% of children with T1D, compared with more than 20% of the general population and is considered to be protective. The genotype combining the two susceptibility haplotypes (DR4-DQ8/DR3-DQ2) contributes the greatest risk of the disease and is most common in children in whom the disease develops very early in life. First-degree relatives of these children are themselves at greater risk of T1D than are the relatives of children in whom the disease develops later.

Candidate gene studies also identified the insulin gene on chromosome 11 as the second most important genetic susceptibility factor, contributing 10% of the genetic susceptibility to T1D.[7] Shorter forms of a variable number tandem repeat in the insulin promoter are associated with susceptibility to the disease, whereas longer forms are associated with protection. Demonstration of increased expression of insulin in the thymus of people with protective repeats suggesting more efficient deletion of insulin-specific T cells provides an attractive potential mechanism for the role of the insulin gene in T1D. Over the last decade, whole genome screens have indicated that there are at least 15 other loci associated with T1D and of those another two genes associated with T-cell activation have been identified. An allele of the gene acting as a negative regulator of T-cell activation, cytotoxic T-lymphocyte antigen 4 (CTLA-4), found on chromosome 2q33, is considered to be the third susceptibility gene for T1D and has been associated with increased levels of soluble CTLA-4 and the frequency of regulatory T cells.[8] A variant of PTPN22, the gene encoding lymphoid phosphatase (LYP), also a suppressor of T-cell activation, has been deemed the fourth susceptibility gene.[9] The observation that the four most important susceptibility genes for T1D can all be represented on a single diagram of antigen presentation to T cells emphasizes the potential importance of current therapeutic strategies targeting this interaction.

Genetic studies have highlighted the importance of large, well-characterized populations in the identification of susceptibility genes for T1D. Recruitment of increasingly large populations of patients with T1D and their families is required to provide statistically powerful cohorts to identify other disease-associated genes. Some genes have a relatively minor individual impact on susceptibility to disease but could nevertheless provide more clues to future preventive therapies.

The presence of autoantibodies to beta cells is the hallmark of T1D. Abnormal activation of the T-cell-mediated immune system in susceptible individuals leads to an inflammatory response within the islets as well as to a humoral response with production of antibodies to beta cell antigens. Islet cell antibodies (ICA) were the first described, followed by more specific autoantibodies to insulin (IAA), glutamic acid decarboxylase (GAD) and the protein tyrosine phosphatase (IA-2), all of which can be easily detected by sensitive radioimmunoassay and are now measured[10] to identify subjects at risk of developing T1D.[11] These autoantibodies are common in both childhood- and adult-onset T1D with many subjects being positive for multiple autoantibodies. The type of immune response is age dependent, but seroconversion to multiple autoantibody positivity usually occurs tightly clustered in time and is associated with genetic risk.

The presence of one or more type of antibody can precede the clinical onset of T1D by years or even decades. These autoantibodies are usually persistent, although a small group of individuals may revert back to being seronegative without progressing to clinical diabetes.[12] The presence and persistence of positivity to multiple antibodies increases the likelihood of progression to clinical disease.

Continuing destruction of beta cells leads to a progressive reduction of insulin secretory reserve and loss of first-phase insulin secretion in response to an intravenous glucose tolerance test, followed by clinical diabetes when insulin secretion falls below a critical amount, and finally, to a state of absolute insulin deficiency.

Supportive evidence for the autoimmune pathogenesis of T1D comes from data showing susceptibility of individuals at risk for T1D to other autoimmune conditions including Hashimoto's thyroiditis, Graves' disease, Addison's disease, coeliac disease, myasthenia gravis, and vitiligo.[13]

Regarding the role of environmental factors, it should be underlined that the increase in incidence of T1D is too rapid to be caused by alterations in the genetic background and is likely to be the result of environmental changes. This is confirmed by recent experiments showing that the increase in T1D has been accompanied by a concomitant widening of the HLA risk profile, which suggests increased environmental pressure on susceptible HLA genotypes. The environmental factors in T1D are difficult to study because the variety of the environmental conditions as well as the possible multiple interactions between putative factors.

What Are the Environmental Factors?

Certain viral infections may play a role in the pathogenesis of human T1D. *Congenital rubella* is the classical example of virus-induced diabetes in human beings, but effective immunization programs have eliminated congenital rubella in most western countries. Currently, the main candidate for a viral trigger of human diabetes are members of the group of *Enterovirus*.[14] They are small non-enveloped RNA viruses, which belong to the Picornavirus family. They consist of more than 60 different serotypes, with the Polioviruses being their best-known representatives. Enterovirus infections are frequent among children and adolescents causing aseptic meningitis, myocarditis, rash, hand-foot-and-mouth disease, herpangina, paralysis, respiratory infections, and severe systemic infections in newborn infants. Most infections, however, are subclinical or manifest with mild respiratory symptoms. The primary replication of the virus occurs in the lymphoid tissues of the pharynx and small intestine, and during the following viremic phase the virus can spread to various organs including the beta cells.

Theoretically, *Enterovirus* could cause beta-cell damage by two main mechanisms. They may infect beta cells and destroy them directly or they may induce an autoimmune response against beta cells.[15] Direct virus-induced damage has been supported by studies showing that *Enterovirus* are present in beta cells in patients who have died from severe systemic *Enterovirus* infection and that the islet cells of these patients are damaged. *Enterovirus* can also infect and damage beta cells in vitro and induce the expression of interferon-alpha and HLA-class I molecules in beta cells, thus mimicking the situation observed in the pancreas of patients affected by T1D. In addition, *Enterovirus* infections may have interactions with other risk factors increasing the immune response to dietary antigens as they replicate in gut-associated lymphoid tissues.[16]

The first reports connecting *Enterovirus* infections to T1D were published more than 30 years ago showing that the seasonal variation in the onset of T1D follows that of *Enterovirus* infections.[17] At the same time antibodies against *Coxsackievirus B* serotypes were found to be more frequent in patients with newly diagnosed T1D than in control subjects.[18] *Enterovirus* have also been isolated from patients with newly diagnosed T1D. In one case report *Coxsackievirus B4* was isolated from the pancreas of a child who had died from diabetic ketoacidosis, and this virus caused diabetes when transferred to a susceptible mouse strain. The beta cells of diabetic patients also express interferon-alpha, a cytokine that is induced during viral infections, suggesting the presence of some virus in the beta cells. Prospective studies are particularly valuable in the evaluation of viral triggers because they cover all stages of the beta-cell damaging process.

Enterovirus are not the only viruses that have been connected to the pathogenesis of T1D. *Mumps, measles, cytomegalovirus,* and *retroviruses* also have been found to be associated with T1D, but the evidence is less convincing than that for *Enterovirus*.

The Role of Cow's Milk

There is evidence that cow's milk proteins can act as triggers for the autoimmune process of beta cell destruction based on studies indicating bottle feeding as triggering factor for an autoimmune response to beta cells.

There are several arguments for the milk hypothesis in T1D including the following (reviewed in ref.[19]):

Epidemiological studies show increased risk for T1D if the breast-feeding period is short and cow's milk is introduced before 3–4 months of age.

Skim milk powder can be "diabetogenic" in diabetes-prone BB rats.

Patients with T1D have increased levels of antibodies against cow's milk constituents.

Milk albumin and beta casein have some structural similarity to the islet autoantigen ICA69 and GLUT2, respectively.

A number of hypotheses have been postulated to explain the pathogenic role of cow's milk. One of the most convincing one is that immature gut mucosa allows the passage of high molecular weight, potentially antigenic proteins which share some molecular mimicry with pancreatic beta cells.[20] Among diabetogenic proteins in cow's milk, beta casein, beta lactoglobulin, and albumin have been implicated as sources of potential antigens.

Casein represents the major protein in cow's milk. Human and bovine beta casein are approximately 70% homologous and 30% identical. There are several reasons why it is thought that beta casein is a good candidate to explain the observed association between cow's milk consumption and T1D:[21] (a) it has several structural differences from the homologous human protein; (b) casein is probably the milk fraction promoting diabetes in the NOD mouse, since a protein-free diet prevents the disease while a diet containing casein as the sole source of protein produces diabetes in the same animals; (c) several sequence homologies exist between bovine beta casein and beta cell autoantigens; (d) specific cellular and humoral immune responses toward bovine beta casein are detectable in most T1D patients at the time of diagnosis,[22] highly suggestive that this protein may participate in the immune events triggering the disease; (e) casein hydrolysate was shown to be nondiabetogenic in the BB rat and NOD mouse models; therefore, it was thought that this dietary intervention might be beneficial in humans as well for disease prevention.

The rationale behind the use of cow's milk hydrolysate for primary prevention of T1D is based on several epidemiological and in vitro studies indicating that intact cow's milk, if given before 3 months of age, may induce an immune response toward beta cells.

The Role of Vitamin D Deficiency

Several epidemiological studies have described an intriguing correlation between geographical latitude and the incidence of T1D and an inverse correlation between monthly hours of sunshine and the incidence of diabetes.[23] A seasonal pattern of disease onset has also been described for T1D, once again suggesting an inverse correlation between sunlight and the disease.[24] Vitamin D is an obvious candidate as a mediator of this sunshine effect.

Dietary vitamin D supplementation is often recommended in pregnant women and in children to prevent vitamin D deficiency. Cod liver oil taken during the first year of life reportedly reduced the risk of childhood-onset T1D, and a multicenter case–control study also showed an association between vitamin D supplementation in infancy and a decreased risk of T1D.[25] A further study found that an intake of 2000 IU of vitamin D during the first year of life diminished the risk of developing T1D and showed that the incidence of childhood diabetes was three times higher in subjects with suspected rickets.[26,27] It remains to be determined whether these observations are the result of supplementation of vitamin D to supraphysiological levels or are simply the result of the prevention of vitamin D deficiency. Observations in animal models suggest the latter, since regular supplements of vitamin D in neonatal and early life offered no protection against T1D in non-obese diabetic (NOD) mice or in BB rats, whereas the prevalence of diabetes is doubled in NOD mice rendered vitamin D deficient in early life.[28] The results of genetic studies investigating a possible relationship between VDR polymorphisms and T1D are inconsistent: a clear correlation exists in some populations, whereas no correlation is observed in others.

Prediction of T1D as the Basis for Disease Prevention

There are different approaches for the identification of individuals at risk for T1D. These approaches are based on family history of T1D, genetic disease markers, autoimmune markers, or metabolic markers of T1D. These alternatives may also be combined in various ways to improve the predictive characteristics of the screening strategy. The importance of understanding the natural history of immune-mediated prediabetes lies in the development of prevention strategies. Several randomized clinical intervention trials have been concluded and the next generation of such trials will rely upon improved and simplified identification of individuals who are at high risk of progression to T1D. This is essential to ensure that trials have sufficient statistical power to detect a given effect of the intervention within the time available for the study. Such understanding is also needed to avoid exposing those who will not develop T1D to the risk of adverse effects of the intervention. In addition there is accumulating evidence that, at the onset of T1D, preservation of even low levels of insulin secretion has multiple benefits in terms of improved glycemic control and prevention of complications.[29]

Prevention of T1D: Current Status

Although the process by which pancreatic beta cells are destroyed is not well understood, several risk factors and immune-related markers are known to accurately identify first-degree relatives of patients with T1D who may develop the disease. Since we now have the ability to predict the development of T1D, investigators have begun to explore the use of intervention therapy to halt or even prevent beta cell destruction in such individuals. The autoimmune pathogenesis of T1D determines the efforts to prevent it. Susceptible individuals are identified by searching for evidence of autoimmune activity directed against beta cells. While direct evaluation of T-cell activity might be preferable, antibody determinations are generally used for screening because these assays are more robust. Antibody titers are often used in combination with an assessment of the genetic susceptibility, primarily evaluated by HLA typing.

Interventions are generally designed to delay or prevent T1D by impacting some phases of the immune pathogenesis of the disease. As discussed below, current trials are attempting to modify the course of disease progress at many points along the presumed pathogenic pathway. Most prevention trials include only relatives of T1D patients, a group in which risk prediction strategies are most established. Trials in genetically at-risk infants evaluate whether avoiding one of the putative environmental triggers for T1D can delay or prevent its onset.

Primary Prevention

Primary prevention identifies and attempts to protect individuals at risk from developing T1D. It can therefore reduce both the need for diabetes care and the need to treat diabetes-related complications.

T1D is relatively easy to prevent in animal models of the disease, including an array of therapies is effective. However, the mechanism of prevention is usually poorly defined, and there is a lack of surrogate assays of the immune response to define which therapies are likely to prevent diabetes in humans. Inability to define surrogate assays probably results from a fine balance of the immune system, so that even with inbred strains of animals, only a subset progresses to diabetes, and thus, relatively small changes in immune function may prevent disease. These observations have led to the hypothesis that identifying children at a very high genetic risk for diabetes, prior to development of measurable beta cell autoimmunity, and treating them at that point may be a more effective means of diabetes prevention. Studies for the primary prevention of T1D, i.e., prior to the expression of islet autoantibodies, are currently being designed and implemented. These studies target young children at a very high genetic risk for T1D and propose treatments that are very safe. These studies require large-scale screening to identify high-risk subjects and a follow-up over a long period of time to observe the outcome of anti-islet autoimmunity as a surrogate marker for the disease and onset of hyperglycemia as final end point.

A large worldwide trial called *TRIGR* and a small one in Italy called *PREVEFIN* aim to answer the question of whether cow's milk administered in early life is diabetogenic and whether the use of cow's milk hydrolysate can protect from the disease (Figs. 49.1 and 49.2). The rationale behind the use of cow's milk hydrolysate for primary prevention of T1D is based on several epidemiological and in vitro studies indicating that intact cow's milk, if given before 3 months of age, may induce an immune response toward beta cells.[30]

TRIGR International

Objective

To determine whether delaying dietary exposure to intact cow's milk proteins can reduce the incidence of type 1 diabetes in genetically predisposed children

Type of Study

Double-blind, randomised controlled trial

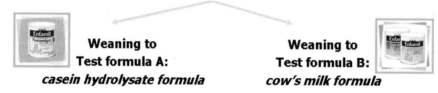

Weaning to Test formula A: *casein hydrolysate formula*   **Weaning to Test formula B:** *cow's milk formula*

Fig. 49.1 Design of the trial to reduce the incidence of type 1 diabetes in the genetically at-risk study (TRIGR study)

TRIGR is a randomized double-blind intervention study with the intention to treat as well as statistically analyze the incidence of predictive islet cell autoantibodies vs. the actual occurrence of clinical diabetes in two treatment groups (Fig. 49.1).[31] This trial, which investigates cow's milk as an environmental factor, has several key features. First, it is designed to intervene specifically in first-degree relatives of T1D patients. The newborns enrolled must have a genotype with diabetogenic HLA alleles without protective alleles and a mother, father, or a sibling who suffers from T1D. Second, the sample size is highly significant since previous trials were considered to estimate the number of newborns necessary to participate. This is an international trial, and recruitment has been carried out during a 2-year period in nine European countries, six major centers in the USA, 12 centers in Canada, and three centers in Australia. Due to statistical considerations, the frequency of the high-risk HLA genotype, consent, and dropout rates, the trial required initial access to 8000 pregnancies which ultimately yielded 5156 infants necessary for randomization. Each formula milk used in the two treatment groups is a nutritionally complete infant formula. The study formula contains extensively hydrolysed casein as the protein source, vegetable oils as fat source, glucose polymers, and modified starch as carbohydrate source.

The control formula is a mixture of a standard commercial cow's milk-based formula powder made by the same company plus casein hydrolysate powder in a 4:1 ratio designed to mask the flavor and smell distinctions between the two study formulas. The major outcome for the first phase is the frequency of T1D-associated islet cell autoantibodies and/or the development of clinical diabetes by the age of 6 years. The outcome of the second phase will be the manifestation of T1D by the age of 10 years. The manifest diabetes outcome will be assessed as the proportion of subjects in each group who develop T1D, as well as age at diagnosis.

In *PREVEFIN*, the first national preventive trial of T1D in Italy, newborns from the general population (over 10,000 screened at birth) screened for the presence of the high-risk genotype HLA-DR/DQ for T1D (DRB1*-DQB1*0201/DRB1*04-DQB1*0302) (Fig. 49.2).[32] This high-risk genotype has been found to have a frequency of only 0.9% in the general Italian population, lower than in other Caucasian populations, thus explaining the

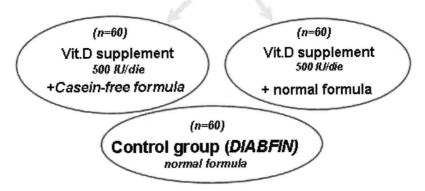

PREVEFIN TRIAL

**A multicenter randomized trial evaluating the efficacy of vitamin D
supplementation and β casein-free diet for the prevention of type 1 diabetes**

Newborns with high risk genotype
(n~120) randomized into 2 groups :

(n=60)
Vit.D supplement
500 IU/die
+Casein-free formula

(n=60)
Vit.D supplement
500 IU/die
+ normal formula

(n=60)
Control group (DIABFIN)
normal formula

Fig. 49.2 Design of the PREVEFIN project: Prevention of type 1 diabetes in the general population

low incidence of T1D in continental Italy. Many centers are participating in the project which will yield information concerning acceptability of and compliance with early childhood intervention to prevent T1D. The HLA screening is performed within the first 2 weeks of life, so that randomization occurs before 1 month of age. High-risk newborns are recruited into two treatment arms from the time mothers have stopped breast-feeding or if they do not breast-feed. Treatment consists of (i) normal cow's milk formula with vitamin D supplementation (500 IU/day) or (ii) cow's milk hydrolysate with vitamin D supplementation (500 IU/day) continued for up to 1 year. Vitamin D supplementation was included following recent evidence in animal models and humans that administration of this vitamin to newborns can reduce T1D incidence later in life. Detection of islet cell autoantibody and later insurgence of diabetes will be used as an end point. Subjects who participate in similar project, called *DIABFIN*,[33] form a control groups, where newborns with the same high-risk HLA genotype as in the *PREVEFIN* trial are being followed for the appearance of islet cell autoantibodies and diabetes. While the proposed trial may not allow all questions to be fully answered, this national collaborative network will provide safety, efficacy, and logistic data necessary to design a phase III trial.

Another pilot study, called *BABYDIET*, is currently underway to determine whether primary intervention through delayed introduction of dietary gluten is feasible and may reduce the incidence of islet autoimmunity in high-risk first-degree relatives of patients with T1D (Fig. 49.3).[34] The study is based on the premise that introduction of foods containing gluten or cereal before the age of 3 months is associated with an increased risk of islet autoimmunity in childhood. Newborn children are eligible if they are younger than 3 months, are offspring or siblings of patients with T1D, and have HLA genotypes that confer a high T1D risk.

Finally, the Diabetes Prediction and Prevention Project (*DIPP Study*)[35] is a longitudinal study on T1D prediction and prevention carried out in the university hospitals of Turku, Tampere, and Oulu (Finland) (Fig. 49.4). The aim of the study is to investigate longitudinally the dietary factors in relation to the development of diabetic autoantibodies and clinical T1D. The diet of the children is followed up by a structured questionnaire and by 3-day dietary records at various ages. A food frequency questionnaire is applied for studying the dietary intake of pregnant and lactating mothers.

The aims of this project are (1) to identify infants at increased genetic risk for T1D from the general population at birth, (2) to monitor such children for the appearance of diabetes-associated autoantibodies, to identify those at high risk to develop clinical disease, and to characterize the natural course of T1D, (3) to identify the environmental factors inducing the seroconversion to autoantibody positivity in children at increased genetic risk; and

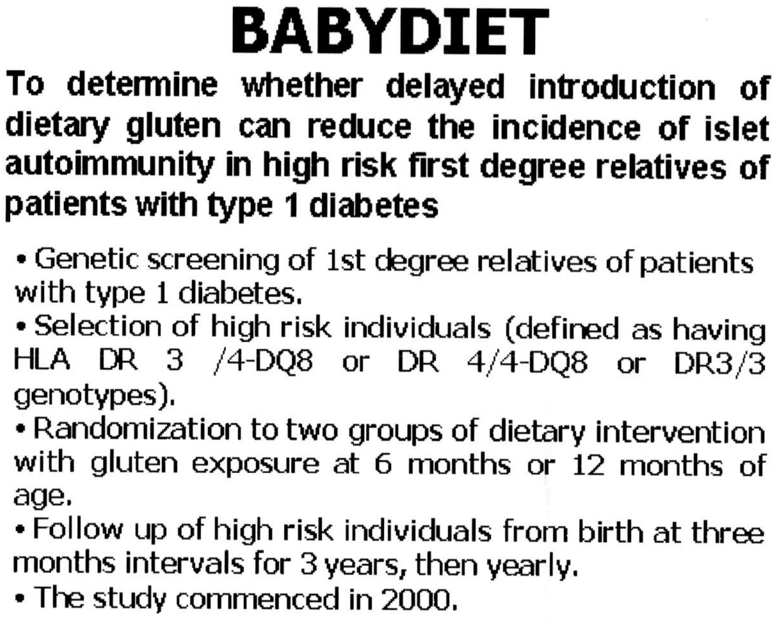

BABYDIET

To determine whether delayed introduction of dietary gluten can reduce the incidence of islet autoimmunity in high risk first degree relatives of patients with type 1 diabetes

- Genetic screening of 1st degree relatives of patients with type 1 diabetes.
- Selection of high risk individuals (defined as having HLA DR 3 /4-DQ8 or DR 4/4-DQ8 or DR3/3 genotypes).
- Randomization to two groups of dietary intervention with gluten exposure at 6 months or 12 months of age.
- Follow up of high risk individuals from birth at three months intervals for 3 years, then yearly.
- The study commenced in 2000.

Fig. 49.3 Design of the BABYDIET study

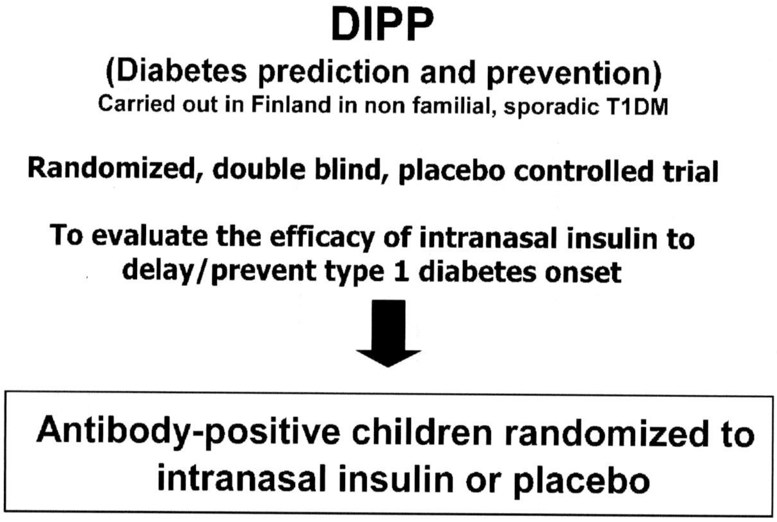

DIPP

(Diabetes prediction and prevention)
Carried out in Finland in non familial, sporadic T1DM

Randomized, double blind, placebo controlled trial

To evaluate the efficacy of intranasal insulin to delay/prevent type 1 diabetes onset

Antibody-positive children randomized to intranasal insulin or placebo

Fig. 49.4 Design of the diabetes prediction and prevention study (DIPP study)

(4) to evaluate whether it is possible to delay or prevent progression to clinical T1D by daily administration of intranasal insulin.

Whereas points 1–4 have been fulfilled and useful information has been obtained, the trial with intranasal insulin did not show any beneficial effect of this treatment in preventing the disease (unpublished data, oral presentation, 9th International Congress of the IDS and ADA Research Symposium, Miami, FL (USA) 14–18 November 2007).

In conclusion, since the failure of *ENDIT* and *DPT1* trials (see section "Secondary Prevention") in preventing the onset of T1D in subjects who are beta cell autoantibody positive, interest has switched to prevention trials starting *before* islet cell autoimmunity has developed. These primary prevention trials of T1D offer an exciting view of how our knowledge of the pathogenesis of this disease can lead to the possibility of intervening at birth. There is still a long way to go; however, the rationale is sound and the prospects seem good.

Secondary Prevention

Secondary prevention aims to reduce the incidence of T1D by stopping progression of beta cell destruction in individuals with signs of such a process. A number of early studies of secondary prevention were carried out, in some cases interesting results were obtained (as in the case of gluten-free diet study), but the majority of these studies suffered from the limitation of the inadequate dimension of the population in the study or an insufficient follow-up time. To this end consortia of investigators have been created, extended to numerous centers, with the objective to generate the required critical mass for the development of studies with sufficient numbers of subjects at risk for T1D.

European Nicotinamide Diabetes Intervention Trial (ENDIT)

The *ENDIT* study conducted predominantly in Europe examined whether nicotinamide could lead to a reduction in the rate of progression to T1D in at-risk relatives of T1D probands. Over 40,000 first-degree relatives aged 5–40 years were screened in centers in Europe and North America. The study was designed to recruit at least 422 subjects with ICA titers ≥ 20 JDF units to be randomized to either a nicotinamide- or a placebo-treated group. With an expected rate of progression to diabetes of 40% in the placebo arm, the proposed 5-year observation period should have allowed a 90% power to observe a 35% reduction in the incidence of disease.[36–38]

The rationale for using nicotinamide was derived from studies conducted in animal models and humans. In both the streptozotocin- and the alloxan-induced models as well as the NOD mouse and BB rat, nicotinamide was shown to protect the animals from diabetes. In human studies, nicotinamide was reported to preserve C-peptide levels, and, in high-risk ICA-positive subjects, to delay progression to T1D.[39] Similarly, in studies of both at-risk relatives and the general population carried out in New Zealand, nicotinamide appeared to have a protective effect on the subsequent development of T1D.[40]

Several mechanisms have been proposed to explain the protective effect of this antioxidant. One model of beta cell death proposes that, whatever the nature of the beta cell insult is (e.g., cytokine/toxin), nitrous oxide is generated leading to DNA strand breaks, activation of poly(ADP) ribose polymerase (PARP), NAD depletion, and cell death. Part of nicotinamide's protective effect is thought to derive from its ability to prevent NAD depletion during DNA repair by inhibiting PARP. In PARP-depleted knockout mice, those susceptible to diabetes were prevented from developing the disease. Other mechanisms, including inhibition of free radical formation, beta-cell regeneration, protection from macrophage-mediated cytotoxicity, suppression of MHC class II expression on islet cells, and suppression of adhesion molecule-1 expression on islet cells, may also be involved.[41]

Despite all these promises based on a sound rationale, nicotinamide treatment at the doses used did not show any significant effect on the primary outcome – progression to T1D. A total of 159 participants developed the disease within 5 years of randomization to treatment, 82 (30%) in the active treatment group and 77 (28%) in the placebo group. The unadjusted Cox proportional hazard estimate showed no difference between the placebo and the nicotinamide groups on an intention to treat basis. Nor any difference was found between groups after adjustment for age at baseline, glucose concentrations at 2-h glucose in the OGTT, and number of islet autoantibodies. The proportion of relatives who developed diabetes within 5 years was almost identical in those treated with nicotinamide and those treated with placebo, and there was no suggestion of a treatment effect in any of the subgroups defined by well-established markers of additional risk.

A useful message of this trial has been that large-scale collaborations were essential to move things forward and that the place for single-center trials was limited.

DPT-1 Trials

The Diabetes Prevention Trial – Type 1 (*DPT-1*) consisted of two clinical trials that sought to delay or prevent T1D. Nine medical centers and more than 350 clinics in the USA and Canada took part in the two trials of the *DPT-1*.[42–44]

Individuals who were eligible for testing were identified as follows: age 3–45 years, with a brother or sister, child or parent with T1D, and age 3–20 years, with a cousin, uncle or aunt, nephew or niece, grandparent, or half sibling with T1D. Those who met these criteria had ICA antibodies measured. To be eligible, a subject had to be positive for ICAs.

Animal research and small studies indicated that small, regular doses of insulin could prevent or delay T1D in subjects at risk. One *DPT-1* trial tested whether low-dose insulin injections could prevent or delay the development of T1D in people at high risk for developing T1D within 5 years. The study was divided into three parts: screening, staging, and intervention. Subjects were recruited from study clinics and through media campaigns.

Screening

First-degree relatives, 3–45 years of age, and second-degree relatives, 3–20 years of age, of patients with T1D were screened for islet cell antibodies. Those with an islet cell antibody titer of 10 JDF units or higher were offered staging evaluations.

Staging

Staging confirmed the presence of islet cell antibodies, measured insulin antibodies, assessed the first-phase insulin response to intravenous glucose, assessed oral glucose tolerance, and determined the presence or absence of HLA-DQA1*0102,DQB1*0602, a protective haplotype, which, if present, excluded subjects from further participation.[43]

Islet cell antibody-positive subjects were then defined as having a high risk of diabetes (a 5-year risk of more than 50%) and were deemed eligible for the parenteral insulin trial if they had a first-phase insulin response below the threshold (as defined below) on two occasions, if their oral glucose tolerance results were not completely normal, or both. Relatives who tested positive for islet cell antibodies and insulin antibodies and who had a first-phase insulin response above the threshold and normal glucose tolerance were defined as having intermediate risk (a 5-year risk of 26–50%) and were deemed eligible for the ongoing oral insulin trial.

Intervention

Subjects identified as having a high risk of T1D were eligible for random assignment to the experimental intervention (parenteral insulin therapy) or to a control group that underwent close observation. Subjects were stratified according to glucose tolerance status (normal vs. impaired or indeterminate) before randomization. Randomization was performed by a central, automated system, was stratified according to baseline glucose tolerance and clinical center, and used blocks of random, variable sizes.

By the time randomization was completed, samples for screening for islet cell antibodies had been obtained from 89,827 relatives. Of these, 84,594 samples were eligible for further study. The remaining samples were excluded because they came from subjects without an identified relative with diabetes or persons whose age was outside the range defined by the protocol. By the end of the enrollment period, 84,228 samples had been analyzed for islet cell antibodies, and 3152 of the subjects (3.7%) were found to be islet cell antibody positive. Of these, 354 (11.2%) were excluded before randomization because they had a fasting plasma glucose level of 126 mg/dl or higher or a glucose level of 200 mg/dl or higher 2 h after oral glucose challenge. These values, if confirmed, are diagnostic of diabetes.

A total of 2103 subjects (66.7% of those who were islet cell antibody positive) underwent staging. On initial intravenous glucose tolerance testing, 535 subjects had a low first-phase insulin response. As staging continued, a total of 372 subjects were classified as having a high risk and were deemed eligible for randomization; of these, 339 underwent randomization (91.1%), 169 were assigned to the intervention, and 170 to observation. There were no statistically significant differences between the treatment groups.

The results demonstrated that insulin, in small doses, can indeed be administered safely to persons who are at risk for T1D. The increase in presumed and definite hypoglycemia among the subjects in the intervention group did not adversely affect cognitive function.

In high-risk relatives of patients with diabetes, the insulin regimen did not delay or prevent the development of T1D.[42] Long-term follow-up to detect any effects on the course of diabetes has begun. There are several potential explanations for the lack of effect observed so far. One is that the intervention took place too late in the disease process to slow down the progression of disease. Studies conducted earlier in the disease process, such as the ongoing DPT-1 oral insulin trial in relatives of patients with T1D who have a projected 5-year risk of 26–50%, may be more successful. Moreover, oral insulin may have a greater immunologic effect, although it does not provide for beta cell rest. In fact, the low-dose insulin used in the trial may have failed to achieve such an effect on beta cells, but the dose was limited by the risk of hypoglycemia. With a different dosing scheme or a different regimen, insulin or insulin-like peptides might alter the course of development of diabetes.

The other study was an oral insulin trial that sought to prevent T1D in subjects with a moderate risk for developing diabetes. The study was divided into three parts: screening, staging, and intervention. Participants were recruited through media campaigns.

Screening

First-degree (ages 3–45 years) and second-degree (ages 3–20 years) relatives of patients with T1D were screened for ICAs. Those with ICA titer ≥ 10 JDF units were invited to undergo staging evaluations.

Staging

Staging confirmed ICA positivity, measured insulin autoantibody (IAA) status, assessed first-phase insulin response (FPIR) to intravenous glucose, assessed oral glucose tolerance (OGT), and determined the presence or absence of HLADQA1* 0102/DQB1*0602 (a protective haplotype that excluded subjects from participation). Relatives who were ICA positive and IAA positive and had normal glucose tolerance were projected to have a 5-year risk of 26–50% ("intermediate risk") and were eligible for the oral insulin trial. The original protocol had an entry criterion of confirmed (on two occasions) IAA level >5 SD above the mean of the normal reference range (i.e., ≥ 80 nU/ml). This criterion was agreed upon after reviewing data from natural history studies suggesting that a sufficient cut off was >3 SD above the mean of the reference range (i.e., IAA ≥ 39 nU/ml).[43]

Intervention

The study was a double-masked, placebo-controlled, randomized clinical trial, in which participants were assigned to receive capsules of either oral insulin, 7.5 mg of recombinant human insulin crystals (Eli Lilly, Indianapolis, IN), or matched placebo. Subjects consumed the capsule (insulin or placebo) as a single daily dose before breakfast each day, either by taking the capsule or, if the subject could not swallow capsules, by sprinkling its contents in juice or on food. Randomization used a central automated system, stratified by clinical center, using random variable block sizes.

By the end of enrollment, 97,273 samples were analyzed for ICA and 3483 (3.58%) relatives were ICA positive. Of these, 458 (13.1% of ICA-positive individuals) were excluded before randomization because they already had diabetes. A total of 2523 (72.4% of ICA-positive individuals) underwent staging. There were 1844 relatives with intravenous glucose tolerance FPIR above threshold. As staging continued, a total of 388 relatives were classified as intermediate risk and eligible for randomization; of these, 372 were randomized (97% of eligible subjects), 186 to each study arm; there were no statistically significant differences between treatment groups.

In the primary analysis of relatives selected and randomized in DPT-1, oral insulin did not delay or prevent development of diabetes. There was greater variability in the IAA assay for values 39–79 nU/ml than for values $\geq$80 nU/ml, particularly in confirmation of a positive result (98.7% overall confirmation for values $\geq$80 nU/ml compared with 70.6% for values 39–79 nU/ml). This prompted comparison of the rate of evolution of diabetes by entry IAA level. The cohort with confirmed IAA $\geq$80 nU/ml (the original entry IAA criterion) progressed to diabetes at a faster rate than those subjects who did not have confirmed IAA $\geq$80 nU/ml. In addition, those with confirmed IAA $\geq$ 80 nU/ml had other risk characteristics that suggested more rapid evolution to diabetes, including younger age, greater likelihood of having other antibodies, and greater loss of beta cell function (lower levels of plasma C-peptide in response to several provocative challenges).[44]

The effect of intervention in each of these two subgroups was further evaluated.

The group with confirmed IAA $\geq$ 80 nU/ml showed a beneficial effect of oral insulin, whereas the group who did not have confirmed IAA $\geq$ 80 nU/ml showed a trend suggesting a detrimental effect of oral insulin.[44] This group also had a much lower overall rate of development of diabetes. Thus, the significance of this finding is unclear but is reminiscent of the adjuvant-induced acceleration of diabetes observed in the BB rat.[45]

In conclusion, neither low-dose insulin injections in subjects at high risk for developing T1D nor insulin capsules taken orally by those at moderate risk for T1D were successful at preventing or delaying the disease.

The two large trials of secondary prevention of T1D (nicotinamide and insulin) did not modify progression to T1D. These trials did however show that large-scale international collaborative prevention trials are possible and that current methods for predicting T1D are accurate. They also prepared the way for a worldwide network to allow intervention trials to be completed as rapidly and efficiently as possible. Continuing on from the basis that it is possible to do high-quality studies to test agents that might potentially prevent diabetes, the National Institutes of Health (NIH) in the USA set up a network of centers across North America and other parts of the world to coordinate a program of prevention studies (*TrialNet*).[46]

Tertiary Prevention

Tertiary prevention is aimed at delaying or preventing the development of complications in subjects who already have T1D. A landmark trial investigating patients with T1D showed that good glycemic control can reduce the likelihood of microvascular complications leading to blindness or kidney disease, but the trend toward a decrease in macrovascular disease was not statistically significant. Diabetes education of health-care professionals and those affected by diabetes plays a key role in the tertiary prevention of the disease. Tertiary prevention is identified by the maintenance of the residual beta cell function present at disease onset and can be realized by immune suppression or immune modulation since the time of clinical diagnosis of T1D.

The best results in this field were obtained 20 years ago with the use of *cyclosporine* [47–49] subsequently abandoned because of transient benefits and undesired adverse effects.

In the following years none of the several treatments that have been proposed has obtained appreciable results except for *nicotinamide*.[50,51]

Clinical trials have demonstrated that, after a year of continuous treatment with nicotinamide, baseline C-peptide levels are slightly higher compared with subjects who did not take this substance.[52] Only recently, experience obtained with the use of the *anti-CD3 monoclonal antibody* in two studies (one in the USA and the other in Europe) has revitalized the interest in this type of interventions.[53,54] The first one was an early-phase clinical trial that tested anti-CD3 in patients with newly diagnosed T1D. The drug, a modified form of anti-CD3 antibody that minimizes first-dose side effects, was studied by comparing 12 subjects aged 7–30 years who were treated with the antibody to an equal number of patients in a control group who did not receive the drug. One year after treatment with anti-CD3, the treated patients produced more insulin and needed less insulin therapy than the untreated patients. Retention of even some insulin production is an important clinical goal in the treatment of patients with T1D, since, in general, most patients with the disease eventually lose the ability to make insulin entirely and need to rely completely on injected insulin to maintain metabolic control. Those who received the antibody treatment also had better HbA1c levels. The anti-CD3 was designed to act on the immune system's T cells in a more specific manner than previous attempts at immune intervention in early diabetes. However, adverse effects of anti-CD3 are quite significant and include fever, rash, anemia, nausea, vomiting, and joint pain. The study's encouraging results have led to new trials involving additional patients.

Recently, there has been growing interest in *vitamin D* and its active metabolites in relation to T1D and its immune pathogenesis. Vitamin D metabolites have been shown to exert several immunomodulatory effects, and 1,25-dihydroxyvitamin D3 [1,25-(OH)2D3] can either prevent or suppress autoimmune encephalomyelitis, inflammatory bowel disease, and T1D.[55]

Recent data in humans demonstrated that reduction in vitamin D supplementation is associated with a higher risk of the disease, whereas its supplementation is associated with a decreased frequency of T1D.[56]

Based on this rationale, an open-label randomized trial was designed to determine whether supplementation with the active form of vitamin D (*calcitriol*) at diagnosis of T1D could improve parameters of glycemic control.[57,58] The secretion of C-peptide as an index of residual pancreatic beta-cell function was the primary end point, with HbA1c and insulin requirement as secondary end points. The aim of this study was to investigate whether supplementation with the active form of vitamin D (calcitriol) in subjects with recent-onset T1D protects residual pancreatic beta-cell function and improves glycemic control (HbA1c and insulin requirement). In this open-label randomized trial, 70 subjects with recent-onset T1D, mean age 13.6 ± 7.6 years, were randomized to calcitriol (0.25 μg on alternate days) or nicotinamide (25 mg/kg daily) and were followed up for 1 year. Intensive insulin therapy was implemented with three daily injections of regular insulin + NPH insulin at bedtime. No significant differences were observed between calcitriol and nicotinamide groups with respect to baseline/stimulated C-peptide or HbA1c 1 year after diagnosis, but the insulin dose at 3 and 6 months was significantly reduced in the calcitriol group. In conclusion, at the dosage used, calcitriol had a modest effect on residual pancreatic beta-cell function and only temporarily reduced the insulin dose.[57]

Another important aspect is related to 25 and 1,25 (OH)2D3 plasma levels in subjects with recent-onset T1D, as low levels of these two compounds have been detected[59] and may influence the effect of calcitriol therapy. Whereas the administration of the former may restore low levels of 25 (OH2)D3, the latter is the compound of choice for beta cell protection because of its immune modulatory action. Based on these data another clinical trial was designed and it is now ongoing. It is a double-blind study in which calcitriol is compared with placebo in recent-onset T1D subjects (less than 6 months from diagnosis) in whom residual C-peptide secretion is still detectable and above 0.3 nM. Primary end point of this trial is to estimate the effectiveness of calcitriol in the protection of beta cell function. Secondary end point is to find out if the administration of calcitriol could determine an improvement of metabolic control with consequent reduction of the insulin dose.

The TrialNet Network (Fig. 49.5)

T1D *TrialNet* is a group of studies which aim to examine the development, prevention, and early treatment of T1D. The goal of TrialNet is to perform intervention studies to preserve insulin-producing cells in individuals at risk for T1D and in those with new-onset T1D and to identify individuals "at risk" for developing this disease. Risk is based on positive islet cell autoantibodies or other autoimmune markers and results of oral and intravenous glucose tolerance tests.

Specific study interventions are determined by TrialNet investigators. Each protocol is thoroughly reviewed by an Institutional Review Board (IRB) before approval is given to start recruitment to make sure that the participant is fully protected and not exposed to unnecessary risks. TrialNet is jointly funded by The National Institute of Diabetes and Digestive and Kidney Diseases (NIDDK), The National Institute of Allergy and Infectious Diseases (NIAID), The National Institute of Child Health and Human Development (NICHD), The National Center for Research Resources at the NIH [which provides support through its General Clinical Research Centers (GCRC)

Ongoing TrialNet studies (see text for details):
The Natural History Study of the Development of Type 1 Diabetes
The Oral Insulin for Prevention of Type 1 Diabetes
The Nutritional Intervention to Prevent Type 1 Diabetes
T1DGC
The Rituximab Study (Anti-CD20)
The MMF/DZB Study

Fig. 49.5 Ongoing TrialNet studies

Program], Juvenile Diabetes Research Foundation International (JDRF), and American Diabetes Association (ADA).

TrialNet conducts multiple clinical trials with investigators from 18 clinical centers in the USA, Canada, Finland, the UK, Italy, Germany, Australia, and New Zealand. Several studies are conducted in patients with newly diagnosed T1D, as well as in relatives of people with T1D who are at greater risk of developing the disease. Two types of studies are envisaged: (a) Natural History Studies which will provide information about risk factors associated with developing T1D and (b) Diabetes Intervention Studies which will test either treatments to delay or prevent the onset of T1D or treatments to preserve remaining insulin secretion in subjects recently diagnosed with T1D.

Ongoing Studies (Fig. 49.5)

(1) *The Natural History Study of the Development of Type 1 Diabetes (currently recruiting)* (http://www2.diabetestrialnet.org/nhx) will study subjects at increased risk for T1D to learn more about how T1D develops. The screening phase of the Natural History Study identifies people at increased risk for developing T1D. Subjects who qualify and choose to participate in the Natural History Study may also be offered an opportunity to enter a diabetes prevention study in the future. To be screened, at least one of the two conditions below must be fulfilled:

  – 1 to 45 years of age and have a brother, sister, child, or parent with T1D
  – 1 to 20 years of age and have a cousin, aunt, uncle, niece, nephew, half sibling, or grandparent with T1D

(2) *The Oral Insulin for Prevention of Type 1 Diabetes Study (currently recruiting)* (http://www2.diabetestrialnet.org/oins) TrialNet has launched a clinical study of oral insulin to prevent or delay T1D in at-risk subjects. The goal is to prevent T1D or to delay it as long as possible. Results from the recently completed study (DPT-1) suggest that oral insulin might delay or prevent T1D in some individuals found to be at high risk. Enrolled subjects will be allocated to one of the two arms of the study – oral insulin or placebo.

(3) *The Nutritional Intervention to Prevent Type 1 Diabetes Study (currently recruiting)* (http://www2.diabetestrialnet.org/nip). The Nutritional Intervention to Prevent Type 1 Diabetes study will help to learn more about a dietary compound, docosahexaenoic acid (DHA), which will be given to pregnant mothers in their third trimester and infants less than 5 months of age. This research is being done as a pilot study, which is a "test run" to find out if it is possible to do a larger study. Pregnant women in their third trimester (more than 24 weeks) may enroll in the study if the baby they are expecting has a relative (mother, father, sister, brother, half sister, or half brother) with T1D. Babies up to 5 months old may also be enrolled in the study if they have a relative with T1D. Pregnant and nursing women will take four capsules a day during the third trimester. Capsules will contain either DHA or a placebo.

(4) *T1DGC (currently recruiting)* (http://www.t1dgc.org/home.cfm). Type 1 Diabetes Genetics Consortium (www.t1dgc.org) is a group of diabetes researchers from around the world who have come together to collect blood samples and information from families with T1D. The T1DGC is a NIH- and EU-funded collaborative effort to develop resources for the scientific community to identify genes influencing a subject's risk

of developing T1D. Network Centers are located in the Asia-Pacific (Melbourne and Australia), European (Copenhagen, Denmark, and Italy), North American (Seattle, WA, USA), and the UK (Cambridge, England) regions. The T1DGC is currently collecting data and blood samples (DNA, plasma, serum and cell lines) on 2800 affected-sibling pair families (two affected siblings, and biological parents and up to two unaffected siblings, if possible). The aims of the study are as follows: (a) to detect the effects of HLA and other candidate regions/genes on the signals from the genome screen, all samples will be genotyped for HLA class II and class I genes (DRB1, DQB1, DPB1, DPA1, A, B, C), INS, and CTLA4 polymorphisms that have previously been implicated in susceptibility to T1D; (b) to refine the localization of the five most promising regions identified from linkage and association studies; and (c) to aid in the confirmation and identification of diabetes susceptibility genes within linked regions, the Consortium will use existing and planned resources of single case families (trios, including an unaffected sibling when available) and sets of T1D cases and nondiabetic controls to carry out detailed disease association analyses.

(5) *The Rituximab Study (anti-CD20) (this study is no longer recruiting patients)* (http://www2 .diabetestrialnet.org/anti). This study is attempting to examine if it is possible to stop or slow down the immune system's attack in newly diagnosed T1D patients, so that remaining beta cells can survive and maintain insulin secretion. The goal of the study is to find out if rituximab can prevent further beta cell destruction. Rituximab has been successfully used in other diseases to slow down the immune response. Patients enrolled in the study are randomly assigned to receive rituximab or placebo once a week during the first 4 weeks in the study. Patients eligible for the rituximab study are those diagnosed with T1D within the past 3 months, ages 8–45 years. They need to be islet cell antibody positive and to have evidence of a residual beta cell function.

(6) *The MMF/DZB Study (this study is no longer recruiting patients)* (http://www2.diabetestrialnet.org/mmf). This study will evaluate whether a combination of two drugs can stop the immune system from destroying beta cells in new-onset T1D patients (within 3 months of diagnosis). The two drugs are mycophenolate mofetil (MMF/CellCept®) and daclizumab (DZB/Zenapax®). They both are immunosuppressive agents acting at different levels. The goal is to protect residual beta cell function and improve long-term metabolic control. The study design includes three arms: (a) MMF alone, (b) MMF and DZB together, or (c) placebo.

Patients enrolled in this study are treated for 2 years. MMF or MMF placebo are given as pills (two or three times a day). DZB or DZB placebo are administered intravenously, twice during the first month of the study. In order to be enrolled in this study, patients must have been diagnosed with T1D within the past 3 months and be 12–35 years of age. They need to be islet cell antibody positive and have residual beta cell function.

Summary

The need to obtain consistent results in the difficult field of T1D prevention requires multicentric studies based on international consortia with the aim of being able to achieve of critical mass, statistical power, adequate time of observation, and financing. Examples already mentioned are TRIGR and TrialNet (http://www2.diabetestrialnet.org), a network financed from the NIH and other agencies that has inherited the net formed in the DPT-1 study.

New clinical trials of secondary and tertiary prevention are planned based on the administration of autoantigens (oral or inhaled insulin or GAD) of immune suppression or immune modulation drugs (mofetil mycophenolate, anti-CD25, anti-CD20, anti-CD3 antibodies, and anti-lymphocytes) and of agents potentially able to stimulate a regeneration of the beta cell mass (GLP-1 and analogous). From all these protocols it is reasonable to expect to obtain not only important information on the effectiveness of several treatments but also to learn more about the pathogenesis of the disease. Therefore, prevention of T1D appears at the moment realistically achievable in a near future. Programs of primary prevention must be directed to subjects with a family history for T1D or to those at high risk from the genetic point of view. Moreover, newborns and young adults with

HLA DR3/DR4 who are antibody positive must be carefully followed up with programs of secondary prevention. All the studies must however assure safety and good compliance.

In conclusion, it is necessary to widen the number of clinical trials aimed to develop techniques for prevention of T1D. These studies, however, must include a greater number of subjects and to involve several international centers to achieve the critical mass required for statistically meaningful results.

Acknowledgments　We would like to thank Juvenile Diabetes Research Foundation (JDRF), National Institute of Health (NIH) Consortia, Centro Internazionale Studi Diabete (CISD), Diabete e Metabolismo (DEM) Foundation, and University Campus Bio-Medico that support clinical research on T1D in our University Hospital.

Useful Websites

http://www2.diabetestrialnet.org
http://www2.diabetestrialnet.org/nhx
http://www2.diabetestrialnet.org/oins
http://www2.diabetestrialnet.org/nip
http://www.t1dgc.org/home.cfm
http://www2.diabetestrialnet.org/anti
http://www2.diabetestrialnet.org/anti
http://trigr.epi.usf.edu/

References

1. Ludvigsson J. Why diabetes incidence increases – a unifying theory. *Ann N Y Acad Sci.* 2006;1079:374–382.
2. White F, Rafique G. Diabetes prevalence and projections in South Asia. *Lancet.* 2002;360:804–805.
3. Fleming DM, Schellevis FG, Van Casteren V. The prevalence of known diabetes in eight European countries. *Eur J Public Health.* 2004;14:10–14.
4. Wild S, Roglic G, Green A, Sicree R, King H. Global prevalence of diabetes: estimates for the year 2000 and projections for 2030. *Diabetes Care.* 2004;27:1047–1053.
5. Rich SS, Concannon P, Erlich H, et al. The Type 1 Diabetes Genetics Consortium. *Ann N Y Acad Sci.* 2006;1079:1–8.
6. Valdes AM, McWeeney S, Thomson G. HLA class II DR-DQ amino acids and insulin-dependent diabetes mellitus: application of the haplotype method. *Am J Hum Genet.* 1997;60:717–728.
7. Bennett ST, Wilson AJ, Cucca F, et al. IDDM2-VNTR-encoded susceptibility to type 1 diabetes: dominant protection and parental transmission of alleles of the insulin gene-linked minisatellite locus. *J Autoimmun.* 1996;9:415–421.
8. Nisticò L, Buzzetti R, Pritchard LE, et al. The CTLA-4 gene region of chromosome 2q33 is linked to, and associated with, type 1 diabetes. Belgian Diabetes Registry. *Hum Mol Genet.* 1996;5:1075–1080.
9. Ladner MB, Bottini N, Valdes AM, Noble JA. Association of the single nucleotide polymorphism C1858T of the PTPN22 gene with type 1 diabetes. *Hum Immunol.* 2005;66:60–64.
10. Bonifacio E, Bingley PJ. Islet autoantibodies and their use in predicting insulin-dependent diabetes. *Acta Diabetol.* 1997;34:185–193.
11. Wasserfall CH, Atkinson MA. Autoantibody markers for the diagnosis and prediction of type 1 diabetes. *Autoimmun Rev.* 2006;5:424–428.
12. Bingley PJ, Williams AJ. Validation of autoantibody assays in type 1 diabetes: workshop programme. *Autoimmunity.* 2004;37:257–260.
13. Devendra D, Eisenbarth GS. Immunologic endocrine disorders. *J Allergy Clin Immunol.* 2003;111:S624–S636.
14. Peng H, Hagopian W. Environmental factors in the development of Type 1 diabetes. *Rev Endocr Metab Disord.* 2006;7:149–162.
15. Tracy S, Drescher KM. Coxsackievirus infections and NOD mice: relevant models of protection from, and induction of, type 1 diabetes. *Ann N Y Acad Sci.* 2007;1103:143–151.
16. Oikarinen M, Tauriainen S, Honkanen T, et al. Detection of enteroviruses in the intestine of type 1 diabetic patients. *Clin Exp Immunol.* 2008;151:71–75.
17. Frisk G, Fohlman J, Kobbah M, et al. High frequency of Coxsackie-B-virus-specific IgM in children developing type I diabetes during a period of high diabetes morbidity. *J Med Virol.* 1985;17:219–227.
18. Gamble DR, Taylor KW, Cumming H. Coxsackie viruses and diabetes mellitus. *Br Med J.* 1973;4:260–262.
19. Vaarala O. Is type 1 diabetes a disease of the gut immune system triggered by cow's milk insulin?. *Adv Exp Med Biol.* 2005;569:151–156.

20. Harrison LC, Honeyman MC. Cow's milk and type 1 diabetes: the real debate is about mucosal immune function. *Diabetes*. 1999;48:1501–1507.

21. Cavallo MG, Fava D, Monetini L, Barone F, Pozzilli P. Cell-mediated immune response to beta casein in recent-onset insulin-dependent diabetes: implications for disease pathogenesis. *Lancet*. 1996;348:926–928.

22. Monetini L, Cavallo MG, Manfrini S, et al. IMDIAB Group. Antibodies to bovine beta-casein in diabetes and other autoimmune diseases. *Horm Metab Res*. 2002;34:455–459.

23. Holick MF. Sunlight and vitamin D for bone health and prevention of autoimmune diseases, cancers, and cardiovascular disease. *Am J Clin Nutr*. 2004;80:1678S–1688S.

24. Chatfield SM, Brand C, Ebeling PR, Russell DM. Vitamin D deficiency in general medical inpatients in summer and winter. *Intern Med J*. 2007;37:377–382.

25. Stene LC, Ulriksen J, Magnus P, Joner G. Use of cod liver oil during pregnancy associated with lower risk of Type I diabetes in the offspring. *Diabetologia*. 2000;43:1093–1098.

26. The EURODIAB Substudy 2 Study Group. Vitamin D supplement in early childhood and risk for type 1 (insulin-dependent) diabetes mellitus. *Diabetologia*. 1999;42:51–54.

27. Hypponen E, Laara E, Reunanen A, Jarvelin MR, Virtanen SM. Intake of vitamin D and risk of type 1 diabetes: a birth-cohort study. *Lancet*. 2001;358:1500–1503.

28. Driver JP, Foreman O, Mathieu C, van Etten E, Sereze DV. Comparative therapeutic effects of orally administered 1,25-dihydroxyvitamin D(3) and 1alpha-hydroxyvitamin D(3) on type-1 diabetes in non-obese diabetic mice fed a normal-calcaemic diet. *Clin Exp Immunol*. 2008;151:76–85.

29. McCarter RJ, Hempe JM, Chalew SA. Mean blood glucose and biological variation have greater influence on HbA1c levels than glucose instability: an analysis of data from the Diabetes Control and Complications Trial. *Diabetes Care*. 2006;29:352–355.

30. Pozzilli P, Manfrini S, Picardi A. Cow's milk and trials for prevention of Type 1 diabetes. *Diabet Med*. 2003;20:871–872.

31. TRIGR Study Group. Study design of the Trial to Reduce IDDM in the Genetically at Risk (TRIGR). *Pediatr Diabetes*. 2007;8:117–137.

32. Lorini R, Minicucci L, Napoli F, Padovani P, Bazzigaluppi E, Tortoioli C, et al. Screening for type 1 diabetes genetic risk in newborns of continental Italy. Primary prevention (Prevefin Italy) – preliminary data. *Acta Biomed Ateneo Parmense*. 2005;76:31–35.

33. Buzzetti R, Galgani A, Petrone A, et al. Genetic prediction of type 1 diabetes in a population with low frequency of HLA risk genotypes and low incidence of the disease (the DIABFIN study). *Diabetes Metab Res Rev*. 2004;20:137–143.

34. Schmid S, Buuck D, Knopff A, Bonifacio E, Ziegler AG. BABYDIET, a feasibility study to prevent the appearance of islet autoantibodies in relatives of patients with type 1 diabetes by delaying exposure to gluten. *Diabetologia*. 2004;47:1130–1131.

35. Kupila A, Sipila J, Keskinen P, et al. Intranasally administered insulin intended for prevention of type 1 diabetes – a safety study in healthy adults. *Diabetes Metab Res Rev*. 2003;19:415–420.

36. The European Nicotinamide Diabetes Intervention Trial (ENDIT) Group. European Nicotinamide Diabetes Intervention Trial (ENDIT): a randomised controlled trial of intervention before the onset of type 1 diabetes. *Lancet*. 2004;363:925–931.

37. The European Nicotinamide Diabetes Intervention Trial (ENDIT) Group. Intervening before the onset of Type 1 diabetes: baseline data from the European Nicotinamide Diabetes Intervention Trial (ENDIT). *Diabetologia*. 2003;46:339–346.

38. Bingley PJ, Gale EA. European Nicotinamide Diabetes Intervention Trial (ENDIT) Group. Progression to type 1 diabetes in islet cell antibody-positive relatives in the European Nicotinamide Diabetes Intervention Trial: the role of additional immune, genetic and metabolic markers of risk. *Diabetologia*. 2006;49:881–890.

39. Pozzilli P, Andreani D. The potential role of nicotinamide in the secondary prevention of IDDM. *Diabetes Metab Rev*. 1993;9:219–230.

40. Elliott RB, Pilcher CC, Fergusson DM, Stewart AW. A population based strategy to prevent insulin-dependent diabetes using nicotinamide. *J Pediatr Endocrinol Metab*. 1996;9:501–509.

41. Kolb H, Burkart V. Nicotinamide in type 1 diabetes. Mechanism of action revisited. *Diabetes Care*. 1999;22(Suppl 2):B16–B20.

42. Diabetes Prevention Trial Type 1 Diabetes Study Group. Effects of insulin in relatives of patients with type 1 diabetes mellitus. *N Engl J Med*. 2002;346:1685–1691.

43. Greenbaum CJ, Schatz DA, Cuthbertson D, Zeidler A, Eisenbarth GS, Krischer JP. Islet cell antibody-positive relatives with human leukocyte antigen DQA1*0102, DQB1*0602: identification by the Diabetes Prevention Trial-type 1. *J Clin Endocrinol Metab*. 2000;85:1255–1260.

44. Skyler JS, Krischer JP, Wolfsdorf J, et al. Effects of oral insulin in relatives of patients with type 1 diabetes: The diabetes prevention trial – type 1. *Diabetes Care*. 2005;28:1068–1076.

45. Bellmann K, Kolb H, Rastegar S, Jee P, Scott FW. Potential risk of oral insulin with adjuvant for the prevention of type 1 diabetes: a protocol effective in NODmice may exacerbate disease in BB rats. *Diabetologia*. 1998;41:844–847.

46. http://www2.diabetestrialnet.org/

47. The Canadian-European Randomized Control Trial Group. Cyclosporin-induced remission of IDDM after early intervention: association of 1 year of cyclosporin treatment with enhanced insulin secretion. *Diabetes*. 1988;37:1574–1582.

48. Martin S, Schernthaner G, Nerup J, et al. Follow-up of cyclosporin A treatment in type 1 (insulin-dependent) diabetes mellitus: lack of long-term effects. *Diabetologia*. 1991;34:429–434.

49. Feutren G, Mihatsch MJ. Risk factors for cyclosporine-induced nephropathy in patients with autoimmune diseases. International Kidney Biopsy Registry of Cyclosporine in Autoimmune Diseases. *N Engl J Med*. 1992;326:1654–1660.

50. Crino A, Schiaffini R, Ciampalini P, et al. IMDIAB Group. A two year observational study of nicotinamide and intensive insulin therapy in patients with recent onset type 1 diabetes mellitus. *J Pediatr Endocrinol Metab*. 2005;18:749–754.

51. Crino A, Schiaffini R, Manfrini S, et al. IMDIAB group. A randomized trial of nicotinamide and vitamin E in children with recent onset type 1 diabetes (IMDIAB IX). *Eur J Endocrinol*. 2004;150:719–724.

52. Pozzilli P. IDDM preventive trials: what's new?. *Diabetes Metab Rev*. 1998;14:260–261.

53. Herold KC, Hagopian W, Auger JA, et al. Anti-CD3 monoclonal antibody in new-onset type 1 diabetes mellitus. *N Engl J Med*. 2002;346:1692–1698.

54. Keymeulen B, Vandemeulebroucke E, Ziegler AG, et al. Insulin needs after CD3- antibody therapy in new-onset type 1 diabetes. *N Engl J Med*. 2005;352:2598–2608.

55. Mathieu C, van Etten E, Decallonne B, et al. Vitamin D and 1,25-dihydroxyvitamin D3 as modulators in the immune system. *J Steroid Biochem Mol Biol*. 2004;89–90:449–452.

56. Harris SS. Vitamin D in type 1 diabetes prevention. *J Nutr*. 2005;135:323–325.

57. Pitocco D, Crinò A, Di Stasio E, et al. IMDIAB Group. The effects of calcitriol and nicotinamide on residual pancreatic beta-cell function in patients with recent-onset Type 1 diabetes (IMDIAB XI). *Diabet Med*. 2006;23:920–923.

58. Pitocco D, Di Stasio E, Crinò A, et al. Age at diagnosis of type 1 diabetes and the effect of immunomodulatory therapies on residual beta cell function. *Horm Metab Res*. 2007;40(1):66-68 Dec 18; (Epub).

59. Pozzilli P, Manfrini S, Crinò A, et al. IMDIAB Group. Low levels of 25-hydroxyvitamin D3 and 1,25-dihydroxyvitamin D3 in patients with newly diagnosed type 1 diabetes. *Horm Metab Res*. 2005;37:680–683.

Chapter 50
Prevention of Type 2 Diabetes Mellitus

Edward S. Horton

Introduction

Both epidemiology and pathophysiology of type 2 diabetes are discussed in detail elsewhere in this textbook (Chapters 8 and 13). For the purpose of this chapter, a brief summary of these topics is provided.

The prevalence of diabetes mellitus is increasing rapidly throughout the world. In 2003 it was estimated that there were 194 million people with diabetes worldwide, with 90–95% having type 2 diabetes. By 2025 the total number of people with diabetes is predicted to reach 333 million, a 72% increase in prevalence.[1] While all areas of the world are affected, the highest rates of increase are occurring in areas undergoing rapid economic growth and development, which are associated with changes in lifestyle, especially changes in diet and physical activity, as well as growth and aging of the population. In the United States, the increased prevalence of type 2 diabetes is closely associated with a sedentary lifestyle and the development of overweight or obesity. Current data indicate that 66% of adult Americans are overweight, as defined by a body mass index (BMI) >25, and 32% are obese with a BMI $\geq$30.[2] Additionally, 24% meet the National Cholesterol Education Program Adult Treatment Panel III (ATP-III) definition of the metabolic syndrome and are considered to be at increased risk for developing cardiovascular disease.[3] There are currently an estimated 24 million people with diabetes in the United States and 57 million with impaired glucose tolerance (IGT), a high-risk condition for progression to overt type 2 diabetes.[2] In this population, cardiovascular disease is the major cause of mortality, accounting for 70–80% of deaths, and microvascular complications, including diabetic retinopathy leading to visual loss, nephropathy leading to end-stage renal disease requiring dialysis or kidney transplantation, and the disabilities associated with diabetic neuropathy are creating a major health burden for people with diabetes and an increased cost to society. In 2002 the total excess costs of diabetes in the United States were $132 billion. Of this, $39 billion (30%) were indirect costs associated with absence from work and lost productivity, whereas $93 billion (70%) were the direct cost of medical care.[4]

The increasing prevalence of type 2 diabetes, which is now also occurring in younger age groups, has become recognized as a major health problem throughout the world and effective strategies for prevention, early detection, and treatment are a high priority.

Pathophysiology of Type 2 Diabetes

To develop effective approaches to the prevention of type 2 diabetes, a better understanding of the underlying pathophysiology of the disease is needed. The regulation of blood glucose concentration is complex and involves factors affecting the digestion and absorption of dietary carbohydrates, the regulation of hepatic glucose uptake

E.S. Horton (✉)
Joslin Diabetes Center and Harvard Medical School, Boston, MA, USA
e-mail: edward.horton@joslin.harvard.edu

L. Poretsky (ed.), *Principles of Diabetes Mellitus*, DOI 10.1007/978-0-387-09841-8_50,
© Springer Science+Business Media, LLC 2010

and production, and the effectiveness of insulin to stimulate glucose uptake in insulin-sensitive tissues, particularly skeletal muscle and adipose tissue. Following meal ingestion, there is a rapid release of insulin from pancreatic beta cells and suppression of glucagon secretion from pancreatic alpha cells. This results in suppression of hepatic glucose production and stimulation of glucose uptake in peripheral tissues, thus modulating the postprandial rise in blood glucose concentration. In the fasting state, blood glucose concentration is maintained by hepatic glucose production. In type 2 diabetes, excessive hepatic glucose production, combined with decreased peripheral glucose utilization, results in fasting hyperglycemia. Following meal ingestion, the rapid "first phase" of insulin secretion is significantly decreased or absent and the suppression of glucagon secretion is impaired. Both of these processes contribute to postprandial hyperglycemia.

Type 2 diabetes is most commonly associated with obesity and insulin resistance. While the cause of insulin resistance is not fully understood, both genetic and environmental factors play a contributing role. Metabolic factors include intra-abdominal obesity, increased hepatic triglyceride content, and increased plasma free fatty acid concentrations. A variety of adipose tissue-derived cytokines, including leptin, adiponectin, retinol-binding protein 4, IL-6, TNF-α, and other inflammatory proteins affect insulin sensitivity and low levels of physical activity and aging also contribute to insulin resistance. Thus, as individuals become older, less physically active, and more obese, insulin resistance increases. However, insulin resistance alone does not result in the development of type 2 diabetes. If pancreatic beta cell function is normal, plasma glucose concentrations are maintained within a normal range, but at the expense of hyperinsulinemia in both the fasting and the postprandial states. If beta cell function is decreased, impaired glucose metabolism results and may progress to overt type 2 diabetes over time.[5] Data from the United Kingdom Prospective Diabetes Study (UKPDS) indicate that people with newly diagnosed type 2 diabetes have already lost approximately 50% of their beta cell function and beta cell function characteristically continues to decrease with increased duration of disease, making type 2 diabetes a "progressive disease" requiring intensification of treatment over time.[6] The mechanism of the loss of beta cell function in the prediabetic state is not well understood. Predisposing genetic factors undoubtedly play a role but are not currently well defined. Other factors such as toxic effects of glucose and free fatty acids may also play a role in regulating beta cell function and mass.

Identification of High-Risk Populations

The prevalence of type 2 diabetes varies across different racial and ethnic groups, as well as in groups of similar genetic and cultural background who are living in different environments. In the United States, type 2 diabetes is more common in the African-American, Hispanic, and Asian populations than in non-Hispanic whites.[7] Native Americans have the highest rates of type 2 diabetes with its prevalence as high as 50% of the adult population in some groups. While these higher rates of diabetes can be explained in part by genetic predisposition, environmental factors are also clearly important.

In screening for high-risk individuals, one of the most important factors is a positive family history for type 2 diabetes, particularly if one or both parents have the disease or if there is a history of type 2 diabetes in a first-degree relative. Women who have polycystic ovary syndrome, a history of large babies ($\geq$9 lbs at birth) or a history of gestational diabetes, are also at high risk. The presence of overweight or obesity also increases risk progressively with increasing BMI and waist circumference.[8,9]

Screening for impaired glucose metabolism or type 2 diabetes is most commonly done by measuring plasma glucose concentration after an overnight fast or 2 h after a 75 g oral glucose tolerance test (OGTT). Impaired glucose tolerance (IGT), defined as a 2 h value on the OGTT of 140–199 mg/dl, is a strong predictor of risk for progression to 2DM with rates of 3–12% per year reported in various studies.[10] The presence of impaired fasting glucose (IFG), defined as a fasting plasma glucose concentration of 100–125 mg/dl, is also an independent predictor of progression to diabetes, although not as strong as IGT. Together, IFG and/or IGT have been termed "prediabetes," indicating the increased risk of progression to overt type 2 diabetes. The presence of the metabolic syndrome, using modified ATP-III criteria, has also been shown to be associated with increased risk for developing type 2 diabetes.[11,12] Thus, people with increased risk factors for type 2 diabetes as outlined above should be screened for type 2 diabetes on a regular basis and appropriate strategies to prevent or delay the progression to overt diabetes should be undertaken if IFG, IGT, or the metabolic syndrome is present.

Strategies for Prevention of Type 2 Diabetes Mellitus

Epidemiological Studies

The association between type 2 diabetes and obesity has long been recognized. As early as in the 1920s, Dr. Elliot Joslin recommended lifestyle modification focusing on weight reduction and increased physical activity to prevent type 2 diabetes.[13] More recent epidemiological studies have confirmed the importance of obesity, a sedentary lifestyle, and the role of both caloric excess and composition of the diet on the development of type 2 diabetes in genetically predisposed people.[14-17] For example, data from the Nurses' Health Study showed that the risk of developing diabetes increases significantly and progressively with an increase in BMI and is inversely related to the level of physical activity.[18,19]

Randomized Controlled Trials

Several early trials were conducted to determine if lifestyle interventions, focusing on weight reduction and increased physical activity, or treatment with available antidiabetic agents (biguanide or sulfonylureas) would reduce the incidence of type 2 diabetes in people with IGT.[20-22] These trials were small and inconclusive but did pave the way for more recent, larger studies that have examined the effects of lifestyle modification or the use of newer antidiabetic or antiobesity medications on the development of diabetes in high-risk populations (see Table 50.1).

Table 50.1 Summary of results of several major prospective trials of lifestyle modification or medications to prevent or delay the development of type 2 diabetes in high-risk subjects. Relative risk reduction (RRR) compared to treatment with placebo

Study name	Subject number	Mean duration (years)	Interventions	RRR (%)
DaQing[23]	577	6	Diet only	31
			Exercise only	46
			Diet+exercise	42
Finnish DPS[24]	522	3.2	Diet+exercise	58
US DPP[27]	3234	2.8	Diet+exercise	58
US DPP[28]	2342	0.9	Troglitazone	75
Indian DPP[36]	531	2.5	Diet+exercise	28.5
			Metformin	26.4
			Combined therapy	28.2
TRIPOD[37]	266	2.5	Troglitazone	55
DREAM[38]	5269	3	Rosiglitazone	60
ACT NOW	602	2.8	Pioglitazone	79
STOP-NIDDM	1429	3.3	Acarbose	25
XENDOS[43]	3305	4	Orlistat	37

The first major study to examine the effects of dietary modification, weight loss, and increased physical activity was conducted in Da Qing, China.[23] In this study, 577 adult men and women with IGT were randomized according to the community clinic they attended to a control group receiving standard care or to one of three active treatment groups which consisted of dietary modification alone, an exercise program alone, or a combined diet plus exercise program. The participants were followed for 6 years with OGTTs done every 2 years to determine rates of conversion to diabetes. The dietary intervention focused on increased dietary use of vegetables and complex carbohydrates, decreased alcohol consumption, and caloric restriction if the BMI was >25.

The exercise program focused on increasing the activities of daily living and maintaining exercise levels equivalent to brisk walking for at least 20 min daily. The combined diet and exercise group was instructed to use both interventions, whereas the control group received their usual care in the participating clinics. After 6 years of follow-up, the incidence of conversion to diabetes was 68% in the control subjects and was significantly lower in all three intervention groups, being 48, 41, and 46% in the diet only, exercise only, and diet plus exercise groups, respectively. There was no evidence for added effect of diet plus exercise in this study.

In another landmark study, The Finnish Diabetes Prevention Study (DPS) examined the effects of an intensive lifestyle modification program in 522 middle-aged overweight men and women with impaired glucose tolerance.[24] The mean age was 55 years and the mean BMI 31 kg/m. Subjects were randomly assigned to either the intervention group or the control group. Each subject in the intervention group received individualized counseling aimed at reducing body weight by decreasing total intake of calories, specifically decreasing intake of total and saturated fat and increasing intake of dietary fiber, and by increasing moderate-intensity physical activity equivalent to brisk walking for at least 4 h each week. An OGTT was performed annually and the diagnosis of diabetes was confirmed by a second test. After a mean follow-up duration of 3.2 years, the cumulative probability of remaining free of diabetes was significantly improved in the lifestyle intervention group, with a relative risk reduction of 58% compared to the control group who did not participate in the lifestyle intervention program (Fig. 50.1). In this study, the risk reduction in the intervention group was found to be directly linked to the lifestyle changes. For example, patients who lost 5% or more of their body weight had a 74% risk reduction and

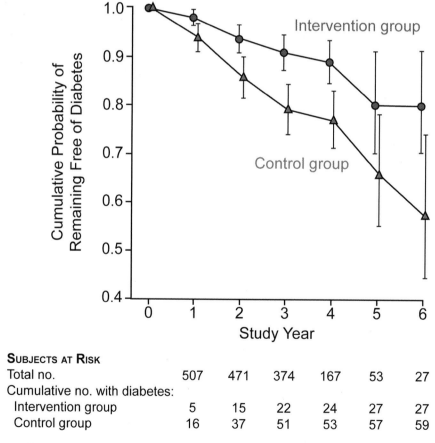

SUBJECTS AT RISK						
Total no.	507	471	374	167	53	27
Cumulative no. with diabetes:						
Intervention group	5	15	22	24	27	27
Control group	16	37	51	53	57	59

Fig. 50.1 The proportion of subjects remaining free of diabetes during the Finnish Diabetes Prevention Trial. From reference[24] with permission

subjects who exceeded the recommended 4 h of exercise per week had an 80% risk reduction. Importantly, the beneficial effects of the lifestyle intervention were maintained after discontinuation of the study. After a median follow-up of 3 years, there was still an overall 43% risk reduction for development of diabetes in the intervention group compared to the control group.[25]

The Diabetes Prevention Program (DPP) is the largest study to date to examine the efficacy of a lifestyle modification program to prevent or delay the development of type 2 diabetes in high-risk individuals with IGT.[26,27] It was conducted in 27 centers in the United States and randomized 3,234 middle-aged overweight men and women to one of the three groups: (1) a program of intensive lifestyle modification focusing on reducing total and saturated dietary fat, increasing dietary fiber, and increasing moderate-intensity exercise for at least 150 min per week; (2) treatment with metformin 850 mg twice daily or (3) a placebo control group. The original study design also included a fourth group of subjects who were treated with troglitazone, 400 mg daily, but this treatment was discontinued before recruitment was completed when it was learned that troglitazone was associated with a significant risk of hepatic toxicity. The DPP recruitment was designed to enroll adult men and women who would be representative of the various racial and ethnic groups in the US population, as well as representative of a wide range of ages, in order to determine the impact of these factors on the efficacy of the interventions. The goal of the lifestyle modification program was to achieve and maintain a weight loss of 7% of initial body weight and to increase physical activity equivalent to brisk walking for at least 150 min each week. Both of these goals were achieved within the first 6 months of treatment. The weight loss was maintained for at least 1 year and then gradually increased, but remained below the baseline weight for the duration of the study. The physical activity levels exceeded the intervention goal and were maintained well throughout the duration of the study. Compliance with metformin was excellent throughout the study. Because of the selection process to recruit subjects at high risk for converting IGT to type 2 diabetes, the control group developed diabetes at a rate of 11.0% per year, whereas the conversion rates were significantly lower in both the metformin and the lifestyle treatment groups, being 7.8 and 4.8% per year, respectively. This represents a 31% risk reduction with metformin treatment and a 58% risk reduction with the lifestyle intervention (Fig. 50.2). In a separate analysis of the group treated with troglitazone, there was a 75% risk reduction compared to the placebo-treated group after a mean of 0.9 years

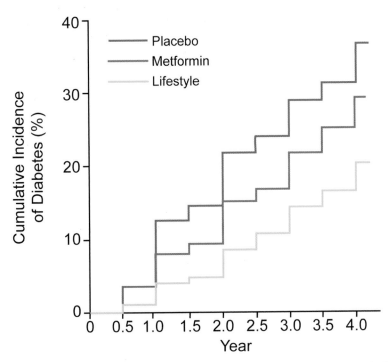

Fig. 50.2 The cumulative incidence of diabetes in the placebo, metformin, and lifestyle treatment groups in the Diabetes Prevention Program. From reference[27] with permission

of treatment (range 0.5–1.5 years). Importantly, during the 3 years after troglitazone withdrawal, there was no demonstrable sustained effect of troglitazone treatment, since the diabetes incidence rate was almost identical to that of the placebo group.[28]

In the DPP there were no differences in the efficacy of the lifestyle or metformin interventions in the various racial and ethnic groups and no differences between men and women. The effectiveness of metformin was least in the older age group (60–85 years) and most effective in the younger age group (25–44 years).[29] Conversely, the lifestyle program was most effective in the older age group and in younger subjects it was approximately equivalent to the effects of treatment with metformin. Metformin was also most effective in those subjects with BMI >36 and least effective in those with BMI <30.[30] The mechanism by which lifestyle intervention reduced risk for progression to diabetes was significantly related to changes in body weight and to improvements in both insulin sensitivity and insulin secretion.[31]

The DPP has also provided an opportunity to examine the effects of lifestyle intervention and treatment with metformin on various cardiovascular risk factors and components of the metabolic syndrome.[32–34] Ongoing studies in the Diabetes Prevention Program Outcome Study (DPPOS) are also examining the impact of the interventions on the development of both microvascular and macrovascular complications of diabetes. At the time of randomization, 53% of the 3234 participants met the original ATP-III criteria for the metabolic syndrome. The prevalence of metabolic syndrome did not vary by gender or age group but did vary by ethnicity, being lowest in Asians (41%) and highest in Caucasians (57%). The lower prevalence in the Asian population most likely represents and underestimate, because population-specific criteria for waist circumference were not used. The prevalence of the individual components did vary by ethnicity and by age group. In those who did not have the metabolic syndrome at randomization, 53% of the subjects in the placebo-treated group had developed it after 3 years. Treatment with metformin resulted in a 17% risk reduction and the lifestyle program resulted in a 41% risk reduction, compared to the control group. Importantly, metformin had significant effects in decreasing the elevated fasting plasma glucose and waist circumference criteria, whereas the lifestyle modification program reduced all the elements of the metabolic syndrome with the exception of improving the serum high-density cholesterol (HDL-C) levels. However, in the total DPP population, the lifestyle program was associated with a significant increase in HDL-C. Furthermore, the lifestyle intervention program resulted in reversal of the metabolic syndrome in 38% of the participants who met the ATP-III criteria at randomization.[32]

Other cardiovascular risk factors were also examined in the DPP study. Hypertension was present in 30% of subjects at baseline and over 3 years it increased in the placebo and metformin treatment groups but significantly decreased in the intensive lifestyle group. Triglycerides decreased in all groups but fell significantly more in the lifestyle group and the lifestyle program also significantly increased HDL-C and decreased the small, dense low-density lipoprotein cholesterol phenotype B. After 3 years of treatment, the use of medications to achieve targets for hypertension was 27–28% less and for dyslipidemia was 25% less in the intensive lifestyle group.[33] In addition, after 1 year of intervention, C-reactive protein decreased by 7–14% in the metformin-treated subjects and by 29–33% in the lifestyle intervention group. These changes correlated mainly with weight loss and not with increased physical activity.[34] Thus, several cardiovascular risk factors were improved by the lifestyle intervention program, which was more effective overall than treatment with metformin.

Other recent diabetes prevention trials have confirmed the effectiveness of lifestyle intervention programs in decreasing the conversion from IGT to type 2 diabetes[35] and one study in India has examined the combination of a lifestyle modification program and treatment with metformin.[36] In this study, weight loss was modest and the dose of metformin used was 250 mg twice daily, less than that in the DPP Study. The relative risk reductions were 28.5% with lifestyle modification and 26.4% with metformin treatment. However, there was no additive effect of combining metformin with lifestyle modification (RRR 28.2%).

Other Pharmaceutical Prevention Trials

Thiazolidinediones

In the TRIPOD study, the effectiveness of troglitazone, 400 mg daily, in decreasing the development of diabetes in Hispanic women with a history of gestational diabetes demonstrated a relative risk reduction of 55%

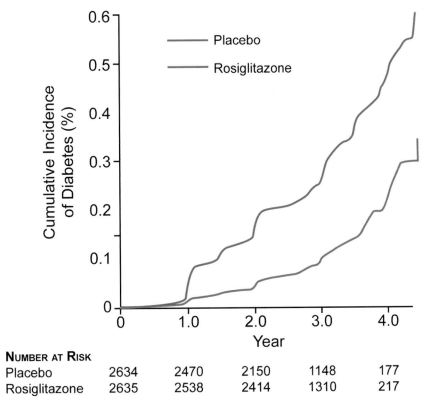

NUMBER AT RISK					
Placebo	2634	2470	2150	1148	177
Rosiglitazone	2635	2538	2414	1310	217

Fig. 50.3 The time to the development of diabetes or death from any cause in the rosiglitazone and placebo-treated subjects in the DREAM Trial. From reference[38] with permission

during this 5-year trial.[37] When studied 8 months after completion of the treatment program, there was a continued beneficial effect of troglitazone treatment, which was associated with improved insulin sensitivity and preservation of beta cell function. A more recent, large, multinational study using rosiglitazone also had very positive results. In this study, the DREAM trial,[38] 5,269 adults, ≥30 years of age, with IFG, IGT, or both were randomized to rosiglitazone, 8 mg daily, or placebo and followed for a median of 3 years. Rosiglitazone was associated with a 60% relative risk reduction for progression to diabetes (Fig. 50.3) and increased the likelihood of regression from impaired glucose metabolism to normoglycemia. The major side effects of treatment were a 2.2 kg increase in weight in the rosiglitazone group and a small increase in congestive heart failure compared to placebo-treated subjects. There was no increase in other cardiovascular events in this study and no increase in bone fractures in women as has been reported in another study with rosiglitazone.[39] A recently completed study using pioglitazone (THE ACT NOW Trial) has also found a 79% risk reduction for conversion from IGT to type 2 diabetes, confirming that thiazolidinediones are very effective in treating these high-risk patients.[40] However, associated fluid retention, weight gain, and increased risk of congestive heart failure or bone fractures with long-term administration of these medications has raised concerns about their use for diabetes prevention.

α-Glucosidase Inhibitors

Based on the concept that impaired first-phase insulin secretion and postprandial hyperglycemia are early manifestations of impaired beta cell function, the use of the α-glucosidase inhibitor acarbose to prevent progression from IGT to type 2 diabetes has been evaluated in some studies.[41] The largest of these is the STOP-NIDDM trial.[42] In this multinational study, 1,429 adult men and women with IGT were randomized to treatment with acarbose, 100 mg three times daily, or placebo and followed for development of type 2 diabetes, using an intent

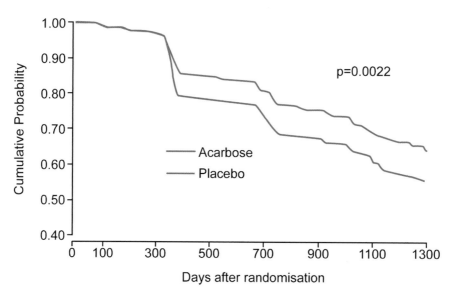

Fig. 50.4 The cumulative probability of remaining free of diabetes with acarbose or placebo treatment in the STOP-NIDDM Trial. From reference[41] with permission

to treat analysis. Despite the fact that subjects were started on a low initial dose of acarbose, which was gradually increased to minimize gastrointestinal side effects, the discontinuation rate was high in both the acarbose (31%) and the placebo groups (19%) and the mean daily dose achieved was 194 mg. Despite these limitations, acarbose treatment resulted in a 25% reduction in risk of progression to diabetes over a mean follow-up period of 3.3 years (Fig. 50.4). In addition, 35% of patients reverted to normal glucose tolerance with acarbose treatment, compared to 31% with placebo. A surprising finding in this study was that acarbose treatment was associated with a 49% relative risk reduction for the development of cardiovascular events, particularly a decrease in the risk of myocardial infarction, and a 34% relative risk reduction for new cases of hypertension. Both of these findings were statistically significant after adjustment for other major cardiovascular risk factors.[43]

Weight Loss Therapies

Various weight loss therapies have also been evaluated for their effectiveness in decreasing the risk of developing diabetes in high-risk populations with obesity. In the XENDOS trial,[44] obese subjects (BMI≥30 kg/m^2) were randomized to treatment with the intestinal lipase inhibitor orlistat, 120 mg three times daily, or matching placebo plus a lifestyle modification program including a calorically restricted diet and increased daily physical activity designed to induce weight loss. Subjects were followed for up to 4 years. In those who completed 4 years of treatment, maximum weight loss occurred after 1 year of treatment and was a mean of 6.2 kg in the control group and 10.6 kg in the orlistat-treated subjects. After 4 years, a partial regain of the weight loss had occurred and was 3.0 kg in the control subjects compared to 5.8 kg in the orlistat-treated subjects. This was associated with a 37% relative risk reduction in the development of type 2 diabetes in this high-risk population.

Another approach to achieving significant weight loss in high-risk obese subjects is the use of bariatric surgery. Pories et al. observed marked improvement and even "cure" of type 2 diabetes following weight reduction surgery in severely obese subjects[45] and this has been confirmed by recent studies using gastric bypass or laparoscopic gastric banding procedures.[46,47] In the follow-up of obese subjects undergoing bariatric surgical procedures, it has also been noted that the development of new cases of diabetes is also significantly reduced.[48] The first major prospective trial to examine this was the Swedish Obese Subjects (SOS) Study,[49] which followed the development of diabetes in a large number of subjects undergoing a variety of surgical procedures for weight reduction and a matched control group who received standard medical care. After 10 years of follow-up, there was a 75% relative risk reduction for the development of diabetes in the surgically treated group, which was clearly related to the degree of weight loss achieved. These results have led to increased interest in using weight reduction surgery for both the treatment and the prevention of type 2 diabetes in severely obese, high-risk subjects. However, the relative risks and benefits of different surgical procedures and long-term effectiveness are still not known.

Recommendation for Screening and Management

People who are at increased risk of developing type 2 diabetes should be identified and screened for impaired glucose metabolism (prediabetes) or features of the metabolic syndrome initially and at least every 2–3 years thereafter. High-risk individuals can be identified based on their personal and family history, physical examination, and routine laboratory tests that can be done as part of an office visit. Key historical and demographic factors include a family history of diabetes or early cardiovascular disease, being a member of a high-risk racial or ethnic group, the presence of overweight or obesity, particularly intra-abdominal obesity, and, in women, a history of gestational diabetes, delivery of a baby weighing more than 9 lb, or a history of polycystic ovary syndrome. It is also important to screen for elements of the metabolic syndrome including hypertension, increased fasting serum triglycerides, low concentrations of HDL-C, and IFG. An OGTT to determine if the patient has normal glucose tolerance, IGT, or previously undiagnosed type 2 diabetes is optional but is recommended every 2–3 years if other risk factors for diabetes are present. The OGTT is more sensitive than the fasting glucose concentration to detect either IGT or previously undiagnosed type 2 diabetes and in several large studies a diagnosis of type 2 diabetes has been established in up to 20% of screened subjects. To establish a diagnosis of type 2 diabetes, a confirmatory test demonstrating increased fasting or 2-h post-glucose challenge plasma glucose concentrations that exceed the diagnostic criteria for diabetes is required.

For people who have prediabetes, defined as IFG, IGT, or both, or who have the metabolic syndrome, appropriate therapies should be implemented to reduce both the risks for progression to type 2 diabetes and the development of cardiovascular disease. Current recommendations from the American College of Endocrinology and the American Association of Clinical Endocrinologists[50] are to implement a program of lifestyle modification as the cornerstone of therapy. Based on the findings of the Diabetes Prevention Program and the Finnish Diabetes Study, overweight individuals should reduce their body weight by 5–10% with long-term maintenance at this level. This should be accomplished by a combination of dietary modification and increased physical activity, achieving 30–60 min of moderate-intensity exercise on at least 5 days a week. The diet should focus on moderate calorie restriction, reduction in total and saturated fat, increased fiber intake, reduced sodium intake, and avoidance of excess alcohol. To assist patients in maintaining these long-term lifestyle changes, support strategies should be provided for long-term success. The use of weight loss medications, such as Orlistat, may be helpful in some people and bariatric surgery can be considered for severely overweight patients (BMI ≥ 35 kg/m^2) who are unable to lose significant amounts of weight through lifestyle modification or medications.

Currently, no medications are approved in the United States for treatment of "prediabetes." While the efficacy of both metformin and acarbose has been demonstrated in randomized controlled trials, their long-term efficacy to prevent or delay progression to type 2 diabetes is not yet known. However, both classes of drugs have been used extensively for the treatment of people with diabetes and their long-term safety is well established. Therefore, it would not be unreasonable to consider either of these medications for treatment of selected patients with IFG or IGT. Although the thiazolidinediones, rosiglitazone and pioglitazone, have also been shown to be very effective in preventing progression from prediabetes to diabetes, several questions remain regarding their side effects and long-term safety, so their use is not currently recommended. Newer classes of antidiabetic medications such as the dipeptidyl peptidase-4 inhibitors or long-acting glucagon-like peptide-1 agonists may eventually prove to be useful for the prevention of type 2 diabetes in high-risk populations, but no clinical trial data are currently available.

Because of the high risk of cardiovascular disease and the frequent presence of features of the metabolic syndrome and other cardiovascular risk factors in this population, appropriate screening and treatment is a high priority. Treatment targets for LDL-C and blood pressure should be equivalent to those used for treating people with established diabetes and antiplatelet therapy, such as low-dose aspirin, should be used unless contraindicated.

Summary

The worldwide prevalence of type 2 diabetes is increasing rapidly and is a major health problem for both developed and developing countries. It is largely due to changes in lifestyle, particularly changes in diet, physical activity, and the development of obesity, as well as to population growth and increased longevity. Type 2 diabetes is a major cause of morbidity and mortality in the population with up to 80% of deaths due to cardiovascular disease. The delay or the prevention of progression to diabetes in high-risk individuals and the early identification of previously undiagnosed diabetes are major health-care goals and high-risk individuals should be identified and screened as part of their routine medical care. This includes screening for impaired glucose metabolism and cardiovascular risk factors, including elements of the metabolic syndrome.

Lifestyle interventions, focusing on a healthy diet, weight reduction, and increased moderate-intensity physical activity, have been demonstrated to significantly reduce the progression from IGT to diabetes and to reduce other associated cardiovascular disease risk factors. However, long-term effects of those interventions on cardiovascular event rates are not yet known. Several classes of antidiabetic medications have also been shown to decrease progression from IGT to type 2 diabetes. Both metformin and the α-glucosidase inhibitor acarbose are effective and safe and may be appropriate for use in some populations. The thiazolidinediones are also very effective but may carry increased risks such as weight gain, fluid retention, and increased risk of congestive heart failure in some individuals. Recently, increased risk of bone fractures has also been noted and there is currently controversy over long-term effects on cardiovascular mortality with rosiglitazone treatment.[51] Weight loss medications and bariatric surgery have also been demonstrated to be effective to prevent, delay, or reverse diabetes in high-risk, obese subjects and may be useful in appropriately selected people. However, long-term efficacy of these treatments is not yet known.

In summary, patients at risk for developing type 2 diabetes should be identified as part of their routine health-care examinations and appropriate preventive strategies implemented to reduce both the risk of diabetes and its long-term complications and to treat associated cardiovascular disease risk factors. Lifestyle modification is the cornerstone of treatment, although several classes of medications have also been demonstrated to be effective. Although not currently recommended, antidiabetic medications with good efficacy and safety profiles may be considered for use in some patients with impaired glucose metabolism. For severely obese patients, weight loss medications and bariatric surgery are also options.

References

1. Diabetes Atlas Committee. *Diabetes Atlas*. 2nd ed. Brussels: International Diabetes Federation; 2003.
2. Centers for Disease Control and Prevention website: www.cdc.gov/diseases
3. Ford ES, Giles WH, Dietz WH. Prevalence of metabolic syndrome among US Adults. *JAMA*. 2002;287:356–359.
4. Hogan P, Dall T, Nikolov P. American Diabetes Association. Economic costs of diabetes in the US in 2002. *Diabetes Care*. 2003;26:917–932.
5. Kahn SE. The relative contributions of insulin resistance and beta-cell dysfunction to the pathophysiology of Type 2 diabetes. *Diabetologia*. 2003;46:3–19.
6. U.K. Prospective Diabetes Study Group. Perspectives in Diabetes. U.K. Prospective Diabetes Study 16. Overview of 6 years' therapy of type II diabetes: a progressive disease. *Diabetes*. 1995;44:1249–1258.
7. Cowie CC, Rust KF, Byrd-Holt DD, et al. Prevalence of diabetes and impaired fasting glucose in adults in the U.S. population: National Health and Nutrition Examination Survey 1999–2002. *Diabetes Care*. 2006;29:1263–1268. [PMID: 16732006] [Abstract/Free Full Text].
8. Chan JM, Rimm EB, Colditz GA, et al. Obesity, fat distribution, and weight gain as risk factors for clinical diabetes in men. *Diabetes Care*. 1994 Sep;17(9):961–969.
9. Colditz GA, Willett WC, Rotnitzky A, et al. Weight gain as a risk factor for clinical diabetes mellitus in women. *Ann Intern Med*. 1995;122:481–486.
10. Knowler WC, Narayan KM, Hanson RL, et al. Preventing non-insulin-dependent diabetes. *Diabetes*. 1995;44:483–488.
11. Wilson WF, Dagostino RB, Parise H, et al. Metabolic syndrome as a precursor of cardiovascular disease and type 2 diabetes mellitus. *Circulation*. 2005;112:3066–3072.
12. Lorenzo C, Williams K, Hunt KJ, et al. National Cholesterol Education Program-Adult Treatment Panel III, International Diabetes federation and WHO Definitions of the Metabolic Syndrome as Predictors of Cardiovascular Disease and Diabetes. *Diabetes Care*. 2007;30:8–13.

13. Joslin E. The prevention of diabetes mellitus. *JAMA*. 1921;76:79–84.
14. Malik VS, Willett WC, Hu FB. Sugar-sweetened beverages and BMI in children and adolescents: reanalyses of a meta-analysis. *Am J Clin Nutr*. 2009 Jan;89(1):438–439.
15. Bazzano LA, Li TY, Joshipura KJ, Hu FB. Intake of fruit, vegetables, and fruit juices and risk of diabetes in women. *Diabetes Care*. 2008 Jul;31(7):1311–1317.
16. Jeon CY, Lokken RP, Hu FB, et al. Physical activity of moderate intensity and risk of type 2 diabetes: a systematic review. *Diabetes Care*. 2007 Mar;30(3):744–752.
17. Qi L, Hu FB, Hu G. Genes, environment, and interactions in prevention of type 2 diabetes: a focus on physical activity and lifestyle changes. *Curr Mol Med*. 2008 Sep;8(6):519–532.
18. Field AE, Willett WC, Lissner L, Colditz GA. Dietary fat and weight gain among women in the Nurses' Health Study. *Obesity*. 2007 Apr;15(4):967–976.
19. Hu FB, Sigal RJ, Rich-Edwards JW, et al. Walking compared with vigorous physical activity and risk of type 2 diabetes in women. *JAMA*. 1999;282:1433–1439.
20. Jarrett RJ, Keen H, Fuller JH, McCartney M. Worsening to diabetes in men with impaired glucose tolerance ("borderline diabetes"). *Diabetologia*. 1979;16:25–30.
21. Keen H, Jarrett RJ, McCartney P. The ten-year follow-up of the Bedford survey (1962–1972): glucose tolerance and diabetes. *Diabetologia*. 1982;22:73–78.
22. Sartor G, Scherstén B, Carlström S, Melander A, Nordén A, Persson G. Ten-year follow-up of subjects with impaired glucose tolerance: prevention of diabetes by tolbutamide and diet regulation. *Diabetes*. 1980;29:41–49.
23. Pan XR, Li GW, Hu YH, et al. Effects of diet and exercise in preventing NIDDM in people with impaired glucose tolerance. The Da Qing IGT and Diabetes Study. *Diabetes Care*. 1997;20:537–544.
24. Tuomilehto J, Lindström J, Eriksson JG, et al. Prevention of type 2 diabetes mellitus by changes in lifestyle among subjects with impaired glucose tolerance. *N Engl J Med*. 2001;344:1343–1350.
25. Lindström J, Ilanne-Parikka P, Peltonen M, et al. Sustained reduction in the incidence of type 2 diabetes by lifestyle intervention: follow-up of the Finnish Diabetes Prevention Study. *Lancet*. 2006;368:1673–1679.
26. The DPP Research Group. Baseline characteristics of the randomized cohort. *Diabetes Care*. 2000;23:1619–1629.
27. The DPP Research Group. Reduction in the incidence of type 2 diabetes with lifestyle intervention or metformin. *N Engl J Med*. 2002;346:393–403.
28. The DPP Research Group. Prevention of type 2 diabetes with troglitazone in the Diabetes Prevention Program. *Diabetes*. 2005;54:1150–1156.
29. The DPP Research Group. Effect of weight loss with lifestyle intervention on risk of diabetes. *Diabetes Care*. 2006;29: 2102–2107.
30. The DPP Research Group. The influence of age on the effects of lifestyle modification and metformin in prevention of diabetes. *J Gerontol A Biol Sci Med Sci*. 2006;61:1075–1081.
31. The DPP Research Group. Role of insulin secretion and sensitivity in the evolution of type 2 diabetes in the diabetes prevention program. *Diabetes*. 2005;54:2404–2414.
32. Orchard TJ, Temprosa M, Goldberg R, et al. The effect of metformin and intensive lifestyle intervention on the metabolic syndrome: the Diabetes Prevention Program randomized trial. *Ann Int Med*. 2005;142: 611–619.
33. The DPP Research Group. Impact of intensive lifestyle and metformin therapy on cardiovascular disease risk factors in the Diabetes prevention Program. *Diabetes Care*. 2005;28:888–894.
34. The DPP Research Group. Intensive lifestyle intervention or metformin on inflammation and coagulation in participants with impaired glucose tolerance. *Diabetes*. 2005;54:1566–1572.
35. Kosaka K, Noda M, Kuzuya T. Prevention of type 2 diabetes by lifestyle intervention: a Japanese trial in IGT males. *Diabetes Res Clin Pract*. 2005;67:152–162.
36. Ramachandran A, Snehalatha C, Mary S, Mukesh B, Bhaskar AD, Vijay V. The Indian Diabetes Prevention Programme shows that lifestyle modification and metformin prevent type 2 diabetes in Asian Indian subjects with impaired glucose tolerance (IDPP-1). *Diabetologia*. 2006;49:289–297.
37. Buchanan TA, Xiang AH, Peters RK, et al. Preservation of pancreatic beta-cell function and prevention of type 2 diabetes by pharmacologic treatment of insulin resistance in high-risk Hispanic women. *Diabetes*. 2002;51: 2796–2803.
38. The DREAM Trial Investigators. Effect of rosiglitazone on the frequency of diabetes in patients with impaired glucose tolerance or impaired fasting glucose: a randomized controlled trial. *Lancet*. 2006;368:1096–1105.
39. Kahn SE, Haffner SM, Heise MA, et al. Glycemic durability of rosiglitazone, metformin, or glyburide monotherapy. *N Engl J Med*. 2006;355:2427–2443.
40. DeFronzo RA, Banerji MA, Bray GA, et al. Actos Now for the prevention of diabetes (ACT NOW) Study. *BMC Endocrine Disorders*. 2009;9:17 .
41. Yang W, Lin L, Qi J, et al. The preventive effect of Acarbose and Metformin on the progression to diabetes mellitus in the IGT population: a 3-year multicenter prospective study. *Chin J Endocrinol Metab*. 2001;17:131–136.
42. Chiasson JL, Josse RG, Gomis R, Hanefeld M, Karasik A, Laakso M. Acarbose for prevention of type 2 diabetes mellitus: the STOP-NIDDM randomised trial. *Lancet*. 2002;359:2072–2077.

43. Chiasson JL. Acarbose for the prevention of diabetes, hypertension, and cardiovascular disease in subjects with impaired glucose tolerance: the Study to Prevent Non-Insulin-Dependent Diabetes Mellitus (STOP-NIDDM) Trial. *Endocr Pract.* 2006;12(Suppl 1):25–30.

44. Torgerson JS, Hauptman J, Boldrin MN, Sjöström L. XENical in the prevention of diabetes in obese subjects (XENDOS) study: a randomized study of orlistat as an adjunct to lifestyle changes for the prevention of type 2 diabetes in obese patients. *Diabetes Care.* 2004;27:155–161.

45. Pories WJ, MacDonald KG Jr, Morgan EJ, et al. Surgical treatment of obesity and its effect on diabetes: 10-y follow-up. *Am J Clin Nutr.* 1992;55:582S–585S.

46. Schauer PR, Burguera B, Ikramuddin S, et al. Effect of laparoscopic rous-en Y gastric bypass on type 2 diabetes mellitus. *Ann Surg.* 2003;238:467–485.

47. Dixon JB, O'Brien PE, Playfair J, et al. Adjustable gastric banding and conventional therapy for type 2 diabetes: a randomized controlled trial. *JAMA.* 2008 Jan 23;299(3):316–323.

48. Sugerman HJ, Wolfe LG, Sica DA, et al. Diabetes and hypertension in severe obesity and effects of gastric bypass-induced weight loss. *Ann Surg.* 2003;237:751–758.

49. Sjöström L, Lindroos AK, Peltonen M, et al. Lifestyle, diabetes, and cardiovascular risk factors 10 years after bariatric surgery. *N Engl J Med.* 2004;351:2683–2693.

50. American College of Endocrinology Task Force on the Prevention of Diabetes. Diagnosis and management of prediabetes in the continuum of hyperglycemia-when do the risks of diabetes begin? A consensus statement from the American College of Endocrinology and the American Association of Clinical Endocrinologists. *Endocrine Practice.* 2008;14:2–14.

51. Nissen SE, Wolski K. Effect of rosiglitazone on the risk of myocardial infarction and death from cardiovascular causes. *N Engl J Med.* 2007;356:2457–2471.

Part X

Chapter 51
Resources for Patients with Diabetes

Marina Krymskaya

Introduction

Modern comprehensive care for patients with diabetes includes many components. One of these is Diabetes Self-Management Education (DSME). DSME empowers patients to control their disease on a daily basis. The best way to arm the patient with the knowledge is to offer comprehensive counseling provided by the diabetes team, which may include physicians, nurses, registered dietitians, exercise physiologists, and other specialists. Often DSME is provided by Certified Diabetes Educators (CDE) – health care professionals who obtained their certification by passing the National Board Examination for Diabetes Educators. Some pre-examination requirements include a minimum of 2 years of professional practice experience in diabetes self-management education and a minimum of 1000 h of diabetes self-management education experience.

The comprehensive education is offered in specialized diabetes centers, yet it may be difficult to receive such education outside of these centers. To help patients who do not have access to specialized comprehensive diabetes programs, various organizations and agencies have developed an array of methods and materials. These organizations include specialty associations, government agencies, outreach programs, pharmaceutical companies, and medical equipment and diabetes supplies manufacturers. All of them are excellent sources of information and can help providers to improve the quality of diabetes care.

One of the main sources of information is the Department of Health and Human Services. The Department has a few agencies accountable for a variety of essential elements of comprehensive diabetes care. These agencies include the Center for Disease Control and Prevention (CDC), the National Institutes of Health (NIH), and the Indian Health Service (IHS). The CDC seeks to promote healthy behaviors by providing accurate health information through its many partnerships. The IHS Diabetes Program concentrates on preventing and controlling diabetes within American Indian and Native Alaskan communities. Two of the institutes within the NIH that deal specifically with diabetes and diabetes-related disease are the National Institute of Diabetes and Digestive and Kidney Diseases (NIDDK) and the National Eye Institute (NEI).

The NIDDK disseminates information on diabetes-related topics through its National Diabetes Clearinghouse. The copies of fact sheets or booklets on topics as varied as devices for taking insulin, complications of diabetes, Medicare coverage, and financial assistance can be ordered here. The NIDDK sponsors research via its Diabetes Research and Training Centers. These centers are involved in diabetes education and community outreach as well.

The NEI was established to protect and prolong the vision of Americans. It conducts its own research and supports research at over 250 medical centers around the country. The NEI also conducts education programs to increase awareness of services and devices that are available for people with vision impairment.

M. Krymskaya (✉)

Division of Endocrinology, Department of Medicine, Gerald J. Friedman Diabetes Institute, Beth Israel Medical Center, New York, NY, USA

e-mail: mkrymska@chpnet.org

L. Poretsky (ed.), *Principles of Diabetes Mellitus*, DOI 10.1007/978-0-387-09841-8_51,
© Springer Science+Business Media, LLC 2010

Another group of agencies includes the voluntary organizations dedicated to educating the public and to improving health. They are the American Heart Association (AHA), the American Diabetes Association (ADA), and the American Dietetic Association. The websites of these agencies include strategies for reducing the risk of cardiovascular and cerebrovascular disease as well as for weight management. Information about recommended books (which can be purchased online) is also found on these websites.

The AHA promotes education and awareness, defines risk factors for heart disease, and emphasizes the importance of screening. AHA also publishes research information, statistics, and clinical guidelines. One of the AHA programs, *The Heart of Diabetes,* was created to help people with type 2 diabetes lower their risk for heart disease and stroke. *The Heart of Diabetes* provides a series of educational tools to help people with diabetes manage the disease and improve their health through physical activity, nutrition, and cholesterol management.

The ADA's mission is to prevent and cure diabetes and to improve the lives of all people affected by the disease. It does this with advocacy programs by funding research and providing information about type 1 and type 2 diabetes via its magazine for patients, *Diabetes Forecast,* and website. Detailed description of medications for diabetes, as well as the reviews of the newest diabetes care products can be found on ADA website. Here one can also obtain such fundamental information as guidelines for laboratory values and monitoring strategies. The website links the consumers with free screenings, education programs, and support groups in their local area.

The American Dietetic Association works at the state, local, and national levels to influence policy on nutrition issues. Some examples are food labeling, medical nutrition therapy, and food programs. The association's website provides dietary advice on multiple topics. One can learn, for example, for how to choose leaner cuts of meat, to reduce fat content of meals, to determine appropriate serving sizes, and to improve the health value of holiday eating. If necessary, the referral to a registered dietitian can be obtained via the American Dietetic Association's website.

Among the charitable organizations for people with type 1 diabetes is Juvenile Diabetes Research Foundation International (JDRF). The mission of JDRF is to find a cure for diabetes and its complications through the support of research. It was founded in 1970 by parents of children with type 1 diabetes, and has funded 700 centers, grants, and fellowships in 20 countries with more than $1.16 billion. JDRF funds research which focuses on restoration of normal blood glucose levels and other therapeutic strategies which allow to avoid and reverse complications of diabetes. JDRF also supports research on prevention of diabetes. The JDRF website provides information about the latest research, the database of the funded research centers and projects, current information about its advocacy efforts, and updated news about the activities of its chapters and affiliates worldwide.

The pharmaceutical industry is another valuable asset that can be utilized in the care of the patients with diabetes. In addition to manufacturing medications, many companies provide educational pamphlets about their products as well as general diabetes education materials and support services. Pharmaceutical companies often have programs which assist indigent patients in obtaining medications. They also organize continuing education programs for health care providers working with these patients.

Manufacturers and suppliers of diabetes equipment donate products to patients that may not be able to afford these supplies. These companies also produce educational materials to enhance understanding of the disease. Home blood glucose-monitoring devices are often donated to diabetes centers. This measure not only relieves the patient of the financial burden of purchasing this device, but also enables the diabetes educator to demonstrate the process of measuring blood glucose and to observe the patient's ability to perform this procedure accurately.

Journals offer information, which can supplement the diabetes education delivered by the health care providers, and offer health tips or guidelines for managing diabetes. An issue may be devoted to heart disease, hyperlipidemia, or foot care and may give suggestions on how to handle some difficult scenarios encountered in daily life. Some journals offer a "pen pal" section where patients can correspond with others who have similar interests.

Other agencies, such as the American Foundation for the Blind and the National Limb Loss Information Center, can assist patients who developed some of the devastating complications of diabetes. These agencies can provide information about support groups and local resources. International associations help meet various needs of the patients with diabetes in a number of countries.

The following list includes some diabetes-related resources (additional websites are listed in Chapter 2). Information obtained from these sources can help to augment patient's understanding of diabetes, but should not be used to replace a comprehensive evaluation by a diabetes team.

Associations

American Association of Clinical Endocrinologists (AACE)
1000 Riverside Avenue, Suite 205
Jacksonville, FL 32304
Phone: (904) 353-7878
Fax: (904) 353-8185
Internet: http://www.aace.com

American Association of Diabetes Educators
444 North Michigan Avenue, suite 1240
Chicago, IL 60611
Phone: (312) 424-2426
Fax: (312) 424-2427
Diabetes Educator Access Line: (800) 832-6874
Internet: http://www.aadenet.org

American Diabetes Association
1660 Duke Street
Alexandria, VA 22314
Phone: (888) 342-2387
Fax: (703) 549-6995
Internet: http://www.diabetes.org

American Dietetic Association
216 West Jackson Boulevard, Suite 800
Chicago, IL 60606-6995
Phone: (312) 899-0040, (800) 342-2383, (800) 366-1655 (consumer nutrition hotline)
Fax: (800) 899-1976
Internet: http://www.eatright.org

American Heart Association
National Center
7272 Greenville Avenue
Dallas, TX 75231
Phone: (214) 373-6300; check individual states for local chapter phone numbers.
Internet: http://www.americanheart.org

American Podiatric Medical Association (APMA)
9312 Old Georgetown Road
Bethesda, MD 20814-1698
Phone: (800) 366-8227
Fax: (301) 530-2752
Internet: http://www.apma.org

Diabetes Education and Camping Association (DECA)
P.O. Box 385Huntsville, AL 35804
Phone: (902) 479-0857
Fax: (902) 431-0680
Internet: http://www.diabetescamps.org/

Diabetes Exercise and Sports Association (DESA)
1647 West Bethany Home Road, #B
Phoenix, AZ 85015
Phone: (800) 898-4322
Fax: (602) 433-9331
Internet: http://www.diabetes-exercise.org

Endocrine Society
4350 East West Highway, Suite 500
Bethesda, MD 20814-4410
Phone: (301) 941-0200
Fax: (301) 941-0259
Internet: http://www.endo-society.org

Juvenile Diabetes Research Foundation International (JDRF)
120 Wall Street, 19th floor
New York, NY 10005
Phone: (800) 533-2873, (212) 785-9500
Fax: (212) 785-9595
Internet: http://www.jdrf.org

National Kidney Foundation
30 East 33rd Street, Suite 1100
New York, NY 10016
Phone: (800) 622-9010
Internet: http://www.kidney.org

Pedorthic Footwear Association (PFA)
7150 Columbia Gateway Drive, Suite G
Columbia, MD 21046-1151
Phone: (800) 673-8447
Fax: (410) 381-1167
Internet: http://www.pedorthics.org

American Foundation for the Blind
15 West 16th Street
NYC, NY 10011
Phone: (800) 232-5463
Internet: http://www.afb.org

National Federation of the Blind
1800 Johnson Street
Baltimore, MD 21230
Phone (410) 659-9314
Internet: http://www.nfb.com

National Limb Loss Information Center
900 East Hill Avenue Suite 285
Knoxville, TN 37915-2568
Phone: (888) 267-5669
Internet: http://www.nllicfo@amputee-coaltion.org

British Diabetic Association
10 Queen Anne Street
London W1G9LH
England
Phone: 020-7323-1531
Internet: http://www.diabetes.org.uk

Canadian Diabetes Association
15 Toronto Street, Suite 800
Toronto, Ontario M5C2E3
Canada
Phone: (416) 363-3373
Internet: http://www.diabetes.ca

Diabetes New Zealand
Wilford House
115 Molesworth Street
Thorndon, Wellington
New Zealand
Phone: 64 4 499 7145
Internet: http://www.diabetes.org.nz

International Diabetes Institute
260 Kooyoong road
Caulfield, Victoria 3162
Australia
Phone: (03) 9258-5050
Internet: http://www.idi.org.au

International Diabetic Athletes Association
1647-B West Bethany Home Road
Phoenix, AZ 85015
Phone: (800) 898-4322; (602) 433-2113

Government Agencies

Centers for Disease Control and Prevention
National Center for Chronic Disease Prevention and Health Promotion
Division of Diabetes Translation
2858 Woodcock Boulevard
Davidson Building
Atlanta, GA 30341-4002
Phone: (877)-232-3422
Internet: http://www.cdc.gov/diabetes

Indian Health Service
Diabetes Program
5300 Homestead Road, N.E.
Albuquerque, NM 87110
Phone: (505) 248-4182
Fax: (505) 248-4188
Internet: http://www.ihs.gov/medicalprograms/diabetes

National Diabetes Education Program
1 Information Way
Bethesda, MD 20892-3560
Phone: (800) 438-5383
Internet: http://ndep.nih.gov

National Diabetes Information Clearinghouse (NDIC)
1 Information Way
Bethesda, MD 20892-3560
Phone: (800) 860-8747
Internet: http://www.niddk.nih.gov/health/diabetes/diabetes.htm

National Eye Institute
National Eye Health Education Program
2020 Vision Place
Bethesda, MD 20892-3633
Phone: (800) 869-2020 (to order materials); (301)-496-5248
Internet: http://www.nei.nih.gov

U.S. Public Health Service
Office of Minority Health Resource Center
P.O. Box 37337
Washington, DC 20013-7337
Phone: (800) 444-6472
Fax: (301) 230-7198
Internet: http://www.niddk-nih.gov/health/diabetes/ndic.htm

Outreach Programs

Diabetes Assistance & Resources Program (DAR)
Phone: (888)-Diabetes
Internet: http://www.diabetes.org/dar

African American Program
Phone: (888)-Diabetes
Internet: http://www.diabetes.org/africanamerican

Awakening the Spirit
Phone: (888)-Diabetes
Internet: http://www.diabetes.org.awakening

Journals

Diabetes Self Management
P.O. Box 52890
Boulder, CO 80322-2890
Phone: (800) 234-0923
Internet: http://diabetes-self-mgmt.com

Diabetes Forecast
1701 North Beauregard Street
Alexandria, VA 22311
Phone: (800) 806-7801
Internet: http://www.diabetes.org/diabetesforecast

Diabetes Interview
6 School Street, Suite 160
Fairfax, CA 94930
Phone: (800) 488-8468
Internet: http://www.diabetes interview.com

Pharmaceutical Companies and Medical Equipment Manufacturers

Abbott Laboratories Inc.
MediSense Products
4A Crosby Drive
Bedford, MA 01730-1402
Phone: (800) 527-3339
Internet: http://www.abbottdiagnostics.com

Amylin Pharmaceuticals
9360 Towne Centre Drive
San Diego, CA 92121
Phone: (858) 552-2200
Fax(858) 552-2212 fax
Internet: http://www.amylin.com

Amira Pharmaceuticals
4742 Scotts Valley Drive
Scotts Valley, CA 95066
Phone: (800) 654-0619
Internet: http://www.amirapharm.com

Animas
590 Lancaster Avenue
Frazer, PA 19355
Phone: (877) 937-7867
Internet: http://www.animascorp.com

Aventis Pharmaceuticals
300 Somerset Corporate Boulevard
P.O. Box 6977
Bridgewater, NJ 08807-0977
Phone: (800) 207-8049 Indigent Program (800) 321-0855
Internet: http://www.diabeteswatch.com

Bayer Pharmaceuticals
400 Morgan Lane
West Haven, CT 06516
Phone: (800) 288-8371 Indigent Patient (800) 998-91080
Internet: http://www.pharma.bayer.com

BD Consumer Healthcare
11 Jennifer drive
Holmdel, NJ 07733
Phone: (800) 316-1611
Internet: http://www.bd.com

Bristol-Myers Squibb
602 White Oak Ridge Road
Short Hills, NJ 07078
Phone: (800) 332-2056 Patient Assistance (800) 437-0994
Internet: http://www.bms.com

Can-Am Care
Cimetra Industrial Park Box 98
Chazy, NY 12921
Phone: (800) 461-4414
Internet: http://www.invernessmedical.com

Cell Robotics Inc.
Personal Lasette
2715 Broadbent Parkway, NE
Albuquerque, NM 87107
Phone: (800) 846-0590 ext. 100
Internet: http://www.cellrobotics.com

Disetronic
5151 Program Avenue
St. Paul, MN 55112
Phone: (800) 280-7801
Internet: http://www.disetronic-usa.com

Eli Lilly and Company
82 Plymouth Avenue
Maplewood, NJ 07040
Phone: (800) 545-5979 Lilly Cares (800) 545-6962
Internet: http://www.lilly.com

Glaxo SmithKline Beecham Pharmaceuticals
45 River Drive South
Jersey City, NJ 07310
Phone: (888) 825-5249 Patient Assistance (888) 825-5249
Internet: http://www.gsk.com

Lifescan
1000 Gibraltar Drive
Milpitas, CA 95035-6312
Phone: (800) 227-8862
Internet: http://www.lifescan.com

Medic Alert Foundation
2323 Colorado Avenue
Turlock, CA 95382
Phone: (888) 633-4298
Internet: http://medicalert.org

Minimed
263 Nob Hill Drive
Elmsford, NY 10523
Phone: (800) 646-4633
International Headquarters Phone: (818) 362-5958
Internet: http://www.minimed.com

Novo Nordisk
100 College Road West
Princeton, NJ 08540
Phone: (800) 727-6500 Indigent Program (800) 727-6500
Internet: http://www.novonordisk.com

Paddock Laboratories Inc.
3940 Quebec Avenue North
Minneapolis, MN 55427
Phone: (800) 328-5113
Fax: (763) 546-4842
Internet: http://paddocklabs.com

Pfizer
Pfizer for Living
P.O. Box 29179
Shawnee Mission, KS 66201-9911
Phone: (888) 999-5657 Pfizer Prescription Assistance
Internet: www.pfizer.com

Roche Diagnostics
9115 Hague Road
P.O. Box 50457
Indianapolis, IN 46256
Phone: (317) 845-2000
Internet: http://www.roche.com

Therasense
1360 South Loop Road
Alameda, CA 94502
Phone: (888) 522-5226
Internet: http://www.therasense.com

Diabetes Product Supply Companies

American Medical Supplies
P.O. Box 294009
Boca Raton, FL 33429-4009
Phone: (800) 575-2345
Internet: http://www.diabeticmedicare.com

Diabetic Express
31128 Vine Street
Phone: (800) 338-4656
Internet: http://www.diabeticexpress.com

Diabetic Care Services
31122 Vine Street
Cleveland, OH 44095
Phone: (800) 633-7167
Fax: (800) 474-8262
Internet: http://www.diabeticcareservices.com

Diabetic Promotions
P.O. Box 5400
Willowick, OH 44095-0400
Phone: (800) 433-1477
Internet: http://www.info@diabeticpromotions.com

Liberty Medical Supply Inc.
10045 South Federal Highway
Port St. Lucie, FL 34952
Phone: (800) 633-2001
Internet: http://www.libertymedical.com

Subject Index

A

Abacavir
  for HIV infection and glucose metabolism
    disturbances, 630
  See also Non-nucleoside reverse transcriptase
    inhibitors (NNRTIs)

Abdominal pain
  gastrointestinal symptoms in diabetic patients, 427
  See also Gastrointestinal manifestations of diabetes

Acanthosis nigricans
  dermatological complications of DM, 462–463
  extreme insulin resistance syndromes clinical
    feature, 264

Accelerator hypothesis
  T1DM and, 190
  See also Insulin resistance

**ACCORD (Action to Control Cardiovascular Risk in
    Diabetes) trial, 11, 504, 652, 731**

Acculturation
  defined, 134
  See also Cultural factors

Acidosis
  glucose production and hepatorenal glucose
    reciprocity, 25
  See also Glucose homeostasis (normal)

Acquired lipodystrophy syndromes
  Barraquer–Simons syndrome (acquired partial
    lipodystrophy), 269
  Lawrence syndrome (acquired generalized
    lipodystrophy), 269
  lipodystrophy in HIV patients, 270
  localized lipodystrophies, 270
  See also Familial lipodystrophy syndromes

Acquired perforating dermatosis, 464
  See also Dermatological complications of DM

Acrochordons (skin tags), 468

Acromegaly
  hyperglycemia and insulin resistance association
    with, 251
  secondary DM cause, 251–252
  See also Secondary diabetes mellitus

Acute fulminant diabetes, 194

Acute hepatitis
  secondary DM cause, 250
  See also Chronic hepatitis; Liver diseases

Acute hyperglycemic syndromes
  diabetic ketoacidosis (DKA), 281–291
  hyperosmolar hyperglycemic syndrome (HHS),
    291–293

Acute liver failure, 566

Acute pancreatitis
  secondary DM cause, 245
  See also Exocrine pancreas diseases

Adenocarcinoma
  esophagus, 582
  See also Diabetes and cancer; Obesity and cancer

Adipokines
  adiponectin, 588
  fatty acid synthase (FAS), 588
  leptin, 587
  See also Cytokines

Adiponectin
  cancer causing obesity and diabetes, 588
  for HIV infection and glucose metabolism
    disturbances, 632
  for peripheral lipoatrophy effects on glucose
    metabolism, 626–627

Adipose tissue
  implant for extreme insulin resistance
    syndromes, 273
  subcutaneous, 537
  visceral (VAT), 538, 627, 632

L. Poretsky (ed.), *Principles of Diabetes Mellitus*, DOI 10.1007/978-0-387-09841-8,
© Springer Science+Business Media, LLC 2010

ISBN 978-0-387-09840-1

EAN

9 780387 098401 >